坎贝尔骨科手术学
儿童骨科

Campbell's Operative Orthopaedics

第 14 版
（影印版）

Frederick M. Azar, MD

James H. Beaty, MD

人民卫生出版社
·北 京·

图书在版编目（CIP）数据

坎贝尔骨科手术学 . 儿童骨科 : 英文 /（美）弗雷德里克·M. 阿扎尔（Frederick M. Azar），（美）詹姆斯·H. 比蒂（James H. Beaty）主编 . —影印本 . —北京：人民卫生出版社，2021.12

ISBN 978-7-117-32516-5

Ⅰ. ①坎⋯ Ⅱ. ①弗⋯ ②詹⋯ Ⅲ. ①骨科学 – 外科手术 – 英文②儿科学 – 骨科学 – 外科手术 – 英文 Ⅳ. ①R68

中国版本图书馆 CIP 数据核字（2021）第 241255 号

| 人卫智网 | www.ipmph.com | 医学教育、学术、考试、健康，购书智慧智能综合服务平台 |
| 人卫官网 | www.pmph.com | 人卫官方资讯发布平台 |

图字：01–2021–6747 号

坎贝尔骨科手术学

儿 童 骨 科

Kanbeier Guke Shoushuxue

Ertong Guke

主　　编：Frederick M. Azar　James H. Beaty
出版发行：人民卫生出版社（中继线 010-59780011）
地　　址：北京市朝阳区潘家园南里 19 号
邮　　编：100021
E - mail：pmph @ pmph.com
购书热线：010-59787592　010-59787584　010-65264830
印　　刷：三河市宏达印刷有限公司（胜利）
经　　销：新华书店
开　　本：889×1194　1/16　印张：36
字　　数：1714 千字
版　　次：2021 年 12 月第 1 版
印　　次：2022 年 1 月第 1 次印刷
标准书号：ISBN 978-7-117-32516-5
定　　价：499.00 元

打击盗版举报电话：010-59787491　E-mail：WQ @ pmph.com
质量问题联系电话：010-59787234　E-mail：zhiliang @ pmph.com

坎贝尔骨科手术学
儿童骨科

Campbell's Operative Orthopaedics

第14版

（影印版）

Frederick M. Azar, MD

Professor

Department of Orthopaedic Surgery and Biomedical Engineering University of Tennessee–Campbell Clinic

Chief of Staff, Campbell Clinic

Memphis, Tennessee

James H. Beaty, MD

Harold B. Boyd Professor and Chair

Department of Orthopaedic Surgery and Biomedical Engineering University of Tennessee–Campbell Clinic

Memphis, Tennessee

Editorial Assistance

Kay Daugherty *and* **Linda Jones**

人民卫生出版社

·北 京·

Elsevier (Singapore) Pte Ltd.
3 Killiney Road,
#08–01 Winsland House I,
Singapore 239519
Tel:（65）6349–0200; Fax:（65）6733–1817

ELSEVIER

This English Reprint of Parts Ⅸ, Ⅹ, and Ⅺ from Campbell's Operative Orthopaedics, 14E by Frederick M. Azar and James H. Beaty was undertaken by People's Medical Publishing House and is published by arrangement with Elsevier (Singapore) Pte Ltd.

Parts Ⅸ, Ⅹ, and Ⅺ from Campbell's Operative Orthopaedics, 14E by Frederick M. Azar and James H. Beaty由人民卫生出版社进行影印，并根据人民卫生出版社与爱思唯尔（新加坡）私人有限公司的协议约定出版。

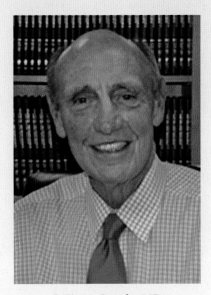

S. Terry Canale, MD

It is with humble appreciation and admiration that we dedicate this edition of *Campbell's Operative Orthopaedics* to Dr. S. Terry Canale, who served as editor or co-editor of five editions. He took great pride in this position and worked tirelessly to continue to improve "The Book." As noted by one of his co-editors, "Terry is probably the only person in the world who has read every word of multiple editions of *Campbell's Operative Orthopaedics*." He considered *Campbell's Operative Orthopaedics* an opportunity for worldwide orthopaedic education and made it a priority to ensure that each edition provided valuable and up-to-date information. His commitment to and enthusiasm for this work will continue to influence and inspire every future edition.

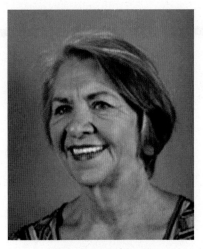

Kay C. Daugherty

It is with equal appreciation and regard that we dedicate this edition to Kay C. Daugherty, the managing editor of the last nine editions *Campbell's Operative Orthopaedics*. Over the last 40 years, she has faithfully and tirelessly edited, reshaped, and overseen all aspects of publication from manuscript preparation to proofing. She has a profound talent to put ideas and disjointed words into comprehensible text, ensuring that each revision maintains the gold standard in readability. Each edition is a testament to her dedication to excellence in writing and education. A favorite quote of Mrs. Daugherty to one of our late authors was, "I'll make a deal. I won't operate if you won't punctuate." We are grateful for her many years of continual service to the Campbell Foundation and for the publications yet to come.

FREDERICK M. AZAR, MD
Professor
Director, Sports Medicine Fellowship
University of Tennessee–Campbell Clinic
Department of Orthopaedic Surgery and
    Biomedical Engineering
Chief-of-Staff, Campbell Clinic
Memphis, Tennessee

JAMES H. BEATY, MD
Harold B. Boyd Professor and Chair
University of Tennessee–Campbell Clinic
Department of Orthopaedic Surgery and
    Biomedical Engineering
Memphis, Tennessee

MICHAEL J. BEEBE, MD
Instructor
University of Tennessee–Campbell Clinic
Department of Orthopaedic Surgery and
    Biomedical Engineering
Memphis, Tennessee

CLAYTON C. BETTIN, MD
Assistant Professor
Director, Foot and Ankle Fellowship
Associate Residency Program Director
University of Tennessee–Campbell Clinic
Department of Orthopaedic Surgery and
    Biomedical Engineering
Memphis, Tennessee

TYLER J. BROLIN, MD
Assistant Professor
University of Tennessee–Campbell Clinic
Department of Orthopaedic Surgery and
    Biomedical Engineering
Memphis, Tennessee

JAMES H. CALANDRUCCIO, MD
Associate Professor
Director, Hand Fellowship
University of Tennessee–Campbell Clinic
Department of Orthopaedic Surgery and
    Biomedical Engineering
Memphis, Tennessee

DAVID L. CANNON, MD
Associate Professor
University of Tennessee–Campbell Clinic
Department of Orthopaedic Surgery and
    Biomedical Engineering
Memphis, Tennessee

KEVIN B. CLEVELAND, MD
Instructor
University of Tennessee–Campbell Clinic
Department of Orthopaedic Surgery and
    Biomedical Engineering
Memphis, Tennessee

ANDREW H. CRENSHAW JR., MD
Professor Emeritus
University of Tennessee–Campbell Clinic
Department of Orthopaedic Surgery and
    Biomedical Engineering
Memphis, Tennessee

JOHN R. CROCKARELL, MD
Professor
University of Tennessee–Campbell Clinic
Department of Orthopaedic Surgery and
    Biomedical Engineering
Memphis, Tennessee

GREGORY D. DABOV, MD
Assistant Professor
University of Tennessee–Campbell Clinic
Department of Orthopaedic Surgery and
    Biomedical Engineering
Memphis, Tennessee

MARCUS C. FORD, MD
Instructor
University of Tennessee–Campbell Clinic
Department of Orthopaedic Surgery and
    Biomedical Engineering
Memphis, Tennessee

RAYMOND J. GARDOCKI, MD
Assistant Professor
University of Tennessee–Campbell Clinic
Department of Orthopaedic Surgery and
    Biomedical Engineering
Memphis, Tennessee

BENJAMIN J. GREAR, MD
Instructor
University of Tennessee–Campbell Clinic
Department of Orthopaedic Surgery and
    Biomedical Engineering
Memphis, Tennessee

JAMES L. GUYTON, MD
Associate Professor
University of Tennessee–Campbell Clinic
Department of Orthopaedic Surgery and
    Biomedical Engineering
Memphis, Tennessee

JAMES W. HARKESS, MD
Associate Professor
University of Tennessee–Campbell Clinic
Department of Orthopaedic Surgery and
    Biomedical Engineering
Memphis, Tennessee

ROBERT K. HECK JR., MD
Associate Professor
University of Tennessee–Campbell Clinic
Department of Orthopaedic Surgery and
    Biomedical Engineering
Memphis, Tennessee

MARK T. JOBE, MD
Associate Professor
University of Tennessee–Campbell Clinic
Department of Orthopaedic Surgery and
    Biomedical Engineering
Memphis, Tennessee

DEREK M. KELLY, MD
Professor
Director, Pediatric Orthopaedic Fellowship
Director, Resident Education
University of Tennessee–Campbell Clinic
Department of Orthopaedic Surgery and
    Biomedical Engineering
Memphis, Tennessee

SANTOS F. MARTINEZ, MD
Assistant Professor
University of Tennessee–Campbell Clinic
Department of Orthopaedic Surgery and
    Biomedical Engineering
Memphis, Tennessee

ANTHONY A. MASCIOLI, MD
Assistant Professor
University of Tennessee–Campbell Clinic
Department of Orthopaedic Surgery and
    Biomedical Engineering
Memphis, Tennessee

BENJAMIN M. MAUCK, MD
Assistant Professor
Director, Hand Fellowship
University of Tennessee–Campbell Clinic
Department of Orthopaedic Surgery and
    Biomedical Engineering
Memphis, Tennessee

MARC J. MIHALKO, MD
Assistant Professor
University of Tennessee–Campbell Clinic
Department of Orthopaedic Surgery and
    Biomedical Engineering
Memphis, Tennessee

WILLIAM M. MIHALKO, MD PhD
Professor, H.R. Hyde Chair of Excellence in
    Rehabilitation Engineering
Director, Biomedical Engineering
University of Tennessee–Campbell Clinic
Department of Orthopaedic Surgery and
    Biomedical Engineering
Memphis, Tennessee

ROBERT H. MILLER III, MD
Associate Professor
University of Tennessee–Campbell Clinic
Department of Orthopaedic Surgery and
    Biomedical Engineering
Memphis, Tennessee

G. ANDREW MURPHY, MD
Associate Professor
University of Tennessee–Campbell Clinic
Department of Orthopaedic Surgery and
    Biomedical Engineering
Memphis, Tennessee

ASHLEY L. PARK, MD
Clinical Assistant Professor
University of Tennessee–Campbell Clinic
Department of Orthopaedic Surgery and
    Biomedical Engineering
Memphis, Tennessee

EDWARD A. PEREZ, MD
Associate Professor
University of Tennessee–Campbell Clinic
Department of Orthopaedic Surgery and
    Biomedical Engineering
Memphis, Tennessee

BARRY B. PHILLIPS, MD
Professor
University of Tennessee–Campbell Clinic
Department of Orthopaedic Surgery and
    Biomedical Engineering
Memphis, Tennessee

DAVID R. RICHARDSON, MD
Associate Professor
University of Tennessee–Campbell Clinic
Department of Orthopaedic Surgery and
    Biomedical Engineering
Memphis, Tennessee

MATTHEW I. RUDLOFF, MD
Assistant Professor
Co-Director, Trauma Fellowship
University of Tennessee–Campbell Clinic
Department of Orthopaedic Surgery and
    Biomedical Engineering
Memphis, Tennessee

JEFFREY R. SAWYER, MD
Professor
Co-Director, Pediatric Orthopaedic
    Fellowship
University of Tennessee–Campbell Clinic
Department of Orthopaedic Surgery and
    Biomedical Engineering
Memphis, Tennessee

BENJAMIN W. SHEFFER, MD
Assistant Professor
University of Tennessee–Campbell Clinic
Department of Orthopaedic Surgery and
    Biomedical Engineering
Memphis, Tennessee

DAVID D. SPENCE, MD
Assistant Professor
University of Tennessee–Campbell Clinic
Department of Orthopaedic Surgery and
    Biomedical Engineering
Memphis, Tennessee

NORFLEET B. THOMPSON, MD
Instructor
University of Tennessee–Campbell Clinic
Department of Orthopaedic Surgery and
    Biomedical Engineering
Memphis, Tennessee

THOMAS W. THROCKMORTON, MD
Professor
Co-Director, Sports Medicine Fellowship
University of Tennessee–Campbell Clinic
Department of Orthopaedic Surgery and
    Biomedical Engineering
Memphis, Tennessee

PATRICK C. TOY, MD
Associate Professor
University of Tennessee–Campbell Clinic
Department of Orthopaedic Surgery and
    Biomedical Engineering
Memphis, Tennessee

WILLIAM C. WARNER JR., MD
Professor
University of Tennessee–Campbell Clinic
Department of Orthopaedic Surgery and
    Biomedical Engineering
Memphis, Tennessee

JOHN C. WEINLEIN, MD
Assistant Professor
Director, Trauma Fellowship
University of Tennessee–Campbell Clinic
Department of Orthopaedic Surgery and
    Biomedical Engineering
Memphis, Tennessee

WILLIAM J. WELLER, MD
Instructor
University of Tennessee–Campbell Clinic
Department of Orthopaedic Surgery and
    Biomedical Engineering
Memphis, Tennessee

A. PAIGE WHITTLE, MD
Associate Professor
University of Tennessee–Campbell Clinic
Department of Orthopaedic Surgery and
    Biomedical Engineering
Memphis, Tennessee

KEITH D. WILLIAMS, MD
Associate Professor
University of Tennessee–Campbell Clinic
Department of Orthopaedic Surgery and
    Biomedical Engineering
Memphis, Tennessee

DEXTER H. WITTE III, MD
Clinical Assistant Professor in
    Radiology
University of Tennessee–Campbell Clinic
Department of Orthopaedic Surgery and
    Biomedical Engineering
Memphis, Tennessee

When Dr. Willis Campbell published the first edition of *Campbell's Operative Orthopaedics* in 1939, he could not have envisioned that over 80 years later it would have evolved into a four-volume text and earned the accolade of the "bible of orthopaedics" as a mainstay in orthopaedic practices and educational institutions all over the world. This expansion from some 400 pages in the first edition to over 4,500 pages in this 14th edition has not changed Dr. Campbell's original intent: "to present to the student, the general practitioner, and the surgeon the subject of orthopaedic surgery in a simple and comprehensive manner." In each edition since the first, authors and editors have worked diligently to fulfill these objectives. This would have not been possible without the hard work of our contributors who always strive to present the most up-to-date information while retaining "tried and true" techniques and tips. The scope of this text continues to expand in the hope that the information will be relevant to physicians no matter their location or resources.

As always, this edition also is the result of the collaboration of a group of "behind the scenes" individuals who are involved in the actual production process. The Campbell Foundation staff—Kay Daugherty, Linda Jones, and Tonya Priggel—contributed their considerable talents to editing often confusing and complex author contributions, searching the literature for obscure references, and, in general, "herding the cats." Special thanks to Kay and Linda who have worked on multiple editions of *Campbell's Operative Orthopaedics* (nine editions for Kay and six for Linda). They probably know more about orthopaedics than most of us, and they certainly know how to make it more understandable. Thanks, too, to the Elsevier personnel who provided guidance and assistance throughout the publication process: John Casey, Senior Project Manager; Jennifer Ehlers, Senior Content Development Specialist; and Belinda Kuhn, Senior Content Strategist.

We are especially appreciative of our spouses, Julie Azar and Terry Beaty, and our families for their patience and support as we worked through this project.

The preparation and publication of this 14th edition was fraught with difficulties because of the worldwide pandemic and social unrest, but our contributors and other personnel worked tirelessly, often in creative and innovative ways, to bring it to fruition. It is our hope that these efforts have provided a text that is informative and valuable to all orthopaedists as they continue to refine and improve methods that will ensure the best outcomes for their patients.

Frederick M. Azar, MD
James H. Beaty, MD

CONTENTS

PART I

CONGENITAL AND DEVELOPMENTAL DISORDERS

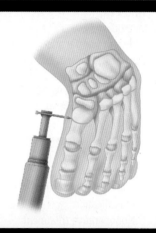

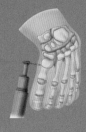

CHAPTER 1

CONGENITAL ANOMALIES OF THE LOWER EXTREMITY

Derek M. Kelly

This chapter describes congenital anomalies of the foot and lower extremity. Congenital anomalies of the hip and pelvis are described in chapter 2, and congenital anomalies of the trunk and upper extremities are described in chapter 3. Congenital anomalies of the spine are discussed in Spine Surgery, and congenital anomalies of the hand are discussed in Hand Surger. Many of the operative techniques described here are useful for other conditions and are found in the references in other chapters.

ANOMALIES OF THE TOES

The most common anomaly of the toes is polydactyly, the presence of supernumerary digits. Others are syndactyly (webbed toes), macrodactyly (enlarged toes), and congenital contracture or angulation. Any of these conditions may require surgery. When surgery is contemplated for anomalies of the toes, several factors must be considered, including cosmesis, pain, and difficulty in fitting shoes, but overall long-term function of the foot is the primary concern. A satisfactory clinical result should correct all of these problems.

POLYDACTYLY

Polydactyly of the toes may occur in established genetic syndromes but occurs most commonly as an isolated trait with an autosomal dominant inheritance pattern and variable expression. The overall incidence of polydactyly is approximately two cases per 1000 live births. Surgical treatment of polydactyly is amputation of the accessory digit. Preoperative radiographs should be obtained to detect any extra metatarsal articulating with the digit, which should be amputated with its associated digit (Fig. 1.1). Occasionally, a combined polydactyly-syndactyly deformity requires more complex surgical correction (Fig. 1.2), such as resection of the more peripheral digit using residual skin for coverage.

Venn-Watson classified polydactyly and directed attention to the difference between preaxial and postaxial types (Fig. 1.3). In preaxial polydactyly, the most medial great toe usually is excised. The remaining great toe should have a careful repair of the capsule if necessary to prevent a progressive hallux varus; Kirschner wire fixation can be used for stability if needed for 4 to 6 weeks. A more recent classification system by Seok et al. focuses on the importance of associated syndactylism, axis deviation, and metatarsal extension, with each of these factors resulting in a higher rate of unsatisfactory results after surgical correction. Good results can be expected regardless of the age at which the amputation is performed; however, most supernumerary digits are excised when the child is between 6 and 18 months of age.

AMPUTATION OF AN EXTRA TOE (SIMPLE POSTAXIAL POLYDACTYLY)

TECHNIQUE 1.1

- At the base of the toe to be amputated, make an oval or racquet-shaped incision through the skin and fascia, preserving extra skin to ensure tension-free closure after amputation of the extra digit (Fig. 1.4).
- Draw the tendons distally as far as possible and divide them.

- Incise the capsule of the metatarsophalangeal joint transversely, dissect it from the metatarsal, and disarticulate the joint.
- With an osteotome or bone-cutting forceps, sharply resect any bone that may have protruded from the metatarsal head.
- If the radiograph has revealed an extra metatarsal, resect it after continuing the incision proximally on the dorsolateral aspect of the foot. A complete extra ray amputation may require transfer of the peroneus brevis tendon insertion with partial resection of the lateral border of the cartilaginous cuboid.

See also Video 1.1.

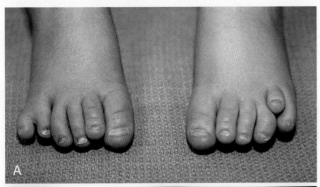
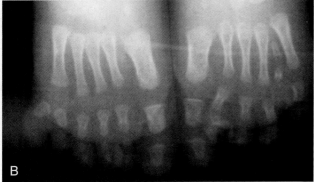

FIGURE 1.1 **A,** Bilateral polydactyly in 6-month-old infant. **B,** Accessory metatarsal of left foot can be seen on radiograph.

SYNDACTYLY

Syndactyly of the toes rarely interferes with function. The same technique is used as for the fingers. Syndactyly is commonly

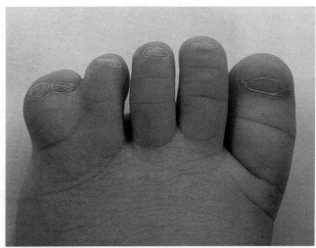

FIGURE 1.2 Complex polydactyly-syndactyly of left fifth toe with bony and soft-tissue syndactyly. (From Lee HS, Park SS, Yoon JO, et al: Classification of postaxial polydactyly of the foot, *Foot Ankle Int* 27:356–362, 2006.)

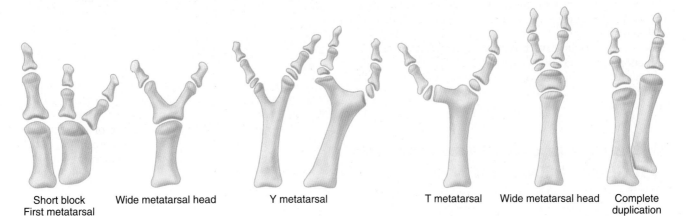

| Short block First metatarsal | Wide metatarsal head | Y metatarsal | T metatarsal | Wide metatarsal head | Complete duplication |

A   B

FIGURE 1.3 Venn-Watson classification of polydactyly. **A,** Preaxial polydactyly. **B,** Postaxial polydactyly.

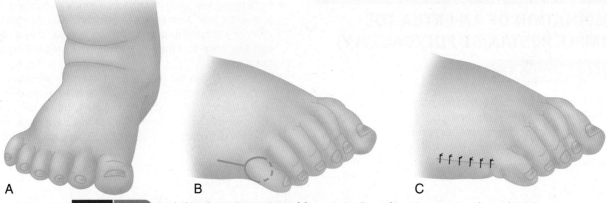

A   B   C

FIGURE **1.4** Polydactyly. **A,** Front view of foot. **B,** Outline of incision passing through web space between fifth and sixth toes and extending in racquet-shaped incision along lateral border of foot. **C,** Surgical excision of supernumerary digit. **SEE TECHNIQUE 1.1.**

associated with polydactyly in the foot, and removal of the more medial or lateral digit is typically preferred.

MACRODACTYLY

Macrodactyly occurs when one or more toes or fingers have hypertrophied and are significantly larger than the surrounding toes or fingers. The most common associated conditions are neurofibromatosis, hemangiomatosis, and congenital lipofibromatosis. Surgery is indicated to relieve functional symptoms, primarily pain or difficulty in fitting shoes. The cosmetic goal is to alter the abnormal appearance of the toes and foot and to achieve a foot similar in size to the opposite foot (Fig. 1.5).

Many operative procedures have been described for the treatment of macrodactyly, including reduction syndactyly, soft-tissue debulking combined with ostectomy or epiphysiodesis, toe amputation, and ray amputation. Soft-tissue debulking combined with ostectomy or epiphysiodesis can be used in the initial treatment of a single digit with macrodactyly; the recurrence rate with this technique is virtually 100%. Ray resection, combined with debulking repeated as necessary has been recommended; however, when the great toe is involved, the result often is only fair, and repeated soft-tissue debulking may be necessary. When enlargement of the toe or forefoot is less severe, epiphysiodesis of the phalangeal physes is recommended when the toe reaches adult size; debulking is repeated as necessary. Ray amputation is indicated in patients with massive enlargement of the bone and soft tissues and is also the procedure of choice for severe recurrence after reduction syndactyly or soft-tissue debulking. Hallux valgus may occur after resection of the second ray and occasionally requires surgical correction during adolescence.

TSUGE RAY REDUCTION

The Tsuge procedure is an additional option for pedal macrodactyly treatment. It is a rare procedure for a rare condition; however, according to the authors, the benefit of this procedure is that it debulks and shortens the toe but maintains good cosmesis by preserving the toenail.

TECHNIQUE 1.2

(TSUGE)
- After administering general anesthesia and placing a tourniquet, make a midaxial fish-mouth incision (Fig. 1.6A).
- Dissect sharply down the plantar aspect of the distal and middle phalanges.
- Disarticulate the distal interphalangeal joint.
- Identify and protect the neurovascular bundles within the dorsal flap. Do not excise or debulk.
- Release the flexor digitorum longus and extensor digitorum longus tendon insertions from the distal phalanx and tag these (maintain and protect the extensor digitorum longus attachment to the middle phalanx).
- Using a microsagittal saw, make a coronal cut along the distal phalanx, excising the plantar portion and leaving approximately a third of the phalanx beneath the nail plate and matrix (Fig. 1.6B).
- Make a transverse cut across the distal phalanx, excising the physis (Fig. 1.6C).
- Skeletonize the middle phalanx dorsally, protecting the extensor attachment.
- Make a similar size-matched coronal cut in the middle phalanx at the one third dorsal to two thirds plantar level.
- Create a transverse osteotomy across the dorsal aspect of the middle phalanx, leaving the physis still attached to the plantar aspect of the residual bone.
- Excise the distal aspect of the dorsal middle phalanx (Fig. 1.6D).
- Shorten the remaining plantar aspect of the middle phalanx if needed to the desired length of the toe.
- Bring the dorsal sliver of the distal phalanx, which contains the nail, proximally and fit it to the plantar portion of the middle phalanx (Fig. 1.6E) and secure the transferred bone with a small Kirschner wire or suture lasso.
- Reattach the flexor digitorum longus tendon to the remaining middle phalanx using Vicryl suture (Ethicon, Somerville, NJ). Reattach the extensor digitorum longus tendon to the middle phalanx.
- Deflate the tourniquet and obtain hemostasis using bipolar electrocautery.

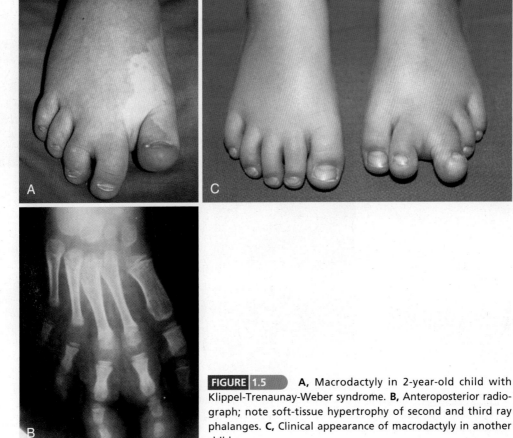

FIGURE 1.5 **A,** Macrodactyly in 2-year-old child with Klippel-Trenaunay-Weber syndrome. **B,** Anteroposterior radiograph; note soft-tissue hypertrophy of second and third ray phalanges. **C,** Clinical appearance of macrodactyly in another child.

- After the bony work, debulk any redundant plantar flap of tissue and fat (Fig. 1.6F) to allow wound closure (Fig. 1.6G).
- Copiously irrigate the wound and close with absorbable suture. As a result of the digital shortening, a dorsal bump just proximal to the nail is created.
- Apply a sterile dressing and a well-padded short leg walking cast.

POSTOPERATIVE CARE The patient is allowed weight bearing as tolerated.

- Fuse the physis at the level of the metatarsal head. If necessary, repeat this process for any phalanges until the ray has been shortened to normal length.
- Insert a smooth, longitudinal Kirschner wire from the tip of the toe to the base of the metatarsal to align the ray.
- Secure hemostasis, close the wound with interrupted sutures, and apply a short leg cast.

POSTOPERATIVE CARE The Kirschner wire is removed at 6 weeks, and a short leg walking cast is worn until any bony procedures have healed.

RAY REDUCTION

TECHNIQUE 1.3

- Outline dorsal skin incisions along the ray to be reduced, with a single long incision or multiple small incisions along the metatarsal and phalanges.
- Debulk any fibrofatty tissue, protecting the digital neurovascular bundles.
- Osteotomize the metatarsal neck and shorten the metatarsal by removing a segment of sufficient length to match this metatarsal to the others.

RAY AMPUTATION

TECHNIQUE 1.4

- Outline the ray to be amputated with skin flaps to include amputation from the tip of the toe to the base of the metatarsal.
- Make dorsal and plantar incisions starting over the metatarsophalangeal joint, with connecting incisions in the web space of adjacent toes. Continue the incisions proximally, dorsally, and plantarward, to the base of the metatarsal to be resected (Fig. 1.7).

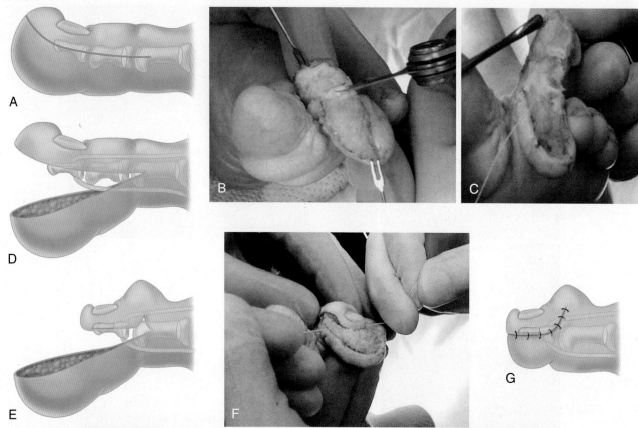

FIGURE 1.6 Tsuge ray reduction procedure. **A,** Fish-mouth incision made to the level of the proximal phalanx. **B,** Coronal osteotomy of the distal phalanx. **C,** Physis is removed by transverse osteotomy from remaining dorsal bone. Plantar portion is removed. **D,** Osteotomy and removal of dorsal middle phalanx. **E,** Dorsal third of distal phalanx is fixed to plantar two thirds of middle phalanx and tendons reattached. **F,** Fibrofatty tissue remains when digit is shortened, creating a dorsal bump. **G,** Excess tissue is debulked. (From Morrell NT, Fitzpatrick J, Szalay EA: The use of the Tsuge procedure for pedal macrodactyly: relevance in pediatric orthopaedics, *J Pediatr Orthop B* 23:260–265, 2014.) **SEE TECHNIQUE 1.2.**

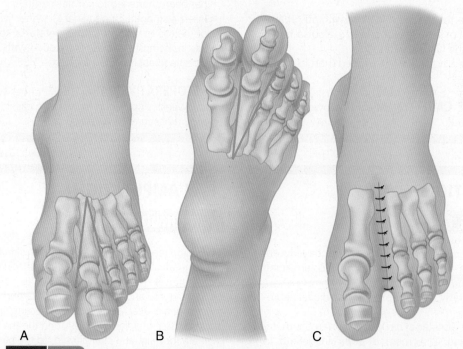

FIGURE 1.7 Ray amputation for macrodactyly. **A,** Incision on dorsal surface of foot. **B,** Plantar incision. **C,** Closed incision after amputation. **SEE TECHNIQUE 1.4.**

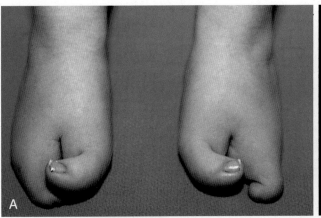
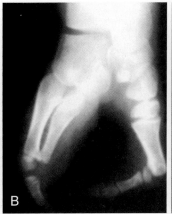
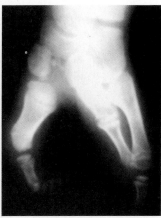

FIGURE 1.8   **A,** Bilateral cleft foot in 4-year-old boy. **B,** Anteroposterior view; note angular deformity of metatarsophalangeal joints of great toe and fifth toe.

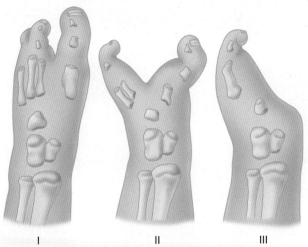

I   II   III

FIGURE 1.9   Clinical classification of cleft foot deformity (see text).

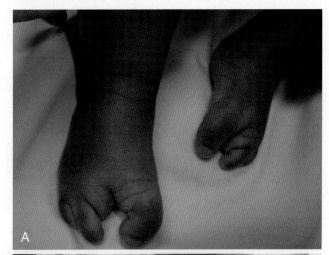
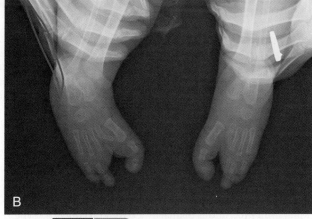

FIGURE 1.10   Type 1 cleft foot.

- Amputate the metatarsal and its associated phalanges and any surrounding hypertrophied soft tissue. Protect the neurovascular bundles that supply adjacent toes.
- After adequate resection of tissue, close the wound with interrupted sutures in the usual manner.

POSTOPERATIVE CARE A short leg cast is applied to protect the wound until healing occurs at 4 to 6 weeks.

CLEFT FOOT (PARTIAL ADACTYLY)

Cleft foot (lobster foot) is an anomaly in which a single cleft extends proximally into the foot, sometimes as far as the midfoot. Generally, one or more toes and parts of their metatarsals are absent, and often the tarsals are abnormal. Although the deformity varies in degree and type, the first and fifth rays are usually present (Fig. 1.8). If a metatarsal is partially or completely absent, its respective toe is always absent. Blauth and Borisch classified the deformities into six types based on the number of metatarsal bones present. Type I and type II are cleft feet with minor deficiencies, both having five metatarsals. The metatarsals are normal in type I and partially hypoplastic

in type II. The number of identifiable metatarsals decreases progressively: type III, four metatarsals; type IV, three metatarsals; type V, two metatarsals; and type VI, one metatarsal.

Abraham et al. described a simplified clinical classification on which they based treatment recommendations (Fig. 1.9). Type I has a central ray cleft or deficiency (usually second or third rays or both) extending up to the midmetatarsal level without splaying of medial or lateral rays (Fig. 1.10). For this type of cleft foot, they recommended soft-tissue

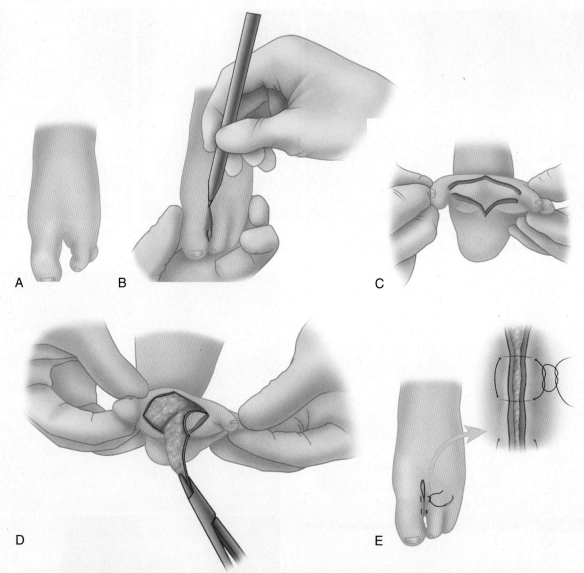

FIGURE 1.11   Syndactylism of cleft. **A-C,** Cleft is manually closed, and cleavage area is marked with sterile ink pen on dorsum and sole of foot. **D,** Skin and some subcutaneous tissue is removed as outlined by ink lines. **E,** Undermined skin edges are approximated with horizontal mattress sutures.

syndactylism with partial hallux valgus correction if needed; however, this type of deformity typically results in little functional limitation and is primarily a cosmetic concern. Type II has a deep cleft up to the tarsal bones with forefoot splaying, for which they recommended soft-tissue syndactylism, with first-ray osteotomy if needed, before age 5 years. Type III is a complete absence of the first through third or fourth rays, for which they did not recommend surgery; Abraham et al. recommended syndactylism for all type II cleft feet in the first 3 years of life while the forefoot is still supple. All of their patients older than 5 years with type II deformities had first ray amputation.

Any surgery for cleft foot should improve function and appearance. When surgical correction is performed, dorsal and plantar flaps are raised from the skin of the apposing surfaces, which are then sutured together (Fig. 1.11). Any bony or joint deformity of the first or fifth ray should be corrected at the time of surgery (Fig. 1.12). This may require capsulotomies and osteotomies of any retained rays. If pin fixation is used for fixation of osteotomies of the phalanges or metatarsals, the pins and short leg cast are removed 6 weeks after surgery, and a short leg walking cast or cast boot may be worn for an additional few weeks.

Wood, Peppers, and Shook described a simplified cleft closure using rectangular flaps. According to these authors, this technique is easier than techniques using multiple triangular flaps and produces superior cosmetic results. They recommended correction of the cleft foot at 6 months old because of fewer anesthesia risks, minimal growth deformities, and malleability of the soft tissues.

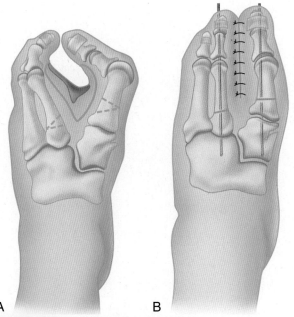

FIGURE 1.12 Correction of cleft foot. **A,** Skin incisions along cleft between abnormal rays of foot. **B,** Artificial syndactyly created after excision of skin cleft, apposition of rays, and osteotomies of metatarsals.

SIMPLIFIED CLEFT CLOSURE

TECHNIQUE 1.5

(WOOD, PEPPERS, AND SHOOK)

- At least two metatarsals must be present for good cleft closure.
- On the lateral side, or fifth ray, raise a rectangular flap, starting from the plantar surface of the foot to the dorsum (Fig. 1.13A). This does not include fascia but includes a fairly thick flap with fat.
- Exactly opposite this flap on the medial side, or first ray, raise a rectangular flap starting on the dorsum of the foot to the plantar aspect. Repeat this two or three times until the skin of the entire cleft is removed (Fig. 1.13B).
- At the longest toe, raise a distally based flap for suturing to the adjacent toe to make a wide web.
- If the toes spring apart, make a closing wedge osteotomy at the base of each metatarsal to centralize the toes (Fig. 1.13C) and stabilize the osteotomies with Kirschner wires (Fig. 1.13D).
- To stabilize the intermetacarpal distance further and unload tension on the surgical flaps, reconstruct the ligament with

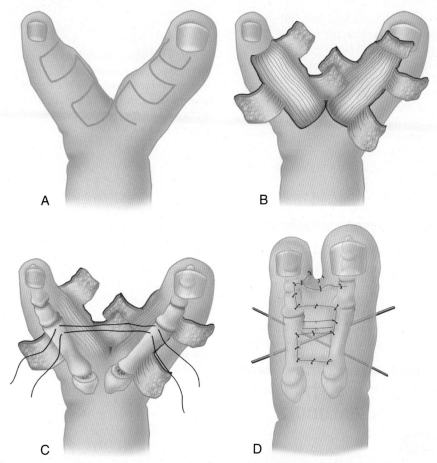

FIGURE 1.13 Cleft foot closure (see text). **A,** Rectangular flaps are raised on both rays. **B,** Flaps are raised until skin of entire cleft is removed. At distal tip of longer toe, flap is raised to suture to adjacent toe to make wide toe web. **C,** If toes spring apart, closing wedge osteotomy is made at base of each metatarsal to centralize bones. **D,** Kirschner wires are inserted to maintain position. **SEE TECHNIQUE 1.5.**

local ligamentous tissue, joint capsule, or tendon obtained from the cleft foot or with autograft plantaris tendon or fascia lata.

■ Close the wound in routine fashion and apply a cast.

POSTOPERATIVE CARE At 3 weeks, weight bearing in a walking cast is allowed. At 6 weeks, the cast is discontinued, and the Kirschner wires are removed.

CONTRACTURE OR ANGULATION OF THE TOES

Congenital contracture, angulation, or subluxation of the fifth toe is a fairly common familial deformity, but rarely causes symptoms. The anomaly is rarely disabling, and surgery usually is indicated only to improve function of the foot or make shoe fitting easier. The direction of angulation of the fifth toe determines the operative procedure. Surgical procedures for the correction of an angulated toe include soft-tissue correction alone, soft-tissue correction with proximal phalangectomy, and amputation.

CORRECTION OF ANGULATED TOE
TECHNIQUE 1.6

■ Approach the fifth metatarsophalangeal joint through a Z-plasty incision. With the toe held in the corrected position, draw the central limb of the Z-plasty along the band of contracted skin to the fourth web space. Create the proximal and distal limbs of the Z-plasty of equal lengths (Fig. 1.14). Make the angle of the Z-plasty 60 degrees, which allows maximal elongation along the longitudinal axis of the Z-plasty when the limbs are transposed.
■ Release the extensor digitorum longus tendon of the fifth toe in a long, oblique fashion.
■ Release the dorsal and medial capsule and place the toe in the corrected position.
■ Transpose the two limbs of the Z-plasty and suture them with interrupted absorbable sutures.

Butler arthroplasty can be done for correction of a dorsally overriding fifth toe. One complication of Butler arthroplasty is the potential for vascular damage caused by excessive tension on the neurovascular bundle. This complication can be prevented by (1) avoiding any tension on the neurovascular bundle, (2) taking care not to manipulate or exert traction on the toe, and (3) avoiding the use of circumferential taping or rigid splinting.

ARTHROPLASTY OF THE FIFTH METATARSOPHALANGEAL JOINT
TECHNIQUE 1.7

(BUTLER)
■ After preparing and draping the foot and applying a tourniquet, make a double-racquet incision, with the dorsal

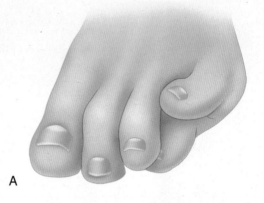

A

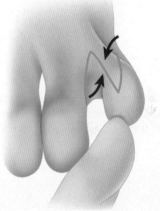

B

FIGURE 1.14 Correction of congenital crossover fifth toe. **A,** Preoperative appearance. **B,** Z-incision with 60-degree angles. *Arrows* indicate direction flaps are transposed to allow lengthening along longitudinal axis of Z-plasty. (From Thordarson DB: Congenital crossover fifth toe correction with soft-tissue release and cutaneous Z-plasty, *Foot Ankle Int* 22:511–512, 2001.) **SEE TECHNIQUE 1.6.**

handle following the extensor longus tendon and the plantar handle inclined laterally to provide a circumferential incision (Fig. 1.15A). For milder deformities, the dorsal limb of the double-racquet incision alone may allow complete correction of the deformity.
■ To expose the contracted extensor tendon, elevate skin flaps by blunt dissection, protecting the neurovascular bundle (Fig. 1.15B).
■ Transect the extensor tendon to the fifth toe and divide the dorsal aspect of the metatarsophalangeal joint capsule (Fig. 1.15C).
■ The toe should now partially rotate downward and laterally into the correct position. In long-standing deformities, the plantar aspect of the capsule is adherent and prevents full reduction of the proximal phalanx on the metatarsal during derotation of the toe.
■ If necessary, separate the adherent plantar capsule by blunt dissection and divide it transversely to allow the toe to lie freely in a fully corrected position (Fig. 1.15D and E). This may require the second limb of the double-racquet incision originally described.
■ Close the skin with multiple interrupted sutures and apply a light dressing to the suture line (Fig. 1.15F and G).

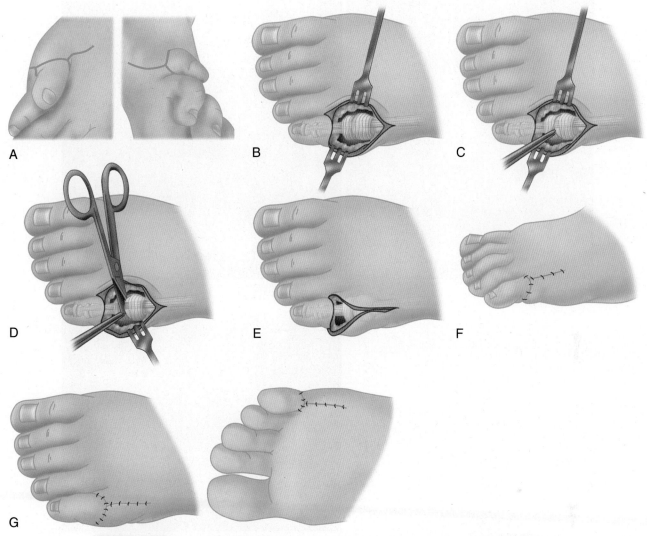

FIGURE 1.15 Butler arthroplasty. **A,** Double-racquet incision. **B,** Exposure of extensor tendon. **C,** Transection of extensor tendon. **D,** Separation of adherent capsule. **E,** Corrected position of toe. **F and G,** Skin closure. **SEE TECHNIQUE 1.7.**

POSTOPERATIVE CARE A short leg cast or postoperative surgical shoe may be worn, with a light dressing only over the fifth toe. Protected activity is allowed as tolerated.

CONGENITAL HALLUX VARUS

Congenital hallux varus is a deformity in which the great toe is angled medially. The varus deformity of the toe varies in severity from only a few degrees to 90 degrees. The hallux varus can occur at the metatarsophalangeal joint with a normal metatarsal or it can occur in association with other deformities of the medial foot such as bracket epiphysis or preaxial polydactyly.

Typically, congenital hallux varus is unilateral and is associated with one or more of the following: (1) a short, thick first metatarsal; (2) accessory bones or toes; (3) varus deformity of one or more of the four lateral metatarsals; and (4) a firm fibrous band that extends from the medial side of the great toe to the base of the first metatarsal (Fig. 1.16). The explanation for this anomaly is that two great toes originate in

utero, but the medial or accessory one fails to develop. Later, the rudimentary medial toe, together with the band of fibrous tissue, acts like a taut bowstring and gradually pulls the more fully developed great toe into a varus position.

The proper treatment for congenital hallux varus depends on the severity of the deformity and the rigidity of the contracted soft structures. A metatarsal epiphyseal bracket can be treated with physiolysis if performed very early or physiolysis combined with corrective osteotomy if performed later for milder hallux varus (Fig. 1.17). An osteotomy without physiolysis has an increased risk of recurrence, and the use of a bone graft increases the risk of fusing the epiphyseal bracket. A fat graft can be used as interposition material; however, Choo and Mubarak noted that fat attaches poorly to the diaphysis. Several of their patients developed a peripheral bar at the proximal metaphyseal-epiphyseal junction causing recurrent deformity. They recommended using polymethyl methacrylate as interposition material.

The Farmer technique is effective in correcting moderate deformity. The operation of Kelikian et al. is also satisfactory for severe deformity with an excessively short first metatarsal

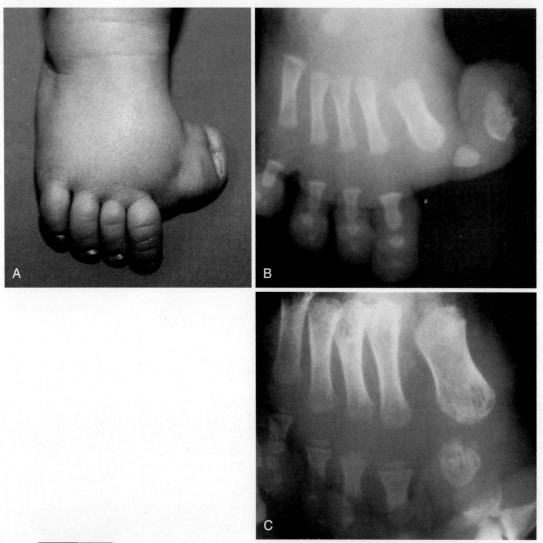

FIGURE 1.16 **A,** Congenital hallux varus of right foot. **B,** Anteroposterior radiograph; note short first metatarsal and accessory distal phalanx. **C,** Appearance after surgical correction.

(Fig. 1.18). Each of these procedures is designed to create a syndactyly between the second toe and the hallux to maintain deformity correction. If the deformity is complicated by traumatic arthritis of the metatarsophalangeal joint, arthrodesis of this joint is indicated. In rare cases, if the deformity is too severe either to be corrected or to undergo arthrodesis, amputation is indicated.

CREATION OF SYNDACTYLY OF THE GREAT TOE AND SECOND TOE FOR HALLUX VARUS

TECHNIQUE 1.8

(FARMER)

- Raise a broad Y-shaped flap of skin and subcutaneous tissue from the dorsal surface of the web between the first and second toes (Fig. 1.19); base the flap dorsally in the space between the first and second metatarsals and include in it the skin contiguous with the web distally along the two toes for one third of their length.
- From the medial edge of the base of the flap, curve the incision medially and slightly distally across the medial aspect of the first metatarsophalangeal joint. Deepen this incision transversely through the medial part of the capsule of the first metatarsophalangeal joint.
- Move the great toe laterally against the second toe and create a syndactyly between these two toes by suturing the apposing skin edges together.
- A smooth longitudinal Kirschner wire can be inserted from the tip of the great toe into the first metatarsal to align the great toe in a neutral position.
- Excise any accessory phalanx or hypertrophic soft tissue from the great toe through a separate dorsomedial incision.
- Swing the Y-shaped flap of skin and subcutaneous tissue medially and suture it in place to cover the defect in the skin on the dorsal and medial aspects of the first metatarsophalangeal joint.

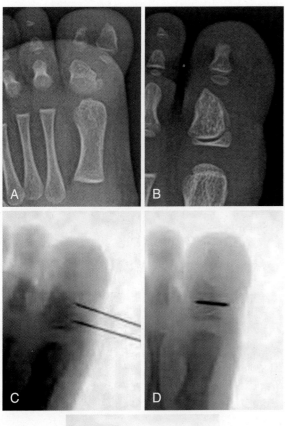

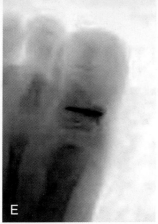

FIGURE 1.17 Epiphyseal bracket. **A,** Foot with preaxial polydactyly had reconstruction. **B,** Several months later an epiphyseal bracket of the proximal phalanx was noted with early ossification. **C,** The patient had excision of the hallux bracket. Intraoperative imaging demonstrating two needles at edges of bracket. **D,** Kirschner wire placed transversely through proximal phalanx. **E,** Polymethyl methacrylate cement was placed around wire. (From Choo AD, Mubarak SJ: Longitudinal epiphyseal bracket, *J Child Orthop* 7:449–454, 2013.)

- In an alternative technique described by Farmer, the Y-shaped flap of skin and subcutaneous tissue is raised from the plantar surface of the foot (Fig. 1.20); the rest of the procedure is the same as already described, with the flap swung medially to cover the defect in the skin at the first metatarsophalangeal joint. Any defect that cannot be closed by the flap either is left open to heal secondarily or is covered by a full-thickness skin graft.

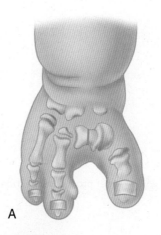

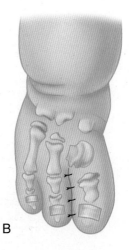

FIGURE 1.18 Kelikian procedure for congenital hallux varus. **A,** Preoperative appearance of foot. **B,** After artificial syndactyly.

POSTOPERATIVE CARE The foot is immobilized in a cast. At 6 weeks, the cast and pins are removed, and full activities are allowed.

CONGENITAL METATARSUS ADDUCTUS

Metatarsus adductus, which consists of adduction of the forefoot in relation to the midfoot and hindfoot, is a common anomaly, often causing intoeing in children. It can occur as an isolated anomaly or in association with clubfoot. Among children with metatarsus adductus, 1% to 5% also have developmental dysplasia of the hip or acetabular dysplasia.

Clinically, metatarsus adductus can be classified as mild, moderate, or severe (Fig. 1.21). In the mild form, the forefoot can be clinically abducted to the midline of the foot and beyond. The moderate form has enough flexibility to allow abduction of the forefoot to the midline, but usually not beyond (Fig. 1.22). In rigid metatarsus adductus, the forefoot cannot be abducted at all. There also may be a transverse crease on the medial border of the foot or an enlargement of the web space between the great and second toes. In general, mild metatarsus adductus resolves without treatment. Moderate or severe metatarsus adductus is best treated initially by serial stretching and casting for 6 to 12 weeks, or until the foot is clinically flexible (Fig. 1.23).

Metatarsus adductus may be seen as a residual deformity in patients previously treated surgically or nonsurgically for congenital clubfoot. This residual metatarsus adductus can be rigid, indicating fixed positioning of the forefoot on the midfoot and hindfoot, or it can be dynamic, caused by imbalance of the anterior tibial tendon during gait. The rigidity or flexibility of the forefoot should be determined before undertaking any surgical correction in an older child. Metatarsus adductus, particularly in its milder forms, is often only a cosmetic concern. However, shoe wear may also become an issue as the child ages.

■ TREATMENT

In a young child, surgery is not indicated until conservative treatment has failed. When a child passes the appropriate age for serial stretching and casting, surgery becomes a reasonable option. Indications for surgery include pain, objectionable appearance, and difficulty in fitting shoes because of

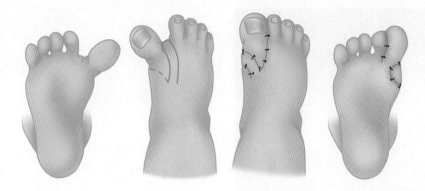

FIGURE 1.19 Farmer procedure for congenital hallux varus (see text). **SEE TECHNIQUE 1.8.**

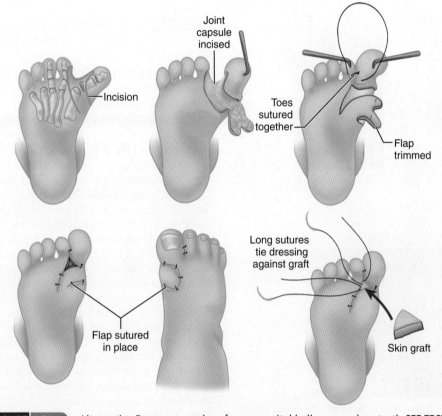

FIGURE 1.20 Alternative Farmer procedure for congenital hallux varus (see text). **SEE TECHNIQUE 1.8.**

residual forefoot adduction. Numerous soft-tissue and bony procedures have been described for correction of metatarsus adductus. The most reliable involved osteotomies at either the tarsal or metatarsal levels as described below.

DOME-SHAPED OSTEOTOMIES OF METATARSAL BASES

Berman and Gartland recommended dome-shaped osteotomies for all five metatarsal bases for resistant forefoot adduction in children 4 years old and older (Fig. 1.24). For a mature foot with uncorrected metatarsus adductus, or if all of the medial soft-tissue structures are contracted, they recommended a laterally based closing wedge osteotomy through the bases of the metatarsals. Correcting the alignment without shortening the lateral border of the foot can cause excessive tension on the skin on the medial border or on the neurovascular bundle posterior to the medial malleolus. Steinmann pins inserted parallel to the medial and lateral borders of the foot are usually necessary to hold the foot in the corrected position until the osteotomies have healed. Without internal fixation, the soft tissue on the medial side may cause recurrence of deformity.

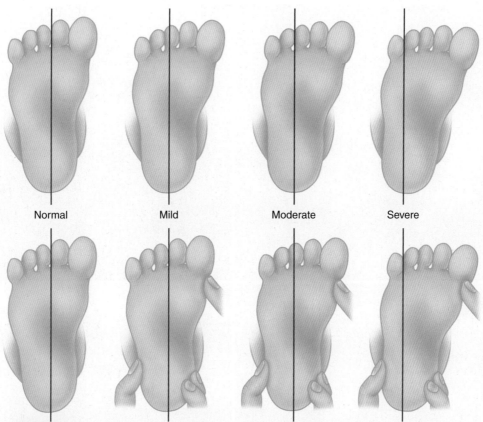

Normal   Mild   Moderate   Severe

FIGURE 1.21 Heel bisector defines relationship of heel to forefoot from left to right: normal (bisecting second and third toes), mild metatarsus adductus (bisecting third toe), moderate metatarsus adductus (bisecting third and fourth toes), and severe metatarsus adductus (bisecting fourth and fifth toes).

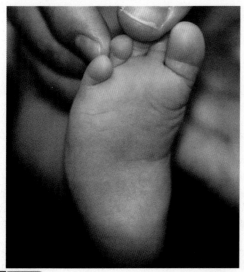

FIGURE 1.22 Congenital metatarsus adductus. Moderate deformity.

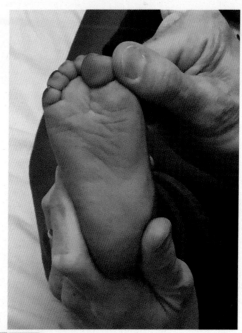

FIGURE 1.23 Stretching for correction of metatarsus adductus deformity.

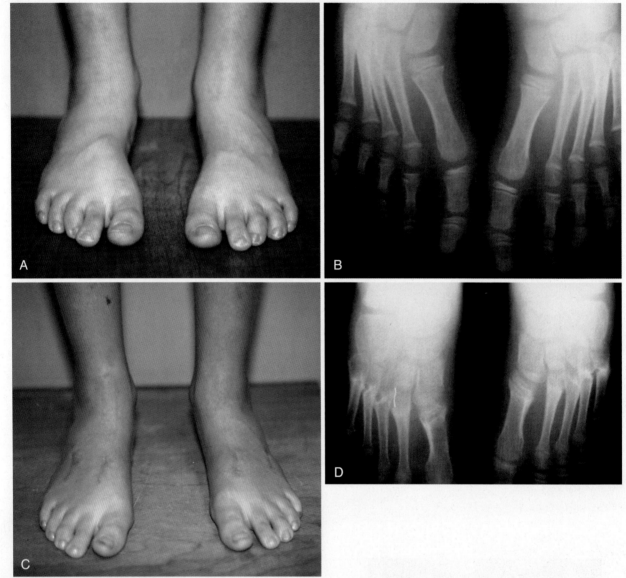

FIGURE 1.24   **A** and **B,** Rigid metatarsus adductus in 8-year-old child. **C** and **D,** After multiple metatarsal osteotomies. **SEE TECHNIQUE 1.9.**

TECHNIQUE 1.9

(BERMAN AND GARTLAND)

- Approach all five metatarsal bases dorsally. Make two longitudinal dorsal incisions, one between the first and second metatarsals and the other overlying the fourth. Protect the extensor tendons and superficial nerves and preserve the superficial veins as much as possible.
- Expose subperiosteally the proximal metaphysis of each metatarsal, and with a small power drill make a dome-shaped osteotomy in each with the apex of the dome proximally (Fig. 1.25). Avoid the physis at the base of the first metatarsal.
- If adequate correction cannot be obtained by these osteotomies, resect small wedges of bone based laterally at the osteotomies as needed.
- Align the metatarsals and transfix the foot in the corrected position with small, smooth Steinmann pins inserted proximally through the shafts of the first and fifth metatarsals cand across the osteotomies in these bones and, if needed, in all five metatarsals. Prevent dorsal or volar angulation and overriding of the fragments.

- Before closing the wound, check the placement of the pins, position of the osteotomies, and forefoot alignment by radiographs (Fig. 1.26). The anteroposterior talus–first metatarsal angle should be corrected to 0 to 10 degrees.

POSTOPERATIVE CARE A short leg cast is applied with the foot in the corrected position. At 6 weeks, the cast and pins are removed, and weight bearing is begun, commonly in a walking cast or cast boot for 2 to 4 weeks.

For the osteotomy portion of the above technique, Knorr et al. described using the Cahuzac technique of percutaneous osteotomies of the metatarsals in children with metatarsus adductus. The approach uses a beaver blade to create two small incisions over the base of the second metatarsal and the third intermetatarsal space. A high-speed surgical burr is used to create a percutaneous osteotomy of the second through fourth metatarsal bases. Percutaneous cuneometatarsal capsulotomy is performed with a 19-gauge needle.

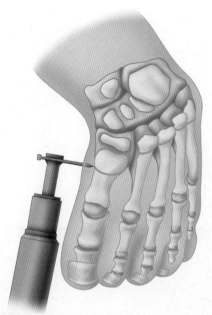

FIGURE 1.25 Berman and Gartland technique for metatarsal osteotomies. Dome-shaped osteotomy is completed at base of each metatarsal. **SEE TECHNIQUE 1.9.**

The forefoot is manipulated and stabilized with an obliquely oriented, percutaneous 2-mm Kirschner wire from the first metatarsal into the tarsal bones.

CUNEIFORM AND CUBOID OSTEOTOMIES

McHale and Lenhart recommended opening wedge osteotomy of the medial cuneiform and closing wedge osteotomy of the cuboid for correction of deformities in the midfoot with severe shortening of the medial column ("bean-shaped" foot).

TECHNIQUE 1.10

(MCHALE AND LENHART)

- With the anesthetized patient supine, make a small longitudinal incision over the cuboid (Fig. 1.27A).
- Remove a 7- to 10-mm wedge with its base in a dorsolateral position (Fig. 1.27B).
- Approach the medial cuneiform by using part of the distal extension of the medial incision (Fig. 1.27A) or a 2-cm incision medially over the medial cuneiform.
- Make the osteotomy in the cuneiform, leaving the anterior tibial tendon attached to the distal piece of bone.
- Spread the medial cuneiform osteotomy with a smooth spreader and insert the wedge of bone removed from the cuboid, with the base of the wedge straight medially (Fig. 1.27C).
- Check clinical correction of the deformity. If the lateral border of the foot still appears prominent (midfoot supination has not been corrected), remove a larger wedge of bone from the cuboid.
- Use two smooth Kirschner wires to fix the foot in the corrected position. Insert one pin through the cuboid, starting in the calcaneus and exiting through the base of the

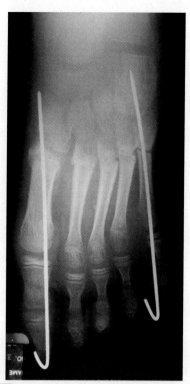

FIGURE 1.26 Completed osteotomies with Steinmann pins inserted to hold corrected position. **SEE TECHNIQUE 1.9.**

fifth metatarsal. Place the other pin through the first web space, through the medial cuneiform and tarsal navicular, and into the talus.
- Confirm the position of the pins and the correction of the bony deformity with radiographs.
- After correct positioning of the foot, the lateral three toes may remain in passively uncorrectable flexion. If so, perform simple flexor tenotomy.
- Close the wounds and apply a short leg cast with thick padding to allow for swelling.

POSTOPERATIVE CARE At 2 weeks, the wounds are checked, and a more form-fitting, non–weight-bearing cast is applied. The pins are removed at 6 weeks, and a weight-bearing cast is applied. A cast or cast boot is worn until bony union is evident on radiographs, usually at 8 to 12 weeks.

ANOMALIES OF THE FOOT
CONGENITAL CLUBFOOT (TALIPES EQUINOVARUS)

The incidence of congenital clubfoot is approximately 1 in every 1000 live births. Although most cases are sporadic occurrences, families have been reported with clubfoot as an autosomal dominant trait with incomplete penetrance. Bilateral deformities occur in 50% of patients. In patients with bilateral deformity, the severity and response to treatment is highly correlated between the 2 feet.

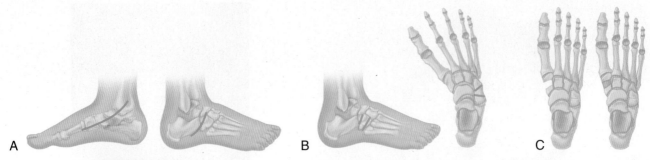

A   B   C

FIGURE 1.27 Osteotomies of medial cuneiform and cuboid for correction of residual deformity. **A,** Lateral and medial incisions. **B,** Removal of dorsolateral wedge from cuboid. **C,** Placement of wedge in osteotomy in medial cuneiform. **SEE TECHNIQUE 1.10.**

Several theories have been proposed regarding the cause of clubfoot, but the underlying cause of clubfoot is still mostly unknown. One theory is that a primary germplasm defect in the talus causes continued plantarflexion and inversion of this bone, with subsequent soft-tissue changes in the joints and musculotendinous complexes. Another theory is that primary soft-tissue abnormalities within the neuromuscular units cause secondary bony changes. There may be a vascular cause because many children with clubfoot have a hypertrophic anterior tibial artery or other vascular anomalies. Several authors have documented abnormal distribution of type I and type II muscle fibers in clubfeet. While the exact cause remains unknown, a number of factors have been correlated with a higher frequency of clubfoot, including maternal and paternal smoking, maternal obesity, family history, amniocentesis, and some selective serotonin reuptake inhibitors.

Multiple studies have demonstrated no correlation between clubfoot and developmental dysplasia of the hip. It is thought that a routine clinical examination screening is all that is needed for the evaluation of hip pathology in children born with a clubfoot deformity.

The pathologic changes caused by congenital clubfoot must be understood if the anomaly is to be treated effectively. The four basic components of clubfoot are cavus, adduction, varus, and equinus. The deformity varies in severity, from a mild positional clubfoot that is passively correctable to near the neutral position to a much more severe clubfoot with extreme, rigid hindfoot equinus and forefoot adduction. The typical deformity is shown in Fig. 1.28. Clubfoot often is accompanied by internal tibial torsion. The ankle, midtarsal, and subtalar joints all are involved in the pathologic process. In unilateral cases, the abnormal foot may be one half to one size smaller in length and width.

Turco attributed the deformity to medial displacement of the navicular and calcaneus around the talus. The talus is forced into equinus by the underlying calcaneus and navicular, whereas the head and neck of the talus are deviated medially. From a three-dimensional perspective, the relationship of the calcaneus to the talus is characterized by abnormal rotation in the sagittal, coronal, and horizontal planes. As the calcaneus rotates horizontally while pivoting on the interosseous ligament, it slips beneath the head and neck of the talus anterior to the ankle joint, and the calcaneal tuberosity moves toward the fibular malleolus posteriorly. The proximity of the calcaneus to the fibula is primarily caused by horizontal rotation of the talocalcaneal joint, rather than by equinus alone. The heel appears to be in varus because the

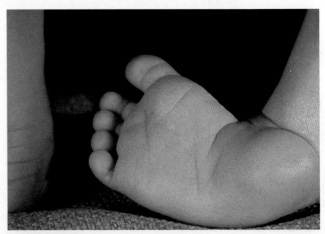

FIGURE 1.28 Congenital clubfoot in newborn. Posterior view—inversion, plantarflexion, and internal rotation of calcaneus and cavus deformity with transverse plantar crease.

calcaneus rotates through the talocalcaneal joint in a coronal plane and horizontally. The talonavicular joint is in an extreme position of inversion as the navicular moves around the head of the talus. The cuboid is displaced medially on the calcaneus.

In a three-dimensional clubfoot computer model, the talar neck has been shown to be internally rotated relative to the ankle mortise, but the talar body is externally rotated in the mortise. The calcaneus is significantly internally rotated with the sloped articular facet of the calcaneocuboid joint causing additional internal rotation of the midfoot.

Contractures or anomalies of the soft tissues exert further deforming forces and resist correction of bony deformity and realignment of the joints. Talocalcaneal joint realignment is opposed by the calcaneofibular ligament, the superior peroneal retinaculum (calcaneal fibular retinaculum), the peroneal tendon sheaths, and the posterior talocalcaneal ligament. Resisting realignment of the talonavicular joint are the posterior tibial tendon, the deltoid ligament (tibial navicular), the calcaneonavicular ligament (spring ligament), the entire talonavicular capsule, the dorsal talonavicular ligament, the bifurcated (Y) ligament, the inferior extensor retinaculum, and occasionally the cubonavicular oblique ligament. Internal rotation of the calcaneocuboid joint causes contracture of the bifurcated (Y) ligament, the long plantar ligament, the plantar calcaneocuboid ligament, the navicular cuboid ligament, the inferior extensor retinaculum (cruciate ligament), the dorsal calcaneocuboid ligament, and occasionally the cubonavicular ligament.

The metatarsals also are often deformed. They may deviate at the tarsometatarsal joints, or these joints may be normal, and the shafts of the metatarsals themselves may be adducted.

If the clubfoot is allowed to remain deformed, many other late adaptive changes occur in the bones. These changes depend on the severity of the soft-tissue contractures and the effects of walking. In untreated adults, some joints may spontaneously fuse, or they may develop degenerative changes secondary to the contractures. The untreated clubfoot is cosmetically, functionally, and psychologically unacceptable. Every effort should be made to correct the deformity.

The initial examination of the foot and the progress of treatment should depend on clinical judgment and occasionally radiographic examination.

■ RADIOGRAPHIC EVALUATION

If the clubfoot deformity is somewhat atypical, is associated with a global genetic or neurologic condition, or appears resistant to initial nonoperative treatment, imaging evaluation should be included. In a nonambulatory child, standard radiographs include simulated weight-bearing anteroposterior and stress dorsiflexion lateral radiographs of both feet. Standing anteroposterior and lateral standing radiographs may be obtained for an older child. Alternatively, ultrasonography has been proposed as a radiation-free imaging modality and could be used in locations familiar with the technique.

Important angles to consider in the evaluation of clubfoot are the talocalcaneal angle on the anteroposterior radiograph and, on the lateral radiograph, the talocalcaneal angle, the tibiocalcaneal angle, and the talus–first metatarsal angle (Fig. 1.29). The anteroposterior talocalcaneal angle in normal children ranges from 30 to 55 degrees (Table 1.1). In clubfoot, this angle progressively decreases with increasing heel varus. On the dorsiflexion lateral radiograph, the talocalcaneal angle in a normal foot varies from 25 to 50 degrees; in clubfoot, this angle progressively decreases with the severity of the deformity to an angle of 0 degrees, or parallelism. The tibiocalcaneal angle in a normal foot is 10 to 40 degrees on the stress lateral radiograph. In clubfoot, this angle generally is negative, indicating equinus of the calcaneus in relation to the tibia. Finally, the talus–first metatarsal angle is a radiographic measurement of forefoot adduction. This is useful in the treatment of metatarsus adductus alone but is equally important in the treatment of clubfoot to evaluate the position of the forefoot. In a normal foot, this angle is 5 to 15 degrees on the anteroposterior view; in clubfoot, it usually is negative, indicating adduction of the forefoot.

■ CLASSIFICATION

Two of the more commonly used classifications by Pirani et al. and Diméglio et al. are based solely on physical examination requiring no radiographic measurements or other special studies. Pirani's system is composed of six different physical examination findings and includes a hindfoot contracture score and a midfoot contracture score, each scored 0 for no abnormality, 0.5 for moderate abnormality, or 1 for severe abnormality. Each foot is assigned a total score, the maximum being 6 points, with a higher score indicating a more severe deformity. In the system of Diméglio et al., four parameters are assessed on the basis of their reducibility with gentle manipulation as measured with a handheld goniometer: (1) equinus deviation in the sagittal plane, (2) varus deviation in the frontal plane, (3) derotation of the calcaneopedal block in the horizontal plane, and (4) adduction of the forefoot relative to the hindfoot in the horizontal plane (Fig. 1.30). One additional point is given for each of the following: a posterior skin crease, a medial skin crease, rigid cavus, and poor muscle condition. In a comparison of the two systems, both were shown to have good interobserver reliability after the initial learning phase. Routine clinical use of one or both of these classification systems can be helpful in determining prognosis and documenting maintenance of correction or recurrence over time.

■ NONOPERATIVE TREATMENT

The initial treatment of clubfoot is nonoperative. Various treatment regimens have been proposed, including the use of corrective splinting, taping, and casting. Although a number of various casting techniques are used, the most widely accepted technique is that described by Ignacio Ponseti and consists of weekly serial manipulation and casting during the first weeks of life.

▌ PONSETI CASTING TECHNIQUE FOR CORRECTION OF CLUBFOOT DEFORMITY

Successful correction of clubfoot deformity generally is reported in more than 90% of children 2 years and younger treated with Ponseti casting even after previous unsuccessful nonoperative treatment. Multiple studies have highlighted the success and reproducibility of the Ponseti method even in developing nations. Achilles tenotomy generally is required, and anterior tibial tendon transfer may be added to the casting routine when necessary. Bleeding complications have been reported after percutaneous tenotomy from injury to the peroneal artery or the lesser saphenous vein; making a small open incision directly over the tendon before severing it, making the tenotomy from medial to lateral (Fig. 1.31), and using a more rounded beaver-eye blade can help avoid vascular injury.

Reported recurrence rates after Ponseti casting range from 10% to 30%; however, many recurrent deformities can be treated successfully with repeat casting, with or without the

TABLE 1.1		
Progression of Foot Angles in Normal Feet Over Average 6-Year Follow-Up		
ANGLE	AVERAGE FIRST VISIT (DEGREES)	AVERAGE LAST VISIT (DEGREES)
ANTEROPOSTERIOR VIEW		
Talocalcaneal	36.3	27.4
Calcaneal–second metatarsal	14.4	12.3
Talus–first metatarsal	16.9	8.1
LATERAL VIEW		
Talocalcaneal	46	44.2
Calcaneal–first metatarsal	150	148
Tibiocalcaneal	61.5	73.2
Talus–first metatarsal	16.3	12.1
Talocalcaneal index	83	71.6

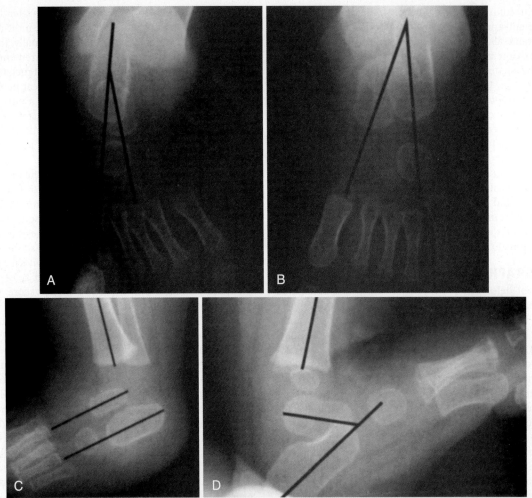

FIGURE 1.29 Radiographic evaluation of clubfoot. **A,** Anteroposterior view of right clubfoot with decrease in talocalcaneal angle and negative talus–first metatarsal angle. **B,** Talocalcaneal angle on anteroposterior view of normal left foot. **C,** Talocalcaneal angle of 0 degrees and negative tibiocalcaneal angle on dorsiflexion lateral view of right clubfoot. **D,** Talocalcaneal and tibiocalcaneal angles on dorsiflexion lateral view of normal left foot.

addition of Achilles tenotomy or anterior tibial tendon transfer. Numerous authors have noted that the most important factor in avoiding recurrent deformity is patient compliance with the postoperative brace wear regimen. Although the Ponseti method is ideally used in newborns, many studies have demonstrated successful use of the Ponseti method in older children or children with recurrent deformities after initial casting treatment. Also, the reported recurrence rates are higher in studies of children with syndrome-associated clubfoot deformities than in children with idiopathic clubfeet. Although the success rates are lower in older children and in those with syndromic clubfeet, nonoperative treatment should still be considered the first line of treatment even in these more challenging situations.

Strict adherence to the principles described by Ponseti is important to achieve optimal results. Only a few modifications to his original technique have demonstrated equivalent results. An accelerated casting program biweekly can result in more rapid correction of the deformity without compromising outcome. Fiberglass casting material has been shown to provide similar results to plaster casts. Bracing up to the age of 4 years may be superior to discontinuing brace treatment at the age of 3 years as originally described.

Application of Ponseti Casts. The Ponseti method consists of two phases: treatment and maintenance. The treatment phase should begin as early as possible, optimally within the first 2 weeks of life; however, older children also can be treated nonoperatively using Ponseti's principles. Gentle manipulation and casting are done weekly, although more frequent cast changes over a shorter period of time have been advocated by some authors. The order of correction by serial manipulation and casting should be as follows: first, correction of forefoot cavus and adduction; next, correction of heel varus; and finally, correction of hindfoot equinus. Correction should be pursued in this order so that a rocker-bottom deformity is prevented by dorsiflexing the foot through the ankle joint rather than the midfoot. Each cast holds the foot in the corrected position, allowing it to reshape gradually. Generally, five to six casts are required to correct the alignment of the foot and ankle fully. Before application of the final cast, most infants require percutaneous Achilles tenotomy to gain adequate lengthening of the Achilles tendon and prevent a rocker bottom deformity.

The first cast application corrects the cavus deformity by aligning the forefoot with the hindfoot, supinating the forefoot

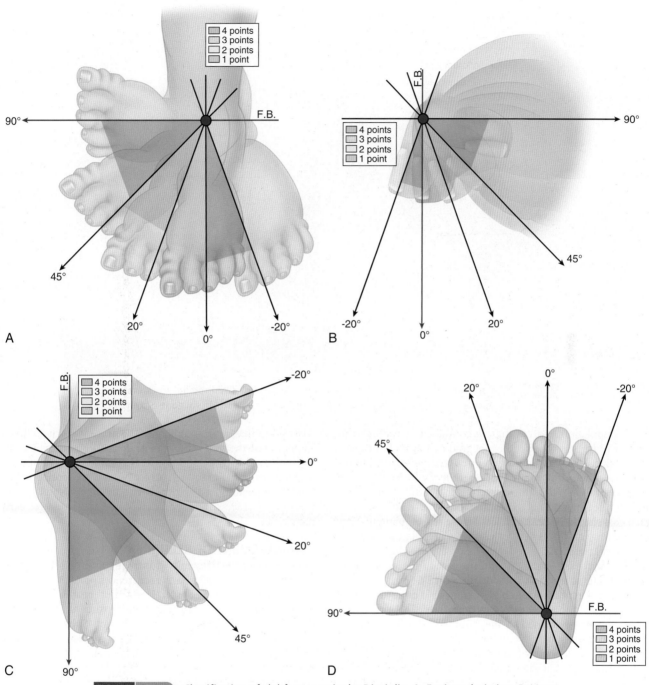

FIGURE 1.30 Classification of clubfoot severity by Diméglio. **A,** Equinus deviation. **B,** Varus deviation. **C,** Derotation. **D,** Adduction. (From Diméglio A, Bensahel H, Souchet P, et al: Classification of clubfoot, *J Pediatr Orthop B* 4:129–136, 1995.)

to bring it in line with the heel, and elevating (dorsiflexing) the first metatarsal (Fig. 1.32A). The casts should be applied in two stages: first, a short leg cast to just below the knee, then extension above the knee when the plaster sets. Long leg casts are essential to maintain a strong external rotation force of the foot beneath the talus, to allow adequate stretching of the medial structures, and to prevent cast slippage.

One week after application, the first cast is removed, and after about 1 minute of manipulation, the next toe-to-groin cast is applied (Fig. 1.32B). Manipulation and casting at this stage are focused on abducting the foot around the head of the talus, with care to maintain the supinated position of the forefoot and avoid any pronation. During these manipulations, the navicular can be felt reducing over the talar head by a thumb placed on the head of the talus. It is crucial that forefoot derotation occur about the talus rather than the calcaneocuboid joint, and the heel should not be directly manipulated. Maintaining forefoot supination throughout the process and correcting the talonavicular subluxation without producing a rocker-bottom deformity will cause the calcaneus to abduct and evert. Final correction of residual calcaneus deformity can then be achieved with a percutaneous Achilles tenotomy.

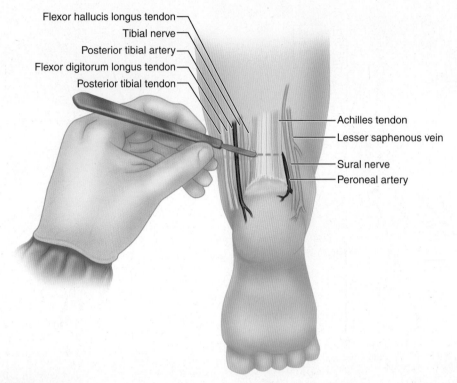

Flexor hallucis longus tendon
Tibial nerve
Posterior tibial artery
Flexor digitorum longus tendon
Posterior tibial tendon

Achilles tendon
Lesser saphenous vein
Sural nerve
Peroneal artery

FIGURE 1.31 Technique of percutaneous Achilles tenotomy from medial to lateral; note proximity of peroneal artery, lesser saphenous vein, and sural nerve to lateral edge of tendon.

Manipulation and casting are continued weekly for the next 2 to 3 weeks to abduct the foot gradually around the head of the talus. The foot should never be actively pronated; however, the amount of supination is gradually decreased over these several casts until the forefoot is in neutral position relative to the longitudinal axis of the foot (Fig. 1.32C). Ideally, each cast should be removed just before repeat manipulation and casting, and a variety of casting materials can be used with similar success.

The final cast is applied with the foot in the same maximally abducted position and dorsiflexed 15 degrees. In most children, a percutaneous Achilles tenotomy is done to prevent development of a rocker-bottom deformity. This procedure can either be performed in the clinic with local skin anesthesia, or in the operating room under sedation or general anesthesia. The benefit of tenotomy in the clinic setting is a reduced need for anesthesia and prolonged fasting; however, the operating room offers the ability to more easily control any excess bleeding that may occur. The foot is casted in the final position of approximately 70 degrees of abduction and 15 degrees of dorsiflexion for 3 weeks (Fig. 1.32D). Five or six casts usually are necessary to correct the clubfoot deformity **(see Video 1.2)**.

Maintenance Phase. When the final cast is removed, the infant is placed in a brace that maintains the foot in its corrected position (abducted and dorsiflexed). The brace (foot abduction orthosis) consists of shoes mounted to a bar in a position of 70 degrees of external rotation and 15 degrees of dorsiflexion. The distance between the shoes is set at about 1 inch wider than the width of the infant's shoulders (Fig. 1.33).

Multiple different types of shoes and bars have been designed and proposed. In some cases, it may be necessary to experiment with different combinations to find a brace that

will lead to maximal compliance. The brace is worn 23 hours each day for the first 3 months after casting and then while sleeping for 3 to 4 years. Brace wear compliance is of upmost importance in maintaining correction and preventing recurrence. Frequent follow-up during the bracing period is essential to encourage continued compliance and to detect early recurrence.

MANAGEMENT OF RECURRENCE

Recurrence of the deformity is infrequent if the bracing protocol is followed closely. Early recurrences (usually mild equinus and heel varus) are best treated with repeat manipulation and casting. The first cast may require some dorsiflexion of the first ray if cavus deformity is present. Subsequent casts abduct the foot around the talar head, correcting the varus and ultimately allowing ankle dorsiflexion. Achilles tendon lengthening may be necessary if dorsiflexion is insufficient; transfer of the anterior tibial tendon may be necessary to help maintain correction, particularly in children with persistent dynamic inversion.

ANTERIOR TIBIAL TENDON TRANSFER

TECHNIQUE 1.11

■ Begin the anterior tibial tendon transfer only if adequate ankle dorsiflexion is present or has been obtained by a lengthening of the gastroc-soleus-Achilles complex (see Technique 5.13).

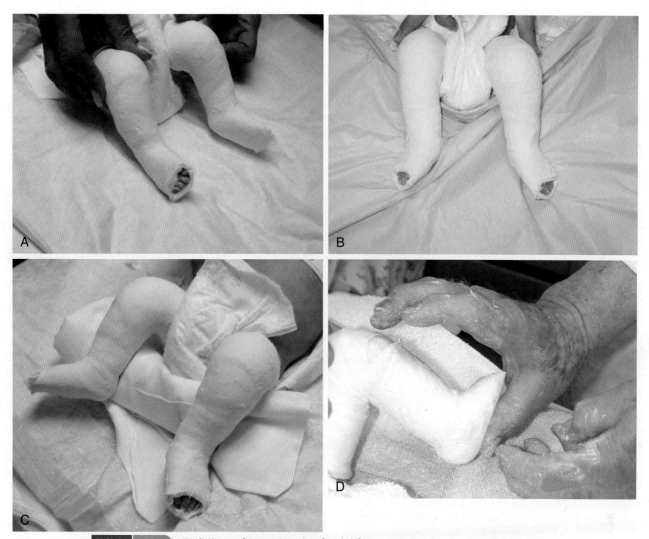

FIGURE 1.32 Technique of Ponseti casting for clubfoot correction (see text). **A,** First cast; note positioning of forefoot to align with heel, with outer edge of foot tilted even farther downward because of Achilles tendon tightness. **B,** Second cast is applied with outer edge of foot still tilted downward and forefoot moved slightly outward. **C,** Third cast; Achilles tendon is stretched bringing outer edge of foot into more normal position as forefoot is turned farther outward. **D,** Final cast; Achilles tendon is stretched more with foot pointed upward. (From Scher DM: The Ponseti method for clubfoot correction, *Oper Tech Orthop* 15:345, 2005.)

- Make a small 1- to 2-cm incision directly over the insertion of the anterior tibial tendon on the dorsomedial aspect of the foot.
- Open the tendon sheath and free the anterior tibial tendon from its insertion sharply, preserving as much length as possible.
- The tendon can then be transferred into the lateral cuneiform by one of two techniques. A two-incision technique moves the tendon directly across the dorsum of the foot and results in a change in direction of the tendon pull at the level of the ankle. A three-incision technique reroutes the tendon through a more proximal incision, resulting in a more direct path to the new insertion site, but the three-incision technique requires an additional incision and more surgical dissection.

- For the three-incision technique, palpate the anterior tibial tendon over the anterior distal third of the tibia and make a small, 1-cm incision.
- Dissect down to the tendon sheath and then open it sharply. Pass a hemostat behind the tendon and pull it firmly into the proximal incision. Some additional dissection may be required from both the proximal and distal wounds to free up the tendon from the sheath.
- Close the distal wound in a standard fashion. Closing each wound, once they are no longer needed, avoids the need to maintain prolonged foot dorsiflexion at the end of the case while all wounds are closed.
- Using a tendon locking stitch, such as a whipstitch, Krakow stitch, or crossing stitch, secure a number 1 Vicryl suture to the tendon, leaving long ends for transfer.

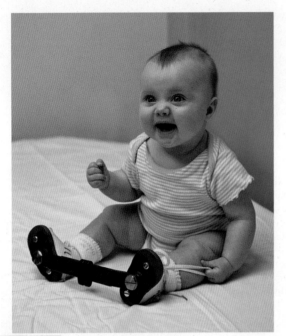

FIGURE 1.33 Foot abduction orthosis consists of shoes mounted to bar in 70 degrees external rotation and 15 degrees dorsiflexion.

- Identify the location of the lateral cuneiform with image intensification. Make a small, 1- to 2-cm incision over that position. Identify and protect any branches of the superficial peroneal nerve.
- Retract the extensor digitorum longus tendons and extensor digitorum muscle belly out of the way of the underlying lateral cuneiform periosteum.
- Create a "trapdoor" of periosteum and capsule directly over the lateral cuneiform. Leave the distal portion of this soft-tissue flap intact.
- Pass a Kelly clamp from the distal-lateral incision deep to the ankle retinaculum and up to the more proximal incision. Spread the Kelly clamp and make two or three passes to make space for the transferred tendon.
- Grasp the tendon sutures with the Kelly clamp and deliver them, along with the tendon, into the distal incision.
- Use image intensification to localize the center of the lateral cuneiform. Create a hole in the bone from dorsal to plantar with a trephine similar in size to that of the tendon.
- Using two straight Keith needles, pass the two limbs of the suture through the bone hole and out the plantar aspect of the foot. Pass the needles through a piece of sterile felt and through the holes of sterile plastic button.
- Have an assistant maintain the foot in a dorsiflexed and everted position. Make sure that the tendon has passed into the trephinated hole in the lateral cuneiform. Secure the suture snuggly against the button.
- Replace the bone plug from the trephine into the space adjacent to the tendon using a plunger.
- Lay the trapdoor flap against the tendon and secure with a horizontal mattress suture.

- Close any remaining wounds and apply a dressing and a short leg cast with the foot in the corrected position.

POSTOPERATIVE CARE The cast is left on for 6 weeks and then removed in the clinic along with the felt and button.

■ OPERATIVE TREATMENT

Surgery in clubfoot is indicated for deformities that do not respond to conservative treatment by serial manipulation and casting and should be attempted only after all other, less-aggressive means have been exhausted. Often in children with a significant rigid clubfoot deformity, the forefoot has been corrected by conservative treatment, but the hindfoot remains fixed in varus and equinus, or the deformity has recurred. Surgery in the treatment of clubfoot must be tailored to the age of the child and to the deformity to be corrected.

Extensive release that includes the posterolateral ligament complex most often is required for severe deformity. The procedure described by McKay takes into consideration the three-dimensional deformity of the subtalar joint and allows correction of the internal rotational deformity of the calcaneus and release of the contractures of the posterolateral and posteromedial foot. A modified McKay procedure through a transverse circumferential (Cincinnati) incision is our preferred technique for the initial surgical management of most clubfeet. In many cases, a complete exposure of the talonavicular joint medially may not be required because partial correction often can be achieved with initial or repeat casting. This selective approach to soft-tissue release is preferred to lessen postoperative stiffness.

TRANSVERSE CIRCUMFERENTIAL (CINCINNATI) INCISION

One option for comprehensive release is the use of the transverse circumferential incision, also known as the Cincinnati incision. This incision provides excellent exposure of the subtalar joint and is useful in patients with a severe internal rotational deformity of the calcaneus. One potential problem with this incision is tension on the suture line when attempting to place the foot in dorsiflexion to apply the postoperative cast. To avoid this, the foot can be placed in plantarflexion in the immediate postoperative cast and then in dorsiflexion to the corrected position at the first cast change when the wound has healed at 2 weeks. This cast change frequently requires sedation or outpatient general anesthesia.

If primary skin closure is difficult in a foot in a fully corrected position, a fasciocutaneous flap closure can be used. The rotation of V-Y flaps allow complete wound closure without any skin tension.

TECHNIQUE 1.12

(CRAWFORD, MARXEN, AND OSTERFELD)
- Begin the incision on the medial aspect of the foot in the region of the naviculocuneiform joint (Fig. 1.34A).

- Dissect the subcutaneous tissue up and down the Achilles tendon to lengthen the tendon at least 2.5 cm in the coronal plane. If sagittal plane lengthening is done, the lateral attachment of the Achilles tendon to the calcaneus should be preserved to aid in correction of hindfoot varus.
- Incise the superior peroneal retinaculum off the calcaneus at the point where it blends with the sheath of the Achilles tendon.
- Dissecting carefully, release the peroneal tendons from their sheaths and protect them with a vessel loop, then separate the calcaneofibular and posterior calcaneotalar ligaments, the thickened superior peroneal retinaculum, and the peroneal tendon sheath.
- Incise the calcaneofibular ligament close to the calcaneus (this ligament is short and thick and attached very close to the apophysis).
- Incise the lateral talocalcaneal ligament and the lateral capsule of the talocalcaneal joint from their attachments to the calcaneocuboid joint to the point where they enter the sheath of the flexor hallucis longus tendon posteriorly. In more resistant clubfeet, the origin of the extensor digitorum brevis, cruciate crural ligament (inferior extensor retinaculum), dorsal calcaneocuboid ligament, and, occasionally, cubonavicular oblique ligament must be dissected off the calcaneus to allow the anterior portion of the calcaneus to move laterally.
- On the medial side, dissect free the neurovascular bundle (medial and lateral plantar nerves and associated vascular components) into the arch of the foot, preserving the medial calcaneal branch of the lateral plantar nerve. Protect and retract the neurovascular bundle with a small Penrose drain or vessel loop. Complete dissection of the medial and lateral neurovascular bundle throughout the arch of the foot.
- Enter the compartment of the medial plantar neurovascular bundle and follow it into the arch of the foot well beyond the cuneiforms; elevate the abductor hallucis muscle to enter the plantar aspect of the foot.
- Enter the sheaths of the posterior tibial tendon, the flexor hallucis longus and flexor digitorum longus tendons, and protect each of these structures.
- Section the narrow strip of fascia between the medial and lateral branches of the plantar nerve to allow the abductor hallucis to slide distally.
- Enter the sheath of the posterior tibial tendon just posterior to and above the medial malleolus. Split the sheath and superficial deltoid ligament up the tibia until the muscle can be identified.
- Lengthen the tendon by Z-plasty at least 2.5 cm proximal from the medial malleolus to the maximal distance allowed by the incision. Starting from the point at which the flexor digitorum longus and the flexor hallucis longus tendons cross, sharply dissect both sheaths from the sustentaculum tali, moving in a proximal direction until the talocalcaneal joint is entered.
- Continue the dissection down and around the navicular, holding the distal segment of the lengthened posterior tibial tendon attached to the bone.
- Open the talonavicular joint by pulling on the remaining posterior tibial tendon attachment and carefully cut the deltoid ligament (medial tibial navicular ligament),

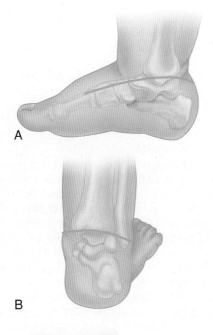

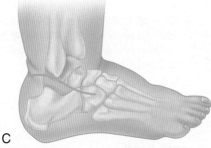

FIGURE 1.34 Transverse circumferential (Cincinnati) incision as described by Crawford et al. **A,** Medial view. **B,** Posterior view. **C,** Lateral view. **SEE TECHNIQUES 1.12 AND 1.21.**

- Carry the incision posteriorly, gently curving beneath the distal end of the medial malleolus and ascending slightly to pass transversely over the Achilles tendon approximately at the level of the tibiotalar joint (Fig. 1.34B).
- Continue the incision in a gentle curve over the lateral malleolus and end it just distal and slightly medial to the sinus tarsi (Fig. 1.34C).
- Extend the incision distally medially or laterally, depending on the requirements of the operation.

EXTENSILE POSTEROMEDIAL AND POSTEROLATERAL RELEASE

TECHNIQUE 1.13

(MCKAY, MODIFIED)
- Incise the skin through a transverse circumferential (Cincinnati) incision, preserving if possible the veins on the lateral side and protecting the sural nerve.

talonavicular capsule, dorsal talonavicular ligament, and plantar calcaneonavicular (spring) ligament close to the navicular.

■ Enter and carefully expose by blunt dissection and retraction the interval between the dorsal aspect of the talonavicular joint and the extensor tendons and neurovascular bundle on the dorsum of the foot. Do not dissect or disturb the blood supply to the dorsal aspect of the talus.

■ Follow through with the dissection, incising the capsule of the talonavicular joint all the way around medially, inferiorly, superiorly, and laterally. Inferior and lateral to the joint is the bifurcated (Y) ligament; incise both ends of this ligament to correct the horizontal rotation of the calcaneus.

■ Complete the release of the talocalcaneal joint ligaments and capsule by incising the remaining medial and posteromedial capsule and superficial deltoid ligament attached to the sustentaculum tali. Do not incise the talocalcaneal ligaments (interosseous ligaments) at this time.

■ Retract the lateral plantar nerve, detach the origin of the quadratus plantae muscle using a periosteal elevator on the medial inferior surface of the calcaneus, and expose the long plantar ligament over the plantar calcaneocuboid ligament and the peroneus longus tendon.

■ At this point, the talus should roll back into the ankle joint, exposing at least 1.5 cm of hyaline cartilage on its body. If this does not happen, incise the posterior talofibular ligament. If the talus still does not roll back into the ankle joint, cut the posterior portion only of the deep deltoid ligament.

■ The decision must be made as to the necessity of dividing the interosseous talocalcaneal ligament to correct the horizontal rotational abnormality through the talocalcaneal joint. This decision depends on the completeness of the correction and the mobility of the subtalar complex, as determined by the position of the foot. The interosseous ligament should be preserved intact if at all possible.

■ Line up the medial side of the head and neck of the talus with the medial side of the cuneiforms and medially push the calcaneus posterior to the ankle joint while pushing the foot as a whole in a posterior direction. Examine the angle made by the intersection of the bimalleolar ankle plane with the horizontal plane of the foot; if the angle is 85 to 90 degrees, the ligament need not be cut. In children older than 1 year of age, such an incision generally is necessary, however, because the ligament usually has become broad and thick, preventing derotation of the talocalcaneal joint.

■ After the foot has been satisfactorily corrected, pass a small Kirschner wire through the talus from the posterior aspect into the middle of the head. Positioning the pin in a slightly lateral direction in the head of the talus is beneficial in older children with more pronounced medial deviation of the talar head and neck because it allows lateral displacement of the navicular and cuneiforms on the head of the talus to eliminate forefoot adduction.

■ Pass the pin through the talonavicular joint and cuneiforms and out the forefoot on either the medial or the lateral side of the first metatarsal. While an assistant inserts the pin, mold the forefoot out of adduction. Cut off the end of the pin close to the body of the talus. The pin can be left out of the skin on the dorsum of the forefoot

or just under the skin requiring a small incision later for removal in the operating room.

■ Check for proper positioning of the foot: The longitudinal plane of the foot is 85 to 90 degrees to the bimalleolar ankle plane, and the heel under the tibia is in slight valgus.

■ If the talocalcaneal ligament has been divided, insert a pin through the calcaneus, burying it deep in the talus from the plantar surface. Do not penetrate the ankle joint.

■ Suture the posterior tibial and Achilles tendons snugly with the foot in slight dorsiflexion. Lengthening of the flexor digitorum longus is rarely required, but the flexor hallucis longus is typically tight with the foot in the corrected position. The flexor hallucis longus tightness can be corrected by a fractional lengthening at the musculotendinous junction, a Z-lengthening of the tendon, transection of the tendon after formal tenodesis to the flexor digitorum longus at the master knot of Henry (preferred technique), or by flexor tenotomy at the level of proximal phalanx of the great toe.

■ Reposition the lengthened posterior tibial tendon in its sheath and repair the sheath beneath the medial malleolus. With the fibrofatty tissue left attached to the calcaneus anterior to the Achilles tendon, cover the lateral aspect of the ankle joint. Keep the peroneal tendons and sheaths from subluxating around the fibula by suturing the sheaths of the peroneal tendons to the fibrofatty flap. Close the subcutaneous tissue and skin with interrupted sutures.

■ Apply nonadherent dressing and, very loosely, apply a padded long leg cast with the foot in plantarflexion and flexed to 90 degrees (Fig. 1.35).

POSTOPERATIVE CARE A long leg cast is applied with the foot in plantarflexion. At 2 weeks, the cast is changed, and the foot is placed in the corrected position. This can be done with sedation or general anesthesia as an outpatient procedure. At 6 weeks, the cast and pins are removed in the operating room (Fig. 1.36). Correction is maintained in an ankle/foot orthosis.

In addition to complete recurrent deformity, special attention should be given to two specific problems in clubfoot. The first is residual hindfoot equinus in children 6 to 12 months old who have obtained adequate correction of forefoot adduction and hindfoot varus. This equinus can be corrected adequately by Achilles tendon lengthening and posterior capsulotomy of the ankle and subtalar joints without an extensive one-stage posteromedial release. Careful intraoperative assessment is necessary to determine if a more extensive release is required instead of a limited procedure that corrects only hindfoot equinus. The heel varus and internal rotation must have been corrected adequately if Achilles tendon lengthening and posterior capsulotomy are to be used alone.

The second specific problem is dynamic metatarsus adductus and forefoot supination caused by overpull of the anterior tibial tendon in older children who have had correction of clubfoot. In these children, the treatment of choice is transfer of the anterior tibial tendon to the lateral cuneiform. The hindfoot and forefoot must be flexible for a tendon transfer to succeed (see Technique 6.9).

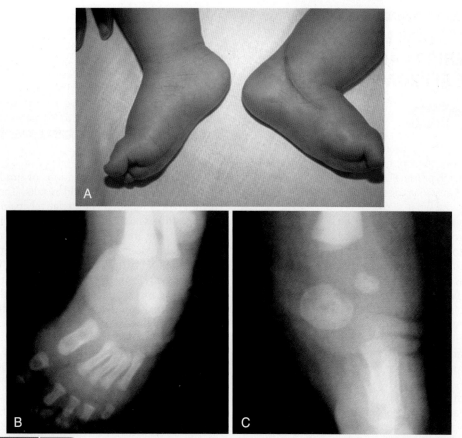

FIGURE 1.35 Modified McKay procedure using Cincinnati incision. **A,** Clinical appearance after correction. **B** and **C,** Preoperative anteroposterior and lateral radiographs. **SEE TECHNIQUE 1.13.**

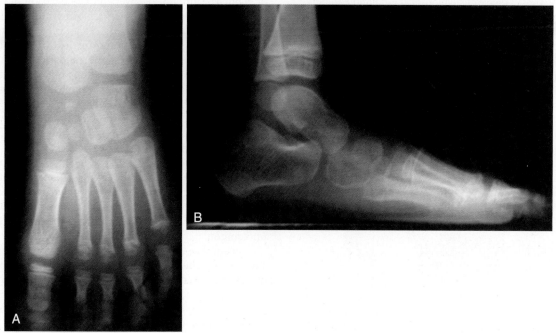

FIGURE 1.36 **A** and **B,** Radiographic appearance of left foot in 6-year-old child who had modified McKay procedures at 6 months of age. **SEE TECHNIQUE 1.13.**

ACHILLES TENDON LENGTHENING AND POSTERIOR CAPSULOTOMY (SELECTIVE APPROACH)

TECHNIQUE 1.14

- Make a straight longitudinal incision over the medial aspect of the Achilles tendon, beginning at its most distal point and extending proximally to 3 cm above the level of the ankle joint. Carry sharp dissection through the subcutaneous tissue.
- Identify the Achilles tendon and make an incision through the peritenon medially. Dissect the Achilles tendon circumferentially to expose it for a length of 3 to 4 cm.
- Perform a tenotomy of the plantaris tendon if it is present.
- Identify medially the flexor hallucis longus, flexor digitorum communis, and posterior tibial tendons and the neurovascular bundle; protect these with Penrose drains.
- Perform a Z-plasty to lengthen the Achilles tendon by releasing the medial half distally and the lateral half proximally for a distance of 2.5 to 4 cm (Fig. 1.37).
- Gently debride pericapsular fat at the level of the subtalar joint.
- Identify the posterior aspect of the ankle joint by gentle plantar flexion and dorsiflexion of the foot. If the ankle joint cannot be easily identified, make a small vertical incision in the midline until synovial fluid exudes from the joint.
- Perform a transverse capsulotomy at the most medial aspect, stopping at the sheath of the posterior tibial tendon and the most lateral articulation of the tibiofibular joint. Do not divide the posterior tibial tendon sheath and its underlying deep deltoid ligament.
- If posterior subtalar capsulotomy is required, enter the subtalar joint at the most proximal aspect of the sheath of the flexor hallucis longus tendon, and extend the capsulotomy medially and laterally as necessary.
- Place the foot in 10 degrees of dorsiflexion and approximate the Achilles tendon to assess tension. Place the foot in plantarflexion and repair the Achilles tendon at the appropriate length.

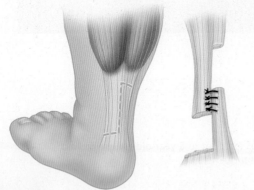

FIGURE 1.37 Achilles tendon lengthening (see text). **SEE TECHNIQUE 1.14.**

- Deflate the tourniquet, obtain hemostasis with electrocautery, and close the wound in layers.
- Apply a long leg, bent-knee cast with the foot in 5 degrees of dorsiflexion.

POSTOPERATIVE CARE The cast is removed 6 weeks after surgery. Postoperative bracing with an ankle-foot orthosis can be used for 6 to 9 months longer.

Several long-term evaluations of surgically treated clubfeet have demonstrated good results. The feet typically are plantigrade, functional, and relatively painless; however, persistent stiffness and mild discomfort with prolonged standing or activity are common. A number of recent studies have compared the long-term outcomes and functionality of clubfeet treated with the Ponseti method to those treated with extensive soft-tissue release. The Ponseti-treated feet had better range of motion, less pain, and less arthritis than the surgically treated feet. Every attempt should be made to avoid extensive surgical release.

■ RECALCITRANT CLUBFEET

Treatment of residual or resistant clubfoot in an older child is one of the most difficult problems in pediatric orthopaedics. The deformity may take many forms, and there are no clear-cut guidelines for treatment. Each child must be evaluated carefully to determine which treatment would best correct his or her particular functional impairment. Thorough physical examination should include careful assessment of the forefoot and hindfoot. Residual forefoot deformity should be determined to be either dynamic (with a flexible forefoot) or rigid. The amount of inversion and eversion of the calcaneus and dorsiflexion and plantarflexion of the ankle should be determined. Any prior surgical procedures causing significant scarring around the foot or loss of motion should be noted. Standing anteroposterior and lateral radiographs should be obtained to assess anatomic measurements; if the clubfoot deformity is unilateral, the opposite foot can be used as a control for measurements. All possible causes of the persistent deformity, including underlying neuropathy, abnormal growth of the bones, or muscle imbalance, should be investigated. Most deformities have been reported to result from undercorrection at the time of the primary operation caused by failure to release the calcaneocuboid joint and plantar fascia and failure to recognize residual forefoot adduction on intraoperative radiographs; however, over-correction with hindfoot valgus or dorsal subluxation of the navicular is not uncommon.

Incomplete correction may not be obvious at the time of surgery, but it becomes apparent with growth as the persistent deformities become more evident (Fig. 1.38). Clubfoot that appears by clinical and radiographic evaluation to be uncorrected may not always require surgery. The functional ability of the child, the severity of symptoms associated with the deformity, and the likelihood of progression if the deformity is left untreated must be considered when treatment decisions are being made. Repeat manipulation and casting should always be considered as an option for the recurrent clubfoot. Many difficult foot deformities can be improved or corrected with a series of repeat manipulations and castings.

Even if the repeat casting does not completely correct the residual or recurrent deformity, parts of the deformity often can be improved, lessening the degree of surgery required for full correction.

The basic surgical correction of resistant, recalcitrant clubfoot includes soft-tissue release and bony osteotomies. The appropriate procedures and combination of procedures depend on the age of the child, the severity of the deformity, and the pathologic processes involved. In general, the older the child, the more likely it is that combined procedures will be required. Children 2 to 3 years old may be candidates for the modified McKay procedure (see Technique 1.13), but if previous soft-tissue release has caused stiffness of the subtalar joint, osteonecrosis of the talus, or severe skin contractures, osteotomies are a better choice. Children older than 5 years almost always require osteotomies for correction of resistant deformity; children 3 to 5 years old constitute a gray area in which treatment guidelines are unclear and careful judgment is required. Common components of resistant clubfoot deformity are adduction or supination, or both, of the forefoot, a short medial column or long lateral column of the foot, internal rotation and varus of the calcaneus, and equinus.

Dorsal bunions that develop after clubfoot surgery have been attributed to muscle weakness, particularly of the triceps surae, wherein a bunion develops as the patient tries to push off with the toe flexors to compensate for the weakness of the triceps, or to imbalance between the anterior tibial muscle and an impaired peroneus longus muscle. Most authors recommend transfer of the flexor hallucis longus to the neck of the first metatarsal, combined with bony correction by plantar closing wedge osteotomy of the first metatarsal.

Correction of the forefoot with residual adduction or supination or both is similar to correction of isolated metatarsus adductus by multiple metatarsal osteotomies or by combined medial cuneiform and lateral cuboid osteotomies, when the deformity is in the forefoot. Because dynamic supination and adduction often are caused by overactivity of the anterior tibial tendon and underactivity of the peroneal tendon, a tendon-balancing procedure may be the most reasonable solution in the flexible foot.

Evaluation of the hindfoot should determine whether the deformity is caused by isolated heel varus, a long lateral column of the foot, or a short medial column. In children younger than 2 or 3 years who have had no previous surgery, residual heel varus may be corrected by extensive subtalar release, but children 3 to 10 years old who have residual soft-tissue and bony deformities usually require combined procedures.

Ankle valgus must be differentiated from hindfoot valgus because the methods and timing of surgical correction are different. For symptomatic ankle valgus, percutaneous medial malleolar epiphysiodesis using a 4.5-mm cortical screw has been recommended.

For isolated heel varus with mild supination of the forefoot, a Dwyer osteotomy with a lateral closing wedge osteotomy of the calcaneus can be performed. Opening wedge osteotomy of the calcaneus occasionally is followed by sloughing of tight skin along the incision over the calcaneus. Consequently, although some height of the calcaneus is lost after a lateral closing wedge osteotomy, most authors now prefer lateral closing wedge osteotomy with Kirschner wire fixation, if necessary. The ideal age for the operation is 3 to 4 years, but there is no upper age limit.

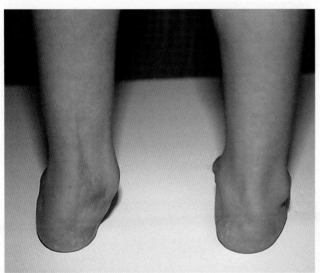

FIGURE 1.38   Overcorrection of left clubfoot deformity apparent in 6-year-old girl.

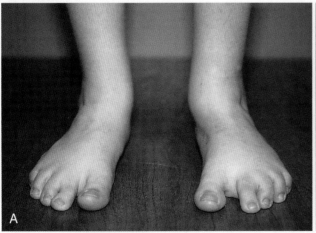
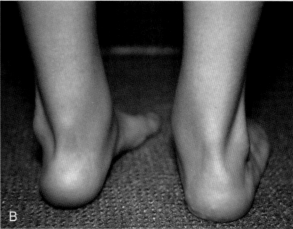

FIGURE 1.39   **A** and **B,** Deformities in 12-year-old boy after undercorrection of left clubfoot. Note metatarsus adductus, heel varus, and internal tibial torsion.

If the hindfoot deformity includes heel varus and residual internal rotation of the calcaneus with a long lateral column of the foot, the Lichtblau procedure may be appropriate. This procedure corrects the long lateral column of the foot by a closing wedge osteotomy of the lateral aspect of the calcaneus or by cuboid enucleation. The best results with this procedure are obtained in children 3 years old or older in whom the calcaneus and lateral column are long relative to the talus. Potential complications include the development of a "Z"-foot, or "skew"-foot, deformity.

Adductus of the forefoot, as measured by the calcaneal–second metatarsal angle has been reported to improve after combined cuboid-cuneiform osteotomy, with no further surgery required.

Residual heel equinus can be corrected by Achilles tendon lengthening and posterior ankle and subtalar capsulotomies in a younger child with a mild deformity. In rare cases, an isolated, fixed equinus deformity in an older child requires a Lambrinudi arthrodesis. Anterior distal tibial hemiepiphysiodesis as a method to correct ankle equinus has been shown to be ineffective in achieving the desired clinical result.

Talonavicular arthrodesis also has been described for residual midfoot deformities with or without lateral column shortening and a calcaneal wedge osteotomy with improvement in symptoms. This should be carefully considered if much of the foot motion is occurring at this joint.

If all three deformities are present in a child older than 10 years (Fig. 1.39), triple arthrodesis may be appropriate. Internal tibial torsion occasionally occurs with resistant clubfoot deformity but rarely requires derotational osteotomy. Before tibial osteotomy is considered, it must be determined absolutely that the pathologic condition is confined to the tibia and is not a resistant deformity in the foot.

Correction using the Ilizarov device, with or without bony procedures, has been described for correction in children with severe soft-tissue and bony deformities.

The principles of Ilizarov correction of severe resistant clubfoot include stable bone fixation to the tibia as well as pin fixation to the talus, calcaneus, and forefoot. Some advocate partial soft-tissue release before gradual correction, but the risk of wound complications is greatly increased by this approach. After correction, soft-tissue release with or without arthrodesis also may be required to maintain correction and prevent recurrence. This approach offers the ability to maintain foot length while achieving a plantigrade position and three-dimensional deformity correction. However, the psychologic impact of Ilizarov treatment must be carefully considered, and rehabilitation can be quite challenging.

FIRST METATARSAL OSTEOTOMY AND TENDON TRANSFER FOR DORSAL BUNION

TECHNIQUE 1.15   *Figure 1.40*

(SMITH AND KUO)

- Through a medial incision, expose the first metatarsal and perform a proximal plantar closing wedge osteotomy.
- Bring the metatarsal into alignment with the forefoot by plantarflexion and insert a Kirschner wire for fixation.
- Carry the incision distally or make a second incision at the metatarsophalangeal joint to allow identification and transection of the flexor hallucis longus tendon.

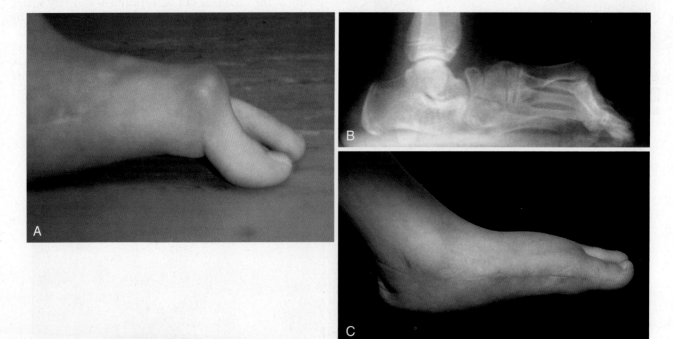

FIGURE 1.40   **A,** Dorsal bunion in 9-year-old boy after clubfoot release at 9 months of age. **B,** Lateral view of dorsal bunion at metatarsophalangeal joint of left great toe. **C,** Postoperative appearance of left foot after plantar closing wedge osteotomy of first metatarsal with transfer of flexor hallucis longus to first metatarsal neck. **SEE TECHNIQUE 1.15.**

- Drill a hole in the distal first metatarsal neck in a dorsal-to-plantar direction.
- Pass the flexor hallucis tendon through the hole and suture it back on itself.
- Close the wounds and apply a short leg, non–weight-bearing cast.

POSTOPERATIVE CARE Non–weight bearing is continued in the cast for 6 weeks, after which the Kirschner wire is removed. A walking cast is worn for 4 weeks. Full activity usually can be resumed at 3 to 4 months.

OSTEOTOMY OF THE CALCANEUS FOR PERSISTENT VARUS DEFORMITY OF THE HEEL

Dwyer reported osteotomy of the calcaneus for relapsed clubfoot using an opening wedge osteotomy medially to increase the length and height of the calcaneus. The osteotomy is held open by a wedge of bone taken from the tibia. A modification of this technique is a laterally based closing wedge osteotomy of the calcaneus.

TECHNIQUE 1.16

(DWYER, MODIFIED)
- Expose the calcaneus through a lateral incision over the calcaneus.

- Expose the lateral surface of the bone subperiosteally and with a wide osteotome resect a wedge of bone based laterally large enough, when removed, to permit correction of the heel varus. Do not injure the peroneal tendons.
- Remove the wedge of bone, place the heel into the corrected position, and close the incision with interrupted sutures.
- If necessary, fix the osteotomy with a Kirschner wire.
- Apply a short leg cast with the foot in the corrected position.

POSTOPERATIVE CARE The Kirschner wire is removed at 6 weeks, and casting is discontinued at 8 to 12 weeks.

MEDIAL RELEASE WITH OSTEOTOMY OF THE DISTAL CALCANEUS

An alternative to calcaneocuboid arthrodesis is lateral closing wedge osteotomy of the calcaneus, as described by Lichtblau (Fig. 1.41). This procedure may prevent the long-term stiffness of the hindfoot seen with the Dillwyn-Evans procedure.

TECHNIQUE 1.17   *Figure 1.42*

(LICHTBLAU)
- If soft-tissue release medially is required, make an incision on the medial aspect of the foot beginning about 1 cm below the medial malleolus, crossing the tuberosity of the navicular, and sloping downward to the base of the first

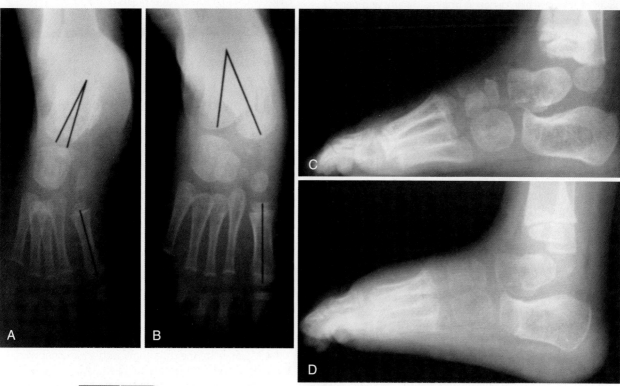

FIGURE 1.41   **A-D,** Severe residual clubfoot deformity in 5-year-old child on anteroposterior (**A**) and lateral (**C**) radiographs. **B** and **D,** After Lichtblau procedure. **SEE TECHNIQUE 1.17.**

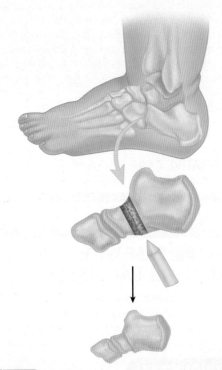

FIGURE 1.42 Lichtblau procedure (see text). **SEE TECHNIQUE 1.17.**

metatarsal. Identify and free the superior border of the abductor hallucis muscle and reflect it plantarward.

■ Isolate the posterior tibial tendon at its insertion on the beak of the navicular, dissect it from its sheath, and perform a Z-plasty about 1 cm from its insertion. Allow the proximal end of the tendon to retract, using the distal end as a guide to the talonavicular joint.

■ Resect the tendon sheath overlying the joint and open it generously on its medial, dorsal, and plantar aspects.

■ Open the flexor tendon sheaths and lengthen them by Z-plasty technique.

■ Make a lateral incision 4 cm long centered over the calcaneocuboid joint.

■ Dissect the origin of the extensor digitorum brevis muscle from the calcaneus and reflect it distally to permit exposure and opening of the calcaneocuboid joint.

■ Identify the distal end of the calcaneus and perform a wedge-shaped osteotomy, removing about 1 cm of the distal and lateral border of the calcaneus and 2 mm of the distal and medial border. Leave the articular surface of the calcaneus intact.

■ Bring the cuboid into contact with the distal end of the calcaneus at the osteotomy site and evaluate the amount of correction of the varus deformity. If the cuboid cannot be closely approximated to the calcaneus, resect more of the calcaneus.

■ A smooth Kirschner wire can be inserted across the calcaneocuboid joint to fix the osteotomy.

■ Repair all soft tissues and close the subcutaneous tissue and skin. Apply a long leg cast with the foot in the corrected position.

Alternatively, the lateral-based, closing wedge can be removed from the cuboid instead of the calcaneus. This often is chosen for a patient with a deformity that seems to be most severe at the level of the midfoot rather than the hindfoot.

POSTOPERATIVE CARE The long leg cast is changed to a short leg cast 3 weeks after surgery. The short leg cast is worn for 6 more weeks. The pin is removed at 8 to 12 weeks.

SELECTIVE JOINT-SPARING OSTEOTOMIES FOR RESIDUAL CAVOVARUS DEFORMITY

Described by Mubarak and Van Valin, selective joint-sparing osteotomies of the foot can be used for multiple etiologies that result in rigid cavus and cavovarus foot deformities, including hereditary motor sensory neuropathies, traumatic brain injury, spinal cord lipoma, and residual or recurrent clubfoot. The technique involves stepwise correction of each aspect of the deformity with a closing wedge osteotomy of the first metatarsal, opening plantar wedge osteotomy of the medial cuneiform, closing wedge osteotomy of the cuboid, osteotomies of the second and third metatarsals, sliding osteotomy of the calcaneus, plantar fasciotomy, and peroneus-to-brevis transfer. Indications for this procedure are rigid cavus or cavovarus deformity, ankle or foot instability symptoms including pain, painful metatarsal heads and callosities, and ankle or foot sprains or fractures.

TECHNIQUE 1.18

(MUBRAK AND VAN VALIN)

■ To correct rigid cavus, make an incision along the medial foot over the first metatarsal and medial cuneiform.

■ Partially free the anterior tibial tendon to expose the cuneiform.

■ Under fluoroscopic guidance, place intraosseous needles or small Kirschner wires in the mid-portion of the medial cuneiform and 1 cm distal to the first metatarsal physis. Take care not to disturb the physis.

■ Perform a dorsal, closing-wedge osteotomy of the first metatarsal by removing a large 20- to 30-degree wedge (Fig. 1.43A). Then create a plantar-based, opening wedge osteotomy of the medial cuneiform and insert the bone wedge (Fig. 1.43B). Stabilize both osteotomies with Kirschner wires.

■ To correct forefoot varus, make a longitudinal lateral incision overlying the cuboid. Identify the calcaneocuboid and cuboid-fifth metatarsal joints with fluoroscopy and protect these joints. Create a laterally based, closing-wedge osteotomy of the cuboid by removing a triangular wedge of bone with a base size of 5 to 10 mm (Fig. 1.43C). Stabilize the osteotomy with a Kirschner wire.

■ If second and third metatarsal head prominence remains after the osteotomies have been completed, dorsal closing wedge osteotomies of the second and third metatarsals

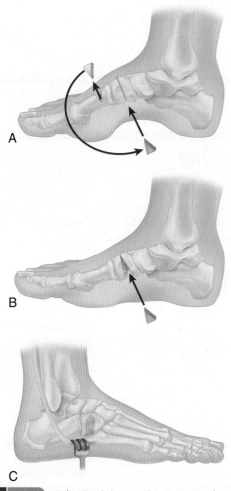

FIGURE 1.43 Selective joint sparing osteotomies (Mubarak and Van Valin). **A,** Dorsal closing-wedge osteotomy of the first metatarsal. **B,** Plantar-based opening-wedge osteotomy of the medial cuneiform. **C,** Laterally-based closing-wedge osteotomy of the cuboid. **SEE TECHNIQUE 1.18.**

are required. Make a single incision overlying the bases of the second and third metatarsals. Create dorsally a slightly lateral based closing wedge osteotomy of the base of each metatarsal and stabilize them with intramedullary Kirschner wires.

■ For rigid hindfoot varus, perform a Dwyer osteotomy of the calcaneus (see Technique 1.16).

■ Next, evaluate the plantar fascia. If this structure is tight, perform a plantar fasciotomy (Technique 83.6 in Tenth Edition).

■ For deformities caused by neurologic conditions, consider a peroneus longus-to-brevis transfer. Through the same incision used for the cuboid osteotomy, release the peroneus longus just under the cuboid and reattach it to the brevis.

■ Close the incision. Apply a bivalved, short leg cast.

POSTOPERATIVE CARE The bivalved cast is closed at 1 week. Non–weight bearing is continued for 4 weeks. Then the pins are removed under sedation anesthesia and a short leg cast is applied. Weight bearing is allowed in the second cast for 4 more weeks.

▌TRIPLE ARTHRODESIS AND TALECTOMY FOR UNCORRECTED CLUBFOOT

Triple arthrodesis and talectomy generally are salvage operations for uncorrected clubfoot in older children and adolescents (Figs. 1.44 and 1.45). Triple arthrodesis corrects the severely deformed foot by a lateral closing wedge osteotomy through the subtalar and midtarsal joints. Functional results generally are improved despite postoperative joint stiffness. Talectomy should be reserved for severe, untreated clubfoot; for previously treated clubfoot that is uncorrectable by any other surgical procedures; and for severe, recalcitrant, neuromuscular clubfoot.

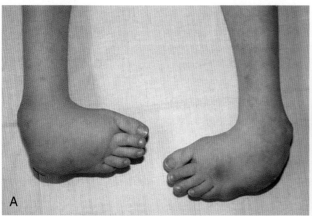
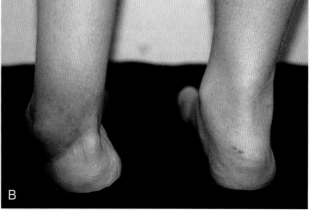

FIGURE 1.44 **A,** Untreated clubfoot in 14-year-old girl. **B,** Recurrent left hindfoot varus in 8-year-old girl.

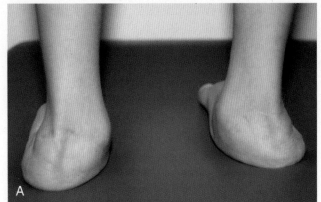

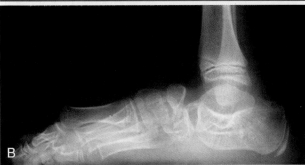

FIGURE 1.45 **A,** Overcorrected clubfoot in 12-year-old boy showing hindfoot valgus, dorsal dislocation of navicular on talus, and dorsal bunion deformity. **B,** Standing lateral radiograph.

TRIPLE ARTHRODESIS

TECHNIQUE 1.19

- Make an incision along the medial side of the foot parallel to the inferior border of the calcaneus.
- Free the attachments of the plantar fascia and of the short flexors of the toes from the plantar aspect of the calcaneus.
- By manipulation, correct the cavus deformity as much as possible.
- Through an oblique anterolateral approach, expose the midtarsal and subtalar joints (Fig. 1.46).
- Resect a laterally based wedge of bone that includes the midtarsal joints. Resect enough bone to correct the varus and adduction deformities of the forefoot.
- Through the same incision, resect a wedge of bone, again laterally based, which includes the subtalar joint. Resect enough bone to correct the varus deformity of the calcaneus. If necessary, include in the wedge the navicular and most of the cuboid and lateral cuneiform and the anterior part of the talus and calcaneus, and in the second wedge include much of the superior part of the calcaneus and the inferior part of the talus.
- Lengthen the Achilles tendon by Z-plasty and perform a posterior capsulotomy of the ankle joint. By manipulating the ankle, correct the equinus deformity.
- Hold the correct position with a Kirschner wire inserted through the calcaneocuboid and talonavicular joints or with staple fixation.

POSTOPERATIVE CARE With the foot in the corrected position and the knee flexed 30 degrees, a long leg cast is applied from the base of the toes to the groin. The Kirschner wire and cast are removed at 6 weeks. A short leg walking cast is worn for 4 more weeks.

TALECTOMY

Trumble et al. described a talectomy for clubfoot deformity in patients with myelomeningocele, but the technique can be modified for treatment of a severe, resistant, idiopathic clubfoot deformity. Outcomes are acceptable with these very severe deformities provided the talus is completely removed and the calcaneus is properly positioned.

TECHNIQUE 1.20

(TRUMBLE ET AL.)
- Expose the talus through an incision parallel to the inferior border of the calcaneus (Fig. 1.47A). If additional soft-tissue release is required, talectomy can be done after circumferential release (see Technique 1.12).
- Carry the dissection to the prominent lateral articular margin of the navicular in the interval between the extensor digitorum longus and peroneus tertius tendons. Invert and plantar flex the forefoot.
- Place a towel clip around the neck of the talus and deliver it into the wound; dissect all of its ligaments (Fig. 1.47B). Excise the talus intact because retained remnants of cartilage may interfere with proper positioning of the foot; these remnants also may grow and cause later deformity and loss of correction.
- Derotate the forefoot and displace the calcaneus posteriorly into the ankle mortise until the navicular abuts the anterior edge of the tibial plafond. The exposed articular surface of the tibial plafond should be opposite the middle articular facet of the calcaneus. If necessary to obtain adequate posterior displacement, excise the tarsal navicular.
- Section the deltoid and the lateral collateral ligaments of the ankle.
- Correct equinus deformity of the hindfoot by sectioning the Achilles tendon and allowing its proximal end to retract.
- In feet with uncorrected, severe equinovarus deformity, the dome of the talus may be extruded anterior to its normal relationship in the ankle mortise. Adaptive narrowing of the mortise may require release of the anterior and posterior tibiofibular ligaments of the syndesmosis to allow proper posterior positioning of the calcaneus.
- In the proper plantigrade position, the long axis of the foot should be aligned at a right angle to the bimalleolar axis of the ankle, not to the axis of the knee joint. This usually requires 20 to 30 degrees of external rotation of the foot.
- When the proper position has been achieved, insert one or two Steinmann pins from the heel through the calcaneus and into the distal tibia.
- Apply a long leg cast with the knee flexed to 60 degrees.

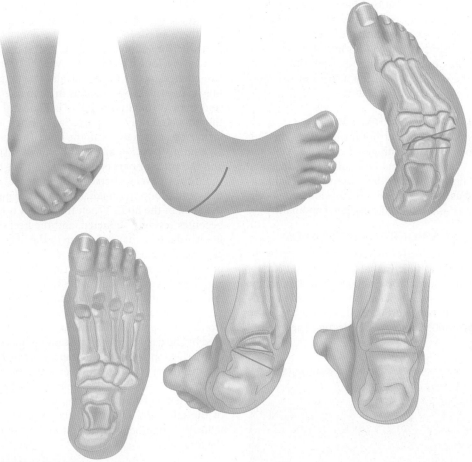

FIGURE 1.46 Arthrodesis for persistent or untreated clubfoot. Area between blue lines represents amount of bone removed from midtarsal region and subtalar joint in moderate fixed deformity. In severe deformity, wedge may include large part of talus and calcaneus and part of cuneiforms. **SEE TECHNIQUE 1.19.**

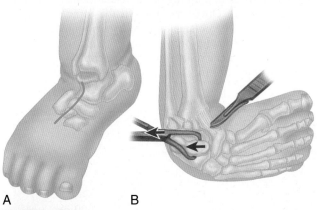

A   B

FIGURE 1.47 Talectomy. **A,** Anterolateral skin incision. **B,** Total talectomy. **SEE TECHNIQUE 1.20.**

POSTOPERATIVE CARE The Steinmann pins are removed at 6 weeks and a below-knee, weight-bearing cast is applied. The cast is worn for 12 more weeks.

CALCANEOVALGUS FOOT

Calcaneovalgus foot deformity is a benign soft-tissue contracture that is present in its mildest form in up to 40% of newborns. The condition is characterized by hindfoot eversion and dorsiflexion without true dislocation of any of the joints of the hindfoot or midfoot. The etiology is consistent with a classic intrauterine "packaging" problem, and it is therefore more common in first-born children.

On physical examination, the foot has a severe flat appearance with hindfoot eversion, and in some cases the dorsum of the foot can rest on the anterior surface of the tibia. In most cases, however, the foot is passively correctable at the time of birth or soon after. In contrast to the more severe and rigid congenital vertical talus, calcaneovalgus foot deformity has no hindfoot equinus (Fig. 1.48).

Imaging rarely is indicated for this condition in the newborn period; however, if there is any question as to the exact diagnosis, a forced dorsiflexion and forced plantarflexion lateral radiograph of the foot can distinguish calcaneovalgus deformity from congenital vertical talus. In calcaneovalgus foot, the forced plantarflexion lateral radiograph will reveal alignment of the first metatarsal with the long axis of the talus; on the forced dorsiflexion image, the hindfoot will dorsiflexion out of equinus.

Treatment involves observation and periodic passive stretching exercises. The foot can be plantarflexed, adducted, and inverted multiple times a day during diaper changes and baths. The condition typically resolves completely by the third to sixth month of life. Casting rarely is indicated. Should casting be required, the deformity is likely a form of the more severe condition, congenital vertical talus.

CONGENITAL VERTICAL TALUS

Congenital vertical talus, rocker-bottom flatfoot, or congenital rigid flatfoot must be distinguished from flexible pes planus commonly seen in infants and children. Congenital vertical talus may be associated with numerous neuromuscular disorders, such as arthrogryposis and myelomeningocele, but it also may occur as an isolated congenital anomaly.

■ CLINICAL AND RADIOGRAPHIC FINDINGS

Congenital vertical talus usually can be detected at birth by the presence of a rounded prominence of the medial and plantar surfaces of the foot produced by the abnormal location of the head of the talus (Fig. 1.49). The talus is so distorted plantarward and medially as to be almost vertical. The calcaneus also is in an equinus position, but to a lesser degree. The forefoot

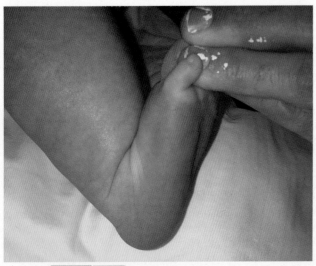

FIGURE 1.48 Calcaneovalgus foot.

is dorsiflexed at the midtarsal joints, and the navicular lies on the dorsal aspect of the head of the talus. The sole is convex, and there are deep creases on the dorsolateral aspect of the foot anterior and inferior to the lateral malleolus.

As the foot develops and weight bearing begins, adaptive changes occur in the tarsals. The talus becomes shaped like an hourglass but remains in so marked an equinus position that its longitudinal axis is almost the same as that of the tibia, and only the posterior third of its superior articular surface articulates with the tibia. The calcaneus remains in an equinus position also and becomes displaced posteriorly, and the anterior part of its plantar surface becomes rounded. Callosities develop beneath the anterior end of the calcaneus and along the medial border of the foot superficial to the head of the talus. When full weight is borne, the forefoot becomes severely abducted, and the heel does not touch the floor. Adaptive changes occur in the soft structures. All the capsules, ligaments, and tendons on the dorsum of the foot become contracted. The posterior tibial and peroneus longus and brevis tendons may come to lie anterior to the malleoli and act as dorsiflexors rather than plantar flexors.

Congenital vertical talus can be difficult to distinguish from severe pes planus, although the two can be differentiated by the use of appropriate radiographs or ultrasound. The plantarflexion lateral radiograph is most helpful to confirm the diagnosis of congenital vertical talus (Fig. 1.50). In the case of pes planus or calcaneovalgus foot deformity, a forced plantarflexion lateral radiograph will demonstrate alignment of the talus and the first metatarsal. In congenital vertical talus, the alignment is not restored by simply plantarflexing the forefoot.

■ TREATMENT

Congenital vertical talus is difficult to correct and tends to recur. Dobbs described the use of outpatient serial casting to achieve relaxation of the dorsolateral structures of the foot and partial or complete reduction of the talonavicular joint followed by percutaneous retrograde pinning or open reduction and retrograde pinning of the talonavicular joint in the operating room. Once the talonavicular joint is stabilized by pin fixation, percutaneous Achilles tenotomy is done to achieve ankle dorsiflexion without persistent rocker-bottom deformity. Excellent results in terms of clinical appearance, function, and deformity correction have been reported by a

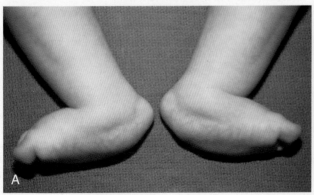
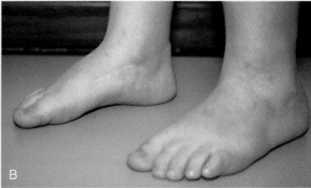

FIGURE 1.49 **A,** Bilateral congenital vertical talus in 14-month-old child. **B,** At 6 years of age, after bilateral operative correction at age 14 months in which transverse circumferential approach was used.

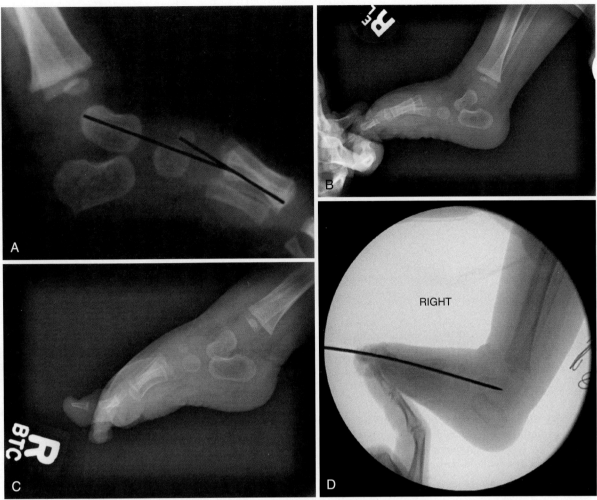

FIGURE 1.50 Plantarflexion lateral stress radiographs in diagnosis of congenital vertical talus. **A,** In normal foot, long axis of first metatarsal passes plantarward to long axis of talus. **B,** Forced plantarflexion lateral demonstrates inability of first metatarsal to line up with the talus. **C,** After 5 weeks of casting the plantarflexion lateral demonstrates good alignment of the first metatarsal and talus. **D,** After percutaneous pinning of talonavicular joint and percutaneous Achilles tenotomy.

number of authors, and this technique has emerged as a viable initial option for many patients with congenital vertical talus **(see Video 1.3)**.

Persistent or recurrent deformity after a trial of casting may necessitate more extensive operative intervention, particularly in children with more severe or rigid deformities.

The exact surgery indicated is determined by the age of the child and the severity of the deformity. Children 1 to 4 years old generally are best treated by open reduction and realignment of the talonavicular and subtalar joints. Occasionally, in children 3 years old or older who have a severe deformity, navicular excision is required at the time of open reduction. Children 4 to 8 years old can be treated by open reduction and soft-tissue procedures combined with extraarticular subtalar arthrodesis. Children 12 years old or older are best treated by triple arthrodesis for permanent correction of the deformity.

Kodros and Dias reported a single-stage procedure in which a threaded Kirschner wire is used as a "joystick" to manipulate the talus into correct position. The corrected position is held with threaded Kirschner wires across the talonavicular and subtalar joints (Fig. 1.51).

For a young child with a mild or moderate deformity, the technique of Kumar, Cowell, and Ramsey is recommended.

OPEN REDUCTION AND REALIGNMENT OF TALONAVICULAR AND SUBTALAR JOINTS

TECHNIQUE 1.21

(KUMAR, COWELL, AND RAMSEY)

■ Make the first of three incisions on the lateral side of the foot, centered over the sinus tarsi, or use the transverse circumferential (Cincinnati) approach (Fig. 1.34), which we prefer.

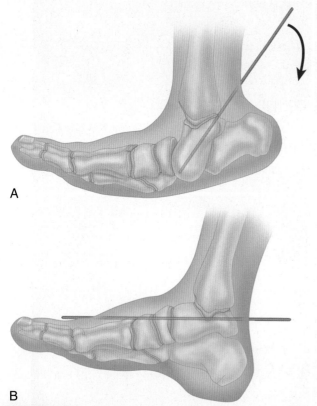

A

B

FIGURE 1.51 Single-stage correction of congenital vertical talus. **A,** After soft-tissue release, a threaded Kirschner wire is placed axially in the vertical talus from posterior and is used as "joystick" to manipulate talus into reduced position. **B,** Wire is advanced across talonavicular joint.

- Expose the extensor digitorum brevis and reflect it distally to expose the anterior part of the talocalcaneal joint.
- Identify the calcaneocuboid joint and release all tight structures around it, including the calcaneocuboid ligament.
- Make the second incision on the medial side of the foot, centered over the prominent head of the talus. This exposes the head of the talus and medial part of the navicular.
- The anterior tibial tendon also is exposed; if the tendon is contracted, lengthen it by Z-plasty. Alternatively, release the anterior tibial tendon from its attachment to the medial cuneiform and first ray and transpose it into the planter aspect of the repaired talonavicular capsule, which is our preferred technique.
- Release all tight structures on the medial and dorsal aspects of the head of the talus and the navicular. Free also the anterior part of the talus from its ligamentous attachments to the navicular and calcaneus. This includes releasing the dorsal talonavicular ligament, the plantar calcaneonavicular ligament, and the anterior part of the superficial deltoid ligament. If necessary, divide part of the talocalcaneal interosseous ligament so that the talus can be easily maneuvered into position by a blunt instrument. If the peroneal, extensor hallucis longus, and extensor digitorum longus tendons remain contracted, expose and lengthen them by Z-plasty. Alternatively, perform a

fractional lengthening of these tendons through an anterior incision at the musculotendinous junction.
- Make a third incision 2 inches long on the medial side of the Achilles tendon. Lengthen this tendon by Z-plasty, and, if necessary, perform a capsulotomy of the posterior ankle and subtalar joints.
- The talus and calcaneus can now be placed in the corrected position, and the forefoot can be reduced on the hindfoot.
- Pass a Kirschner wire through the navicular and into the neck of the talus to maintain the reduction. Obtain anteroposterior and lateral radiographs to confirm reduction of the vertical talus (Fig. 1.52). This pin can be advanced into the dorsum of the foot and cut flush with the back of the talus and can be removed weeks later through a small dorsal incision.
- Reconstruct the talonavicular ligament, repair any lengthened tendons, transfer the anterior tibial tendon to the plantar aspect of the talonavicular joint capsule, and close the wound in layers.
- Apply a long leg cast with the knee flexed and the foot in proper position.

POSTOPERATIVE CARE At 8 weeks, the cast and Kirschner wire are removed. A new long leg cast is applied, and this type of cast is worn for 1 month. A short leg cast is worn for an additional month. The foot is supported in an ankle-foot orthosis for another 3 to 6 months.

OPEN REDUCTION AND EXTRAARTICULAR SUBTALAR FUSION

Coleman et al. described open reduction and extraarticular subtalar fusion in older children with severe or recurrent deformities. This technique combines the procedure of Kumar et al. with a Grice-Green fusion performed 6 to 8 weeks later. Dennyson and Fulford modified this technique by using screw fixation across the talocalcaneal joint.

TECHNIQUE 1.22

(GRICE-GREEN)
- Make a short curvilinear incision on the lateral aspect of the foot directly over the subtalar joint.
- Carry the incision down through the soft tissues to expose the cruciate ligament overlying the joint. Split this ligament in the direction of its fibers and dissect the fatty and ligamentous tissues from the sinus tarsi.
- Dissect the short toe extensors from the calcaneus and reflect them distally. The relationship of the calcaneus to the talus now can be determined, and the mechanism of the deformity can be shown.
- Place the foot in equinus and invert it to position the calcaneus beneath the talus.
- A severe, long-standing deformity may require division of the posterior capsule of the subtalar joint or removal of a small piece of bone laterally from beneath the anterosuperior articular surface of the calcaneus.

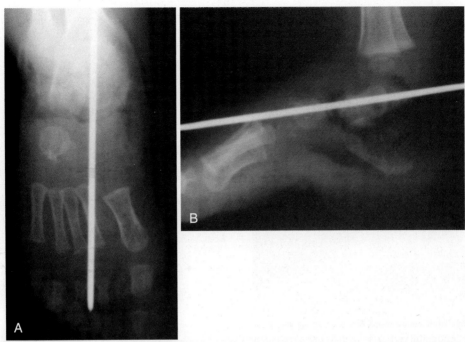

FIGURE 1.52 Intraoperative radiographs after correction of congenital vertical talus through transverse circumferential approach. **A,** Anteroposterior view shows correction of talocalcaneal and talus–first metatarsal angles. **B,** Lateral view shows corrected position of talus and reduction of navicular and forefoot after fixation with single Steinmann pin. **SEE TECHNIQUE 1.21.**

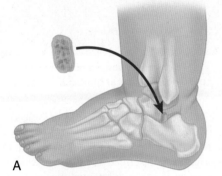
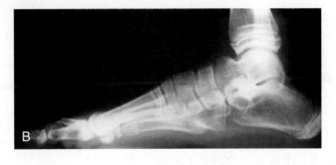

FIGURE 1.53 Grice-Green subtalar fusion. **A,** Preparation of graft bed and placement of graft in lateral aspect of subtalar joint. **B,** Lateral view of 10-year-old patient who had open reduction and Grice-Green fusion for congenital vertical talus at 3 years of age. **SEE TECHNIQUE 1.22.**

- Insert an osteotome or broad periosteal elevator into the sinus tarsi and block the subtalar joint to evaluate the stability of the graft and its proper size and position.
- Prepare the graft beds by removing a thin layer of cortical bone from the inferior surface of the talus and superior surface of the calcaneus (Fig. 1.53).
- Make a linear incision over the anteromedial surface of the proximal tibial metaphysis, incise the periosteum, and take a block of bone large enough for two grafts (usually 3.5 to 4.5 cm long and 1.5 cm wide). As an alternative to tibial bone, a short segment of the distal fibula or a circular segment of the iliac crest can be used.
- Cut the grafts to fit the prepared beds. Use a rongeur to shape the grafts so that they can be countersunk into cancellous bone to prevent lateral displacement.

- With the foot held in a slightly overcorrected position, place the grafts in the sinus tarsi. Evert the foot to lock the grafts in place.
- If a segment of the fibula or iliac crest is used, a smooth Kirschner wire can be used to hold the graft in place for 12 weeks, or a screw can be inserted anteriorly from the talar neck into the calcaneus for rigid fixation (Fig. 1.54).
- The foot should be stable enough to allow correction of equinus deformity by Achilles tendon lengthening if necessary.
- Apply a long leg cast with the knee flexed, the ankle in maximal dorsiflexion, and the foot in the corrected position.

POSTOPERATIVE CARE The long leg cast is worn for 12 weeks, and weight bearing is not allowed. The Kirschner wire is removed, and a short leg walking cast is worn for 4 more weeks.

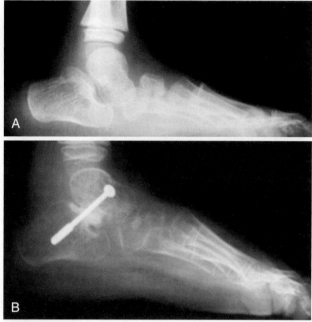

FIGURE 1.54 **A,** Congenital vertical talus in 6-year-old child. **B,** Corrected position of talus fixed with screw through neck of talus into calcaneus, as described by Dennyson and Fulford. Bone graft in middle and posterior aspects of subtalar joint. **SEE TECHNIQUE 1.22.**

▌TRIPLE ARTHRODESIS

Older children (>12 years) with uncorrected vertical talus who have pain or difficulty with shoe wear can be treated with triple arthrodesis. The procedure generally requires medial and lateral incisions and adequate osteotomies to place the foot in a plantigrade position, a technique similar to that used for correction of a severe tarsal coalition deformity.

ANOMALIES OF THE LEG
CONGENITAL ANGULAR DEFORMITIES OF THE LEG

Congenital angular deformities of the leg are primarily of two kinds: deformities in which the apex of the angulation is anterior and deformities in which it is posterior. In both, the tibia often is bowed not only anteriorly or posteriorly, but also medially or laterally. Anterior bowing of the tibia is commonly associated with neurofibromatosis.

Posterior angular deformities of the tibia tend to improve with growth (Fig. 1.55). A limb-length discrepancy also may be present, ranging from several millimeters to several centimeters. Children with these deformities should be examined yearly for any potential limb-length discrepancy that may require limb equalization, usually by an appropriately timed epiphysiodesis or limb lengthening in severe deformities.

Anterior angular deformities of the tibia are more worrisome because of their potential association with congenital pseudarthrosis of the tibia. Occasionally, these tibias maintain a normal medullary canal and show no evidence of narrowing or of the sclerotic "high-risk tibia." If any indication of narrowing of the medullary canal is present or develops in an

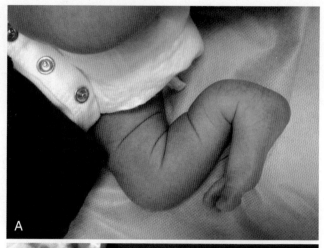

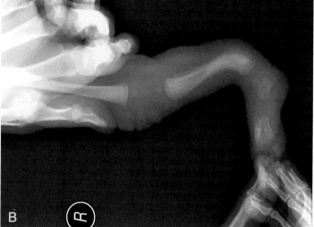

FIGURE 1.55 Congenital posteromedial bowing of right tibia. **A,** Clinical appearance. **B,** Radiographic appearance.

anteriorly bowed tibia, the limb should be braced until skeletal maturity is reached.

Unilateral anterior bowing of the tibia with duplication of the great toe has been described as a distinct syndrome, which should be considered in the differential diagnosis of anterolateral tibial bowing and should not be mistaken for congenital pseudarthrosis. Associated conditions, in addition to duplication of the great toe, include shortening of the tibia, which results in significant leg-length discrepancy, clinodactyly, and anomalous maturation of the carpal bones and metacarpals.

POSTEROMEDIAL BOWING OF THE TIBIA

This form of congenital tibial bowing is believed to result from intrauterine positioning. It is marked by severe distal tibial dorsiflexion at a level just above the ankle joint. The dorsal surface of the foot often contacts the anterior surface of the tibia. Many patients also have some characteristics of calcaneovalgus foot deformity. Imaging can help quickly distinguish isolated calcaneovalgus foot deformity from posteromedial bowing (Fig. 1.55B). Early treatment includes observation with anticipation that the deformity will resolve with time and growth (Fig. 1.56). Families often need considerable reassurance that such a striking condition will resolve in time without aggressive intervention. Appropriately timed epiphysiodesis can help resolve the expected limb-length inequality. Rarely, lengthening may be considered for marked leg length discrepancy.

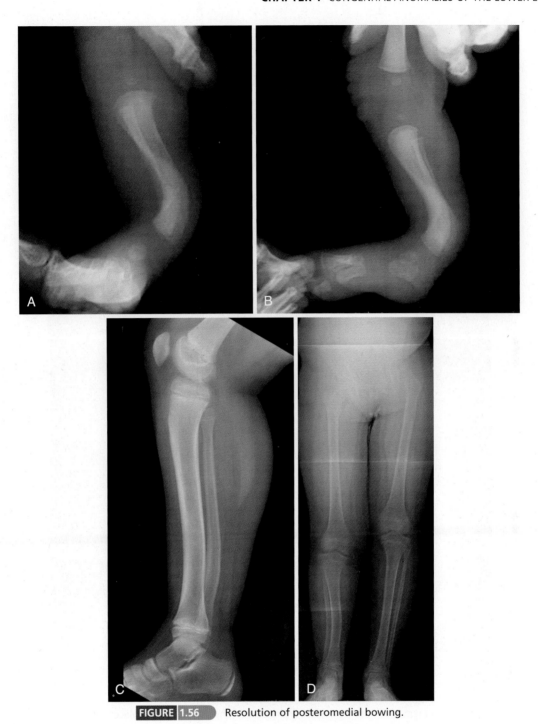

FIGURE 1.56   Resolution of posteromedial bowing.

CONGENITAL PSEUDARTHROSIS OF THE FIBULA AND TIBIA

Congenital pseudarthrosis is a specific type of nonunion that at birth is either present or incipient. Its cause is unknown, but it occurs often enough in patients with either neurofibromatosis or related stigmata to suggest that neurofibromatosis, if not the cause of congenital pseudarthrosis, is closely related to it. Congenital pseudarthrosis most commonly involves the distal half of the tibia and often that of the fibula in the same limb. The true cause of the poor healing potential of the bone at the pseudarthrosis site is unknown; however, hamartomatous thickened fibrous

tissue with limited vascular ingrowth is seen universally at the site of the pseudarthrosis (Fig. 1.57).

▓ FIBULA

Congenital pseudarthrosis of the fibula often precedes or accompanies the same condition in the ipsilateral tibia. Several grades of severity of this pseudarthrosis are seen: bowing of the fibula without pseudarthrosis, fibular pseudarthrosis without ankle deformity, fibular pseudarthrosis with ankle deformity, and fibular pseudarthrosis with latent pseudarthrosis of the tibia. Sometimes it even develops between the time of successful bone grafting of a pseudarthrosis of the tibia and skeletal maturity;

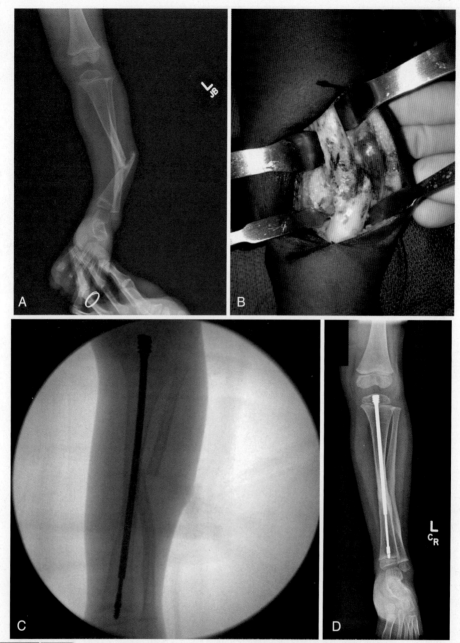

FIGURE 1.57 Congenital pseudarthrosis. **A,** Radiograph of 3-year-old child with established nonunion present since birth. **B,** Intraoperative photo of hamartomatous tissue. **C,** Postoperative radiograph demonstrating stabilization of tibia using telescoping intramedullary rod following surgical debridement, iliac crest bone graft, and bone morphogenetic protein placement. **D,** Healed nonunion 10 months postoperatively.

because the lateral malleolus becomes displaced proximally, a progressive valgus deformity of the ankle develops.

Until skeletal maturity is reached, the ankle can be stabilized by an ankle-foot orthosis. At maturity, any significant deformity can be treated by supramalleolar osteotomy made through essentially normal bone, and union of the osteotomy can be expected. Langenskiöld devised an operation for children, however, to prevent this valgus deformity or halt its progression. He created a synostosis between the distal tibial and fibular metaphyses. Because in congenital pseudarthrosis securing union by bone grafting may be as difficult in the fibula as in the tibia, an operation that prevents the ankle deformity without grafting in fibular pseudarthrosis is useful (Fig. 1.58).

TIBIOFIBULAR SYNOSTOSIS

TECHNIQUE 1.23

(LANGENSKIÖLD)

- Make a longitudinal incision anteriorly over the distal fibula.
- Divide the fibula 1 to 2 cm proximal to the level of the distal tibial physis and excise the cone-shaped part of the distal fibular shaft.
- In the lateral surface of the tibia, at the level of the cut surface of the fibula, and at the attachment of the

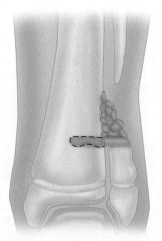

FIGURE 1.58 Langenskiöld technique for creating synostosis between distal tibial and fibular metaphyses to prevent valgus deformity of ankle in congenital pseudarthrosis of fibula (see text). **SEE TECHNIQUE 1.22**.

interosseous membrane, make a hole as wide as the diameter of the fibula. Proximal to the hole, remove the periosteum and interosseous membrane from the tibia over an area of several square centimeters.
- From the ilium, obtain a bone graft the same width as that of the hole in the tibia and long enough to extend from the lateral surface of the fibula into the spongy bone of the tibial metaphysis.
- Insert the graft perpendicular to the long axis of the limb so that it rests on the cut surface of the fibula and extends into the slot in the tibial cortex.
- Pack spongy iliac bone in the angle between the proximal surface of the graft and the lateral surface of the tibia.
- Apply a cast from below the knee to the base of the toes.

POSTOPERATIVE CARE At 2 months, full weight bearing in the cast is allowed, and at 4 months, the cast is discontinued.

■ TIBIA

Congenital pseudarthrosis of the tibia is rare, with an incidence of approximately 1 in 250,000 live births. Most large series report 50% to 90% association of this disorder with the stigmata of neurofibromatosis, including skin and osseous lesions.

■ CLASSIFICATION

Multiple classification systems have been created to describe congenital pseudarthrosis of the tibia. These classification systems tend to be more descriptive of the radiographic appearance of the lesion at a particular course in the disease and often provide little insight into the correct type of treatment or prognosis. Nevertheless, a descriptive classification can be helpful for communication between treating physicians and is important from a historical standpoint. We prefer the Boyd classification of congenital pseudarthrosis of the tibia:

Type I pseudarthrosis occurs with anterior bowing and a defect in the tibia present at birth. Other congenital deformities also may be present.

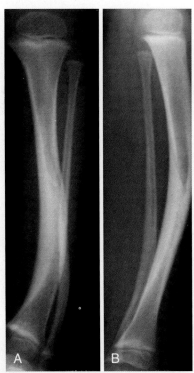

FIGURE 1.59 Type II congenital pseudarthrosis of tibia. **A,** Anteroposterior view of left tibia. **B,** Lateral view. Note anterior bowing and narrow, sclerotic medullary canal.

Type II pseudarthrosis occurs with anterior bowing and an hourglass constriction of the tibia present at birth. Spontaneous fracture, or fracture after minor trauma, commonly occurs before 2 years of age. This is the so-called high-risk tibia. The tibia is tapered, rounded, and sclerotic, and the medullary canal is obliterated. This type is the most common, is often associated with neurofibromatosis, and has the poorest prognosis. Recurrence of the fracture is common during the growth period but decreases in frequency with age and generally ceases to occur after skeletal maturation (Fig. 1.59).

Type III pseudarthrosis develops in a congenital cyst, usually near the junction of the middle and distal thirds of the tibia. Anterior bowing may precede or follow the development of a fracture. Recurrence of the fracture after treatment is less common than in type II, and excellent results after only one operation have been reported to last well into adulthood (Fig. 1.60).

Type IV pseudarthrosis originates in a sclerotic segment of bone in the classic location without narrowing of the tibia. The medullary canal is partially or completely obliterated. An "insufficiency" or "stress" fracture develops in the cortex of the tibia and gradually extends through the sclerotic bone. With completion of the fracture, healing fails to occur, and the fracture widens and becomes a pseudarthrosis. The prognosis for this type generally is good, especially when it is treated before the insufficiency fracture becomes complete (Fig. 1.61).

Type V pseudarthrosis of the tibia occurs with a dysplastic fibula. A pseudarthrosis of the fibula or tibia or both may develop. The prognosis is good if the lesion is confined to the fibula. If the lesion progresses to a tibial

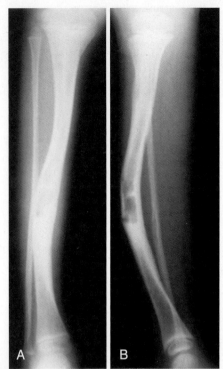

FIGURE 1.60   Type III congenital pseudarthrosis of tibia. **A,** Anteroposterior view of right tibia. **B,** Lateral view. Note cyst formation in middle third of tibia with anterior bowing and narrow medullary canal distal to cyst.

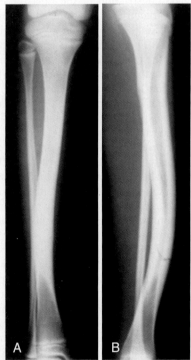

FIGURE 1.61   Type IV congenital pseudarthrosis of tibia. **A,** Anteroposterior view of right tibia. **B,** Lateral view. Note fracture in anterior cortex in distal third of tibia.

pseudarthrosis, the natural history usually resembles that of type II pseudarthrosis.

Type VI pseudarthrosis occurs as an intraosseous neurofibroma or schwannoma that results in a pseudarthrosis. This is extremely rare. The prognosis depends on the aggressiveness and treatment of the intraosseous lesion.

A more recent and simplified classification system proposed by Johnston et al. could guide treatment and prognosis. This classification scheme includes (1) the presence or absence of a fracture and (2) age of first fracture, before or after age 4 years. Under this classification scheme, fractured tibias require surgical treatment while intact tibias can be treated with observation and splinting.

For those tibias that require surgery, the treatment involves first resecting the entire pseudarthrosis, leaving a bone gap and soft-tissue defect that must be treated regardless of the descriptive radiographic classification before surgical resection.

■ TREATMENT

Treatment of congenital pseudarthrosis of the tibia depends on the age of the patient and the presence or absence of a fracture. Before walking age, little treatment is required for a pseudarthrosis, but once the child begins to ambulate, the leg should be immobilized in a clamshell orthosis and protected. If no fracture is present, the child can be treated in a brace until skeletal maturity with close follow-up. Once a true pseudarthrosis of the tibia develops, it cannot be expected to heal when treated by casting or bracing alone.

Initial surgical management of tibial pseudarthrosis involves resection of the entire pseudarthrosis and surrounding hamartomatous tissue, restoration of mechanical alignment, and intramedullary fixation. These three basic principles often are augmented by a combination of primary shortening, bone transport, supplemental bone grafting, and bone morphogenetic protein. Osseous union probably is more difficult to obtain in this condition than in any other (31% to 56% reported successful treatment). Even when union is obtained, it often is transient, and refracture, leg-length discrepancy, and malalignment may require further surgical management and possibly amputation.

Amputation is rarely, if ever, considered in the initial management of congenital pseudarthrosis of the tibia; however, amputation is frequently required and should be discussed early as a possible outcome of attempted treatment. Factors favoring amputation include anticipated shortening of more than 2 or 3 inches (5 to 7.5 cm), a history of multiple failed surgical procedures, and stiffness and decreased function of a limb that would be more useful after an amputation and prosthetic fitting.

▮ INTRAMEDULLARY FIXATION

Although many techniques have been described, the most commonly used is the intramedullary rodding technique described by Anderson et al. The pseudarthrosis is often quite distal in the tibia, making intramedullary fixation alone inadequate and unstable. Therefore the ankle joint often must be crossed by the rod to provide additional stability in these very distal pseudarthroses. The rod can migrate with growth, resulting in restoration of some ankle motion over time or can be surgically advanced to a position above the ankle once solid union has been achieved. For those lesions that appear more proximal in the tibia, it might be possible to avoid this protein have been used. In each series, BMP was used in conjunction with other accepted forms of bony stabilization such as intramedullary fixation. Early union rates have been favorable, but long-term follow-up and prospective comparative studies are needed to better understand the long-term efficacy and safety of these treatments. Because the treatment of congenital pseudarthrosis of the tibia is challenging, BMPs should be considered as an adjunct to treatment.

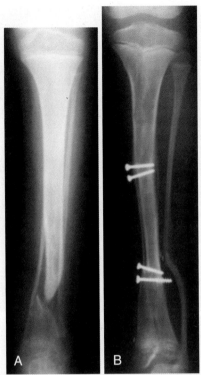

FIGURE 1.62 Congenital pseudarthrosis of tibia treated with vascularized fibular bone graft. **A,** Preoperative radiograph of tibia with established distal pseudarthrosis after multiple failed surgical procedures. **B,** Three years after repair with vascularized fibular graft.

crossing the ankle joint (Fig. 1.57). In these cases, larger rod diameter or an interlocking option could aid in stability.

VASCULARIZED GRAFT

Resection of the pseudarthrosis with reconstruction using a free vascularized bone graft with either fibular or iliac crest grafts (Fig. 1.62) also has been described with good results. The procedure requires experience with microvascular techniques, however, and two surgical teams are advantageous, one to harvest the graft while the second prepares the pseudarthrosis site to receive the graft. Vascularized fibular grafts may be indicated for pseudarthroses with gaps of more than 3 cm and for pseudarthroses in which multiple surgical procedures have failed.

ILIZAROV TECHNIQUE

In addition, good preliminary results were reported with the Ilizarov technique, but problems have included difficulty transporting the proximal tibia, "docking" malalignment, and poor quality of regenerated bone, leading to refracture. For most established pseudarthroses, initial treatment should be intramedullary rodding and bone grafting. The Ilizarov approach with bone transport does offer the advantage of maintaining or gaining tibial length.

BONE MORPHOGENETIC PROTEIN

Multiple reports have documented the successful use of recombinant human bone morphogenetic protein (rhBMP) in the treatment of congenital pseudarthrosis of the tibia. Both currently available forms (rhBMP-2 and rhBMP-7) of

---

INSERTION OF WILLIAMS INTRAMEDULLARY ROD AND BONE GRAFTING

TECHNIQUE 1.24   *Figure 1.63*

(ANDERSON ET AL.)

- Position the patient supine on a radiolucent operating table and apply a tourniquet to the thigh.
- Expose the ipsilateral iliac crest and harvest as much cancellous bone and bone from the outer table as can be obtained safely.
- Approach the tibia through an anterior incision that is centered over the pseudarthrosis and just lateral to the tibial crest. Divide the deep fascia of the anterior compartment at this level.
- Subperiosteally, expose the normal bone of the tibial shaft just proximal and distal to the pseudarthrosis.
- Completely excise the bone and fibrous tissue at the pseudarthrosis until normal medullary bone of both tibial fragments is exposed. Resection generally results in tibial shortening of 1 to 3 cm.
- Tibial union may be difficult to achieve in patients with a normal fibula; therefore a fibular osteotomy should be considered to allow adequate approximation of the two ends of the tibia.
- Ream the medullary canals of both tibial fragments with a drill or small curet or both.
- The Williams device consists of an indwelling rod and an insertion rod. The indwelling rod is smooth and cylindrical and varies in diameter. The proximal end is machined to a diamond tip, and the distal blunt end is threaded internally for approximately 15 mm so that a second (insertion) rod of equal outside diameter can be attached to it temporarily. The insertion rod is machined proximally so that its external threads screw into the distal end of the indwelling rod, and it is machined distally to a diamond tip. Alternatively, other intramedullary devices can be used, such as the telescoping Fassier-Duval Telescoping IM System (PEGA Medical-Laval Canada).
- To determine the Williams rod length needed, make a lateral radiograph to determine the expected length of the leg after the affected bone and fibrous tissues have been removed, and the angular deformity has been corrected.
- Drive the coupled rods into the distal part of the tibia at the site of the osteotomy, across the ankle and subtalar joints, and out the sole through the heel pad. When the rod is placed across the ankle joint, it is important to correct

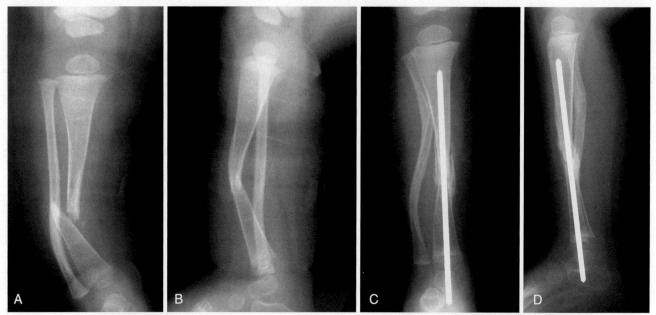

FIGURE 1.63   Insertion of Peter Williams rod for congenital pseudarthrosis of tibia, as described by Anderson et al. **A,** Anteroposterior view of type II congenital pseudarthrosis of tibia in 16-month-old child. **B,** Lateral view. **C,** Postoperative anteroposterior view. **D,** Postoperative lateral view. **SEE TECHNIQUE 1.24.**

valgus deformity of the ankle and dorsiflexion deformity of the foot, which are the inevitable consequences of weight bearing on an anterolaterally bowed tibia. Fluoroscopy is helpful during this part of the procedure.

- Approximate the tibial fragments and drive the rod retrograde into the region of the proximal tibial metaphysis, nearly to the tibial physis, but not encroaching on it. Unscrew the insertion rod a single full turn and verify the junction of the rod on a lateral radiograph.
- Fully disassemble (unscrew) the insertion rod and remove it, leaving the distal end of the implanted rod in the calcaneus.
- Pack the autologous corticocancellous bone strips from the iliac crest around the osteotomy and secure them with circumferential sutures of fine stainless steel or, as have been used more recently, absorbable sutures.
- Prophylactic fasciotomies often are required before wound closure.
- Close the subcutaneous tissue and skin and apply a long leg cast.

POSTOPERATIVE CARE The duration of immobilization and the type of cast are determined by the amount of healing noted on clinical and radiographic examinations. When healing is sufficient, the cast is discontinued. Removal of the cast and institution of progressive weight bearing usually are possible several months after surgery. A knee-ankle-foot orthosis or patellar tendon–bearing brace is worn until skeletal maturity is reached.

■ COMPLICATIONS
▌ STIFFNESS OF THE ANKLE AND HINDFOOT
A stiff ankle should be expected until the distal tip of the rod is proximal to the ankle joint after longitudinal growth of the

distal end of the tibia. Even if stiffness persists, it rarely hampers functional results.

▌ REFRACTURE
Refracture is common in patients with pseudarthroses, despite apparently solid clinical and radiographic union. Refracture can be managed with casting or removal and replacement of the intramedullary rod with additional bone grafting. Because of the likelihood of refracture, removal of the rod after union is not recommended until skeletal maturity has been reached.

▌ VALGUS ANKLE DEFORMITY
The distal tibial fragment must be fixed so that valgus deformity of the ankle is corrected at the time of placement of the intramedullary rod. Intraoperative fluoroscopy is useful for monitoring this procedure. Long-term bracing is mandatory during the growth years to minimize progressive valgus ankle deformity, or surgical treatment with the Langenskiöld procedure may be indicated.

Valgus deformity has been found to be significantly more frequent when the fibula is left intact than when fibular osteotomy is done (with or without fibular fixation). In addition, the presence of fibular insufficiency (fracture or prepseudarthrotic lesion) appears to be highly prognostic for subsequent valgus deformity, whether or not the fibula eventually healed.

▌ TIBIAL SHORTENING
Tibial shortening should be anticipated in almost all these children. The maximal projected shortening in the patients of Anderson et al. was 4 cm. In selected patients, tibial shortening can be treated by a well-timed contralateral epiphysiodesis or limb lengthening of the proximal tibia. The Ilizarov technique may be useful initially in severe cases with significant shortening and a wide nonunion or in patients in whom medullary nailing and standard bone grafting procedures fail. If Ilizarov techniques are used to gain length in a shortened tibia with

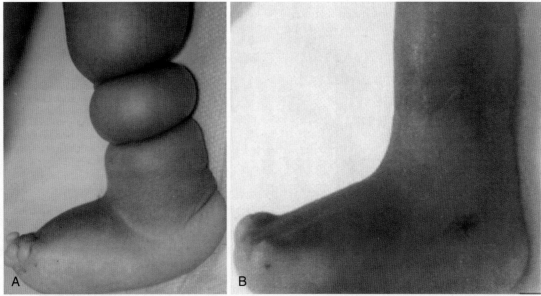

FIGURE 1.64   **A,** Congenital constriction of leg and congenital vertical talus. **B,** Appearance after excision of constricting bands. (From Gabos PG: Modified technique for the surgical treatment of congenital constriction bands of the arms and legs of infants and children, *Orthopedics* 29:401–404, 2006.)

persistent anterolateral bowing or if healing followed surgical management of the pseudarthrosis, the lengthening should focus on the uninvolved proximal tibial metaphysis well away from the pseudarthrosis site.

CONSTRICTIONS OF THE LEG

A congenital circumferential constriction, or "Streeter" band of the soft tissues of the leg (Fig. 1.64) is rare, occurring in 1 per 10,000. These lower extremity bands often are associated with other anomalies, such as absent digits, foot deformities, constriction bands on the upper extremity, cleft palate, and heart defects.

The deep fascia may be affected, and usually the lymphatic vessels and superficial circulation are partially obstructed. Distal to the constriction there may be persistent pitting edema that may or may not be cured by excising the constriction. Fractures of the tibia and fibula at the level of the constriction have been reported. In marked contrast to congenital pseudarthrosis, after successful treatment of the constriction, the fractures typically heal promptly without surgery. However, cases of persistent pseudarthrosis at the level of the constriction band have been reported.

Traditionally, constriction bands have been released in two or three stages to prevent vascular compromise of the distal part of the extremity. More recently, however, several authors have reported good results with one-stage release. The advantages of a one-stage release include easier postoperative care, especially in infants, and avoidance of a second or third operation with additional periods of anesthesia.

Hennigan and Kuo divided 135 constriction bands in 73 patients into four zones (Fig. 1.65). Most (50%) were in zone 2, between the knee and ankle. They also classified the bands according to severity: grade 1 bands involved subcutaneous tissue, grade 2 bands extended to the fascia, grade 3 bands extended to the fascia and required release, and grade 4 bands were congenital amputations.

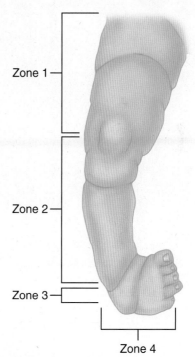

FIGURE 1.65   Zones of constricting bands described by Hennigan and Kuo (see text).

Amputation may be the only treatment option for severe type 3 bands (Fig. 1.66). The prevalence of clubfoot in patients with congenital constricting bands ranges from 12% to 56%.

All neurologic deficits were in children with grade 3 bands in zone 2, and clubfoot in these children required numerous and more extensive surgeries, with poorer results than those in children with no neurologic deficits. These authors suggested early complete soft-tissue release, along with consideration of tendon transfers, and noted that bony surgery eventually becomes necessary, and prolonged bracing will be needed to prevent recurrence.

ONE-STAGE OR TWO-STAGE RELEASE OF CIRCUMFERENTIAL CONSTRICTING BAND

TECHNIQUE 1.25

(GREENE)
- Excise a 1- to 2-mm margin of normal skin and subcutaneous tissue to minimize the risk of recurrence. For a two-stage procedure only excise 180 degrees.

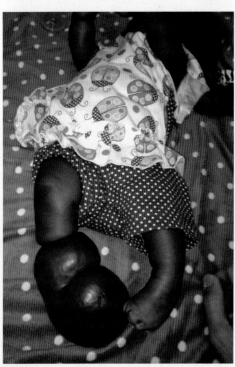

FIGURE 1.66   Amputation may be the only treatment option for severe type 3 bands.

- Resect all constricted fascia and muscle that have been converted to dense fibrous connective tissue.
- After resection of the dermal layers within the constriction band, identify the vascular and neurologic structures proximal and distal to the band by careful dissection as the skin and subcutaneous tissue are undermined.
- If subcutaneous tissue is excessive, especially on the dorsum of the fingers, debulking should be done.
- Close the skin with multiple Z-plasties, fashioning fairly large flaps at an angle of 60 degrees (Fig. 1.67).

POSTOPERATIVE CARE A pressure bandage is applied from proximal to the area of surgery to the distal end of the limb. With young children, a cast or plaster splint is applied and worn for 2 to 3 weeks until the incision has healed.

CONGENITAL HYPEREXTENSION AND DISLOCATION OF THE KNEE

Congenital hyperextension of the knee is only the lowest grade of an abnormality that is divided into three grades according to severity: grade 1, congenital hyperextension; grade 2, congenital hyperextension with anterior subluxation of the tibia on the femur; and grade 3, congenital hyperextension with anterior dislocation of the tibia on the femur (Fig. 1.68). Congenital hyperextension or dislocation of the knee usually is associated with skeletal abnormalities elsewhere in the extremity such as hip dysplasia (Fig. 1.69).

It has been postulated that the basic defect in congenital dislocation of the knee is absence or hypoplasia of the cruciate ligaments, although others consider these findings a result of the dislocation.

The pathologic condition usually varies with the severity of the deformity, but always the anterior capsule of the knee and the quadriceps mechanism are contracted. As the severity of the anterior displacement of the tibia increases, other findings include intraarticular adhesions and other abnormalities within the joint and hypoplasia or absence of the patella. Fibrosis and loss of bulk of the vastus lateralis muscle have been noted, as well as obliteration of the suprapatellar pouch from the adherent quadriceps tendon and lateral displacement of the patella. In severe anterior dislocation, the collateral ligaments have been shown to course anteriorly

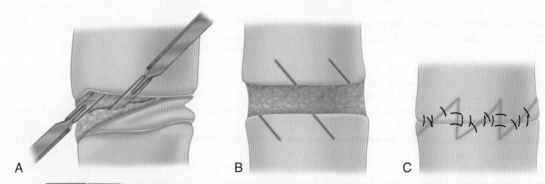

FIGURE 1.67   Congenital constriction release and Z-plasty. **A,** Excision of constriction band and undermining of skin edges. **B,** Z-plasty incisions at 60 degrees. **C,** Repair of Z-plasties with simple or mattress sutures. **SEE TECHNIQUE 1.25.**

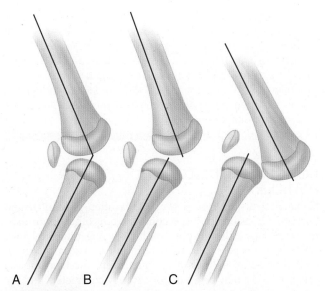

FIGURE 1.68 **A,** Congenital hyperextension of the knee. **B,** Subluxation of knee. **C,** Dislocation of knee.

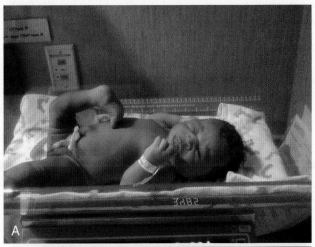

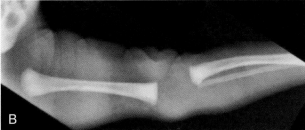

FIGURE 1.69 Congenital dislocation of knee. **A,** Clinical photograph of a child with congenital hyperextension deformity of the knee. **B,** Lateral radiograph after partial correction of the deformity demonstrates persistent anterior subluxation of the tibia. (Courtesy of Jay Cummings, MD.)

from their femoral attachments and anterior subluxation of the hamstring muscles in some patients to function as extensors of the knee in this deformed position.

The treatment of congenital hyperextension of the knee depends on the severity of the subluxation or dislocation and the age of the patient. In a newborn with mild-to-moderate

hyperextension or subluxation, conservative treatment methods, such as the use of and serial casting to increase knee flexion followed by a Pavlik harness for a few weeks to prevent early recurrence are likely to succeed. Roach and Richards proposed two criteria for successful nonoperative treatment of congenital knee dislocation: radiographic evidence of reduction and knee flexion to 90 degrees or more. According to most authors, nonoperative treatment can be continued for 3 months. In children who do not respond to conservative measures, the use of skeletal traction for correction is an option, but the deformity is difficult to correct with this method. In older children with moderate or severe subluxation or dislocation, surgery is indicated. In a child with congenital dislocation of the knee and congenital dislocation of the hip, surgical correction of the knee first is advisable. However, Johnston et al. described a single-stage correction for both deformities with similar outcomes to staged reconstructions.

Curtis and Fisher described a procedure for correction of congenital dislocation of the knee that is recommended for children 6 to 18 months old. The technique combines anterior capsular release, lengthening of the quadriceps mechanism, and release of intraarticular adhesions. Occasionally, the articular surfaces of the knee remain abnormal if the deformity recurs. Ideally, a functional range of motion can be obtained. In rare cases, osteotomy of the femur or tibia may be required in an older child. When needed, femoral shortening can be a good adjunct to quadricepsplasty with good midterm to long-term function.

Joseph et al. proposed some modifications to the Curtis and Fisher procedure that includes a laterally based incision, a more extensive, tongue-type release of the quadriceps tendons, and avoidance of dissection up to and including the collateral ligaments. These modifications were designed to correct specific problems such as anterior wound dehiscence, inadequate quadriceps tendons length, and postoperative knee instability caused by a collateral transection, respectively.

Dobbs proposed a less invasive treatment of congenital dislocation of the knee that involves serial casting and miniopen tenotomy of the quadriceps with additional anterior capsulotomy if required. This protocol resulted in successful deformity correction in 14 of 16 knees, with two knees requiring additional surgery. Longer follow-up is needed to determine the lasting effects of this treatment.

CAPSULAR RELEASE AND QUADRICEPS LENGTHENING FOR CORRECTION OF CONGENITAL KNEE DISLOCATION

TECHNIQUE 1.26

(CURTIS AND FISHER)

- Make a long anterior midline incision starting superomedially at the level of the middle third of the femur and extending inferolaterally to the tibial tuberosity. Alternatively, Joseph described exposure through a lateral incision with fewer wound complications.

- Expose the anterior thigh muscles and divide the quadriceps mechanism superior to the patella by either an inverted V-shaped incision (Fig. 1.70) or a Z-plasty. The former incision provides a tongue of tissue superior to the patella that is suitable for attachment of the proximal muscle mass after the extensor mechanism has been lengthened. Joseph modified this step to include a tongue-type separation of the quadriceps tendon from the vastus medialis and lateralis.
- Divide the anterior capsule transversely and extend the incision posteriorly to the tibial and fibular collateral ligaments. Mobilize and displace these ligaments posteriorly as the knee is flexed. In some, dissection to the level of the collateral ligaments can be avoided as long as they can be displaced posteriorly.
- If the patella is displaced laterally, release the lateral part of the patellar tendon and the vastus lateralis so that the patella can be moved to its proper location on the femoral condyles.
- Release any tight iliotibial band and lengthen the fibular collateral ligament if needed.
- Mobilize all normal-appearing quadriceps muscle and align it in the long axis of the femur to exert a direct pull on the patella.
- Suture the lengthened quadriceps mechanism with repair of the vastus medialis muscle to the lengthened rectus femoris.
- Evaluate tracking of the patella from extension to 90 degrees of flexion.
- Close the wound and apply a long leg cast with the knee flexed 30 degrees.

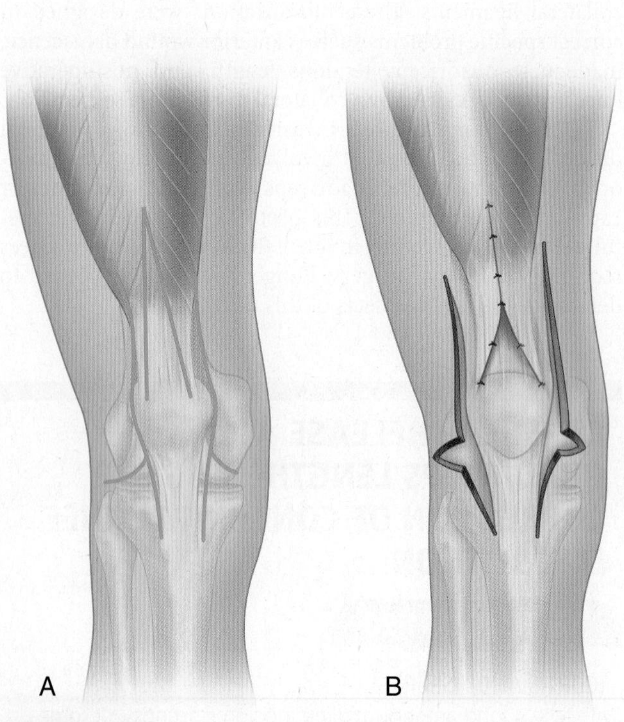

FIGURE 1.70 Curtis and Fisher technique for congenital dislocation of knee. **A,** Lines of incision to release anterior capsule medially and laterally and medial and lateral retinaculum of quadriceps mechanism. **B,** Correction after soft-tissue release and lengthening of rectus femoris muscle. **SEE TECHNIQUE 1.26.**

POSTOPERATIVE CARE If the anterior skin is under excessive tension, the cast can be changed at 2 weeks with the use of outpatient anesthesia. At 4 to 6 weeks, the cast is removed, and active and passive exercises are begun. In older patients, continuous passive motion can be used to regain motion during the first 3 to 6 weeks after surgery, and a long leg brace is worn for 6 to 12 months to prevent hyperextension of the knee.

CONGENITAL DISLOCATION OF THE PATELLA

Congenital dislocation of the patella often is familial and bilateral. Occasionally, it is accompanied by other abnormalities, especially arthrogryposis multiplex congenita and Down syndrome. It is persistent and irreducible and usually accompanied by abnormalities of the quadriceps mechanism. The vastus lateralis may be absent or severely contracted, and the patella may be dislocated laterally and attached to the anterior aspect of the iliotibial band. Often the patella is small and misshapen and in an abnormal location in the quadriceps mechanism. Genu valgum and external rotation of the tibia on the femur commonly develop. The capsule on the medial side of the knee is stretched, the lateral femoral condyle is flattened, or the insertion of the patellar tendon is located more laterally than normally.

Eilert noted that two clinical syndromes have been described in the literature: congenital dislocation of the patella or fixed lateral dislocation of the patella and habitual dislocation of the patella, which he suggested should be more accurately termed "obligatory dislocation" of the patella. These two syndromes have different clinical presentations (Table 1.2), and the timing of surgical correction is different.

The diagnosis of congenital dislocation of the patella often is difficult to make before the patient is 3 to 4 years old because of lack of ossification of the patella; however, more

TABLE 1.2

Two Types of Congenital Dislocation of the Patella

PERSISTENT DISLOCATION	OBLIGATORY DISLOCATION
Patella is dislocated lateral and persistent in that location	Patella dislocates and reduces spontaneously with flexion and extension of knee joint
Often obvious in infancy	Usually present at 5–10 years old
Frequently associated with generalized syndrome	Usually isolated anomaly
Knee flexion contracture is present	Range of knee motion usually normal
Nearly always produces little functional disability	May be well tolerated with little functional disability
Early surgical correction	Surgical correction can be delayed until patient is symptomatic

Adapted from Eilert RE: Congenital dislocation of the patella, *Clin Orthop Relat Res* 389:22–29, 2001.

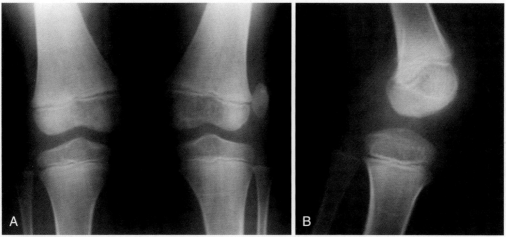

FIGURE 1.71 Untreated congenital dislocation of left patella in 5-year-old boy. **A,** Antero-posterior view shows fixed lateral dislocation. **B,** On lateral view, patella appears absent because of superimposed femoral condyles.

severe cases, with associated knee flexion contractures, can be diagnosed soon after birth. Magnetic resonance imaging (MRI) can show the cartilaginous patella lying lateral to the femur and can confirm the diagnosis when congenital lateral patellar dislocation is suspected. Several authors have described the use of ultrasound to define the position of the cartilaginous patella. Because the severity of the deformity is directly related to the length of time that the deformity is allowed to remain uncorrected, surgery can be done as soon as the diagnosis is made to try to prevent a valgus, flexion, or external rotation deformity of the knee (Fig. 1.71).

The underlying pathologic condition of congenital or habitual dislocation of the patella is contracture of the quadriceps mechanism, which is more severe in patients with congenital dislocations. Operative techniques vary according to the extent and degree of these operative findings. The primary objective is release of the contracted structures on the lateral side of the patella (the lateral capsule, iliotibial band, and lateral portion of the quadriceps) to allow reduction of the patella. Medial plication of the lax capsule is necessary to stabilize the reduced patella. In most patients, especially younger children, extensive lateral release and capsular plication are sufficient to obtain patellofemoral congruency. In older children, advancement of the vastus medialis often is necessary to tighten the muscle and improve muscle action. In addition to these steps, in their 1976 article, Stanisavijevic et al. described adding a Roux-Goldthwait patellar tendon procedure. A more recent study on the Stanisavijevic procedure has demonstrated promising results.

LATERAL RELEASE AND MEDIAL PLICATION
TECHNIQUE 1.27

(BEATY; MODIFIED FROM GAO ET AL. AND LANGENSKIÖLD)
- Make a midline incision from the distal aspect of the femur to the tibial tuberosity. Perform a full-thickness skin dissection over the patella to expose the medial and lateral aspects of the knee joint and the quadratus femoris muscle.
- Release the vastus lateralis from its most proximal muscle origin in the quadratus femoris to the level of the joint. This may require release of the iliotibial band laterally to the intermuscular septum.
- Because a midline surgical incision over the patella tends to heal with more proliferative scarring in children than in adults, Eilert suggested making the surgical incision over the anterolateral knee so that the scar is not under direct pressure against the patella. The incision must be long enough to expose a sufficient portion of the quadriceps muscle so that it can be realigned, and in an infant with congenital patellar dislocation, the incision may extend halfway up the thigh.
- Occasionally, the rectus femoris must be dissected and lengthened by a Z-plasty.
- Incise the vastus medialis obliquus from its origin proximally and distally from the patella, the medial capsule, and the patellar tendon.
- Reduce the patella into the femoral groove.
- Reattach laterally and distally the vastus medialis obliquus to the patellar tendon and medial retinaculum to secure the patella in the femoral groove.
- When the initial suture has been placed distally, move the knee through a gentle range of motion to assess reduction and tracking of the patella in the femoral groove. If the tension is too tight on the vastus medialis obliquus, remove the suture and transfer the muscle slightly proximally. If the tension is too lax, attach the vastus medialis obliquus farther distally and laterally.
- Occasionally, the patella is so unstable that the gracilis or semitendinosus tendon must be divided at the musculotendinous junction and transferred into the patella as a checkrein for added stability. The vastus medialis obliquus is sutured to the remaining retinaculum of the patella and the quadratus femoris.
- Continue the repair of the vastus medialis obliquus proximally and distally.

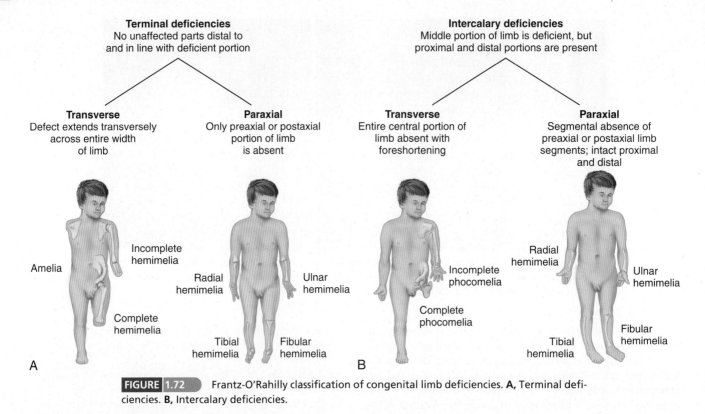

Terminal deficiencies
No unaffected parts distal to
and in line with deficient portion

Transverse
Defect extends transversely
across entire width
of limb

Paraxial
Only preaxial or postaxial
portion of limb
is absent

Amelia

Incomplete
hemimelia

Radial
hemimelia

Ulnar
hemimelia

Complete
hemimelia

Tibial
hemimelia

Fibular
hemimelia

A

Intercalary deficiencies
Middle portion of limb is deficient, but
proximal and distal portions are present

Transverse
Entire central portion of
limb absent with
foreshortening

Paraxial
Segmental absence of
preaxial or postaxial limb
segments; intact proximal
and distal

Incomplete
phocomelia

Complete
phocomelia

Radial
hemimelia

Ulnar
hemimelia

Tibial
hemimelia

Fibular
hemimelia

B

FIGURE 1.72 Frantz-O'Rahilly classification of congenital limb deficiencies. **A,** Terminal deficiencies. **B,** Intercalary deficiencies.

- Move the knee again through a range of motion to ensure reduction of the patella in the femoral groove and normal tracking during flexion and extension.
- Deflate the tourniquet and obtain hemostasis with electrocautery. Insert a drain deep into the wound and close the subcutaneous tissue and skin.
- Apply a long leg cast with the knee in 30 degrees of flexion.

POSTOPERATIVE CARE The cast is removed approximately 6 weeks after surgery, and active and passive range-of-motion exercises are begun.

CONGENITAL DEFICIENCIES OF THE LONG BONES

The first scientific approach to the problem of congenital long bone deficiencies was devised by Frantz and O'Rahilly in 1961. Their widely-used classification system described deficiencies as terminal or intercalary. In terminal deficiencies, there is an amputation with no body parts distal to the site (Fig. 1.72A). In intercalary deficits, a middle segment is missing, but the distal segments are present (Fig. 1.72B). Terminal and intercalary deficiencies are defined further as transverse or longitudinal. The complete absence of a hand at the wrist is a terminal transverse deficiency. A complete hand without a radius or ulna is an intercalary transverse deficiency. An example of a terminal longitudinal deficiency is fibular hemimelia, in which the lateral two rays also are missing. Fibular hemimelia in which the foot is normal is an intercalary longitudinal, or paraxial, deficiency.

■ TIBIAL HEMIMELIA

Since the disorder was first described by Otto in, tibial hemimelia has been known by a variety of names, including congenital longitudinal deficiency of the tibia, congenital dysplasia of the tibia, paraxial tibial hemimelia, tibial dysplasia, and congenital deficiency or absence of the tibia. This condition actually represents a spectrum of deformities, ranging from total absence of the tibia (the most severe form) to mild hypoplasia of the tibia (the least severe form). The incidence has been estimated at one in 1 million live births, and the condition may be bilateral in 30% of patients. It usually occurs sporadically, although familial cases with either autosomal dominant or recessive transmission patterns have been reported. There are multiple distinct syndromes that have tibial hemimelia as a component including polydactyly–triphalangeal thumb syndrome (Werner syndrome), tibial hemimelia diplopodia, tibial hemimelia–split hand/foot syndrome, tibial hemimelia–micromelia–trigonal brachycephaly syndrome, and femoral bifurcation-tibial hemimelia-hand ectrodactyly (Gollop-Wolfgang Complex). The exact cause is multifactorial, and a variety of gene defects have been discovered. However, it does not appear that one particular gene mutation or one inheritance pattern can be used to explain all cases.

The involved leg is short, and the fibular head is palpable if it is proximally displaced. The foot is often held in severe equinovarus, and the hindfoot is stiff (Fig. 1.73). In older children, the proximal tibial anlage may be palpable, even if it is not radiographically visible. The knee is generally flexed, and in more severe deformities, quadriceps insufficiency causes a lack of knee extension. Careful clinical evaluation of the quadriceps extensor mechanism is important because this has significant prognostic value regarding the potential for reconstruction of the knee. Femoral hypoplasia may be seen.

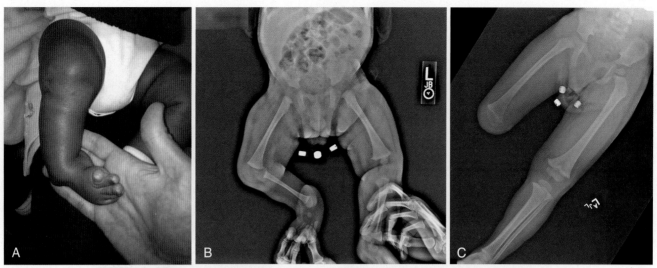

FIGURE 1.73   **A,** Jones type I deformity with rigid foot deformity and absent quadriceps function. **B,** Complete radiographic absence of the tibia. **C,** Radiograph after knee disarticulation.

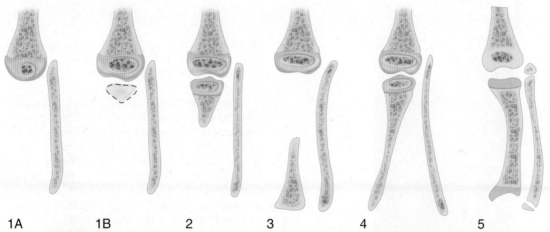

1A   1B   2   3   4   5

FIGURE 1.74   Classification of tibial hemimelia. In type 1A, fibula is dislocated proximally, tibia is not radiographically evident, and distal femoral epiphysis is smaller than on normal side. In type 1B, fibula is dislocated proximally, and proximal tibial anlage may be visible at birth on ultrasound or magnetic resonance imaging, but not on plain radiographs. Type 2 deformity has proximal dislocation of fibula and radiographically visible proximal tibia with normal-appearing knee joint. In type 3 deformity, fibula is dislocated proximally, distal tibia is radiographically visible, but proximal tibia is not seen. In rare type 4 deformity, fibula has migrated proximally, with diastasis of distal tibiofibular joint. Type 5 Birch modification of Jones classification to include global shortening of the tibia relative to the fibula.

CLASSIFICATION

The most widely used classification scheme for tibial hemimelia is that of Jones, Barnes, and Lloyd-Roberts (Fig. 1.74), which is based on the early radiographic presentation. Treatment recommendations are given for each type.

In type 1A deformity, there is a complete radiographic absence of the tibia and a hypoplastic distal femoral epiphysis (compared with the normal side). In type 1B deformity, there also is no radiographic evidence of a tibia, but the distal femoral epiphysis appears more normal in size and shape. This difference is crucial because the type 1B deformity has a proximal tibial cartilaginous anlage that can be expected to ossify with time. Arthrography, ultrasound, and MRI have shown this cartilaginous anlage in type 1B deformities (Fig. 1.75B, *right*). In time,

the proximal tibial anlage of a type 1B deformity may ossify to become a type 2 lesion.

In type 2 deformity, a proximal tibia of varying size is present at birth. The fibula usually is normal in size, but the head is proximally dislocated (Fig. 1.75A and B, *left*).

Type 3 deformity, in which the proximal tibia is not radiographically visible, is rare. The distal tibial epiphysis sometimes is visible, along with a mature distal metaphysis; however, there may be only a diffuse calcified density within the distal tibial anlage. The distal femoral epiphysis usually is well formed, but the upper end of the fibula is proximally dislocated. Although the distal femoral epiphysis usually is of normal size, the knee generally is unstable.

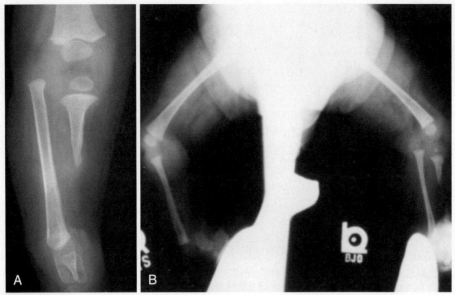

FIGURE 1.75 **A,** Congenital tibial hemimelia type 1A. **B,** Bilateral tibial hemimelia (right type 1B and left type 2).

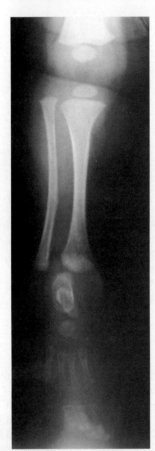

FIGURE 1.76 Newborn with congenital diastasis of ankle representing type 4 tibial hemimelia; note absence of first ray.

In type 4 deformity, which is rare, the tibia is shortened, and there is a proximal migration of the fibula with distal tibial fibular diastasis (Fig. 1.76). This deformity also has been called congenital diastasis of the ankle joint and congenital tibiofibular diastasis. Clinton and Birch, in their 37-year review of 125 limbs with tibial hemimelia, noted no true type 3 deformities. They also proposed the addition of a Jones type 5, which involves global tibial shortening relative to the fibula of varying severity.

A more recent classification takes into account the MRI, ultrasonographic, and intraoperative findings of the cartilaginous anlage both proximally and distally. This classification includes seven types, with "a" and "b" subtypes depending on the presence or absence of cartilaginous portions (Fig. 1.77). This classification includes global shortening of the tibia, which was previously not classified in the Jones system. Although not currently widely used, this system may become more mainstream in the years to come.

In tibial hemimelia, the superficial peroneal nerve may terminate at the level of the ankle. Leg muscles that normally insert on the plantar surface of the foot tend to blend into a common tendon sheath. The talus and calcaneus frequently are congenitally fused. The anterior tibial artery is absent, and the plantar arterial arch is incomplete. Similar vascular findings in clubfoot and tibial hemimelia suggest reduced vascular flow as a cause. Associated anomalies generally are most severe when the tibia is least developed. In type 4 deformities, the distal tibial epiphysis may be absent.

TREATMENT

As with all congenital lower limb deficiencies, the goal of treatment is a functional limb equal in length to the normal limb. The type of surgical treatment depends on the radiographic classification and clinical appearance. For severe deficiencies, amputation and prosthetic rehabilitation are the most practical means of treatment.

Jones Type 1A Tibial Hemimelia. The two options for treatment of type 1A deformities are knee disarticulation and knee reconstruction (with or without foot amputation). The easiest and frequently most effective option is knee disarticulation followed by fitting with an above-knee prosthesis. This option provides a definitive solution with one operation and is indicated when there is no intact quadriceps-patellar tendon

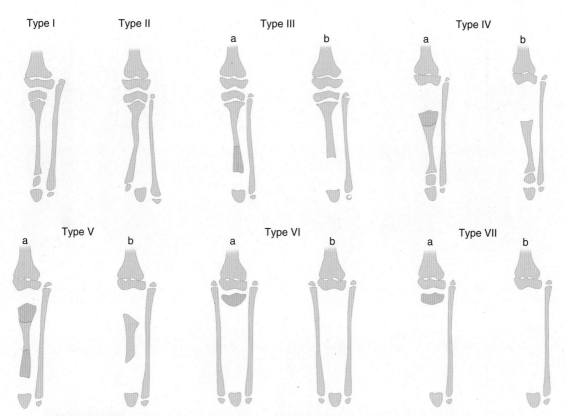

FIGURE 1.77   Weber classification of tibial hemimelia based on severity in a higher maturation level. Type I, hypoplasia; type II, diastasis; type III, distal aplasia; type IV, proximal aplasia; type V, bifocal aplasia; type VI, agenesia with double fibula; type VII, agenesia with single fibula. (Type *[a]* is with cartilaginous anlage and *[b]* is without cartilaginous anlage; *tan* represents bone, and *blue* represents cartilage). (From Weber M: New classification and score for tibial hemimelia, *J Child Orthop* 2:169–175, 2008.)

complex (Fig. 1.73). Knee disarticulation is preferred over above-knee amputation because above-knee amputation for type 1A deformity may result in skin problems from bony stump overgrowth. Because the ultimate femoral growth often is diminished, the end result of a knee disarticulation may be a functional above-knee amputation level. Children treated in this manner are almost uniformly active, functional prosthetic users. Attempts to correct the equinovarus and absent knee joint frequently result in repeated operations and eventual failure. The Brown procedure, transfer of the proximal fibula under the distal femur in type 1A deformities, has not produced stable long-term results. It may be reasonable to preserve the foot in bilateral deformities because limb-length discrepancy is not a consideration but attempts to reconstruct the knee in conjunction with foot amputation have produced mixed results.

Jones Type 1B and 2 Tibial Hemimelia. In type 1B and type 2 deformities, a functional knee joint exists, and knee disarticulation is not required if the quadriceps mechanism is present and functional. A proximal tibiofibular synostosis combined with a Syme amputation or distal reconstruction is the treatment of choice (Fig. 1.78).

Putti used a side-to-side configuration (Fig. 1.79C), but most authors now prefer end-to-end alignment between the tibial remnant and the fibula. Although it would seem preferable to wait until the proximal tibial anlage ossifies, stability can be achieved even when the proximal tibia is purely cartilaginous. At a second stage, the foot is amputated to make prosthetic

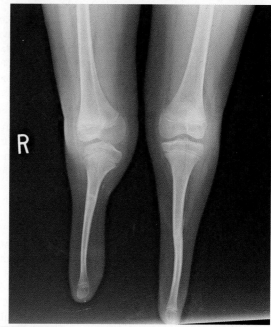

FIGURE 1.78   Follow-up after fibula to tibia transfer and Syme amputation. **SEE TECHNIQUE 1.29.**

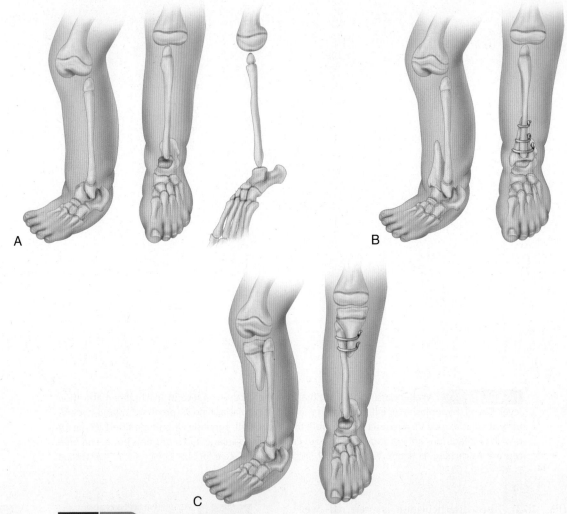

FIGURE 1.79 Variations of Putti procedure for reconstruction of congenital absence of tibia. **A,** Fibula is inserted into hindfoot with foot in severe equinus to lengthen limb. Fibula also has been transferred to intercondylar notch. **B,** Fibula has been transferred to intercondylar notch, and distal tibiofibular synostosis has been created. **C,** Type 2 deficiency. Fibula has been synostosed to proximal tibia and inserted into hindfoot with foot positioned in equinus to obtain additional length. End-to-end synostosis is preferred; if side-to-side synostosis is performed, transverse screw can be used for fixation.

rehabilitation easier. Retention of the foot during the proximal tibial reconstruction is helpful because it serves as a fixation point for a long leg cast. Making a synostosis between the fibula and tibia creates a more uniform, in-line, weight-bearing mechanical axis. When the fibula is not transferred to the tibia, a peculiar, curved, hypertrophied fibula develops, causing a secondary deformity. Fusing the fibula underneath the tibia encourages its transformation into a more tibia-like bone. The Syme amputation is preferred to a through-bone amputation to prevent transdiaphyseal problems of bony stump overgrowth and to preserve maximal length of the stump. Another option, if the tibial segment is long enough, involves the creation of a synostosis between the distal tibia and fibula (Fig. 1.79B). The Ertl amputation results in a functional transtibial amputation with a proposed decreased risk of bone overgrowth (Fig. 1.80).

Authors have attempted to treat types 1B and 2 tibial hemimelia with surgical equalization of leg length, production of a plantigrade foot, and creation of a stable knee. Traditional leg-lengthening procedures, soft-tissue reconstruction, and casting have not reliably achieved these goals in patients with tibial hemimelia; however, the Ilizarov method offers a viable option for reconstruction in selected cases. These decisions can be quite difficult. Amputation is an undesirable option for many families who hope for a normal limb. Therefore the expected function of the reconstructed limb, the multiple surgical procedures required, and the prolonged time in an external fixator frame must be weighed carefully against the function that can be obtained with timely amputation and prosthetic management. Other ingenious procedures have been used for reconstruction in children with tibial hemimelia.

In patients with tibial hemimelia and ipsilateral femoral deficiency, arthrodesis of the fibula to the distal femur can be performed or, in younger children, chondrodesis, aligning the fibula directly with the femur and the intercondylar notch. Combining this with a Syme amputation significantly lengthens the effective lever arm of the femur.

Although Syme and Boyd amputations have been the accepted treatments to make prosthetic rehabilitation easier,

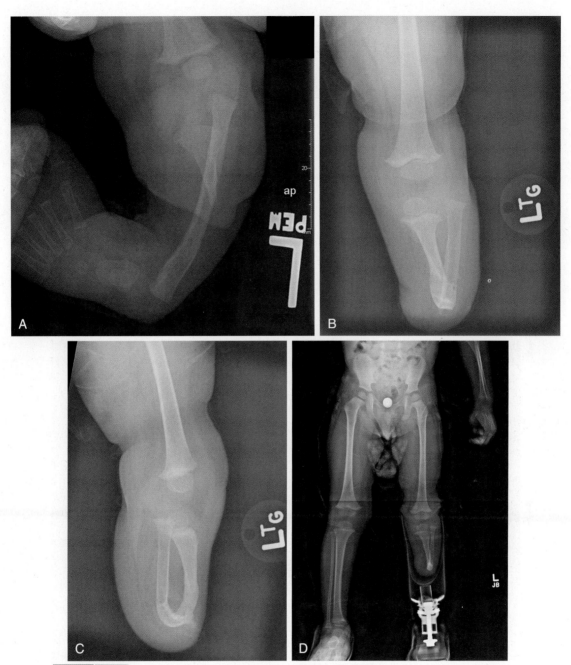

FIGURE 1.80   **A,** Jones type II hemimelia with significant tibial shortening and rigid foot deformity. **B,** Posterior Ertl amputation (anteroposterior view). **C,** Lateral view. **D,** Prosthetic fitting.

other alternatives have been described. If a family is absolutely opposed to amputation of the foot, an acceptable alternative is reconstruction of the foot and ankle complex by implanting the distal fibula into the talus in an extreme equinus position to increase the length of the limb (Fig. 1.79A). Prostheses can be constructed to take advantage of this extra length while accommodating the foot.

Some authors recommend knee disarticulation even in type 2 deficiencies if severe knee flexion contractures are present before surgery. Finally, proximal tibiofibular synostosis is not absolutely indicated for all type 2 deformities; the literature contains reports of satisfactory prosthetic rehabilitation after Syme amputation alone; however, if the fibula is transferred under the tibial remnant, it can be expected to remodel reliably and form into a large, tibia-like bone eventually.

Jones Type 3 Tibial Hemimelia. Type 3 deficiencies are extremely rare and in the limited reports available have been treated with a variety of amputations. In some patients, tibiofibular synostosis may be possible.

Jones Type 4 Tibial Hemimelia. For patients with type 4 deficiencies, treatment must be individualized. Syme amputation provides excellent function (Fig. 1.81). Customized reconstruction of the ankle joint to retain the foot and ankle also has been described. Most patients can be treated with combinations of distal tibiofibular synostosis and distal fibular epiphysiodesis. Equinovarus deformities of the foot, if present, require soft-tissue releases.

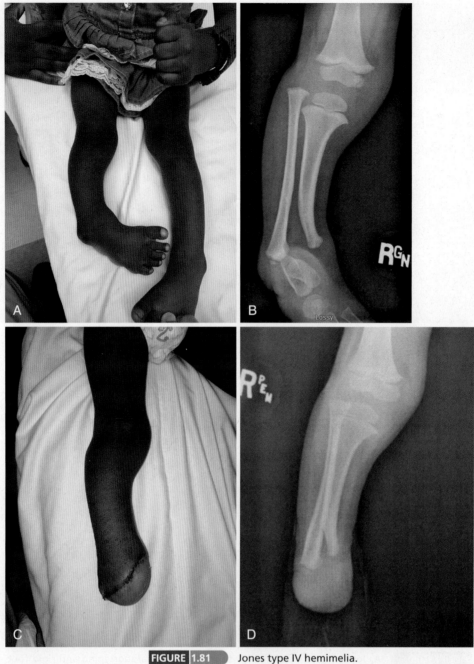

FIGURE 1.81 Jones type IV hemimelia.

DISTAL FIBULOTALAR ARTHRODESIS

TECHNIQUE 1.28

- Place the patient supine on the operating table.
- Approach the distal fibulotalar articulation anterolaterally to expose both bones.
- Dissect soft tissue to allow central placement of the body of the talus onto the distal end of the fibula.

- Create a trough through the dome of the talus into which the distal fibula is placed plantigrade and in neutral alignment with the foot.
- If necessary, fix the fibulotalar articulation with longitudinal and crossed Kirschner wires.
- Remove the cartilage from the distal fibular epiphysis and from the dome of the talus to allow bone-to-bone contact.
- Close the wound and apply a long leg, bent-knee cast.

POSTOPERATIVE CARE The cast is worn until the arthrodesis has united, usually at 12 to 16 weeks.

PROXIMAL TIBIOFIBULAR SYNOSTOSIS

TECHNIQUE 1.29 *See Figure 1.78*

- Make an anterolateral incision beginning at the proximal tibia and extending distally and anteriorly to the middle third of the tibia. Identify and protect the peroneal nerve.
- Dissect a sufficient portion of the anterior compartment musculature from the proximal medial tibia to expose the proximal tibial cartilaginous anlage (in type 1B deficiency) or the bony proximal tibia (in type 2 deficiency).
- Leave the proximal attachments of the fibula intact but perform a subperiosteal dissection of the fibula.
- At an appropriate point opposite the distal end of the proximal tibial anlage, perform an osteotomy of the fibula.
- Drill a Steinmann pin of appropriate size distally through the medullary canal of the fibula out the plantar aspect of the foot.
- Reduce the fibula on the proximal tibia and drive the medullary pin retrograde into the proximal tibial remnant.
- If necessary, pass the pin into the distal femur for stability.
- Distally, bend the pin 90 degrees and cut it off below the level of the skin to be removed 6 to 8 weeks later. Immobilize the leg in a cast. Alternative fixation techniques can include screws, cross pins, and cerclage wires.

At a later date, the foot may be amputated. In some patients, the foot may be salvaged with a combination of soft-tissue release, Ilizarov technique, and talectomy or arthrodesis as needed. The tip of the proximal tibial remnant should be sectioned sufficiently to create a wide surface for either chondrodesis or synostosis with the fibula. The periosteum of the fibula should be sutured to the proximal tibial remnant, if possible, to prevent reformation of the fibula to its proximal remnant.

◼ FIBULAR HEMIMELIA

Fibular hemimelia, also known as congenital absence of the fibula, congenital deficiency of the fibula, paraxial fibular hemimelia, and aplasia or hypoplasia of the fibula, is the most common long bone deficiency (followed by aplasia of the radius, femur, tibia, ulna, and humerus). Whether or not dysgenesis and relative ischemia affect the developing mesenchyme and cause the skeletal dysplasia seen in fibular hemimelia is still conjectural. There are no clear genetic or toxic pathogenetic mechanisms. Fibular hemimelia consists of a spectrum of anomalies, the least severe being mild fibular shortening and the most severe being total absence of the fibula associated with defects in the foot, tibia, and femur. Because of the myriad anomalies associated with even mild fibular deficiency, postaxial hypoplasia may be a more descriptive designation for this condition.

The clinical presentation depends on the specific classification and associated anomalies. Generally, there is leg-length discrepancy with equinovalgus deformity of the foot, flexion contracture of the knee, femoral shortening, instability of the knee and ankle, and a stiff hindfoot with absent lateral rays

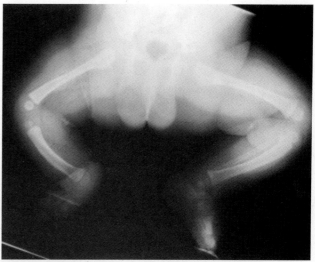

FIGURE 1.82 Radiograph of infant with classic fibular hemimelia. Femur and tibia are both short, and foot is in valgus with absent lateral rays.

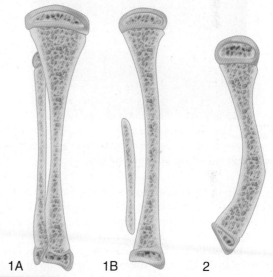

1A   1B   2

FIGURE 1.83 Achterman and Kalamchi classification of fibular hemimelia. Type 1A: proximal fibular epiphysis is more distal, and distal fibular epiphysis is more proximal than normal. Type 1B: more severe deficiency of fibula with at least 30% to 50% of fibula missing and no distal support to ankle joint. Type 2: complete absence of fibula with bowing and shortening of tibia.

(Fig. 1.82). Although equinovalgus is the most common foot deformity, equinovarus and calcaneovalgus also have been reported. Clinical problems are leg-length inequality and foot and ankle instability. In bilateral involvement, the leg-length discrepancy generally is manifested as disproportionate dwarfism because both sides usually are affected to a similar degree.

CLASSIFICATION

A useful classification scheme proposed by Achterman and Kalamchi (Fig. 1.83) distinguishes a type 1 deformity (hypoplasia of the fibula) from a type 2 deformity (complete absence of the fibula). Type 1 deformities are subdivided further into type 1A and type 1B. In type 1A, the proximal fibular epiphysis is distal to the proximal tibial epiphysis, and the distal

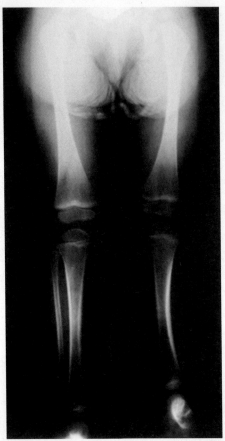

FIGURE 1.84 Achterman and Kalamchi type 1B fibular hemi-melia with very hypotrophic, faintly visible fibula; mild shortening of femur; and moderate shortening of tibia.

TABLE 1.3	
Fibular Deficiency: Functional Classification and Treatment Guidelines (Birch)	
CLASSIFICATION	**TREATMENT**
TYPE I: FUNCTIONAL FOOT	
IA: 0%–5% inequality	Orthosis, epiphysiodesis
IB: 6%–10% inequality	Epiphysiodesis ± limb lengthening
IC: 11%–30% inequality	1 or 2 limb-lengthening procedures or amputation
ID: >30% inequality	>2 limb-lengthening procedures or amputation
TYPE II: NONFUNCTIONAL FOOT	
IIA: Functional upper limb	Early amputation
IIB: Nonfunctional upper limb	Consider limb salvage procedure

current percentage of shortening. Generally, because the percentage of shortening in an infant remains relatively constant throughout childhood, reasonable predictions of final leg-length discrepancy can be made based on very early radiographs. The function of the foot also is assessed as described. For a patient with a functional foot and minimal limb-length inequality (≥5%), the goals of treatment are equalization of limb length and correction of the foot deformity. Shoe lifts are prescribed during the growth period, and epiphysiodesis of the normal leg is performed at the appropriate time so that leg lengths are equal at the end of skeletal growth. If contralateral epiphysiodesis or shortening would result in unacceptable overall diminution of height, the physician is faced with a difficult decision: either the short leg is lengthened, or the foot is amputated, and length is equalized with a prosthesis.

For inequality of 6% to 10%, appropriately timed epiphysiodesis can be used with or without limb lengthening in patients with a functional foot. Stevens and Arms recommended combining limb lengthening with hemiepiphysiodesis of the distal femur or ankle or both to correct valgus alignment. They also suggested that adjunctive contralateral epiphysiodesis might be preferable to repeated limb lengthening, emphasizing the multiple procedures that may be required for associated deformities. For patients with 11% or more limb-length inequality and a functional foot, a difficult decision must be made whether to undertake limb salvage with multiple lengthening or amputation. If limb salvage is chosen, a stable plantigrade foot and ankle are necessary and should be created through a combination of soft-tissue releases and osteotomies before lengthening procedures. McCarthy et al. found that patients who had amputations were able to perform more activities, had less pain, were more satisfied, had a lower complication rate, and had undergone fewer surgical procedures than patients with tibial lengthenings; however, the decision to proceed with amputation is often a difficult one for families to make. For more severe deformities of the foot, those with less than three rays or rigid equinovalgus, early amputation and prosthetic reconstruction usually are considered the best options for these nonfunctional feet; however, if the upper limbs also are severely affected, salvage of the deformed foot may be beneficial to maintain global function.

fibular epiphysis is proximal to the talar dome. In type 1B, the deficiency of the fibula is more severe, with 30% to 50% of the length missing, and no distal support for the ankle joint (Fig. 1.84). Abnormalities of the femur are common, as is hypoplasia of the patella and lateral femoral condyle. The cruciate ligaments also are clinically unstable. Angulation of the tibia is found most often in patients with type 2 deficiencies. Ball-and-socket ankle joints are present in most patients with type 1A deficiencies, and more severe foot and ankle problems are found in patients with type 2 deformities. Some patients with type 2 deformities have relatively stable ankle joints, however, despite the absence of a fibula, and others have complete instability of the tibiotalar articulation. Tarsal coalitions and absence of the lateral rays are common.

Another classification by Birch et al. takes overall limb-length inequality and foot function into account when determining treatment (Table 1.3).

The foot is considered functional if it can be made plantigrade and has three or more rays. Limb-length inequality is determined by a full-length radiograph or scanogram. The percentage of shortening remains constant in 85% of fibular deficiency patients. If both limbs are involved, the longer limb is considered "normal" and the percentage of shortening is measured relative to the "normal" limb.

TREATMENT

At the initial evaluation, the physician should attempt to predict the ultimate limb-length discrepancy, based on the

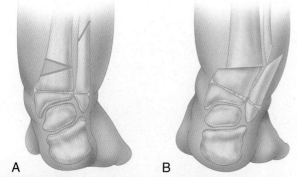

FIGURE 1.85 **A** and **B**, Closing wedge technique can result in translation deformity with prominent medial malleolus (**B**).

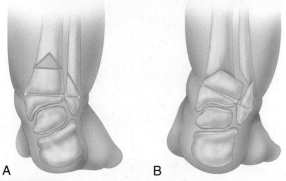

FIGURE 1.86 Wiltse varus osteotomy for valgus ankle deformity. This osteotomy corrects translation that occurs during closing wedge osteotomy. **A**, Translatory shift occurs because deformity is present in ankle joint, and osteotomy is done more proximally in metaphysis. **B**, Translating distal fragment laterally results in more natural contour of ankle. **SEE TECHNIQUE 1.30.**

Choi et al. noted that the distal tibial epiphysis in patients with fibular hemimelia often is wedge-shaped, and they found that the severity of the wedging was predictive of the severity of foot deformity after tibial lengthening. In patients with mildly wedged epiphyses (type I), varying degrees of mild growth retardation and minimal foot deformity should be anticipated; in patients with moderately wedged epiphyses (type II), worsened asymmetric growth retardation and progressive foot deformity should be expected; and in patients with severely wedged epiphyses (type III), severe growth retardation and severe foot deformities should be expected.

When the foot is to be salvaged, various reconstructive procedures have been described. For equinovalgus deformity, posterior and lateral releases are required. The Achilles tendon and the fibrocartilaginous anlage of the absent fibula must be released. In older children, ankle valgus can be corrected with a dome or varus supramalleolar osteotomy. Varus osteotomy shortens the limb but also eliminates the medial prominence associated with a simple closing wedge osteotomy (Fig. 1.85). A Wiltse osteotomy corrects the translational deformity (Fig. 1.86).

When the foot is amputated, Syme amputation is typically performed. At the time of amputation any residual bowing of the tibia can be corrected with an osteotomy, or this angular correction can be postponed to an older age. Although a Boyd

amputation offers greater length than a Syme procedure, it should be used cautiously in very young children because the Boyd amputation leaves a remnant of calcaneus that can migrate posteriorly (Fig. 1.87). Prophylactic sectioning of the Achilles tendon should be considered when amputation is performed for congenital limb deficiencies. Cruciate deficiency is common in patients with fibular hemimelia. However, the treatment of anterior cruciate ligament deficient knees remains controversial. Some authors have found good function and health status relative to age-matched controls over long-term follow-up in patients with anterior cruciate ligament deficient knees and a wide variety of fibular hemimelia severity and treatments.

Others have suggested that anterior cruciate ligament reconstruction should be considered for athletes with fibular hemimelia and anterior cruciate ligament insufficiency, with expectation of good results and function after reconstruction.

VARUS SUPRAMALLEOLAR OSTEOTOMY OF THE ANKLE

TECHNIQUE 1.30

(WILTSE)

- Make an anterior approach to the distal tibia and a lateral approach to the distal fibula.
- Create a triangular osteotomy, removing a segment of bone that can be used for bone grafting (Fig. 1.86A). Make the base of the triangle parallel to the floor, but not parallel to the ankle joint.
- Make an oblique osteotomy of the distal fibula.
- Displace the distal segments proximally and laterally to avoid excessive prominence of the medial malleolus (Fig. 1.86B).
- Fix the osteotomy with Steinmann pins and apply a long leg cast.

POSTOPERATIVE CARE Weight bearing is not allowed until the osteotomies have healed adequately.

▓ PROXIMAL FEMORAL FOCAL DEFICIENCY

Similar to many other congenital longitudinal and transverse deficiencies, proximal femoral focal deficiency (PFFD) includes a broad spectrum of defects. Mild forms result in minor hypoplasia of the femur, whereas severe involvement may result in near complete agenesis of the femur (Fig. 1.88). Most commonly, PFFD consists of a partial skeletal defect in the proximal femur with a variably unstable hip joint, shortening, and associated other anomalies. Most patients with PFFD, especially patients with bilateral involvement, have associated anomalies, the most common of which are fibular hemimelia and agenesis of the cruciate ligaments of the knee. A variety of other congenital anomalies have been reported in association with PFFD, including clubfoot, talocalcaneal coalitions, congenital heart anomalies, spinal dysplasia, and facial dysplasias.

The incidence of PFFD has been reported to be 1 per 50,000 live births. Maternal diabetes has been implicated in femoral hypoplasia.

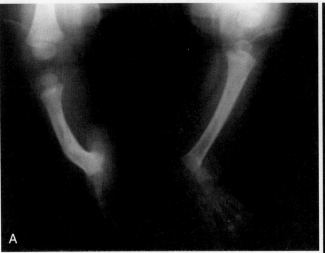

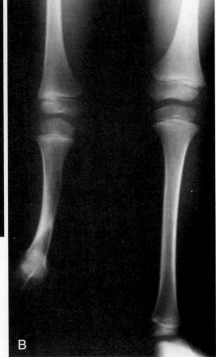

FIGURE 1.87 **A,** Bilateral type 2 deficiencies affecting right side more severely than left side—four rays on left foot and only three on right. **B,** After Boyd amputation on right and foot centralization on left. (Courtesy Robert N. Hensinger, MD.)

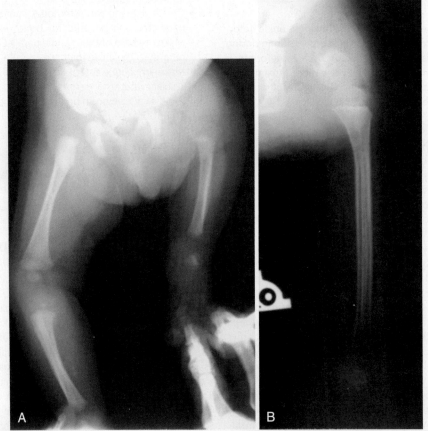

FIGURE 1.88 **A,** Infant with severe proximal femoral focal deficiency. In addition to absent femur, tibia is short and lateral ray is absent. **B,** At 5 years of age, after Boyd amputation. Distal femoral epiphysis is seen, but there is no femoral shaft or head. Acetabulum shows no sign of development. Cartilaginous anlage of distal femoral epiphysis was present at birth but not yet radiographically evident.

▌CLASSIFICATION

Aitken's four-part classification scheme (classes A, B, C, and D) is one of the earliest attempts to provide a systematic taxonomy of this condition (Table 1.4).

In class A, there is a normal acetabulum and femoral head with shortening of the femur and absence of the femoral neck on early radiographs. With age, the cartilaginous neck ossifies, although this frequently is associated with a pseudarthrosis. This may heal, but the usual radiographic picture shows severe coxa vara with significant shortening of the limb. Class B is similar to class A in that an acetabulum and femoral head are present; however, there is no bony connection between the proximal femur and the femoral head, and a pseudarthrosis is present. In class C, there is further degradation in the formation of the hip, characterized by a dysplastic acetabulum, absent femoral head, and short femur. A small, separate ossific tuft can be seen at the proximal end of the femur. In class D, the acetabulum, femoral head, and proximal femur are totally absent, and, in contrast to class C, there is no ossified tuft capping the proximal femur. Class D patients often have bilateral anomalies.

Other authors have expanded the definition of PFFD to include lesser expressions of femoral malformation. In his

TABLE 1.4				
Proximal Focal Femoral Deficiency (Aitken Classification)				
TYPE	**FEMORAL HEAD**	**ACETABULUM**	**FEMORAL SEGMENT**	**RELATIONSHIP AMONG COMPONENTS OF FEMUR AND ACETABULUM AT SKELETAL MATURITY**
A	Present	Normal	Short	Bony connection between components of femur Femoral head in acetabulum Subtrochanteric varus angulation, often with pseudarthrosis
B	Present	Adequate or moderately dysplastic	Short, usually proximal bony tuft	No osseous connection between head and shaft Femoral head in acetabulum
C	Absent or represented by ossicle	Severely dysplastic	Short, usually proximally tapered	May be osseous connection between shaft and proximal ossicle No articular relation between femur and acetabulum
D	Absent	Absent Obturator foramen enlarged Pelvis squared in bilateral cases	Short, deformed	None

Modified from Herring JA: *Tachdjian's pediatric orthopaedics*, ed 4, Philadelphia, 2014, Elsevier.

evaluation of 125 patients with PFFD, Pappas described nine classes that ranged in severity from complete absence of the proximal femur (class I) to mild femoral aplasia (class IX). The Pappas class II corresponds to the Aitken class D, the Pappas class III corresponds to the Aitken class B, and the Pappas class IV and class V may be correlated with the Aitken class A (Table 1.5). Kalamchi et al. developed a simplified classification scheme for congenital deficiency of the femur that included five groups: group I, short femur and intact hip joint; group II, short femur and coxa vara of the hip; group III, short femur, but well-developed acetabulum and femoral head; group IV, absent hip joint and dysplastic femoral segment; and group V, total absence of the femur. Group III is further subdivided into type A (bony defect of the femoral neck eventually ossifies) and type B (bony defect does not ossify and results in a persistent pseudarthrosis).

Gillespie and Torode identified two major groups for treatment purposes. Group I patients had a hypoplastic femur in which the hip and the knee were reconstructible, and leg equalization was sometimes possible. Group II patients exhibited a "true" PFFD in which the hip joint was markedly abnormal. Although some of these patients had tenuous connections between the femoral head and the proximal femur, the alignment and surrounding musculature were markedly abnormal. Also, these legs were too shortened, rotated, and marred by flexion contractures of the hip and knee to be reconstructible. These patients required only reconstructive procedures that make prosthetic fitting easier.

TREATMENT

The major problems with PFFD are limb-length inequality and variable inadequacy of the proximal femoral musculature

TABLE 1.5

Nine Pappas Classes of Congenital Abnormalities of the Femur

	CLASS I 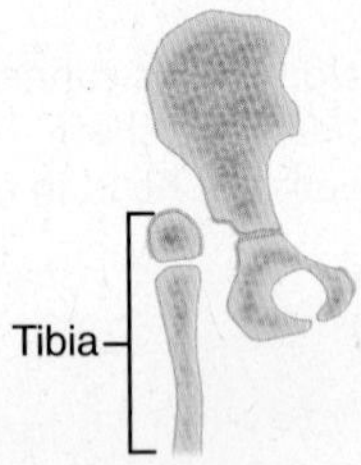	CLASS II (AITKEN D) 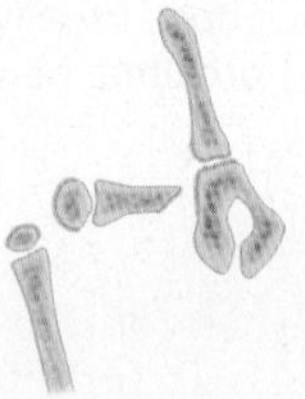	CLASS III (AITKEN B) 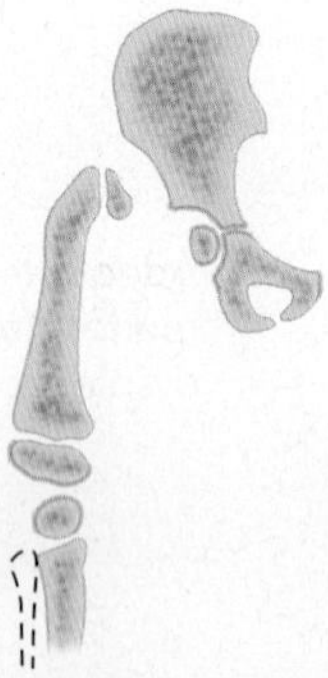	CLASS IV (AITKEN A) 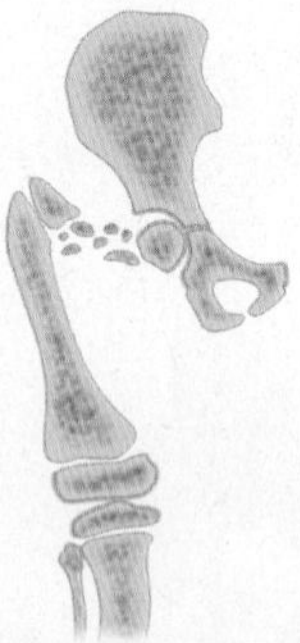
Femoral shortening (%)		70-90	45-80	40-67
Femoropelvic abnormalities	Femur absent Ischiopubic bone structures underdeveloped and deficient Lack of acetabular development	Femoral head absent Ischiopubic bone structures delayed in ossification	No osseous connection between femoral shaft and head Femoral head ossification delayed Acetabulum may be absent Femoral condyles maldeveloped Irregular tuft on proximal end of femur (rare)	Femoral head and shaft joined by irregular calcification in fibrocartilaginous matrix
Associated abnormalities	Fibula absent	Tibia shortened Fibula, foot, knee joint, and ankle joint abnormal	Tibia shortened 0%–40% Fibula shortened 5%–100% Patella absent or small and high riding Knee joint instability common Foot malformed	Tibia shortened 0%–20% Fibula shortened 4%–60% Knee joint instability frequent Foot small with infrequent malformations
Treatment objectives	Prosthetic management	Pelvic-femoral stability through prosthetic management	Union between femoral shaft and hip for stability Prosthetic management	Union between femoral head, neck, and shaft Prosthetic management

(In the illustration row, the leftmost bracket is labeled "Tibia")

From Pappas AM: Congenital abnormalities of the femur and related lower-extremity malformations: classifications and treatment, *J Pediatr Orthop* 3(1):45–60, 1983.

and hip joint. Treatment is highly individualized and ranges from amputation and prosthetic rehabilitation to limb salvage, lengthening, and hip reconstruction. The natural history of the particular variant and the limitations of surgical reconstruction must be considered.

Often no surgical reconstruction of any kind is indicated. Bilateral PFFD is best treated nonoperatively (Fig. 1.89). These patients can walk well without prostheses, but for social or cosmetic reasons extension prostheses may be provided. The patients learn to accept their short stature and are quite functional. Foot surgery may be required to correct other anomalies. Limb lengthening is not indicated in these patients because extreme lengthening would be necessary, and the hips are unstable. Knee fusion is not indicated because the knee functions in conjunction with the hip pseudarthrosis to provide useful motion.

Most children with PFFD can learn to walk without a prosthesis, but a prosthesis helps equalize leg lengths. For selected patients, prosthetic management that incorporates the patient's foot without surgical treatment can be used for PFFD, but, more commonly, this type of prosthetic management is used as a temporary solution in a younger patient until definitive surgery is performed (Fig. 1.90). An alternative approach is to use the prosthesis to mold the foot into equinus so that it fits into an above-knee amputation prosthetic socket. The socket is fashioned to include the entire femur. Later an arthrodesis can be done, if necessary, to make prosthetic fitting easier. It is possible, however, that some knee motion within the stump of the prosthesis may serve as a protective mechanism for the abnormal proximal hip. If a knee arthrodesis is performed, the potential benefits in gait and prosthetic fitting may be outweighed by the increased stress placed on the

CLASS V (AITKEN A)	CLASS VI	CLASS VII	CLASS VIII	CLASS IX
48-85	30-60	10-50	10-41	6-20
Femur incompletely ossified, hypoplastic, and irregular Midshaft of femur abnormal	Distal femur short, irregular, and hypoplastic Irregular distal femoral diaphysis	Coxa vara Hypoplastic femur Proximal femoral diaphysis irregular with thickened cortex Lateral femoral condyle deficiency common Valgus distal femur	Coxa valga Hypoplastic femur Femoral head and neck smaller Proximal femoral physis horizontal Abnormality of femoral condyles common, with associated bowing of shaft and valgus of distal femur	Hypoplastic femur
Tibia shortened 4%–27% Fibula shortened 10%–100% Knee-joint instability common Severe malformations of foot common	Single-bone lower leg Patella absent Foot malformed	Tibia shortened <10%–24% Fibula shortened <10%–100% Lateral and high-riding patella common	Tibia shortened 0%–36% Fibula shortened 0%–100% Lateral and high-riding patella common Foot malformed	Tibia shortened 0%–15% Fibula shortened 3%–30% Additional ipsilateral and contralateral malformations common
Prosthetic management	Prosthetic management	Extremity length equality Improved alignment of (a) proximal and (b) distal femur	Extremity length equality Improved alignment of (a) proximal and (b) distal femur	Extremity length equality

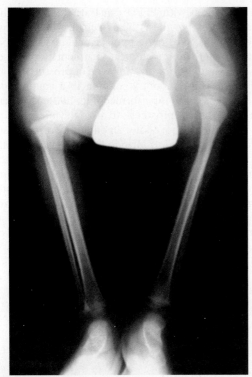

FIGURE 1.89 Severe (Aitken class D) bilateral proximal femoral focal deficiency in 3-year-old boy; note total lack of formation of acetabulum.

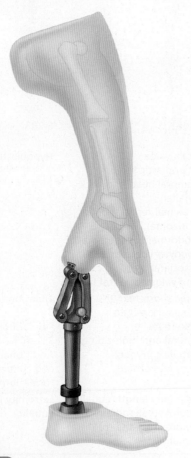

FIGURE 1.90 Prosthesis incorporating foot.

proximal femur and proximal hip articulation and pseudar-throsis, if present.

Once it is determined that surgical treatment is neces-sary, two key factors must be assessed: stability of the hip joint and percentage of limb-length inequality. For patients with a stable hip and predicted length of more than 50% of the contralateral limb, limb lengthening (as described later in this chapter) should be considered. Knee fusion and Syme ampu-tation or knee fusion and rotationplasty are indicated for patients with a stable hip and limb length less than 50% of the contralateral extremity. Finally, if the hip is unstable, stability can be achieved with a Steel or Brown fusion of the femur to the pelvis followed by Syme amputation or rotationplasty.

Stable Hip and Minimal Shortening. When there is a stable hip and relatively little shortening (<50% predicted length), salvage of the limb often is preferred. For patients with a femoral head and an acetabulum (Aitken class A and class B), many authors have recommended surgery to establish con-tinuity between the femoral head and the femur. Because of poor bone stock, surgery is best delayed until ossification of the femoral head and proximal metaphysis is adequate; even then supplemental autogenous bone grafting may be needed at the pseudarthrosis site. Although the radiographic picture may be improved with correction of the proximal pseudarthrosis, it remains to be shown that function is improved. Many patients treated nonoperatively have good motion and reasonably good function. For less severe PFFD (Pappas class VII, class VIII, and class IX), hip reconstruction is limited to osteotomies that improve biomechanical alignment. Care must be taken not to damage the proximal femoral physis in these children who already have problems with diminished growth of the femur.

Surgical limb lengthening, with or without contralateral shortening, should be considered only if the femur is intact. Ten to 12 cm has been recommended as the maximal amount of lengthening possible in a single long bone with congenital deficiency and, combined with contralateral shortening, 17 to 20 cm as the maximal amount of inequality that can be cor-rected. Limb lengthening should be done only in a femur with more than 50% of predicted femoral length or less than 20 cm of projected shortening; other prerequisites for lengthening include hip stability and a stable, plantigrade foot. Regardless of technique, limb lengthening in patients with PFFD is dif-ficult, with the ever-present danger of knee and hip subluxa-tion. For large discrepancies, lengthening can be done in stages: one at 4 or 5 years of age, a second at 8 or 9 years, and a third during adolescence. Depending on the predictions of the patient's overall height based on the normal leg, a contra-lateral epiphysiodesis may be indicated.

Limb lengthening procedures place stress on the hip and knee. Bowen et al. emphasized the importance of avoiding hip subluxation and dislocation during femoral lengthening in patients with unilateral femoral shortening. They identified several factors that predict progressive subluxation or disloca-tion of the hip during femoral lengthening: (1) type of defor-mity (Kalamchi classification), (2) the combined abnormality of coxa vara plus the varus bow of the femoral shaft, and (3) acetabular dysplasia present before lengthening. No hip abnor-malities occurred after lengthening in patients with Kalamchi type I or II deficiencies, but progressive subluxation or dislo-cation of the hip occurred in patients with type IIIA femurs with a combined coxa vara plus varus bow of the femoral shaft of less than 115 degrees and an acetabular index of more

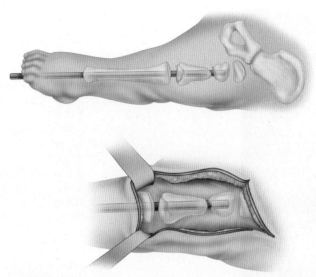

FIGURE 1.91 When proximal femur is small, with pseudarthrosis between femoral neck and shaft, it can be stabilized to create better lever arm. Simultaneous knee arthrodesis can be performed to create one-bone leg. If possible, medullary fixation should stop just short of proximal femoral epiphysis.

than 25 degrees. They recommended correction of the varus bow of the femur and the neck-shaft angle to 120 degrees and the acetabular index to less than 25 degrees before lengthening of type IIIA femurs.

Stable Hip and Severe Shortening. Knee arthrodesis (Fig. 1.91) with foot amputation, rather than limb lengthening, often is the preferred treatment for patients with severe shortening and stable hips (Figs. 1.92 and 1.93). Knee arthrodesis as described by King serves to create a single bony segment from the tibia and shortened femur to function as an above-knee amputation after foot amputation.

Unstable Hip. For more severe deformities in which the hip is unstable and there is no femoral head or acetabulum (Aitken class C and class D or Pappas class II and class III), many authors recommend that no attempt be made at hip reconstruction, although there are notable exceptions. Steel iliofemoral fusion (Fig. 1.94), which requires a simultaneous Chiari osteotomy to create a suitable bony bed to receive the small femoral remnant, allows the knee joint to assume the function of the hip joint. The femoral fragment is fused in a 90-degree flexed position relative to pelvis so that knee extension now serves as hip flexion. Additional bone graft to ensure fusion has been recommended for Steel fusions. Closing wedge osteotomies can be used to eliminate the anterior bowing of the femur and allow additional hip flexion for sitting. The Brown modification (Fig. 1.95) of the Steel fusion partially addresses this concern by rotating the femoral fragment 180 degrees. With this technique, the femoral segment is fused to the pelvis in the extended position. In this position, former knee flexion now functions as hip flexion and former ankle dorsiflexion now functions as knee flexion. Iliofemoral fusion may limit mobility of the limb. Even with a certain amount of instability, the knee generally functions as a hinge, providing flexion and extension only. Rotation and abduction are lost after iliofemoral arthrodesis.

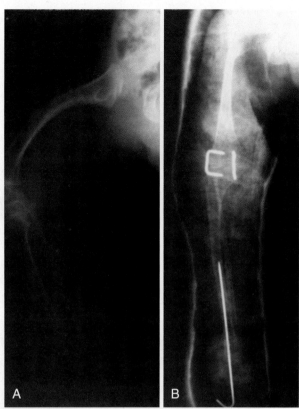

FIGURE 1.92 **A,** Proximal femoral focal deficiency in 7-year-old child; femur is severely shortened, and tibia is relatively hypoplastic. **B,** After Boyd ankle amputation, stabilization with medullary Steinmann pin, and staple arthrodesis of knee joint, patient can be rehabilitated as after knee disarticulation.

KNEE FUSION FOR PROXIMAL FEMORAL FOCAL DEFICIENCY

TECHNIQUE 1.31

(KING)

- Make an S-shaped incision to expose the distal femur and proximal tibia anteriorly.
- With an oscillating saw remove the proximal aspect of the proximal tibial epiphysis until the ossific nucleus is seen. Then remove the entire distal femoral epiphysis. The remaining tibial epiphysis and distal femoral metaphysis will be approximated and stabilized to achieve fusion.
- Insert an intramedullary rod into the proximal tibia in an antegrade fashion until it exits the plantar surface of the foot. Alternatively, the fusion can be stabilized with a plate and screws if the anatomy of the two bones will not accommodate an intramedullary implant (see Fig. 1.93).
- Completely excise the patella to prevent patellofemoral symptoms later in life.
- Next, approximate the two bony surfaces, taking care to ensure proper rotational alignment while maintaining a straight segment.

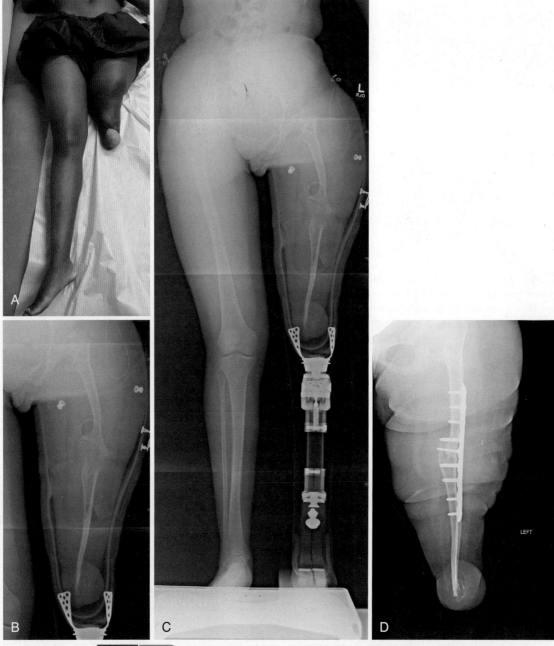

FIGURE 1.93 Proximal femoral focal deficiency treated with fusion. **SEE TECHNIQUE 1.31.**

- Advance the rod retrograde into the intramedullary canal of the femoral segment.
- Close the wound in routine manner and apply a hip spica cast.

POSTOPERATIVE CARE The spica cast and rod are removed in the operating room when bony union at the arthrodesis site is achieved, usually at 6 weeks. Amputation of the foot often is done at the time of rod removal.

For removal of the foot, ankle disarticulation, Syme amputation, or Boyd amputation can all be used. The heel pad is stabilized by either the Syme or the Boyd amputation, an advantage over simple ankle disarticulation. The Boyd amputation saves the entire calcaneus and provides a slightly more bulbous stump and additional length. If the combined length of the tibia, femoral remnant, and foot is greater than the femur on the opposite side, however, taking into account potential growth, there is no advantage in the small increase and additional length provided by the Boyd amputation.

Prosthetic reconstruction can be made easier in severe cases by a Syme amputation. The child is observed with serial scanograms until sufficient data have been collected to construct a working Moseley straight-line graph; then further surgery can be planned. If knee arthrodesis is selected to improve fitting of a prosthesis and gait, the physes around the knee can be epiphysiodesed if necessary to ensure that the prosthetic knee is at the same level as the contralateral normal knee when the child reaches skeletal maturity. Precise predictions

Anteroposterior view   **Lateral view**

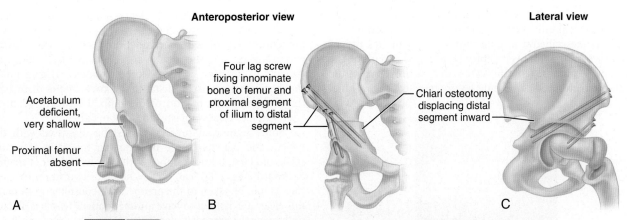

Acetabulum deficient, very shallow

Proximal femur absent

Four lag screw fixing innominate bone to femur and proximal segment of ilium to distal segment

Chiari osteotomy displacing distal segment inward

A   B   C

FIGURE 1.94   Steel iliofemoral fusion. **A,** Proximal femur is absent. **B,** The femur has been shortened to just above the distal physis and rotated 180 degrees so that popliteal fossa now faces anteriorly. A Chiari pelvic osteotomy has been fixed with two screws; this is optional depending on bony contact of the femur to the pelvis. The femur is fixed to the pelvis with several screws. **C,** Lateral view of the final position of the femur. It is important that the femur be shortened as much as possible and that the femoral epiphysis be ablated.

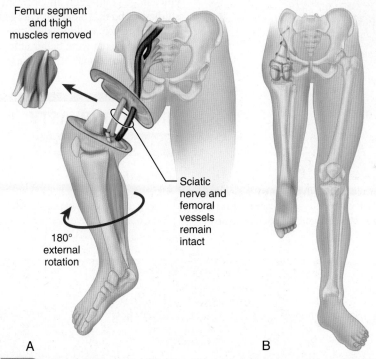

Femur segment and thigh muscles removed

Sciatic nerve and femoral vessels remain intact

180° external rotation

A   B

FIGURE 1.95   Rotationplasty and femoropelvic arthrodesis (see text). **A,** Proximal part of femur (with hypoplastic head) and surrounding thigh muscles are removed, and leg is rotated 180 degrees. **B,** Limb is rotated, and residual femur is attached to pelvis.

are unnecessary because small amounts of additional shortening in the involved leg can be readily accommodated by the prosthesis. If the involved femorotibial unit is longer than the contralateral normal femur, however, the prosthetic knee must be placed in either a very proximal or a very distal position, which is less cosmetically desirable (Fig. 1.96). Although this can be treated with a leg-shortening procedure at skeletal maturity, a simpler preventive procedure, such as a well-timed epiphysiodesis during the growing years, is preferable.

Rotationplasty. Rotationplasty (Van Nes procedure) can be used as an alternative to knee arthrodesis and amputation. This reconstruction should be considered in patients who,

because of significant femoral shortening, are not candidates for femoral lengthening. The procedure combines arthrodesis of the knee with rotation of the distal tibia 180 degrees externally so that the ankle joint becomes a functional knee joint: ankle plantarflexion becomes "knee" extension, and ankle dorsiflexion becomes "knee" flexion. A reasonably stable hip joint and a well-functioning ankle are required for this technique. Many patients with PFFD also have fibular hemimelia, with a poorly functioning ankle joint. An arc or ankle motion of at least 90 degrees is required for rotationplasty reconstruction to be beneficial. The femur, knee, and tibia should equal the length of the opposite femur, but this usually is not the case, so ipsilateral knee epiphysiodesis is done to equalize the reconstructed femoral unit and the contralateral normal femur.

Brown described a modification of the Van Nes procedure in which the limb is completely detached except for the sciatic nerve and the femoral vessels, the proximal part of the dysplastic femur and some muscles are resected, the residual

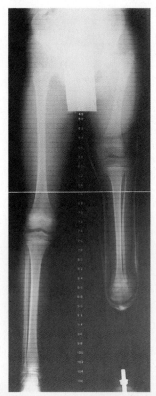

FIGURE 1.96 Twelve-year-old child with previous Boyd amputation but no knee arthrodesis. Prosthetic management is that of below-knee amputation, but result is cosmetically poor because of extremely long "tibia."

limb is externally rotated 180 degrees, and the rotated distal part of the femur is fused to the pelvis (see Fig. 1.95). With this procedure, the rotated knee functions as a hip with flexion and extension, and the rotated ankle acts as a knee, allowing patients to function as below-knee amputees. Brown noted that because the muscles distal to the knee are not disturbed, the problem of derotation of the limb, a frequent problem after Van Nes rotationplasty, does not occur.

Some significant problems must be discussed with the patient and parents before undertaking this type of reconstruction. First, the appearance of the leg, with the foot rotated backward (Fig. 1.97), can be psychologically disturbing; great care should be taken in the preoperative consultation to make this clear. It is helpful to have another patient who has already undergone the procedure demonstrate how the prosthesis functions. If such a patient is unavailable, the family should be shown photographs and drawings of a rotationplasty. Another problem, especially in young children, is derotation of the surgically rotated foot, which has been reported to occur in as many as 50% of patients. Compared with a Syme amputation, rotationplasty has been shown to result in a slightly more (10%) energy-efficient gait, although an electromyographic and gait analysis study showed that older patients generally had lower functional scores, shorter walking distances, and worse gait patterns. Younger patients were better able to adapt to the altered anatomic and functional situation and to develop good function.

ROTATIONPLASTY

TECHNIQUE 1.32   *Figure 1.98*

(VAN NES)
- Position the patient supine and drape the entire limb free so that the skin is exposed from the toes to the iliac crest. Place a small towel under the sacrum.

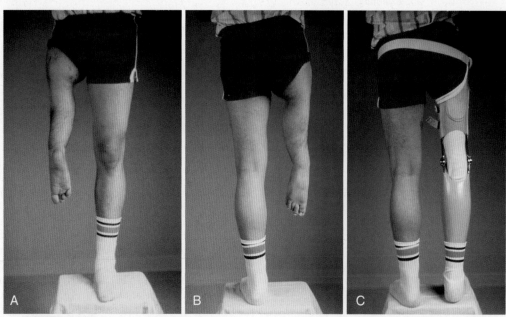

FIGURE 1.97 Appearance of limb after Van Nes rotationplasty: front view (**A**), back view (**B**), and with prosthesis (**C**).

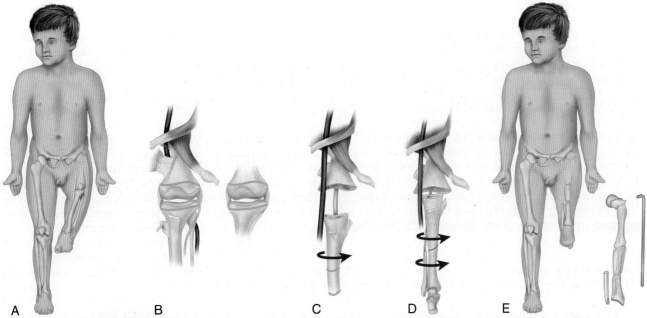

FIGURE 1.98 Van Nes rotationplasty. Preoperatively, ankle joint of shortened extremity is approximately at level of opposite knee joint. **A,** Long incision on lateral aspect of leg extends from hip to midshaft of tibia. **B,** Quadriceps and sartorius tendons are taken down distally to expose adductor hiatus and femoral artery; peroneal nerve is dissected free. **C,** After resection of knee joint and freeing of femoropopliteal artery, tibia is externally rotated 140 degrees. **D,** Further rotation of 40 degrees more is possible after tibial osteotomy, allowing stretch on soft tissues to spread over greater distance. External rotation is preferred to internal rotation to prevent stretching of peroneal nerve. **E,** Fixation with medullary Rush rod. **SEE TECHNIQUE 1.32.**

- Begin the incision proximal and lateral to the knee and extend it across the knee distally along the subcutaneous crest of the tibia.
- Elevate the flaps medially and laterally to expose the knee capsule and patellar tendon.
- Divide the patellar tendon and open the knee capsule transversely.
- Apply traction on the capsule proximally and distally to expose the knee joint fully by dividing the collateral ligaments and the anterior, medial, and lateral capsule.
- On the medial side, carefully dissect out the insertion of the adductor magnus up to the level of the femoral artery.
- Divide the adductor magnus to enable the artery to derotate anteriorly and to limit postoperative derotation.
- Trace the femoral artery distally and posteriorly as it becomes the popliteal artery.
- Divide the medial hamstring muscles at their insertion.
- On the lateral side, carefully dissect out the peroneal nerve. If the fibula is deficient, the anatomic relationship between the peroneal nerve and the proximal fibular head may be abnormal. To prevent damage to the peroneal nerve, trace the nerve proximally to its point of origin on the sciatic nerve. Release any fascial attachments distally over the peroneal nerve.
- After the major neurovascular structures have been completely identified and protected, divide the posterior knee capsule, and section the origins of the gastrocnemius heads.

- The only remaining attachments from the femur to the tibia are the skin, subcutaneous tissues, and neurovascular structures. Release the lateral hamstrings.
- With an osteotome or oscillating saw, remove the articular cartilage of the proximal tibia down to the level of the proximal tibial epiphysis. Do not damage the proximal tibial physis.
- If the leg needs to be shortened, shorten the femur by removing the distal femoral epiphysis and physis.
- Insert an intramedullary Rush rod through the distal femur proximally, exiting through the piriformis fossa into the buttock. If necessary, ream the femur with a drill to prevent comminution during nail insertion.
- Make a small incision in the buttock where the nail exits.
- Remove the nail and reinsert it from proximal to distal through the femur and into the tibia, stopping short of the distal tibial physis. While the nail is being inserted, rotate the tibia externally to relax the peroneal nerve.
- Gently transfer the femoral popliteal artery anteriorly through the adductor hiatus.
- If the leg cannot be comfortably rotated through the knee resection, obtain additional rotation through a separate osteotomy in the midshaft of the tibia, which also is stabilized by the intramedullary nail.
- Additional shortening can be performed through the tibia if necessary. In such instances, a fibular osteotomy also is performed.

- Attempt to rotate the extremity 180 degrees. If the rotation places too much torque on the vascular structures, and the distal pulses are lost, derotate the leg through the knee until the pressure on the vessels is relieved.
- Close the wounds and apply a spica cast that maintains rotation.

POSTOPERATIVE CARE If derotation of the foot was required to relieve vascular pressure, the foot is rotated serially using successive hip spica casts to turn the foot on the axis of the intramedullary nail. When the osteotomies have healed, the child is fitted with a modified below-knee prosthesis. Although it is possible to amputate the toes to make the foot look more like a below-knee stump and less like a "backward" foot, most patients decline this option.

Amputations. Although most of the basic surgical principles of amputation in adults apply to children, there are important differences. Most amputations in children are performed for congenital conditions. Either the child is born without a portion of the limb, or an amputation is performed to make reconstruction and prosthetic rehabilitation easier in a deficient limb. Trauma accounts for most acquired amputations in children. In contrast to typical adult dysvascular patients, children may tolerate skin grafts over stumps and, to a certain extent, tension at the suture line. Most revision surgeries in children with congenital amputations involve the lower extremity. Revision amputation surgery in upper extremity limb deficiencies rarely is required.

Prosthetic fitting after amputation in children should begin after complete wound healing and standard stump preparation. A rigid postoperative plaster dressing that is bivalved to allow for swelling is preferred. When the wounds are sufficiently healed, stump wrapping with elastic bandages is begun to prepare the stump for a prosthesis. Phantom pain and phantom sensations are problems in child amputees, especially after tumor surgery. Neuroma formation is rare, but gentle handling of the nerves and sectioning with a sharp knife without applying excessive traction on the nerves should be routine in all amputation surgery in children.

In planning amputation surgery, maximal length should be preserved to provide maximal lever arm strength for powering a prosthesis. Physes should be preserved whenever possible to ensure continued growth of the limb. This is especially true for the physes around the knee, which provide most of the growth in the lower extremity, and the physes around the shoulder and wrist, which provide most of the longitudinal growth of the upper extremity. Although amputation through a long bone in a growing child can result in appositional terminal overgrowth, this is not an adequate reason for sacrificing length. In below-knee amputations in young children, it is highly likely that the fibula, and to a lesser extent the tibia, will overgrow, but this can be satisfactorily remedied by revision surgery. Although knee disarticulation would prevent overgrowth, it is far more important to preserve the knee joint to power a below-knee prosthesis than to prevent overgrowth of the stump. Even short below-knee segments should be preserved if possible in growing children. Because the proximal tibial physis contributes most of the growth of the tibia, an initially short stump has the potential to become a longer,

more functional stump. In older children, it is possible to lengthen a short below-knee stump using the Ilizarov technique to provide a more functional stump in selected patients. Involving the prosthetist in the decision-making process can be helpful in making the decision between knee disarticulation and preservation of a very short proximal tibia.

Terminal overgrowth has been reported most frequently in the humerus, followed by the fibula, tibia, and femur. Because it seems to be caused by appositional periosteal bone formation distally and not by epiphyseal growth proximally (Fig. 1.99), epiphysiodesis does not prevent stump overgrowth. A variety of techniques have been devised to prevent stump overgrowth, but none has been completely successful. Small bone spurs that form at the edge of the transected bone do not constitute true overgrowth and rarely require surgical removal. Stump overgrowth occurs in congenital and traumatic amputations.

Patellar dislocations and patella alta are common problems in adolescents with below-knee amputations, presumably caused by the force of the patellar tendon-bearing prosthesis against the lower surface of the patella. Elongation of the patellar tendon might be prevented by earlier modification of the prosthesis to distribute the force around a greater area rather than concentrating it on the patellar tendon.

Ankle Disarticulation. Although standard amputation techniques are described in other chapter, important variations of amputations around the ankle exist for reconstruction in children with congenital limb deficiencies. The two most common reconstructive amputations performed for these children are the Syme and Boyd procedures. The Syme amputation is a modified ankle disarticulation. The Boyd procedure amputates all of the foot bones except the calcaneus and fuses the calcaneus to the distal tibia.

Many studies have documented excellent results with both procedures, and there are pros and cons to each. There is no clear consensus in the literature regarding the preferred technique. The problems encountered in Syme amputations in children have been overgrowth of retained portions of calcaneal apophyses, heel pad migration, and formation of exostoses. The advantages of the Boyd operation are the additional length gained and the prevention of the posterior displacement of the heel pad, which occurs in many patients with Syme amputations. In the Boyd amputation, it is important to align the calcaneus properly. If the calcaneus is not aligned correctly, it angulates into equinus and interferes with weight bearing.

A problem common to the Syme and the Boyd amputations is the flare of the distal tibial metaphysis, which gives a bulbous shape to the distal stump and necessitates a special prosthesis with a removable medial window. In children with congenital limb deficiencies, such as tibial or fibular hemimelia, the distal ankle is relatively hypoplastic, however, so a bulbous stump usually is not a problem.

SYME AMPUTATION

TECHNIQUE 1.33

- Make a fish-mouth incision beginning at the lateral malleolus, extending over the dorsum of the foot, and ending 1 cm distal to the medial malleolus (Fig. 1.100A). The

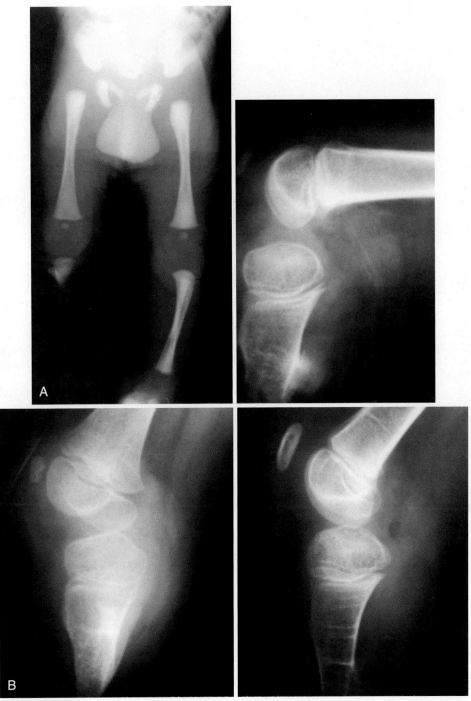

FIGURE **1.99**   **A,** Newborn with congenital amputation through proximal tibia. **B,** At 5 years of age, continued growth of distal stump and penciling resulted in protrusion of bone from skin. (Courtesy Robert N. Hensinger, MD.)

plantar portion should extend distally enough to allow adequate skin closure anteriorly.

- Place the foot in as much equinus as possible to expose the anterior ankle capsule and divide it.
- Divide the deltoid ligament between the talus and the medial malleolus, but do not damage the nearby posterior tibial vessels.
- Section the lateral ligament between the calcaneus and the fibula.

- Grasp the talus with a large clamp and force it further into equinus to permit dissection of the posterior ankle capsule.
- Make a subperiosteal dissection of the posterior aspect of the calcaneus through the ankle joint.
- Cut the Achilles tendon at its point of insertion into the calcaneus, but do not "button hole" it through the skin.
- Place further traction on the hindfoot and further hyperflexion into equinus and dissect the soft tissues with a

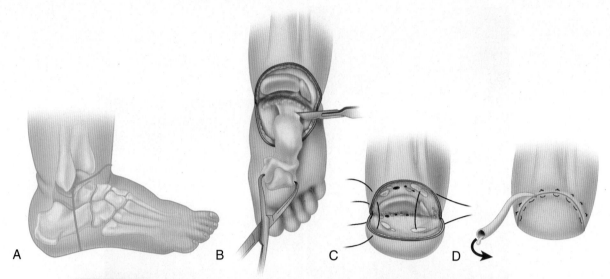

A **B** **C** **D**

FIGURE 1.100 Syme amputation. **A,** Fish-mouth incision. **B,** Enucleation of talus and calcaneus. **C,** Plantar flap sutured to distal tibia. **D,** Completed closure with drain in place. **SEE TECHNIQUE 1.32.**

periosteal elevator and a knife, staying in the subperiosteal plane to avoid damaging the heel pad.

- Continue the dissection until the entire calcaneus has been excised (Fig. 1.100B).
- To anchor the heel pad, drill holes in the anterior aspect of the distal tibia and use stout sutures from the distal aspect of the heel pad, anchoring it in the aponeurosis of the distal tibia (Fig. 1.100C).
- In children, it is unnecessary to remove the cartilage of the distal tibia, but if desired the flare of the medial malleolus and distal fibula can be trimmed to create a more even weight-bearing surface.
- Pull the flexor tendons distally, transect them, and allow them to retract.
- Ligate the posterior and anterior tibial arteries as far distally as possible to prevent ischemic necrosis of the flaps.
- Insert suction drains in the wound and close the skin in layers (Fig. 1.100D).
- Apply a rigid plaster dressing to diminish pain after surgery; bivalve the cast to allow for swelling.

POSTOPERATIVE CARE Weight bearing on the stump in a cast is delayed until the wound has healed adequately.

BOYD AMPUTATION

TECHNIQUE 1.34

- Make a fish-mouth incision as described for the Syme amputation.
- Elevate the skin flaps proximally and amputate the forefoot through the midtarsal joints.
- Excise the entire talus, using sharp dissection.
- With an oscillating saw or osteotome, transect the distal end of the calcaneus (Fig. 1.101A).

- In a similar manner, remove the articular surface of the subtalar joint on the calcaneus perpendicular to the long axis of the tibia.
- Resect an adequate amount of the distal tibial articular cartilage so that the bony epiphysis of the distal tibia is exposed (Fig. 1.101B).
- Shape the calcaneus to fit accurately against the surface of the distal tibial epiphysis. Stabilize this with a smooth Steinmann pin that enters the heel pad and provides fixation to the tibia by crossing the distal tibial physis into the metaphysis.
- Occasionally, the Achilles tendon must be severed to allow accurate positioning of the calcaneus.
- Shift the calcaneus anteriorly before fixing it with the Steinmann pin (Fig. 1.101C).
- Section the medial and lateral plantar nerves and allow them to retract.
- Section the posterior and anterior tibial arteries as far distally as possible to prevent wound necrosis.
- Close the wound over drains and apply a plaster cast. A hip spica cast may be necessary for young children.

POSTOPERATIVE CARE The pin usually can be removed at 6 weeks, and a new cast is applied and worn for an additional 6 weeks. After this, the stump usually has healed sufficiently for prosthetic rehabilitation.

LIMB-LENGTH DISCREPANCY

Limb-length equality in the lower extremity is not only a cosmetic concern, but also a functional concern. The short leg gait is awkward, increases energy expenditure because of the excessive vertical rise and fall of the pelvis or compensatory ankle movements and may result in back pain from long-standing significant discrepancies. Compensatory scoliosis and decreased spinal mobility also have been reported with discrepancies of 1.2 to 5.2 cm; however, it

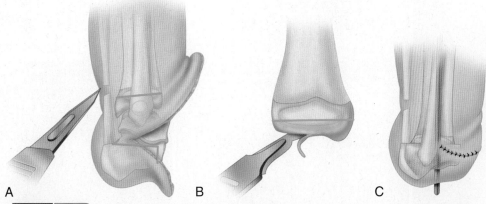

FIGURE 1.101 Boyd amputation. **A,** Fish-mouth incision; shaded areas represent resected bone. **B,** Cartilage of distal tibia is removed by shaving gradually until bony epiphysis is reached; calcaneus is shifted anteriorly, and Achilles tendon is sectioned to prevent it from migrating proximally. **C,** Fixation with smooth medullary pin aids fusion of calcaneus to distal tibial epiphysis. **SEE TECHNIQUE 1.34.**

should be noted that limb-length inequalities of 0.5 to 2 cm are common in the normal, asymptomatic population.

Limb-length inequality of more than 2.5 cm has traditionally been considered significant, with an increased likelihood of knee, hip, and lumbar spine pain; however, support for this exact value is lacking in the literature. The management of a patient with limb-length inequality is quite complex, and multiple factors including cause of the discrepancy, associated conditions, pain, and patient/family expectations must be taken into account along with the measured difference before treatment is undertaken.

Limb-length inequality may be acquired and result from trauma or infection that damages the physis, from asymmetric paralytic conditions (e.g., poliomyelitis or cerebral palsy), or from tumors or tumor-like conditions that affect bone growth by stimulating asymmetric growth, such as occurs with juvenile rheumatoid arthritis or postfracture hypervascularity. Idiopathic unilateral hypoplasia and hyperplasia are other common causes of limb-length discrepancy. Finally, congenital conditions such as femoral or fibular deficiency or tibial hemimelia can cause the inequality.

The treatment of limb-length discrepancy must be tailored to the specific conditions and needs of the individual patient. Treatment plans can be formulated only after a careful evaluation that includes assessment of the chronologic and skeletal ages of the patient, the current and predicted discrepancy in the limb lengths, the predicted adult height, the cause of the discrepancy, the functional status of the joints, and the social and psychologic background of the patient and family.

■ CLINICAL ASSESSMENT

Clinical evaluation should include assessment for any rotational and angular deformities, foot height differences, scoliosis, pelvic obliquity, and joint mobility and function. In certain paralytic conditions, particularly spastic diplegia, flexion contractures of the knee and hip make the limb appear shorter than it really is on clinical and radiographic examinations; however, mild shortness of the paralytic side can improve gait by allowing the paralytic foot to clear the floor more easily during the swing phase of gait.

The simplest means of measuring limb-length discrepancy is to place wooden blocks of known heights under the short leg until the pelvis is level (Fig. 1.102); however, asymmetric pelvic development or pelvic obliquity can cause miscalculation. Measurement also can be made from the anterior superior iliac spine to the medial malleolus, but this measurement may not be accurate because of patient positioning. Supine and prone Galeazzi measurements can help to localize the discrepancy to the femoral or tibial segment respectively.

■ RADIOGRAPHIC ASSESSMENT

Radiographic measurements are an essential part of the evaluation of limb-length inequality, and they are important for accuracy because clinically palpable landmarks may be inaccurate. Two traditional, commonly-used radiographic techniques for measuring lower limb-length discrepancy are the standing orthoradiograph and the scanogram. The orthoradiograph is made on a long cassette that includes the hip, knee, and ankle on a single exposure. A magnification marker placed on the leg at the level of the bone minimizes magnification error. The scanogram uses separate exposures of the hip, knee, and ankle, so there is little parallax error (Figs. 1.103 and 1.104).

However, it does require that the child remain still for all three exposures. Although the parallax error is greater with standing orthoradiographs, they do offer the additional benefit of showing limb alignment, as well as reducing the exposure to ionizing radiation. With either study, it is imperative that the legs be positioned with the patellae facing forward. Skeletal age is an important factor to include when making treatment decisions. A view of the left wrist is obtained to estimate skeletal age from the Greulich and Pyle atlas; however, this is unnecessary for children younger than 5 years old because the skeletal and chronologic ages are not significantly different in these children. Although the use of the Greulich and Pyle atlas is an important part of the overall assessment of skeletal age, it should be noted that the standard deviation for this atlas is one page either way.

CT scanograms have been proposed as an improvement over standard scanograms because the radiation exposure is

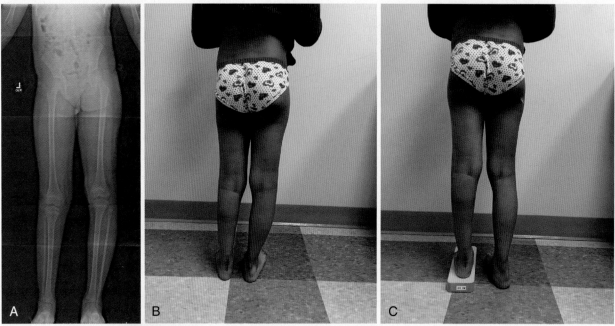

FIGURE 1.102 Block test for evaluation of limb length discrepancy.

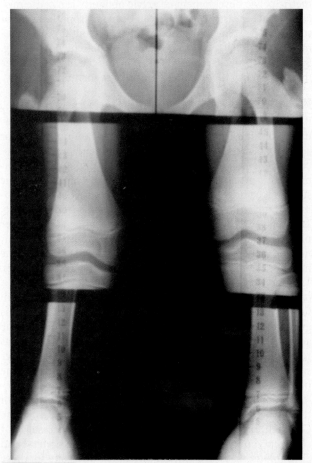

FIGURE 1.103 Scanogram obtained for evaluation of limb-length discrepancy in 12-year-old boy with fibular hemimelia on right.

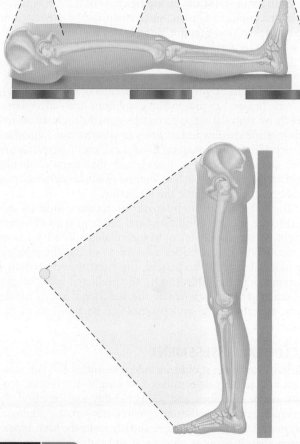

FIGURE 1.104 Scanogram compared with standing orthoradiograph.

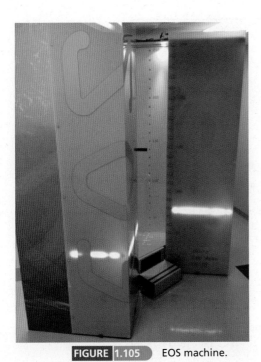

FIGURE 1.105 EOS machine.

less, and accuracy is not compromised. On lateral CT scanograms, accurate measurement can be made of even a limb with a flexion deformity. On biplanar CT scanograms, foot height also can be measured. EOS slot scanning technology (EOS Imaging, Paris, France) offers an alternative in some centers (Fig. 1.105). Benefits include simultaneously obtained biplanar, upright images of the entire length of both lower extremities with little to no magnification error, and lower radiation exposure. To avoid motion artifact, the child must remain still throughout the short scan time. This technology has been shown to provide greater accuracy and reliability over more traditional imaging modalities.

■ TECHNIQUES FOR PREDICTING GROWTH REMAINING

Multiple techniques are used to predict growth and to help the surgeon determine the timing of limb equalization procedures. One is the Green-Anderson growth-remaining chart. Proper use of this chart requires the clinician to estimate the percentage of growth inhibition for the patient by taking two interval measurements separated by at least 3 months. The growth difference between the involved limb and the normal limb is multiplied by 100, and that result is divided by the growth of the normal limb. Moseley simplified the Green-Anderson chart by mathematically manipulating the original data to allow it to fit on a straight-line graph that is visually graphic and easier to apply (Fig. 1.106). It avoids the need for mathematical calculations of growth inhibition and provides a ready prediction of the results of epiphysiodesis, lengthening, and shortening (Box 1.1). Reference slopes are provided for predicting future limb growth after epiphysiodesis of the distal femur, the proximal tibia, or both. The difference between the slopes of the normal leg and the short leg is the growth inhibition. Lengthening of the short leg in a growing child can be depicted by a sharp vertical rise, followed by a continued gradual slope equivalent to the slope of growth before lengthening (Fig. 1.107).

One criticism of the Green-Anderson tables and the Moseley straight-line graph for limb-length discrepancy is that they do not include an estimation for foot height. A discrepancy of 4 cm by radiographic scanograms may be 5 cm by the clinical block technique if the short leg also has a small foot and ankle unit.

There are some fundamental problems with the Green-Anderson and the Moseley methods. The original data for growth and height may not be applicable to modern children. The skeletal age according to Greulich and Pyle's atlas is at best an approximation. Human growth is not always mathematically predictable because it is influenced by nutritional, metabolic, hormonal, and socioeconomic factors as well as the cause of the leg-length discrepancy. Limb-length discrepancy in some children with juvenile rheumatoid arthritis and Perthes disease may follow an upward slope/downward slope pattern in which the discrepancy corrects itself. In overgrowth after a femoral fracture, the pattern of growth may level off, and after a short period the discrepancy remains constant. Despite these atypical patterns, most leg-length discrepancies follow the traditional growth prediction curves.

Simpler methods of predicting growth are available. The Menelaus method is convenient because it requires no special charts or graphs and relies on chronologic age rather than skeletal age. Menelaus assumes that in adolescents older than 9 years of age, the distal femur grows ⅜ inch (9 mm) per year, the proximal tibia grows ¼ inch (6 mm) per year, and growth ceases at age 14 years in girls and at age 16 years in boys. Using his technique, Menelaus achieved a final limb-length discrepancy of less than ¾ inch in 94 patients who underwent epiphysiodesis.

Paley, Bhave, Herzenberg, and Bowen developed a "multiplier" method for predicting limb-length discrepancy at skeletal maturity. Using available databases, they divided femoral and tibial lengths at skeletal maturity (L_m) by femoral and tibial lengths (L) at each age for each percentile group. The resultant number was called the multiplier (M). This multiplier is used in formulas to predict limb-length discrepancy and the amount of growth remaining and to calculate the timing of epiphysiodesis. According to these authors, the multiplier method allows for a quick calculation of predicted limb-length discrepancy at skeletal maturity, without the need to plot graphs, and is based on one or two measurements. A simple chart of multipliers and several formulas are all that is required (Table 1.6).

The multiplier method can be applied to total limb-length discrepancy, including femoral, tibial, and foot-height differences. Clinical data in their study confirmed that the multiplier method correlated closely with the Moseley method. Smartphone applications are now available that can quickly and reliably provide treatment recommendations based on the multiplier method. The surgeon must understand the underlying assumptions of the multiplier method before relying completely on the application.

In a group of patients with limb lengthenings, there was no difference in the accuracy of the two methods; in a group with epiphysiodeses, the multiplier method was more accurate. In two later clinical validation studies, Aguilar et al. showed the multiplier method to be more accurate than the Moseley and Anderson methods; the multiplier method also was quicker and simpler to use, requiring only one data point for predicting limb length at maturity. No matter the method used, all are, at best, approximations. A final clinical

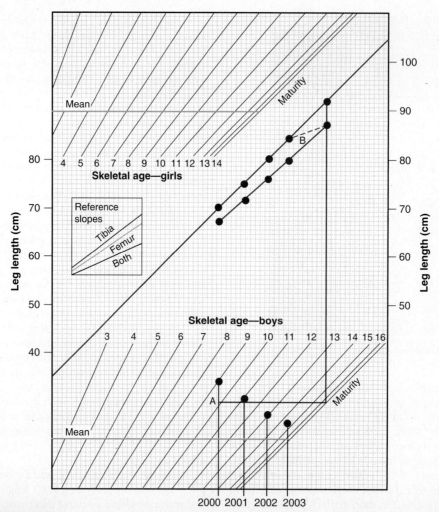

FIGURE 1.106 Moseley straight-line graph. Example shown is boy with idiopathic hemiatrophy observed clinically for 4 consecutive years. In 2000, longer leg measured 70 cm, shorter leg was 67 cm, and bone age was 9 years. Additional scanograms and bone age radiographs are plotted as shown. Horizontal straight line *(A)* extends to maturity line with equal number of skeletal ages above and below line. At skeletal maturity, longer leg is projected to measure 92 cm, and shorter leg is projected to measure 87 cm. Broken line *(B)* represents projected growth of longer leg if epiphysiodeses of distal femur and proximal tibia are performed when longer leg reaches 84 cm in length, obtaining limb equalization by skeletal maturity.

discrepancy of 1 to 1.5 cm after treatment should be considered an excellent outcome.

■ TREATMENT

The goals of treatment are a balanced spine and pelvis, equal limb lengths, and a correct mechanical weight-bearing axis. In patients with rigid scoliosis and an oblique lumbosacral take-off, some degree of limb-length discrepancy may be desirable to preserve a balanced spine. By convention, the term epiphysiodesis is used to describe the arrest of growth of a particular physis. It should be noted that physeal, rather than epiphyseal, growth is halted through this process, and the term physiodesis might be a more accurate term. Nevertheless, in keeping with convention, epiphysiodesis is used through the remainder of the chapter when discussing cessation of physeal growth.

Four types of treatment are available for limb-length equalization: shoe lift or prosthetic conversion, epiphysiodesis of the long leg, shortening of the long leg (in patients too old for epiphysiodesis), and lengthening of the short leg. Judicious combinations of ipsilateral lengthening and contralateral epiphysiodesis can be used for significant discrepancies to reduce the amount of lengthening required.

For small discrepancies of 1.5 cm or less, no treatment is necessary. If a patient desires, a 1-cm shoe lift can be provided to wear inside the shoe. The lift need not compensate for the entire discrepancy because people rarely stand erect with both knees and hips straight, and many people have small (1 cm) differences that are functionally insignificant. The degree of discrepancy that can be compensated for with an internal shoe lift is limited, however, and for differences of 2 to 4 cm, a lift on the outside of the shoe is necessary. For small discrepancies, a heel lift can be used, and for larger differences, a full-sole lift is needed (Fig. 1.108). A shoe lift can be used for large discrepancies if the patient declines shortening or lengthening. Lifts of 5 to 10 cm are unsightly and unstable, however, and may require additional uprights or an ankle-foot orthosis to help support the ankle.

BOX 1.1

Instructions for Using Moseley Straight-Line Graph for Leg-Length Inequality

Depiction of Past Growth
- At each office visit, obtain three values:
  - Length of the normal leg measured by orthoradiograph from the most superior part of the femoral head to the middle of the articular surface of the tibia at the ankle
  - Length of the short leg
  - Radiographic estimate of skeletal age
- Place the point for the normal leg on the normal leg line of the appropriate length.
- Draw a vertical line through that point the entire height of the graph and through the skeletal age "scalar" area of either boys or girls; this line represents the current skeletal age.
- Place the point for the short leg on the current skeletal age line of the correct length.
- Mark the point where the current skeletal age line intersects that sloping "scalar" in the skeletal age area that corresponds to the radiographic estimate of skeletal age.
- Plot successive sets of three points in the same fashion.
- Draw the straight line that best fits the points plotted previously for successive lengths of the short leg.
- *Discrepancy* is represented by the vertical distance between two growth lines.
- *Inhibition* is represented by the difference in the slope between the two growth lines, taking the slope of the normal leg as 100.

Prediction of Future Growth
- Extend to the right growth line of the short leg.
- Draw the horizontal straight line that best fits the points plotted previously in the skeletal age area.
- *Growth percentile* is represented by the position of that horizontal line and indicates whether the child is taller or shorter than the mean.
- *Skeletal age scale* is represented by the intersections of this horizontal line with the scalars in the skeletal age area. The maturity point is the intersection of the line with the maturity scale.
- Draw a vertical line through the maturity point. This line represents maturity and the cessation of growth. Its intersection with the growth lines of the two legs represents their anticipated lengths at maturity.
- In keeping a child's graph up to date, it is recommended that these lines be drawn in pencil. The addition of further data

makes this method more accurate and may require slight changes in the positions of these lines.

Effects of Surgery
Epiphysiodesis
- Ascertain the length of the normal leg just before surgery, and mark that point on the normal leg line.
- From that point, draw a line parallel to the reference point for the particular physis fused. This is the new growth line for the normal leg (contribution of physes to total growth of leg: distal femur, 37%; proximal tibia, 28%; both, 65%).
- The percentage decrease in slope of the new growth line (taking the previous slope as 100%) exactly represents the loss of the contribution of the fused physis or physes.

Lengthening
- Draw the growth line for the lengthened leg exactly parallel to the previous growth line but displaced upward by a distance exactly equal to the length increase achieved. Because the physes are not affected, the growth rate is not affected and thus the slope of the line is unchanged.

Timing of Surgery
Epiphysiodesis
- Project the growth line of the short leg to intersect the maturity line, taking into account the effect of a lengthening procedure if necessary.
- From the intersection with the maturity line, draw a line whose slope is equal to the reference slope for the proposed surgery.
- The point at which this line meets the growth line of the normal leg indicates the point at which surgery should be done. This point is defined not in terms of the calendar but in terms of the length of the normal leg.

Lengthening
- Because lengthening procedures do not affect the rate of growth, the timing of this procedure is not critical and is governed by clinical considerations.

Postoperative Follow-Up
- Draw the new growth line of the normal leg as explained under Effects of Surgery.
- Data are plotted exactly as before except that the length of the short leg is plotted first and is placed on the growth line previously established for the short leg.

Many children reject shoe lifts on reaching adolescence, preferring instead to walk with compensatory mechanisms, including ankle equinus, pelvic tilt, and contralateral knee flexion. Nevertheless, shoe lifts often are beneficial in this age group as a trial to allow the patient to assess the potential benefits of a proposed surgical option. Extension prostheses are "modified shoe lifts" in that the foot is not amputated. Instead, the foot is forced into an equinus position and is fitted into a custom prosthesis that has a prosthetic foot distal to the natural foot (Fig. 1.90). Conversion with a Syme or Boyd amputation is preferred, however, to make prosthetic fitting easier.

OPERATIVE TREATMENT
Theoretically, lengthening of the short limb is the optimal treatment, but technical difficulty and frequent complications of lengthening procedures have made epiphysiodesis a more attractive option for small discrepancies. For growing children, epiphysiodesis is a relatively simple procedure with reasonably low morbidity and fast recovery. In adolescents too old for effective epiphysiodesis, limb shortening is accurate, safe, and simple, with a complication rate only slightly higher than epiphysiodesis. Joint stiffness after shortening is rare because the muscles are made slack by shortening of the limb, in contrast to lengthening, which frequently results in permanent joint stiffness and subluxation.

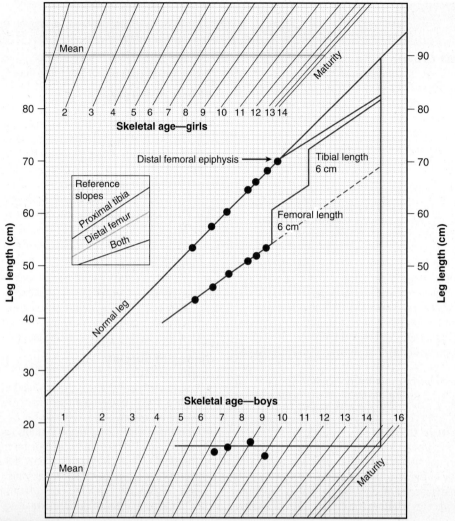

FIGURE 1.107 Moseley graph of patient with congenitally short femur and fibular hemimelia shows plan of femoral lengthening, tibial lengthening, and distal femoral epiphysiodesis.

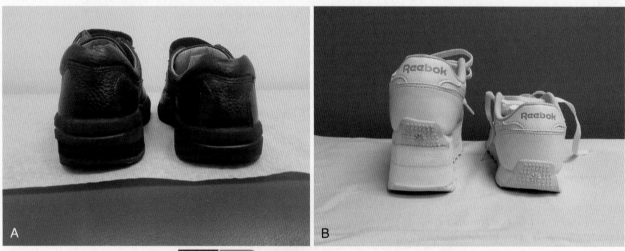

FIGURE 1.108 Shoe lifts for mild leg-length discrepancy.

TABLE 1.6

Lower Limb Multipliers for Boys and Girls

AGE	MULTIPLIER	
(YEAR + MONTH)	BOYS	GIRLS
Birth	5.080	4.630
0 + 3	4.550	4.155
0 + 6	4.050	3.725
0 + 9	3.600	3.300
1 + 0	3.240	2.970
1 + 3	2.975	2.750
1 + 6	2.825	2.600
1 + 9	2.700	2.490
2 + 0	2.590	2.390
2 + 3	2.480	2.295
2 + 6	2.385	2.200
2 + 9	2.300	2.125
3 + 0	2.230	2.050
3 + 6	2.110	1.925
4 + 0	2.000	1.830
4 + 6	1.890	1.740
5 + 0	1.820	1.660
5 + 6	1.740	1.580
6 + 0	1.670	1.510
6 + 6	1.620	1.460
7 + 0	1.570	1.430
7 + 6	1.520	1.370
8 + 0	1.470	1.330
8 + 6	1.420	1.290
9 + 0	1.380	1.260
9 + 6	1.340	1.220
10 + 0	1.310	1.190
10 + 6	1.280	1.160
11 + 0	1.240	1.130
11 + 6	1.220	1.100
12 + 0	1.180	1.070
12 + 6	1.160	1.050
13 + 0	1.130	1.030
13 + 6	1.100	1.010
14 + 0	1.080	1.000
14 + 6	1.060	NA
15 + 0	1.040	NA
15 + 6	1.020	NA
16 + 0	1.010	NA
16 + 6	1.010	NA
17 + 0	1.000	NA

MULTIPLIER METHOD FOR PREDICTING LOWER LIMB–LENGTH DISCREPANCIES

Length at Skeletal Maturity

$Lm = L \times M$

This formula can be used to determine the length of the femur, tibia, femur and tibia, or entire lower limb, including the foot height. It applies equally to the short and long limbs.

Continued

Lower Limb Multipliers for Boys and Girls—cont'd		
AGE		**MULTIPLIER**
(YEAR + MONTH)	BOYS	GIRLS

Congenital Limb-Length Discrepancy

$\Delta m = \Delta \times M$

This formula can be used to determine limb-length discrepancy in patients with congenital short femur, fibular hemimelia, hemihypertrophy, or hemiatrophy.

Developmental Limb-Length Discrepancy

$\Delta m = \Delta + (I \times G)$

where $I = 1 - (S - S)/(L - L)$ and $G = L(M - 1)$. This formula can be used to determine limb-length discrepancy in patients with Ollier disease, poliomyelitis, or growth arrest. It also can be used to determine discrepancy in patients with a congenital discrepancy. It also is useful in predicting the growth-remaining discrepancy in patients who have already undergone one or more limb-lengthening procedures.

Timing of Epiphysiodesis

$L\varepsilon = Lm - G\varepsilon$

and

$M\varepsilon = Lm/L\varepsilon$

Look in the multiplier table for the value of $M\varepsilon$ and determine which age corresponds to this multiplier value. This is the age of the patient at the time of epiphysiodesis.

G, Amount of growth remaining; I, amount of growth inhibition; L, current length of long limb; L, length of long limb as measured on previous radiographs (preferably made at least 6 or 12 months before current radiographs); Lm, length of femur or tibia at skeletal maturity; M, multiplier; S, current length of short limb; S, length of short limb as measured on previous radiographs (preferably made at least 6 or 12 months before current radiographs); Δ, current limb-length discrepancy; Δm, limb-length discrepancy at skeletal maturity; ε, desired correction following epiphysiodesis; $G\varepsilon$, amount of femoral or tibial growth remaining at age of epiphysiodesis ($G\varepsilon = \varepsilon/0.71$ for femur and $\varepsilon/0.57$ for tibia); $L\varepsilon$, desired length of bone to undergo epiphysiodesis at time of epiphysiodesis; $M\varepsilon$, multiplier at age of epiphysiodesis.

NA, Not applicable.
From Paley D, Bhave A, Herzenberg JE, et al: Multiplier method for predicting limb-length discrepancy, *J Bone Joint Surg* 82A:1432–1446, 2000.

Shortening and epiphysiodesis have several disadvantages: (1) the normal limb is operated on rather than the pathologic limb, and if there is a deformity in the short limb, a second operation may be necessary to correct that deformity; (2), the resulting body proportions may be cosmetically displeasing after shortening; (3) the degree of shortening possible is limited because of the inability of the muscles to adapt to shortening of more than 5 cm; and (4) the final height after shortening or epiphysiodesis may be unacceptably low.

EPIPHYSIODESIS

Phemister described epiphysiodesis in 1933, and his original technique, with minor modifications, has been widely used for limb-length equalization. Most authors recommend epiphysiodesis when 2 to 5 cm of shortening is required; however, Menelaus and others recommended epiphysiodesis for discrepancies of 8 to 10 cm to avoid the complications of limb lengthening. Currently, epiphysiodesis is not recommended for shortening of more than 5 cm. Although typically a safe procedure with predictable results, epiphysiodesis can have complications; the most common complication in recent large series of patients was unintended angular deformity.

A newer technique of epiphysiodesis involves the use of percutaneous instrumentation to obliterate the physis through small, cosmetically pleasing incisions (Technique 1.36).

Angled curets can be used instead of high-speed burrs to scrape the epiphyseal cartilage. It should be noted that normal physeal anatomy often contains multiple undulations or peaks and valleys. Care should be taken to obliterate as much

of the physis as possible so that growth arrest is complete and predictable.

Métaizeau et al. described a technique for percutaneous epiphysiodesis using transphyseal screws (PETS) (Technique 1.37). In 32 patients with leg-length discrepancies, PETS reduced the final discrepancy to less than 1 cm in 82% and to 5 mm or less in 56%. PETS has also shown success in the correction of angular deformities of the lower extremity. Multiple authors have cited as advantages of PETS simplicity of the technique, short operating time, rapid postoperative rehabilitation, and potential reversibility (Fig. 1.109). However, there seems to be a lag time before the PETS technique produces the desired effect; therefore the epiphysiodesis should be performed up to 1 year before the time predicted for a formal open procedure.

PHYSEAL EXPOSURE AROUND THE KNEE

TECHNIQUE 1.35

(ABBOTT AND GILL, MODIFIED)
- Flex the knee 30 degrees to relax the hamstring muscles and make a lateral incision 6.5 cm proximal to the lateral femoral condyle, continuing distally between the biceps tendon and iliotibial band to the fibular head and extending anteriorly over the lateral aspect of the tibia. Such a

In general, femoral shortening is tolerated better than tibial shortening because the soft-tissue muscular envelope is much larger, making skin closure easier, offering a better cosmetic result, and ensuring prompt union of the osteotomy. If the discrepancy is largely confined to the tibia, however, tibial shortening is preferred to make the knee heights level.

Wagner recommended metaphyseal osteotomy if angular or rotational correction is required, and diaphyseal osteotomy if shortening alone is necessary. Proximal metaphyseal osteotomy of the femur has fewer complications than distal osteotomy, which may compromise knee motion. Additionally, proximal femoral shortening has less negative effect on the strength of the quadriceps. Distal femoral metaphyseal osteotomy should be avoided unless necessary for correction of angular deformity. The development of interlocking intramedullary fixation has made diaphyseal shortening preferable to metaphyseal osteotomy in the femur, even if rotational correction is needed. Shortening over an intramedullary rod should be delayed until complete skeletal maturity has been reached, or the entry portal of the nail should be the greater trochanter instead of the piriformis fossa to decrease the risk of femoral head osteonecrosis.

PROXIMAL FEMORAL METAPHYSEAL SHORTENING

TECHNIQUE 1.39   *Figure 1.115*

(WAGNER).
- Before surgery, plan the osteotomy to provide the needed angular correction
- Through a proximal lateral incision, split the fascia lata and elevate the vastus lateralis and the periosteum.

- Fashion an insertion site for the right-angle blade plate or hip screw according to the preoperative plan.
- Mark the bone to control rotation and remove the proscribed segment with an oscillating saw. Leave a spike of medial cortex and lesser trochanter intact to act as a buttress.
- Remove the segment and bring the distal fragment into direct apposition with the proximal segment.
- Apply the osteosynthesis plate and insert the screws to create compression across the osteotomy.

DISTAL FEMORAL METAPHYSEAL SHORTENING

TECHNIQUE 1.40   *Figure 1.116*

(WAGNER).
- Before surgery, make a careful plan for the resection and angular correction.
- Make a lateral incision through the fascia lata and elevate the vastus lateralis anteriorly, avoiding the knee joint.
- Use the blade plate seating device to prepare the entrance for the blade plate.
- With an oscillating saw, make the proximal osteotomy and then the distal osteotomy. For added stability, try to preserve a medial spike of bone with the distal fragment.
- Impact the two fragments and apply the blade under compression or insert a distal femoral sliding screw and fixation plate device.

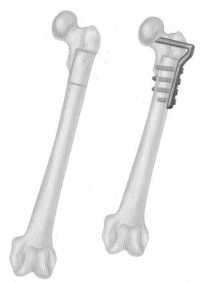

FIGURE 1.115   Wagner technique for proximal femoral metaphyseal shortening. **SEE TECHNIQUE 1.39.**

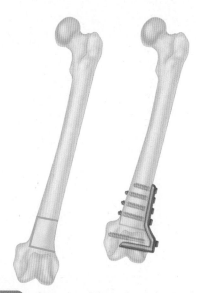

FIGURE 1.116   Wagner technique for distal femoral metaphyseal shortening. **SEE TECHNIQUE 1.40.**

PROXIMAL TIBIAL METAPHYSEAL SHORTENING

TECHNIQUE 1.41   *Figure 1.117*

(WAGNER).

- Through a lateral incision, resect a portion of the fibula at the junction of the proximal and middle thirds.
- Make a separate anterior incision to expose the proximal tibia subperiosteally.
- Resect the desired amount of bone (no more than 4 cm except in unusual circumstances) below the tibial tuberosity with an oscillating saw.
- Hold the two bone ends under compression with a T-plate.
- Perform a prophylactic fasciotomy.
- Wound closure may be difficult because of the nature of the skin around the proximal tibia.

TIBIAL DIAPHYSEAL SHORTENING

TECHNIQUE 1.42

(BROUGHTON, OLNEY, AND MENELAUS)

- Make a longitudinal incision over the anteromedial surface of the tibia.
- Perform a subperiosteal dissection and make a step-cut osteotomy, removing the desired amount of bone and allowing for 5 to 7.5 cm of overlap after shortening.
- Through a separate incision, remove an equivalent amount of bone from the midshaft of the fibula (Fig. 1.118A).
- Shorten the leg and fix the step-cut osteotomy with two lag screws (Fig. 1.118B) or, in mature patients, with an intramedullary nail (Fig. 1.119). This is the only technique indicated in skeletally immature patients.

CLOSED FEMORAL DIAPHYSEAL SHORTENING

TECHNIQUE 1.43

(WINQUIST, HANSEN, AND PEARSON)

- Position the patient on a fracture table in the supine "scissor" position.
- Use the standard techniques for closed medullary nailing and ream to the desired width in 0.5-mm increments. Consider venting the distal metaphyseal-diaphyseal junction with a 4.8-mm cannulated drill bit to prevent fat embolism.
- Adjust the saw for the appropriate depth according to the preoperative plan and insert the saw until, with the

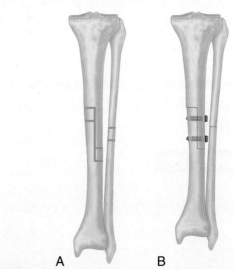

FIGURE 1.118   **A** and **B,** Technique for tibial diaphyseal shortening in skeletally immature patients. **SEE TECHNIQUE 1.42.**

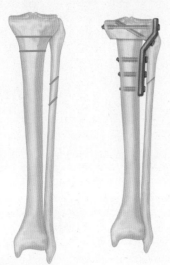

FIGURE 1.117   Wagner technique for proximal tibial metaphyseal shortening. **SEE TECHNIQUE 1.41.**

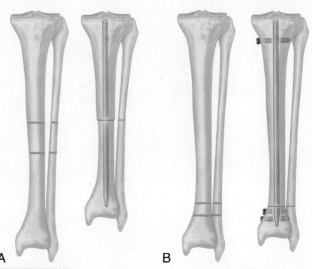

FIGURE 1.119   **A,** Diaphyseal shortening with medullary fixation. **B,** Distal tibial shortening with locked intramedullary nail. **SEE TECHNIQUE 1.42.**

blade fully retracted, the measuring device is seated firmly against the greater trochanter.

- While an assistant applies pressure to hold the measuring device in place for the proximal and the distal cuts, deploy the saw blade in increments, making complete revolutions (Fig. 1.120A). If necessary, back up one index notch to repeat the cuts if the blade is getting stuck.
- Slowly continue cutting until the final index mark is reached, at which point the blade is fully deployed. The most difficult area to cut is posteriorly in the linea aspera. If necessary, complete the cut percutaneously with a thin osteotome. The next larger size blade and cam can be inserted to get a larger cutting diameter, but this can be difficult if the canal is not reamed widely enough.
- After completing the first cut, retract the blade fully.
- Remove the foot from the fracture table and angulate the distal femur 60 to 70 degrees in all directions to complete the osteotomy; replace the traction.
- Advance the measuring device handle distally while holding the locking nut in place. The distance that develops between these two components should equal the amount of femur to be resected.
- Spin the locking nut distally to lock the measuring device handle.
- With an assistant holding the measuring device firmly against the greater trochanter, make the second (proximal) osteotomy in the same fashion as the first.

- After completing the second osteotomy, retract the blade fully and remove the saw. The resected bone should be subtrochanteric rather than diaphyseal to lessen the effect on the quadriceps mechanism.
- Insert an internal chisel of appropriate size, hook the medial aspect of the intercalary segment, and pound on the handle backward with a tuning-fork hammer to split the bone (Fig. 1.120B).
- Repeat this maneuver at least one more time on the lateral segment.
- Use the hook of the chisel to push the fragments away from the canal.
- Have the unscrubbed assistant again remove the foot from the fracture table and impact the osteotomy, displacing the segmental fragments to either side, using the chisel to manipulate the fragments if necessary.
- In some cases, splitting of the "napkin ring" resected bone piece is unsuccessful. Should this occur, make a small lateral incision to remove the intercalary segment.
- Pass a nail-driving guidewire across the osteotomy and insert an appropriate-size nail for fixation while the unscrubbed assistant maintains rotational alignment.
- Lock the nail proximally and distally for rotational control and to prevent inadvertent lengthening postoperatively (Fig. 1.121).
- Steinmann pins can be inserted into the lateral aspect of the femoral condyle and the greater trochanter just

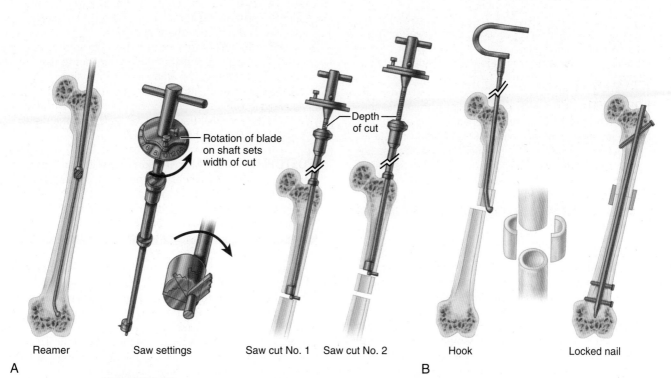

Reamer Saw settings Saw cut No. 1 Saw cut No. 2 Hook Locked nail

Rotation of blade on shaft sets width of cut

Depth of cut

A B

FIGURE 1.120 Closed femoral diaphyseal shortening, as described by Winquist et al. (see text). **A,** Medullary canal is reamed with standard cannulated reamer. Special medullary saw is inserted into reamed canal. One or two rotations are made with saw at each setting, and saw is progressively opened until blade is completely exposed. **B,** After both saw cuts have been made, intercalary segment is split using back-cutting chisel. Rotational alignment and distraction can be controlled with locked medullary nail. **SEE TECHNIQUE 1.43.**

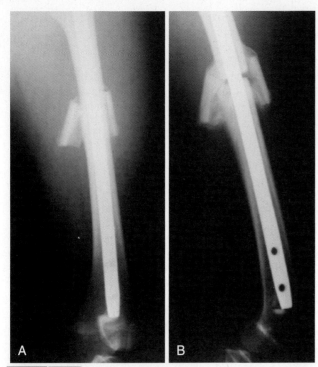

FIGURE 1.121   **A,** Sixteen-year-old girl underwent 4-cm closed femoral shortening. Shortly after surgery, intercalary fragment is seen around site of osteotomy, acting as bone graft. **B,** Osteotomy has healed 8 weeks later. At least 4 mm of distraction occurred after osteotomy. Locking of nail is recommended to preserve alignment and length, if necessary. **SEE TECHNIQUE 1.43.**

before the first osteotomy to serve as references for rotational alignment control.
- Check rotational alignment before leaving the operating room.

POSTOPERATIVE CARE A knee splint is used to stabilize the shortened quadriceps mechanism, and a vigorous strengthening program is begun. Rehabilitation is faster if the patient has participated in a quadriceps-strengthening and hamstring-strengthening program before surgery. Rotation or distraction at the osteotomy site may occur if a locked nail is not used.

▌LIMB LENGTHENING

A limb-lengthening program requires a patient and family fully committed to maximal participation in an extended project. The success of limb lengthening depends largely on the patient's efforts in physical therapy and the care of the external fixator. Although technical improvements have reduced the frequency with which major complications associated with limb lengthening occur, the process remains difficult and should be performed by surgeons with appropriate experience.

Shortening procedures are preferable for many patients who are candidates for limb lengthening. Patients who are unable to participate in frequent follow-up or who do not have the support to care for the fixator properly and to undergo vigorous physical therapy are best treated by means other than lengthening. Candidates for limb lengthening and

their parents benefit from meeting other patients in various stages of the lengthening process.

Acute long bone lengthening seldom is indicated; however, Salter described acute distraction and interposition grafting through the innominate bone. Millis and Hall reported a modification of this technique; they achieved an average lengthening of 2.3 cm in 20 patients with acetabular dysplasia with femoral shortening, pure limb-length inequality, decompensated scoliosis, and primary intrapelvic asymmetry. This technique may be useful in patients who also require acetabular reconstruction, but epiphysiodesis or gradual distraction lengthening techniques are more reliable alternatives for isolated limb-length discrepancy.

TRANSILIAC LENGTHENING

TECHNIQUE 1.44

(MILLIS AND HALL)
- Use the anterior ilioinguinal approach to the pelvis described for the Salter innominate osteotomy (see chapter 2).
- Use a Gigli saw to make the osteotomy from the sciatic notch to the anterior inferior iliac spine (Fig. 1.122A).
- Insert a lamina spreader into the anterior aspect of the osteotomy.
- Have an assistant apply caudally directed pressure on the iliac crest to prevent displacement of the proximal fragment by shear force through the sacroiliac joint, while another assistant applies traction to the femur, keeping the knee flexed to relax the sciatic nerve.
- Fashion a full-thickness block of iliac crest into a trapezoid. The height of the graft directly superior to the acetabulum determines the amount of lengthening.
- Wedge the iliac graft into the distraction site (Fig. 1.122B) and hold it with two large, threaded Steinmann pins that transfix the proximal fragment, the graft, and the distal supraacetabular fragment (Fig. 1.122C).

POSTOPERATIVE CARE Traction is applied for 5 days. Range-of-motion exercises are begun at 3 days, and touch-down weight bearing is allowed at 7 days. Full weight bearing is delayed until graft incorporation is evident on radiographs, usually at 3 to 6 months.

Lengthening by callotasis (or low-energy corticotomy followed by gradual distraction of the bone fragments with a mechanical apparatus) has been the basic procedure for limb lengthening since Putti's report of the technique in 1921. Osteotomy and fixation techniques have been modified by several authors, but the principles remain the same. The corticotomy should be made by low-energy methods, usually multiple percutaneous drill holes connected by an osteotome, with care taken to avoid significant disruption of the surrounding soft tissues. Distraction should begin after a brief latent period of 1 to 3 weeks to allow for early callous formation. The rate of distraction should be approximately 1 mm/day divided over four 0.25-mm increments. The formation of the distraction regenerate should be closely monitored with

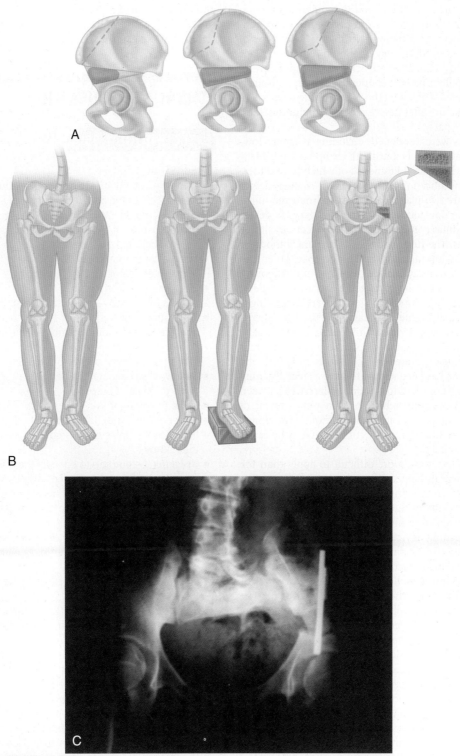

FIGURE 1.122   **A,** Acute transiliac lengthening accomplished by modification of Salter technique. Instead of triangular graft, square or trapezoidal graft is used. Lengthening is greater with larger grafts. **B,** Acetabular dysplasia and mild limb-length inequality. Pelvic obliquity results in compensatory scoliosis. In middle figure, block has been placed beneath shorter leg. Although this balances pelvis and straightens spine, it causes acetabulum to be even more vertical. On right, transiliac lengthening has been performed to improve femoral acetabular coverage and regain length. **C,** Transiliac lengthening with trapezoidal graft. **SEE TECHNIQUE 1.44.**

frequent radiographic assessment, and the rate of distraction should be altered accordingly to avoid premature consolidation or poor regenerate formation. No matter what type of external apparatus is used, the device should remain in place for 1 month for every 1 cm of length achieved. Despite careful technique and excellent patient cooperation, high complication rates are reported with all methods, including deep infection, nonunion, fracture after device removal, malunion, joint stiffness, and nerve palsy.

Several fixators were developed, including Wagner's low-profile, monolateral fixator, DeBastiani's Orthofix, the Ilizarov device, and the Taylor Spatial Frame, all of which have undergone numerous modifications. The original Wagner device is adjustable in only two planes, and the Hoffman modification is adjustable in one additional plane. DeBastiani's device (Orthofix) has modular components that allow certain simple angular corrections. The Ilizarov device is extremely modular and can be adapted with extensions and hinges to lengthen and correct angular and translational deformities simultaneously. Rotational deformities can be corrected either at the time of fixator application or later by applying outriggers to the rings.

The Taylor Spatial Frame also has been used for deformity correction and lengthening. This frame uses the slow correction principles of the Ilizarov system but adds a six-axis deformity analysis incorporated in a computer program. The Taylor Spatial Frame has been shown to have a steep learning curve and has a high cost. In addition, no differences between the Taylor and Ilizarov frames have been noted in terms of lengthening index and complication rate, although rotational, translational, and residual deformity correction may be easier with the Taylor frame.

The circular devices are more difficult to apply than the monolateral fixators, and extensive training and experience are recommended before using them. For detailed descriptions of the components of these fixators, preoperative planning, and frame construction and application, see other chapter.

Internal lengthening devices were developed to eliminate the problems associated with pin track infection and soft-tissue transfixation, to maintain mechanical alignment and stability during lengthening and consolidation, and to improve patient comfort and tolerance. Lengthening of these devices may be initiated by rotation of the involved limb (Albizzia nail; DePuy Australia Pty Ltd, Mount Waverly, Australia); controlled rotation, ambulation, and weight bearing (Intramedullary Skeletal Kinetic Device; Orthofix, McKinney, TX); an implanted electrically activated motorized drive (Fitbone; Wittenstein Igersheim, Germany); or an externally applied magnetic field (PRECICE Nail, Ellipse Technologies, Inc., Irvine, CA, or the PHENIX M2 Lengthening nail; Phenix Medical, France).

These intramedullary devices do not allow for gradual correction of angular deformities because they can only lengthen in one plane; therefore any angular deformities must be corrected at the time of nail insertion or by other means after lengthening. There are a number of studies demonstrating difficulty in controlling rate of growth using the Intramedullary Skeletal Kinetic Device (ISKD) nail, and many authors are suggesting alternative devices.

Finally, some authors have reported the use of an intramedullary nail or submuscular plate in addition to an external fixator for distraction osteogenesis.

With most of these techniques, distraction osteogenesis is done with the use of an external device as described above, and the submuscular plate or intramedullary nail is then used to stabilize the regenerate as it consolidates, allowing earlier removal of the external device.

TIBIAL LENGTHENING

TECHNIQUE 1.45

(DEBASTIANI ET AL.)
- Place the patient supine on a radiolucent table.
- Resect 2 cm of the distal fibula through a lateral approach.
- Use the mated Orthofix drills, drill guides, and screw guides to insert the conical, self-tapping cortical and cancellous screws.
- Insert a cancellous screw 2 cm distal to the medial aspect of the knee, parallel to the knee joint.
- Place the appropriate rigid template parallel to the diaphysis of the tibia and insert the distalmost screw.
- Go to the proximal part of the template and insert the next screw in the fourth template hole distal to the upper screw. The last screw to be placed is in the distal template, in the hole farthest away from the distalmost screw.
- Remove the template and perform a corticotomy just distal to the tibial tuberosity.
- Incise the anterior skin and periosteum longitudinally.
- Under direct vision, drill a series of unicortical holes in the tibia. Set the drill stop at 1 cm to prevent penetration of the marrow.
- Use a thin osteotome to connect the drill holes and to divide along the posteromedial and posterolateral cortices as much as can be done safely.
- Flex the tibia at the corticotomy to crack the posterior aspect of the tibia.
- Apply the Orthofix lengthener. If the fracture fixation device is used, fix the ball joint rigidly with a small amount of methylmethacrylate.
- Suture the periosteum and close the skin over drains.

POSTOPERATIVE CARE Partial weight bearing and physical therapy are begun immediately. Distraction is delayed until callus is visible on radiographs, usually by 10 to 15 days. Distraction is begun at 0.25 mm every 6 hours but can be reduced if pain or muscle contraction occurs. Radiographs are made 1 week after distraction begins to ensure a complete corticotomy and are made at 4-week intervals thereafter. If the regenerated callus is of poor quality, distraction is stopped for 7 days. Recompression is indicated for gaps in the callus and for evidence of excessive neurovascular distraction. When the desired length is obtained, the body-locking screw mechanism is tightened, and the distraction mechanism is removed from the fixator. Full weight bearing is allowed until good callus consolidation is seen, then the body-locking screw is unlocked to allow dynamic axial compression. The fixator is removed when corticalization is complete. If stability is confirmed, the screws are removed. If there is any doubt as to stability of the bone, the fixator is replaced for an additional period.

TIBIAL LENGTHENING

TECHNIQUE 1.46   *Figure 1.123*

(ILIZAROV, MODIFIED)

- Frame preconstruction involves assembling a frame consisting of four equal Ilizarov rings sized to the patient; use the smallest diameter rings that leave sufficient space for swelling after surgery. There should be one fingerbreadth of space between the proximal ring and the tibial tuberosity and two fingerbreadths posteriorly at the largest diameter of the posterior calf muscles (Fig. 1.124A). The most proximal ring can be a ⅝-inch ring to allow more knee flexion after surgery, especially if the ipsilateral femur is to be lengthened at the same time, because full rings would touch each other with relatively little knee flexion.
- Connect the upper two rings with 20-mm threaded, hexagonal sockets for better stability. In small patients, there may be room proximally for only one ring and a drop wire (Fig. 1.124B). The distal two rings can be spaced farther apart than the top two rings for better stability, but for significant lengthening it is better to have the distal two-ring construct relatively farther away from the intended proximal metaphyseal corticotomy site; such an arrange-

ment maximizes the amount of soft tissue available for stretching, contributing to the overall lengthening.
- For initial preconstruction, use only two connections between each pair of rings, one anteriorly and one directly posteriorly. Plan the frame so that the central connection bolts are centered directly over the tibial tuberosity and the anterior crest of the tibia.
- Assemble all rings symmetrically.
- To compensate for the anterior and valgus angulation that often occurs during tibial lengthening, some surgeons connect the upper two-ring set to the lower set with anterior and posterior threaded rods attached to the lower of the proximal two rings with conical washer couples. These allow a tilt of 7 degrees to be built into the system.
- Adjust the frame so that the proximal rings are higher anteriorly and medially. The frame is applied in this "cockeyed" position, but after the corticotomy is made, the conical washer bolts are removed and all four rings are brought into parallel alignment, placing the tibia in about 5 degrees of prophylactic recurvatum and varus.
- More often, a symmetrically aligned frame is used without any prophylactic positioning. Instead, careful attention is paid to the follow-up radiographs during lengthening. If axial deviations are found at the end of

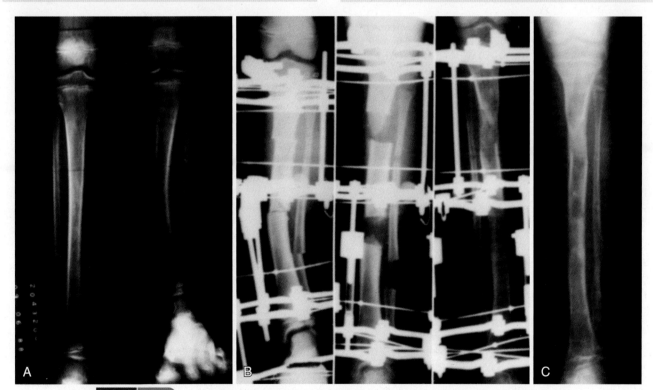

FIGURE 1.123 **A,** Congenital posteromedial bowing of tibia in 11-year-old girl. Although deformity largely corrected spontaneously, child is left with 6 cm of shortening and valgus angulation in midshaft of tibia. **B,** Double-level tibial lengthening. Lower corticotomy is made at apex of angular deformity in midshaft, and upper corticotomy could have been made more proximally in metaphyseal region. After distraction with appropriately placed hinge, more distal corticotomy not only opens up for elongation but also corrects valgus deformity. **C,** Final result after removal of fixator shows excellent regenerated bone in gaps. This 6-cm lengthening required 4 ½ months in fixator. Premature consolidation of proximal fibular osteotomy resulted in spontaneous proximal fibular epiphysiolysis. **SEE TECHNIQUE 1.46.**

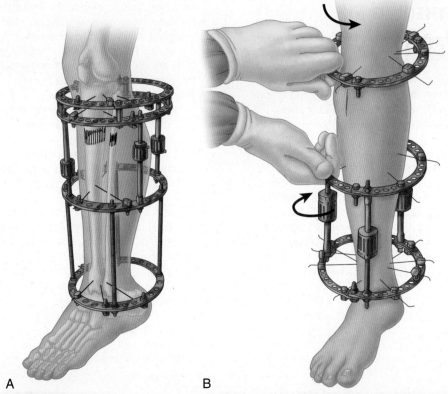

A B

FIGURE 1.124 Typical Ilizarov frame for moderate tibial lengthening. **A,** In skeletally immature child with intact physes, proximal segment would not have enough room for two rings. Single ring distal to proximal tibial epiphysis is used with drop wire for additional segmental stabilization of proximal segment. For significant amount of lengthening, third ring can be placed more distally to allow greater mass of soft tissue for recruitment into lengthening process. **B,** If necessary, Ilizarov rings can be used to complete the posterior aspect of the corticotomy by externally rotating the distal segment. **SEE TECHNIQUE 1.46.**

lengthening, corrective hinges are placed onto the ring to obtain proper alignment.
- For frame application, position the patient on a radiolucent table and apply a tourniquet to the upper thigh.
- Through a lateral incision, expose the midfibula by subperiosteal dissection and transect it with an oscillating saw.
- Release the tourniquet and close the fibular wound in layers.
- Under fluoroscopic control, insert a reference wire from medial to lateral, perpendicular to the long axis of the tibia (for a normally aligned leg), just below the proximal tibial physis. Use 1.8-mm wires in large children and adolescents and 1.5-mm wires in smaller children.
- Attach the preassembled frame to this reference wire.
- Place another wire from the fibula to the tibia just proximal to the distal tibial physis. Use the standard Ilizarov principles of wire insertion and fixation at all times.
- Wires should be pushed or gently tapped through the soft tissues rather than drilled, especially when exiting close to neurovascular structures.
- When passing wires through the anterior compartment muscles, hold the foot dorsiflexed for the same reason.

- Incise the skin to allow passage of olive wires.
- Never pull or bend a wire to the ring. Instead, build up to the wire with washers or posts as necessary to avoid undue torque and undesirable moments on the tibia.
- Tension the wires to 130 kg, unless the wire is suspended off a ring, in which case 50 to 60 kg of tension is used to prevent warping of the ring. It is best to use two wire tensioners to tighten two wires simultaneously on the same ring, if possible, to prevent warping of the ring.
- After tensioning and securing the wires, cut the ends long (about 4 cm) and curl the ends of the wire directly over the wire-fixation bolt to allow later retensioning, if necessary. Bend the cut wire points into available ring holes so that they do not injure the patient or staff members.
- After the first two wires have been attached to the frame and tensioned, the frame can act as a drill guide for placement of the remaining wires. The wires in the first ring are the initial transverse reference wire and a medial face wire that is parallel to the medial surface of the tibia.
- Place a third wire from the fibular head into the tibia to prevent dissociation of the proximal tibiofibular joint during lengthening. This wire does not risk damage to the peroneal nerve if the fibular head is readily palpable. Do not use an olive wire because it would compress the proximal

tibiofibular joint. Ideally, this wire should be proximal to the proximal fibular physis.

- In the second ring, place a transverse wire and another medial face wire, avoiding the pes anserinus tendons, if possible.
- Because there is a strong tendency to valgus during proximal tibial lengthening, place olive wires on the top and bottom rings laterally and on the middle two rings medially to function as fulcrums for bending the tibia into varus. Half-pins (5 mm or 6 mm) are now used more frequently, especially in the diaphysis.
- For corticotomy, remove the two threaded rods connecting the proximal fixation block with the distal fixation block.
- Make a 2-cm incision over the crest of the tibia just below the tibial tuberosity.
- Incise the periosteum longitudinally and insert a small periosteal elevator.
- Elevate a narrow portion of periosteum the width of the small periosteal elevator along the medial and lateral surfaces of the tibia.
- Insert a 1.2-cm (½ inch) osteotome transversely into the thick anterior cortex.
- Use a 5-mm (¼ inch) osteotome to score the medial side and then the lateral side. The periosteal elevator can be placed flush along the bone to act as a directional guide for the osteotome.
- The corticotomy is guided by feel and by hearing the sound change when the osteotome exits the back cortex. On the medial side, no important structures are at risk; on the lateral cortex, the posterior tibial muscle belly is between the tibia and the deep neurovascular structures.
- After cutting the medial and lateral cortices, withdraw the osteotome and reinsert it along the medial cortex.
- Turn the osteotome 90 degrees to spread the cortices and crack the posterior cortex. Repeat this maneuver at the lateral cortex, if needed.
- Although Ilizarov recommended not violating the medullary canal, most Western surgeons have adopted DeBastiani's method of making several front-to-back drill holes to weaken the posterior cortex. The corticotomy also can be completed by externally rotating the distal tibia, but do not internally rotate the tibia for fear of stretching the peroneal nerve.
- For proximal or distal tibial metaphyseal "corticotomies," a Gigli saw makes a smooth osteotomy without risk of fracture into adjacent pin sites. The Gigli saw method requires two transverse incisions, one anteriorly and one posteromedially. Subperiosteal dissection with a small elevator is done on all three sides of the tibia. Right-angle and curved clamps are used to pass a heavy suture, which is tied to the Gigli saw. The suture can be passed before frame application and the Gigli saw after completion of the fixation. When activating the saw, assistants must retract the skin edges. Care is taken to protect the medial face periosteum at the final part of the osteotomy.
- For frame assembly, reduce the fracture, and insert four distraction rods or graduated telescopic rods, approximately 90 degrees apart, between the middle two rings.
- Close the corticotomy site, over a drain if necessary, and apply compressive dressings.

- Dress the wire sites with foam sponges held in place by plastic clips or rubber stoppers. If rubber stoppers are used, put them on before fixing the wires to the rings.

POSTOPERATIVE CARE Physical therapy and crutch walking with partial weight bearing are begun immediately. Distraction is delayed for 5 to 7 days. In children, the distraction rate is 0.25 mm four times per day. The patient and family are taught to care for the pins before discharge from the hospital, usually 5 to 7 days after surgery. Radiographs are made 7 to 10 days after distraction is begun to document separation at the corticotomy site. Regenerated bone should be seen in the gap by 4 to 6 weeks, although linear streaks of regenerated bone usually are visible before then, especially in younger children. If the regenerated bone formation is insufficient, the rate of distraction should be slowed, stopped, or in some instances temporarily reversed. Weight bearing and functional activity of the limb aid in maturation of the regenerated bone. During distraction, knee flexion contractures and ankle equinus contractures can be prevented with prophylactic splints and orthoses. The fixator is removed when there is evidence of corticalization of the regenerated bone, and the patient is able to walk without aids.

For significant lengthening, especially when ankle mobility is abnormal before surgery, the foot can be fixed into the lengthening device by inserting an olive wire from each side of the calcaneus at divergent angles to one another. These are attached to an appropriate-size half-ring. This half-ring must be within 2 cm of the back of the heel to capture the obliquely placed wires anteriorly. The heel ring is connected to the lowest ring of the lengthening frame with short plates and threaded rods. The heel ring and wires can be removed after lengthening is complete to prevent subtalar stiffness. A custom orthosis can be constructed to accommodate the foot construct.

For lengthening of more than 6 cm, double-level lengthening speeds the process and reduces the time in fixation by about 40%. In this modification, three rings are used, with a drop wire off each ring to give "bilevel" fixation at each segment (Fig. 1.124). The fibula should have one wire transfixing it at each of the three rings. Two fibular osteotomies and two corticotomies are required, one of each just below the proximal ring and one of each just above the distal ring. A heel ring and wires are added to prevent equinus of the ankle. The bottom two rings can be connected to provide a stable handle on the distal segments to complete the proximal corticotomy, and the top two rings can be connected to complete the distal corticotomy.

If a fixed knee contracture develops during lengthening, the physical therapy treatments should be done more often. If the knee contracture does not respond to physical therapy and splinting, the frame can be extended proximally to the thigh with a cuff cast incorporating a ring and a hinge incorporated at the approximate axis of rotation of the knee. The device can be used to distract and correct the knee contracture slowly.

To correct other deformities of the tibia while lengthening, the Ilizarov frame can be modified with hinges to effect angular and translational correction simultaneously. Internal rotation can be corrected distally by osteotomy at the time of fixator application. Proximally, internal rotation should be corrected gradually after lengthening is complete but before the regenerated bone is solid. Use of the Ilizarov device for multiplane corrections should be attempted only by surgeons with experience in these techniques.

TIBIAL LENGTHENING OVER INTRAMEDULLARY NAIL (PRECICE INTRAMEDULLARY LENGTHENING SYSTEM, ELLIPSE TECHNOLOGIES, IRVINE, CA)

TECHNIQUE 1.47

(HERZENBERG, STANDARD, GREEN)
- Preoperative planning is essential to determine the amount of lengthening required, the correct nail length, and correct location for the tibial corticotomy.
- Place the patient supine, with the hip and knee flexed and the affected leg hanging vertically down over a padded bar or sterile triangle, avoiding any pressure on the fibular head (common peroneal nerve). Patient positioning for the PRECICE procedure is the same as that for other intramedullary nailing procedures.
- Create an osteotomy of the fibula through a separate incision to allow distraction of the tibial osteotomy. Consider prophylactic fasciotomies as well as a gastrocsoleus recession if indicated (Chapter 5).

VENTING OF INTRAMEDULLARY CANAL
- Drill two or three 4-mm or 5-mm diameter holes in the tibia, across both cortices and into the intramedullary canal. Position the vent at the level of the planned corticotomy. Venting reduces intramedullary pressure during reaming.
- Reamings from the vent holes will serve as additional bone graft.

SYNDESMOSIS SCREW
- A cannulated screw should be placed across the tibia and fibula distal to the tip of the nail (see syndesmotic screw placement).
- Syndesmotic screw fixation ensures that the fibula lengthens with the tibia.
- Place a proximal syndesmotic screw (if needed) after final nail insertion.

NAIL INSERTION
- Make a 5-cm vertical skin incision in the midline, centered at the level of the tibial plateau. Ensure that the entry portal is no more than 1 cm distal to the anterior edge of the tibial plateau; a more distal entry point may result in damage to the posterior cortex.
- Reflect the skin and subcutaneous tissues medially until the medial border of the patellar tendon is visible, make an incision medial to the tendon and proximal to the tibial tuberosity, and retract the tendon laterally to allow

identification of the midpoint of the anterior margin of the tibial plateau.
- Use an awl or cannulated opening reamer over a guidewire to open the medullary canal in the midline. Use image intensification in the sagittal and frontal planes to confirm that the tip of the reamer and guide pin are in the line of the tibial canal.
- Insert the ball-tipped guidewire until its tip sits 3 to 4 cm beyond the planned distal end of the nail.
- Reaming begins with an 8-mm flexible reamer and increases in 0.5-mm increments. Ream 2.0 mm beyond the planned implant diameter.
- Connect the appropriate diameter and length PRECICE nail to the proximal guide arm. Verify correct alignment of the proximal interlocking screws by passing a drill bit through the guide and screw hole in the implant.
- Advance the nail to just above the level of the planned osteotomy.
- Remove the guide rod to complete the corticotomy.

OSTEOTOMY
- Complete the osteotomy at the level of the vent holes. The appropriate osteotomy level is commonly at the junction of the upper and middle thirds of the tibia (Fig. 1.125).
- To make the osteotomy, create additional drill holes at the level of the previously placed vent holes. Preserve the periosteum to protect the blood supply to the regenerated bone. Complete the osteotomy with multiple passes with a small osteotome. The posterior cortex may be difficult to cut and can be broken through osteoclasis by rotating the limb.

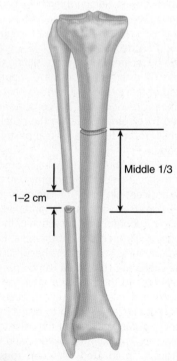

FIGURE 1.125 Location of osteotomies for tibial lengthening with intramedullary skeletal kinetic distractor (see text). (From Cole JD: Intramedullary skeletal kinetic distractor: tibial surgical technique: technique manual, Orthofix, McKinney, TX.) **SEE TECHNIQUE 1.47.**

- Test that the two bone segments rotate freely and independently of each other.
- Advance the nail beyond the osteotomy to the desired level.
- Using the proximal screw guide, place two bicortical locking screws.
- With a freehand technique, insert two distal locking screws.

CLOSURE

- After careful irrigation to remove any remaining bone fragments from the proximal wound, insert closed suction drainage, close the incisions in layers in the usual fashion, and apply firm dressings to prevent hematoma formation.

INTRAOPERATIVE EXTERNAL REMOTE CONTROL (ERC) DISTRACTION

- Locate the center of the magnet with image intensification and mark the skin. The mark should be frequently refreshed postoperatively.
- Place the ERC in a sterile bag and place over the skin mark.
- Activate the ERC to distract the PRECICE nail 1.0 to 2.0 mm to verify correct functioning of the system. It takes 7 minutes for 1.0 mm of lengthening. It is not necessary to retract the device.

POSTOPERATIVE CARE The drains are removed at 24 to 48 hours after surgery. Partial weight bearing with crutches is allowed at 1 week and is continued throughout the lengthening and consolidation phases. Full weight bearing is not allowed until cortication of the regenerated bone is evident in three of four cortices during the end of the consolidation phase. Isometric exercises for the whole limb are encouraged early. Gentle knee mobilization can be started after about 4 days within the limits of comfort. Lengthening should be initiated 7 to 8 days after surgery. Daily lengthenings are typically 0.5 to 1.0 mm divided into two to four sessions. The physician and his staff should properly train the patient on use of the ERC. Weekly radiographic evaluation is important to monitor progress. Removal of the PRECICE is recommended 12 to 18 months after radiographic evidence of full bony consolidation.

FEMORAL LENGTHENING

TECHNIQUE 1.48

(DEBASTIANI ET AL.)
- Place the patient supine on a radiolucent table.
- Use the mated drills, drill guides, and screw guides to insert the conical self-tapping cortical and cancellous screws.
- Insert a cortical screw at the level of the lesser trochanter, perpendicular to the shaft of the femur.
- Attach the rigid template and insert the distalmost screw, lining the template up parallel to the shaft of the femur.

- Return to the proximal end of the template and insert the next screw into the fourth template hole distal to the upper screw. The last screw to be placed is in the distal template, in the hole farthest away from the distalmost screw.
- Remove the template and perform a corticotomy 1 cm distal to the proximal two screws (just distal to the iliopsoas insertion).
- Incise the anterior thigh skin longitudinally and dissect bluntly between the sartorius muscle and the tensor fasciae latae muscle and through the substance of the vastus intermedius and rectus femoris muscles. Incise the periosteum longitudinally and elevate it laterally and medially.
- Under direct vision, drill a series of 4.8-mm unicortical holes in the visible aspect of the anterior two thirds of the circumference of the femur (Fig. 1.126A). Set the drill stop at 1 cm to prevent penetration of the marrow.
- Use a thin osteotome to connect the drill holes without violating the marrow. Flex the femur at the corticotomy to crack the posterior cortex, completing the corticotomy. Do not use the Orthofix pins as handles to complete the corticotomy, or they may loosen.
- Reduce the fracture and apply the Orthofix lengthener. If the Orthofix fracture-fixation device is used, fix the ball joint rigidly with a small amount of methylmethacrylate. The Orthofix slide-lengthening device can be used with or without swivel clamps.
- If swivel clamps are used, blocking them with methylmethacrylate should be considered. The slide lengthener is especially useful for double-level lengthening.

Price recommended acute valgus of a few degrees for subtrochanteric lengthening to help prevent the common problem of varus at this level. Adductor tenotomy also is advised. Suture the periosteum and close the skin over drains. The use of six pins has been recommended for femoral lengthening to gain stability and to resist a tendency for varus deviation (Fig. 1.126B).

POSTOPERATIVE CARE Postoperative care is the same as that for tibial lengthening (Technique 1.46).

FEMORAL LENGTHENING

TECHNIQUE 1.49

(ILIZAROV, MODIFIED)
- Frame preconstruction includes the following considerations. The standard femoral lengthening frame consists of a proximal fixation block made of two arcs, a distal fixation block made of two identically sized rings, and an "empty" middle ring (usually one size larger than the distal rings) to link the two fixation blocks.
- Preconstruct the frame before surgery to reduce the time spent in the operating room.
- Use the smallest diameter rings that leave sufficient space for swelling after surgery because smaller rings give a more mechanically stable construct. There should be one

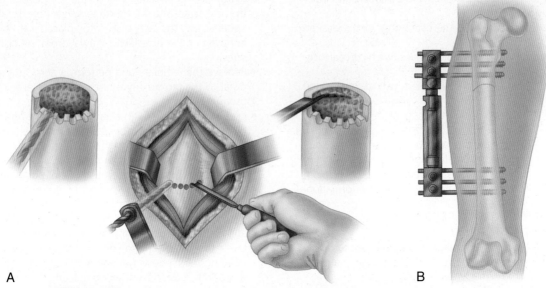

A   B

FIGURE 1.126 **A,** DeBastiani technique for corticotomy. Using limited open exposure and a 4- or 5-mm drill, multiple holes are drilled in anterior half of bone. These are connected with 5-mm osteotome, which also is used to complete corticotomy posteriorly. **B,** Orthofix device for femoral lengthening. To control varus deviation, three screws are used proximally and three distally, or frame can be applied with prophylactic valgus built into construct. **SEE TECHNIQUES 1.48 AND 1.49.**

fingerbreadth of space between the distal ring and the anterior thigh and two fingerbreadths posteriorly at the largest diameter of the posterior calf muscles. The distal-most ring can be a ⅝-inch ring to allow more knee flexion after surgery. This is especially important if there is to be a simultaneous lengthening of the ipsilateral tibia with proximal tibial rings. (Full rings would touch each other after relatively little knee flexion, limiting knee mobility.)

- Connect the bottom two rings initially with two 20-mm or 40-mm threaded hexagonal sockets for better stability, one positioned directly anteriorly and one directly posteriorly. With newer carbon fiber rings, it is possible to "cut out" the back portion of the distal ring as needed to improve knee flexion and to prevent impingement against a tibial construct. Appropriate reinforcement to the nearest ring is required before the carbon fiber ring is cut. In small patients, there may be room distally for only one ring and a drop wire.
- Plan the frame so that the central connection bolts are centered directly over the anterior and posterior midlines.
- Choose two parallel arcs to match the contour of the proximal lateral thigh, usually a 90-degree arc most proximally and a 120-degree arc below it; this causes less impingement of the proximal end of the fixator against the lower abdomen and pelvis during hip flexion.
- Connect the two arcs with two 40-mm hexagonal sockets. The reach of the 120-degree arc can be extended by attaching two oblique supports off the first and last holes on the arc.
- Attach the oblique support to the empty middle ring, which does not hold any wires but allows a more even 360-degree push-off between the distal and proximal fixation blocks.

- Connect the empty middle ring to the distal fixation block with two threaded rods, one placed anteriorly and one medially, to align the empty ring with the distal ring block anteriorly and medially where the soft-tissue sleeve of the thigh is minimal, and the larger, empty ring placed laterally and posteriorly where extra skin clearance is required. It may be necessary later to build out from the distal block laterally and posteriorly with short connection plates to have additional threaded rods or graduated telescopic rods in these locations.
- For placement of reference wires, position the patient supine with a folded sheet under the ipsilateral buttock. A radiolucent table that splits at the lower extremities, allowing removal of the part of the table under the involved leg, is helpful. Place the foot on a Mayo stand or other small table to permit flexion and extension of the knee and hip to allow assessment of acceptable placement of the wires in the soft tissues around the knee.
- Use fluoroscopy to guide insertion of the distal reference wire. In the distal femur, use 1.8-mm wires, and in the proximal femur, use 5-mm conical self-drilling, self-tapping screws. If preferred, other heavy-gauge half-pins, especially those designed to be predrilled, can be substituted. When using conical pins, be careful not to back them out once they have been inserted, or they will loosen.
- Under fluoroscopic control, insert as the distal reference wire an olive wire from lateral to medial, almost perpendicular to the mechanical axis of the femur, parallel to the knee joint, but slightly higher on the medial side at the level of the adductor tuberosity.
- For the proximal reference pin, insert a half-pin just distal to the level of the greater trochanter, parallel to an imaginary line drawn from the tip of the greater trochanter to

the center of the femoral head, normally within 3 degrees of parallel to the axis of the knee joint.

- The distal reference wire should be perpendicular to the mechanical axis of the femur, not perpendicular to the anatomic axis (Fig. 1.127A). This is important because lengthening should occur along the mechanical axis rather than the shaft axis. Failure to adhere to this principle disrupts the normal mechanical axis and causes medialization of the knee.
- Secure the preassembled frame to the top reference pin and bottom reference wire and ensure that clearance between the skin and the frame is adequate, and that all connections are tight.
- Tension the wires to 130 kg of force after fixing the olive end of the wire to the distal ring. Ensure adequate soft-tissue clearance and use the frame as a guide to insert the proximal half-pin secured with either a monopin fixation clamp or a buckle clamp (Fig. 1.127B and C).
- For fixation, insert two oblique smooth wires on the distal ring and one medial olive wire and an oblique smooth wire on the ring above.
- Some important technical points must be remembered while inserting the wires. When inserting a wire from the anterior to the posterior thigh, first flex the knee 45 degrees as the wire penetrates the anterior skin. Then flex the knee 90 degrees as the wire penetrates the quadriceps muscle. Drill the wire through the femur just to the opposite cortex. Tap the wire through the soft tissue, keeping the knee fully extended as the wire traverses the hamstrings; flex the knee to 45 degrees as the wire exits the skin.
- After each wire has been inserted, move the knee from full extension to 90 degrees of flexion. The wire should "float" in the soft tissue and should not be pulled by the muscle or cause tenting of the skin. This technique of wire placement helps minimize skin irritation and joint contractures.
- If a wire does not exit directly in the plane of the ring, build the ring up to the level of the wire with washers or posts. Do not bend the wire in any plane to make it lie closer to the ring.
- In the proximal arc, add one more pin anteriorly, on the opposite side of the arc, to avoid the reference pin. Do not insert this pin any more medially than the anterior superior iliac spine, or the femoral nerve will be at risk.
- On the second arc, place two additional pins, one on each side of the arc, in the oblique plane between the two top pins. The ideal mechanical placement of wires and pins should approach 90 degrees when viewed axially, within anatomic limits. A 90-degree fixation spread within a given ring or fixation block resists bending moments in a more uniform manner. Olive wires add mechanical strength to the construct but should not be overused. The olive wires function as fulcrums, acting on the bone to resist or correct axial deviation. Lengthening around the knee tends to angulate into valgus, whereas lengthening near the ankle and hip tends to angulate into varus. All sites are prone to anterior angulation. The olive wires in the femoral construct are placed strategically to resist valgus angulation. An additional olive wire can be placed opposite the lateral olive wire of the distal ring to lock the distal ring into place, if desired. More recently, an alternative method of distal ring fixation has been used, consisting of one transverse reference wire and two half-pins, one posteromedial and one posterolateral.

- For corticotomy, remove the anterior and medial connecting rods from between the empty ring and the distal fixation block.
- Make a ½-inch incision in the lateral skin just proximal to the distal fixation block. Incising the fascia lata transversely makes the lengthening process easier and diminishes the tendency for valgus angulation.
- Dissect bluntly down to the femur with Mayo scissors and insert a small, sharp periosteal elevator down to the lateral cortex of the femur.
- With a knife, make a longitudinal incision through the periosteum and use the elevator to strip a thin, 1-cm wide section of periosteum anterior and posterior, as much as can be reached.
- Transect the lateral cortex with a ½-inch osteotome; cut the anterior and posterior cortices, including the linea aspera, with a ¼-inch osteotome. Do not violate the medullary canal. Alternatively, make the corticotomy as described by DeBastiani (Fig. 1.126).
- To prevent medial cortex comminution and fracture extension into the distal wires, predrill three 3.2-mm holes in the medial cortex, inserting the drill from the lateral wound.
- Fracture the most medial cortex by bending the femur. Ensure that the fragments show enough motion to indicate complete corticotomy, but do not widely displace them.
- Reduce the fracture and align the proximal and distal fixation blocks parallel to each other.
- Use four upright, threaded rods or short, graduated, telescopic tubes to connect the distal fixation block to the empty ring (Fig. 1.127C). Complete the frame by adding components until there are four connectors between every arc or ring in the frame (Fig. 1.127D).
- Close the skin over a drain if needed and apply a pressure dressing to the lateral wound.
- Dress the wire and pin sites with sponges. Apply rubber stoppers to each wire and pin site before attaching them to the frame. The stoppers help maintain slight pressure on the pin dressings and minimize pin-skin interface motion, which is a prelude to pin site infection. Wrap the proximal four pins tightly with stretch gauze to minimize skin motion over these pins.

POSTOPERATIVE CARE Physical therapy and protected weight bearing with crutches are begun immediately. Knee flexion of at least 45 to 75 degrees is encouraged, but the knee is splinted in extension at night. Lengthening is begun at 4 to 6 days after surgery, depending on the age of the child, and progresses at a rate of 0.25 mm four times daily. The patient and family are taught how to lengthen before discharge from the hospital, and a record of lengthening should be maintained. Although lengthening at precisely every 6 hours is desirable, it is far more practical to lengthen at breakfast, lunch, dinner, and bedtime. A preoperative lateral view of the knee is essential to help judge early signs of subluxation, especially during large lengthenings in patients with congenital deficiencies of the femur. Radiographs should be made 7 to 10 days after lengthening is begun to ensure distraction of the corticotomy. If insufficient regenerated bone is present after 4 to 6 weeks, the rate of distraction can be adjusted.

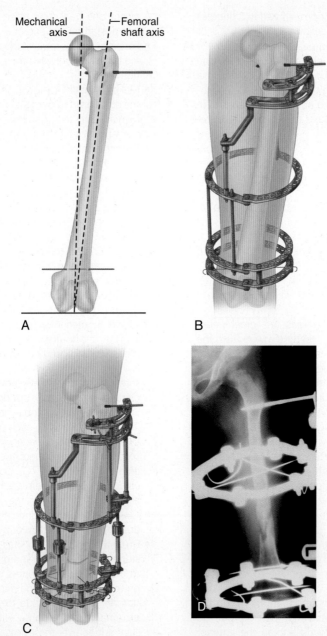

FIGURE 1.127 Application of Ilizarov frame (see text). **A,** Frame is applied perpendicular to mechanical axis, not femoral shaft axis. Distally, reference wire is placed parallel to femoral condyles. Proximally, reference pin is drilled perpendicular to mechanical axis. **B,** Ilizarov femoral lengthening frame is constructed on proximal and distal reference pins. Middle ring is larger in diameter than distal two rings to accommodate conical shape of thigh. **C,** Completed femoral frame. Graduated telescopic distractors are placed in alternating up-down position for greater stability. Olive wires add greater stability to construct. "Empty" middle ring serves as even push-off point. **D,** Modified Ilizarov frame in place after femoral corticotomy for lengthening. **SEE TECHNIQUE 1.49.**

When the desired length has been achieved, the fixator is kept in place until there is corticalization of the regenerated bone. Some surgeons "train" the regenerated bone before fixator removal by placing it under slight compression or by retensioning the wires. Weight bearing and fixator stability are crucial factors in producing healthy regenerated bone. At the time of fixator removal, the knee can be manipulated if necessary, but only before removal of the device. Protected weight bearing and vigorous physical therapy are continued, and activity is increased gradually. When lengthening is complete, knee motion typically is limited to about 40 degrees, but after the frame is removed, motion usually is regained at the rate of 10 to 15 degrees a month.

The Ilizarov frame and application can be modified to correct deviation of the mechanical axis or deformity of the proximal femur. Hinges can be placed at the lengthening corticotomy site to effect angular correction. Proximal deformities can be immediately corrected by percutaneous osteotomy between the two proximal arcs. The arcs are initially angulated relative to one another, the osteotomy is performed, and the arcs are immediately brought into parallel alignment to effect the desired correction. Rotational corrections are best done acutely through a proximal (subtrochanteric) osteotomy at the time of initial frame application. The Taylor Spatial Frame also may be used for distraction osteogenesis.

FEMORAL LENGTHENING OVER INTRAMEDULLARY NAIL (PRECICE)

TECHNIQUE 1.50

(STANDARD, HERZENBERG, AND GREEN)
- Venting of the femur is done as described for tibial lengthening (see Technique 1.47).
- Place the patient supine or in the lateral decubitus position, depending on surgeon preference and prepare and drape the leg from the anterior superior iliac spine to the proximal tibia.
- Make an osteotomy at the junction of the proximal and middle thirds of the femur unless preexisting bony deformity requires particular positioning of the osteotomy for acute angular correction. As with the tibial technique, do not make the osteotomy in the proximal or distal metaphyseal areas (Fig. 1.128).
- Trochanteric and piriformis entry nails are available. Piriformis entry should be used only on skeletally mature patients because of the risk of osteonecrosis. Alternatively, retrograde nailing combined with distally placed corticotomy can be used (Fig. 1.129).
- Make a 7- to 10-mm incision proximal to the greater trochanter; continue dissection until the tip of the greater trochanter can be palpated. Divide the fibers of the iliotibial band exactly in the middle of the trochanter.
- Check the dimensions of the trochanter by palpation to locate the insertion in the midline; the ideal position is in the piriformis fossa, close to its lateral wall, just medial to the greater trochanter. To avoid injury to the circumflex femoral artery, ensure that the insertion site is not too medial.

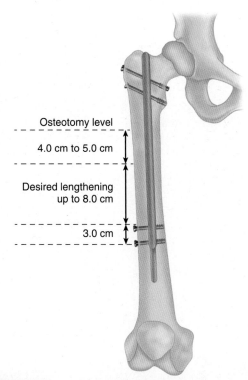

Osteotomy level

4.0 cm to 5.0 cm

Desired lengthening up to 8.0 cm

3.0 cm

FIGURE 1.128 Osteotomies for femoral lengthening with intramedullary skeletal kinetic distractor (see text). (From Cole JD: Intramedullary skeletal kinetic distractor: femoral surgical technique: technique manual, Orthofix, McKinney, TX.) **SEE TECHNIQUE 1.50.**

- Using a Kirschner wire and cannulated reamer, create the entry to the piriformis fossa just medial to the trochanter, insert the reamer 1 to 2 cm, and check its position with image intensification to ensure that the tip of the reamer is directly in line with the axis of the diaphysis in the frontal and the sagittal planes.
- When correct position is verified, using gentle pressure and rotational movement, advance the reamer into the femoral canal for 3 to 4 cm, keeping the straight part of the handle in line with the diaphysis.
- Position the guidewire centrally and drive it down until its tip sits in the subchondral bone exactly on the roof of the intercondylar notch, midway between the femoral condyles.
- Starting with an 8-mm reamer, ream the medullary canal with increasingly larger reamers (0.5-mm increments) until a width of 2 mm larger than the proposed lengthener diameter has been obtained.
- Insert the PRECICE nail to the level of the corticotomy.
- Perform the corticotomy as described for the tibial nail (see Technique 1.47).
- Insert the distal and proximal locking screws as described for the tibial nail (see Technique 1.47).

INTRAOPERATIVE EXTERNAL REMOTE CONTROL DISTRACTION
- Perform intraoperative external remote control (ERC) distraction as described for the tibial nail (see Technique 1.47).

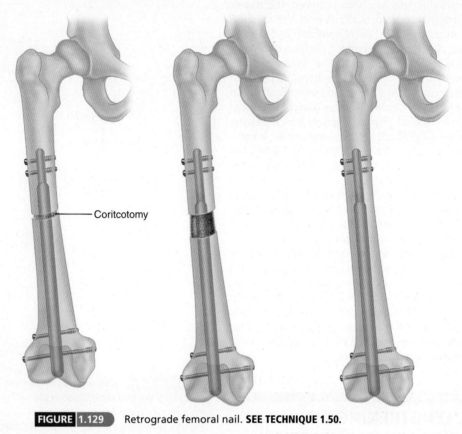

Coritcotomy

FIGURE 1.129 Retrograde femoral nail. **SEE TECHNIQUE 1.50.**

■ Remove the drill guide and close the incisions in usual fashion. Generally, suction drainage is needed in only the proximal incision (entry portal). Apply a compression dressing and an elastic bandage wrapped around the hip, starting from the foot, to avoid wound seroma.

POSTOPERATIVE CARE The drain is removed at 24 to 48 hours after surgery. Partial weight bearing with crutches is allowed after 1 week; full weight bearing is not allowed until cortication of the regenerated bone is visible in three of four cortices during the end of the consolidation phase (Fig. 1.130). Isometric exercises are begun early, and gentle knee mobilization can be initiated at about 4 days. Lengthening is initiated 5 to 7 days after surgery (see Postoperative Care for Technique 1.47).

Complications of Lengthening. All types of limb-lengthening devices and techniques have some complications in common, but certain complications are more or less likely to occur with a given device.

Pin Track Infection. The most common problem is pin track infection, which can be minimized by careful pin insertion. Thin wires should be inserted through the skin directly at the level that the wire enters bone to prevent tenting of the skin. At the end of the procedure, moving the nearby joints through a full range of motion identifies skin tenting over wires, and the sites can be released with a scalpel. The thin transfixion wires may cause fewer problems than the large half-pins, but skin and muscle motion over any wire or pin should be minimized by special dressing techniques. For thin-wire fixators, commercially available 1-inch foam cubes with a slit are placed around the pin site. The slit is stapled to hold the cube in place. Finally, a clip or previously applied rubber stopper is lowered onto the foam to apply mild pressure on the skin. Excessive pressure should be avoided, however, because it can cause ulcerations, especially over bony prominences. For large pins, especially in the thigh, surgical gauze can be wrapped snugly around two or more neighboring pins to apply pressure to the skin around the pins. All wire and pin care should include daily sterilization with an antiseptic, such as povidone-iodine (Betadine) or chlorhexidine gluconate (Hibistat), but only a small amount (1 mL per pin) should be used to avoid skin irritation. If the skin becomes irritated, the solution can be diluted, or a nonirritating antibiotic ointment, such as polymyxin B sulfate-neomycin sulfate (Neosporin), can be used.

At the first sign of pin track infection, broad-spectrum antibiotics should be given, local pin care should be intensified, and the pin site should be incised to promote drainage if necessary. If the infection does not improve with these measures, the pin may have to be removed. If pin removal jeopardizes the stability of the frame, a replacement pin should be inserted. With the Ilizarov apparatus, this is relatively simple: a wire can be placed in a nearby hole or dropped off the ring on a post to avoid the infected pin site. With monolateral fixators, insertion of a replacement pin away from the infected site is more difficult. The Orthofix supplemental screw device can be useful for inserting additional half-pins off-axis. Severe infection usually requires curettage of the pin track and bone.

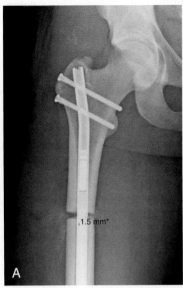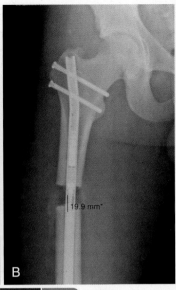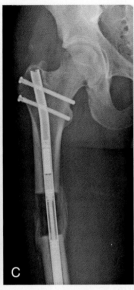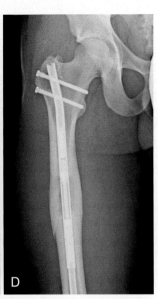

A   B   C   D

FIGURE **1.130**   Distraction osteogenesis with Precice nail.

Muscular Problems. The most difficult complications that occur during lengthening are related to the muscles. Theoretically, the bones can be lengthened by any amount, but the muscles have a limited ability to stretch. Typically, the muscles that cause the most problems are the triceps surae during tibial lengthening and the quadriceps or hamstrings during femoral lengthening. Decreased knee flexion or obligate lateral patellar dislocation with knee flexion after femoral lengthening may require a quadricepsplasty if therapy alone proves insufficient to achieve the desired range of motion. Knee flexion contracture is common during tibial lengthening and can be prevented with prophylactic splinting, especially at night. Custom orthoses or commercially available Dynasplints (Dynasplint Systems, Severna Park, MD) are helpful, and vigorous, frequent physical therapy is crucial. Prophylactic treatment should be started within 1 week of the original surgery. For tibial lengthenings of more than 4 to 5 cm, the foot should be fixed in neutral position by applying a posterior splint for monolateral fixators or by placing two wires in the heel and connecting them to a ring attached to the frame of a thin-wire circular fixator. The heel pins should be removed as soon as possible after lengthening is complete (provided that the knee is not contracted) to allow the subtalar and ankle joints to regain motion. Lengthening of the Achilles tendon should be considered if residual contracture persists. Any preoperative contracture of the Achilles tendon should be corrected before or during tibial lengthening. Muscular contracture and tightness may be improved with botulinum toxin A, which has shown promise as adjunct treatment during lengthening to decrease pain and reduce the number of pin-site infections.

Joint Problems. Joint subluxation or dislocation has been reported during femoral lengthening, especially if either the hip or the knee joint is unstable before surgery (as is frequently the case in patients with PFFD). In patients with congenital deformities, prophylactic tenotomies of the rectus femoris proximally, the adductors, and sometimes the hamstrings can be useful. For hips with varus deformities, corrective valgus osteotomy should be delayed until after lengthening. As a general rule, the hip radiograph should show a center-edge angle of at least 15 to 20 degrees before femoral lengthening is considered;

otherwise, a preliminary pelvic osteotomy may be necessary. The cruciate ligaments generally are deficient in patients with PFFD, making knee subluxation more likely, and prophylactic fixation of the knee joint with a mobile hinge is possible with the Ilizarov apparatus. A posteriorly dislocated tibia can be slowly pulled anteriorly with a mobile Ilizarov hinge on a rail to reduce the dislocation and allow knee motion. With monolateral fixators, these options are unavailable. For hip subluxation, traction and bed rest usually are sufficient.

Neurovascular Problems. Neurovascular complications usually are related to faulty pin placement but may result from stretching during lengthening. If the rate of distraction is 1 mm/d, neurovascular tissues almost always are able to stretch to accommodate the lengthening. Decreasing or temporarily stopping the distraction usually is sufficient. If a cutaneous nerve is tented over a wire or pin, removal of the pin is indicated. Peroneal nerve dysfunction that occurs during tibial lengthening should be treated by nerve decompression at the fibular head, extending proximally 5 to 7 cm and distally into the anterior compartment.

Bony Problems. Bony complications of distraction osteogenesis include premature consolidation and delayed consolidation. In Wagner lengthening, common problems are deep infection, pseudarthrosis, plate breakage, and malunion. With distraction osteogenesis by either the Ilizarov or the DeBastiani technique, delayed or premature consolidation usually can be resolved without compromising a satisfactory result. Premature consolidation is caused by an excessive latency period. For femoral lengthening in children, a latency period of 5 days is recommended, and for tibial lengthening, 7 days is recommended. For older patients and patients with compromised vascularity to the limb, longer latency periods may be appropriate. Premature consolidation of the fibula in tibial lengthenings can be prevented by using a standard open osteotomy of the fibula instead of a corticotomy. In some reports of premature consolidation, patients reported successively difficult lengthening until finally a "pop" was felt, followed by brief but intense pain, indicating spontaneous rupture through the consolidated regenerated bone. The bone ends should be brought back to the level of apposition before the rupture, and after a brief latency period, lengthening is resumed. Failure to "back up" can result in cyst formation and nonunion.

Delayed consolidation is more common with diaphyseal lengthening than with metaphyseal corticotomy. Contributing factors include frame instability, overly vigorous corticotomy with excessive periosteal stripping, and a distraction rate that is too rapid, especially after too brief a latency period. Gigli saw osteotomies in thick diaphyseal cortical bone can lead to delayed healing. Underlying medical or nutritional problems and lack of exercise are other contributing factors. In addition to correcting these factors, distraction can be slowed or stopped, the bone can be compressed, or the bone can be alternately compressed and lengthened. Walking and normal use of the limb should always be encouraged. In adults and older children, the best regenerated bone develops in patients who are active and use analgesics sparingly. Autologous cancellous bone grafting of the gap is a final resort, although recent studies have demonstrated some efficacy with an injection of autologous bone marrow aspirate combined with platelet rich plasma.

Extra precautions should be taken during the preparation and draping of the fixator because the pin sites may harbor bacteria. With Wagner lengthening, bone grafting of the gap is expected, but it is easier to drape the monolateral fixators out of the sterile operative site.

Malunion and Axial Deviation. Malunion and axial deviation can be avoided with careful preoperative planning to prevent the introduction of deformity during the lengthening. It is important to remember that intramedullary devices lengthen along the anatomic axis of the bone rather than the mechanical axis of the limb, and this should be taken into consideration when planning the rod insertion, osteotomy level, and direction of initial osteotomy displacement. Malunion also can occur with bending of the regenerate. This often can be avoided by maintaining the rod or external device until adequate consolidation has occurred or with the use of supplemental plate fixation or rodding after the desired length has been obtained in the case of external ring fixator lengthening procedures.

REFERENCES

ANOMALIES OF THE TOES

Bor N, Rozen N, Rubin G: Treatment of longitudinal epiphyseal bracket by excision and polymethylmethacrylate insertion at the preossified disease state, *J Foot Ankle Surg* 54:1136, 2015.

Choo AD, Mubarak SJ: Longitudinal epiphyseal bracket, *J Child Orthop* 7:449, 2013.

Hop MJ, van der Biezen JJ: Ray reduction of the foot in the treatment of macrodactyly and review of the literature, *J Foot Ankle Surg* 50:434, 2011.

Downey-Carmona FJ, Lagares A, Farrington-Rueda D, et al.: Island nail flap in the treatment of foot macrodactyly of the first ray in children: report of two cases, *J Child Orthop* 9:281, 2015.

Kubat O, Anticevic D: Does timing of surgery influence the long-term results of foot polydactyly treatment? *Foot Ankle Surg* 24:353, 2018.

Morrell NT, Fitzpatrick J, Szalay EA: The use of the Tsuge procedure for pedal macrodactyly: relevance in pediatric orthopedics, *J Pediatr Orthop B* 23:260, 2014.

Seok HH, Park JU, Kwo ST: New classification of polydactyly of the foot on the basis of syndactylism, axis deviation, and metatarsal extent of extra digit, *Arch Plast Surg* 40:232, 2013.

ANOMALIES OF THE FOOT

CONGENITAL METATARSUS ADDUCTUS.

Aiyer AA, Shariff R, Ying L, et al.: Prevalence of metatarsus adductus in patients under going hallux valgus surgery, *Foot Ankle Int* 35:1292, 2014.

Dawoddi AI, Perera A: Radiological assessment of metatarsus adductus, *Foot Ankle Surg* 18:1, 2012.

Herzenberg JE, Burghardt RD: Resistant metatarsus adductus: prospective randomized trial of casting versus orthosis, *J Orthop Sci* 19:250, 2014.

Knörr J, Soldado F, Pham TT, Torres A, Cahuzac JP, De Gauzy JS: Percutaneous correction of persistent severe metatarsus adductus in children. *J Pediatr Orthop.*; 34:447, 2014.

CLUBFOOT

Agarwal A, Gupta N: Does initial Pirani score and age influence number of Ponseti casts in children? *Int Orthop* 38:569, 2014.

Ahmed AA: The use of the Ilizarov method in management of relapsed club foot, *Orthopedics* 33:881, 2010.

Al-Aubaidi Z, Lundgaard B, Pedersen NW: Anterior distal tibial epiphysiodesis for the treatment of recurrent equinus deformity after surgical treatment of clubfeet, *J Pediatr Orthop* 31:716, 2011.

Alkar F, Louahem D, Bonnet F, et al.: Long-term results after extensive soft tissue release in very severe congenital clubfeet, *J Pediatr Orthop* 37:500, 2017.

Bashi RH, Baghdadi T, Shirazi MR, et al.: Modified Ponseti method of treatment for correction of neglected clubfoot in older children and adolescents—a preliminary report, *J Pediatr Orthop B* 25:99, 2016.

Bhargava SK, Tandon A, Prakash M, et al.: Radiography and sonography of clubfoot: a comparative study, *Indian J Orthop* 46:229, 2012.

Brazell C, Carry PM, Jones A, et al.: Dimeglio score predicts treatment difficulty during Ponseti casting for isolated clubfoot, *J Pediatr Orthop* 39:e402, 2019.

Chand S, Mehtani A, Sud A, et al.: Relapse following use of Ponseti method in idiopathic clubfoot, *J Child Orthop* 12:566, 2018.

Chen C, Kaushal N, Scher DM, et al.: Clubfoot etiology: a meta-analysis and systematic review of observational and randomized trials, *J Pediatr Orthop* 38:e462, 2018.

Chu A, Labar AS, Sala DA, et al.: Clubfoot classification: correlation with Ponseti cast treatment, *J Pediatr Orthop* 30:695, 2010.

Dragnoi M, Farsetti P, Vena G, et al.: Ponseti treatment of rigid residual deformity in congenital clubfoot after walking age, *J Bone Joint Surg Am* 98:1706, 2016.

El-Adwar KL, Taha Kotb H: The role of ultrasound in clubfoot treatment: correlation with the Pirani score and assessment of the Ponseti method, *Clin Orthop Relat Res* 468:2495, 2010.

El-Sherbini MH, Omran AA: Midterm follow-up of talectomy for severe rigid equinovarus feet, *J Foot Ankle Surg* 54:1093, 2015.

Faizan M, Jilani LZ, Abbas M, et al.: Management of idiopathic clubfoot by Ponseti technique in children presenting after one year of age, *J Foot Ankle Surg* 54:967, 2015.

Ferreira GF, Stéfani KC, Haje DP, et al.: The Ponseti method in children with clubfoot after walking age—systematic review and meta-analysis of observational studies, *PLoS One* 13:e0207153, 2018.

Ganesan B, Luximon A, Al-Jumaily A, et al.: Ponseti method in the management of clubfoot under 2 years of age: a systematic review, *PLoS One* 12:e0178299, 2017.

Ganger R, Radler C, Handlbauer A, Grill F: External fixation in clubfoot treatment—a review of the literature, *J Pediatr Orthop B* 21:52, 2012.

Gao R, Tomlinson M, Walker C: Correlation of Pirani and Dimeglio scores with number of Ponseti casts required for clubfoot correction, *J Pediatr Orthop* 34:639, 2014.

Graf A, Hassani S, Krzak J, et al.: Long-term outcome evaluation in young adults following clubfoot surgical release, *J Pediatr Orthop* 30:379, 2010.

Gray K, Barnes E, Gibbons P, et al.: Unilateral versus bilateral clubfoot: an analysis of severity and correlation, *J Pediatr Orthop B* 23:397, 2014.

Gray K, Gibbons P, Little D, Burns J: Bilateral clubfeet are highly correlated: a cautionary tale for researchers, *Clin Orthop Relat Res* 472:3517, 2014.

Harnett P, Freeman R, Harrison WJ, et al.: An accelerated Ponseti versus the standard Ponseti method: a prospective randomised controlled trial, *J Bone Joint Surg* 93:404, 2011.

Hassan FO, Jabaiti S, El tamimi T: Complete subtalar release for older children who had recurrent clubfoot deformity, *Foot Ankle Surg* 16:38, 2010.

Hsu LP, Dias LS, Swaroop VT: Long-term retrospective study of patients with idiopathic clubfoot treated with posterior medial-lateral releases, *J Bone Joint Surg* 95:e27, 2013.

Hui C, Joughin E, Nettel-Aguirre A, et al.: Comparison of cast materials for the treatment of congenital idiopathic clubfoot using the Ponseti method: a prospective randomized controlled trial, *Can J Surg* 57:247, 2014.

Jain S, Ajmera A, Solanki M, et al.: Interobserver variability in Pirani clubfoot severity scoring system between the orthopedic surgeons, *Indian J Orthop* 51:81, 2017.

Jeans KA, Karol LA, Erdman AL, et al.: Functional outcomes following treatment for clubfoot: ten-year follow-up, *J Bone Joint Surg Am* 100:2018, 2015.

Josse A, Fraisse B, Marleix S, et al.: Correlations between physical and ultrasound findings in congenital clubfoot at birth, *Orthop Traumatol Surg Res* 104:651, 2018.

Jowett CR, Morcuende JA, Ramachandran M: Management of congenital talipes equinovarus using the Ponseti method: a systematic review, *J Bone Joint Surg* 93:1160, 2011.

Little Z, Yeo A, Gelfer Y: Poor evertor muscle activity is a predictor of recurrence in idiopathic clubfoot treated by the Ponseti method: a prospective longitudinal studyd with a 5-year follow-up, *J Pediatr Orthop* 39(6):e467, 2019.

Mahan ST, Spencer SA, Kasser JR: Satisfactory patient-based outcomes after surgical treatment for idiopathic clubfoot: includes surgeon's individualized technique, *J Pediatr Orthop* 34:631, 2014.

Mandlecha P, Kanojia RK, Champawat VS, et al.: Evaluation of modified Ponseti technique in treatment of complex clubfeet, *J Clin Orthop Trauma* 10:599, 2018.

Maripuri SN, Gallacher PD, Bridgens J, et al.: Ponseti casting for club foot—above—or below-knee?: A prospective randomised clinical trial, *Bone Joint J* 95B:1570, 2013.

McKay SD, Dolan LA, Morcuende JA: Treatment results of late-relapsing idiopathic clubfoot previously treated with the Ponseti method, *J Pediatr Orthop* 32:406, 2012.

Merrill LJ, Gurnett CA, Siegel M, et al.: Vascular abnormalities correlate with decreased soft tissue volumes in idiopathic clubfoot, *Clin Orthop Relat Res* 469:1442, 2011.

Miron MC, Grimard G: Ultrasound evaluation of foot deformities in infants, *Pediatr Radiol* 46:193, 2016.

Morgenstein A, Davis R, Talwalkar V, et al.: A randomized clinical trial comparing reported and measured wear rates in clubfoot bracing using a novel pressure sensor, *J Pediatr Orthop* 35:185, 2015.

Saghieh S, Bashoura A, Berjawi G, et al.: The correction of the replaced club foot by closed distraction, *Strategies Trauma Limb Reconstr* 5:127, 2010.

Smith PA, Kuo KN, Graf AN, et al.: Long-term results of comprehensive clubfoot release versus the Ponseti method: which is better? *Clin Orthop Relat Res* 472:1281, 2014.

Thapa MM, Pruthi S, Chew FS: Radiographic assessment of pediatric foot alignment: review, *AJR Am J Roentgenol* 194:S51, 2010.

Thomas HM, Sangiorgio SN, Ebramzadeh E, et al.: Relapse rates in patients with clubfoot treated using the Ponseti method increase with time: a systematic review, *JBJS Rev* 7:e6, 2019.

Tripathy SK, Saini R, Sudes P, et al.: Application of the Ponseti principle for deformity correction in neglected and relapsed clubfoot using the Ilizarov fixator, *J Pediatr Orthop B* 20:26, 2011.

Van Bosse HJ: Treatment of the neglected and relapsed clubfoot, *Clin Podiatr Med Surg* 30:513, 2013.

Xu RJ: A modified Ponseti method for the treatment of idiopathic clubfoot: a preliminary report, *J Pediatr Orthop* 31:317, 2011.

Zhang W, Richards BS, Faulks ST, et al.: Initial severity rating of idiopathic clubfeet is an outcome predictor at age two years, *J Pediatr Orthop B* 21:16, 2012.

CONGENITAL VERTICAL TALUS

Alaee F, Boehm S, Dobbs MB: A new approach to the treatment of congenital vertical talus, *J Child Orthop* 1:165, 2007.

Aslani H, Sadigi A, Tabrizi A, et al.: Primary outcomes of the congenital vertical talus correction using the Dobbs method of serial casting and limited surgery, *J Child Orthop* 6:307, 2012.

Chalayon O, Adams A, Dobbs MB: Minimally invasive approach for the treatment of nonisolated congenital vertical talus, *J Bone Joint Surg* 94:e73, 2012.

David MG: Simultaneous correction of congenital vertical talus and talipes equinovarus using the Ponseti method, *J Foot Ankle Surg* 50:494, 2011.

Eberhardt O, Fernandez FF, Wirth T: The talar axis-first metatarsal base angle in CVT treatment: a comparison of idiopathic and nonidiopathic cases treated with the Dobbs method, *J Child Orthop* 6:491, 2012.

Merrill LJ, Gurnett CA, Connolly AM, et al.: Skeletal muscle abnormalities and genetic factors related to vertical talus, *Clin Orthop Relat Res* 469:1167, 2011.

Miller M, Dobbs MB: Congenital vertical talus: etiology and management, *J Am Acad Orthop Surg* 23:604, 2015.

Thometz JG, Zhu H, Liu XC, et al.: MRI pathoanatomy study of congenital vertical talus, *J Pediatr Orthop* 30:360, 2010.

Wright J, Coggings D, Maizen C, Ramachandran M: Reverse Ponseti-type treatment for children with congenital vertical talus: comparison between idiopathic and teratological patients, *Bone Joint J* 96B:274, 2014.

Yang JS, Dobbs MB: Treatment of congenital vertical talus: comparison of minimally invasive and extensive soft-tissue release procedures at minimum five-year follow-up, *J Bone Joint Surg Am* 97:1354, 2015.

TARSAL COALITION

Bauer T, Golano P, Hardy P: Endoscopic resection of a calcaneonavicular coalition, *Knee Surg Sports Traumatol Arthrosc* 18:669, 2010.

Birisik F, Demirel M, Bilgili F, et al.: The natural course of pain in patients with symptomatic tarsal coalitions: a retrospective clinical study, *Foot Ankle Surg* 26(2):228, 2020.

Crim J: Imaging of tarsal coalition, *Radiol Clin North Am* 46:1017, 2008.

Docquier PL, Maldaque P, Bouchard M: Tarsal coalition in paediatric patients, *Orthop Traumatol Surg Res* 105(1S):S123, 2019.

Edmonds WB, Wiley K, Panas K: Technique article: Tarsal coalition resection using Kirschner wires across the subtalar joint in a two-incision approach, *J Foot Ankle Surg* 58:337, 2019.

Guignand D, Journeau P, Mainrad-Simard L, et al.: Child calcaneonavicular coalitions: MRI diagnostic value in a 19-case series, *Orthop Traumatol Surg Res* 97:67, 2011.

Klammer G, Espinosa N, Iselin LD: Coalitions of the tarsal bones, *Foot Ankle Clin* 23:435, 2018.

Masquijo JJ, Jarvis J: Associated talocalcaneal and calcaneonavicular coalitions in the same foot, *J Pediatr Orthop B* 19:507, 2010.

Zaw H, Calder JD: Tarsal coalitions, *Foot Ankle Clin* 15:349, 2010.

CONGENITAL ANGULAR DEFORMITIES OF THE LEG AND CONGENITAL PSEUDARTHROSIS

Kesireddy N, Kheireldin RK, Lu A, et al.: Current treatment of congenital pseudarthrosis of the tibia: a systematic review and meta-analysis, *J Pediatr Orthop B* 27:541, 2018.

Kaufman SD, Fagg JA, Jones S, et al.: Limb lengthening in congenital posteromedial bow of the tibia, *Strategies Trauma Lim Reconstr* 7:147, 2012.

Paley D: Congenital pseudarthrosis of the tibia: biological and biomechanical considerations to achieve union and prevent refracture, *J Child Orthop* 13:120, 2019.

Richards BS, Anderson TD: rhBMP-2 and intramedullary fixation in congenital pseudarthrosis of the tibia, *J Pediatr Orthop* 38:230, 2018.

Richards BS, Oetgen ME, Johnston CE: The use of rhBMP-2 for the treatment of congenital pseudarthrosis of the tibia: a case series, *J Bone Joint Surg* 92:177, 2010.

Shah H, Joseph B, Nair BVS, et al.: What factors influence union and refracture of congenital pseudarthrosis of the tibia? A multicenter long-term study, *J Pediatr Orthop* 38:e332, 2018.

Vanderstappen J, Lammens J, Berger P, et al.: Ilizarov bone transport as a treatment of congenital pseudarthrosis of the tibia: a long-term follow-up study, *J Child Orthop* 9:319, 2015.

Westberry DE, Carpenter AM, Tisch J, et al: Amputation outcomes in congenital pseudarthrosis of the tibia, *J Pediatr Orthop* 38:e475, 2018.

Zhu GH, Mei HB, He RG, et al.: Effect of distraction osteogenesis in patients with tibial shortening after initial union of congenital pseudarthrosis of the tibia (CPT): a preliminary study, *BMC Musculoskeletal Disord* 16:216, 2015.

CONSTRICTIONS OF THE LEG

Anathan A, Athalye JG, Du Plessis J, et al.: Amniotic band syndrome with pseudarthrosis of the tibia and fibula: a case report, *Ir Med J* 11:570, 2017.

Das SP, Sahoo P, Mohanty R, Das S: One-stage release of congenital constriction band in lower limb from new born to 3 years, *Indian J Orthop* 44:198, 2010.

Habenicht R, Hülsemann W, Lohmeyer JA, Mann M: Ten-year experience with one-step correction of constriction rings by complete circular resection and linear circumferential skin closure, *J Plast Reconstr Aesthet Surg* 66:1117, 2013.

Koskimies E, Syvänen J, Nietosvaara Y, et al.: Congenital constriction band syndrome with limb defects, *J Pediatr Orthop* 35:100, 2015.

CONGENITAL HYPEREXTENSION AND DISLOCATION OF THE KNEE, CONGENITAL DISLOCATION OF THE PATELLA

Johnston 2nd CE: Simultaneous open reduction of ipsilateral congenital dislocation of the hip and knee assisted by femoral diaphyseal shortening, *J Pediatr Orthop* 31:732, 2011.

Oetgen ME, Walick KS, Tulchin K, et al.: Functional results after surgical treatment for congenital knee dislocation, *J Pediatr Orthop* 30:216, 2010.

Sever R, Fishkin M, Hemo Y, et al.: Surgical treatment of congenital and obligatory dislocation of the patella in children, *J Pediatr Orthop,* 39(8):436, 2019.

Stewart D, Cheema A, Szalay EA: Dual 8-plate technique is not as effective as ablation for epiphysiodesis about the knee, *J Pediatr Orthop* 33:843, 2013.

Sud A, Kumar N, Mehtani A: Femoral shortening in the congenital dislocation of the knee joint: results of mid-term follow-up, *J Pediatr Orthop B* 22:440, 2013.

Tercier S, Shah H, Joseph B: Quadricepsplasty for congenital dislocation of the knee and congenital quadriceps contracture, *J Child Orthop* 6:397, 2012.

Youssef AO: Limited open quadriceps release for treatment of congenital dislocation of the knee, *J Pediatr Orthop* 37:192, 2017.

CONGENITAL LONG BONE DEFICIENCIES

TIBIAL AND FIBULAR HEMIMELIA, PROXIMAL FEMORAL FOCAL DEFICIENCY.

Birch JG, Lincoln TL, Mack PW, Birch CM: Congenital fibular deficiency: a review of thirty years' experience at one institution and a proposed classification system based on clinical deformity, *J Bone Joint Surg* 93B:1144, 2011.

Carvalho DR, Santos SC, Oliveira MD, Speck-Martins CE: Tibial hemimelia in Langer-Giedion syndrome in 8q23.1-q24.12 interstitial deletion, *Am J Med Genet A* 155A:2784, 2011.

Catagni MA, Radwan M, Lovisetti L, et al.: Limb lengthening and deformity correction by the Ilizarov technique in type III fibular hemimelia: an alternative to amputation, *Clin Orthop Relat Res* 469:1175, 2010.

Cho TJ, Baek GH, Lee HR, et al.: Tibial hemimelia-polydactyly-five –fingered hand syndrome associated with a 404 G>A mutation in a distant sonic hedgehog cis-regulator (ZRS): a case report, *J Pediatr Orthop B* 22:219, 2013.

Clinton R, Birch JG: Congenital tibial deficiency: a 37-year experience at 1 institution, *J Pediatr Orthop* 35:385, 2015.

Crawford DA, Tompkins BJ, Baird GO, Caskey PM: The long-term function of the knee in patients with fibular hemimelia and anterior cruciate ligament deficiency, *J Bone Joint Surg* 94:328, 2012.

Kowalczyk B, Kuznik-Buziewica A: Outcomes and subjective assessment of rotation-plasty in patients with proximal femoral focal deficiency, *J Pediatr Orthop B* 27:503, 2018.

Mascarenhas R, Simon D, Forsythe B, Harner CD: ACL reconstruction in a teenage athlete with fibular hemimelia, *Knee* 21:613, 2014.

Mishima K, Kitoh H, Iwata K, et al.: Clinical results and complications of lower limb lengthening for fibular hemimelia: a report of eight cases, *Medicine (Baltimore)* 95:e3787, 2016.

Paley D: Tibial hemimelia: new classification and reconstructive options, *J Child Orthop* 10:529, 2016.

Paley D: Surgical reconstruction for fibular hemimelia, *J Child Orthop* 10:557, 2016.

Radhakrishna VN, Madhuri V, Palocaren T: Optimizing the use of fibula in type II tibial hemimelia: early results, *J Pediatr Orthop B* 28:144, 2019.

Szymczuk VL, Hammouda AI, Gesheff MG, et al.: Lengthening with monolateral external fixation versus magnetically motorized intramedullary nail in congenital femoral deficiency, *J Pediatr Orthop* 39(9):458, 2019.

Wada A, Nakamura T, Fujii T, et al.: Limb salvage treatment for Gollop-Wolfgang complex (femoral bifurcation complete tibial hemimelia, and hand ectrodactyly), *J Pediatr Orthop B* 22:457, 2013.

Wada A, Nakamura T, Urano N, et al.: Foot centralization for tibial hemimelia, *J Pediatr Orthop B* 24:147, 2015.

LIMB-LENGTH DISCREPANCY

Bayhan IA, Karatas AF, Rogers KJ, et al.: Comparing percutaneous physeal epiphysiodesis and eight-plate epiphysiodesis for the treatment of limb length discrepancy, *J Pediatr Orthop* 37:323, 2017.

Burghardt RD, Herzenberg JE, Specht SC, Paley D: Mechanical failure of the intramedullary skeletal kinetic distractor in limb lengthening, *J Bone Joint Surg* 93:6839, 2011.

Burghardt RED, Specht SC, Herzenberg JE: Mechanical failures of eight-PlateGuided Growth System for temporary hemiepiphysiodesis, *J Pediatr Orthop* 30:594, 2010.

Cha SM, Shin HD, Kim KC, Song JH: Plating after tibial lengthening: unilateral monoaxial external fixator and locking plate, *J Pediatr Orthop B* 22:571, 2013.

Escott BG, Ravi B, Weathermon AC, et al.: EO low-dose radiography: reliable and accurate upright assessment of lower-limb lengths, *J Bone Joint Surg* 95A:e1831, 2013.

Gordon JE, Manske MC, Lewis TR, et al.: Femoral lengthening over a pediatric femoral nail: results and complications, *J Pediatr Orthop* 33:730, 2013.

Hammouda AI, Jauregui JJ, Gesheff MG, et al.: Treatment of post-traumatic femoral discrepancy with PRECICE magnetic-powered intramedullary lengthening nails, *J Orthop Trauma* 31:369, 2017.

Harbacheuski R, Fragomen AT, Rozbruch SR: Does lengthening and then plating (LAP) shorten duration of external fixation? *Clin Orthop Relat Res* 470:1771, 2012.

Hubbard EW, Liu RW, Iobst CA: Understanding skeletal growth and predicting limb-length in equality in pediatric patients, *J Am Acad Orthop Surg* 27:312, 2019.

Journeau P, Lascombes P, Barbier D, et al.: Residual bone growth after lengthening procedures, *J Child Orthop* 10:613, 2016.

Kenawey M, Krettek C, Liodakis E, et al.: Leg lengthening using intramedullary skeletal kinetic distraction: results of 57 consecutive applications, *Injury* 42:150, 2011.

Lee DH, Ryu KJ, Kim JW, et al.: Bone marrow aspirate concentrate and platelet-rich plasma enhanced bone healing in distraction osteogenesis of the tibia, *Clin Orthop Relat Res* 472:3789, 2014.

Lee DH, Ryu KJ, Song HR, Han SH: Complications of the intramedullary skeletal kinetic distractor (ISKD) in distraction osteogenesis, *Clin Orthop Relat Res* 472:3852, 2014.

Martin BD, Cherkashin AM, Tulchin K, et al.: Treatment of femoral lengthening-related knee stiffness with a novel quadricepsplasty, *J Pediatr Orthop* 33:446, 2013.

Park HW, Kim HW, Kwak YH, et al.: Ankle valgus deformity secondary to proximal migration of the fibula in tibial lengthening with use of the Ilizarov external fixator, *J Bone Joint Surg* 93:294, 2011.

Popkov D, Popkov A, Haumont T, et al.: Flexible intramedullary nail use in limb lengthening, *J Pediatr Orthop* 30:910, 2010.

Poutawera V, Stott NS: The reliability of computed tomography scanograms in the measurement of limb length discrepancy, *J Pediatr Orthop B* 19:42, 2010.

Schiedel F, Elsner U, Gosheger G, et al.: Prophylactic titanium elastic nailing (TEN) following femoral lengthening (lengthening then rodding) with one or two nails reduces the risk for secondary interventions after regenerate fractures: a cohort study in monolateral vs. bilateral lengthening procedures, *BMC Musculoskelet Disord* 14:302, 2013.

Shabtai L, Herzenberg JE: Limits of growth modulation using tension band plates in the lower extremities, *J Am Acad Orthop Surg* 24:691, 2016.

The complete list of references is available online at Expert Consult. com.

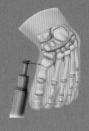
DEVELOPMENTAL DYSPLASIA OF THE HIP

Developmental dysplasia of the hip (DDH) generally includes subluxation (partial dislocation) of the femoral head or complete dislocation of the femoral head from the true acetabulum and acetabular dysplasia. In a newborn with true congenital dislocation of the hip, the femoral head can often be dislocated and reduced into and out of the true acetabulum. In an older child, the femoral head remains dislocated and secondary changes develop in the femoral head and acetabulum.

Historically, the incidence of DDH has been estimated to be approximately 1 in 1000 live births. A meta-analysis of the literature estimated the incidence of DDH to be 8.6 per 1000 revealed by physical examination by pediatricians; 11.5 per 1000 revealed by orthopaedic screening; and 25 per 1000 revealed by ultrasound examination. and for ultrasound examination, 25 per 1000. The estimated odds ratio for DDH for breech delivery was 5.5, for female sex, 4.1 and for positive family history, 1.7. Ultrasound screening of 18,060 hips detected 1001 that deviated from normal (incidence of 55.1 per 1000); however, only 90 hips remained abnormal at repeat examinations at 2 and 6 weeks, for a true DDH incidence of 5 per 1000. None of the other hips with "sonographic DDH" developed true DDH during 12-month follow-up. The left hip is more commonly involved than the right, and bilateral involvement is more common than involvement of the right hip alone.

Several risk factors should arouse suspicion of DDH. The disorder is more common in girls than in boys—in many series five times more common. Breech deliveries constitute 3% to 4% of all deliveries, and the incidence of DDH is significantly increased in this patient population. MacEwen and Ramsey in a study of 25,000 infants found the combination of female infants and breech presentation to result in DDH in one out of 35 such births. DDH is more common in firstborn children than in subsequent siblings. A family history of DDH increases the likelihood of this condition to approximately 10%. Ethnic background plays some role in that DDH is more common in white children than in black children. Other reported examples include the high incidence among Navajo Indians and the relatively low incidence among Chinese.

A strong association also exists between DDH and other musculoskeletal abnormalities, such as congenital torticollis, metatarsus adductus, and talipes calcaneovalgus. The coexistence rate of congenital muscular torticollis and DDH is approximately 8%, with boys nearly five times as likely to have both as girls. The relationship between DDH and clubfoot is controversial; however, multiple studies have demonstrated very little association between the presence of clubfoot and DDH. We recommend careful screening by performing hip physical examination in every infant who has a clubfoot deformity. Although we do not perform ultrasound routinely on all these babies, we have a low threshold to obtain a screening hip ultrasound evaluation in this patient population.

Several theories regarding the cause of DDH have been proposed, including mechanical factors, hormone-induced joint laxity, primary acetabular dysplasia, and genetic inheritance. Breech delivery, with the mechanical forces of abnormal flexion of the hips, can easily be seen as a cause of dislocation of the femoral head. The most common intrauterine position places the left hip of the fetus against the maternal sacrum. This could partially explain the increased incidence of DDH in the left hip. Prematurity is likely not an independent risk factor for DDH, but postnatal mechanical factors could play a role. An increased incidence of DDH has been reported in cultures that swaddle infants with the hip in constant extension.

Several authors have proposed ligamentous laxity as a contributing factor in DDH. The theory is that the influence of the maternal hormone relaxin, which produces relaxation of the pelvis during delivery, may cause enough ligamentous laxity in the child in utero and during the neonatal period to allow dislocation of the femoral head. This theory has credibility because relaxin has been shown to cross the placenta, and DDH is more common in females who are presumably more susceptible to the influences of relaxin.

Studies have demonstrated a familial occurrence of hip dysplasia. Therefore, hip dysplasia in a first- or second-degree relative should be considered an additional risk factor for DDH.

DIAGNOSIS AND CLINICAL PRESENTATION

The clinical presentation of DDH varies according to the age of the child. In newborns (<6 months old), it is especially important to perform a careful clinical examination because radiographs are not always reliable in making the diagnosis of developmental dysplasia in this age group.

The infant should be calm, relaxed, and pacified during the examination, and only one hip should be examined at a time. The hips should first be examined for limited abduction. In a child with a unilateral dislocation, hip abduction will be limited compared to the contralateral side. For the instability examination, the examiner places his or her hand around the infant's knees so that the thumb lies on the inner thigh and the index and long fingers lie along the lateral thigh near the level of the greater trochanter. The Ortolani test is performed by gently abducting the flexed hip while applying an anteromedially directed force to the greater trochanter to detect any reduction of the femoral head into the true acetabulum. The provocative maneuver of Barlow detects any potential subluxation or posterior dislocation of the femoral head by direct pressure on the longitudinal axis of the femur while the hip is in adduction. A palpable, rather than an audible, clunk is felt as the femoral head reduces into or subluxes out of the acetabulum (Fig. 2.1).

A child may be born with acetabular dysplasia without dislocation of the hip, and the latter may develop weeks or months later. Westin et al. reported the late development of

dislocation of the hip in children with normal neonatal clinical and radiographic examinations; they termed this *developmental dysplasia* as opposed to *congenital dysplasia* of the hip, as it was previously known.

As the child reaches age 6 to 18 months, several factors in the clinical presentation change. When the femoral head is dislocated and the ability to reduce it by abduction has disappeared, several other clinical signs become obvious. The first and most reliable is a decrease in the ability to abduct the dislocated hip because of a contracture of the adductor musculature (Fig. 2.2A). Asymmetric skin folds are commonly mentioned as a sign to look for, but this sign is not always reliable because normal children may have asymmetric skin folds and children with dislocated hips may have symmetric folds. In general, the rate of DDH is much higher in hips with at least one abnormal clinical finding than in hips without any. Limitation of abduction and asymmetric skin folds are the two most common findings.

The Galeazzi sign is noted when the femoral head becomes displaced not only laterally but also proximally, causing an apparent shortening of the femur on the side of the dislocated hip (Fig. 2.2B). Bilateral dislocations may appear symmetrically abnormal.

In a child of walking age with an undetected dislocated hip, families describe a "waddling" type of gait, indicating dislocation of the femoral head and a Trendelenburg gait pattern. Parents also may describe difficulty in abducting the hip during diaper changes.

SCREENING

The American Academy of Pediatrics recommends routine screening examination of all infants but does not recommend routine ultrasound evaluation of all newborns, although routine ultrasound screening is practiced in some health care systems in other countries. Research on universal ultrasound screening programs has found mixed results. Some studies suggest that children are treated earlier and have fewer surgeries when part of a universal screening program; however, other studies have suggested that many children received unnecessary referrals and treatments when universal screening programs were in place. Currently, referral to an orthopaedist is recommended with a positive newborn examination or a positive result at 2-week follow-up examination. Ultrasound is recommended for physical examination findings or risk factors that raise suspicion for DDH when the Ortolani and Barlow tests are negative; however, the ultrasound may be delayed until 6 weeks of age to decrease the chances of a false positive result in infants in whom the physical examination is normal and DDH is suspected solely on the basis of risk factors

The American Academy of Orthopaedic Surgeons developed clinical practice guidelines in 2014 for the detection and nonoperative management of pediatric DDH in infants up to 6 months of age. Their recommendations related to screening and imaging include the following:

1. Moderate evidence supports not performing universal ultrasound screening of newborn infants.
2. Moderate evidence supports performing an imaging study before 6 months of age in infants with one or more of the following risk factors: breech presentation, family history, or history of clinical instability.

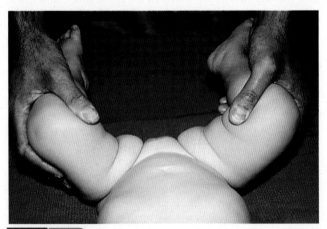

FIGURE 2.1 Ortolani maneuver for routine screening of congenital dislocation of hip. Examiner gently stabilizes infant's left hip and lower extremity and places left hand around right thigh and index and middle fingers over greater trochanter.

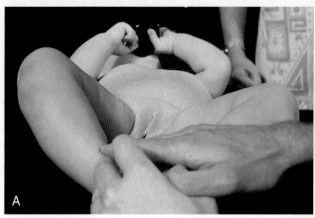

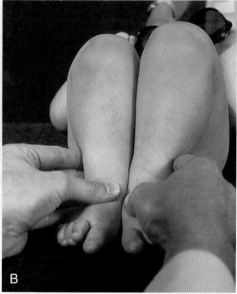

FIGURE 2.2 Clinical signs of congenital dislocation of hip in 13-month-old infant. **A,** Decrease in abduction of right hip with adduction contracture. **B,** Positive Galeazzi sign with apparent shortening of right lower extremity.

3. Limited evidence supports that the practitioner might obtain an ultrasound in infants younger than 6 weeks of age with a positive instability examination to guide the decision to initiate brace treatment.
4. Limited evidence supports the use of an anteroposterior pelvic radiograph instead of an ultrasound to assess DDH in infants beginning at 4 months of age.
5. Limited evidence supports that a practitioner reexamine infants previously screened as having a normal hip examination on subsequent visits prior to 6 months of age.
6. Limited evidence supports that the practitioner perform serial physical examinations and periodic imaging assessments (ultrasound or radiograph based on age) during management for unstable infant hips.

IMAGING

Many reports have evaluated the use of ultrasound screening of newborns for early diagnosis of DDH. The most comprehensive accounts of the anatomy of the infant hip by ultrasound are by Graf of Austria, who described the ultrasonographic anatomy of the newborn hip and devised an ultrasonographic classification for hip dysplasia (Fig. 2.3). Although ultrasound is noninvasive and relatively simple to use, many authors have emphasized that the examination is highly observer dependent and that it is easy to overdiagnose "dysplasia." In addition, ultrasound findings before 6 weeks of age can be questionable because of ligamentous laxity in the early newborn period; treatment before 6 weeks of age should be based on physical examination rather than ultrasound findings alone. Ultrasound diagnosis of "acetabular dysplasia" with a stable hip examination in the early postnatal period may result in unnecessary treatment. Nevertheless, ultrasound can be a useful adjunct to the physical examination and often is helpful in measuring and documenting the response of the hip to Pavlik harness treatment.

Although radiographs are not always reliable in making the diagnosis of DDH in newborns, screening radiographs may reveal any severe acetabular dysplasia or findings of a teratologic dislocation. As a child with a dislocated hip ages and the soft tissues become contracted, radiographs become more reliable and helpful in diagnosis and treatment (Fig. 2.4). The most commonly used lines of reference are the vertical line of Perkins and the horizontal line of Hilgenreiner, both used to assess the position of the femoral head. In addition, the Shenton line is disrupted in an older child with a dislocated hip. Normally, the metaphyseal beak of the proximal femur lies within the inner lower quadrant of the reference lines noted by Perkins and Hilgenreiner. The International Hip Dysplasia Institute (IHDI) has further refined this measurement, and various studies have shown excellent inter- and intra-rater reliability of this technique (Fig. 2.5). The acetabular index in a newborn generally is 30 degrees or less. Any significant increase in this measurement may be a sign of acetabular dysplasia. Three-dimensional imaging provides little diagnostic benefit for a newborn or toddler with DDH. However, CT or MRI can be helpful in preoperative planning or to evaluate the success of surgical intervention in older patients. Indications for three-dimensional imaging will be discussed with the various treatment options below.

TREATMENT

The treatment of DDH is age-related and tailored to the specific pathologic condition. Five age-related treatment groups have been designated: newborn (birth to 6 months old), infant (6 to 18 months old), toddler (18 to 36 months old), child (3 to 8 years old), and adolescent and young adult (>8 years old). There can be overlap in these age groups that requires modification of treatment plans.

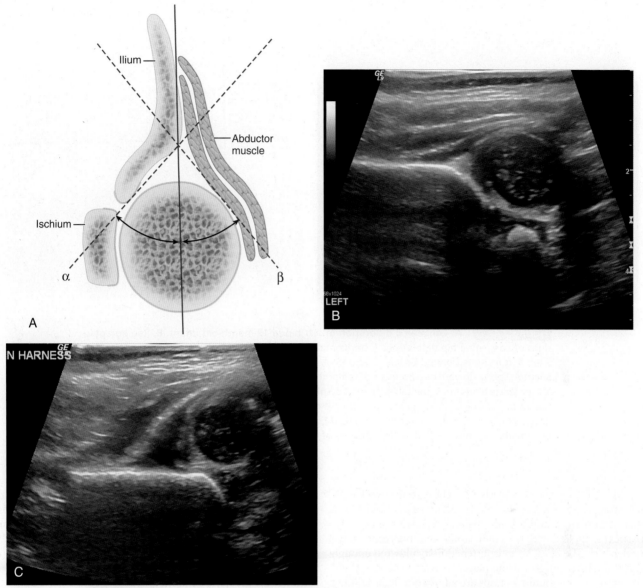

FIGURE 2.3 Ultrasonographic classification of hip dysplasia. **A,** Image is rotated 90 degrees clockwise to resemble a hip in the anteroposterior plane in a standing or supine child. Angle α is formed by the intersection of the baseline and the acetabular roofline; it is normally greater than 60 degrees. Angle β is formed by the intersection of the baseline and the inclination line; it is normally less than 55 degrees. In a normal hip, the baseline should bisect the femoral head. **B,** Ultrasound appearance of a normal hip: α angle of 60 degrees and baseline bisects the femoral head. **C,** Dislocated hip.

■ NEWBORN (BIRTH TO 6 MONTHS)

From birth to approximately 6 months old, treatment is directed at stabilizing the hip that has a positive Ortolani or Barlow test or reducing the dislocated hip with a mild-to-moderate adduction contracture. When the diagnosis has been made, either clinically or radiographically, it is essential to carefully evaluate the direction of dislocation, hip stability, and the reducibility of the hip before treatment. A success rate of 85% to 95% has been reported in children treated in the Pavlik harness during the first few months of life. As the child ages and soft-tissue contractures develop, along with secondary changes in the acetabulum, the success rate of the Pavlik harness decreases.

Attention to detail is required in the use of this harness because the potential complications include osteonecrosis of the femoral head, although this appears to occur in less than 1% of patients.

When properly applied and maintained, the Pavlik harness is a dynamic flexion-abduction orthosis that can produce excellent results in the treatment of dysplastic and dislocated hips in infants during the first few months. The harness is difficult to use in children who are crawling or who have fixed soft-tissue contractures and a fixed hip dislocation. If a teratologic dislocation is present, the Pavlik harness is unlikely to be successful, and other treatment options should be used.

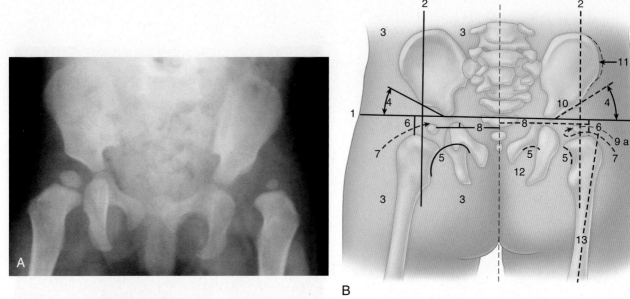

FIGURE 2.4 **A,** Congenital dislocation of left hip in 13-month-old infant. **B,** Radiographic signs of congenital hip dislocation. *1,* horizontal line (Hilgenreiner line); *2,* vertical line (Perkins line); *3,* quadrants (formed by lines *1* and *2*); *4,* acetabular index (Kleinberg and Lieberman); *5,* Shenton line; *6,* upward displacement of femoral head; *7,* lateral displacement of femoral head; *8,* Y coordinate (Ponseti); *9,* capital epiphyseal dysplasia (*a,* delayed appearance of center of ossification of femoral head; *b,* irregular maturation of center of ossification); *10,* bifurcation (furrowing of acetabular roof in late infancy, Ponseti); *11,* hypoplasia of pelvis (ilium); *12,* delayed fusion (ischiopubic juncture); *13,* adduction attitude of extremity.

The Pavlik harness consists of a chest strap, two shoulder straps, and two stirrups. Each stirrup has an anteromedial flexion strap and a posterolateral abduction strap. The harness is applied with the child supine and in a comfortable undershirt. The chest strap is fastened first, allowing enough room for three fingers to be placed between the chest and the harness. The shoulder straps are adjusted to maintain the chest strap at the nipple line. The feet are placed in the stirrups one at a time. The hip is placed in flexion (90 to 110 degrees), and the anterior flexion strap is tightened to maintain this position. Finally, the lateral strap is loosely fastened to limit adduction, not to force abduction. Excessive abduction to ensure stability is unacceptable. The knees should be 3 to 5 cm apart at full adduction in the harness (Fig. 2.6).

A radiograph of the patient in the harness can help to confirm that the femoral neck is directed toward the triradiate cartilage, but a radiograph is not routinely necessary because clinical examination and ultrasound usually are sufficient to monitor the success of treatment. During the first few weeks of harness wear, when the hip feels stable clinically, ultrasound evaluation is appropriate to confirm reduction of the hip.

Four basic patterns of persistent dislocation have been observed after application of the Pavlik harness: *superior, inferior, lateral,* and *posterior.* If the dislocation is superior, additional flexion of the hip is indicated. If the dislocation is inferior, a decrease in flexion is indicated. A lateral dislocation in the Pavlik harness should be observed initially. As long as the femoral neck is directed toward the triradiate cartilage, as

confirmed by radiograph or ultrasound, the head may gradually reduce and "dock" into the acetabulum. A persistent posterior dislocation is difficult to treat if it continues for more than a few weeks, and Pavlik harness treatment frequently is unsuccessful. Posterior dislocation is usually accompanied by tight hip adductor muscles and may be diagnosed by palpation of the greater trochanter posteriorly.

If any of these patterns of dislocation or subluxation persist for more than 3 to 6 weeks, treatment in the Pavlik harness should be discontinued and a new program initiated; in most patients, this consists of closed or open reduction and casting. Some studies, however, have demonstrated successful reduction in a rigid abduction orthosis when Pavlik harness treatment has failed (Fig. 2.7). The Pavlik harness should be worn 23 to 24 hours per day until stability is attained, as determined by negative Barlow and Ortolani tests. During this time, the patient is examined at 1- to 2-week intervals and the harness straps are adjusted to accommodate growth. The family is instructed in care of the child in the harness, including bathing, diapering, dressing, and the avoidance of restrictive swaddling. One study noted no difference in success rates between 23- and 24-hour per day brace wear, allowing for removal of the brace once a day for bathing with the compliant family.

Quadriceps function should be noted at each examination to detect a femoral nerve palsy, and families should be instructed to remove the legs from the brace daily to ensure that the infant is able to actively extend the knee against gravity. If a femoral nerve palsy develops, the brace should be

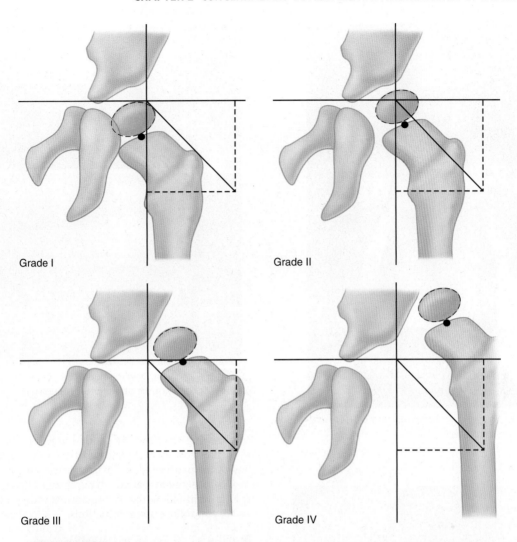

Grade I

Grade II

Grade III

Grade IV

FIGURE 2.5 The International Hip Dysplasia Institute (IHDI) Classification System utilizes the Hilgenreiner and Perkins lines to create four quadrants. The lower outer quadrant is then subdivided into two regions by a 45-degree line. The center of the proximal femoral metaphysis is used as the reference point that allows for utilization of the IHDI Classification before ossification of the ossific nucleus. Grade I is considered normal. Grades II to IV indicate varying degrees of subluxation or dislocation. (Redrawn from Narayanan U, Mulpuri K, Sankar WN, et al: Reliability of a new radiographic classification for developmental dysplasia of the hip, *J Pediatr Orthop* 35(5):478, 2015.)

discontinued until full motor function returns. The duration of treatment depends on the patient's age at diagnosis and the degree of hip instability. There are very few guidelines for brace discontinuation. Recommendations vary from abrupt discontinuation of the Pavlik harness 6 weeks after clinical stability has been obtained, to weaning of up to 2 hours per week until the brace is worn only at night, to transitioning to a nighttime abduction orthosis for additional weeks or months.

Radiographic or ultrasound documentation can be used throughout the treatment period to verify the position of the hip. Ultrasonographic evaluation is useful at the following times: immediately after the initiation of treatment, after any major adjustment in the harness, when the hip examination is stable after beginning Pavlik harness treatment, and 6 weeks after the hip stabilizes clinically or at the time weaning begins. Radiographs are useful at the age of 6 months old as well as at 1 year (Fig. 2.8).

Suggested risk factors for Pavlik harness failure include absent Ortolani sign at initial evaluation (irreducible dislocation), bilateral hip dislocations, the development of a femoral nerve palsy during Pavlik treatment, an acetabular angle of 36 degrees or more on a radiograph, irreducible hips, initial coverage of less than 20% (as determined by ultrasound), and delay of Pavlik harness treatment beyond 7 weeks of age. Failure of Pavlik harness management of developmental dislocation of the hip commonly indicates a need for closed or open reduction and a more dysplastic acetabulum. However, a trial with a rigid abduction orthosis can be attempted for a few weeks in patients in whom Pavlik harness treatment has failed, with some studies indicating occasional successful reduction in these patients.

In multiple series of dislocated hips reduced with the use of the Pavlik harness, the more severe the dislocation, the higher the rates of failed reduction and osteonecrosis,

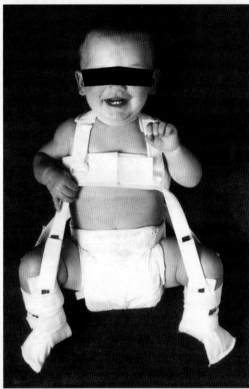

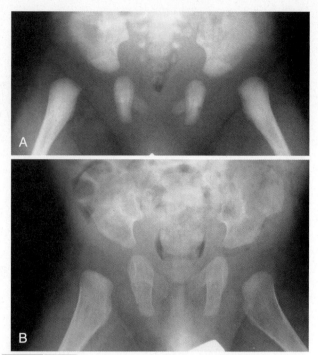

FIGURE 2.8 **A,** Developmental dislocation of hip in 2-month-old boy. **B,** At 5 months of age after reduction in Pavlik harness.

FIGURE 2.6 Properly applied Pavlik harness (see text). (Courtesy Wheaton Brace, Carol Stream, IL.)

emphasizing the need for gentle reduction and progression to further treatment when the harness fails. Long-term follow-up of patients with Pavlik harness treatment is necessary because many patients have changes in the acetabulum at long-term follow-up despite normal radiographs at 3-year and 5-year follow-up examinations.

■ INFANT (6 TO 18 MONTHS)

When a child reaches crawling age (6 to 10 months old), success with the Pavlik harness decreases significantly. A 6- to 18-month-old infant with a dislocated hip is likely to require either closed or open reduction.

Children in this age group are often seen initially with a shortened extremity, limited passive abduction, and a positive Galeazzi sign. If the child is walking, a Trendelenburg gait may be present. Radiographic changes include delayed ossification of the femoral head, lateral and proximal displacement of the femoral head, and a shallow, dysplastic acetabulum.

With persistent dysplasia, the femoral head eventually moves superiorly and laterally with weight bearing. The capsule becomes permanently elongated, and anteriorly the psoas tendon may obstruct reduction of the femoral head into the true acetabulum. The limbus acetabuli may hypertrophy along the periphery of the acetabulum, and the ligamentum teres hypertrophies and elongates. The femoral head becomes reduced in size with posteromedial flattening, and coxa valga and excessive anteversion are noted. The true acetabulum is characteristically shallow and at surgery appears small because of the anterior capsular constriction, the hypertrophied limbus, and constriction of the deep acetabular ligament.

Treatment in this age group may include preoperative traction, adductor tenotomy, and closed reduction and arthrogram or open reduction in children with a failed closed reduction. Femoral shortening may be needed in a hip with

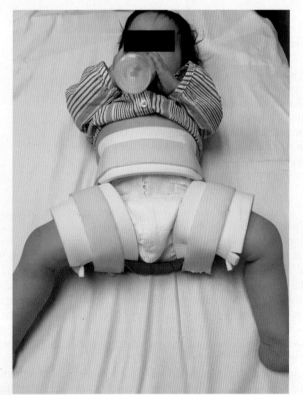

FIGURE 2.7 A rigid abduction orthosis such as pictured here can be used successfully in some children in whom a Pavlik harness has failed to produce a stable reduction (Rhino "Cruiser" hip abduction brace, Cascade Orthopedic Supply, Inc., Chico, CA).

a high proximal dislocation. Preoperative traction, adductor tenotomy, and gentle reduction with an acceptable "safe zone" are especially helpful in the prevention of osteonecrosis of the femoral head.

PREOPERATIVE TRACTION

The role of preliminary traction in reducing the incidence of osteonecrosis and in improving reduction is controversial. Disagreement exists about whether skin or skeletal traction should be used, whether home or in-hospital traction is preferable, the amount of weight that should be used, the most beneficial direction of pull, and the duration of traction. Although controversial, some suggest that if traction decreases the risk of osteonecrosis even slightly it may be considered. However, a large retrospective study of over 300 children younger than 3 years of age failed to demonstrate any benefit of preoperative traction in improving the rate of successful closed reduction or in decreasing the rate of osteonecrosis. Although skin traction could be an option for some centers, skeletal traction is not indicated, and primary femoral shortening is now routinely used in older children. The objectives of traction or primary femoral shortening are to bring the laterally and proximally displaced femoral head down to and below the level of the true acetabulum to allow a gentler reduction with less risk of osteonecrosis.

ADDUCTOR TENOTOMY

A percutaneous adductor tenotomy under sterile conditions can be performed for a mild adduction contracture. For a more severe adduction contracture or one of long duration, an open adductor tenotomy through a small transverse incision is preferable (see Technique 5.1).

ARTHROGRAPHY AND CLOSED REDUCTION

Arthrography and gentle closed reduction are accomplished with the child under general anesthesia.

The interposition of soft tissue in the acetabulum may be suggested by lateralization of the femoral head. Because the radiograph of the hip in an infant or young child cannot yield all the information desired in diagnosing or treating DDH, arthrography is helpful in determining (1) whether mild dysplasia is present, (2) whether the femoral head is subluxated or dislocated, (3) whether manipulative reduction has been or can be successful, (4) to what extent any soft-tissue structures within the acetabulum may interfere with complete reduction of the dislocation, (5) the condition and position of the acetabular labrum (the limbus), and (6) whether the acetabulum and femoral head are developing normally during treatment. Because arthrograms are not always easy to interpret, the surgeon must be thoroughly familiar with the normal and abnormal signs they may reveal and with the technique of making arthrograms (Video 2.1).

An arthrogram of the hip is beneficial in all children, regardless of age, who are given a general anesthetic for closed reduction, unless closed reduction is obviously impossible. It is most helpful to determine when manipulative reduction is unstable or when the femoral head is not concentrically seated within the acetabulum. The most important factor that determines outcome of closed treatment of developmental hip dislocation is the quality of the initial reduction. Proposed criteria for accepting a reduction are a medial dye

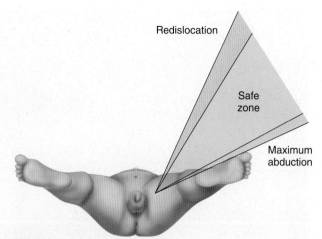

FIGURE 2.9 Safe zone used to determine acceptability of closed reduction of congenital dislocation of hip.

pool of 5 mm or less and maintenance of reduction in an acceptable "safe zone."

The use of image intensification in arthrography makes insertion of the needle much easier. The danger of damaging the articular surfaces and the possibility of injecting the contrast medium into areas other than the hip joint are decreased. This improves the safety of the procedure and decreases the likelihood of improper injection of the contrast material into an area that will obscure the surgeon's view.

The findings of the clinical examination and of arthrography at the time of attempted closed reduction determine if the hip will be stable or may require open reduction. A clinical finding that usually indicates an acceptable closed reduction is the sensation of a "clunk" as the femoral head reduces in the true acetabulum. The "safe zone" concept of Ramsey, Lasser, and MacEwen can be used in determining the zone of abduction and adduction in which the femoral head remains reduced in the acetabulum. A wide safe zone (minimum of 20 degrees, preferably 45 degrees) (Fig. 2.9) is desirable, and a narrow safe zone implies an unstable or unacceptable closed reduction. Forceful abduction to maintain a closed reduction is to be avoided, to decrease the likelihood of osteonecrosis. Osteonecrosis after closed reduction has been reported to be as high as 25% in some studies. A careful clinical evaluation of the reduction should be made before and after adductor tenotomy and before the arthrogram because, when the hip capsule is distended with dye, clinical examination becomes more difficult. An increase in the knee flexion angle (popliteal angle) is another indicator of a successful closed reduction.

ARTHROGRAPHY OF THE HIP IN DDH

TECHNIQUE 2.1

- Place the child supine after a general anesthetic has been administered. Perform sterile preparation and draping of the hip.
- With a gloved fingertip, locate the hip joint immediately inferior to the middle of the inguinal ligament and one

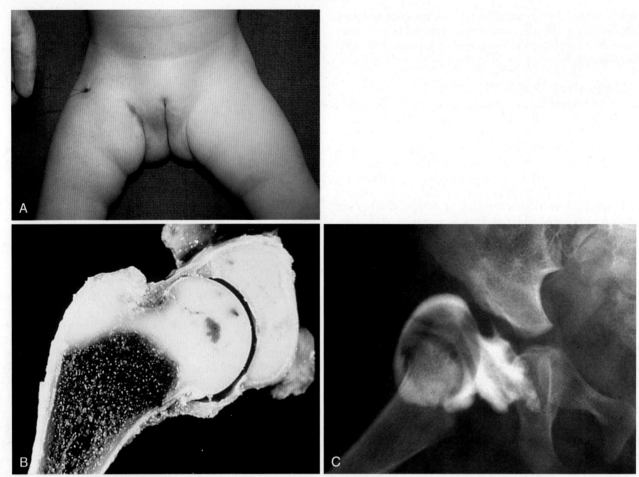

FIGURE 2.10 Arthrography of the hip. **A,** Insertion of 22-gauge spinal needle one fingerbreadth lateral to femoral artery and immediately inferior to anterior superior iliac spine for arthrography. **B,** In necropsy specimen, areas of hip in which dye may be easily injected: beneath acetabular labrum, in medial or lateral capsular pouch, and at junction of ossified and cartilaginous portion of femoral head. **C,** Irreducible hip with medial dye pool. (Courtesy John Ogden, MD.) **SEE TECHNIQUE 2.1.**

fingerbreadth lateral to the pulsating femoral artery (Fig. 2.10). Alternatively, insert the needle medially, just behind the adductor longus.

- With the assistance of image intensification, insert a 22-gauge spinal needle, to which is attached a 5-mL syringe filled with normal saline solution, until it enters the hip joint; resistance is met as the needle passes through the joint capsule.
- Inject the saline solution into the joint; this is easy at first but becomes more difficult as the joint becomes distended and the hip gradually flexes.
- Release the plunger of the syringe; if the joint has been successfully entered, the saline solution that is under pressure in it reverses the plunger and fluid escapes into the syringe.
- Aspirate the saline solution from the joint and remove the syringe from the needle.
- Fill the syringe with 5 mL of a 25% strength medically approved contrast agent such as diatrizoate or iohexol

solution and inject 1 to 3 mL through the needle into the joint with image intensification.

- Rapidly withdraw the needle and begin the examination under image intensification as the contrast agent will begin to clear soon after injection.
- Bring the hip through a full range of motion, performing provocative maneuvers of Barlow and Ortolani to gauge the ability to achieve a closed reduction and the stability of that reduction once achieved. Identify any and all obstacles to a deep, stable closed reduction (Video 2.1).
- Use image intensification to evaluate the reduction and safe zone. Alternatively, if image intensification is not available, obtain plain film arthrogram images with portable radiography in both the dislocated and reduced positions. When arthrograms are to be made of both hips, insert a needle into each, ensuring that both are within the joints before either joint is injected. Inject both hips as described here and make arthrograms of both (Video 2.1).

APPLICATION OF A HIP SPICA CAST

After confirmation of a stable reduction, a hip spica cast is applied with the hip joint in 95 degrees of flexion and 40 to 45 degrees of abduction. Salter advocated this "human position" as best for maintaining hip stability and minimizing the risk of osteonecrosis. Kumar described an easily reproducible and simple technique for applying a hip spica cast. Fiberglass can be used in place of plaster, but the technique is described in its original form. Although this technique is useful, good results can be obtained with modifications of the spica cast as described as long as the surgeon adheres to key principles: (1) the cast should be well-fitted and well-molded, particularly along the greater trochanter; (2) there should be appropriate space for toileting and hygiene to avoid cast soiling; (3) excessive abduction beyond the safe zone should be avoided but with enough hip flexion and abduction to maintain reduction.

TECHNIQUE 2.2

(KUMAR)

- Place the anesthetized child on the spica frame. Abduct the hip to 40 to 45 degrees and flex it to about 95 degrees (Fig. 2.11A). The amount of hip flexion and abduction required to keep the hip in the most stable position should be determined clinically and checked by radiographs.
- After the correct position of flexion and abduction for stability is determined, place a small towel in front of the abdomen.
- Cover the pelvis and extremities with stockinette. Roll 2-inch (5-cm) Webril from the level of the nipples down to the ankles (Fig. 2.11B). Pad around the bony points with 2-inch (5-cm) standard felt. Apply the first pad over the proximal end of the spica, near the nipple line (Fig. 2.11C).

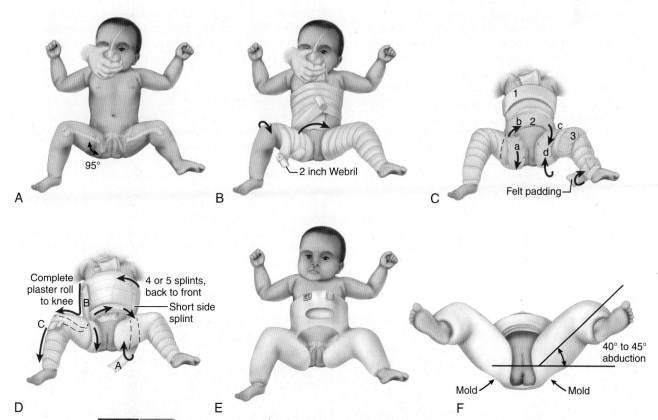

FIGURE 2.11   A to F, Technique of application of hip spica cast for congenital dislocation of hip. Note positioning of patient in "human" position. (Redrawn from Kumar SJ: Hip spica application for the treatment of congenital dislocation of the hip, *J Pediatr Orthop* 1:97, 1981.) **SEE TECHNIQUE 2.2.**

- Start a second piece of the same size felt at the level of the right groin and carry it posteriorly across the gluteal fold, over the right iliac crest, in front of the abdomen, over the lateral aspect of the left thigh, and to the left inguinal area (Fig. 2.11C).
- Apply a third piece of felt over the knee (Fig. 2.11C) and a fourth piece above the ankle over the distal leg. Place similar pieces of felt over the opposite knee and leg.
- Apply the plaster in two sections—a proximal section from the nipple line to the knees and a distal section from the knees to the ankles.
- Apply a single layer of 4-inch (10-cm) plaster roll from the nipple line to the level of the knees on both sides. Apply four or five plaster splints back to front from the nipple line to the back of the sacrum to reinforce the back of the cast. At the same time, apply a short, thick splint over the anterolateral aspect of the inguinal area (Fig. 2.11D).
- Apply another splint. Starting from the right inguinal area, carry it posteriorly across the gluteal region, the iliac crest, the front of the abdomen, and back the same way on the opposite thigh (Fig. 2.11D). This is a reinforcing splint that attaches the thigh to the upper segment.
- Apply another long splint from the level of the knee across the anterolateral aspect of the inguinal area and up the chest wall (Fig. 2.11D). This splint is one of the main anchors of the thigh to the body segment.
- Follow this by a roll of 4-inch (10-cm) plaster from the nipple line to the knees. This completes the proximal section of the spica.
- Complete the cast from the knees down to the ankles. Do this by applying on both sides a single roll of 3-inch (7.5-cm) plaster from the knee to the ankle level and reinforcing this by two splints over the medial and lateral aspects of the thigh, knee, and leg.
- Follow this by another roll of 3-inch (7.5-cm) plaster. (Fig. 2.11E).
- Because the cast is reinforced laterally around the hips, a wide segment can be removed from the front of the hips

without weakening the cast. This permits better radiographs of the hips (Fig. 2.11E).

The final inferior view of the spica cast should appear as shown in Figure 2.11F, with about 40 to 45 degrees of abduction. The amount of abduction is determined by the position of hip stability. Excessive abduction should be avoided. We have found that the hips are always flexed less than they appear to be and are abducted more than they appear. A gentle cast mold over the greater trochanter can aid in maintaining hip reduction.

POSTOPERATIVE CARE Spica cast immobilization is continued for 3 to 4 months. The cast can be changed at the midpoint with the patient under general anesthesia. Radiographs or arthrograms can be obtained to ensure that the femoral head is reduced anatomically into the acetabulum. Clinical and radiographic follow-up is essential until the hip is considered normal.

■ THREE-DIMENSIONAL IMAGING AFTER CLOSED REDUCTION

CT or MRI is useful in the postoperative period to assess reduction. These studies can be obtained under the same anesthetic as the closed reduction, or they can be delayed 24 to 28 hours to allow time for the child to become more active. A comparison of MRI and CT in the evaluation of reduction of DDH found sensitivity of 100% for both CT and MRI and specificity of 96% for CT and 100% for MRI. CT required less time (3 minutes) than MRI (10 minutes) and was less expensive but exposes the child to ionizing radiation. In contrast to routine radiography, a cast does not alter the image of an axial CT or MRI (Figs. 2.12 and 2.13), but because of the radiation exposure of CT, the number of cuts should be limited. Fast MRI hip sequences have been proposed to allow for acquisition of MRI data without additional anesthesia. Long-term follow-up is recommended after successful closed reduction to monitor for resubluxation and acetabular remodeling. If stable closed reduction is achieved early in life, acceptable acetabular remodeling often results; however, if

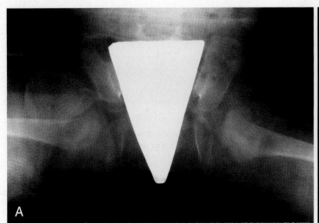
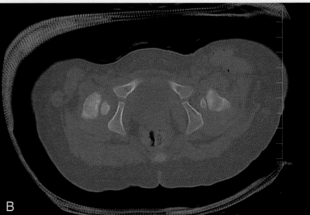

FIGURE 2.12 **A,** Anteroposterior radiograph of pelvis obtained with patient in hip spica cast after closed reduction. Note difficulty in assessing position of femoral head. **B,** CT scan of pelvis to confirm bilateral reduction of femoral head into true acetabulum.

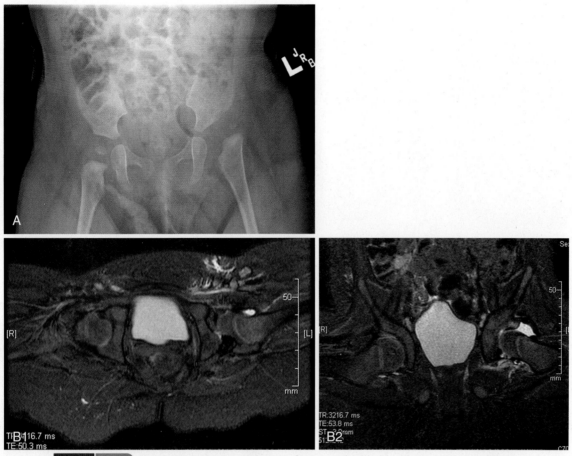

FIGURE 2.13 **A,** Plain anteroposterior view of a 9-month-old girl with persistent hip dislocation. **B,** Axial and coronal MRI of hip after arthrogram, successful closed reduction, and spica cast application.

there is a delay in diagnosis and treatment of a dysplastic hip, the completeness of acetabular remodeling is not ensured, and additional surgical correction of acetabular dysplasia may be required.

OPEN REDUCTION

In children in whom efforts to reduce a dislocation without force have failed, open reduction is indicated to correct the interposed soft-tissue structures and to reduce the femoral head concentrically in the acetabulum. This surgical option is indicated by pathology rather than by age because open reduction may be required in children younger than 6 months and closed reduction occasionally can be successful in children 18 months of age. Open reduction can be performed through an anterior or medial approach; the choice depends on the experience of the surgeon and the particular dislocation.

Regardless of the approach chosen, open reduction of the dislocated and dysplastic hip should correct as many of the blocks to reduction as possible, which may include hourglass constricted capsule, iliopsoas tendon, hypertrophied limbus, inverted labrum, hypertrophied and elongated ligamentum teres, transverse acetabular ligament, and excess fibrofatty pulvinar. The surgeon should strive to correct all aspects of the deformity in a single surgical event because revision surgery often is challenging.

The anterior approach requires more anatomic dissection but provides greater versatility because the pathologic condition in the anterior and lateral aspects is easily reached and pelvic osteotomy can be performed through this approach if necessary.

The medial (Ludloff) approach utilizes the interval between the iliopsoas and the pectineus. This approach places the medial circumflex vessels at a higher risk and has been reported to be associated with a higher incidence of osteonecrosis (10% to 20%) in some studies and similar rates of osteonecrosis in others. Although the medial approach allows removal of the impediments to reduction, it does not allow capsulorrhaphy and is, therefore, generally recommended in infants 6 to 18 months old.

ANTERIOR APPROACH

TECHNIQUE 2.3

(BEATY; AFTER SOMERVILLE)

- Make an anterior bikini incision from the middle of the iliac crest to a point midway between the anterior superior iliac spine and the midline of the pelvis. The anterior superior iliac spine should be at the midpoint of the incision, which can be placed 1 cm below the iliac crest (Fig. 2.14A).

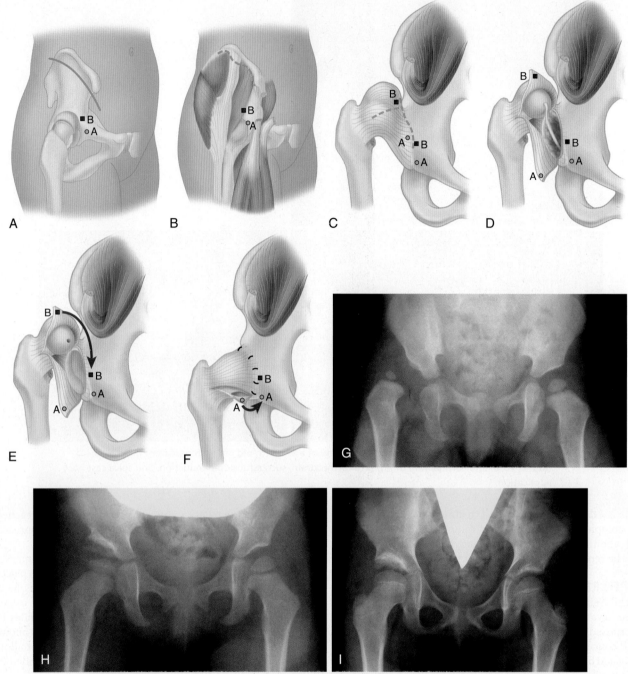

FIGURE 2.14 Technique of anterior open reduction in congenital dislocation of hip. **A,** Bikini incision. **B,** Division of sartorius and rectus femoris tendons and iliac epiphysis. **C and D,** T-shaped incision of capsule. **E,** Capsulotomy of hip and use of ligamentum teres to find true acetabulum. **F,** Reduction and capsulorrhaphy after excision of redundant capsule. **G,** Developmental dislocation of right hip. **H,** After anterolateral open reduction. **I,** At age 7 years; note remodeling of femoral head and acetabulum. **SEE TECHNIQUE 2.3.**

- Carry sharp dissection through the subcutaneous tissue to the deep fascia.
- Identify and enter the interval between the sartorius and tensor fasciae latae muscles, protecting the lateral femoral cutaneous nerve by retracting it with a Penrose drain during the entire procedure. The presence of inguinal lymph nodes in the most medial dissection indicates the proximity of the neurovascular bundle.
- Detach the iliac apophysis from the ilium, beginning at the anterior superior iliac spine and extending 4 cm posteriorly along the ilium. Alternatively, the iliac apophysis can be split sharply.

- Subperiosteally dissect the tensor fasciae latae laterally to expose the ilium and the full extent of the anterolateral capsule.
- Identify the origin of the sartorius muscle at the anterior superior iliac crest, divide it, and allow it to retract distally.
- Dissect the tensor fasciae latae origin to the anterior inferior iliac spine.
- Place a retractor along the medial aspect of the anterior inferior iliac spine onto the superior pubic ramus.
- Identify the psoas tendon in its groove on the superior pubic ramus and perform a recession tenotomy to facilitate placement of a right-angle retractor in the groove on the superior pubic ramus normally occupied by the iliopsoas tendon. The retractor protects the psoas muscle and neurovascular bundle anteriorly and assists in medial exposure.
- Identify the origins of the direct and oblique heads of the rectus femoris muscle and perform a tenotomy approximately 1 cm distal to the anterior inferior iliac spine (Fig. 2.14B). Tag the distal segment and allow the tendon to retract distally.
- Identify the capsule of the hip joint anteriorly, medially, and laterally. A large amount of redundant capsule may be present laterally in the region of a false acetabulum.
- Make a T-shaped incision from the most medial aspect of the capsule to the most lateral and continue the incision along the anterior border of the femoral head and neck (Fig. 2.14C,D). For more exposure, use Kocher clamps to retract the capsule.
- Identify the femoral head and the ligamentum teres; detach the ligamentum teres from the femoral head and place on it a Kocher clamp. Trace the ligamentum teres to the true acetabulum and excise with a rongeur or sharp dissection any pulvinar in the true acetabulum (Fig. 2.14E).
- Gently expose the bony articular surface of the acetabulum with its circumferential cartilage.
- Expose the acetabulum laterally, superiorly, medially, and inferiorly to the level of the deep transverse acetabular ligament, which should be divided to enlarge the most inferior aspect of the acetabulum. Enlarge the entrance to the acetabulum by excision of the fat from the innermost aspect of the acetabulum until the entrance is large enough to allow reduction of the femoral head without difficulty.
- After reducing the femoral head into the acetabulum, move the hip through a complete range of motion (including flexion, extension, adduction, and abduction) to determine the "safe zone" of reduction.
- If the reduction is concentric and stable, reduce the femoral head and close the capsule, suturing the lateral flap of the T-shaped incision as far medially as possible to eliminate any redundant capsule in the region of the false acetabulum (Fig. 2.14F). An adequate capsulorrhaphy significantly improves stability of the hip. Place sutures in the tips of the "T" and along the superior border of the acetabulum.
- When capsulorrhaphy is completed, suture the rectus femoris tendon to its origin and the iliac apophysis to the fascia of the tensor fasciae latae along the iliac crest.
- Close the superficial fascial layers, the subcutaneous tissues, and the skin. Apply a double spica cast with the hips

in 90 to 100 degrees of flexion and 40 to 55 degrees of abduction.

POSTOPERATIVE CARE Radiography, CT, or MRI can be used to confirm reduction of the femoral head into the acetabulum. The spica cast is changed in the operating room at 5 to 6 weeks with final removal at 10 to 12 weeks. Sequential radiographs are used to assess development of the femoral head and acetabulum (Fig. 2.14G to I); these are obtained on a regular basis until the child reaches skeletal maturity.

MEDIAL APPROACH

TECHNIQUE 2.4

(LUDLOFF)
- Make a transverse incision centered at the anterior margin of the adductor longus, approximately 1 cm distal and parallel to the inguinal ligament (Fig. 2.15).
- Open the fascia along the superior border of the adductor longus. Isolate this muscle, divide it close to its insertion on the pelvis, and retract it distally to expose the adductor brevis muscle in the inferior part of the wound and the pectineus muscle in the superior part of the wound.
- Identify the branches of the anterior obturator nerve on the surface of the adductor brevis muscle and with blunt dissection follow this nerve beneath the pectineus muscle. Free the posterior border of the pectineus muscle proximally to its origin on the pelvis.
- Place a retractor beneath the pectineus muscle and retract it superiorly. Identify by palpation the lesser trochanter

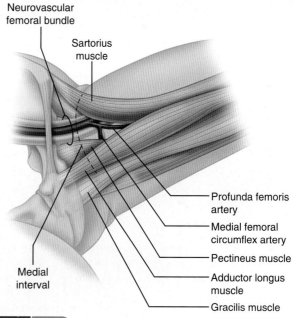

FIGURE 2.15 Incision for medial (Ludloff) approach and open reduction. **SEE TECHNIQUE 2.4.**

and the iliopsoas tendon. Open the fascial layer surrounding the tendon, pull the tendon into the wound with a right-angle clamp, and sharply divide it.

■ With blunt dissection clear the pericapsular fat from the capsule. Dissect free the small branch of the medial circumflex artery that crosses the capsule inferiorly and preserve it.

■ Incise the capsule in the direction of the femoral neck. Identify the transverse acetabular ligament and section it.

■ If needed for reduction, perform additional release of the capsule. Reduce the hip in 90 to 100 degrees of flexion and 40 to 60 degrees of abduction.

■ When the optimal position is determined, close the deep fascia and skin in routine fashion and apply a double spica cast. Some studies have suggested that repair of the iliopsoas tendon could be helpful to preserve long-term muscle strength, although spontaneous reattachment is common.

■ Consider obtaining three-dimensional imaging after cast application to confirm reduction of the femoral head.

POSTOPERATIVE CARE Postoperative care is similar to that after closed reduction and varies according to the age of the child. Generally, 8 to 12 weeks of cast immobilization is sufficient.

Three-dimensional imaging should be considered after successful closed or open reduction. See the section, "Three-Dimensional Imaging After Closed Reduction" for a discussion on the timing, cost, anesthesia, and radiation considerations for the various options.

▌CONCOMITANT OSTEOTOMY

The use of a concomitant osteotomy of the ilium, acetabulum, or femur at the time of open reduction remains controversial. Innominate osteotomy, acetabuloplasty, proximal femoral varus derotation osteotomy, or femoral shortening osteotomy might increase the stability of open reduction. However, in younger children (<12 months), acetabular remodeling potential could render these procedures unnecessary.

Conversely, inadequate remodeling after open reduction may necessitate a return to the operating room at a later date for a bony procedure.

Zadeh et al. used concomitant osteotomy at the time of open reduction to maintain stability of the reduction in which the following test of stability after open reduction was used.

1. Hip stable in neutral position—no osteotomy
2. Hip stable in flexion and abduction—innominate osteotomy
3. Hip stable in internal rotation and abduction—proximal femoral derotational varus osteotomy
4. "Double-diameter" acetabulum with anterolateral deficiency—Pemberton-type osteotomy

Aside from the need for osteotomy at the time of open reduction to maintain stability, there also are concerns about residual acetabular dysplasia. Better results have been reported in children younger than 30 months of age who were treated with combined open reduction and Salter osteotomy than in those treated with a staged procedure.

Concomitant osteotomy, particularly a femoral shortening osteotomy with or without derotation, should be done at the time of open reduction when necessary to maintain a safe, stable reduction. If open reduction is stable without an osteotomy, a bony procedure for residual deformity should be considered at the time of the open reduction in an older child (>18 months) and used with caution even in younger infants.

▌TERATOLOGIC DISLOCATIONS

A teratologic dislocation of the hip is one that occurs at some time before birth, resulting in significant anatomic distortion and resistance to treatment. It often occurs with other conditions, such as arthrogryposis, Larsen syndrome, myelomeningocele, and diastrophic dwarfism.

The anatomic changes in teratologic dislocations are much more advanced than the changes in a typical developmental hip dislocation in a child of the same age. The acetabulum is small, with an oblique or flattened shape; the ligamentum teres is thickened, and the femoral head is of variable size and may be flattened on the medial side (Fig. 2.16). The hip joint is usually stiff and irreducible, and radiographs show superolateral displacement.

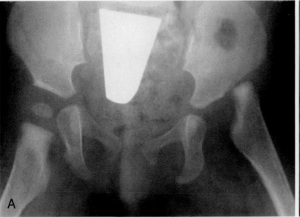
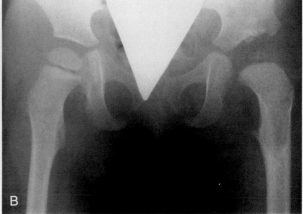

FIGURE 2.16 **A,** Teratologic dislocation of left hip in 18-month-old girl. **B,** Appearance at 3 years of age after primary femoral shortening, anterior open reduction, and innominate osteotomy.

Most authors agree that closed reduction is ineffective and that open reduction is necessary, but indications for treatment are unclear. Most agree that unilateral dislocations should be treated more aggressively than bilateral dislocations, and the ambulatory potential of the patient is probably the most important consideration in deciding whether to treat bilateral dislocations. The difficulty of successfully treating teratologic dislocations is reflected in the results of Gruel et al., who found that of the 27 hips in their series, 44% had poor results and 70% had complications. Osteonecrosis occurred in 48% of hips, redislocation occurred in 19%, and subluxation occurred in 22%. Anterior open reduction and femoral shortening produced the best results with the fewest complications, whereas the worst results and most complications occurred in the hips treated by closed reduction.

Although multiple procedures may be required, good results can be obtained and a stable hip can be achieved in properly selected patients. Open reduction through a medial approach has been recommended for children 3 to 6 months old combined with surgical correction of congenital contractures of the knee and foot. In older children, primary femoral shortening and anterior open reduction, with or without pelvic osteotomy, is preferred.

▌OSTEONECROSIS

The most serious complication associated with treatment of DDH in early infancy is the development of osteonecrosis. Estimated rates of osteonecrosis vary widely, ranging from less than 5% to almost 50%. Proposed risk factors for osteonecrosis include open reduction with concomitant osteotomies, redislocation after surgical correction, or the need for secondary procedure after initial closed or open reduction. Although the rate of osteonecrosis after closed reduction is lower than after open reduction, the rate is still as high as 10% to 35% after closed treatment. Some authors have suggested that osteonecrosis is more frequent when reduction is done before the appearance of the ossific nucleus of the femoral head, whereas others have stated that waiting until the ossific nucleus appears does not seem to affect the development of osteonecrosis. Most recently, meta-analyses have indicated that the presence of the ossific nucleus provides little protective benefit against osteonecrosis after closed or open reduction, and Luhmann et al. found that delaying reduction of a dislocated hip until the appearance of the ossific nucleus more than doubled the need for future surgery. Despite a slight increase in the rate of osteonecrosis after reduction of hips without an ossific nucleus, they advocated early reduction to optimize development of the hip with the minimal number of operations.

Potential sequelae of osteonecrosis include femoral head deformity, acetabular dysplasia, lateral subluxation of the femoral head, relative overgrowth of the greater trochanter, and limb-length inequalities; osteoarthritis is a common late complication. Bucholz and Ogden and Kalamchi and MacEwen proposed classification systems based on morphologic changes in the capital femoral epiphysis, the physis, and the proximal femoral metaphysis (Fig. 2.17). These classifications are useful in determining proper treatment and prognosis for a particular patient; however, the proper classification may not be identifiable on radiographs until the child is 4 to 6 years old. The prognostic ability of the Bucholz and

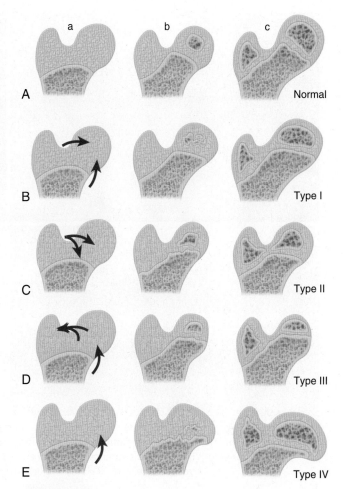

FIGURE 2.17 Bucholz and Ogden classification of osteonecrosis of femoral head in congenital dislocation of hip. **A,** Normal femoral head at 2 months (*a*), 1 year (*b*), and 9 years (*c*) of age. **B,** Type I: *a*, sites of temporary vascular occlusion; *b*, irregular ossification in secondary center; *c*, normal epiphyseal contour, slight decrease in height of capital femoral ossification center. **C,** Type II: *a*, probable primary site of vascular occlusion; *b*, metaphyseal and epiphyseal irregularities; *c*, premature fusion of lateral metaphysis and epiphysis. **D,** Type III: *a*, sites of temporary vascular occlusion; *b*, impaired longitudinal growth of capital femoral epiphysis; *c*, irregularly shaped femoral head. **E,** Type IV: *a*, sites of temporary vascular occlusion; *b*, impaired longitudinal and latitudinal growth; *c*, premature epiphyseal closure. (Redrawn from Bucholz RW, Ogden JA: Patterns of ischemic necrosis of the proximal femur in nonoperatively treated congenital hip disease. In *The hip: Proceedings of the Sixth Open Scientific Meeting of the Hip Society*, St Louis, Mosby, 1978.)

Ogden classification system has been brought into question by an interrater reliability study; the authors concluded that a new classification scheme is needed. A simplification of the Kalamchi and MacEwen classification scheme has been proposed that combines groups II, III, and IV into a single group B. By classifying osteonecrosis cases into group A or group B, the authors were able to demonstrate that the type of reduction (closed with traction versus open without femoral shortening) was a factor in the development of osteonecrosis.

Treatment should be directed toward the clinical problems associated with each radiographic classification group.

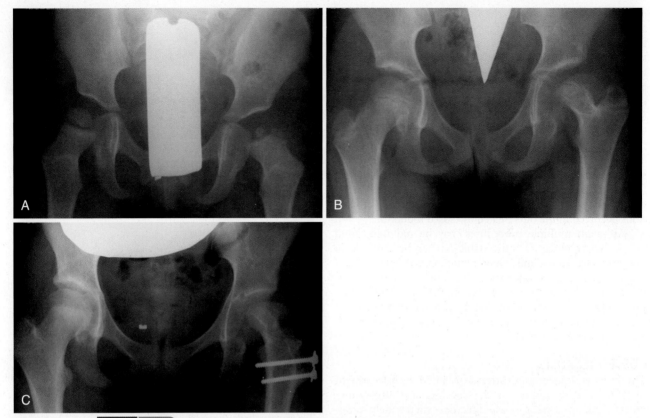

FIGURE 2.18 **A,** Osteonecrosis of left femoral head in 4-year-old girl after closed reduction of left congenital dislocation of hip at 6 months of age. **B,** At 10 years of age, now type II osteonecrosis is present, with premature lateral epiphyseal arrest and relative trochanteric overgrowth. **C,** At 13 years of age, after transfer of trochanter distally and anteriorly.

Many patients do not require any treatment during adolescence and young adulthood. In a few, femoral head deformity and acetabular dysplasia that predisposes the hip joint to incongruity and persistent subluxation can be treated with femoral osteotomy or appropriate pelvic osteotomy or both.

Children with osteonecrosis after treatment of developmental dislocation of the hip should be followed to maturity with serial orthoradiographs. Significantly better results have been reported in patients treated early (1 to 3 years after the ischemic insult) with innominate osteotomy than in patients treated later (5 to 10 years after the ischemic insult) and patients without pelvic osteotomy. Patients treated early also had less pain and fewer gait disturbances and required fewer additional procedures for limb-length inequality or greater trochanteric overgrowth. Early innominate osteotomy has been suggested to induce spherical remodeling of the femoral head, with a resultant congruous hip joint, whereas with later osteotomy the femoral head was already deformed, with little potential for remodeling. Significant limb-length inequality can be corrected by appropriate techniques, usually a well-timed epiphysiodesis. Symptomatic overgrowth of the greater trochanter can be treated in older patients with greater trochanteric advancement, which increases the abductor muscle resting length and increases the abductor lever arm (Fig. 2.18).

TROCHANTERIC ADVANCEMENT

TECHNIQUE 2.5

(LLOYD-ROBERTS AND SWANN)

- Approach the trochanter through a long lateral incision. Place a Gigli saw deep to the gluteus medius and minimus muscles and divide the trochanter at its base. Alternately, remove the lateral two thirds of the greater trochanter with an oscillating saw or large osteotome. Protect the lateral ascending cervical artery medial to the piriformis fossa.
- Mobilize the gluteus muscles anteriorly and posteriorly as they are dissected off the joint capsule and strip them for a short distance from the ilium above.
- Displace the detached trochanter with its attached muscles distally to the lateral cortex of the femur while the hip is abducted.
- Bevel the femoral cortex to help reduce tension and improve placement of the trochanter.
- Secure the trochanter to the femur with screws and suture the femoral periosteum and vastus lateralis muscle.

The top of the greater trochanter now should be positioned at the level of the center of the femoral head on an anteroposterior radiograph. The trochanter usually requires advancement anteriorly and distally.

Trochanteric advancement also can be performed following the surgical approach description.

POSTOPERATIVE CARE The hip is protected by a spica cast in abduction for 3 to 6 weeks. A physical therapy program is begun for rehabilitation of the hip abductor musculature.

■ TODDLER (18 TO 36 MONTHS)

Because of widespread screening of newborns, it is becoming less common for DDH to go undetected beyond the age of 1 year. An older child with this condition has a wide perineum, shortened lower extremity, and hyperlordosis of the lower spine as a result of femoropelvic instability. For these children with well-established hip dysplasia, open reduction with femoral or pelvic osteotomy, or both, often is required. Persistent dysplasia can be corrected by a redirectional proximal femoral osteotomy in very young children. If the primary dysplasia is acetabular, pelvic redirectional osteotomy alone is more appropriate. Many older children require femoral and pelvic osteotomies, however, if significant deformity is present on both sides of the joint.

▌ FEMORAL OSTEOTOMY IN DYSPLASIA OF THE HIP

Surgeons who recommend femoral osteotomies advise an operation on the pelvic side of the joint only after (1) the femoral head has been concentrically seated in the dysplastic acetabulum by such an osteotomy, (2) the joint has failed to develop satisfactorily, and (3) the growth potential of the acetabulum no longer exists. Opinions differ widely as to the age at which the acetabulum loses its ability to develop satisfactorily over a femoral head concentrically located, although 8 years appears to be most frequently cited upper age limit after which little benefit is derived from femoral osteotomy alone. Femoral osteotomy is most frequently indicated with primary femoral shortening, but the technique is included here for completeness.

VARUS DEROTATIONAL OSTEOTOMY OF THE FEMUR IN HIP DYSPLASIA, WITH PEDIATRIC HIP SCREW FIXATION

TECHNIQUE 2.6

- Place the patient supine on a radiolucent operating table. Image intensification in the anteroposterior projection is desirable.

- Prepare and drape the affected extremity, leaving the unaffected leg draped free to allow intraoperative radiographs or imaging.
- Make a lateral incision from the greater trochanter distally 8 to 12 cm, incise the iliotibial band, and reflect the vastus lateralis muscle to expose the lateral aspect of the femur.
- Make a transverse line in the femoral cortex with an osteotome to mark the level of the osteotomy at the level of the lesser trochanter or slightly distal. Correct positioning of the osteotomy can be verified with image intensification.
- Make a longitudinal orientation line on the anterior femoral cortex to determine correct rotation. Additional rotational orientation can be obtained by placing small Kirschner wires both just inside the anterior femoral neck and across the distal femoral epicondylar access.
- Drill a hole just distal to the greater trochanter and check its placement with the image intensifier.
- This osteotomy can be stabilized with a pediatric hip screw, an angled blade plate, or a proximal femoral locking plate. The description presented uses a pediatric hip screw.
- Place an appropriate guide pin of the proper length in the femoral neck with the aid of an adjustable angle guide (see Fig. 36.113A).
- Check the placement of the guide pin with image intensification. When the guide pin is placed, use a percutaneous direct measuring gauge to determine the lag screw length.
- Set the adjustable positive stop on the combination reamer for the lag screw length determined by the percutaneous direct measuring gauge.
- Place the reamer over the guide pin and ream until the positive stop reaches the lateral cortex (see Fig. 36.113C). It is prudent to check periodically the fluoroscopic image during reaming to ensure that the guide pin is not inadvertently advancing proximally into the epiphysis.
- Set the adjustable positive stop on the lag screw tap to the same length that was reamed. Tap until the positive stop reaches the lateral cortex. Screw the appropriate intermediate compression screw over the guide pin (see Fig. 36.113D, E).
- Take the plate chosen during preoperative planning and insert its barrel over the barrel guide and onto the back of the lag screw. The plate angle ultimately determines the final hip angle.
- Remove the barrel guide and insert a compressing screw to prevent the plate from disengaging during the reduction maneuver. Use the slotted screwdriver for the pediatric compressing screw or the hex screwdriver for the intermediate compressing screw. If the plate obscures the osteotomy site, loosen the screw and rotate the side plate.
- Make the osteotomy cut at the transverse line on the cortex in a transverse or oblique direction, depending on the correction desired. If rotational, in addition to angular, correction is desired, complete the osteotomy through the medial cortex. Using the longitudinal mark in the femoral cortex as a guide, rotate the femur as needed to correct femoral anteversion (usually 15 to 30 degrees). Because the deformity is more rotational than angulatory, evaluate the position of the femur with radiographs or image intensification before continuing with varus correction. To achieve varus angulation, remove an appropriate wedge

of bone from the medial cortex to effect a neck-shaft angle of 120 to 135 degrees.

- To achieve compression, insert a drill or tap guide into the distal portion of the most distal compression slot. Drill through the medial cortex. If less compression is required, follow the same steps just detailed in the distal portion of either the second or the third distal slots for 2.5 mm of compression.
- Select the appropriate length bone screw and insert it using the screwdriver. Use the self-holding sleeve to keep the screw from disengaging from the screwdriver (see Fig. 8.113F).
- Finally, in the most proximal slot, the intermediate combination drill/tap guide can be angled proximally so that the drill and ultimately the bone screw cross the osteotomy line. Positioning the proximal bone screw in this way can provide additional stability at the osteotomy site.
- Insert screws into any remaining screw holes.
- The lag screw can be inserted farther to provide more compression. To insert the lag screw for approximately 5 mm of compression, stop when the lateral cortex is midway between the two depth calibrations (see Fig. 8.113G). To insert the lag screw for approximately 10 mm of compression, stop when the second depth calibration meets the lateral cortex (see Fig. 8.113H).
- Confirm the position of the fixation device and the proximal and distal fragments with an anteroposterior radiograph or image intensification.
- Irrigate the wound and close it in layers, inserting a suction drain if needed. Apply a one and one half spica cast.

POSTOPERATIVE CARE The spica cast is worn for 6 to 8 weeks until union of the osteotomy occurs; however, longer immobilization may be required if simultaneous open reduction was performed. The internal fixation should be removed at 12 to 24 months.

■ CHILD (3 TO 8 YEARS)

The management of untreated developmental dislocation of the hip in a child older than 3 years of age is difficult. Even when surgical reduction is achieved and when bony corrections have been made, secondary procedures are common in this age group. By this age, adaptive shortening of the periarticular structures and structural alterations in the femoral head and the acetabulum have occurred. Dislocated hips in this age group require open reduction. Preoperative skeletal traction should not be used as the only means of achieving reduction because of the high frequencies of osteonecrosis (54%) and redislocation (31%) reported with its use alone. Femoral shortening aids in the reduction and decreases the potential for complications but is technically demanding, as is treatment of the dislocated hip, in this older age group.

▌PRIMARY FEMORAL SHORTENING

Since the early 1990s, the combination of primary open reduction and femoral shortening, usually with pelvic osteotomy, has been an accepted method of treatment of DDH in older children. This approach avoids expensive in-hospital traction, obtains predictable reduction, and results in a lower rate of osteonecrosis (Figs. 2.19 and 2.20).

Primary femoral shortening, anterior open reduction, and capsulorrhaphy, with or without pelvic osteotomy as indicated, have been recommended in children 3 years old or older. Certain circumstances, such as teratologic hip dislocation or a failed traction program or need for assistance in hip reduction, may make the procedure appropriate for younger children. A completely dislocated hip in an older child becomes fixed in a position superior to the true acetabulum. The degree of this superior migration ranges from severe subluxation (inferior head still adjacent to labrum), to dislocation with formation of a false acetabulum just superior to the true acetabulum, to severe dislocation with the femoral head high in the abductor musculature without formation of a false acetabulum. The extent of proximal migration determines the degree of deformation of the capsule and the extent of soft-tissue reconstruction required to correct the deformity.

The capsular abnormality in a developmentally dislocated hip must be recognized and corrected to achieve successful open reduction. The methods for bony correction are well defined, perhaps because the techniques can be clearly illustrated and documented radiographically, but the soft-tissue abnormalities and methods for their correction are not well described. As a result, a hip that appears reduced immediately after surgery may subluxate or redislocate with weight bearing, even though the bony procedure appears radiographically faultless.

The dislocation of the hip leads to adaptive enlargement of the hip capsule, with the capsule becoming nearly twice the normal size in the completely dislocated hip. The ligamentum teres hypertrophies and often becomes a partial weight-bearing structure. In older children, this ligament occasionally avulses from the femoral head, retracting and reattaching to the inferior capsule and forming a mass of tissue that may impede reduction. The fibrocartilaginous labrum is flattened superolaterally, with the attached hypertrophied capsule protruding into the overlying abductor muscle mass, which adheres to the displaced capsule. If the capsule is not separated adequately from the adherent overlying muscles, reduction is difficult and the chance of redislocation is increased.

In a high, severely dislocated hip, the abductor muscles have contracted, and occasionally, despite prior traction or femoral shortening, these contracted muscles and fascia make it difficult to pull the proximal femur distal enough to reduce the femoral head fully. In rare instances, this requires release of the piriformis insertion or release of the anteriormost gluteus minimus fibers, or both, to allow adequate distal movement of the femoral head after femoral shortening. The middle and inferior portions of the capsule are predictably constricted by the overlying psoas tendon. The transverse acetabular ligament, crossing the base of the horseshoe-shaped true acetabulum, is contracted and thickened.

The following description of the technique for primary femoral shortening is a modification of the techniques described by Klisíc et al. and by Wenger and includes anterior open reduction (Technique 2.3) and varus derotational osteotomy (Technique 2.6) along with soft-tissue management. These techniques should be reviewed carefully before primary femoral shortening is performed (Fig. 2.21).

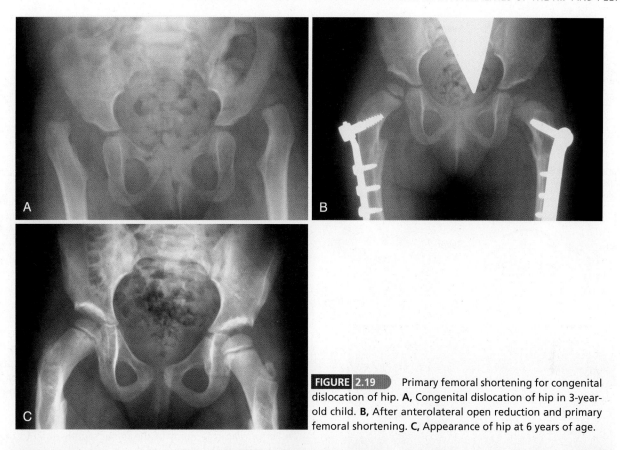

FIGURE 2.19 Primary femoral shortening for congenital dislocation of hip. **A,** Congenital dislocation of hip in 3-year-old child. **B,** After anterolateral open reduction and primary femoral shortening. **C,** Appearance of hip at 6 years of age.

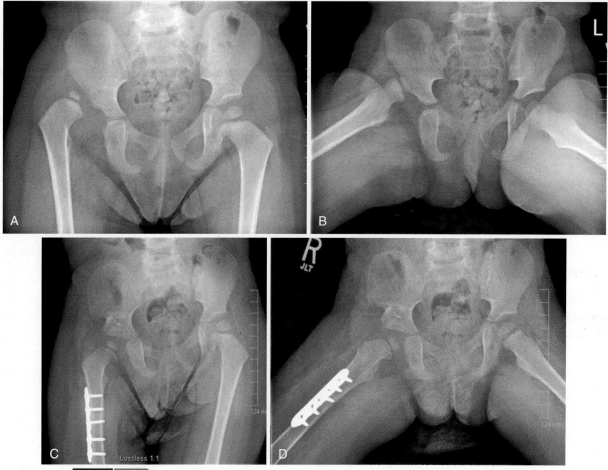

FIGURE 2.20 **A** and **B,** Four-year-old child with dislocated hip and severe dysplasia. **C** and **D,** Postoperative radiographs 3 months after primary femoral shortening, open reduction with capsulorrhaphy, and Pemberton acetabuloplasty.

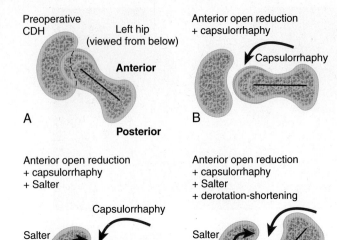

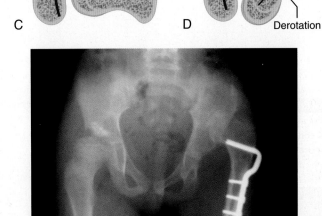

FIGURE 2.21 **A,** Anteverted femur and acetabulum in preoperative developmental dislocation of hip. **B,** Redirection of femoral neck by snug anterior capsulorrhaphy. **C,** Capsulorrhaphy and Salter innominate osteotomy. **D,** Capsulorrhaphy, Salter innominate osteotomy, and full femoral derotation. Combined in excess, this sequence can produce posterior dislocation. **E,** Open reduction, primary femoral shortening, derotation osteotomy, and Salter osteotomy produced fixed posterior hip dislocation in 5-year-old girl. (**A to D,** Redrawn from Wenger DR: Congenital hip dislocation: techniques for primary open reduction including femoral shortening, *Instr Course Lect* 38:343, 1989.) **SEE TECHNIQUE 2.7.**

PRIMARY FEMORAL SHORTENING

TECHNIQUE 2.7

- Place the patient supine on the operating table with a small radiolucent pad beneath the affected hip. Prepare and drape the extremity in the usual manner to allow exposure of the pelvis and femur.
- Two incisions are made—an anterior ilioinguinal incision as described for anterior open reduction (Technique 2.3) and a straight lateral incision. Through the anterior

ilioinguinal incision, perform anterior open reduction as described in Technique 2.3, continuing the dissection to the point where capsulorrhaphy normally would be performed.
- Proceed to the femoral shortening. Make a straight lateral incision from the tip of the greater trochanter to the distal third of the femoral shaft.
- If varus correction is not needed, the femoral shortening and derotation can be performed at the level of the femoral shaft rather than the intertrochanteric level. This shaft osteotomy can be stabilized with a one third tubular plate or a standard compression plate.
- Expose the shaft by dissection through the tensor fasciae latae muscle, iliotibial band, and vastus lateralis muscle.
- Make a transverse mark on the femoral shaft at the level of the lesser trochanter to indicate the osteotomy site and make a longitudinal mark on the anterior border of the proximal shaft to orient derotation of the femur.
- Insert a lag screw into the femoral neck in the usual manner.
- Estimate the amount of shortening that will be necessary from preoperative radiographs, measuring from the most proximal aspect of the femoral head to the triradiate cartilage. The amount of shortening generally required varies from 1 to 3 cm. Conversely, the correct amount of bony resection can be "dialed in" as bone is removed until the femoral head can be reduced into the acetabulum without undue tension.
- Perform an osteotomy of the femur slightly distal to the lag screw in the femoral neck.
- Make a second transverse osteotomy at the appropriate distance distal from the first. Angle the osteotomy to allow for varus if needed. Remove the measured segment of the femoral shaft (Fig. 2.22).
- If the iliopsoas tendon prevents the proximal fragment from a caudal reduction to the level of the acetabulum, consider carefully incising subperiosteally the iliopsoas attachment to the lesser trochanter and the capsule attached to the medial femoral neck, avoiding the medial circumflex artery.
- Gently reduce the femoral head into the acetabulum. Derotation of the proximal fragment of 15 to 45 degrees usually is required.
- Appose the two segments of the femur and stabilize with a side plate and screws. Use radiographs or image intensification to evaluate the femoral shortening and reduction of the femoral head.
- At this point, a Salter or Pemberton osteotomy, if indicated to correct acetabular dysplasia, can be performed. A thorough and meticulous capsulorrhaphy should be performed as previously described. The most lateral flap of the capsule should be transposed medially to eliminate the redundant capsule of the false acetabulum.
- Irrigate both wounds and close them in the usual manner. Suction drains can be inserted if necessary.
- Apply a spica cast with the extremity in neutral rotation and slight flexion and abduction.

POSTOPERATIVE CARE The drains are removed 24 to 48 hours after surgery. The spica cast is removed at 8 to 12 weeks. Sequential radiographs are obtained to

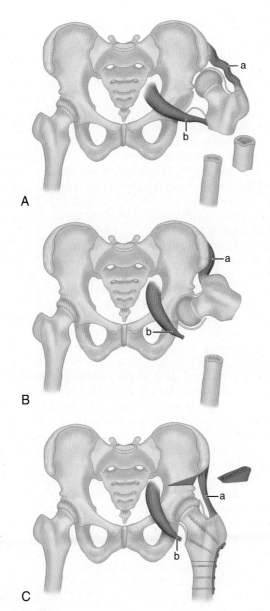

FIGURE 2.22 Technique for open reduction, primary femoral shortening, and Salter osteotomy. **A,** Femoral head is dislocated. Gluteal muscles *(a)* are retracted and slightly shortened. Iliopsoas muscle *(b)* is intact. Capsule is interposed between femoral head and ilium. Segment of femur is resected. **B,** Proximal femur is abducted; iliopsoas tendon *(b)* is divided if needed to mobilize the proximal fragment. Capsule is incised on inferior surface parallel to femoral neck. **C,** Operation is complete. Gluteal muscles *(a)* are tight. Salter osteotomy is completed with graft in place. Femoral fragments are fixed with pediatric hip screw. **SEE TECHNIQUE 2.7.**

evaluate development of the femoral head and acetabulum. Additionally, axial imaging can be obtained with either MRI or limited CT in the immediate postoperative period to assess the adequacy of reduction. Limb-length discrepancy may be evaluated annually by clinical evaluation and radiography.

PELVIC OSTEOTOMY

Operations on the pelvis, alone or combined with open reduction, are useful in developmental dysplasia or dislocation of the hip to ensure or to increase stability of the joint. The operations most often used are (1) osteotomy of the innominate bone (Salter), (2) acetabuloplasty (Pemberton), (3) osteotomies that free the acetabulum (Steel triple innominate osteotomy or Ganz acetabular osteotomy), (4) shelf operation (Staheli), and (5) innominate osteotomy with medial displacement of the acetabulum (Chiari). In an older child, one of these operations can be combined with femoral osteotomy to correct femoral and acetabular abnormalities.

Osteotomy of the innominate bone, an operation devised by Salter, is useful only when any subluxation or dislocation has been reduced or can be reduced by open reduction at the time of osteotomy in a child 18 months to 6 years old. The entire acetabulum together with the pubis and ischium is rotated as a unit, with the symphysis pubis acting as a hinge. The osteotomy is held open anterolaterally by a wedge of bone, and the roof of the acetabulum is shifted more anteriorly and laterally. The osteotomy is contraindicated in patients with nonconcentric hips or severe dysplasia.

Acetabuloplasty is also useful only when any subluxation or dislocation has been reduced or can be reduced by open reduction at the time of operation in children at least 18 months old and up to the age when the triradiate cartilage closes. In acetabuloplasty, the inclination of the acetabular roof is decreased by an osteotomy of the ilium made superior to the acetabulum. Pemberton described a *pericapsular osteotomy of the ilium* in which the osteotomy is made through the full thickness of the bone from just superior to the anterior inferior iliac spine anteriorly to the triradiate cartilage posteriorly; the triradiate cartilage acts as a hinge on which the acetabular roof is rotated anteriorly and laterally. This procedure decreases the volume of the acetabulum and produces joint incongruity that requires remodeling.

Osteotomies that free the acetabulum have been devised by Steel, Eppright, and Ganz. These operations free part of the pelvis, creating a movable segment of bone that includes the acetabulum. They are indicated in older children, adolescents, and skeletally mature adults with residual dysplasia and subluxation in whom remodeling of the acetabulum can no longer be anticipated. These operations are useful because they place articular cartilage over the femoral head. The shelf operation and the operation of Chiari interpose capsular fibrous tissue between the femoral head and the reconstructed acetabulum.

In the triple innominate osteotomy (Steel), the ischium, the superior pubic ramus, and the ilium superior to the acetabulum all are divided and the acetabulum is repositioned and stabilized by a bone graft and metal pins. In the pericapsular dial osteotomy of the acetabulum (Eppright), the entire acetabulum superiorly, posteriorly, inferiorly, and anteriorly is freed by osteotomy and as a single segment of bone is redirected to cover the femoral head appropriately. The Bernese periacetabular osteotomy (Ganz) creates a free acetabular segment through a series of osteotomies in the ischium, superior pubic ramus, and ilium while preserving the posterior column of the pelvis.

The *shelf* procedure (Staheli) is useful for subluxations and dislocations that have been reduced and in which no other osteotomy would establish a congruous joint with apposition of the articular cartilage of the acetabulum to the femoral head. In a classic shelf operation, the acetabular roof is extended laterally, posteriorly, or anteriorly, either by a graft or by turning distally over the femoral head the acetabular roof and part of the lateral cortex of the ilium superior to it.

Innominate osteotomy with medial displacement of the acetabulum, an operation devised by Chiari for patients older than 4 years old, is a modified shelf operation that places the femoral head beneath a surface of bone and joint capsule and corrects the pathologic lateral displacement of the femur. An osteotomy is made at the level of the acetabulum, and the femur and the acetabulum are displaced medially. The inferior surface of the proximal fragment forms a roof over the femoral head. General recommendations for all of these osteotomies are summarized in Table 2.1.

TABLE 2.1

Recommended Osteotomies for Congenital or Developmental Dislocation of the Hip

OSTEOTOMY	AGE	INDICATIONS
Salter innominate osteotomy	18 months to 6 years	Congruous hip reduction; <10 to 15 degrees correction of acetabular index required
Pemberton acetabuloplasty	18 months to 10 years	>10 to 15 degrees of correction of acetabular index required; small femoral head, large acetabulum
Steel or Ganz osteotomy	Late adolescence to skeletal maturity	Residual acetabular dysplasia; symptoms; congruous joint
Shelf procedure or Chiari osteotomy	Any age possible, but typically for older children or adolescents	Incongruous joint; symptoms; other osteotomy not possible

SALTER INNOMINATE OSTEOTOMY

During open reduction of developmental dislocations of the hip, Salter observed that the entire acetabulum faces more anterolaterally than normal. When the hip is extended, the femoral head is insufficiently "covered" anteriorly, and when it is adducted, there is insufficient coverage superiorly. Salter's osteotomy of the innominate bone redirects the entire acetabulum so that its roof "covers" the femoral head anteriorly and superiorly. If indicated to correct acetabular dysplasia, any dislocation or subluxation must be reduced concentrically before this operation is performed; if not, open reduction is done at the time of osteotomy. During the operation, any contractures of the adductor or iliopsoas muscles are released by tenotomy, and, in dislocations when the capsule is elongated, a capsulorrhaphy is done.

Salter recommended his osteotomy in the primary treatment of developmental dislocation of the hip in children 18 months to 6 years old and in the primary treatment of developmental subluxation in early adulthood. He also recommended it in the secondary treatment of any residual or recurrent dislocation or subluxation after other methods of treatment within the age limits described (Fig. 2.23).

The following are prerequisites for the success of this operation:
1. The femoral head must be positioned opposite the level of the acetabulum. This may require a period of traction before surgery or primary femoral shortening.
2. Contractures of the iliopsoas and adductor muscles must be released. This is indicated in subluxations and dislocations. Open reduction is performed for hip dislocation but usually is unnecessary for hip subluxation.
3. The femoral head must be reduced into the depth of the true acetabulum completely and concentrically. This generally requires careful open reduction and excision of any soft tissue, exclusive of the labrum, from the acetabulum.
4. The joint must be reasonably congruous.
5. The range of motion of the hip must be good, especially in abduction, internal rotation, and flexion.

In a cadaver study, Birnbaum et al. identified several structures that are at risk of injury during a Salter innominate osteotomy:

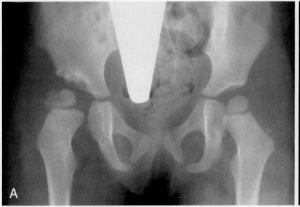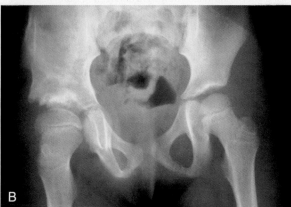

FIGURE 2.23 Salter osteotomy for congenital dislocation of hip. **A,** Residual acetabular dysplasia and subluxation of right hip in 4-year-old girl in whom open reduction had been performed at 9 months of age. **B,** One year after repeat open reduction and Salter innominate osteotomy.

1. The lateral femoral cutaneous nerve may be injured during an anterior approach. Ensuring that the skin including the lateral femoral cutaneous nerve is pulled anteriorly avoids this.
2. The nutrient vessels to the tensor fasciae latae muscle can be injured if retraction is too prolonged.
3. The sciatic nerve can be crushed or irritated by an inadequate subperiosteal approach during the pull on the Hohmann retractor.
4. An inadequate subperiosteal application of the medial Hohmann retractor can damage the obturator nerve.
5. Too prolonged retraction of the iliopsoas muscle can cause compression of the femoral nerve.

Because of the narrow spatial connection between the anatomic pathways and the osteotomy area, strict subperiosteal dissection and careful use of retractors are essential to prevent nerve and vessel injuries.

INNOMINATE OSTEOTOMY INCLUDING OPEN REDUCTION

TECHNIQUE 2.8

(SALTER)

- Place the patient supine on the operating table with the thorax on the affected side elevated by a radiolucent sandbag. Drape the trunk on the affected side to the midline anteriorly and posteriorly and to the lower rib cage superiorly. Drape the lower extremity so that it can be moved freely during the operation.
- Release the adductor muscles by subcutaneous or open tenotomy.
- Make a skin incision beginning just inferior to the middle of the iliac crest, extending anteriorly to just inferior to the anterior superior iliac spine and continuing to about the middle of the inguinal ligament. Decrease bleeding by applying pressure with sponges to the wound edges.
- Bluntly dissect between the tensor fasciae latae muscle laterally and the sartorius and rectus femoris medially and expose the anterior superior iliac spine.
- Dissect the rectus femoris from the underlying joint capsule and release its reflected head.
- Make a deep incision separating the iliac apophysis along the crest from the posterior end of the skin incision to the anterior superior iliac spine anteriorly and then turning distally to the anterior inferior iliac spine.
- Reflect the lateral part of the iliac apophysis and the periosteum from the lateral surface of the iliac crest in a continuous sheet inferiorly to the superior edge of the acetabulum and posteriorly to the greater sciatic notch.
- Free any adhesions of the joint capsule from the lateral surface of the ilium and from any false acetabulum.
- Expose the capsule anteriorly and laterally by dissecting bluntly the interval between it and the abductor muscles.
- Pack the dissected spaces with large sponges to control bleeding and to increase the interval between the reflected periosteum and the sciatic notch.

- If concentric reduction of the femoral head into the acetabulum is impossible, open the capsule superiorly and anteriorly, parallel with and about 1 cm distal to the rim of the acetabulum.
- Excise the ligamentum teres if it is hypertrophied.
- Gently reduce the femoral head into the acetabulum. Never excise the limbus. Incise the distal flap of capsule at right angles to the first incision, creating a T-shaped incision, and resect the inferolateral triangular flap so created. Test the stability of the joint; if the head becomes displaced superiorly from the acetabulum when the hip is adducted or anteriorly when it is extended or externally rotated, osteotomy of the innominate bone is performed.
- Allow the hip to redislocate and then strip the medial half of the iliac apophysis from the anterior half of the iliac crest and strip the periosteum from the medial surface of the ilium posteriorly and inferiorly to expose the entire medial aspect of the bone to the sciatic notch.
- Pack the surfaces exposed with sponges to control the loss of blood and to enlarge the interval between the periosteum and the bone.
- Expose the tendinous part of the iliopsoas muscle at the level of the pelvic brim. With scissors, separate the tendinous part from the muscular part and divide the former while protecting the muscle.
- Pass a curved forceps subperiosteally medial to the ilium into the sciatic notch and with it grasp one end of a Gigli saw. Gently retract the curved forceps to pass the Gigli saw into the sciatic notch. Alternatively, a large suture or umbilical tape can be passed first and then attached to the Gigli saw to aid in passage.
- Retract the tissues medially and laterally from the ilium and divide the bone with the saw in a straight line from the sciatic notch to the anterior inferior iliac spine.
- Remove a full-thickness graft from the anterior part of the iliac crest (Fig. 2.24A) and trim it to the shape of a wedge. If a primary femoral shortening was performed concurrently, the removed femoral bone segment can be used as structural autograft bone. Make the base of the wedge about as wide as the distance between the anterior superior and anterior inferior iliac spines.
- With towel clips, grasp each fragment of the osteotomized ilium.
- Insert a curved elevator into the sciatic notch and, by levering it anteriorly and by exerting traction on the towel clip that grasps the inferior fragment, shift this fragment anteriorly, inferiorly, and laterally to open the osteotomy anterolaterally. Ensure that the osteotomy remains closed posteriorly (Fig. 2.24B). Placing the limb in a figure-of-four position makes displacement of the distal fragment easier.
- Do not apply traction in a cephalad direction on the proximal fragment because this may dislocate the sacroiliac joint.
- Insert the bone graft into the osteotomy and release the traction on the inferior fragment.
- Drill a strong Kirschner wire through the remaining superior part of the ilium, through the graft, and into the inferior fragment (Fig. 2.24C). Ensure that the Kirschner wire does not enter the acetabulum but that it does traverse all three fragments.

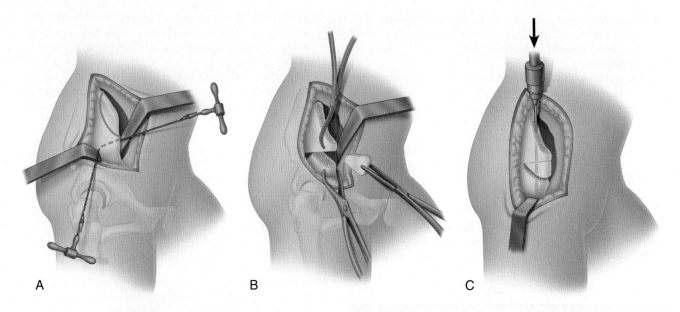

A   B   C

FIGURE 2.24 **A to C,** Salter technique of osteotomy of innominate bone, including open reduction. **SEE TECHNIQUE 2.8.**

- If needed for stability, drill a second Kirschner wire parallel with the first, using the same precautions.
- Reduce the femoral head again into the acetabulum and reevaluate its stability. Reduction should now be stable with the hip either in adduction or in slight external rotation.
- While closing the wound, have an assistant hold the knee flexed and the hip slightly abducted, flexed, and internally rotated.
- Obliterate any residual pocket of capsule by performing a capsulorrhaphy.
- Move the distal half of the lateral flap of capsule medially beyond the anterior inferior iliac spine. This brings the capsular edges together and increases the stability of reduction by keeping the hip internally rotated. Repair the capsule with interrupted sutures.
- Suture the sartorius and rectus femoris tendons to their origins.
- Suture together over the iliac crest the two halves of the iliac apophysis.
- Cut the Kirschner wires so that their anterior ends lie within the subcutaneous fat.
- Close the skin with a continuous subcuticular suture.
- With the hip held in the same position as during closure, apply a single spica cast.

POSTOPERATIVE CARE At 8 to 12 weeks, the spica cast is removed and, with the patient under general or local anesthesia, the Kirschner wires are also removed. The positions of the osteotomy and of the hip are checked by radiographs.

┃ PEMBERTON ACETABULOPLASTY

The term *acetabuloplasty* designates operations that redirect the inclination of the acetabular roof by an osteotomy of the ilium superior to the acetabulum followed by levering of the roof inferiorly. Pemberton devised an acetabuloplasty that he called *pericapsular osteotomy of the ilium,* in which an osteotomy is made through the full thickness of the ilium, using the triradiate cartilage as the hinge around which the acetabular roof is rotated anteriorly and laterally. After a review of 115 hips in 91 patients followed for at least 2 years after surgery, Pemberton recommended this procedure for any dysplastic hip in patients between the age of 1 year and the age when the triradiate cartilage becomes too inflexible to serve as a hinge (about 12 years old in girls and 14 years old in boys), provided that any subluxation or dislocation has been reduced or can be reduced at the time of osteotomy (Fig. 2.25).

One advantage of pericapsular over innominate osteotomies is that internal fixation is not always required, and a second, although minor, operation (implant removal) is avoided. A greater degree of correction can be achieved with less rotation of the acetabulum in the pericapsular osteotomy because the fulcrum, the triradiate cartilage, is nearer the site of desired correction; however, Pemberton's operation is technically more difficult to perform. In addition, it alters the configuration and capacity of the acetabulum and can result in an incongruous relationship between it and the femoral head; consequently, some remodeling of the acetabulum is required. Overcorrection should be avoided to decrease the chances of femoroacetabular impingement (FAI) later in life, although a 10-year follow-up study of over 150 Pemberton acetabuloplasties revealed that FAI is uncommon after this procedure.

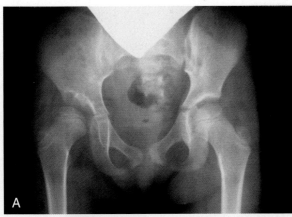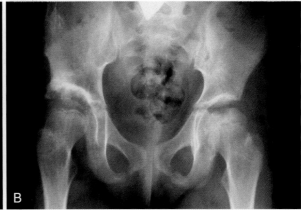

FIGURE 2.25 Pemberton acetabuloplasty. **A,** Symptomatic residual acetabular dysplasia in 8-year-old girl after treatment of congenital dislocation of right hip. **B,** After Pemberton acetabuloplasty.

PERICAPSULAR OSTEOTOMY OF THE ILIUM

TECHNIQUE 2.9

(PEMBERTON)

- Place the patient supine with a small radiolucent sandbag beneath the affected hip and expose the hip through an anterior iliofemoral approach.
- Make the superior part of the incision distal to and parallel with the iliac crest and extend it from the anterior superior iliac spine anteriorly to the middle of the crest posteriorly. Extend the distal part of the incision from the anterior superior iliac spine inferiorly for 5 cm parallel with the inguinal crease.
- Beginning at the crest, strip the gluteus and the tensor fasciae latae muscles subperiosteally from the anterior third of the ilium distally to the joint capsule and posteriorly until the greater sciatic notch is exposed.
- With a sharp elevator, separate the iliac apophysis with its attached abdominal muscles from the anterior third of the iliac crest and strip the muscles subperiosteally from the medial aspect of the ilium until the sciatic notch is again exposed.
- Open the capsule of the hip and remove any soft tissue that restricts reduction (Open Reduction Technique 2.3).
- Reduce the hip under direct vision and ensure that it is well seated; redislocate it until the osteotomy has been made and propped open with a graft.
- Insert two flat retractors subperiosteally into the sciatic notch—one along the medial surface of the ilium and one along the lateral surface to keep the anterior third of the ilium exposed medially and laterally. Image intensification can be helpful in visualizing the location and direction of the osteotomy. Both anteroposterior and oblique views of the ilium can be used to guide the osteotome.
- With a narrow curved osteotome, cut through the lateral cortex of the ilium as follows. Start slightly superior to the anterior inferior iliac spine and curve the osteotomy

posteriorly about 1 cm proximal to and parallel with the joint capsule until the osteotome is seen to be well anterior to the retractor resting in the sciatic notch. Image intensification aids in confirming correct placement of the osteotomy (Fig. 2.26A).

- From this point, when driven farther the blade of the osteotome disappears from sight, and it is important to direct its tip sufficiently inferiorly so that it does not enter the sciatic notch but instead enters the ilioischial rim of the triradiate cartilage at its midpoint (Fig. 2.26B).
- After directing the osteotome properly, drive it 1.5 cm farther to complete the osteotomy of the lateral cortex of the ilium.
- With the same osteotome, make a corresponding cut in the medial cortex of the ilium, starting anteriorly at the same point just superior to the anterior inferior iliac spine. Direct this cut posteriorly parallel with that in the lateral cortex until it reaches the triradiate cartilage (Fig. 2.27A).
- The direction in which the acetabular roof becomes displaced after the osteotomy is controlled by varying the position of the posterior part of the osteotomy of the medial cortex. The more anterior this part of the osteotomy, the less the acetabular roof rotates anteriorly; conversely, the more posterior this part of the osteotomy, the more the acetabular roof rotates anteriorly.
- After completing the osteotomy of the two cortices, insert a wide curved osteotome into the anterior part of the osteotomy and lever the distal fragment distally until the anterior edges of the two fragments are at least 2 to 3 cm apart. Alternatively, a laminar spreader can be used (Fig. 2.26C).
- The acetabular roof should be turned inferiorly far enough to correct the dysplasia. The exact degree of correction can be difficult to determine. Multiple radiographic images should be obtained and compared to the normal hip to determine adequate femoral head coverage while avoiding extreme overcorrection. Cut a narrow groove in the anteroposterior direction in each raw surface of the ilium.
- Resect a wedge of bone from the anterior part of the ilium including the anterior superior iliac spine; with a lamina

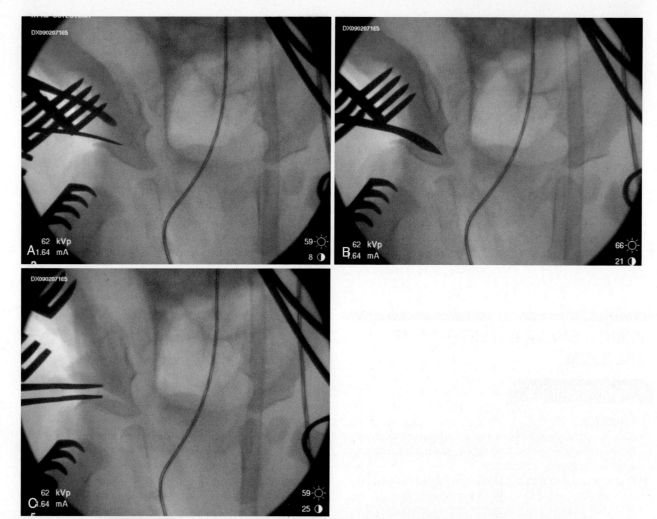

FIGURE 2.26 Intraoperative anteroposterior fluoroscopic image of the pelvis. **A,** Note placement of thin curved osteotome just above anterior inferior iliac spine, directed toward open triradiate cartilage. **B,** Osteotomy continued toward the triradiate cartilage. **C,** Laminar spreader is used to open the completed osteotomy to the desired level of correction where it is stabilized while the graft is inserted. **SEE TECHNIQUE 2.9.**

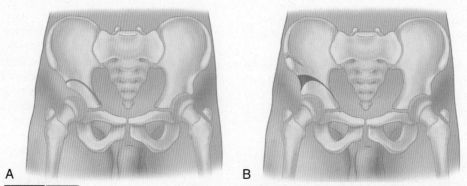

FIGURE 2.27 Pemberton pericapsular osteotomy. **A,** Line of osteotomy beginning slightly superior to anterior inferior iliac spine and curving into triradiate cartilage. **B,** Completed osteotomy with acetabular roof in corrected position and wedge of bone impacted into open osteotomy site. **SEE TECHNIQUE 2.9.**

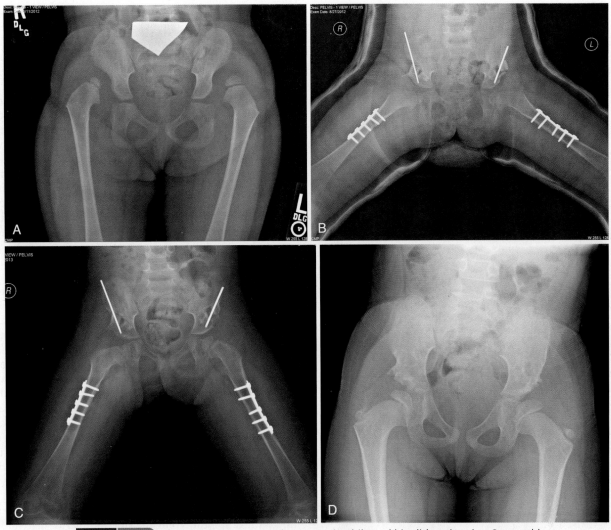

FIGURE 2.28   **A,** Preoperative image demonstrating bilateral hip dislocations in a 2-year-old patient. **B,** Anteroposterior pelvic view after staged open reductions, capsulorrhaphies, primary femoral shortenings, and Pemberton acetabuloplasties using resection femoral segment for pelvic bone grafting. **C,** Postoperative anteroposterior pelvis after spica cast removal. **D,** Two-year follow-up view reveals healing and maintenance of hip reduction. Some residual dysplasia exists, particularly on the left hip. **SEE TECHNIQUE 2.9.**

spreader, separate the osteotomy fragments and place the wedge of bone in the grooves made in the surfaces of the ilium; drive the wedge into place and firmly impact it. The acetabular roof should remain fixed in the corrected position (Fig. 2.27B). Alternatively, a segment of femur can be used when a concurrent primary femoral shortening procedure has been performed (Fig. 2.28).
- Hold the correction with a Kirschner wire, if necessary.
- If the hip has remained dislocated during the osteotomy, reduce it at this time.
- Perform a meticulous capsulorrhaphy for additional soft-tissue stability.
- Suture the iliac apophysis over the remaining ilium and close the wound.

POSTOPERATIVE CARE With the hip in neutral position (or in slight abduction and internal rotation, if this has been found the most favorable position for closure of the wound), a spica cast is applied from the nipple line to the toes on the affected side and to above the knee on the opposite side. At 8 to 12 weeks, the cast is removed and the osteotomy is checked by radiographs.

STEEL OSTEOTOMY

The Pemberton pericapsular osteotomy is limited by the mobility of the triradiate cartilage, and hinging on this cartilage can cause premature physeal closure. Although the Salter innominate osteotomy can be used in older patients, its results depend on the mobility of the symphysis pubis, and the amount of femoral head coverage is limited. Other, more complex osteotomies, such as those of Steel and Eppright, can provide more correction and improve femoral head coverage.

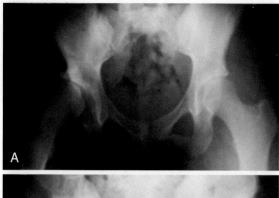

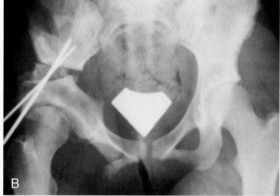

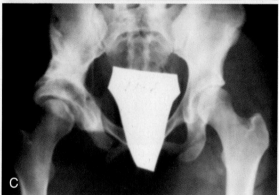

FIGURE 2.29 Steel triple innominate osteotomy. **A,** Sixteen-year-old girl with painful right hip, subluxation, and acetabular dysplasia. **B,** After Steel osteotomy. **C,** One year after surgery. (Courtesy Randal Betz, MD, and Howard Steel, MD.)

In the *triple innominate osteotomy* developed by Steel, the ischium, the superior pubic ramus, and the ilium superior to the acetabulum all are divided, and the acetabulum is repositioned and stabilized by a bone graft and pins. The objective of this procedure is to establish a stable hip in anatomic position for dislocation or subluxation of the hip in older children when this is impossible by any one of the other osteotomies (Fig. 2.29). For the operation to be successful, the articular surfaces of the joint must be congruous or become so when the acetabulum has been redirected so that a functional, painless range of motion is achieved and a Trendelenburg gait is absent. Steel reviewed 45 patients in whom 52 of his osteotomies had been performed. The results were satisfactory in 40 hips and unsatisfactory in 12. The unsatisfactory hips were painful and easily fatigued; in two, the Trendelenburg test was positive, and in one, significant motion had been lost.

Lipton and Bowen modified the Steel osteotomy by (1) resecting 1.0 to 1.5 cm of bone after the ischial osteotomy to facilitate medialization and rotation of the acetabulum, (2) resecting a triangular wedge of bone from the outer cortex of the proximal part of the ilium to create a slot that serves as an abutment into which the distal posterior aspect of the ilium fits, and (3) using two 7.3-mm cannulated screws instead of Steinmann pins for fixation of the iliac osteotomy. The procedure is done through two incisions: an ischial incision and a bikini-type iliofemoral incision. Primary advantages of this technique include better coverage of the femoral head by articular cartilage of the acetabulum, better hip joint stability for weight bearing, and no need for spica cast immobilization. Disadvantages include the technical difficulty of the procedure; it does not change the size of the acetabulum, and it distorts the pelvis such that natural childbirth may be impossible in adulthood. Femoral shortening may be performed, and, if necessary, any contracted muscles around the hip are released surgically.

Using three-dimensional CT, Frick et al. identified excessive (>10 degrees) external rotation of the acetabulum after triple innominate osteotomy in five hips, which included two with pubic osteotomy nonunions, two with ischial nonunions, and one with marked external rotation of the leg. They cautioned that the surgical technique for triple innominate osteotomy should be designed to avoid excessive external rotation of the acetabular fragment, which can result in (1) excessive external rotation of the lower limb, (2) decreased posterior coverage, (3) increased gaps at the pubic and ischial osteotomy sites with resultant higher rates of nonunion, and (4) lateralization of the joint center. Technique modifications by Frick et al. include avoidance of the figure-of-four maneuver to mobilize the acetabulum (they believe this promotes external rotation of the acetabulum); strict attention to the intraoperative landmarks of the proximal ilium and anterior inferior iliac spine, keeping the anterior inferior iliac spine in line with the plane of the proximal ilium to prevent external rotation; and use of a temporary Schanz screw in the acetabular segment to serve as a handle to guide the acetabulum into the correct position. Careful evaluation of the transverse plane acetabular position before and after provisional fixation is recommended to aid in preventing rotational malunions.

TRIPLE INNOMINATE OSTEOTOMY

TECHNIQUE 2.10

(STEEL)
- Place the patient supine on the operating table and flex the hip and knee 90 degrees. Keep the hip in neutral abduction, adduction, and rotation.
- Drape the posterior aspect of the proximal thigh and the buttock, leaving the ischial tuberosity exposed.
- Make a transverse incision perpendicular to the long axis of the femoral shaft 1 cm proximal to the gluteal crease.
- Retract the gluteus maximus muscle laterally and expose the hamstring muscles at their ischial origin.

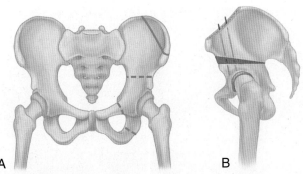

FIGURE 2.30   Steel triple innominate osteotomy. **A,** Osteotomies to be performed in iliac wing and superior and inferior pubic rami. Note wedge of bone to be taken as graft from superiormost portion of ilium. **B,** Lateral view showing graft in place and fixation with two Kirschner wires. **SEE TECHNIQUE 2.10.**

- By sharp dissection, free the biceps femoris, the most superficial muscle in the area, from the ischium and expose the interval between the semimembranosus and the semitendinosus muscles. The sciatic nerve lies far enough laterally not to be endangered.
- Insert a curved hemostat in the interval between the origins of the semimembranosus and the semitendinosus deep to the ischium and into the obturator foramen.
- Elevate the origins of the obturator internus and externus and bring the tip of the hemostat out at the inferior margin of the ischial ramus. Ensure that the hemostat remains in contact with the bone during its passage deep to the ramus.
- With an osteotome directed posterolaterally and 45 degrees from the perpendicular, divide completely the ischial ramus. Allow the origin of the biceps femoris to fall into place.
- Suture the gluteus maximus to the deep fascia and close the skin.
- Change gowns, gloves, and instruments, and begin in the iliopubic area the second stage of the operation. As an alternative, the superior and inferior pubic rami can be dissected and divided through a medial adductor approach. If a posterior incision was chosen, however, proceed with a full skin preparation medially to the midline and superiorly to the costal margin and drape the extremity free.
- Through an anterior iliofemoral approach, reflect the iliac and gluteal muscles from the wing of the ilium.
- Detach the sartorius and the lateral attachments of the inguinal ligament from the anterior superior iliac spine and reflect them medially.
- Reflect the iliacus and psoas muscles subperiosteally from the inner surface of the pelvis; this protects the femoral neurovascular bundle.
- Divide the tendinous part of the origin of the iliopsoas and expose the pectineal tubercle. Detach the pectineus muscle subperiosteally from the superior pubic ramus and expose the bone 1 cm medial to the pubic tubercle.
- Pass a curved hemostat superior to the superior pubic ramus into the obturator foramen near the bone. With this hemostat, penetrate the obturator fascia so that the tip of the hemostat is brought out inferior to the ramus. If the

bone is especially thick, pass a second hemostat inferior to the ramus and direct it superiorly to contact the first one.
- Direct an osteotome posteromedially and 15 degrees from the perpendicular and perform an osteotomy of the pubic ramus.
- The obturator artery, vein, and nerve are protected by the hemostat or a blunted Hohmann retractor. Using the technique as described by Salter for innominate osteotomy, divide the ilium with a Gigli saw. When this osteotomy has been completed, free the periosteum and fascia from the medial wall of the pelvis to free the acetabular segment (Fig. 2.30).
- If the femoral head is subluxated or dislocated, open the capsule at this time and remove any tissue obstructing reduction. Reduce the femoral head as near as possible to the center of the triradiate cartilage and close the capsule.
- With a towel clip, grasp the anterior inferior iliac spine and rotate the acetabular segment in the desired direction, usually anteriorly and laterally, until the femoral head is covered. In an older child, use a lamina spreader to open the osteotomy because the sacroiliac joint usually is more stable in this age group and is not likely to be subluxated.
- With the acetabular fragment in proper position, stabilize it with a triangular bone graft removed from the superior rim of the ilium.
- Transfix the graft with two pins that penetrate the inner wall of the ilium.
- Allow the pectineus and iliopsoas muscles to fall into place.
- Reattach the sartorius and the lateral end of the inguinal ligament to the anterior superior iliac spine and close the wound in layers.

POSTOPERATIVE CARE A spica cast is applied with the hip in 20 degrees of abduction, 5 degrees of flexion, and neutral rotation. At 8 to 10 weeks, the cast and pins are removed and active and passive motion of the hip are started. All three osteotomies usually unite by 12 weeks after surgery, at which time progressive weight bearing on crutches is started.

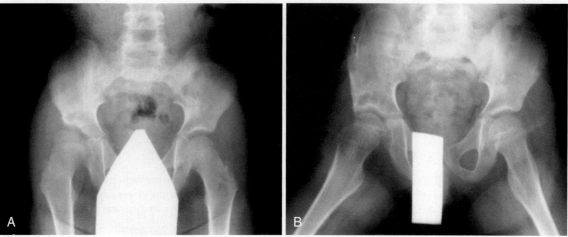

FIGURE 2.31 Before **(A)** and after **(B)** Dega transiliac osteotomy.

▌DEGA OSTEOTOMY

In 1969, Dega described a transiliac osteotomy for the treatment of residual acetabular dysplasia secondary to developmental hip dysplasia or dislocation. This incomplete transiliac osteotomy involves osteotomy of the anterior and middle portions of the inner cortex of the ilium, leaving an intact hinge posteriorly consisting of the intact posteromedial iliac cortex and sciatic notch.

Because of the variable hinge location, the Dega osteotomy can be done with either an open or a closed triradiate cartilage, although it is usually done before closure of the triradiate cartilage. This osteotomy is only one component of the comprehensive, complicated surgery required to treat severe DDH in children of walking age. It must be accompanied by a satisfactory open reduction and an appropriate correction of proximal femoral deformity when needed (Fig. 2.31).

TRANSILIAC (DEGA) OSTEOTOMY

TECHNIQUE 2.11

(GRUDZIAK AND WARD)

- Position the patient supine with the involved hip tilted up 30 to 40 degrees by a bump placed at the midlumbar level.
- Make an extended anterolateral incision starting 1 cm inferior and posterior to the anterior superior iliac spine and extending distally over the proximal part of the femur, centered over the greater trochanter. Alternatively, this procedure can be performed through a standard ilioinguinal approach at the time of open reduction of the hip.
- Develop the interval between the tensor fasciae latae muscles posteriorly and the sartorius muscle anteriorly and release the sartorius from its origin on the anterior superior iliac spine.
- Sharply reflect the abductor muscles off of the lateral wall of the ilium just distal to the iliac apophysis, but do not split the apophysis itself. Completely separate the abductor muscles and periosteum from the ilium and the hip capsule back to the sciatic notch, which is fully exposed, and insert an adult-size blunt Hohmann retractor into the notch. Do not dissect either the muscles or the periosteum off of the inner wall of the ilium.

- Separate the reflected head of the rectus femoris muscle from the hip capsule and incise it. Detach the tendon of the straight head of the rectus femoris muscle from the anterior inferior iliac spine only when necessary for proper exposure of the capsule.
- Isolate the tendinous portion of the iliopsoas muscle from the capsule and transect it either over the anteromedial aspect of the capsule just distal to the pelvic brim or more distally near its insertion.
- If required, reduce the hip and perform a femoral osteotomy with shortening and rotation to correct excessive anteversion.
- Make the Dega osteotomy to decrease acetabular dysplasia and to enhance containment of the femoral head.
- Mark the orientation of the osteotomy on the lateral cortex of the ilium (Fig. 2.32A). The direction of the osteotomy is curvilinear when viewed from the lateral cortex, starting just above the anterior inferior iliac spine, curving gently cephalad and posteriorly to reach a point superior to the midpoint of the acetabulum, and then continuing posteriorly to end 1.0 to 1.5 cm in front of the sciatic notch. The most cephalad extent of the osteotomy is in the middle of the acetabulum, at a point on the ilium determined by the steepness of the acetabulum. Very steep acetabular inclinations require a correspondingly higher midpoint.
- Insert a guidewire under fluoroscopic control at the most cephalad point of the curvilinear marking line, directing it caudally and medially to ensure that the osteotomy exits at the appropriate level just above the horizontal limb of the triradiate cartilage.
- Use a straight ¼- inch or ½-inch osteotome to make the bone cut, which extends obliquely medially and inferiorly, paralleling the guidewire to exit through the inner cortex just above the iliopubic and ilioischial limbs of the triradiate cartilage (Fig. 2.32B), leaving the posterior one third of the inner cortex intact (Fig. 2.32C).

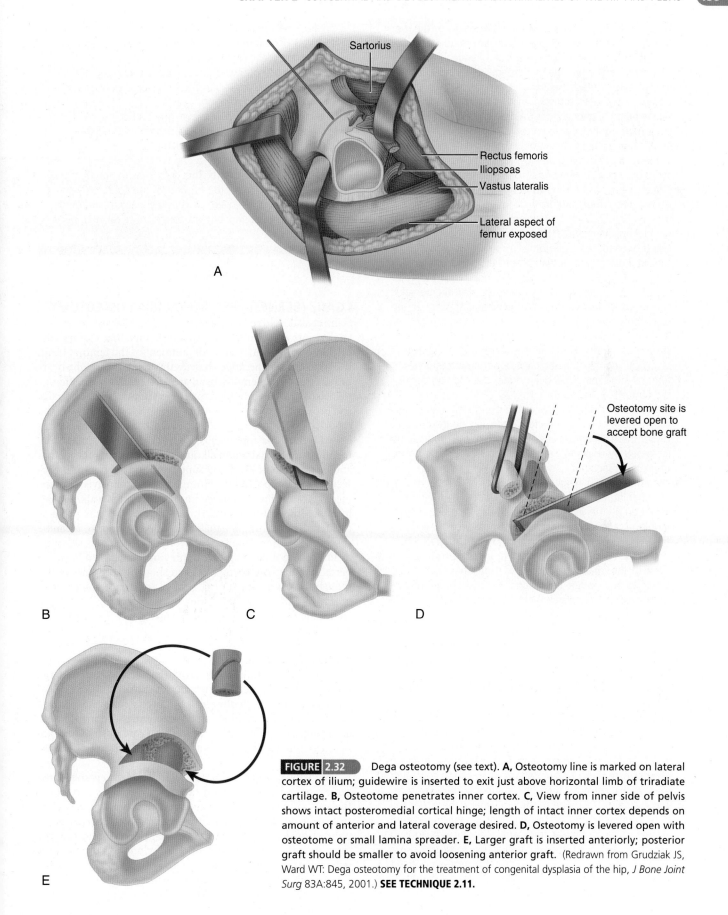

Sartorius

Rectus femoris

Iliopsoas

Vastus lateralis

Lateral aspect of
femur exposed

A

Osteotomy site is
levered open to
accept bone graft

B

C

D

E

FIGURE 2.32 Dega osteotomy (see text). **A,** Osteotomy line is marked on lateral cortex of ilium; guidewire is inserted to exit just above horizontal limb of triradiate cartilage. **B,** Osteotome penetrates inner cortex. **C,** View from inner side of pelvis shows intact posteromedial cortical hinge; length of intact inner cortex depends on amount of anterior and lateral coverage desired. **D,** Osteotomy is levered open with osteotome or small lamina spreader. **E,** Larger graft is inserted anteriorly; posterior graft should be smaller to avoid loosening anterior graft. (Redrawn from Grudziak JS, Ward WT: Dega osteotomy for the treatment of congenital dysplasia of the hip, *J Bone Joint Surg* 83A:845, 2001.) **SEE TECHNIQUE 2.11.**

- If predominantly anterior coverage is desired, cut the medial (inner) cortex over the anterior and middle portion, leaving only the posterior sciatic notch hinge intact.
- If more lateral coverage is desired, leave more of the medial cortex intact, resulting in a posteromedial hinge based on the posteromedial inner cortex and the entire sciatic notch. Generally, approximately one fourth to one third of the inner pelvic cortex is left intact posteriorly. With experience, the osteotomy cut might be done safely without fluoroscopic guidance, as in Dega's original description; however, we prefer to use fluoroscopy.
- Use a ½-inch osteotome to gently lever open the osteotomy site either anteriorly or laterally in a controlled manner (Fig. 2.32D). A small lamina spreader also is useful for this maneuver. Often, while the osteotomy site is being opened, the osteotomy cut on the outer cortex of the ilium propagates toward the sciatic notch as a greenstick fracture. Because the posterior portion of the inner cortex is still intact, however, the outer cortical greenstick fracture does not weaken the recoil and stability at the osteotomy site.
- Keep the osteotomy site open by inserting two correctly sized bone grafts (Fig. 2.32E). Fashion the grafts from a bicortical segment of iliac crest bone, or, alternatively, if femoral shortening has been done, use the segment of the femur that was removed.
- If there is a substantial gap at the osteotomy site, an autogenous femoral or iliac crest graft may be insufficient. Under these circumstances, the height of the graft can be increased by using freeze-dried fibular allograft cut into trapezoidal sections.
- The correct graft height is determined by simply noting the opening of the osteotomy gap created by the lamina spreader or the levering osteotome. In developmental dysplasia, acetabular deficiency is most pronounced anteriorly, mandating placement of the larger graft more anteriorly. Wedge a smaller graft more posteriorly, just in front of the intact sciatic notch. Ensure that both grafts are of an appropriate height and that the amount of correction of the dysplastic acetabulum provides enough coverage of the femoral head.
- After the grafts have been inserted, they are stable because of the inherent recoil at the osteotomy site produced by the intact sciatic notch. Metallic internal fixation is unnecessary. Variations in the graft size and placement, extent of the outer and inner cortical cuts, and thickness of the acetabular fragment make it possible to reorient and reshape the acetabulum. The more posterior the extent of the outer cortical cut, and the greater the amount of the inner cortex left intact, the more lateral the tilt of the acetabulum. A more cephalad starting point and a steeper osteotomy angle produce more lateral coverage. A more extensive cut through the inner cortex allows for more anterior coverage of the hip. Finally, the closer the osteotomy is to the acetabulum, the thinner and more pliable is the acetabular fragment, theoretically allowing for more reshaping and less redirection to occur. These three-dimensional changes in the osteotomy are difficult to quantify, as is the true anatomic nature of a dysplastic hip. An experienced orthopaedic surgeon who is familiar with the spectrum of dysplastic hip pathology and who applies the principles described should be able to perform an osteotomy, however, that is precisely suited to the unique pathology of a given dysplastic hip.
- When the osteotomy is done, satisfactory femoral head coverage can be appreciated and the hip should be stable during flexion and rotation.
- After closure, apply a one and one half spica cast with the hip in neutral extension, approximately 20 degrees of internal rotation and 20 to 30 degrees of abduction.

POSTOPERATIVE CARE The cast is worn for 8 to 12 weeks, depending on the healing of the osteotomy site. After the cast is removed, progressive walking and range of motion are begun but no formal physical therapy is prescribed.

GANZ (BERNESE) PERIACETABULAR OSTEOTOMY

Ganz et al. developed a triplanar periacetabular osteotomy for adolescents and adults with dysplastic hips that require correction of congruency and containment of the femoral head. If significant degenerative changes involving the weight-bearing surface of the femoral head are present, a proximal femoral osteotomy can be added to provide uninvolved acetabular and proximal femoral weight-bearing surfaces (Fig. 2.33). The reported advantages of periacetabular osteotomy are as follows: (1) only one approach is used; (2) a large amount of correction can be obtained in all directions, including the medial and lateral planes; (3) blood supply to the acetabulum is preserved; (4) the posterior column of the hemipelvis remains mechanically intact, allowing immediate crutch walking with minimal internal fixation; (5) the shape of the true pelvis is unaltered, permitting normal child delivery; and (6) it can be combined with trochanteric osteotomy if needed. Although technically more demanding in previously operated hips, the periacetabular osteotomy has been shown to provide similar radiographic and functional results as periacetabular osteotomy in patients without prior hip surgery (Fig. 2.34). The technique for Ganz periacetabular osteotomy is described in other chapter.

SHELF OPERATIONS

Shelf procedures commonly have been performed to enlarge the volume of the acetabulum; however, pelvic redirectional and displacement osteotomies have largely replaced this type of operation. The redirectional osteotomies are inappropriate in hips in which the femoral head and acetabulum are misshapen but still congruent because redirection can cause incongruity.

Staheli described a slotted acetabular augmentation procedure to create a congruous acetabular extension in which the size and position of the augmentation can be easily controlled. A deficient acetabulum that cannot be corrected by redirectional pelvic osteotomy is the primary indication for this operation. Contraindications include dysplastic hips with spherical congruity suitable for redirectional osteotomy, hips requiring concurrent open reduction that must have supplementary stability, and patients unsuited for spica cast immobilization.

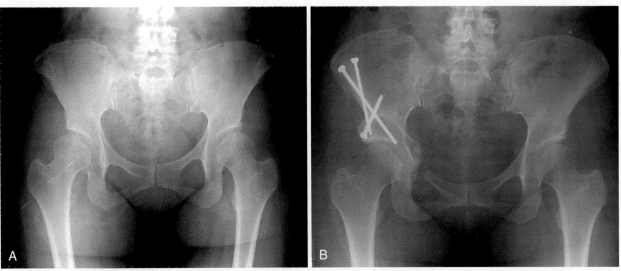

FIGURE 2.33   **A,** Twenty-eight-year-old woman with painful bilateral acetabular dysplasia. **B,** After Ganz osteotomy of right hip. (Courtesy James Guyton, MD.)

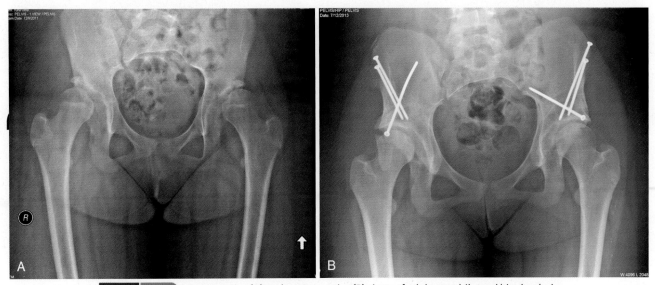

FIGURE 2.34   Preoperative **(A)** and postoperative **(B)** views of adolescent bilateral hip dysplasia in a 14-year-old girl. The patient was treated with bilateral, staged periacetabular osteotomies.

SLOTTED ACETABULAR AUGMENTATION

TECHNIQUE 2.12

(STAHELI)

- Before surgery, determine the center-edge angle of Wiberg from anteroposterior standing pelvic radiographs and superimpose a normal center-edge angle (about 30 to 35 degrees) on the image. Measure the additional width necessary to extend the existing acetabulum to achieve the normal angle (Fig. 2.35). This determines the width of the augmentation; this measurement added to the depth of the slot gives the total graft length.

- Position the patient supine on a radiolucent operating table with a small bump under the affected hip.
- Make a straight bikini-line skin incision 1 cm below and parallel to the iliac crest.
- Expose the hip joint through a standard iliofemoral approach.
- Divide the tendon of the reflected head of the rectus femoris muscle anteriorly and displace it posteriorly. If the capsule is abnormally thick (>6 mm), thin it by "filleting" with a scalpel.
- The placement of the acetabular slot is the most critical part of the procedure; the slot must be created *exactly at the acetabular margin*. Determine the position of the slot by placing a probe into the joint to palpate the position of the acetabulum. Place a drill in the selected site and verify correct position with image intensification. The floor of

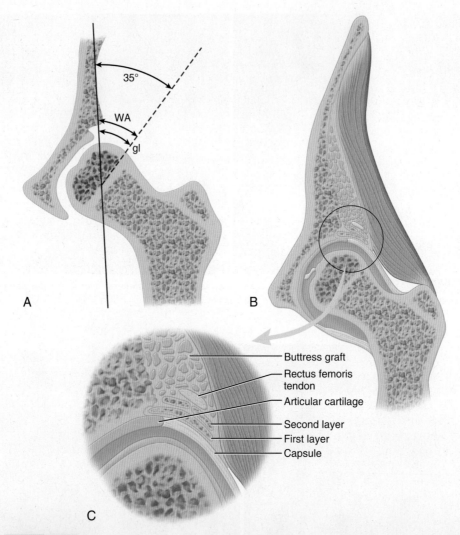

FIGURE 2.35 Slotted acetabular augmentation of Staheli. **A,** Width of augmentation *(WA)* is determined preoperatively from standing anteroposterior radiograph of pelvis. Center-edge angle and 35-degree angle are drawn. Graft length *(gl)* is sum of WA and slot depth. **B,** Objective of procedure is to provide congruous extension of acetabulum. **C,** Details of extension. **SEE TECHNIQUE 2.12.**

the slot should be acetabular articular cartilage and little bone; the end and roof of the slot should be cancellous bone. The slot should be 1 cm deep.

- Make the slot by drilling a series of holes with a {5/32}-inch (4.5-mm) bit and join them with a narrow rongeur. Determine the length of the slot intraoperatively by the need for coverage. If excessive femoral anteversion is present, extend the slot anteriorly. If the acetabulum is deficient posteriorly, extend the slot in that direction.
- Take thin strips of cortical and cancellous bone from the lateral surface of the ilium; cut these as long as possible.
- Extend the shallow decortication inferiorly from the iliac crest to the superior margin of the slot to ensure rapid fusion of the graft to the ilium. Do not remove the inner table of the ilium because this may change the contour of the pelvis.
- Measure the depth of the slot and add this to the width of the augmentation as determined preoperatively.

- Select thin strips (1 mm) of cancellous bone and cut them into rectangles about 1 cm wide and of the appropriate length. Assemble these rectangular pieces on a moist sponge, cutting enough to provide a single layer the length of the augmentation.
- Apply the first layer radially from the slot with the concave side down to provide a congruous extension.
- Select longer cancellous strips for the second layer and cut them to the length of the extension. Place these at right angles to the first layer and parallel to the acetabulum. They may be a little thicker (2 mm), especially the most lateral strip, to provide a well-defined lateral margin of the extension. Both layers must be of appropriate width and length. The augmentation should not extend too far anteriorly to avoid blocking hip flexion.
- Secure these two layers of cancellous grafts by bringing the reflected head of the rectus femoris forward over the grafts and suturing it in its original position.

A capsular flap can be substituted if this tendon is unavailable.

■ Cut the remaining grafts into small pieces and pack them above, but not beyond, the initial layer. They are held in place by the reattached abductor muscles. Some authors have described the use of a piece of structural allograft as the shelf bone. This technique avoids harvesting the iliac crest, provides a more structurally sound graft, and allows for stabilization with a plate and screws.

■ Confirm the position and width of the graft by radiographs.

■ After closure, apply a single hip spica cast with the hip in 15 degrees of abduction, 20 degrees of flexion, and neutral rotation.

POSTOPERATIVE CARE The cast is removed after 6 weeks, and crutch walking is permitted with partial weight bearing on the affected side until the graft is incorporated, usually at 3 to 4 months (Fig. 2.36).

▌INNOMINATE OSTEOTOMY WITH MEDIAL DISPLACEMENT OF THE ACETABULUM (CHIARI)

The Chiari osteotomy is a capsular interposition arthroplasty and should be considered only in situations in which other reconstructions are impossible, such as when the femoral head cannot be centered adequately in the acetabulum or in painfully subluxated hips with early signs of osteoarthritis. This procedure deepens the deficient acetabulum by medial displacement of the distal pelvic fragment and improves superolateral femoral coverage.

The Chiari procedure is an operation that places the femoral head beneath a surface of cancellous bone with the capacity for regeneration and corrects the lateral pathologic displacement of the femur. An osteotomy of the pelvis is performed at the superior margin of the acetabulum, and the pelvis inferior to the osteotomy along with the femur is displaced medially (Fig. 2.37). The superior fragment of the osteotomy then becomes a shelf, and the capsule is interposed between it and the femoral head.

After using this operation on more than 600 patients, 400 of whom had been observed for more than 2 years, Chiari recommended the operation in the following situations: (1) for congenital subluxations in patients 4 to 6 years old or older, including adults (including subluxations that persist after conservative treatment of dislocations and subluxations previously not treated); (2) for untreated congenital dislocations in patients older than 4 years old, soon after open or closed reduction; (3) for dysplastic hips with osteoarthritis; (4) for paralytic dislocations caused by muscular weakness or spasticity; and (5) for coxa magna after Perthes disease or osteonecrosis after treatment of congenital dysplasia. These indications are broader than the indications usually accepted by most pediatric orthopaedists. For children younger than 10 years old, the osteotomy is not recommended in subluxations or in dislocations that can be reduced surgically or conservatively and in which osteotomy of the innominate bone, acetabuloplasty, or osteotomies that free the acetabulum would result in a competent acetabulum. Some surgeons recommend the operation for

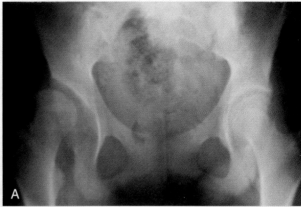

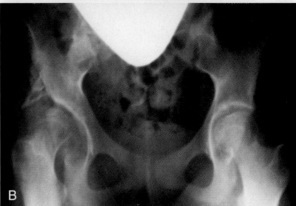

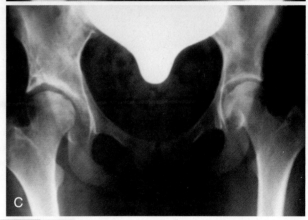

FIGURE 2.36   Staheli slotted acetabular augmentation. **A,** Fourteen-year-old girl with painful right acetabular dysplasia. **B,** Four months after operation. **C,** One year after operation, excellent graft incorporation. (Courtesy Lynn Staheli, MD.)

patients older than 10 years who have symptomatic early subluxation of the hip with acetabular dysplasia too severe to be treated by other pelvic osteotomies; for them, innominate osteotomy with medial displacement is preferred to a shelf operation.

Chiari's operation is a capsular arthroplasty because the capsule is interposed between the newly formed acetabular roof and the femoral head. Because the biomechanics of the hip is improved by displacing the hip nearer the midline, a Trendelenburg limp often is eliminated.

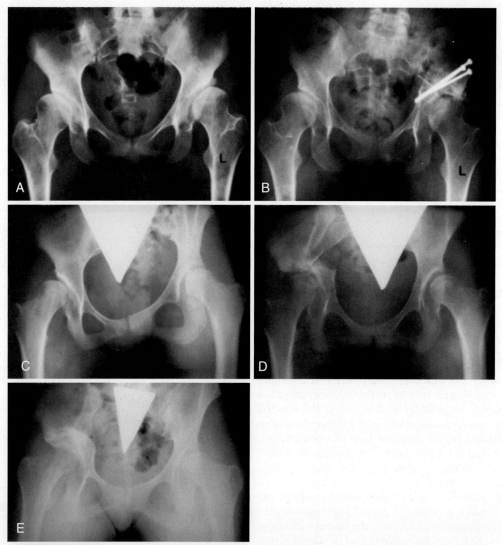

FIGURE 2.37 Chiari osteotomy. **A,** Young adult with painful, bilateral acetabular dysplasia, greater on left than on right. **B,** After Chiari osteotomy of left hip. Note optional internal fixation and medial bone grafting. **C,** Bilateral acetabular dysplasia in 12-year-old girl. **D,** After surgery, right hip is completely displaced. **E,** One year after Chiari osteotomy. (A and B, Courtesy Randal Betz, MD.)

CHIARI OSTEOTOMY

TECHNIQUE 2.13

- Place the patient supine on a fracture table with the feet attached to the traction plate. Slightly abduct and externally rotate the affected hip.
- Make an anterolateral bikini-line incision about 10 cm long. Develop the interval between the tensor fasciae latae and the sartorius muscles and laterally retract the former.
- Incise the iliac apophysis in line with the iliac crest. With a periosteal elevator, detach the lateral half of the apophy-

sis along with the tensor fasciae latae muscle and the anterior part of the gluteus medius muscle.
- Dissect these muscles subperiosteally and retract them posteriorly.
- Insert a periosteal elevator between the capsule of the hip and the gluteus minimus.
- Dissect subperiosteally posteriorly to the point where the pelvis curves inferiorly.
- With a curved periosteal elevator, dissect subperiosteally farther posteriorly until the sciatic notch is reached. Replace this elevator with a flexible metal ribbon retractor 3 cm wide. This completes the dissection posteriorly.
- Return anteriorly to the medial aspect of the ilium. With a periosteal elevator, strip the iliacus muscle and the underlying periosteum posteriorly to the sciatic notch.

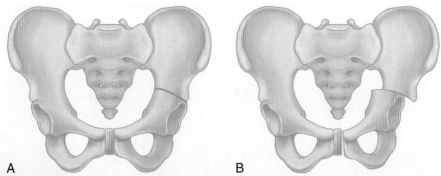

FIGURE 2.38   Chiari medial displacement osteotomy. **A,** Line of osteotomy extending from immediately superior to lip of acetabulum into sciatic notch. Osteotomy can be curved to facilitate femoral head coverage. **B,** Completed osteotomy with medial displacement of distal fragment for interpositional capsular arthroplasty. **SEE TECHNIQUE 2.13.**

- When the sciatic notch is reached, replace the elevator with a flexible metal ribbon retractor that touches and overlaps the ribbon retractor already in the notch.
- With curved scissors, separate the rectus muscle and its reflected head from the capsule of the hip joint. Divide the reflected head.
- The osteotomy should be made with a Hohmann retractor precisely between the insertion of the capsule and the reflected head of the rectus, following the capsular insertion in a curved line and ending distal to the anterior inferior iliac spine anteriorly and in the sciatic notch posteriorly. Do not open or damage the capsule of the joint.
- After the line of the osteotomy has been determined, start the osteotomy with a straight, narrow osteotome, opening the lateral table of the ilium along this line.
- Determine the exact position of the osteotome at the beginning by image intensification or by radiographs. Direct the osteotomy superiorly approximately 20 degrees toward the inner table of the ilium (Fig. 2.38A). Change the position of the osteotome as necessary to make the osteotomy curve superiorly. Do not direct the osteotomy more than 20 degrees superiorly because it might enter the sacroiliac joint.
- When the osteotomy has been completed, displace the hip medially by releasing the traction on the extremity and by forcing the limb into abduction. The distal fragment displaces medially, hinging at the symphysis pubis (Fig. 2.38B). If the adductor muscles are extremely relaxed, however, it may be necessary to manipulate the head manually or to displace the distal fragment with an instrument. Ensure that the distal fragment is displaced far enough medially (if necessary, 100% of the width of the ilium) so that the proximal fragment completely covers the femoral head.
- Internal fixation can be inserted to secure and maintain adequate displacement.
- After the displacement has been completed, decrease the abduction of the limb to about 30 degrees.
- If the capsule is loose, perform a capsulorrhaphy.
- Check the position of the hip and the osteotomy by image intensification or by radiographs.
- Replace and suture the iliac apophysis and close the wound.
- Apply a spica cast with the hip in 20 to 30 degrees of abduction, neutral rotation, and neutral extension.

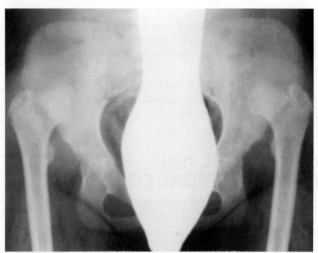

FIGURE 2.39   Bilateral untreated congenital dislocation of hip in 12-year-old girl.

POSTOPERATIVE CARE In children and adults, the cast is removed at 6 to 8 weeks, and active and passive exercises of the hip are started. Partial weight bearing on crutches is allowed and progressed as tolerated.

■ ADOLESCENT AND YOUNG ADULT (>8 YEARS)

In children older than 8 years old or in young adults in whom the femoral head cannot be repositioned distally to the level of the acetabulum, only palliative salvaging operations are possible. Rarely, a femoral shortening combined with a pelvic osteotomy could be considered, but the chances of creating a hip to last a lifetime are minimal. Reduction of a unilateral dislocation should be strongly considered, even in children 6 years old. After some years, degenerative arthritic changes develop in the hip joint. When these changes cause enough pain or limitation of motion to require additional surgery, a reconstructive operation, such as a total hip arthroplasty, may be indicated at the appropriate age. Arthrodesis is now rarely indicated for old unreduced dislocations and is contraindicated for bilateral dislocations. In bilateral dislocations in this age group, the hips should be left unreduced (Fig. 2.39),

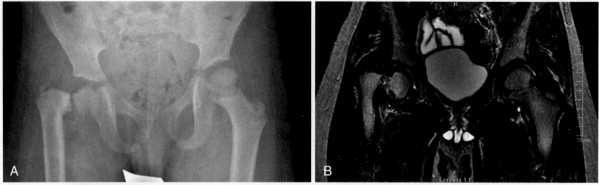

FIGURE 2.40 **A,** Plain anteroposterior radiograph of a 4-year-old boy with congenital coxa vara of the right hip. **B,** Coronal MRI section of the same patient demonstrates irregularity and widening of the physis.

and total hip arthroplasties may be done during adulthood. Degenerative joint disease is more likely to develop in early adulthood in a dislocated hip with a false acetabulum in the wing of the ilium than in a dislocated hip without formation of a false acetabulum. Patients with reduced femoral heads but painful acetabular dysplasia can be treated with an appropriate pelvic osteotomy (see Table 2.1).

CONGENITAL AND DEVELOPMENTAL COXA VARA

The term *congenital coxa vara* has been applied to two types of coxa vara seen in infancy and childhood. The first type is present at birth, is rare, and is associated with other congenital anomalies, such as proximal femoral focal deficiency or anomalies in other parts of the body such as cleidocranial dysostosis or spondyloepiphyseal dysplasia. The second type, usually not discovered until the child is walking, is more common than the first and is associated with no other abnormality.

Coxa vara, often bilateral, is characterized by a progressive decrease in the angle between the femoral neck and shaft, a progressive shortening of the limb, and the presence of a defect in the medial part of the neck (Fig. 2.40). Microscopically, the tissue in this defect consists of cartilage and resembles an abnormal physis; the arrangement of its cells is irregular and ossification within it is atypical. The adjacent metaphyseal bone is osteoporotic, its trabeculae being atrophic, and occasionally it contains large groups of cartilage cells. When walking is begun, the forces that the femoral neck must withstand are increased, and because the neck is weak, varus deformity gradually develops.

As the patient becomes older and heavier, the deformity increases until the greater trochanter eventually lies superior to the femoral head; pseudarthrosis of the femoral neck may develop. In adults, the trochanter may come to lie several inches superior to the femoral head, and if pseudarthrosis is present, the femoral head may be widely separated from the femoral neck. After age 8 years, the likelihood of obtaining a hip that would function normally rapidly diminishes.

The treatment of choice for correction of developmental coxa vara is subtrochanteric osteotomy to place the femoral neck and head in an appropriate valgus position with the shaft of the femur. Surgery can be delayed until the child is 4

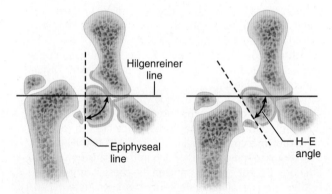

H–E Angle

<45°	Good prognosis
45°–59°	Monitor closely for progression
>60°	Poor prognosis; high risk of progression; surgery is indicated

FIGURE 2.41 Hilgenreiner-epiphyseal *(H-E)* angle of more than 60 degrees is an indication for surgical treatment of congenital coxa vara.

or 5 years old to make internal fixation easier. Surgical treatment is indicated when coxa vara deformity is progressive, painful, unilateral, or associated with leg-length discrepancy or when the Hilgenreiner-epiphyseal (H-E) angle is greater than 60 degrees (Fig. 2.41). Surgery also is indicated when the neck-shaft angle is 110 degrees or less. The subtrochanteric osteotomy is fixed internally with either a blade plate or screw and plate combination (Fig. 2.42). Although biomechanically this may provide enough rigid internal fixation to eliminate the need for postoperative immobilization, a spica cast can be worn until union is complete.

Regardless of the method of osteotomy, the deformity can recur, so children should be examined periodically after surgery until their growth is complete. The risk of recurrence can be lessened by improving the H-E angle to less than 38 degrees. In addition to monitoring for recurrence of the varus deformity, a significant number of children with coxa vara have associated femoral hypoplasia and limb-length discrepancy, which also require monitoring and may ultimately require limb-length equalization. Long-term studies of operative correction have demonstrated that functional outcomes are commonly poor to fair, and persistent gait disturbances are common.

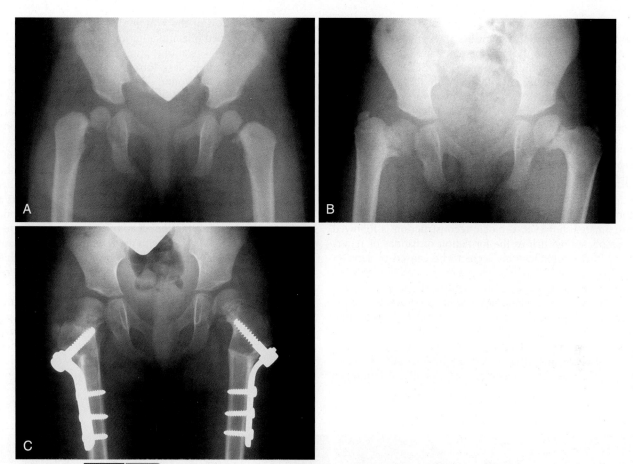

FIGURE 2.42 Congenital coxa vara. **A,** Two-year-old girl with congenital coxa vara. **B,** Preoperative radiograph shows neck-shaft angle of less than 90 degrees bilaterally at age 5 years. **C,** After bilateral subtrochanteric osteotomies and internal fixation with pediatric hip screws.

VALGUS OSTEOTOMY FOR DEVELOPMENTAL COXA VARA

TECHNIQUE 2.14

- Perform an adductor tenotomy through a small medial incision.
- Expose the greater trochanter and proximal shaft of the femur through an 8- to 10-cm lateral, longitudinal incision.
- If a screw and side plate device is used for internal fixation, insert the screw in the midline of the femoral neck as determined by image intensification or anteroposterior and lateral radiographs. Insert the screw as close as possible to the trochanteric apophysis without entering it. If possible, center the screw in the femoral neck distal to the abnormal physis. If this is technically impossible, center the screw in the femoral head. Alternatively, if a proximal femoral plating system is used, place the guide pin for the system just superior to the center position on the anteroposterior view of image intensification and centered on the lateral view. Again, take care to avoid the greater trochanteric apophysis.

- Make a transverse osteotomy slightly distal to the screw at about the level of the lesser trochanter.
- If necessary, take a small lateral wedge of bone to correct the neck-shaft angle to 140 to 150 degrees.
- Fix the side plate to the femoral shaft in the usual manner.
- Irrigate the wound and close it in layers, inserting irrigation-suction drainage if desired.
- Apply a one and one half spica cast.

POSTOPERATIVE CARE The cast is removed at 8 to 12 weeks, when radiographic union of the osteotomy has occurred. Regular follow-up includes assessment of possible recurrence of the deformity and the development of progressive limb-length discrepancy that requires additional treatment.

EXSTROPHY OF THE BLADDER

Exstrophy of the bladder occurs as a result of a congenital failure of fusion of the tissues of the midline of the pelvis. The major anomaly is a maldevelopment of the lower part of the abdominal wall and the anterior wall of the bladder so that the anterior surface of the posterior wall of the bladder is exposed to the exterior. Hernias and other defects of the anterior abdominal wall also may be present more proximally. The orthopaedic surgeon becomes involved in treatment because of the diastasis of the symphysis pubis, the lateral flare of the innominate bones, and the resultant lateral displacement and external rotation of the acetabula. Other orthopaedic anomalies may be present along with exstrophy of the bladder, including congenital dislocation or dysplasia of the hip and myelomeningocele.

ANTERIOR ILIAC OSTEOTOMIES AND APPROXIMATION OF THE SYMPHYSIS PUBIS

Because most of the urologic structures are present or bifid, reconstruction is possible. Unless the symphysis pubis is approximated, however, urologic reconstruction is followed by complications such as the formation of fistulas or recurrences. These complications seem to be caused by tension placed on the soft tissues during closure, and this tension can be relieved by repair of the symphysis pubis. There is some controversy, as some authors have reported successful bladder closure and repair without pelvic osteotomies. However, failure to address the abnormal morphology of the pelvis can have other consequences for the child, such as a wide-based, waddling, externally rotated gait. O'Phelan described the results of bilateral posterior iliac osteotomies

and approximation of the symphysis (Fig. 2.43). Sponseller et al. recommended bilateral anterior iliac osteotomies, with internal or external fixation, citing advantages of increased mobility of the pubis, less intraoperative blood loss, and increased correction. Wound dehiscence or bladder prolapse occurred in 4% of patients, and the only important complication of the osteotomies was transient palsy of the left femoral nerve in seven children. Children who were older at the time of the osteotomy maintained better correction over time. In a later report, Okubadejo et al. reviewed the records of 624 patients who had bladder exstrophy repair and found that orthopaedic complications occurred in 26 (4%). They divided the complications into five categories: bony complications at the osteotomy site, neurologic complications at the osteotomy site, complications of traction, deep infection, and late infection. Proper immobilization with modified Buck traction and external fixation and an immobilization time for more than 4 weeks have been shown to decrease failure rates in a recent study by Sirisreetreerux et al.

In their report on bladder exstrophy, Kasat and Borwankar identified 11 important factors in obtaining a successful primary closure: (1) proper patient selection, (2) a staged approach, (3) anterior approximation of the pubic bones with placement of the bladder and urethra in the true pelvis, (4) posterior bilateral iliac osteotomies when indicated, (5) double-layered

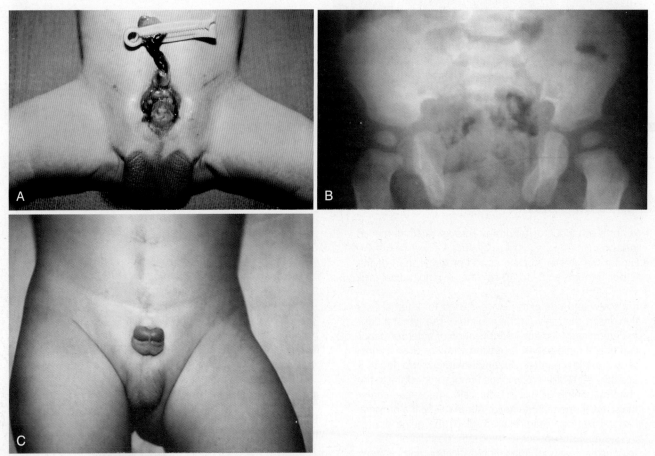

FIGURE 2.43 **A,** Congenital exstrophy of bladder in newborn boy. **B,** Note pubic diastasis on radiograph at 1 year of age. **C,** After bilateral posterior iliac osteotomies and anterior reconstruction.

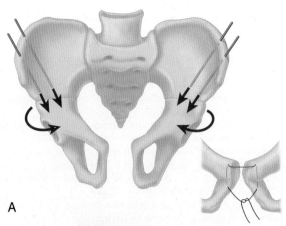

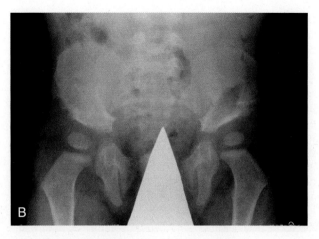

A

B

FIGURE **2.44** **A,** Technique for reconstruction in exstrophy of bladder (see text). *Inset* shows suturing of pubic bones. **B,** Postoperative radiograph after bilateral anterior Salter innominate osteotomies.

closure of the bladder, (6) 2 weeks of proper ureteric catheter drainage, (7) prevention of infection, (8) prolonged and proper postoperative immobilization, (9) prompt treatment of bladder prolapse, (10) prevention of abdominal distention postoperatively, and (11) ruling out bladder outlet obstruction before removing the bladder catheter.

The three steps are performed as one operative procedure: (1) the anterior iliac osteotomies, (2) repair of the anterior structures by a urologic surgeon, and (3) repair of the symphysis pubis. A heavy, nonabsorbable suture or biodegradable implants can be substituted for wire fixation. Although described for treatment of older children or children with recurrent deformities, we prefer this technique for early initial treatment and for older children (Fig. 2.44).

BILATERAL ANTERIOR ILIAC OSTEOTOMIES

TECHNIQUE 2.15

(SPONSELLER, GEARHART, AND JEFFS)
- Place the patient supine on the operating table and circumferentially prepare and drape the entire body below the umbilicus. Elevate the sacrum on folded towels.
- Make an anterior iliofemoral approach to the pelvis, similar to that used for a Salter osteotomy; both sides can be exposed simultaneously.
- Widely expose the medial iliac cortex and carefully elevate the periosteum posteriorly around the sciatic notch, using curved elevators and gauze sponges.
- With a Gigli saw, perform Salter innominate osteotomies. If the saw is difficult to pass, it can be threaded through on a leader of umbilical tape. In children younger than 6 months old, use an oscillating saw because the force applied to the Gigli saw can cause preferential separation of the triradiate cartilage.

- Make the osteotomies from 5 mm above the anterior inferior iliac spine to the most cranial portion of the sciatic notch to leave a sizable inferior segment for internal fixation.
- Rotate the freed ischiopubic segments 30 to 45 degrees to bring the pubic rami together.
- In children older than 6 months, a small external fixator, such as that used in the upper extremity, can be used with 2-mm pins for fixation. Increase the pin size to 4 mm for children 4 to 10 years old and to 5 mm for children older than 10 years old.
- Insert two pins in each iliac wing and two in each distal fragment. Predrilling may be necessary to prevent splitting of the bone in small infants.
- Place one distal fragment pin from the anterior inferior iliac spine to the notch, parallel and 5 to 10 mm inferior to the osteotomy, ensuring that the pin engages the deep posterior cortex of the notch.
- Insert another threaded pin just below this pin but externally angled 30 degrees.
- Close the wounds.
- Have the urologic surgeon prepare the operative field and identify the abnormal bladder and urethral structures.
- Use a single suture of 2-0 nylon in a horizontal mattress stitch to suture the pubic bones; tie it anterior to the neourethra and bladder neck while an assistant rotates the greater trochanters medially.
- Place heavy sutures of polyglactin in the rectus fascia just superficial to the pubic closure.
- After the pelvic ring is closed anteriorly, apply the external fixator. Good subperiosteal exposure is mandatory to ensure accurate pin placement away from the hip and triradiate cartilage.
- The procedure can be modified to exclude external fixation by fixing both osteotomies with Kirschner wires and applying a spica cast to be worn for 8 to 12 weeks, or by applying a biodegradable plate and screws to the symphysis rather than a wire or suture.

POSTOPERATIVE CARE Light Buck traction or a spica cast can be used for 1 to 2 weeks to maintain comfort and bed rest, although a longer period of immobilization (>4 weeks) may be associated with improved outcomes. This is mandatory in children younger than 1 year because they have relatively less cortical bone for fixation, but older children can be discharged from the hospital earlier if good external fixation is obtained. External fixation is continued for 4 weeks in children younger than 2 years and for 6 weeks in older children. Gradual resumption of activities is then allowed. No formal physical therapy program is necessary, but a walker is helpful during the first week of ambulation in older children. Children should be followed for developmental dysplasia of the hip.

REFERENCES

DEVELOPMENTAL DYSPLASIA OF THE HIP

Agus H, Bozoglan M, Kalenderer Ö, et al.: How are outcomes affected by performing a one-stage combined procedure simultaneously in bilateral developmental hip dysplasia? *Int Orthop* 38(6):1219, 2014.

Alassaf N, Abuhaimed J, Almahmoujd N, Binkhulaif R: The added value of postoperative axial imaging in developmental dysplasia of the hip, *Open Orthop J* 11:567, 2017.

American Academy of Orthopaedic Surgeons: Detection and nonoperative management of pediatric developmental dysplasia of the hip in infants up to six months of age. Evidence-based clinical practice guideline. http://www.aaos.org/Research/guidelines/DDHGuidelineFINAL.pdf.

Anderton MJ, Hastie GR, Paton RW: The positive predictive value of asymmetrical skin creases in the diagnosis of pathological developmental dysplasia of the hip, *Bone Joint J* 100-B(5):675, 2018.

Arslan H, Sucu E, Ozkul E, et al.: Should routine pelvic osteotomy be added to the treatment of DDH after 18 months? *Acta Orthop Belg* 80:205, 2014.

Baki ME, Baki C, Aydin H, Ari B, Özcan M: Single-stage medial open reduction and Pemberton acetabuloplasty in developmental dysplasia of the hip, *J Pediatr Orthop B* 25(6):504, 2016.

Bayhan IA, Abousamra O, Rogers KJ, et al.: Valgus hip osteotomy in children with spondyloepiphyseal dysplasia congenita: midterm results, *J Pediatr Orthop*, 39(6):282, 2019.

Bolland BJ, Wahed A, Al-Halloa S, et al.: Late reduction in congenital dislocation of the hip and the need for secondary surgery: radiologic predictors and confounding variables, *J Pediatr Orthop* 30:676, 2010.

Bradley CS, Perry DC, Wedge JH, Murnaghan ML, Lelley SP: Avascular necrosis following closed reduction for treatment of developmental dysplasia of the hip: a systematic review, *J Child Orthop* 10(6):627, 2016.

Carroll KL, Schiffern AN, Murray KA, et al.: The occurrence of occult acetabular dysplasia in relatives of individuals with developmental dysplasia of the hip, *J Pediatr Orthop* 36(1):96, 2016.

Chang CH, Yang WE, Kao HK, et al.: Predictive value for femoral head sphericity from early radiographic signs in surgery for developmental dysplasia of the hip, *J Pediatr Orthop* 31:240, 2011.

Chen C, Doyle S, Green D, et al.: Presence of the ossific nucleus and risk of osteonecrosis in the treatment of developmental dysplasia of the hip: a meta-analysis of cohort and case-control studies, *J Bone Joint Surg* 99-A(9):760, 2017.

Chin MS, Betz BW, Halanski MA: Comparison of hip reduction using magnetic resonance imaging or computed tomography in hip dysplasia, *J Pediatr Orthop* 31:525, 2011.

Chou DT, Ramachandran M: Prevalence of developmental dysplasia of the hip in children with clubfoot, *J Child Orthop* 7(4):263, 2013.

Ö Çiçekli, Doğan M: Evaluation of surgical outcome in advanced age patients with developmental hip dysplasia, *Int J Surg* 52:44, 2018.

Cooke SJ, Rees R, Edwards DL, et al.: Ossification of the femoral head at closed reduction for developmental dysplasia of the hip and its influence on the long-term outcome, *J Pediatr Orthop B* 19:22, 2010.

De Hundt M, Viemmix F, Bais JM, et al.: Risk factors for developmental dysplasia of the hip: a metaanalysis, *Eur J Obstet Gynecol Reprod Biol* 165:8, 2012.

De La Rocha A, Sucato DJ, Tulchin K, Podeszwa DA: Treatment of adolescents with a periacetabular osteotomy after previous pelvic surgery, *Clin Orthop Relat Res* 470:2583, 2012.

Ertürk C, Altay MA, Isikan UE: Femoral segment graft is suitable alternative to stabilize pelvic osteotomies in developmental dysplasia of the hip: a comparative study, *J Pediatr Orthop B* 21:200, 2012.

Firth GB, Robertson SJ, Schepers A, Fatti L: Developmental dysplasia of the hip: open reduction as a risk factor for substantial osteonecrosis, *Clin Orthop Relat Res* 468:2485, 2010.

Fox AE, Paton RW: The relationship between mode of delivery and developmental dysplasia of the hip in breech infants: a four-year prospective cohort study, *J Bone Joint Surg* 92B:1695, 2010.

Fujii M, Nakashima Y, Yamamoto T, et al.: Acetabular retroversion in developmental dysplasia of the hip, *J Bone Joint Surg Am* 92:895, 2010.

Fukuda A, Fukiage K, Futami T, Miyati T: Ultrafast MRI in non-sedated infants after reduction with spica casting for developmental dysplasia of the hip: a feasibility study, *J Child Orthop* 10(3):193, 2016.

Gardner RO, Bradley CS, Sharma OP, et al.: Long-term outcome following medial open reduction in developmental dysplasia of the hip: a retrospective cohort study, *J Child Orthop* 10(3):179, 2016.

Gholve PA, Flynn JM, Garner MR, et al.: Predictors for secondary procedures in walking DDH, *J Pediatr Orthop* 32:282, 2012.

Gokharman FD, Aydin S, Fatihoglu E, et al.: Optimizing the time for developmental dysplasia of the hip screening: earlier or later?, *Ultrasound Q* 35(2):130, 2019.

Gould SW, Grissom LE, Niedzielski A, et al.: Protocol for MRI of the hips after spica cast placement, *J Pediatr Orthop* 32:504, 2012.

Heesakkers NA, Witbreuk MM, Beeselaar PP, Van Der Sluijs JA: Retrospective radiographic evaluation of treatment results of developmental dysplasia of the hip in walking-age children, *J Pediatr Orthop B* 22:427, 2013.

Harcke HT, Karatas AF, Cummings S, Bowen JR: Sonographic assessment of hip swaddling techniques in infants with and without DDH, *J Pediatr Orthop* 36(3):232, 2016.

Hines AC, Neal DC, Beckwith T, et al.: A comparison of Pavlik harness treatment regimens for dislocated but reducible (Ortolani+) hips in infantile developmental dysplasia of the hip, *J Pediatr Orthop*, 39(10):505, 2019.

Iyetin Y, Turkmen I, Saglam Y, et al.: A modified surgical approach of the hip in children: is it safe and reliable in patients with developmental hip dysplasia, *J Child Orthop* 9(3):199, 2015.

Joiner ER, Andras LM, Skaggs DL: Screening for hip dysplasia in congenital muscular toricollis: is physical exam of enough? *J Child Orthop* 8:114, 2014.

Kaneko H, Kitoh H, Mishima K, et al.: Long-term outcome of gradual reduction using overhead traction for developmental dysplasia of the hip over 6 months of age, *J Pediatr Orthop* 33:628, 2013.

Laborie LB, Engesaeter IO, Lehmann TG, et al.: Screening strategies for hip dysplasia: long-term outcome of a randomized controlled trial, *Pediatrics* 132:492, 2013.

Mahan ST, Yazdy MM, Kasser JR, Werler MM: Is it worthwhile to routinely ultrasound screen children with idiopathic clubfoot for hip dysplasia? *J Pediatr Orthop* 33:847, 2013.

Miao M, Cai H, Hu L, Wang Z: Retrospective observational study comparing the International Hip Dysplasia Institute classification with the Tonnis classification of developmental dysplasia of the hip, *Medicine (Baltimore)* 96(3):e5902, 2017.

Molony DC, Harty JA, Burke TE, D'Souza LG: Popliteal angle as an indicator for successful closed reduction of developmental dysplasia of the hip, *J Orthop Surg (Hong Kong)* 19:46, 2011.

Murhaghan ML, Browne RH, Socato DJ, Birch J: Femoral nerve palsy in Pavlik harness treatment for developmental dysplasia of the hip, *J Bone Joint Surg* 93A:493, 2011.

Narayanan U, Mulpuri K, Sankar WN, et al.: Reliabiltiy of a new radiographic classification for developmental dysplasia of the hip, *J Pediatr Orthop* 35(5):478, 2015.

Novais EN, Hill MK, Carry PM, Heyn PC: Is age or surgical approach with osteonecrosis in patients with developmental dysplasia of the hip? A meta-analysis, *Clin Orthop Relat Res* 474(5):1166, 2016.

Okanoue Y, Kawakami T, Izumi M, et al.: Less invasive modified Spitzy shelf procedure for patients with dysplasia of the hip, *Eur J Orthop Surg Traumatol* 25(4):789, 2015.

Orak MM, Onay T, Gümüstas SA, et al.: Is prematurity a risk factor for developmental dysplasia of the hip? A prospective study, *Bone Joint J* 97-B(5):716, 2015.

Ortiz-Neira CL, Paolucci EO, Donnon T: A meta-analysis of common risk factors associated with the diagnosis of developmental dysplasia of the hip in newborns, *Eur J Radiol* 81:e344, 2012.

Paton RW: Screening in developmental dysplasia of the hip (DDH), *Surgeon* 15(5):290, 2017.

Paton RW, Choudry QA, Jugdey R, Hughes S: Is congenital talipes equinovarus a risk factor for pathological dysplasia of the hip? A 21-year prospective, longitudinal observational study, *Bone Joint J* 96-B:1553, 2014.

Perry DC, Tawfig SM, Roche A, et al.: The association between clubfoot and developmental dysplasia of the hip, *J Bone Joint Surg* 92B:1586, 2010.

Pollet V, Percy V, Prior HJ: Relative risk and incidence for developmental dysplasia of the hip, *J Pediatrics* 181:202, 2017.

Pospischill R, Weninger J, Ganger R, et al.: Does open reduction of the developmental dislocated hip increase the risk of osteonecrosis? *Clin Orthop Relat Res* 470:250, 2012.

Ramani N, Patil MS, Mahna M: Outcome of surgical management of developmental dysplasia of hip in children between 18 and 24 months, *Indian J Orthop* 48:458, 2014.

Ramo BA, De La Rocha A, Sucato DJ, Jo CH: A new radiographic classification system for developmental hip dysplasia is reliable and predictive of successful closed reduction and late pelvic osteotomy, *J Pediatr Orthop* 38(1):16, 2018.

Rhodes AM, Clarke NM: A review of environmental factors implicated in human developmental dysplasia of the hip, *J Child Orthop* 8:375, 2014.

Roberts DW, Saglam Y, De La Rocha A, et al.: Long-term outcomes of operative and nonoperative treatment of congenital coxa vara, *J Pediatr Orthop* 38(4):193, 2018.

Roposch A, Liu LQ, Hefti F, et al.: Standardized diagnostic criteria for developmental dysplasia of hip in early infancy, *Clin Orthop Relat Res* 469:3451, 2011.

Roposch A, Odeh O, Doria AS, Wedge JH: The presence of an ossific nucleus does not protect against osteonecrosis after treatment of developmental dysplasia of the hip, *Clin Orthop Relat Res* 469:2838, 2011.

Roposch A, Wedge JH, Riedl G: Reliability of Bucholz and Ogden classification for osteonecrosis secondary to developmental dysplasia of the hip, *Clin Orthop Relat Res* 40:3499, 2012.

Sankar WN, Gornitzky AL, Clarke NM, et al.: Closed reduction for developmental dysplasia of the hip: early-term results from a prospective, multicenter cohort, *J Pediatr Orthop* 39(3):111, 2019.

Sankar WN, Neubuerger CO, Moseley CF: Femoral anteversion in developmental dysplasia of the hip, *J Pediatr Orthop* 30:558, 2010.

Sankar WN, Young CR, Ling AG, et al.: Risk factors for failure after open reduction for DDH: a matched cohort analysis, *J Pediatr Orthop* 31:232, 2011.

Sardelli M, Tashjian RZ, MacWilliams BA: Functional elbow range of motion for contemporary tasks, *J Bone Joint Surg Am* 93:471, 2011.

Sarkissian EJ, Sankar WN, Zhu X, et al.: Radiographic follow-up of DDH in infants: are x-rays necessary after a normalized ultrasound, *J Pediatr Orthop* 36(6):551, 2015.

Schur MD, Lee C, Arkader A, et al.: Risk factors for avascular necrosis after closed reduction for developmental dysplasia of the hip, *J Child Orthop* 10(3):185, 2016.

Sewell MD, Eastwood DM: Screening and treatment in developmental dysplasia of the hip-where do we go from here? *Int Orthop* 35:1359, 2011.

Shin CH, Yoo WJ, Park MS, et al.: Acetabular remodeling and role of osteotomy after closed reduction of developmental dysplasia of the hip, *J Bone Joint Surg* 98-A(11):952, 2016.

Shorter D, Hong T, Osborn DA: Cochrane review: screening programmes for developmental dysplasia of the hip in newborn infants, *Evid Base Child Health* 8:11, 2013.

Studer K, Williams N, Studer P, et al.: Obstacles to reduction in infantile developmental dysplasia of the hip, *J Child Orthop* 11(5):358, 2017.

Sucato DJ, De La Rocha A, Lau K, Ramo BA: Overhead Bryant's traction does not improve the success of closed reduction or limit AVN in developmental dysplasia of the hip, *J Pediatr Orthop* 37(2):e108, 2017.

Tarassoli P, Gargan MF, Atherton WG, Thomas SR: The medial approach for the treatment of children with developmental dysplasia of the hip, *Bone Joint J* 96B:406, 2014.

Walton MJ, Isaacson Z, McMillan D, et al.: The success of management with the Pavlik harness for developmental dysplasia of the hip using a United Kingdom screening programme and ultrasound-guided supervision, *J Bone Joint Surg* 92B:1013, 2012.

Wang YJ, Yang F, Wu QJ, et al.: Association between open or closed reduction and avascular necrosis in developmental dysplasia of the hip: a PRISMA-compliant meta-analysis of observational studies, *Medicine* 95(29):e4276, 2016.

Wenger DR: Surgical treatment of developmental dysplasia of the hip, *Instr Course Lect* 63:313, 2014.

Westacott DJ, Butler D, Shears E, et al.: Universal versus selective ultrasound screening for developmental dysplasia of the hip: a single-centre retrospective cohort study, *J Pediatr Orthop B*, 27(5):387, 2018.

Westacott DJ, Mackay ND, Watson A, et al.: Staged weaning versus immediate cessation of Pavlik harness treatment for developmental dysplasia of the hip, *J Pediatr Orthop B* 23:103, 2014.

White KK, Sucato DJ, Agrawal S, Browne R: Ultrasonographic findings in hips with a positive Ortolani sign and their relationship to Pavlik harness failure, *J Bone Joint Surg Am* 92:113, 2010.

Wilf-Miron R, Kuint J, Peled R, et al.: Utilization of ultrasonography to detect developmental dysplasia of the hip: when reality turns selective screening into universal use, *BMC Pediatr* 17(1):136, 2017.

Wu KW, Wang TM, Huang SC, et al.: Analysis of osteonecrosis following Pemberton acetabuloplasty in developmental dysplasia of the hip: long-term results, *J Bone Joint Surg* 92A:2083, 2010.

Xu RJ, Li WC, Ma CX: Slotted acetabular augmentation with concurrent open reduction for developmental dysplasia of the hip in older children, *J Pediatr Orthop* 30:554, 2010.

Yilmaz S, Aksahin E, Duran S, Bicimoglu A: The fate of iliopsoas muscle in the long-term follow-up after open reduction of developmental dysplasia of the hip by medial approach. Part 1: MRI evaluation, *J Pediatr Orthop* 37(6):392, 2017.

Yilmaz S, Aksahin E, Ersoz M, Bicimoglu A: The fate of the iliopsoas muscle in long-term follow-up after open reduction with a medial approach in developmental dysplasia of the hip. Part 2: isokinetic muscle strength evaluation, *J Pediatr Orthop* 37(6):398, 2017.

CONGENITAL AND DEVELOPMENTAL COXA VARA

Chotigavanichaya C, Leeprakobboon D, Eamsobhana P, Kaewpornsawan K: Results of surgical treatment of coxa vara in children: valgus osteotomy with angle blade plate fixation, *J Media Assoc Thai* (Suppl 9):S78, 2014.

Günther CM, Komm M, Jansson V, Heimkes B: Midterm results after subtrochanteric end-to-side valgization osteotomy in severe infantile coxa vara, *J Pediatr Orthop* 33:353, 2013.

EXSTROPHY OF THE BLADDER

Kajbafzadeh AM, Talab SS, Elmi A, et al.: Use of biodegradable plates and screws for approximation of symphysis pubis in bladder exstrophy: applications and outcomes, *Urology* 77:1248, 2011.

Mundy A, Kushare I, Jayanthi VR, et al.: Incidence of hip dysplasia associated with bladder exstrophy, *J Pediatr Orthop* 36(8):860, 2016.

Mushtag I, Garriboli M, Smeulders N, et al.: Primary bladder exstrophy closure in neonates: challenging the traditions, *J Urol* 193, 2014.

Shnorhavorian M, Song K, Samil pa I, et al.: Spica casting compared to Bryant's traction after complete primary repair of exstrophy: safe and effective in a longitudinal cohort study, *J Urol* 184:669, 2010.

Sirisreetreerux P, Lue KM, Ingviya T, et al.: Failed primary bladder exstrophy closure with osteotomy: multivariable analysis of a 25-year experience, *J Urol* 197:1138, 2017.

Wild AT, Sponseller PD, Stec AA, Gearhart JP: The role of osteotomy in surgical repair of bladder exstrophy, *Semin Pediatr Surg* 20:71, 2011.

The complete list of references is available online at Expert Consult.com.

CHAPTER 3

CONGENITAL ANOMALIES OF THE TRUNK AND UPPER EXTREMITY

Benjamin M. Mauck

This chapter discusses congenital elevation of the scapula, congenital torticollis, and congenital pseudarthrosis of the clavicle, radius, and ulna. Congenital anomalies of the hand and certain other anomalies of the forearm are discussed in other chapter. Congenital conditions of the spine are discussed in other chapters.

CONGENITAL ELEVATION OF THE SCAPULA (SPRENGEL DEFORMITY)

First described by Eulenberg in 1863, Sprengel deformity is characterized as a congenital upward elevation of the scapula in relation to the thoracic cage. The scapula is commonly hypoplastic and misshapen (Fig. 3.1). Other congenital anomalies may be present, such as cervical ribs, malformations of ribs, and anomalies of the cervical vertebrae (Klippel-Feil syndrome); rarely, one or more scapular muscles are partly or completely absent. The presence of this deformity can often indicate abnormalities in other organ systems. The severity of the functional impairment typically is related to the severity of the deformity (Table 3.1). If the deformity is mild, the scapula is only slightly elevated and is a bit smaller than normal and its motion is only mildly limited; however, if the deformity is severe, the scapula is very small and can be so elevated that it almost touches the occiput. The patient's head is often deviated toward the affected side. The primary limitation of shoulder motion is abduction secondary to diminished scapulothoracic motion. In about half of patients, an extra ossicle, the omovertebral bone, is present; this is a rhomboidal plaque of cartilage and bone lying in a strong fascial sheath that extends from the superior angle of the scapula to the spinous process, lamina, or transverse process of one or more lower cervical vertebrae. Recognition of this abnormality is essential to surgical management. A similar osseous structure has also been reported extending from the medial border of the scapula to the occiput. Sometimes a well-developed joint is found between the omovertebral bone and scapula; sometimes it is attached to the scapula by fibrous tissue only. A solid osseous ridge between the spinous processes and the scapula is rare.

Radiographic workup is essential to surgical planning. Plain radiographs should be obtained to assess the level of the scapula in relation to vertebrae and in comparison to the contralateral side. Radiographs also can help recognize the presence of associated abnormalities such as the omovertebral bone.

In a morphometric analysis using three-dimensional CT, Cho et al. found that most of the affected scapulae in 15 patients with Sprengel deformity had a characteristic shape, with a decrease in the height-to-width ratio. An inverse relationship was found between scapular rotation and superior displacement; no significant difference was found in glenoid version. Cho et al. suggested that the point of tethering of the omovertebral connection, when present, may determine the shape, rotation, and superior displacement of the scapula and that three-dimensional CT can be helpful in delineating the deformity and planning scapuloplasty.

If deformity and impairment are mild, no treatment is indicated; if they are more severe, surgery may be indicated, depending on the age of the patient and the severity of any associated deformities. Because the deformity is more than just simple scapular elevation, the results of surgical treatment of Sprengel deformity can vary. The long-term function of the shoulder and cosmetic appearance must be carefully measured against the surgical risk and natural history of the deformity. A 26-year review of 22 patients with Sprengel deformity treated by either observation or surgical repair suggested that surgically treated patients had almost 40 degrees more abduction than their nonsurgical counterparts, with a subjective improvement in cosmesis.

An operation to bring the scapula inferiorly to near its normal position is ideally attempted soon after 3 years of age, because the operation becomes more difficult as the child grows. In older children, an attempt to bring the scapula inferiorly to its normal level can injure the brachial plexus.

Numerous operations have been described to correct Sprengel deformity. Green described surgical release of muscles from the scapula along with excision of the supraspinatus portion of the scapula and any omovertebral bone. The scapula is moved inferiorly to a more normal position, and the muscles are reattached. Other modifications include suturing the scapula into a pocket in the latissimus dorsi after rotating the scapula and moving it caudad to a more normal position, and avoiding dissection of the serratus anterior muscle so that mobilization is begun immediately postoperatively. Wada et al. performed a morphometric analysis and reported

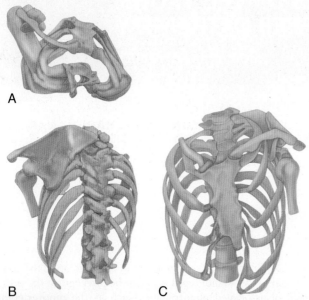

FIGURE 3.1 Elevated, malrotated, and malformed scapula with bony connection to spine. **A,** Axial. **B,** Posterior. **C,** Anterior. (Redrawn from Harvey EJ, Bernstein M, Desy NM, et al. Sprengel deformity: pathogenesis and management, *J Am Acad Orthop Surg* 20:177, 2012.)

TABLE 3.1

Cavendish Classification

Grade 1	Very mild	Shoulders are level; deformity not visible when patient is dressed
Grade 2	Mild	Shoulders are almost level; deformity is visible as a lump in the web of neck when patient is dressed
Grade 3	Moderate	Shoulders elevated 2-5 cm; deformity easily seen
Grade 4	Severe	Shoulder grossly elevated; superior angle of scapula lies near occiput

Information from Cavendish ME: Congenital elevation of the scapula, *J Bone Joint Surg* 54:395, 1972.

23 scapulae in 22 patients treated with the modified Green procedure. At 4-year follow-up the patients demonstrated a 63-degree increase in range of motion.

Woodward, in 1961, described transfer of the origin of the trapezius muscle to a more inferior position on the spinous processes. Greitemann et al. recommended the Woodward procedure for patients with impaired function; for patients with only cosmetic problems, resection of part of the superior angle of the scapula was preferred. They suggested that better results are obtained with the Woodward procedure because (1) the muscles are incised farther from the scapula, which lowers the risk of formation of a scar-keloid that may fix the scapula in poor position; (2) a larger mobilization is possible; and (3) the postoperative scar is not as thick as with Green's procedure. Borges et al. added excision of the prominent superomedial border of the scapula to the Woodward procedure. In a series of patients with long-term follow-up at an average of 14.7 years, Walstra

et al. demonstrated improvement of Cavendish grade 3 to 1 or 2 and significant improvement in overall shoulder abduction and improved contrast; Disability of the Arm, Shoulder, and Hand (DASH) and Simple Shoulder Test (SST) scores also improved. No long-term complications were reported. We generally prefer the Woodard procedure (see later) (Fig. 3.2).

To improve function of the shoulder and the cosmetic appearance, Mears developed a procedure that includes partial resection of the scapula, removal of any omovertebral communication, and release of the long head of the triceps from the scapula. In the eight patients in whom this technique was used, average flexion improved from 100 to 175 degrees and abduction improved from 90 to 150 degrees. In two patients, hypertrophic scars formed at the curvilinear incision; this problem was eliminated by the use of a transverse incision in subsequent patients. Mears observed that a contracture of the long head of the triceps seems to represent a significant inhibition to full abduction in patients with Sprengel deformity and that release of this contracture allows increased abduction. Early postoperative active and active-assisted motion exercises of the shoulder are used to improve function.

Brachial plexus palsy is the most severe complication of surgery for Sprengel deformity. The scapula in this deformity is hypoplastic compared with the normal scapula. During surgery, attention should be directed to placing the spine of the scapula at the same level as that on the opposite side, rather than aligning exactly the inferior angles of the scapulae. To avoid brachial plexus palsy, several authors recommended morcellation of the clavicle on the ipsilateral side as a first step in the operative treatment of Sprengel deformity. This is not a routine part of surgical treatment but is recommended in severe deformity or in children who show signs of brachial plexus palsy after surgical correction. In patients older than 8 years of age, a 2-cm midclavicular osteotomy is recommended to decompress the brachial plexus and first rib before scapular resection. In a younger patient, a 1-cm resection osteotomy is considered for severe deformity. Others have suggested the use of intraoperative somatosensory evoked potentials to monitor brachial plexus function during surgical correction.

WOODWARD OPERATION

TECHNIQUE 3.1

- Place the patient prone on the operating table and prepare and drape both shoulders so that the involved shoulder girdle and the arm can be manipulated and the uninvolved scapula can be inspected in its normal position.
- Make a midline incision from the spinous process of the first cervical vertebra distally to that of the ninth thoracic vertebra (Fig. 3.3A). Undermine the skin and subcutaneous tissues laterally to the medial border of the scapula.
- Identify the lateral border of the trapezius in the distal end of the incision and by blunt dissection separate it from the underlying latissimus dorsi muscle.
- By sharp dissection, free the fascial sheath of origin of the trapezius from the spinous processes.

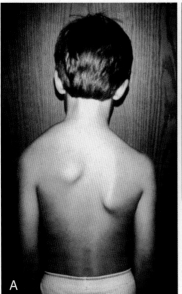
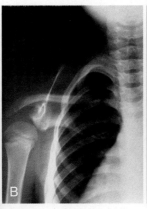
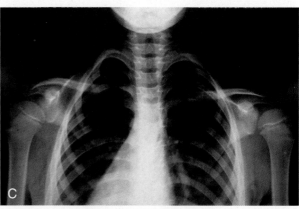

FIGURE 3.2 **A,** Sprengel deformity (left sided) in 5-year-old boy. **B,** Posteroanterior radiograph shows congenital elevation of left scapula. **C,** Posteroanterior radiograph after Woodward procedure.

- Identify the origins of the rhomboideus major and minor muscles and by sharp dissection free them from the spinous processes.
- Free the rhomboids and the superior part of the trapezius from the muscles of the chest wall anterior to them.
- Retract the freed sheet of muscles laterally to expose any omovertebral bone or fibrous bands attached to the superior angle of the scapula.
- By extraperiosteal dissection, excise any omovertebral bone, or if the bone is absent, excise any fibrous band or contracted levator scapulae; avoid injuring the spinal accessory nerve, the nerves to the rhomboids, and the transverse cervical artery.
- If the supraspinous part of the scapula is deformed, resect it along with its periosteum; this releases the levator scapulae (if not already excised), allowing the shoulder girdle to move more freely (Fig. 3.3B).
- Divide transversely the remaining narrow attachment of the trapezius at the level of the fourth cervical vertebra.
- Displace the scapula along with the attached sheet of muscles distally until its spine lies at the same level as that of the opposite scapula (Fig. 3.3C).
- While holding the scapula in this position, reattach the aponeuroses of the trapezius and rhomboids to the spinous processes at a more inferior level.
- In the distal part of the incision, create a fold in the origin of the trapezius and either excise the excess tissue or incise the fold and overlap and suture in place the resultant free edges.

POSTOPERATIVE CARE A Velpeau bandage is applied and is worn for about 2 weeks. Active and passive range-of-motion exercises are begun.

MORCELLATION OF THE CLAVICLE

TECHNIQUE 3.2

- Make a straight incision over the clavicle extending from 1.5 cm lateral to the sternoclavicular joint to 1.5 cm medial to the acromioclavicular joint.
- Expose the clavicle subperiosteally.
- Divide the bone 2 cm from each end, remove it, and cut it into small pieces (morcellate).
- Replace the pieces in the periosteal tube and close the tube with interrupted sutures.
- Close the subcutaneous tissues and skin in a routine manner.

CONGENITAL MUSCULAR TORTICOLLIS

Congenital muscular torticollis (CMT), present in as many as 3.92% of neonates, is caused by fibromatosis within the sternocleidomastoid muscle. A mass either is palpable at birth or becomes so, usually during the first 2 weeks. Congenital muscular torticollis is more common on the right side than on the left side. It may involve the muscle diffusely, but more often it is localized near the clavicular attachment of the muscle. The mass attains maximal size within 1 or 2 months and may remain the same size or become smaller; usually, it diminishes and disappears within 1 year. If it fails to disappear, the muscle becomes permanently fibrotic and contracted and causes torticollis, which also is permanent unless treated (Fig. 3.4).

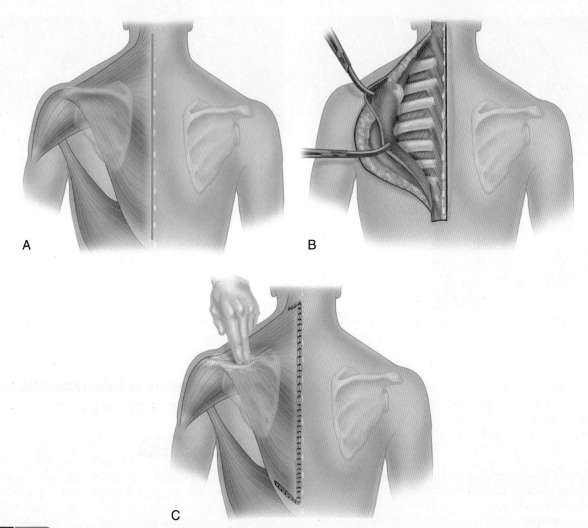

FIGURE 3.3 Woodward operation for congenital elevation of scapula. **A,** Elevation of scapula, extensive origin of trapezius, and skin incision are shown. **B,** Skin has been incised in midline. Origins of trapezius and of rhomboideus major and minor have been freed from spinous processes, and these muscles have been retracted laterally. Levator scapulae, any omovertebral bone, and any deformed superior angle of scapula are to be excised. **C,** Remaining narrow attachment of trapezius superiorly has been divided at level of C4. Scapula and attached sheet of muscles have been displaced inferiorly, and aponeuroses of trapezius and rhomboids have been reattached to spinous processes at more inferior level. A redundant fold of trapezius aponeurosis is formed inferiorly. Fold of trapezius aponeurosis has been incised, and resultant free edges have been overlapped and sutured in place. Free superior edge of trapezius also has been sutured. (Modified from Woodward JW: Congenital elevation of the scapula: correction by release and transplantation of muscle origins: a preliminary report, *J Bone Joint Surg* 43A:219, 1961.) **SEE TECHNIQUE 3.1.**

Although CMT has been recognized for centuries, its cause remains unclear. Clinical studies have shown that infants with CMT are more often the product of a difficult delivery and have an increased incidence of associated musculoskeletal disorders, such as metatarsus adductus, developmental dysplasia of the hip, and talipes equinovarus. There is a reported incidence of congenital dislocation of the hip or dysplasia of the acetabulum ranging from 7% to 20% in children with CMT. Careful hip screening and, if necessary, ultrasound evaluation are indicated.

Various hypotheses of the cause of CMT include malposition of the fetus in utero, intrauterine constraint, birth trauma, infection, and vascular injury. Davids et al. found that MRI of 10 infants with CMT showed signals in the

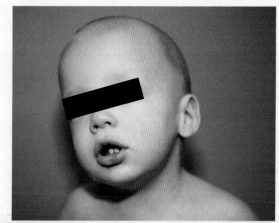

FIGURE 3.4 Congenital torticollis in 14-month-old boy.

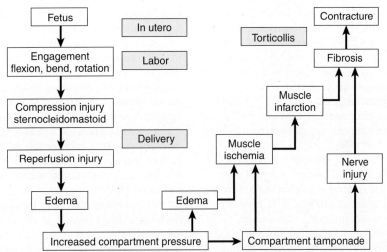

FIGURE 3.5 Pathophysiology of congenital muscular torticollis proposed by Davids, Wenger, and Mubarak, who suggested that congenital muscular torticollis may represent sequela of intrauterine or perinatal compartment syndrome.

sternocleidomastoid muscle similar to signals observed in the forearm and leg after compartment syndrome. Further investigation included cadaver dissections and injection studies that defined the sternocleidomastoid muscle compartment; pressure measurements of three patients with CMT that confirmed the presence of this compartment in vivo; and clinical review of 48 children with CMT that showed a relationship between birth position and the side affected by contracture. These findings led the authors to postulate that CMT may represent the sequela of an intrauterine or perinatal compartment syndrome (Fig. 3.5).

A palpable nodule is present in the affected sternocleidomastoid muscle at birth or within the first few weeks of life. The patient may also have associated plagiocephaly and facial asymmetry. The presence of the characteristic fibrotic nodule typically confirms the diagnosis, rendering further radiographic evaluation unnecessary in most cases. When the diagnosis remains in doubt, or in the presence of neurologic findings, cervical spine radiographs or advanced imaging is appropriate. Ultrasonography also has been advocated for the evaluation and management of congenital muscular torticollis.

When CMT is seen in early infancy, it is impossible to tell whether or not the mass causing it will disappear spontaneously. Lin and Chou reported that ultrasonography was useful in predicting which infants would require surgical treatment. Those patients in whom fibrotic change was limited to only the lower third of the sternocleidomastoid muscle recovered without surgery, whereas 35% of patients with whole muscle involvement required surgical release. Han et al. found several differences between patients with a sternocleidomastoid lesion identified with ultrasound and those without a lesion. Those without a lesion generally were seen later but had a better prognosis and a shorter treatment duration. A head rotation/tilting pattern in which both occurred in the same direction was observed only in patients without a lesion, and head tilting was more limited than head rotation. These findings suggest that pathophysiologic mechanisms may differ between patients with CMT with and without a sternocleidomastoid lesion.

Only conservative treatment is indicated during infancy. The parents should be instructed to stretch the sternocleidomastoid muscle by manipulating the infant's head manually. The child's chin is rotated toward the shoulder on the side of the affected sternocleidomastoid muscle while the head is tilted toward the opposite shoulder. Excising the lesion during early infancy is unjustified; surgery should be delayed until evolution of the fibromatosis is complete, and then, if necessary, the muscle can be released at one or both ends. CMT typically resolves with a home stretching program during the first year of life. Some authors suggest a strong correlation between sternocleidomastoid (5-cm) thickness to duration of and response to stretching exercises. Canale et al. found that CMT did not resolve spontaneously if it persisted beyond the age of 1 year. Children who were treated during the first year of life had better results than children treated later, and an exercise program was more likely to be successful if the restriction of motion was less than 30 degrees and there was no facial asymmetry or if the facial asymmetry was noted only by the examiner. Nonoperative therapy after age 1 year was rarely successful. Regardless of the type of treatment, established facial asymmetry and limitation of motion of more than 30 degrees at the beginning of treatment usually precluded a good result.

Early intervention for infants with CMT, initiated before 3 to 4 months of age, results in excellent outcomes, with 92% to 100% achieving full passive neck rotation and 0 to 1% requiring surgical intervention. The earlier intervention is started, the shorter the duration of intervention, and the need for later surgical intervention is significantly reduced. Petronic et al. found that when treatment was initiated before 1 month of age, 99% of infants with CMT achieved excellent clinical outcomes (no head tilt, full passive cervical rotation), with an average treatment duration of 1.5 months, but if initiated between 1 and 3 months of age, only 89% of infants achieved excellent outcomes with treatment duration averaging 6 months. When initiated between 3 and 6 months of age, 62% of infants achieved excellent outcomes with treatment duration averaging 7.2 months. When intervention was initiated between 6 and 12 months of age, 19% of infants achieved excellent outcomes, with an average treatment duration of 8.9 months. In contrast to recommendations to provide stretching instruction to the parents when CMT is identified at birth and only refer to a physical therapist at 2 months of age if the condition does not resolve, more recent studies suggest that early physical therapy reduces the time to resolution compared with parent-only stretching, that stretching becomes more difficult in infants as they age and develop neck control, and that earlier intervention can negate the need for later surgery.

For more rigid deformities that persist beyond the age of 1 year or despite 6 months of physical therapy, surgical correction has historically been the treatment of choice. Continued physical therapy alone in more resistant CMT, even when performed carefully, can result in injury. Botulinum toxin (BTX) type A injection has been suggested to improve the results of physical therapy. The goal of BTX injections in CMT is to relax the tight soft-tissue structures enough so that a trained physical therapist can gain further correction of the contracture and also work on strengthening to maintain correction. Limpaphayon et al. reported that guided stretching of resistant CMT along with BTX type A injection resulted in resolution of deformity and maintenance of correction, with clinical improvement noted by 92% of caregivers. Sinn and Renaldi described successful treatment with BTX in 82 (61%) of 134 children.

Any permanent torticollis slowly becomes worse during growth. The head becomes inclined toward the affected side and the face toward the opposite side. If the deformity is severe, the ipsilateral shoulder becomes elevated and the frontooccipital diameter of the skull may become less than normal. Such severe deformity could and should be prevented by surgery during early childhood. Ideally, surgery is performed just before school age so that sufficient growth remains for remodeling of facial asymmetry while giving enough time for the growth of the structures to make surgical dissection and release easier. Many patients are first seen only after the deformities have become fixed, and the remaining growth potential is insufficient to correct them (Fig. 3.6). Nevertheless, many authors have suggested that surgical release in older children can be successful and should be attempted even if the child presents later. The clinical results are significantly less successful in children who have finished growth than in children who still have growth remaining; however, most patients have marked improvement in neck motion and head tilt, with satisfactory functional and cosmetic results. Lee et al. reported marked improvement in craniofacial deformity after surgical release in 80 patients with CMT. Improved results were demonstrated if the release was performed before the patient reached 5 years of age. In their study of 31 patients older than 7 years with late-presenting CMT, Lepetsos et al. obtained 84% excellent and 16% good results with operative treatment, and Seyhan et al. reported marked improvements in neck motion and head tilt in patients between the ages of 6 and 23 years who had bipolar release.

Several operations have been devised to release the sternocleidomastoid muscle at the clavicle. Unipolar release of the muscle distally is appropriate for mild deformity. Bipolar release proximally and distally may be indicated for moderate and severe torticollis. Endoscopic release of the sternocleidomastoid muscle has been described, with suggested advantages of precise division of the muscle fibers, preservation of the neurovascular structures, and an inconspicuous scar; we have no experience with this technique and no large series have been reported.

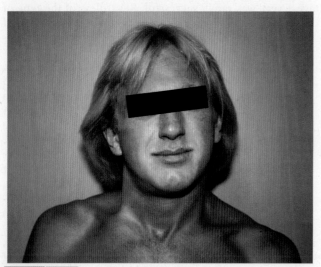

FIGURE 3.6 Untreated torticollis (right side) in 19-year-old man; note limited rotation and plagiocephaly.

UNIPOLAR RELEASE

Open unipolar tenotomy of the sternocleidomastoid muscle could be followed by tethering of the scar to the deep structures, reattachment of the clavicular head or the sternal head of the sternocleidomastoid muscle, loss of contour of the muscle, failure to correct the tilt of the head, or failure of facial asymmetry to correct. Tethering of the scar to the deep structures is more common in younger patients; therefore, the operation should be postponed until after 4 years of age.

TECHNIQUE 3.3

- Make an incision 5 cm long just superior to and parallel to the medial end of the clavicle (Fig. 3.7) and deepen it to the tendons of the sternal and clavicular attachments of the sternocleidomastoid muscle.
- Incise the tendon sheath longitudinally and pass a hemostat or other blunt instrument posterior to the tendons.
- By traction on the hemostat, draw the tendons outside the wound and superior and inferior to the hemostat; clamp them and resect 2.5 cm of their inferior ends. If it is contracted, divide the platysma muscle and adjacent fascia.
- With the child's head turned toward the affected side and the chin depressed, explore the wound digitally for any remaining bands of contracted muscle or fascia; and if any are found, divide them under direct vision until the deformity can, if possible, be overcorrected.
- If after this procedure overcorrection is not possible, make a small transverse incision inferior to the mastoid process and carefully divide the muscle near the bone. Avoid damaging the spinal accessory nerve.
- Close the wound and apply a bulky dressing that holds the head in the overcorrected position.

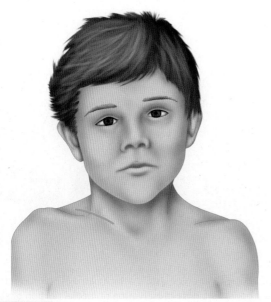

FIGURE 3.7 Unipolar release for torticollis. Note line of skin incision.

POSTOPERATIVE CARE At 1 week postoperatively, physical therapy, including manual stretching of the neck to maintain the overcorrected position, is begun. Manual stretching should be continued three times daily for 3 to 6 months; the use of plaster casts or braces usually is unnecessary (Fig. 3.8).

BIPOLAR RELEASE

Surgical correction in children with severe deformity or after failed operation usually requires a bipolar release of the sternocleidomastoid muscle. Ferkel et al. described a modified bipolar release and Z-plasty of the muscle for use in these circumstances. This approach lessens the sunken or hollow appearance of the distal end of the sternocleidomastoid that often occurs with a simple tenotomy, thereby giving the patient a better cosmetic result.

TECHNIQUE 3.4

(FERKEL ET AL.)

- Make a short transverse proximal incision behind the ear (Fig. 3.9A) and divide the sternocleidomastoid muscle insertion transversely just distal to the tip of the mastoid process. With this limited incision, the spinal accessory nerve is avoided, although the possibility that the nerve may take an anomalous route should be considered.
- Make a distal incision 4 to 5 cm long in line with the cervical skin creases, a fingerbreadth proximal to the medial end of the clavicle and the sternal notch.
- Divide the subcutaneous tissue and platysma muscle, exposing the clavicular and sternal attachments of the sternocleidomastoid muscle. Carefully avoid the anterior and external jugular veins and the carotid vessels and sheath during the dissection.
- Cut the clavicular portion of the muscle transversely and perform a Z-plasty on the sternal attachment so as to preserve the normal V-shaped contour of the sternocleidomastoid muscle in the neckline (Fig. 3.9B). Alternatively, release the clavicular head directly from the clavicle while transecting the sternal head proximal to its insertion by 1 to 2 cm. Then suture the two ends together side to side or end to end (Fig. 3.9C).
- Obtain the desired degree of correction by manipulating the head and neck during the release.
- Release of additional contracted bands of fascia or muscle occasionally is necessary before closure.
- Close both wounds with subcuticular sutures.

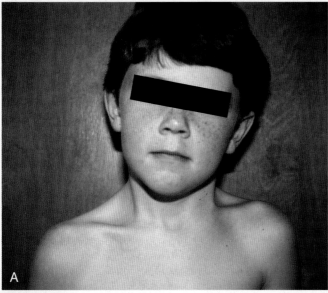
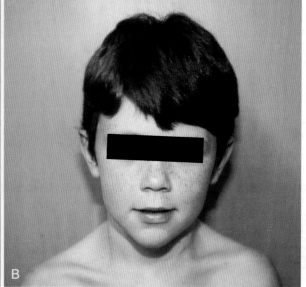

FIGURE 3.8 Seven-year-old boy with left congenital muscular torticollis. **A,** Before unipolar supraclavicular release. **B,** After unipolar release; note scar superior to clavicle in transverse line of skin crease. **SEE TECHNIQUE 3.3.**

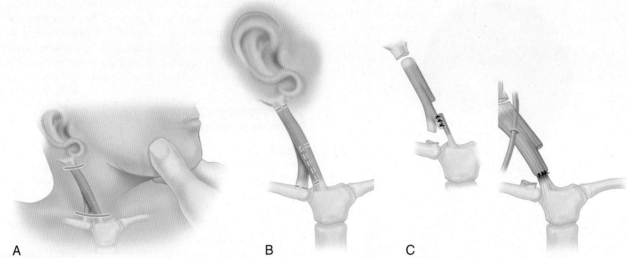

FIGURE 3.9   Bipolar Z-plasty operation for torticollis. **A,** Skin incisions. **B,** Clavicular and mastoid attachments of sternocleidomastoid muscle are cut, and Z-plasty is performed on sternal origin. **C,** Completed operation; note preservation of medial portion of sternal attachment. (Redrawn from Ferkel RD, Westin GW, Dawson EG, et al: Muscular torticollis: a modified surgical approach, *J Bone Joint Surg* 65A:894, 1983.) **SEE TECHNIQUE 3.4.**

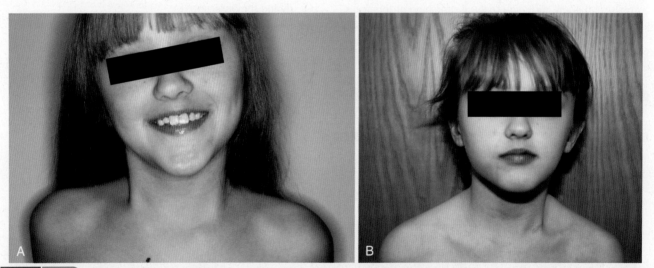

FIGURE 3.10   Bipolar release for congenital torticollis. **A,** Severe congenital torticollis (right side) in 8-year-old girl. **B,** After bipolar release. **SEE TECHNIQUE 3.4.**

POSTOPERATIVE CARE Physical therapy, consisting of stretching, muscle strengthening, and active range-of-motion exercises, is instituted in the early postoperative period. Head-halter traction or a cervical collar also can be used during the first 6 to 12 weeks after surgery (Fig. 3.10).

CONGENITAL PSEUDARTHROSIS OF THE CLAVICLE

Congenital pseudarthrosis of the clavicle is rare. Several theories concerning its cause have been proposed. Because the clavicle develops in two separate masses by medial and lateral ossification centers, pseudarthrosis could be explained by failure of ossification of the precartilaginous bridge that would normally connect the two ossification centers. Alternatively, direct pressure from the subclavian artery on the immature clavicle may be the cause. Congenital pseudarthrosis of the clavicle occurs almost invariably on the right; bilateral involvement occurs in approximately 10% of patients. In a series of 60 unilateral lesions, 59 were on the right, and in the one patient with a pseudarthrosis on the left, dextrocardia was found. Pseudarthrosis of the clavicle is present at birth and usually is in the middle third of the clavicle (Fig. 3.11). Differential diagnoses include cleidocranial dysostosis and rarely nonunion after clavicular fracture.

Congenital pseudarthrosis of the clavicle may require treatment, not because of pain or hypermobility of the shoulder girdle, but usually because of an unacceptable appearance or occasionally because of pain in adolescent

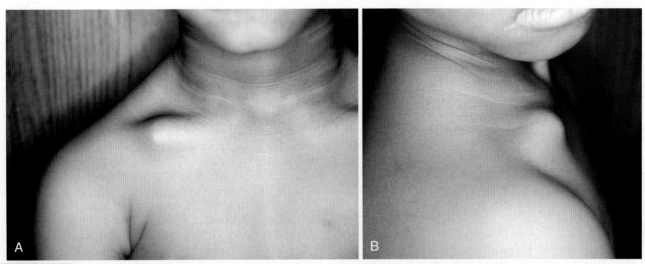

FIGURE 3.11 Congenital pseudarthrosis of clavicle. **A,** Subcutaneous prominence in middle third of right clavicle in 4-year-old child. **B,** Lateral view.

patients. Sales de Gauzy et al. described thoracic outlet syndrome in an adolescent with congenital pseudarthrosis of the clavicle. Hyperabduction of the arm caused compression of the subclavian artery by the medial end of the lateral clavicular fragment. After resection of the pseudarthrosis, iliac bone grafting, and plate fixation, the patient was pain free with total functional recovery. Although congenital pseudarthrosis of the clavicle is asymptomatic in childhood, surgical treatment can restore normal morphology and prevent functional or vascular problems in adolescence and adulthood. Spontaneous union is unknown, and consequently any desired union requires surgical treatment. Most surgeons agree that the ideal time for grafting is between ages 3 and 5 years. Although grafting can be done at any age, with increasing patient age, successful grafting becomes less likely. Simple resection is not recommended because it results in prominent, painful bone ends, prominence of the ends during movements of the shoulder, and asymmetry of the shoulder girdles. Simple resection of the fibrous pseudarthroses and sclerotic bone ends, followed by careful dissection and preservation of the periosteal sleeve to maintain continuity, and approximation of bone ends, without bone grafting or internal fixation has been shown to be successful in children younger than the age of 6 years. Nevertheless, most authors recommend excision of the pseudarthrosis, bone grafting, and fixation with a small reconstruction plate or an intramedullary Kirschner wire.

Union is easier to obtain in congenital pseudarthrosis of the clavicle than in that of the tibia. Almost any type of bone grafting suitable for traumatic nonunion of the clavicle has been satisfactory in pseudarthrosis, but open reduction and internal fixation with plate and screws and autogenous iliac bone grafting have produced the best results with higher rates of union, less time to union, and fewer complications when compared with Kirschner wire fixation. This is especially true if performed in older children (Fig. 3.12). In 2017 Studer et al. demonstrated a high rate of union and good functional results at a mean follow-up of 7 years after nonvascularized iliac crest bone grafts and plate fixation in children with a mean age of 7.1 years.

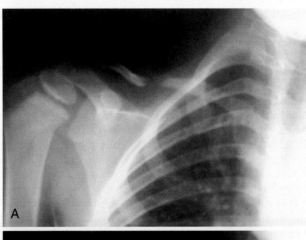

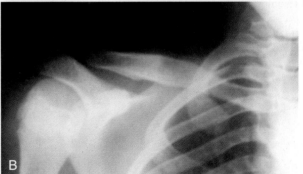

FIGURE 3.12 **A,** Congenital pseudarthrosis of right clavicle before plating and bone grafting. **B,** At 7 years of age after plate removal.

OPEN REDUCTION AND ILIAC BONE GRAFTING FOR CONGENITAL PSEUDARTHROSIS OF THE CLAVICLE

TECHNIQUE 3.5

- Make a transverse 3-inch (7.5-cm) incision centered over the body of the clavicle, approximately a fingerbreadth above the superior border of the bone.

- Carry sharp dissection through the subcutaneous tissue to expose the clavicle medially and laterally in the central third in the area of the pseudarthrosis.
- Expose the bone subperiosteally, protecting the underlying neurovascular structures.
- Debride the site of the pseudarthrosis of all fibrous and cartilaginous tissue down to normal bone medially and laterally.
- Bend a four-hole plate (semitubular, dynamic compression, or acetabular reconstruction) to fit the contours of the bone.
- Fix the plate to the clavicle in the usual manner.
- Obtain autogenous iliac grafts and place them on the superior, inferior, and posterior aspects of the pseudarthrosis.
- Close the wound in layers and the skin with subcuticular sutures.

POSTOPERATIVE CARE A collar and cuff sling is worn for 2 to 3 weeks. The plate can be removed at 12 to 24 months or when radiographic union occurs.

CONGENITAL DISLOCATION OF THE RADIAL HEAD

Congenital dislocation of the radial head, the most common congenital anomaly of the elbow, is rare but should be suspected when the radial head has been dislocated for a long time, there is no evidence that the ulna has been fractured, and the radial head appears abnormally small and misshapen. The radiographic findings are fairly characteristic. The radial shaft is abnormally long, and the ulna usually is abnormally bowed. The radial head is dislocated, frequently posteriorly but sometimes anteriorly; is rounded, showing little if any depression for articulation with the capitellum; and usually is smaller than normal. Occasionally, there is an area of ossification in the tissues around the radial head. The capitellum also may be small, and the radial notch of the ulna that should articulate with the radial head may be small or absent (Fig. 3.13). Although bilaterality has been listed in older studies as a criterion for diagnosis of congenital dislocation of the radial head, more recent reports have confirmed the existence of unilateral dislocations. Congenital dislocation of the radial head may be familial, especially on the paternal side, and may be associated with chondroosteodystrophy, achondroplasia, hypochondroplasia, Larsen syndrome, nail-patella syndrome, and hereditary multiple exostosis.

A congenitally dislocated radial head is irreducible manually or surgically because of adaptive changes in the soft tissues and the absence of normal surfaces for articulation with the ulna and humerus. Consequently, open reduction of the dislocation and reconstruction of the annular ligament in childhood are not advised. Any impairment of function usually is caused by restriction of rotation of the forearm; in children, physical therapy to improve this motion is the only treatment indicated. If pain persists into adulthood, the radial head and neck can be excised. Any resection of the radial head should be postponed until growth is complete, but even then it may not improve motion because of the contractures of the soft tissues. Nevertheless, excision of the radial head should be considered for pain in an older patient and may achieve some improvement in range of motion. Bengard et al. reviewed intermediate and long-term follow-up of both operatively and nonoperatively treated patients with congenital radial head dislocation. The authors showed that operatively treated patients had significant reduction in pain and improved overall satisfaction with minimal gains of motion. However, over 25% of operatively treated patients required additional surgery for wrist pain. Furthermore, nonoperatively treated patients had no loss of motion, development of pain, or the need for further surgical intervention. Radial and ulnar osteotomies have been suggested to treat congenital and chronic radial head dislocation; however, further studies are needed to determine their efficacy.

CONGENITAL PSEUDARTHROSIS OF THE RADIUS

Congenital pseudarthrosis of the radius is extremely rare. In patients with neurofibromatosis, the pseudarthrosis develops from a cyst in the radius, and patients usually have skin

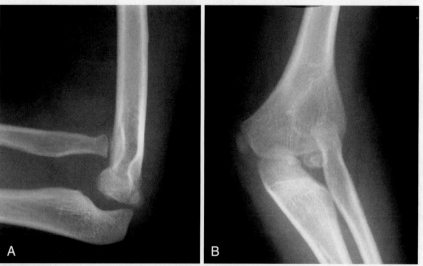

FIGURE 3.13 Congenital dislocation of radial head. **A,** Lateral view. **B,** Anteroposterior view.

manifestations of neurofibromatosis or a strong family history of the disease.

In each instance reported, pseudarthrosis of the radius occurred in the distal third of the bone and the distal fragment was quite short. Because the lesion is near the distal radial physis, the ends of the bone are attenuated and the ulna is relatively long. The treatment of choice is dual-onlay bone grafting. This operation restores length, provides a viselike grip on the osteoporotic distal fragment, increases the size of the distal end of the proximal fragment, and usually results in satisfactory union (Fig. 3.14).

Others have reported good results after complete resection of the involved radius, with the surrounding periosteum and soft tissue, and free vascularized fibular transfer. This operation can be delayed until skeletal maturity, with the arm supported by a forearm brace until surgery is performed. Alternatively, vascularized fibular grafting has been performed in younger patients, but obtaining stable internal fixation can be challenging in this group. Plate and screw fixation risks damage to the vascular supply of the periosteum around the fibular graft, but unstable fixation with only intramedullary and crossed Kirschner wires might lead to delayed union. In their review of the English-language literature, Witoonchart et al. found that free vascular fibular grafting obtained the best union rate among the reported procedures: it was successful in 18 of 19 ulnar or radial pseudarthroses reported. Vascular fibular grafting is described in other chapter.

CONGENITAL PSEUDARTHROSIS OF THE ULNA

Congenital pseudarthrosis of the ulna also is extremely rare. It typically occurs in the patients with neurofibromatosis, and associated congenital pseudarthrosis of the radius is not uncommon. Ulnar pseudarthrosis produces angulation of the radius, shortening of the forearm, and dislocation of the radial head (Fig. 3.15).

Various treatment methods have been described for congenital ulnar pseudarthrosis, including nonvascularized bone grafting with and without internal fixation, creation of a one-bone forearm, free vascularized fibular grafting, and the Ilizarov compression-distraction technique. Bone grafting of congenital pseudarthrosis of the ulna usually has failed, but because significant bowing of the radius develops in very young children, early surgery is indicated. If the pseudarthrosis has developed through a cystic lesion, early curettage of the cyst, internal fixation of the bone, and bone grafting usually are successful. In established pseudarthrosis with tapering of the ends of the bone, the distal ulna should be excised early to relieve its tethering effect on the radius; then the forearm is fitted with a suitable brace. If the radial head dislocates, it should be excised, and a synostosis (one-bone forearm) should be produced between the radius and ulna (Fig. 3.16). Osteotomy of the distal radius to correct bowing also may be indicated. Use of the Ilizarov device has been reported in patients with small pseudarthrosis "gaps" and bony fragments of acceptable quality. Bae et al. reported successful free vascularized fibular grafting in four children with congenital ulnar pseudarthrosis. In two of the children (3 and 5 years old), the proximal fibular epiphysis was included in the graft and continued growth was present at 6 and 3 years, respectively, after surgery.

CONGENITAL RADIOULNAR SYNOSTOSIS

Congenital radioulnar synostosis is a rare malformation in which there is an abnormal connection between the radius and ulna due to an embryologic failure of separation. Congenital radioulnar synostosis usually involves the proximal ends of the radius and ulna, most often fixing the forearm in pronation. It is more often bilateral than unilateral. Familial predisposition is frequent, and the deformity seems to be transmitted on the paternal side of the family. Wilkie noted two types. In the first

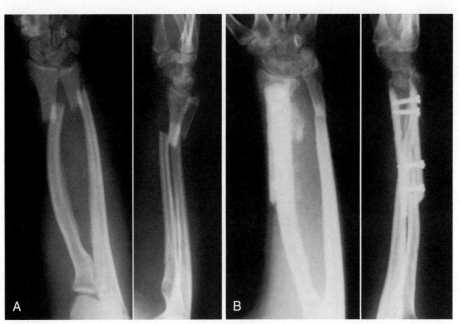

FIGURE 3.14 Congenital pseudarthrosis of radius. **A,** Closed fractures of radius and ulna in child with manifestations of neurofibromatosis. **B,** Union of radius after dual-onlay bone grafting.

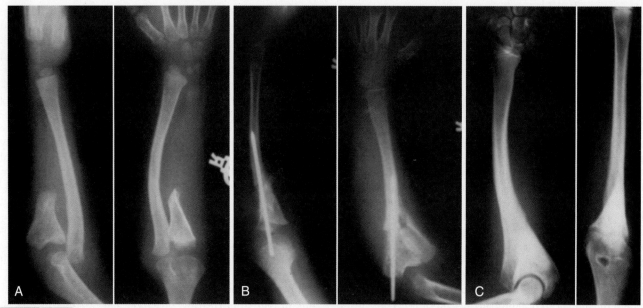

FIGURE 3.15 Congenital pseudarthrosis of ulna with dislocation of radial head. **A,** Before surgery. **B,** After excision of radial head, creation of synostosis between proximal radius and ulna and fixation with medullary nail. **C,** Final appearance of one-bone forearm.

type, the medullary canals of the radius and ulna are joined. The proximal end of the radius is malformed and is fused to the ulna for several centimeters (see Fig. 3.16). The radius is longer and larger than the ulna, and its shaft arches anteriorly more than normally. In the second type, the radius is fairly normal, but its proximal end is dislocated either anteriorly or posteriorly and is fused to the proximal ulnar shaft; the fusion is neither as extensive nor as intimate as in the first type. Wilkie stated that the second type often is unilateral and that sometimes another deformity, such as a supernumerary thumb, absence of the thumb, or syndactylism, also is present.

Two other classifications classify the deformity based on the presence or absence of an associated radial head dislocation and the existence of a fibrous or osseous synostosis (Box 3.1). These two classification systems highlight the association with radial head dislocation that might represent a spectrum of disease beginning in the early embryologic period. Early embryologic development of radioulnar synostosis also explains its association with many other congenital syndromes such as Apert syndrome, Klinefelter syndrome, Carpenter syndrome, arthrogryposis, and others.

Congenital radioulnar synostosis is difficult to treat. Fortunately, the majority of patients do not require surgical intervention. The fascial tissues are short and their fibers are abnormally directed, the interosseous membrane is narrow, and the supinator muscles may be abnormal or absent. The anomalies in the forearm may be so widespread that sometimes no rotation would be possible, even if the radius and ulna were separated and the interosseous membrane split throughout its length. Three-dimensional analysis of congenital radioulnar synostosis showed significant flexion deformities of the radius and internal rotation deformities of the radius and ulna, which would likely impede forearm rotation after corrective surgery. Additionally, patient and parent expectations of improved motion after surgical treatment often lead to disappointment if surgery is attempted. Simply excising the fused part of the radius never improves function. It is inadvisable to perform any operation with the hope of obtaining pronation and supination. Surgery is not recommended for most patients because the

deformity typically is not disabling enough to justify an extensive operation. Motion of the shoulder, especially when the elbow is extended, compensates well for the deformity in most children.

Osteotomy occasionally is indicated in children with bilateral hyperpronation, but the exact position of the forearm is controversial. Some have suggested positioning one forearm in neutral rotation to assist in hygiene. However, modern widespread use of keyboards and hand-held communication devices makes slight pronation more attractive in developed nations. In Asian cultures, it has been suggested that eating habits of holding a bowl in the nondominant hand may necessitate slight supination. Simcock et al. evaluated the safety and efficacy of a proximal derotational osteotomy through the ulnar metaphysis in 31 forearms. They determined their method to be safe and effective but advocated for meticulous surgical technique, including control of the osteotomy site, judicious pin fixation, and prophylactic fasciotomies. They did, however, experience a 12% complication rate owing primarily to transient nerve palsies (anterior interosseous and radial nerves) in large rotational corrections.

Seitz et al. reported the use of a small external fixation device after derotational osteotomy in a 2-year-old child with congenital radioulnar synostosis. They cited as advantages to this technique precise rotational correction, adequate stabilization, and avoidance of cast immobilization.

Lin et al. described a two-stage technique for correction of severe forearm rotational deformities, including congenital radioulnar synostosis. Percutaneous drill-assisted osteotomies of the radius and the ulna are performed and are followed 10 days later by manipulation of the forearm into the desired functional position. No internal or external fixation is used; long arm cast immobilization is used for 6 to 8 weeks. These authors reported functional improvement in 25 of 26 forearms, including all 12 forearms with congenital radioulnar synostosis. Although the range of motion was not significantly changed, the arc of motion was in a more functional hand position. Rotational osteotomy performed in a single stage has been described with the addition of segmental bone resection. Early results have shown promise as a safe technique. Here we describe a two-stage osteotomy.

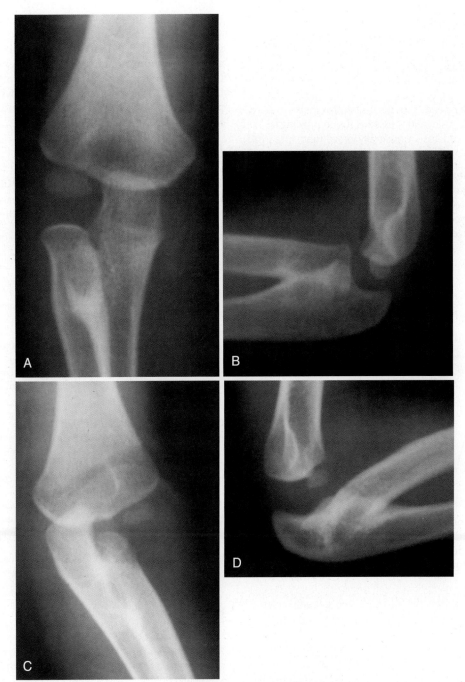

FIGURE 3.16 Congenital radioulnar synostosis. **A** and **B,** First type: proximal radius and ulna are fused for 3 cm, and radius is enlarged. **C** and **D,** Second type: radius is dislocated posteriorly and laterally.

RADIAL AND ULNAR OSTEOTOMIES FOR CORRECTION OF CONGENITAL RADIOULNAR SYNOSTOSIS (TWO-STAGE)

TECHNIQUE 3.6

(LIN ET AL.)

- Under tourniquet control, make a 1- to 2-cm incision over the dorsolateral ridge of the distal third of the radius (Fig. 3.17A).

- Expose the bone subperiosteally and mark the osteotomy site with several fine drill holes that penetrate both cortices.
- Make a second small incision over the subcutaneous aspect of the proximal third of the ulna and similarly expose and drill this bone (Fig. 3.17B).
- Use a sharp osteotome to complete the division of the radius and then the ulna.
- Make no attempt at this point to change the position of the arm.
- Deflate the tourniquet and obtain adequate hemostasis. Irrigate the wounds and close them with subcuticular sutures. Place a long arm cast over sterile dressings.

BOX 3.1

Classifications of Congenital Radioulnar Synostosis

Tachdjian
Type I: Absent radial head, osseous fusion proximally
Type II: Radial head dislocation, osseous fusion proximally
Type III: Fibrous synostosis proximally preventing forearm rotation

Cleary and Omer
Type I: Fibrous synostosis
Type II: Osseous synostosis, reduced radial head
Type III: Osseous synostosis, posteriorly dislocated radial head
Type IV: Osseous synostosis, anteriorly dislocated radial head

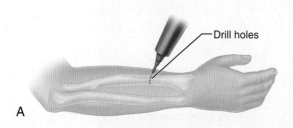

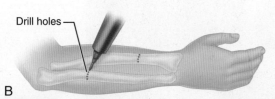

FIGURE 3.17 Correction of congenital radioulnar synostosis with percutaneous drill-assisted osteotomies of radius **(A)** and ulna **(B)**. Ten days later, forearm is manipulated to more functional position. **SEE TECHNIQUE 3.6.**

- Ten days later, remove the cast with the patient under general anesthesia and supinate or pronate the forearm into the desired position.
- Obtain anteroposterior and lateral radiographs to confirm bony apposition and alignment. Generally, affected dominant extremities should be placed in 20 to 30 degrees of pronation and nondominant extremities should be placed in 20 degrees of supination.
- Check pulses carefully after manipulation and monitor the extremity closely to detect signs of compartment syndrome.
- Apply a long arm cast, which is worn for 6 to 8 weeks to allow complete healing of the osteotomies.

Kanaya and Ibaraki described a technique for mobilization of congenital radioulnar synostosis with use of a free vascularized fascia-fat graft to prevent recurrent ankylosis. The graft was obtained from the lateral aspect of the ipsilateral arm, and the authors reported minimal donor site morbidity and no difficulty with closure. The seven patients in whom this procedure was done all had marked

improvements in supination and pronation; at an almost 4-year average follow-up, no patients had recurrent ankylosis or loss of the flap. Kanaya and Ibaraki found that adding a radial osteotomy to the procedure prevented dislocation of the radial head and increased the arc of motion (83 degrees in patients with osteotomy compared with 40 degrees in patients without osteotomy). We have no experience with this technique.

REFERENCES

CONGENITAL ELEVATION OF THE SCAPULA
Dhir R, Chin K, Lambert S: The congenital undescended scapula syndrome: Sprengel and celithrum: a case series and hypothesis, *J Shoulder Elbow Surg* 27:252, 2018.

Elzohairy MM, Salama AM: Congenital elevation of the scapula (Sprengel deformity), *Eur J Orthop Surg Traumatol* 29:37, 2019.

Harvey EJ, Bernstein M, Desy NM, et al.: Sprengel deformity: pathogenesis and management, *Am Acad Orthop Surg* 20:177, 2012.

Jiang Y, Guo Y, Zhu Z, et al.: Surgical management of Sprengel's deformity by a modification of Green's procedure: a single center experience, *Orthopä* 49:255, 2020.

Wada A, Nakamura T, Fujii T, et al.: Sprengel deformity: morphometric assessment and surgical treatment by the modified Green procedure, *J Pediatr Orthop* 34:55, 2014.

Walstra FE, Alta TD, van der Eijken JW, et al.: Long-term follow-up of Sprengel's deformity treated with the Woodward procedure, *J Shoulder Elbow Surg* 22:752, 2013.

CONGENITAL MUSCULAR TORTICOLLIS
Boyko N, Eppinger MA, Straka-DeMarco D, et al.: Imaging of congenital torticollis in infants: a retrospective study of an institutional protocol, *J Neurosurg Pediatr* 20:191, 2019.

Han MH, Kang JY, Don HJ, et al.: Comparison of clinical findings of congenital torticollis between patients with and without sternocleidomastoid lesions as determined by ultrasonography, *J Pediatr Orthop* 39:226, 2019.

Han JD, Kim SH, Lee SJ, et al.: The thickness of the sternocleidomastoid muscle as a prognostic factor for congenital muscular torticollis, *Ann Rehabil Med* 35:361, 2011.

Kaplan SL, Couter C, Sargent B: Physical therapy management of congenital muscular torticollis: a 2018 evidence-based clinical practice guideline from the Academy of Pediatric Physical Therapy, *Pediatr Phys Ther* 30:240, 2018.

Keklicek H, Uygur F: A randomized controlled study on the efficiency of soft tissue mobilization in babies with congenital muscular torticollis, *J Back Musculoskeletal Rehab* 31:315, 2018.

Kim HJ, Ahn HS, Yim SY: Effectiveness of surgical treatment for neglected congenital muscular torticollis: a systematic review and meta-analysis, *Plast Reconstr Surg* 136:67e, 2015.

Lee KS, Chung EG, Lee BH: A comparison of outcomes of asymmetry in infants with congenital muscular torticollis according to age upon starting treatment, *J Phys Ther Sci* 29:543, 2017.

Lee YT, Cho SK, Yoon K, et al.: Risk factors for intrauterine constraint are associated with ultrasonographically detected severe fibrosis in early congenital muscular torticollis, *J Pediatr Orthop* 46:514, 2011.

Lepetsos P, Anastasopoulos PP, Leonidou A, et al.: Surgical management of congenital torticollis in children older than 7 years with an average 10-year follow-up, *J Pediatr Orthop B* 26:580, 2017.

Limpaphayon N, Kohan E, Huser A, et al.: Use of combined botulinum toxin and physical therapy for treatment of resistant congenital muscular torticollis, *J Pediatr Orthop* 39:3343, 2019.

Matusezewski L, Pietrzyk D, Kandzierski G, et al.: Bilateral congenital torticollis: a case report with 25 years of follow-up, *J Pediatr Orthop B* 26:585, 2017.

Min KJ, Park EJ, Yim DY: Effectiveness of surgical release in patients with neglected congenital muscular torticollis according to age at the time of surgery, *Ann Rehabil Med* 40:34, 2016.

Petronic I, Brdar R, Cirovic D, et al.: Congenital muscular torticollis in children: distribution, treatment duration, and outcome, *Eur J Phys Rehabil Med* 46:153, 2010.

Seyhan N, Jasharllari L, Keskin M, Savaci N: Efficacy of bipolar release in neglected congenital muscular torticollis patients, *Musculoskelet Surg* 96(1):55, 2012.

Sinn CN, Rinaldi RJ: Treatment with botulinum toxin type A in infants with refractory congenital muscular torticollis, a 10-year retrospective study, *PMR* 8:S152, 2016.

CONGENITAL PSEUDARTHROSES OF THE CLAVICLE, RADIUS, AND ULNA

Chandran P, George H, James LA: Congenital clavicular pseudarthrosis: comparison of two treatment methods, *J Child Orthop* 5:1, 2011.

Studer K, Baker MP, Krieg AH: Operative treatment of congenital pseudarthrosis of the clavicle: a single-centre experience, *J Pediatr Orthop B* 26(3):245, 2017.

CONGENITAL DISLOCATION OF THE RADIAL HEAD

Bae DS, Canizares MF, Miller PE, et al.: Intraobserver and interobserver reliabilty of the Oberg-Manske-Tonkin (OMT) classification: establishing a registry on congenital upper limb differences, *J Pediatr Orthop* 38:69, 2018.

Bengard MJ, Calfee R, Steffen JA, Goldfarb CA: Intermediate-term to long-term outcome of surgically and nonsurgically treated congenital, isolated radial head dislocation, *J Hand Surg [Am]* 37:2495, 2012.

Gogoi P, Dutta A, Sipani AK, Daolagupu AK: Congenital deficiency of distal ulna and dislocation of the radial head treated by single bone forearm procedure, *Case Rep Orthop* 2014:Article ID 526719, 4 pages, 2014, https://doi.org/10.1155/2014/526719.

Jo AH, Jung ST, Kim MS, et al.: An evaluation of forearm deformities in hereditary multiple exostoses: factors associated with radial head dislocation and comprehensive classification, *J Hand Surg Am* 42:292, 2017.

Kim HT, Ahn TY, Jang JH, et al.: A graphic overlay method for selection of osteotomy site in chronic radial head dislocation: an evaluation of 3D-printed bone models, *J Pediatr Orthop* 37:388, 2017.

Liu R, Miao W, Mu M, et al.: Ulnar rotation osteotomy for congenital radial head dislocation, *J Hand Surg Am* 40:1769, 2015.

Song KS, Ramnani K, Cho CH: Long term follow-up of open realignment procedure for congenital dislocation of the radial head, *J Hand Surg Eur* 36:161, 2011.

CONGENITAL RADIOULNAR SYNOSTOSIS

Elliott AM, Kibria L, Reed MH: The developmental spectrum of proximal radioulnar synostosis, *Skeletal Radiol* 39:49, 2010.

Ezaki M, Oishi SN: Technique of forearm osteotomy for pediatric problems, *J Hand Surg [Am]* 37:2400, 2012.

Hwang JH, Kim HW, Lee DH, et al.: One-stage rotational osteotomy for congenital radioulnar synostosis, *J Hand Surg Eur* 40:855, 2015.

Nakasone M, Nakasone S, Kinjo M, et al.: Three-dimensional analysis of deformities of the radius and ulna in congenital proximal radioulnar synostosis, *J Hand Surg Eur* 43(78):739, 2018.

Shingade VU, Shingade RV, Ughade SN: Results of single-staged rotational osteotomy in a child with congenital proximal radioulnar synostosis: subjective and objective evaluation, *J Pediatr Orthop* 34:63, 2014.

Simcock X, Shah AS, Waters PM, Bae DS: Safety and efficacy of derotational osteotomy for congenital radioulnar synostosis, *J Pediatr Orthop* 35(8):838, 2015.

The complete list of references is available online at ExpertConsult.com.

CHAPTER 4

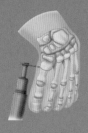

OSTEOCHONDROSIS OR EPIPHYSITIS AND OTHER MISCELLANEOUS AFFECTIONS

Benjamin W. Sheffer

LEGG-CALVÉ-PERTHES DISEASE

The cause of Legg-Calvé-Perthes disease is unknown but has provoked considerable controversy. Previously, some authors thought that an inherited thrombophilia promoted thrombotic venous occlusion in the femoral vein, causing bone death in the femoral head and ultimately leading to Legg-Calvé-Perthes disease. More recent studies have not found an inherited hypercoagulability or a deficiency in protein C activity, however, indicating that inherited thrombophilia is not associated with the osteonecrosis of Legg-Calvé-Perthes disease. Although research continues, it seems that coagulation disorders are not conclusive etiologic factors in Legg-Calvé-Perthes disease. As noted by Hosalkar and Mulpuri, even after 100 years the etiology of Legg-Calvé-Perthes disease remains unclear and its treatment is still controversial.

DIAGNOSIS

The initial diagnosis of Legg-Calvé-Perthes can be difficult if symptoms have not been present for some time. Children with Legg-Calvé-Perthes disease have symptoms present for an average of 6 weeks before the diagnosis is made. This may be longer if the pain is mild and patients delay initial evaluation. Legg-Calvé-Perthes disease occurs three times more frequently in boys than in girls, and the average age of patients with Legg-Calvé-Perthes disease is 7 years, although it can occur in children significantly

younger. Radiographic changes of the femoral head (condensation and sclerosis) generally are delayed but occur 6 weeks after initial symptoms. Therefore, if a child presents early with hip pain and radiographs are normal, a follow-up radiograph should be obtained at 6 weeks if the child is still symptomatic. Radiographic findings of Legg-Calvé-Perthes have been described by Waldenström (Table 4.1), with further modifications by the Perthes Study Group that show good intraobserver and interobserver reliability and may be used in further clinical study.

Meyer dysplasia can be easily mistaken for Legg-Calvé-Perthes disease and lead to unnecessary diagnostic procedures and treatment. Meyer dysplasia has been found to be more common in boys younger than 4 years old and more likely to be bilateral. Characteristic findings included delayed or smaller ossification centers on radiograph, a separated or cracked epiphysis, cystic changes, and mild pain and limping. Condensation, subchondral fractures, fragmentation, and subluxation usually are not present with Meyer dysplasia.

■ CLASSIFICATION

When the diagnosis is established, the primary aim of treatment of Legg-Calvé-Perthes disease is containment of the femoral head within the acetabulum. If this is achieved, the femoral head can re-form in a concentric manner by what Salter has termed *biologic plasticity*.

TABLE 4.1

Stages of Legg-Calvé-Perthes (Waldenström)

Initial	■ Infarction produces a smaller, sclerotic epiphysis with medial joint space widening	■ Radiographs may remain occult for 3-6 months
Fragmentation	■ Femoral head appears to fragment or dissolve ■ Result of a revascularization process and bone resorption producing collapse and subsequent increased density	■ Hip-related symptoms are most prevalent ■ Lateral pillar classification based on this stage
Reossification	■ Ossific nucleus undergoes reossification as new bone appears as necrotic bone is resorbed	■ May last up to 18 months
Healing or remodeling	■ Femoral head remodels until skeletal maturity	■ Begins once ossific nucleus is completely reossified trabecular pattern returns

TABLE 4.2

Catterall Classification

Group I	■ Involvement of the anterior epiphysis only
Group II	■ Involvement of the anterior epiphysis with a clear sequestrum
Group III	■ Only a small part of the epiphysis is not involved
Group IV	■ Total head involvement
	■ Based on degree of head involvement
	■ At-risk signs (indicate a more severe disease course) ■ Gage sign—V-shaped radiolucency in the lateral portion of the epiphysis and/or adjacent metaphysis ■ Calcification lateral to the epiphysis ■ Lateral subluxation of the femoral head ■ Horizontal proximal femoral physis ■ Metaphyseal cyst—added later to the original four at-risk signs described by Catterall

TABLE 4.3

Salter-Thompson Classification

Class A	■ Crescent sign involves <½ of femoral head
Class B	■ Crescent sign involves >½ of femoral head
Based on radiographic crescent sign	

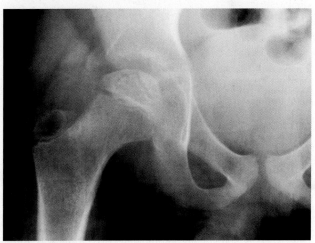

FIGURE 4.1 Type B subchondral fracture involving more than 50% of femoral head.

Historically, Catterall et al. classified patients with this disease into groups according to the amount of involvement of the capital femoral epiphysis: group I, partial head or less than half head involvement; groups II and III, more than half head involvement and sequestrum formation; and group IV, involvement of the entire epiphysis (Table 4.2). They noted that certain radiographic signs described as "head at risk" correlated positively with poor results, especially in patients in groups II, III, and IV. These head-at-risk signs include (1) lateral subluxation of the femoral head from the acetabulum, (2) speckled calcification lateral to the capital epiphysis, (3) diffuse metaphyseal reaction (metaphyseal cysts), (4) a horizontal physis, and (5) the Gage sign, a radiolucent V-shaped defect in the lateral epiphysis and adjacent metaphysis. Catterall recommended containment by femoral varus derotational osteotomy for older children in groups II, III, and IV with head-at-risk signs. Contraindications include an already malformed femoral head and delay of treatment of more than 8 months from onset of symptoms. Surgery is not recommended for any group I children or any child without the head-at-risk signs.

Salter and Thompson advocated determining the extent of involvement by describing the extent of a subchondral

fracture in the superolateral portion of the femoral head. If the extent of the fracture (line) is less than 50% of the superior dome of the femoral head, the involvement is considered type A, and good results can be expected (Table 4.3). If the extent of the fracture is more than 50% of the dome, the involvement is considered type B, and fair or poor results can be expected (Fig. 4.1). According to Salter and Thompson, this subchondral fracture and its entire extent can be observed radiographically earlier and more readily than trying to determine the Catterall classification (8.1 months average). According to these authors, if the femoral head is graded as type B, probably an operation such as an innominate osteotomy should be carried out. The extent of the subchondral fracture line, when present, has been suggested to be more accurate in predicting the extent of necrosis than is the extent of necrosis seen on MRI. In our experience, however, subchondral fractures are present early in the course of the disease in only a third of patients, and although this classification is a reliable indicator

TABLE 4.4

Lateral Pillar (Herring) Classification

Group A	▪ Lateral pillar maintains full height with no density changes identified	▪ Uniformly good outcome
Group B	▪ Maintains >50% height	▪ Poor outcome in patients with bone age >6 years
Group B/C border	▪ Lateral pillar is narrowed (2-3 mm) or poorly ossified with approximately 50% height	▪ Recently added to increase consistency and prognosis of classification
Group C	▪ Less than 50% of lateral pillar height is maintained	▪ Poor outcomes in all patients

- ▪ Determined at the beginning of fragmentation stage
- ▪ Usually occurs 6 months after the onset of symptoms
- ▪ Based on the height of the lateral pillar of the capital femoral epiphysis on anteroposterior imaging of the pelvis
- ▪ Has best interobserver agreement
- ▪ Designed to provide prognostic information
- ▪ Limitation is that final classification is not possible at initial presentation due to the fact that the patient needs to have entered into the fragmentation stage radiographically

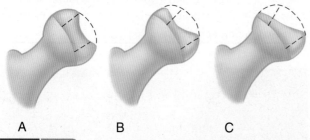

FIGURE 4.2 **A** to **C,** Lateral pillar classification based on height of lateral pillar.

in the group with fractures, it has little to offer in early treatment decisions for the other two thirds of patients.

Presently, the most used classification is by Herring et al. (Table 4.4). They described a classification based on the height of the lateral pillar: group A, no involvement of the lateral pillar; group B, at least 50% of lateral pillar height maintained; and group C, less than 50% of lateral pillar height maintained (Fig. 4.2). A statistically significant correlation was found between the final outcome (Stulberg classification) and the loss of pillar height. Patients in group A had uniformly good outcomes; patients in group B who were younger than 8 to 9 years old at onset had good outcomes, but patients older than age 8 to 9 years had less favorable results; patients in group C had the worst results, with most having aspherical femoral heads, regardless of age at onset or type of treatment. Reproducibility of this classification system was confirmed by 78% of members of the study group who used it. A patient with a pillar group B may progress to a pillar group C or may be in a "gray" area and designated as pillar group B/C border. Herring et al. noted that the advantages of this classification are (1) it can be applied easily during the active stages of the disease and (2) the high correlation between the lateral pillar height and the amount of femoral head flattening at skeletal maturity allows accurate prediction of the natural history and treatment methods. Price has challenged the concept that a lateral pillar sign allows accurate prediction of the natural history and treatment. He noted that the sign may change from A to C in the course of the disease and that containment may no longer be beneficial. The lateral pillar sign may help guide treatment for some patients; however, a prognostic indicator

to assist decision-making in the early stages of the disease may be necessary.

◼ BILATERAL INVOLVEMENT

Reports in the literature indicate that those with bilateral Legg-Calvé-Perthes disease, which occurs in approximately 10% of patients, have more severe involvement than patients with unilateral disease because most have a Catterall III or IV or a Herring B or C classification, and 48% rate as a Stulberg 4 or 5 at skeletal maturity. Bilateral involvement can be confused with multiple epiphyseal dysplasia of the hip. Radiographs of the other joints and a wrist radiograph to determine bone age (which is delayed in Legg-Calvé-Perthes disease) help to distinguish the two. Concerning sex, boys and girls who have the same Catterall classification or lateral pillar classification at the time of initial evaluation can be expected to have similar outcomes according to the classification system of Stulberg, Cooperman, and Wallensten.

◼ IMAGING EVALUATION

In the past, diagnosis often was delayed because plain radiographic changes are not apparent until 6 weeks or more from the clinical onset of Legg-Calvé-Perthes disease. Scintigraphy and MRI can establish the diagnosis much earlier.

MRI seems to be superior to scintigraphy for depicting the extent of involvement in the early or evolutionary stage of Legg-Calvé-Perthes disease. Perfusion MRI has been used at our institution to determine the extent of involvement, the classification, and treatment planning. A limitation of both the Catterall and lateral pillar classifications is that a definitive prediction cannot be made until well into mid-fragmentation stage, thus delaying treatment during this wait and see period (4 to 6 months). Gadolinium-enhanced subtraction MRI (perfusion MRI) has been used at the initial fragmentation (earlier) stage to determine the extent of lateral pillar involvement, thereby allowing initiation of constraint treatment (Fig. 4.3). Although no serious complications have been reported with perfusion MRI for Perthes, approximately 50% of children have to be sedated or given general anesthesia. The Perthes Study Group reported promising results using MRI perfusion for early classification of lateral pillar signs. However, the routine use of perfusion MRI has been challenged by some authors (Schoenecker et al.) who believe that

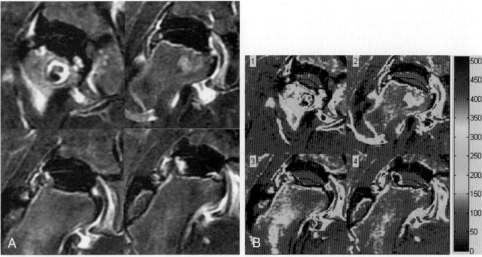

FIGURE 4.3 **A,** Perfusion MRI at initial disease showing lack of perfusion *(black area)* in most of the epiphysis except in *gray area* in lateral aspect *(right lower panel).* **B,** Corresponding HipVasc images showing level of perfusion in epiphysis. *Blue* as shown on color scale indicates absence of perfusion. (From Kim HK, Wiesman KD, Kulkarni V, et al. Perfusion MRI in early stage of Legg-Calvé-Perthes disease to predict lateral pillar involvement: A preliminary study, *J Bone Joint Surg* 96A:1152–1160, 2014.)

knowing early the extent of head and pillar involvement may not be that essential in treatment or ultimate results. A subsequent study of serial perfusion MRIs showed that during the active stage reperfusion of the femoral head progresses at a highly variable rate and in a horseshoe-type pattern, starting posterior and progressing to medial and lateral before converging anteriorly and centrally.

TREATMENT

Treatment depends on where the child is in the course of the disease. Most treatment is during the active process (early fragmentation). The problem again is to determine early the severity or ultimate involvement of the femoral head (Caterall II, IV, lateral pillar B/C, C, Salter-Thompson B). Treatment in the residual phase is reconstructive to prevent a malformed hip from progressing to osteoarthritis at an early age.

Many procedures have been described for both the active and residual phases of the disease. We have used a variety of treatments over the decades, including noncontainment treatments and containment-based treatments such as abduction orthoses, varus osteotomy, and Salter, Pemberton, or pelvic osteotomies when indicated, all with a vigorous hip range of motion program. Current consensus is that containment of the femoral head within the acetabulum throughout the disease process is the goal to allow remodeling of the femoral head.

In the early stage (active phase), our current treatment protocol for children age 4 years and older begins with explaining to the parents the natural history and expected duration of the disease (24 to 36 months). Children 2 to 3 years old can be observed and do not need aggressive treatment. Once synovitis resolves, a daily home physical therapy program, including active and active-assisted range-of-motion and muscle stretching exercises to the hip and knee, is recommended to try to maintain a normal hip range of motion.

Loss of motion at any time indicates a significant change in prognosis. If loss of motion is significant, and subluxation

laterally is occurring, bed rest, skin traction, progressive passive and active physical therapy, abduction exercises, pool therapy, or bracing if possible, are indicated. If there is no improvement, we recommend closed reduction with the patient under general anesthesia and percutaneous adductor longus tenotomy, followed by an ambulatory abduction cast (Petrie) for 6 weeks or more.

If possible, we avoid surgery for Legg-Calvé-Perthes in the active phase of the disease because of the complications possible after major hip surgery, whether it be a varus derotational osteotomy or an innominate osteotomy; however, if containment of the femoral head in the acetabulum is at risk and the femoral head subluxes laterally, surgery may be indicated. Which procedure to use, however, is controversial. Historically, Salter, Thompson, Canale et al., Coleman, and others achieved "containment" by pelvic osteotomy above the hip joint, whereas Axer, Craig, Somerville, and Lloyd-Roberts et al. advocated varus derotational osteotomy. More recently, many studies have emphasized the importance of the timing and the indications for surgery, rather than the type of procedure, recommending that operative intervention be done in the early fragmentation stage before re-formation of a malformed femoral head can occur. Both varus derotational and innominate osteotomies have shown good outcomes at long-term follow-up, with patients who are older with more severe disease having worse outcomes.

Operative treatment may not produce better results than nonoperative treatment in younger patients, but, in general, better results have been reported in older children treated operatively than in children treated nonoperatively when femoral head involvement was severe (lateral pillar B, B/C).

Varus derotational osteotomy and innominate osteotomy have advantages and disadvantages. Varus derotational osteotomy theoretically allows more coverage; however, if too much correction (varus) occurs, and if the capital femoral physis closes prematurely as a result of the disease, excessive varus deformity may persist. Theoretically, a mild increase in length can occur with innominate osteotomy, whereas mild shortening may occur with a varus osteotomy. Compression of an already compromised femoral head also can occur with innominate osteotomy. A second operation to remove the implant is required after many procedures, and both have complications similar to any large operation on the hip. Neither procedure has been shown to accelerate the healing process of the disease. Although numerous authors recommend one procedure over the other, until there is conclusive evidence of superiority, it seems that the choice should be dictated by the surgeon's familiarity and expertise with a particular procedure.

Shelf arthroplasty (lateral labral support) has been advocated for severe Legg-Calvé-Perthes disease (Catterall III or IV; lateral pillar B, BC, C) in the early stages (fragmentation), with incorporation of the shelf graft into the pelvis as a result of continued growth of the lateral acetabular structures. Although acetabular coverage and size may be increased in children younger than 8 years old, these changes are seen at short-term follow-up, and the amount of coverage at long-term follow-up is similar to that obtained by innominate osteotomy.

Distraction of the hip joint (arthrodiastasis) by an external fixator for an average of 4 months has been described in older children with active and severe Legg-Calvé-Perthes disease. Complications, such as pin breakage and pin track infections, have been reported with this procedure, and presently its use seems to be limited to the most severe cases.

MRI before surgery is indicated to determine (1) if any flattening of the femoral head is already present that would contraindicate most osteotomies of any type and (2) how much subluxation is present and how much surgical containment is necessary.

A combined osteotomy (pelvic osteotomy and varus femoral osteotomy) used as a salvage procedure for severe Legg-Calvé-Perthes disease has the theoretical advantage of obtaining maximal femoral head containment while avoiding the complications of either procedure alone, such as limb shortening, extreme neck-shaft varus angulation, and associated abductor weakness. Stevens et al. described guided growth of the trochanteric apophysis using a "tether" with an eight-plate and soft-tissue release as part of a nonosteotomy management strategy for select children with progressive symptoms and related radiographic changes (Fig. 4.4).

In the residual-stage, indications for reconstructive surgery in Legg-Calvé-Perthes disease are (1) a malformed head causing femoroacetabular impingement or "hinge" abduction in which surgical hip dislocation or hip arthroscopy can be used for osteochondroplasty (cheilectomy) or a varus, valgus, or femoral head osteotomy can be performed; (2) coxa magna for which a shelf augmentation would provide coverage; (3) a large malformed femoral head with subluxation laterally, for which a pelvic osteotomy may be considered; and (4) capital femoral physeal arrest for which trochanteric advancement or arrest can be performed for relative lengthening of the femoral neck. External fixation across the pelvis and hip has been used to reduce the femoral head to avoid hinge abduction and persistent subluxation. All of these are procedures for an already malformed hip, and when used a high percentage of unsatisfactory results should be expected.

■ INNOMINATE OSTEOTOMY

The advantages of innominate osteotomy (Figs. 4.5 and 4.6) include anterolateral coverage of the femoral head,

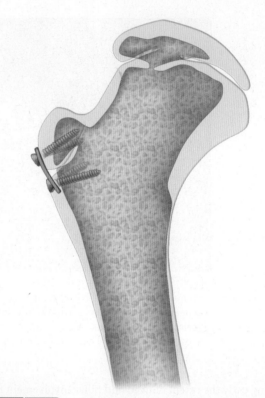

FIGURE 4.4 Tethering of greater trochanter and lack of change to neck-shaft angle after guided growth technique of trochanteric apophysis with soft-tissue release. (Redrawn from Stevens PM, Anderson LA, Gililland JM, et al: Guided growth of trochanteric apophysis combined with soft-tissue release for Legg-Calvé-Perthes disease, *Strategies Trauma Limb Reconstr* 9:37–43, 2014.)

lengthening of the extremity (possibly shortened by the avascular process), and avoidance of a second operation for plate removal. The disadvantages of innominate osteotomy include the inability sometimes to obtain adequate containment of the femoral head, especially in older children; an increase in acetabular and hip joint pressure that may cause further avascular changes in the femoral head; and an increase in leg length on the operated side compared with the normal side that may cause a relative adduction of the hip and uncover the femoral head. Innominate osteotomy as described by Salter is included in the discussion of congenital deformities (see chapter 2). Salter's procedure includes iliopsoas release. Other pelvic osteotomies such as the Pemberton osteotomy (Chapter 2), the Dega osteotomy (Chapter 2), the Bernese osteotomy, or the Ganz periacetabular osteotomy if needed in the residual phase can be used.

INNOMINATE OSTEOTOMY FOR LEGG-CALVÉ-PERTHES DISEASE

TECHNIQUE 4.1

(CANALE ET AL.)

■ Through a Smith-Petersen approach to the hip , release the sartorius, tensor fasciae latae, and rectus femoris

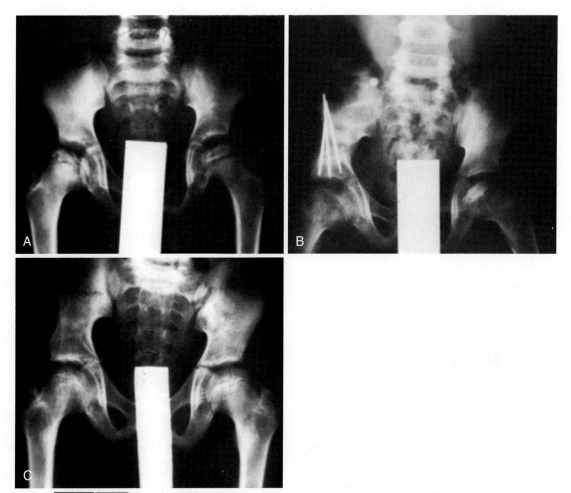

FIGURE 4.5   Innominate osteotomy for Legg-Calvé-Perthes disease. **A,** Seven-year-old child with bilateral Catterall group III involvement with "head-at-risk" signs of lateral calcification (subluxation) and metaphyseal cyst on *right*. **B,** Eight weeks after innominate osteotomy with fixation using three pins. **C,** Three years after innominate osteotomy. Femoral head is contained without evidence of subluxation. Center-edge angle is 28 degrees, and femoral head is concentric but slightly enlarged.

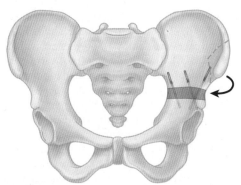

FIGURE 4.6   Innominate osteotomy using quadrangular graft (see text) for Legg-Calvé-Perthes disease. (From Canale ST, D'Anca AF, Cotler JM, et al: Innominate osteotomy in Legg-Calvé-Perthes disease, *J Bone Joint Surg* 54A:25–40, 1972.) **SEE TECHNIQUE 4.1**.

and expose the anterior inferior iliac spine.
- Release the psoas tendon from its insertion, and dissect subperiosteally on the inner and outer walls of the ilium down to the sciatic notch. Using retractors in the sciatic notch, with a right-angle clamp pass a Gigli saw through the notch. With the saw, carefully cut horizontally and anteriorly through the ilium as close as possible to the capsular attachment of the acetabulum.
- Maximally flex the knee and flex and abduct the hip to open the osteotomy. Use a towel clip to pull the distal fragment of the osteotomy anteriorly and laterally.
- Take a full-thickness quadrilateral graft 2 × 3 cm from the wing of the ilium according to the size of the space produced by opening the osteotomy (see Fig. 4.6). Predrill or precut the outline of the graft on the surfaces of the ilium to prevent fracture of the inner and outer cortices. Shape the quadrilateral graft carefully to fit the space produced, and impact it into the osteotomy site.

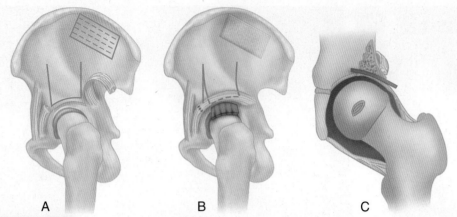

FIGURE 4.7 **A** to **C,** Operative technique for lateral shelf acetabuloplasty (see text) in Legg-Calvé-Perthes disease. **SEE TECHNIQUE 4.2.**

- Use one or more threaded pins for fixation, and leave the ends subcutaneous so that they can be removed later with local or general anesthesia.
- Use the center-edge angle of Wiberg in the weight-bearing position at this time to assess by radiography the coverage and containment of the femoral head.

POSTOPERATIVE CARE The patient is immobilized for 10 to 12 weeks in a spica cast before the pins are removed. Range-of-motion exercises and full weight-bearing ambulation are started, and radiographic evaluation is repeated.

■ LATERAL SHELF PROCEDURE

Except in the active stage of the disease, lateral shelf acetabuloplasty can be used for older children who are not candidates for femoral osteotomy because of insufficient remodeling capacity and the likelihood that shortening of the femur would cause a persistent limp. Recently, it has been suggested to be indicated in the active early stages. Proponents of doing the labral support procedure early argue that it has three beneficial effects: (1) lateral acetabular growth stimulation, (2) prevention of subluxation, and (3) shelf resolution after femoral epiphyseal reossification. Advocates of the shelf procedure in active disease report results as good as those after varus osteotomy or innominate osteotomy of Salter. It is simple to perform (mini-incision with or without a dry arthroscope) and does not induce a permanent deformity in the proximal femur or acetabulum.

LATERAL SHELF PROCEDURE FOR LEGG-CALVÉ-PERTHES DISEASE

TECHNIQUE 4.2

(WILLETT ET AL.)

- Make a curved incision below the iliac crest, passing 1.5 cm below the anterior superior iliac spine to avoid the lateral cutaneous nerve of the thigh. Strip the glutei subperiosteally from the outer table of the ilium to the level

of insertion of the joint capsule. Mobilize and divide the reflected head of the rectus femoris.
- Create a trough in the bone immediately above the insertion of the capsule (Fig. 4.7A). Raise a bony flap 3 cm wide × 3.5 cm long superiorly from the outer cortex of the ilium.
- Cut strips of cancellous graft from the ilium above the flap, and insert them into the trough so that they form a canopy on the superior surface of the hip joint (Fig. 4.7B). Pack the web-shaped space between the flap and the graft canopy with cancellous bone graft (Fig. 4.7C).
- Repair the reflected head of the rectus femoris over the created shelf.
- Close the wound in the usual manner, and apply a spica cast.

POSTOPERATIVE CARE The spica cast is worn for 8 weeks. Protective weight bearing in a single spica cast is continued for 6 additional weeks.

■ VARUS DEROTATIONAL OSTEOTOMY

The advantages of varus derotational osteotomy of the proximal femur include the ability to obtain maximal coverage of the femoral head, especially in an older child, and the ability to correct excessive femoral anteversion with the same osteotomy (Fig. 4.8). The disadvantages of varus derotational osteotomy include excessive varus angulation that may not correct with growth (especially in an older child), further shortening of an already shortened extremity, the possibility of a gluteus lurch produced by decreasing the length of the lever arm of the gluteal musculature, the possibility of nonunion of the osteotomy, and the requirement of a second operation to remove the internal fixation. Premature closure of the capital femoral physis may cause further varus deformity. Aksoy et al. reported poor results in children with pillar group C hips, especially after the age of 9 years. A varus derotational osteotomy is the procedure of choice when containment of the femoral head is necessary but cannot be achieved with a brace for psychosocial or other reasons, when the child is 8 to 10 years old and without leg-length inequality, when on arthrogram or MRI most of the femoral head is uncovered and the angle of Wiberg is decreased, and when there

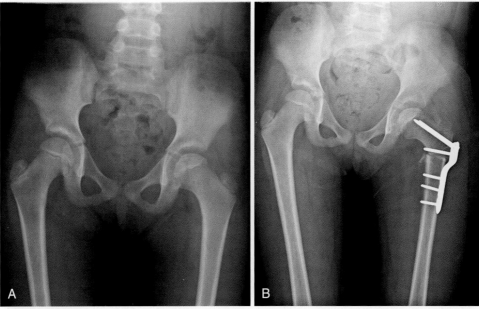

FIGURE **4.8**   Legg-Calvé-Perthes disease. **A,** Preoperative radiograph. **B,** After varus osteotomy and fixation.

is a significant amount of femoral anteversion. An anteroposterior radiograph of the pelvis is taken with the lower extremities in internal rotation and parallel to each other (no abduction). If satisfactory containment of the femoral head is noted, derotational osteotomy alone is carried out. The degree of derotation is roughly estimated from the amount of internal rotation of the extremity, but further adjustments are made during the operation.

When internal rotation is seriously limited and remains so preoperatively after 4 weeks of bed rest with traction, varus osteotomy is carried out with the addition of extension that is produced by a slight backward tilt of the proximal fragment. When internal rotation is sufficient, abduction of the extremity brings about the desired containment of the femoral head. The degree of abduction is expressed by the angle formed by the shaft of the femur and a vertical line parallel to the midline of the pelvis. This angle represents the desired angle of the osteotomy (see Technique 4.2). Herring et al. stated that contrary to conventional belief greater varus angulation does not necessarily produce better preservation of the femoral head after osteotomy. Their recommendation was to achieve 0 to 15 degrees of varus correction for hips that are in the early stages of Perthes.

Reliable information on acetabular containment of the femoral head, the size of the head, the flattening of the epiphysis, and the width of the medial joint space can be obtained from preoperative arthrography or MRI. The osteocartilaginous head of the femur should be covered adequately by the acetabular roof as the femur is abducted and the flattened segment of the femoral head is rotated into the depths of the acetabular fossa. We use a varus (medial closing wedge) osteotomy fixed with an adolescent or pediatric hip screw (Fig. 4.9). According to the recent literature, fracture after plate removal for osteotomies is 5% in patients with Perthes. These data suggest that the time to implant removal should be extended beyond radiographic union to at least 6 months or more after the osteotomy.

VARUS DEROTATIONAL OSTEOTOMY OF THE PROXIMAL FEMUR FOR LEGG-CALVÉ-PERTHES DISEASE

TECHNIQUE 4.3

(STRICKER)
- Place the patient supine on the operating table with image intensification, positioned in the anteroposterior projection; however, make sure with "scout" imaging, that the C-arm can obtain a lateral image of the hip. Prepare and drape the affected extremity, leaving it free to allow for intraoperative radiographs or imaging.
- Make a lateral incision from the greater trochanter distally 8 to 12 cm, and reflect the vastus lateralis to expose the lateral aspect of the femur.
- Identify the femoral insertion of the gluteus maximus, and make a transverse line in the femoral cortex with an osteotome to mark the level of the osteotomy at the level of the lesser trochanter or slightly distal (Fig. 4.9A). Correct positioning of the osteotomy site can be verified with image intensification.
- After the lateral portion of the trochanter and the proximal lateral femur have been exposed, place a guide pin outside the capsule, anterior to the neck. Using the fluoroscopic image, determine the direction of the neck. Set the adjustable angle guide to 120 degrees, and position it against the lateral cortex. Attach the guide to the shaft with the plate clamp. Insert the guide pin through the cannulated portion of the adjustable angle guide and into the femoral neck (Fig. 4.9B). Predrilling the lateral cortex with the twist drill can aid in placing the guide pin. Ensure that the guide pin is placed in the center of the femoral neck

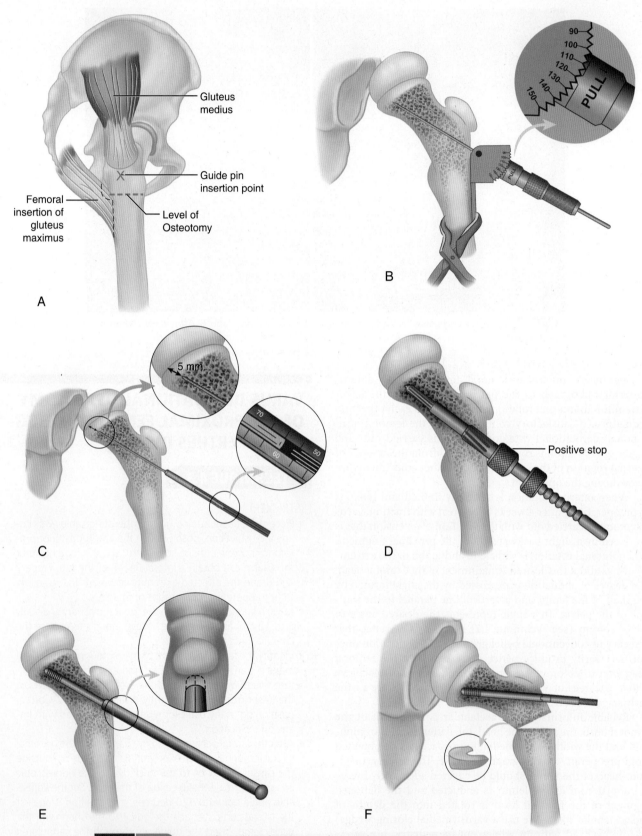

FIGURE **4.9** Varus derotational osteotomy (see text) in Legg-Calvé-Perthes disease. **A,** Level of osteotomy. **B** and **C,** Insertion of guide pin. **D,** Reaming of femur. **E,** First depth marking flush with lateral cortex. **F,** Removal of wedge to customize fit.

Continued

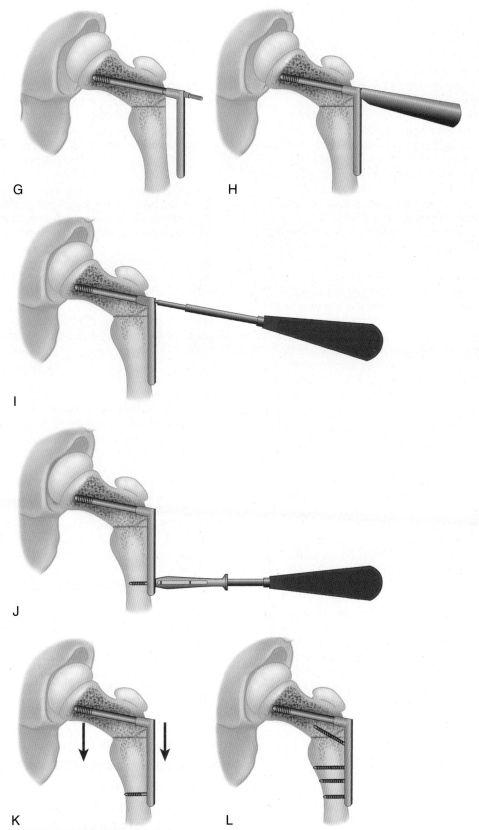

FIGURE 4.9, Cont'd **G-I,** Plate and compression screw application. **J-L,** Insertion of bone screws. (Redrawn from Stricker S: *Intermediate and pediatric osteotomy systems: technique manual*, Memphis, Smith & Nephew Orthopaedics, 2005.) **SEE TECHNIQUE 4.2**.

within 5 mm of the proximal femoral physis without violating it or the trochanteric apophysis (Fig. 4.9C, *inset 1*). Verify guide pin placement in the anteroposterior and lateral views on the image.

- When the guide pin is placed within 5 mm of the physis, use the percutaneous direct measuring gauge to determine the lag screw length (Fig. 4.9C, *inset 2*).
- Set the adjustable positive stop on the combination reamer to the lag screw length determined by the percutaneous direct measuring gauge. Place the reamer over the guide pin and ream until the positive stop reaches the lateral cortex (Fig. 4.9D). Do not violate the physis. It is prudent to check the fluoroscopic image periodically during reaming to ensure that the guide pin is not inadvertently advancing into the femoral epiphysis.
- Set the adjustable positive stop on the lag screw tap to the same length that was reamed. Tap until the positive stop reaches the lateral cortex.
- Insert the selected lag screw into the distal end of the insertion/removal wrench. Place it over the guide pin and into the reamed or tapped hole. The lag screw is at the proper depth when (1) the insertion or removal wrench's first depth marking is flush with the lateral cortex (Fig. 4.9E), and (2) the handle of the insertion or removal wrench is perpendicular to the shaft of the femur, with the longitudinal key line facing proximally. This positioning ensures that the plate barrel and lag screw shaft are properly keyed for rotational stability (Fig. 4.9F). Remove the guide pin when the lag screw is at the appropriate length.
- With the lag screw in place, perform the osteotomy (20-degree transverse osteotomy is illustrated). Make the cut as proximal as possible, just below the lag screw entry point, because the proximal metaphyseal bone usually heals better than the cortical subtrochanteric bone. In addition, the correction of the proximal femoral deformity is best accomplished close to the deformity (i.e., as close to the femoral head as possible).
- Insert the barrel guide into the back of the implanted lag screw to help position the proximal femur. The desired correction can be accomplished by tilting the head into valgus or, in this case, varus, removing wedges to customize the fit if needed (Fig. 4.9G). Iliopsoas tenotomy or recession also may facilitate positioning of the osteotomy.
- Take the plate chosen during preoperative planning (100 degrees × 76 mm × 4 holes in this case), and insert its barrel over the barrel guide and onto the back of the lag screw (Fig. 4.9H). If necessary, insert the cannulated plate tamper over the barrel guide and tap it several times to seat the plate fully (Fig. 4.9I).
- Remove the barrel guide, and insert a compressing screw to prevent the plate from disengaging during the reduction maneuver. Use the slotted screwdriver for the pediatric compressing screw or the hex screwdriver for the intermediate compressing screw (Fig. 4.9J).
- Reduce the osteotomy, and secure the plate to the femur using the plate clamp. Check the rotational position of the lower extremity in extension.
- A range of 2.5 to 6.5 mm of femoral shaft compression is possible with the use of an intermediate osteotomy hip screw. To achieve 6.5 mm of compression, insert the drill guide end of the intermediate combination drill or tap guide into the distal portion of the most distal compres-

sion slot. Drill through to the medial cortex using the twist drill. If less compression is required, follow the same steps detailed previously in the distal portion of either the second or third distal slots for 2.5 mm of compression. If no compression is needed, follow the same steps listed previously except begin by placing the intermediate combination drill/tap guide in the proximal portion of the slot instead of the distal portion used for compression.

- Insert the tap guide end of the intermediate combination drill or tap guide into the slot, and insert the bone screw tap.
- Insert the depth gauge through the slot and into the drilled or tapped hole. Ensure that the nose of the guide is inserted fully into the plate's slot. Insert the needle of the depth gauge, and hook it on the medial cortex. Read the bone screw length measurement directly off of the depth gauge.
- Select the appropriate length bone screw, and insert it using the hex screwdriver. Use the self-holding sleeve to keep the screw from disengaging from the screwdriver. In cases in which compression is being applied, the bone screw abuts the inclined distal aspect of the slot as it is being seated, forcing the plate and the attached proximal fragment slightly distally until resisted by compression of the osteotomy (Fig. 4.9K). Follow the same steps for the remaining two slots.
- In the most proximal slot, the intermediate combination drill or tap guide can be angled proximally so that the drill, and ultimately the bone screw, crosses the osteotomy line. Positioning the proximal bone screw in this way can provide additional stability at the osteotomy site (Fig. 4.9L).
- Irrigate the wound and close in layers, inserting a suction drain if needed. Apply a one and one-half spica cast.

POSTOPERATIVE CARE The spica cast is worn for 8 to 12 weeks, until union is achieved. The internal fixation can be removed 12 to 24 months after the osteotomy if desired.

◼ LATERAL OPENING WEDGE OSTEOTOMY

Axer described a lateral opening wedge osteotomy for children 5 years of age and younger in which a prebent plate is used to hold the cortices apart laterally the measured amount. The defect laterally fills in rapidly in young children, but the open wedge may result in delayed union or nonunion in children older than 5 years. Because few children younger than 5 years are operated on for Legg-Calvé-Perthes disease in the United States, indications for this procedure are rare.

REVERSED OR CLOSING WEDGE TECHNIQUE FOR LEGG-CALVÉ-PERTHES DISEASE

TECHNIQUE 4.4

- After calculating from Table 4.5 the height of the base of the wedge to be removed, hold the extremity in internal

TABLE 4.5

Calculating Height of Base of Wedge to be Removed for Varus Osteotomy*

DESIRED ANGULATORY CHANGE (DEGREES)	FEMORAL SHAFT WIDTH AT OSTEOTOMY SITE (MM)												
	10	12.5	15	17.5	20	22.5	25	27.5	30	32.5	35	37.5	40
10	1.5	2	2.5	3	3.5	4	4.5	5	5.5	6	6.5	7	7.5
15	2	3	4	4.5	5	6	6.5	7.5	8	9	10	10.5	11.5
20	3	4	5	6	7	8	9	10	11	12	13	14	15
25	4.5	5	6.5	7.5	9	10	11.5	12.5	14	15	16	17.5	18.5
30	5.5	6.5	8	10	11.5	12.5	14	15.5	17	18.5	20	22	23
35	6.5	8	10	12	13.5	14	17	18.3	21	22	24	26	27.5
40	8	10	12.5	14.5	16.5	18.5	20	23	25	27	29	31.5	33.5

*The height of the base of the wedge in millimeters is read at the junction of the horizontal axis (desired degrees of angulatory change) and the vertical axis (width of the femoral shaft at the osteotomy site).
Credited to Orkan and Roth. Data from A. Axer, personal communication, 1978.

rotation at the hip and mark a wedge. Close the wedge if a reverse wedge is being used.

- Take a wedge half the height over the anterior surface of the femur with the base medially.
- Remove the wedge with an oscillating saw, rotate the distal fragment externally to the desired degree, turn the bone wedge 180 degrees, and insert it in the osteotomy with its base lateral or reversed. Because its base now is lateral, the varus angle obtained equals the angle that would be obtained with complete removal of a full-height bone wedge medially.
- Fix the bone fragments with the prebent plate as previously described with all cortices in contact. When the reversed bone wedge is not stable enough, fix it to the distal or proximal fragment with small Kirschner wires.

POSTOPERATIVE CARE A double spica plaster cast is applied and removed after 6 weeks or when union is confirmed by radiography. The child is encouraged to walk, in water initially if increased joint stiffness is noted. No restrictions are imposed on the child except for follow-up every 3 months in the first year.

■ ARTHRODIASTASIS

The rationale behind arthrodiastasis is that distraction of the joint not only widens but also unloads the joint space, reduces the pressure on the femoral head, allows fibrous repair of articular cartilage defects, and preserves congruency of the femoral head. The articulated fixator allows 50 degrees of hip flexion. Recent reports have described significant complications with this procedure; it should not be taken lightly and used only for the most severely involved hips with severe subluxation.

ARTHRODIASTASIS FOR LEGG-CALVÉ-PERTHES DISEASE

TECHNIQUE 4.5

(SEGEV ET AL.)
- Place the patient supine on a transparent operating table. Obtain a hip arthrogram medially to assess cartilage architecture and the extent of hinged abduction.
- Tenotomize the adductor and iliopsoas tendons through a medial approach.
- Using image intensification, insert a 1.6-mm Kirschner wire into the femoral head at the center of rotation of the hip while keeping the leg in 15 degrees of abduction with the patella pointing forward.
- Using the articulated body for the hip Orthofix external fixation device (Bussolengo, Italy; Fig. 4.10), apply it onto the Kirschner wire and attach a standard model "kit body" to the hinge distally.
- Fix the proximal part to the supraacetabular area with a T-clamp using two or three 5- to 6-mm Orthofix screws. The procedure is done using a template that is replaced by the aforementioned parts.
- Immediately distract the joint space 4 to 5 mm under image intensification. Continue distraction at 1 mm per day until the Shenton line is overcorrected.

POSTOPERATIVE CARE Flexion and extension exercises are encouraged with the fixator in place, and the patient is kept non–weight bearing. The fixator is left in place for 4 to 5 months until lateral pillar reossification appears. The fixator is removed in the operating room, and a hip arthrogram is obtained. After removal of the frame, the patient continues protective non–weight bearing and intensive physical therapy and hydrotherapy for an additional 6 weeks. At this stage, full weight bearing is allowed with continued physiotherapy for another 6 months.

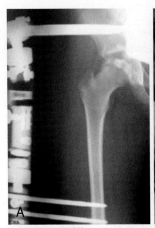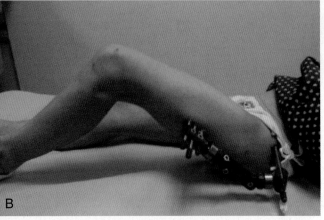

FIGURE 4.10 Radiographic (**A**) and clinical (**B**) appearance of hinged external fixator (Orthofix, Verona, Italy) for hip arthrodiastasis in a patient with Legg-Calvé-Perthes disease. (From Aguado-Maestro I, Abril JC, Banuelos Diaz A, et al: Hip arthrodiastasis in Legg-Calvé-Perthes disease, *Rev Eso Cir Ortop Traumatol* 60:243–250, 2016.)

RECONSTRUCTIVE SURGERY
■ OSTEOCHONDROPLASTY (CHEILECTOMY)

Hip arthroscopy and surgical dislocation of the hip have been used to treat certain types of femoral acetabular impingement (FAI) and other intraarticular lesions caused by Perthes disease. One type of FAI develops in the malformed femoral head; terms such as pincer and cam effect are now replacing terms such as hinge-abduction and "trench." These newer techniques, surgical hip dislocation and arthroscopy, can eliminate intraarticular deformity and other lesions, such as labral tears, osteochondral or chondral lesions, loose bodies, or a torn ligamentum teres, and at the same time they can be combined with previously described extraarticular (extra capsular) procedures that provide coverage of the femoral head, increase acetabular coverage, or change the configuration of the femoral neck by advancing the greater trochanter.

Surgical dislocation of the femoral head has been used to treat FAI, and contrary to previous opinion can be done safely with few or no complications including osteonecrosis, myositis ossificans, or decreased motion secondary to soft-tissue reaction and scarring. Ganz and others popularized this technique and have performed chondroplasties, labral chondral tear or impingement excision, greater trochanteric advancement, and downsizing osteotomy of the mushroomed femoral head. Care must be taken, however, to protect the lateral epiphyseal arteries that are present in a narrow anatomic window on the femoral neck, but as noted by Millis, these are fewer in number in Legg-Calvé-Perthes disease.

Arthroscopy of the hip has become more refined and thus allows osteochondroplasty (cheilectomy) of the hip for FAI (cam and pincer lesions), loose bodies, and chondral and osteochondral defects (OCDs). Although arthroscopy is easier to perform than surgical dislocation and is less traumatic, it is not as extensive. Techniques for hip arthroscopy are found in other chapter. A combined approach of hip arthroscopy and limited open osteochondroplasty by Clohisy and others is described in other chapter.

OSTEOCHONDROPLASTY SURGICAL DISLOCATION OF THE HIP

Ganz, after reviewing the anatomy of the medial circumflex artery, described a technique of surgical dislocation of the hip without compromising the blood supply to the femoral head. Surgical hip dislocation should probably not be carried out when the head is in the early fragmentation phase of the disease. Most of the pathology can be identified at surgery; however, MRI may be helpful as well as hip abduction, adduction, and flexion radiographs to assess for FAI and anterior coverage of the femoral osteotomy. A dynamic, three-dimensional reformation CT scan can be obtained to determine the extent of FAI. The approach for surgical hip dislocation as described by Ganz et al. is in other chapter. Ganz's algorithm for surgical treatment (Fig. 4.11) offers a structured way to identify the problem and the surgical treatment to correct structural abnormalities.

TECHNIQUE 4.6

(GANZ)

- Complete the approach for surgical dislocation of the hip, including an osteotomy of the greater trochanter.
- Reevaluate range of motion for intraarticular sources of FAI, such as femoral neck asphericity or acetabular rim prominence. Trim the head and neck as necessary, starting with the femoral head. Trim the acetabular rim if any FAI persists.
- Check for any impingement of the lesser trochanter (with the ischium or posterior acetabulum).
- Determine the exact location of the chondral damage on the femoral head by dividing the head into eight sections, four anterior, and four posterior (Fig. 4.12). Include articular cartilage lesions, labral lesions, OCD lesions, and incongruent protrusions that were resected.

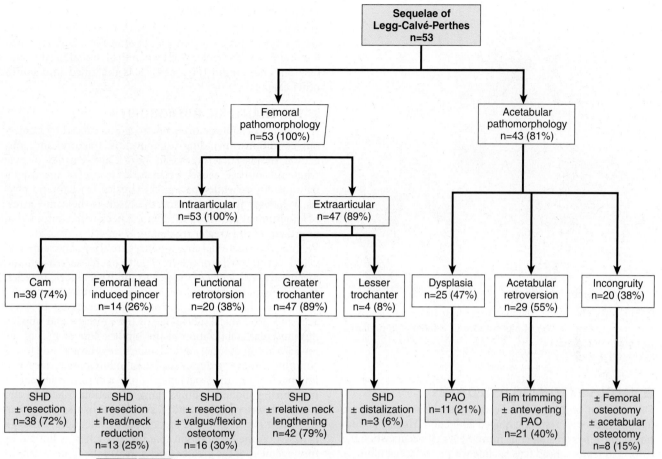

FIGURE 4.11 Morphologic analysis with corresponding surgical treatment algorithm of hips with pathomorphologic sequelae of Legg-Calvé-Perthes disease. *PAO*, Periacetabular osteotomy, *SHD*, surgical hip dislocation. (From: Albers CE, Steppacher SD, Ganz R, et al: Joint-preserving surgery improves pain, range of motion, and abductor strength after Legg-Calvé-Perthes disease. *Clin Orthop Relat Res* 470:2450–2461, 2012.)

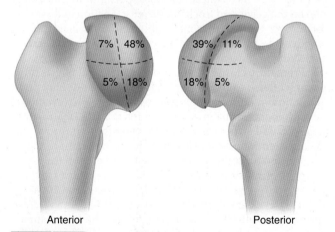

Anterior   Posterior

FIGURE 4.12 Percentages represent frequency of chondral damage found in each of the eight sectors in study by Albers et al. (From Albers CE, Steppacher SD, Ganz R, et al: Joint-preserving surgery improves pain, range of motion, and abductor strength after Legg-Calvé-Perthes disease, *Clin Orthop Relat Res* 470:2450–2461, 2012.) **SEE TECHNIQUE 4.6.**

- Check functional radiographs intraoperatively to determine any joint incongruity and to determine if a proximal femoral osteotomy needs to be performed. Indications for a valgus osteotomy are a nonspherical femoral head with good congruency in an adducted view.
- Check the amount of correction that could be obtained by a pelvic acetabular osteotomy. An indication for a pelvic acetabular osteotomy is an associated secondary acetabular dysplasia (defined as a lateral center-edge angle of less than 25 degrees).
- Perform trochanteric advancement for relative lengthening of the femoral neck (see Technique 4.8).
- Perform a valgus osteotomy (Fig. 4.13) or a pelvic acetabular osteotomy (Technique 4.1) as indicated.
- Reduce the hip and place in a neutral position in a soft splint.

POSTOPERATIVE CARE Remove suction drains at 48 hours. Mobilize the patient with crutches and partial weight bearing (15 kg). Restrict active and passive abduction and adduction to protect the trochanteric osteotomy. Use low-molecular-weight heparin for 8 weeks to avoid deep vein thrombosis.

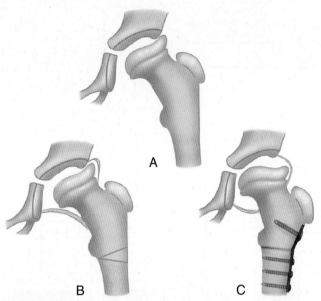

FIGURE 4.13   **A** to **C,** Valgus osteotomy to reduce hinge abduction and increase flexion of hip; osteotomy is fixed with pediatric screw and side plate.

■ VALGUS EXTENSION OSTEOTOMY

One residual of Legg-Calvé-Perthes disease is a malformed femoral head with resulting hinged abduction. Hinged abduction of the hip is an abnormal movement that occurs when the deformed femoral head fails to slide within the acetabulum. A trench is formed laterally, adjacent to a large uncovered portion of the deformed head anterolaterally. Raney et al. described valgus subtrochanteric osteotomy for malformed femoral heads with hinge abduction. All were classified Catterall III and IV with previous failed treatment. At 5-year follow-up, 62% had satisfactory results. We use a valgus extension osteotomy, as described by Catterall, fixed with a pediatric screw and side plate (Fig. 4.13) to relieve this obstruction.

■ VALGUS FLEXION INTERNAL ROTATION OSTEOTOMY

Kim and Wenger, using three-dimensional CT in Legg-Calvé-Perthes disease, noted "functional retroversion" rather than femoral anteversion. As a result, they recommended a valgus flexion, internal rotation femoral osteotomy plus a simultaneous acetabuloplasty in patients with severe femoral head deformity. The combined procedure (1) corrects the functional coxa vara and hinge abduction (valgus osteotomy); (2) establishes a more normal articulation between the posteromedial portion of the true femoral head and the acetabulum, while moving the anterolateral protruding portion of the femoral head away from the anterolateral acetabular margin (valgus-flexion osteotomy); (3) corrects external rotation deformity of the distal limb (internal rotation osteotomy); and (4) improves joint congruity and anterolateral femoral head coverage in hips with associated acetabular dysplasia.

■ SHELF PROCEDURE

If the hip is congruous, a Staheli or Catterall shelf augmentation procedure is performed for coxa magna and lack of acetabular coverage for the femoral head.

■ CHIARI OSTEOTOMY

We have used the pelvic osteotomy described by Chiari as a salvage procedure to accomplish coverage of a large flattened femoral head in an older child when the femoral head is subluxating and painful (Fig. 4.14). It is described in detail in other chapter.

■ TROCHANTERIC OVERGROWTH

Although trochanteric overgrowth can be caused by numerous conditions, including osteomyelitis, fracture, and congenital dysplasia, it occurs in Legg-Calvé-Perthes disease when the disease causes premature closure of the capital femoral physis while sparing the greater trochanteric physis. Whatever the mechanism, the result is the same: arrest of longitudinal growth of the femoral neck with continuation of growth of the greater trochanter (Fig. 4.15). According to Wagner, the functional consequences are always the same: elevation (overgrowth) of the trochanter decreases tension and mechanical efficiency of the pelvic and trochanteric muscles; shortening of the femoral neck moves the greater trochanter closer to the center of rotation of the hip, decreasing the lever arm and mechanical advantage of the muscles, and impairing muscular stabilization of the hip; the line of pull of the muscles becomes more vertical, increasing the pressure forces concentrated over a diminished area of hip joint surface; and impingement of the trochanter on the rim of the acetabular roof during abduction limits range of motion. Macnicol and Makris described a "gear stick" sign of trochanteric impingement that is useful in the preoperative evaluation. This sign is based on the observation that hip abduction is limited by impingement of the greater trochanter on the ilium when the hip is extended but full abduction is possible when the hip is fully flexed. The "gear stick" sign is especially useful for differentiating between trochanteric impingement and other causes of limited abduction. Transfer of the greater trochanter distally restores normal tension to the trochanteric muscles and improves mechanical efficiency, puts a more horizontal pull on the pelvic and trochanteric muscle action to distribute forces over the hip joint more uniformly, and increases the length of the femoral neck to increase abduction and decrease acetabular impingement.

Premature closure of the proximal femoral physis often occurs after Legg-Calvé-Perthes disease and may limit abduction and produce gluteal insufficiency. Trochanteric advancement has been advocated for the late treatment of Legg-Calvé-Perthes disease and is thought to improve gluteal efficiency and increase the range of abduction, which was limited by impingement of the trochanter on the ilium. With surgical dislocation of the hip, the greater trochanter is routinely osteotomized. If trochanteric advancement is necessary, Ganz et al. have described an extended retinacular soft-tissue flap that protects the blood supply to the femoral head and allows for a relative lengthening of the femoral neck. The greater trochanter is advanced distally such that its tip is in line with the center of the femoral head. Fixation is secured with two or three 3.5- or 4.5-mm screws (see Technique 4.7). Alternative methods of treatment include abduction valgus osteotomy of the femur and trochanteric epiphysiodesis. Trochanteric epiphysiodesis does not appear to change the radiographic appearance but according to some authors reduces the Trendelenburg gait.

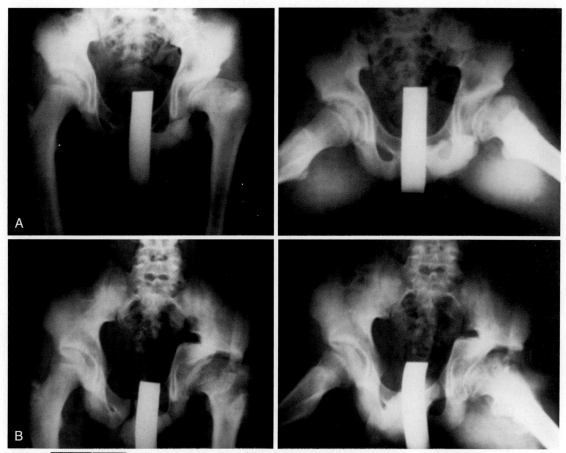

FIGURE 4.14 Chiari osteotomy for residual Legg-Calvé-Perthes disease. **A,** Residual Legg-Calvé-Perthes disease (coxa plana) and subluxation in hip on right. **B,** Eight months after Chiari osteotomy with good coverage of femoral head.

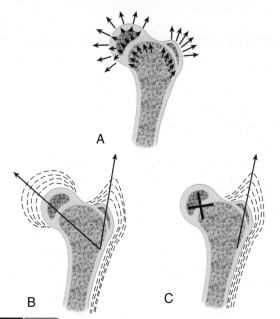

FIGURE 4.15 **A** and **B,** Growth of proximal femur; *arrows* indicate site and direction of growth. **C,** If growth potential is impaired, longitudinal growth is arrested but greater trochanter continues to grow.

TROCHANTERIC ADVANCEMENT FOR TROCHANTERIC OVERGROWTH

TECHNIQUE 4.7

(WAGNER)

- With the patient supine, approach the hip through a lateral incision. Incise the fascia lata longitudinally and release the vastus lateralis from the greater trochanter.
- Retract the gluteus medius muscle posteriorly, and insert a Kirschner wire superiorly, parallel to the femoral neck and greater trochanteric physis and pointing toward the trochanteric fossa (Fig. 4.16A). Confirm the placement of the guidewire by image intensification. Internally rotating the hip slightly aids placement of the wire and allows better imaging.
- Make the osteotomy parallel to the Kirschner wire with a low-speed oscillating saw, completing it proximally with a flat osteotome (Fig. 4.16B). Pry open the osteotomy until the medial cortex fractures (Fig. 4.16C and D).
- Mobilize the greater trochanter first cephalad, and with dissecting scissors remove any adhesions, joint capsule,

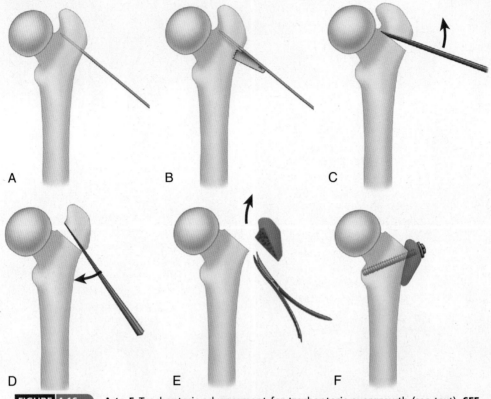

FIGURE 4.16 **A to F,** Trochanteric advancement for trochanteric overgrowth (see text). **SEE TECHNIQUE 4.7.**

and soft-tissue flush with the medial surface of the trochanter, sparing the blood vessels in the trochanteric fossa (Fig. 4.16E).

- When the greater trochanter is freed, transfer it distally and laterally. If excessive anteversion is present, it also can be transferred anteriorly.
- Using an osteotome, freshen the lateral femoral cortex to which the trochanter is to be attached. Place the trochanter against the lateral femoral cortex and check the position with image intensification. According to Wagner, the tip of the greater trochanter should be level with the center of the femoral head, and the distance between them should be 2 to 2.5 times the radius of the femoral head.
- When proper position is confirmed, fix the greater trochanter with two screws inserted in a cephalolateral to caudad direction (Fig. 4.16F). These screws, with washers, should compress an area of bony contact between the trochanter and femur. Bury the screw heads by retracting all soft tissues to prevent soft-tissue necrosis and local mechanical irritation from occurring postoperatively. Wagner uses a supplemental strong tension band suture that he believes helps absorb tensile forces from the pelvic and trochanteric muscles and prevents trochanteric avulsion; we have not found this suture to be necessary.
- No postoperative immobilization is required if the patient is compliant and the fixation is secure.

POSTOPERATIVE CARE Ambulation on crutches is begun at 7 days, but active exercises of the pelvic and trochanteric muscles are not permitted until 3 weeks. Sitting upright and flexing the hip also should be avoided because overpull of the gluteus medius muscle may cause loss of fixation.

TROCHANTERIC ADVANCEMENT FOR TROCHANTERIC OVERGROWTH

TECHNIQUE 4.8

(MACNICOL AND MAKRIS)

- Approach the greater trochanter through a straight lateral incision under lateral image intensification.
- With a power saw, divide the base of the trochanter in line with the upper border of the femoral neck. Mobilize the trochanteric fragment and the gluteal muscles from their distal soft-tissue attachment.
- Remove a thin wedge of bone from the posterolateral femoral cortex (Fig. 4.17) to provide a cancellous bone bed for the transferred trochanter and to ensure that the trochanter does not project too far laterally. Any undue prominence would cause friction of the fascia lata and produce discomfort and bursitis.
- Fix the trochanter with two compression screws to prevent rotation of the fragment and to allow early partial weight bearing.

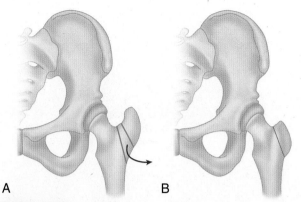

FIGURE 4.17 **A** and **B,** After initial osteotomy of greater trochanter, trapezoidal wedge of bone is removed. (Redrawn from Macnicol MF, Makris D: Distal transfer of the greater trochanter, *J Bone Joint Surg* 73B:838–841, 1991.) **SEE TECHNIQUE 4.8**.

POSTOPERATIVE CARE A spica cast is not used, but patients walk with crutches by the end of the first postoperative week. Exercises to promote movement are introduced gradually, but upright sitting, abduction, flexion, and internal rotation are not forced.

GREATER TROCHANTERIC EPIPHYSIODESIS FOR TROCHANTERIC OVERGROWTH

TECHNIQUE 4.9

- Approach the physis of the greater trochanter through a lateral incision, and determine its location and orientation by inserting a Keith needle. If necessary, use radiographs to confirm its position.
- Use a small drill bit to outline the four corners of a rectangle that spans the lateral portion of the greater trochanteric epiphysis. Remove this lateral rectangle of cortical bone with osteotomies.
- Curet the physis, reverse the rectangle of bone, and replace it in its bed.
- Internal fixation is unnecessary.

POSTOPERATIVE CARE Postoperative cast immobilization is not required unless curettage has been so vigorous that the physis of the greater trochanter has been excessively disrupted. Weight bearing is progressed as tolerated.

OSTEOCHONDROSIS OR EPIPHYSITIS

The terms *osteochondrosis* and *epiphysitis* designate disorders of actively growing epiphyses. The disorder may be localized to a single epiphysis or occasionally may involve two or more epiphyses simultaneously or successively. The cause generally is unknown, but evidence indicates a lack of vascularity that

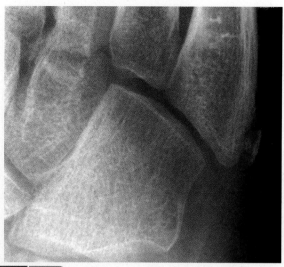

FIGURE 4.18 Ossification of epiphysis on fifth metatarsal shaft.

may be the result of trauma, infection, overuse, vitamin D deficiency, or congenital malformation.

In some epiphyses, osteochondrosis is distinctive enough to be recognized easily as a distinct clinical entity. Osteochondrosis of some intraarticular epiphyses may closely resemble other diseases, however, and requires careful diagnostic study. Only disorders of the epiphyses that frequently present to the orthopaedist, or sometimes require surgical treatment, are discussed in this chapter.

TRACTION EPIPHYSITIS OF THE FIFTH METATARSAL BASE (ISELIN DISEASE)

In the German literature in 1912, Iselin described a traction epiphysitis of the base of the fifth metatarsal occurring in young adolescents at the time of appearance of the proximal epiphysis of the fifth metatarsal. This secondary center of ossification is a small, shell-shaped fleck of bone oriented slightly obliquely with respect to the metatarsal shaft and located on the lateral plantar aspect of the tuberosity (Fig. 4.18). Anatomic studies have shown that this bone is located within the cartilaginous flare onto which the peroneus brevis inserts. It usually is not visible on anteroposterior or lateral radiographs but can be seen on the oblique view. It appears in girls at about age 10 years and in boys at about age 12 years; fusion occurs about 2 years later.

Iselin disease causes tenderness over a prominent proximal fifth metatarsal. Weight bearing produces pain over the lateral aspect of the foot. Participation in sports requiring running, jumping, and cutting, causing inversion stresses on the forefoot, is a common factor. The affected area over the tuberosity is larger on the involved side, with soft-tissue edema and local erythema. The area is tender to palpation at the insertion of the peroneus brevis, and resisted eversion and extreme plantar flexion and dorsiflexion of the foot elicit pain. Oblique radiographs show enlargement and often fragmentation of the epiphysis (Fig. 4.19) and widening of the cartilaginous-osseous junction. Nonunion of the fifth metatarsal (Fig. 4.20) has been reported in several adults as a result of Iselin disease and failure of fusion of the epiphysis.

The un-united epiphysis should not be mistaken for a fracture, and a fracture should not be mistaken for the

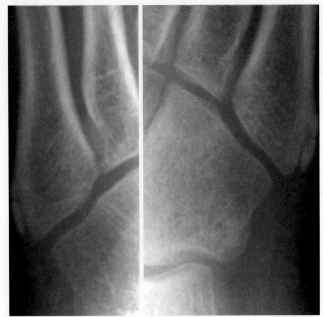

FIGURE 4.19 Enlargement and fragmentation of epiphysis (Iselin disease).

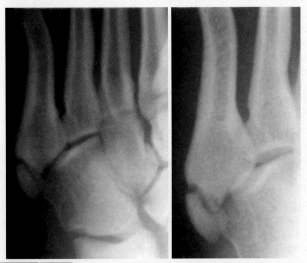

FIGURE 4.20 Nonunion of fifth metatarsal as result of Iselin disease.

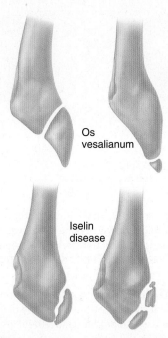

FIGURE 4.21 Os vesalianum must be distinguished from Iselin disease.

epiphysis. This frequently can be determined clinically based on a history of trauma or the absence thereof, as well as tenderness to palpation over the base of the fifth metatarsal. Os vesalianum, a sesamoid in the peroneus brevis (Fig. 4.21), and traction epiphysitis with widening of the epiphysis also must be distinguished from Iselin disease.

Treatment is aimed at prevention of recurrent symptoms. For acute symptoms, initial treatment should decrease the stress reaction and acute inflammation caused by overpull of the peroneus brevis tendon. For mild symptoms, limitation of sports activity, application of ice, and administration of nonsteroidal antiinflammatory medication usually are sufficient. For severe symptoms, cast immobilization may be required. Occasionally, for chronic symptoms, an arch support that wraps around the base of the fifth metatarsal is used. Internal fixation of the epiphysis is not indicated.

OSTEOCHONDROSIS OF THE METATARSAL HEAD (FREIBERG INFRACTION)

Freiberg infraction, also known as Freiberg disease, usually occurs in the head of the second metatarsal but also may occur in the third (Fig. 4.22), fourth, and fifth metatarsals in adolescent patients. Surgery is not recommended during the acute stage, which may persist for 6 months to 2 years. It may be indicated later because of pain, deformity, and disability. Occasionally, a loose body is present (Fig. 4.23), and simply removing it may relieve the symptoms. Other procedures used include scraping the sclerotic area and replacing it with cancellous bone (Smillie procedure), osteochondral plug transplantation (Fig. 4.24), dorsal wedge osteotomy, temporary joint spacer, and total joint arthroplasty (Fig. 4.25). The surgical treatment of this disorder is discussed in other chapter.

OSTEOCHONDROSIS OF THE NAVICULAR (KÖHLER DISEASE)

Osteochondrosis of the tarsal navicular originally was described by Köhler in 1908. Ossification centers of the navicular appear between the ages of 1.5 and 2 years in girls and 2.5 and 3 years in boys. Abnormalities of ossification vary from minor irregularities in the size and shape of the navicular to gross changes indistinguishable from osteochondrosis. These abnormal ossifying nuclei are more common in late-appearing ossification centers of the navicular. The blood supply to the navicular consists of numerous penetrating vessels in children and adults. The development of the ossific nucleus is associated most frequently with a single artery, but the incorporation of other penetrating vessels as part of the vascular supply varies; occasionally a single vessel is the sole supply until the age of 4 to 6 years. Delayed ossification has been suggested to be the earliest event in the changes leading to irregular ossification because the lateness of ossification of the navicular subjects it to more pressure than the bony structures can withstand. Abnormal ossification may be a response of the unprotected,

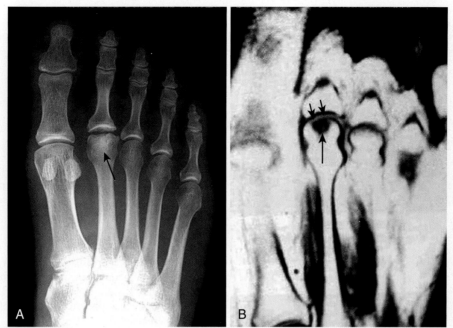

FIGURE 4.22 Freiberg disease. **A,** Elongated second metatarsal enduring stress. **B,** Chronic damage is shown by low-signal intensity on T1 MRI. (From Shane A, Reeves C, Wobst G, et al: Second metatarsophalangeal joint pathology and Freiberg diseases, *Clin Podiatr Med Surg* 30:313–325, 2013.)

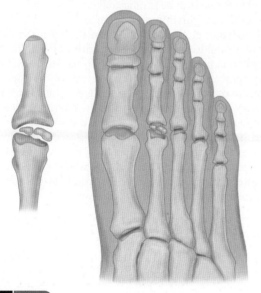

FIGURE 4.23 Freiberg infraction of second metatarsal with two loose bodies.

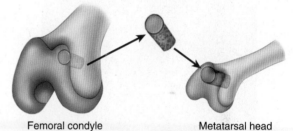

Femoral condyle   Metatarsal head

FIGURE 4.24 Diagram of harvested osteochondral plug from a non–weight bearing site on the upper lateral femoral condyle of the ipsilateral knee, and transplantation of the plug to the bone in the second metatarsal head. (Redrawn from Miyamoto W, Takao M, Uchio Y, et al: Late-stage Freiberg disease treated by osteochondral plug transplantation: a case series, *Foot Ankle Int* 29:950–955, 2008.)

growing nucleus to normal stresses of weight bearing. If osseous vessels are compressed as they pass through the junction between cartilage and bone, ischemia results and leads to reactive hyperemia and pain. The diagnosis of Köhler disease is a clinical one requiring the presence of pain and tenderness in the area of the tarsal navicular associated with radiographic changes of sclerosis and diminished size of the bone, including collapse of the navicular (Fig. 4.26). The appearance of multiple ossification centers without an increase in density should not be confused with Köhler disease, and radiographic findings similar to Köhler disease in an asymptomatic foot should be considered an irregularity of ossification.

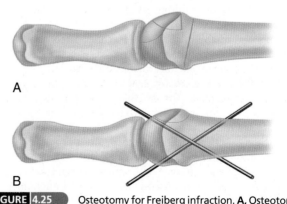

FIGURE 4.25 Osteotomy for Freiberg infraction. **A,** Osteotomy of bony wedge. **B,** Closure and fixation of osteotomy.

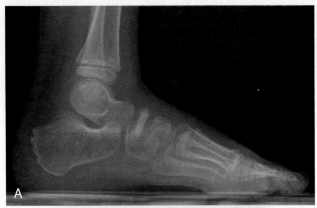

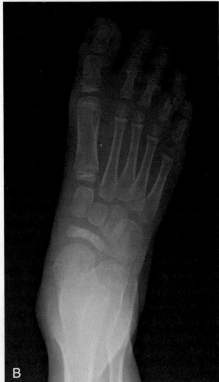

FIGURE 4.26   Lateral **(A)** and oblique **(B)** radiographs show smaller and more sclerotic navicular characteristic of Köhler disease.

Cast boot immobilization with protected weight bearing has been reported to produce quicker resolution of symptoms. This is a self-limiting condition, and operative treatment rarely is indicated.

Pain and disability rarely develop after osteochondrosis if the navicular becomes distorted and sclerotic, the head of the talus becomes flattened, the articular surfaces of the two bones become fibrillated, and osteophytes form along the margin of the articular surfaces. Though this is not common, surgery rarely may be indicated when disabling symptoms persist. In this case arthrodesis is the only operation of value, and the calcaneocuboid joint is included because most of its function is lost when the talonavicular joint is fused. The midtarsal joints (talonavicular and calcaneocuboid) can be arthrodesed by a technique similar to that used for deformities in poliomyelitis (see chapter 6). The results of this operation usually are excellent; most patients become symptom free but may notice loss of lateral movements of the foot, though there are concerns about

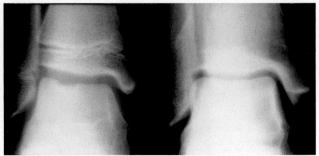

FIGURE 4.27   *Left,* Osteochondritis dissecans in child with open distal tibial physes. *Right,* Three years later, physes closed, patient was asymptomatic, and osteochondritis dissecans lesion was no longer present.

the long-term effects on adjacent joints. When symptoms arise from the naviculocuneiform joints also, these joints should be included in the fusion. Here arthrodesis is difficult to secure; metallic internal fixation and inlay grafts of autogenous cancellous bone are helpful.

OSTEOCHONDRITIS OF THE ANKLE

Osteochondritis of the ankle in adults is discussed in other chapter. The natural history of this lesion in children with open physes seems to be similar to that of osteochondrosis of the knee in that, with immobilization, the lesion heals in most children. Bauer et al., in a long-term (≥20 years) follow-up study of 30 children with osteochondritis of the ankle, found that only one patient developed severe arthritis. Only minor radiographic changes occurred in the rest of the patients, in contrast to osteochondritis of the knee, in which osteoarthritis is frequent. Two of the lesions in their series were located on the joint surfaces of the distal tibia, a site previously unreported. Bauer et al. noted that the lesions in children are indistinguishable from those in adults; however, because the lesions in children heal, there may be some variance in ossification of the talus (Fig. 4.27). Regardless of the cause, the initial treatment should be nonoperative.

APOPHYSITIS OF THE TIBIAL TUBEROSITY (OSGOOD-SCHLATTER DISEASE)

Osgood-Schlatter disease is an apophysitis of the tibial tuberosity that is the result of persistent traction on the apophysis of the tibial tuberosity caused by overuse. It occurs in boys aged 12 to 15 years and girls aged 9 to 13 years and frequently occurs in those who play basketball and volleyball, although it can also affect those who participate in other activities requiring frequent jumping and squatting. It typically occurs at the time that the apophysis has started to ossify but before it has fused to the remaining proximal tibial epiphysis and the remainder of the proximal tibia.

Clinically, patients complain of anterior knee pain and swelling over the tibial tubercle. Radiographs may show widening of the physis between the apophysis and the proximal tibia, irregularity of the tibial tubercle apophysis, or even fragmentation of the apophysis with separate ossicles.

A strong association has been noted between Osgood-Schlatter disease and patella alta, and, in particular, a shortened rectus femoris has been noted. The increase in patellar height may require an increase in the force by the quadriceps to achieve full extension, which could be responsible for the apophyseal lesion. It can be argued, however, that the patella alta is the result of chronic avulsion of the bony tuberosity. Robertsen et al. noted on histologic examination a pseudarthrosis covered with cartilage and no sign of inflammation. A pseudarthrosis may indicate the disease is traumatic in origin. They suggested that persistent symptoms of Osgood-Schlatter disease for more than 2 years warrant exploration. Krause et al. concluded that symptoms of Osgood-Schlatter disease resolve spontaneously in most patients and that patients who continue to have symptoms are likely to have distorted tibial tuberosities associated with fragmentation of the apophysis with ossicles on radiographs. Lynch and Walsh described premature fusion of the anterior part of the upper tibial physis in two patients with Osgood-Schlatter disease who were treated nonoperatively, and they recommended screening for this rare complication.

Surgery rarely is indicated for Osgood-Schlatter disease; the disorder usually is self-limiting or becomes asymptomatic with simple conservative measures, such as the restriction of activities, bracing, or cast immobilization for 3 to 6 weeks. Surgery may be considered if symptoms are persistent and severely disabling. Insertion of bone pegs into the tibial tuberosity (Bosworth procedure) is simple and almost always relieves the symptoms by causing fusion of the apophysis to the remaining tibia; however, an unsightly prominence remains after this operation and is rarely used. The bony prominence can be excised (ossicle resection and tibial tubercleplasty) through a longitudinal incision in the patellar tendon or arthroscopic removal of the ossicle and tibial tubercle debridement. Reported complications of Osgood-Schlatter disease whether treated surgically or not, include subluxations of the patella, patella alta, nonunion of the bony fragment to the tibia, and premature fusion of the anterior part of the epiphysis with resulting genu recurvatum. Because of the possibility of genu recurvatum, surgery should be delayed until the apophysis has fused. We have removed only the ossicle with satisfactory results; we believe the tuberosity should be excised only if it is significantly enlarged and the apophysis is closed. The amount to be excised (debrided) should be determined preoperatively as described by Pihlajamäki et al. (Fig. 4.28).

Sinding-Larsen-Johansson disease is a clinical entity similar to Osgood-Schlatter disease except that the focus is the inferior pole of the patella (Fig. 4.29). Symptoms are similar but pain is in the superior portion of the patellar tendon rather than over the tibial tubercle. Nonoperative treatment is similar and involves rest, stretching, and antiinflammatories.

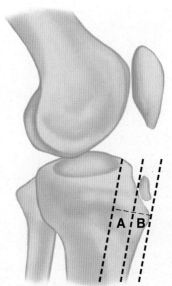

FIGURE 4.28 The tibial tuberosity index assesses the relative thickness of the tuberosity on radiographs. The line through the base of the tibial tuberosity is parallel to the midvertical tibial line. The midvertical tibial line is determined by measuring the middle of the projection of the tibia from four points located at various vertical levels of the cortex of the proximal part of the tibial cortex. The height of the tuberosity is measured from the line running parallel to the midvertical tibial line and passing through the base of the tuberosity. The base of the tubercle is determined by adjusting the line through the estimated base of the tibial tuberosity so that it is parallel to the midvertical tibial line and delineates the tibial tuberosity from the anterior tibial cortex. The tibial tuberosity index is the ratio of the distance from the top of the tuberosity (*dotted line farthest to the right*) to the parallel line of the anterior tibial cortex (*middle dotted line B*) to the distance from the top of the tibial tuberosity to the tibial midline (*dotted line farthest to the left A + B*). The tibial tuberosity index is calculated by dividing the length of the horizontal line B by the sum of the horizontal lines A and B. (Redrawn from Pihlajamäki HK, Mattila VM, Parviainen M, et al: Long-term outcome after surgical treatment of unresolved Osgood-Schlatter disease in young men, *J Bone Joint Surg* 91A:2350–2358, 2009.)

TIBIAL TUBEROSITY AND OSSICLE EXCISION

TECHNIQUE 4.10

(PIHLAJAMÄKI ET AL.)
- Place the patient supine on the operating table.
- Make a vertical 5-cm incision over the center of the distal part of the patellar tendon, 1 cm proximal to the tibial tuberosity, and over the center of the tibial tuberosity (Fig. 4.30A).

- Divide the distal patellar tendon longitudinally, and elevate the tendon laterally and medially to expose the superior part of the tibial tuberosity (Fig. 4.30B and C).
- With an osteotome and rongeur, remove the prominent tibial tuberosity and, if present, the posterior intratendinous ossicles, which may be firmly attached to the patellar tendon. Remove the osteocartilaginous fragments with or without resecting the tibial tuberosity prominence. Make sure all fragments are removed.
- Resect the tibial tuberosity down to the insertion of the tendon and smooth with a file. Drilling is unnecessary. Try not to disturb the peripheral and distal margins of the patellar tendon insertion.
- Close the wound in layers, and apply a light compressive dressing to the whole limb.
- As an alternative, a 5-cm transverse incision can be made, centered over a point 1 cm proximal to the tibial

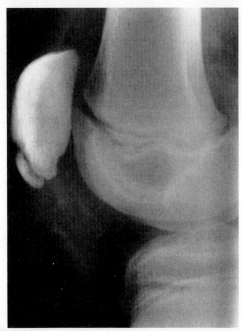

FIGURE 4.29 Sinding-Larsen-Johansson disease is a clinical entity similar to Osgood-Schlatter disease except that the focus is the inferior pole of the patella.

tuberosity (Fig. 4.31A). In this technique, the lateral soft-tissue attachments are released longitudinally, leaving the patellar tendon intact. It is then elevated to remove the osteocartilaginous fragments. The rest of the procedure is as described earlier, with care taken to not disturb the lateral and distal margins of the patellar tendon insertion.

POSTOPERATIVE CARE On the first day after surgery, quadriceps-setting exercises are started and crutches are used for a short period of time. Adequate quadriceps function should be emphasized, but all strenuous activity should be avoided for 6 to 12 weeks.

EXCISION OF UNUNITED TIBIAL TUBEROSITY FRAGMENT FOR OSGOOD-SCHLATTER DISEASE

TECHNIQUE 4.11

(FERCIOT AND THOMSON)
■ Make a longitudinal incision centered over the tibial tuberosity.
■ Expose the patellar tendon, and incise it longitudinally (Fig. 4.32). Elevate the tendon laterally and medially, and

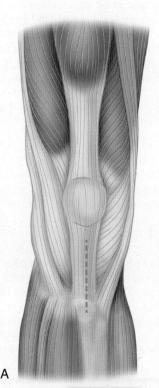
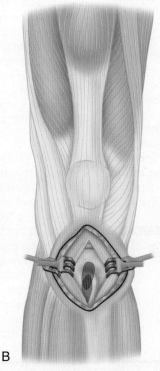
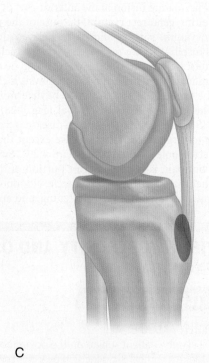

A B C

FIGURE 4.30 Pihlajamäki et al. technique for Osgood Schlatter disease. **A**, Skin incision. **B** and **C**, Patellar tendon is split and retracted to expose tibial tuberosity. (Redrawn from Pihlajamäki HK, Visuri TI: Long-term outcome after surgical treatment of unresolved Osgood-Schlatter disease in young men: surgical technique, *J Bone Joint Surg* 92[Suppl 1]:258–264, 2010.) **SEE TECHNIQUE 4.10.**

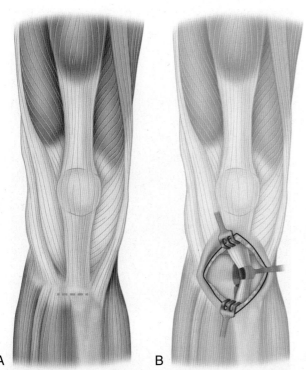

FIGURE 4.31 Pihlajamäki et al. alternative technique for Osgood Schlatter disease. **A,** Skin incision. **B,** Longitudinal incision in lateral soft tissue attachments of patellar tendon, which is elevated to expose tibial tuberosity. (Redrawn from: Pihlajamäki HK, Visuri TI: Long-term outcome after surgical treatment of unresolved Osgood-Schlatter disease in young men: surgical technique, *J Bone Joint Surg* 92[Suppl 1]:258–264, 2010.) **SEE TECHNIQUE 4.10**.

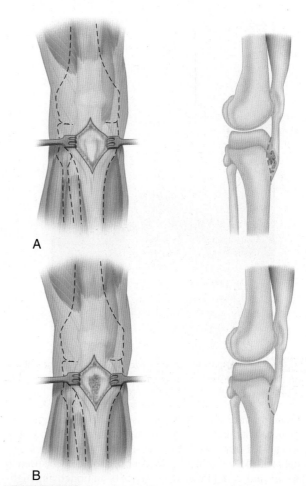

FIGURE 4.32 Ferciot and Thomson excision of ununited tibial tuberosity. **A,** Tibial tuberosity has been exposed. **B,** Bony prominence has been excised. **SEE TECHNIQUE 4.11**.

excise any loose fragments of bone and enough tibial cortex, cartilage, and cancellous bone to remove any bony prominence completely. Do not disturb the peripheral and distal margins of the insertion of the patellar tendon.
- Close the wound.

POSTOPERATIVE CARE A cylinder walking cast is applied and worn for 2 to 3 weeks. Exercises are then begun.

staying anterior to these structures, aggressively debride into the anterior tibial slope.
- Shell out the bony lesions from their soft-tissue attachments.
- Remove small and loose fragments with a pituitary rongeur; remove larger fragments with an arthroscopic burr. Extending the knee and taking tension off the patellar tendon facilitate the debridement along the anterior tibial slope.

POSTOPERATIVE CARE Patients are allowed full weight bearing and unrestricted range of motion after surgery.

ARTHROSCOPIC OSSICLE AND TIBIAL TUBEROSITY DEBRIDEMENT FOR OSGOOD-SCHLATTER DISEASE

TECHNIQUE 4.12

- Make standard knee arthroscopy portals.
- To improve the view of the anterior interval, raise the location of the inferomedial and lateral parapatellar tendon portals slightly.
- Using a mechanical shaver and radiofrequency ablation device, perform an anterior interval release. Viewing the meniscal anterior horns and intermeniscal ligament and

OSTEOCHONDRITIS DISSECANS OF THE KNEE

Osteochondritis dissecans of the knee usually is unilateral and may be painful. Histologic findings suggest a failure of ossification secondary to ischemia of the developing cartilage in the epiphysis. Although there are no specific physical findings diagnostic of osteochondritis dissecans of the knee, the lesions frequently are seen on radiographs and are classically located on the medial femoral condyle, though they may occur in the lateral condyle or the trochlea. Patients may complain of pain or mechanical symptoms. MRI is a highly sensitive method for detection of osteochondritis dissecans and can aid in

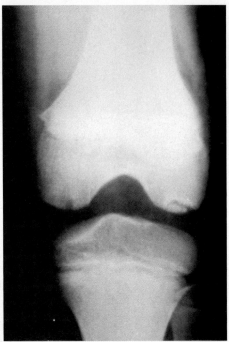

FIGURE 4.33 Bilateral (medial and lateral) anomalous ossification centers in posterior aspect of femoral condyles (not osteochondritis dissecans).

determining if a lesion is stable or unstable. Several recent studies of instability, comparing MRI with arthroscopic findings have reported less specificity and sensitivity than previously thought with MRI, noting that MRI alone should not be used to determine lesion stability. The presence of an underlying high-signal intensity line between the lesion and underlying bone, a cystic area, or a focal articular defect indicates instability and may help in preoperative planning. Furthermore, age seems to be a risk factor for instability, with older children more likely to have unstable lesions. Osteochondritis dissecans of the knee in children should not be confused with anomalous ossification centers. Because these ossification centers may be present in both condyles and in both knees, comparison radiographs of the affected and unaffected knees are advised (Fig. 4.33). MRI findings seem to be different for anomalous ossification centers and osteochondritis dissecans.

Osteochondritis dissecans of the knee in children with open physes usually heals when treated with cast immobilization or protected weight bearing. This treatment is preferable to excising the fragment early in life and creating a crater (Fig. 4.34). If gross instability is present, results generally are better after operative than after conservative treatment. Lesions with increased size, associated swelling, and mechanical symptoms are less likely to heal.

Nonoperative treatment always should be considered in patients with open physes; specific indications for operative treatment of osteochondritis dissecans in children are prolonged pain without evidence of healing during a 6-month period, an unhealed lesion in which symptoms persist after physeal closure, a sclerotic lesion in the crater (unstable lesion), and a troublesome loose body (Fig. 4.35). In skeletally mature individuals, surgery is necessary to evaluate the lesion and implement treatment. Kraus et al. noted that up to 12 months of conservative treatment might be successful if the cyst-like lesions are less than 1.3 mm in length as seen on an MRI.

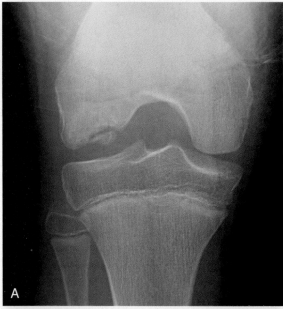

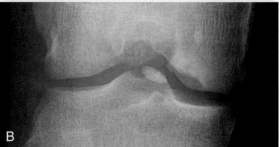

FIGURE 4.34 **A** and **B,** Osteochondritis dissecans of medial femoral condyle.

Whether the lesion is drilled (retrograde or transarticular), excised, curetted, replaced and pinned, including loose fragments, or bone grafted depends on the size, stability, and weight-bearing nature of the lesion, which can be determined only at surgery (Fig. 4.36). A discussion of surgical procedures, indications, and complications in children and adolescents can be found in the chapter on knee injuries.

EXTRAARTICULAR DRILLING FOR STABLE OSTEOCHONDRITIS DISSECANS OF THE KNEE

TECHNIQUE 4.13

(DONALDSON AND WOJTYS)

- Place the patient supine and examine the knee arthroscopically to determine the stability of the articular cartilage.
- Make 1- to 2-cm incisions over the affected femoral condyle distal to the femoral physis. For medial lesions, the incision should be just anterior to the medial collateral ligament, and for lateral lesions it should be just anterior to the lateral collateral ligament.
- With the lower extremity in the anatomic position and the knee in full extension, drill appropriate-size Kirschner

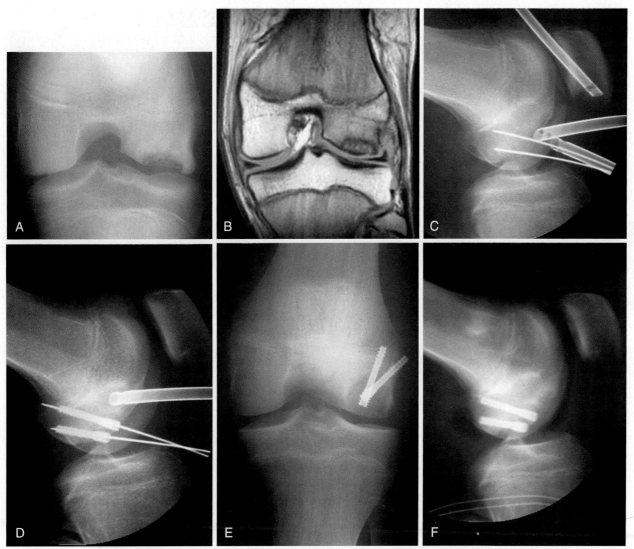

FIGURE 4.35 **A** and **B,** Large osteochondritis dissecans defect on lateral femoral condyle seen on radiograph and MR image. Chondroblastoma was ruled out in this patient with physes still open. **C** and **D,** After 9 months of unsuccessful conservative treatment, arthroscopy and Herbert screw fixation were performed. At time of arthroscopy, lesion was hinged but attached. This procedure requires use of image intensifier for correct guide pin placement and to avoid the physis with the Herbert screws. **E** and **F,** Postoperative anteroposterior and lateral radiographs with Herbert screws in acceptable position.

wires into the lesion from proximal to distal, avoiding the physis. Direct the Kirschner wires toward the lesion in the anteroposterior plane. Anteroposterior lateral C-arm imaging should be used to guide the drilling into the defect so as not to penetrate the knee joint or violate the articular cartilage. Arthroscopy is extremely helpful in obtaining appropriate guidewire placement. The success of the procedure is related to perforating the cortical shell of the lesion. If this is not done, revascularization probably will not occur.

POSTOPERATIVE CARE The knee is wrapped in a soft dressing after surgery. Motion is encouraged and the patients are kept at toe-touch weight bearing on crutches for 6 weeks. Physical therapy should be focused on range-of-motion exercises and low-resistance strength training.

OSTEOCHONDRITIS DISSECANS OF THE PATELLA

Osteochondritis dissecans of the patella is a rare entity that affects the subchondral bone and articular surface and the cartilage overlying the surface of the patella. It may appear as an elliptical fragment within a crater. It rarely occurs bilaterally. It is frequently painful and quite debilitating. Boys age 10 to 15 are most commonly affected.

Osteochondritis dissecans of the patella should be differentiated from a dorsal defect of the patella so that surgical treatment is not carried out on an asymptomatic defect (Table 4.6). The differences between the two are subtle but present. In contrast to osteochondritis dissecans of the patella (Fig. 4.37A), a dorsal defect is a simple, asymptomatic, subchondral defect in the superolateral portion of the patella that does not involve the articular cartilage and usually is an incidental

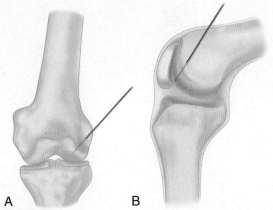

FIGURE 4.36 Anteroposterior **(A)** and lateral **(B)** illustration showing pin placement in osteochondritis dissecans of the knee in skeletally immature patients. (Redrawn from Donaldson LD, Wojtys EM: Extraarticular drilling for stable osteochondritis dissecans in the skeletally immature knee, *J Pediatr Orthop* 28:831–835, 2008.) **SEE TECHNIQUE 4.13**.

TABLE 4.6

Differentiation of Osteochondritis Dissecans of the Patella from Dorsal Defect of the Patella

OSTEOCHONDRITIS DISSECANS OF THE PATELLA	DORSAL DEFECT OF THE PATELLA
Usually symptomatic	Usually asymptomatic
Separation of chondral or osteochondral fragment from subchondral bone	Incidental finding on radiograph
Involves articular cartilage	Does not involve articular cartilage
Rarely bilateral	Round subchondral defect in superolateral portion of patella; occasionally sclerotic border; 20%-40% bilateral occurrence
Bone scan hot	Bone scan cold

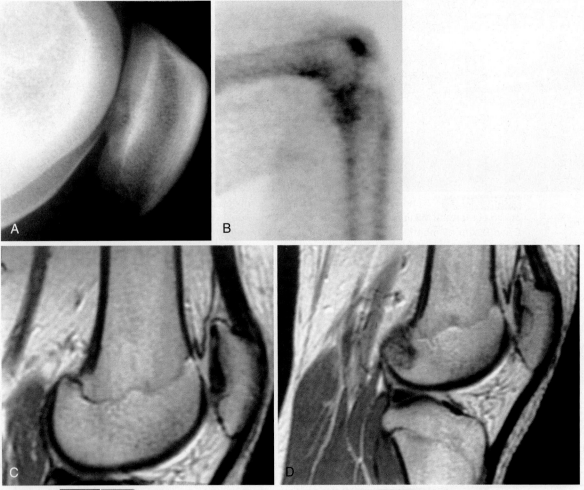

FIGURE 4.37 Osteochondritis dissecans of patella. **A,** Lateral radiograph. **B,** Bone scan. **C** and **D,** MR images showing osteocartilaginous fragment including articular cartilage within crater.

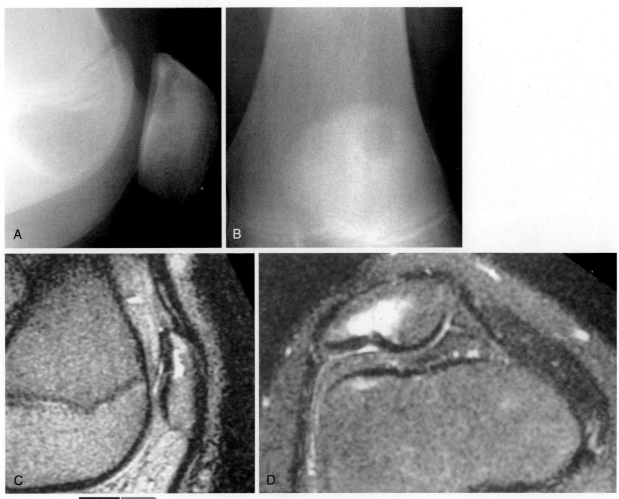

FIGURE 4.38 **A** and **B,** Radiographs of dorsal defect of patella in superolateral quadrant. **C** and **D,** MRI reveals dorsal defect of patella with cystic defect noted but not involving articular cartilage.

finding on radiograph (Fig. 4.38A and B). A sclerotic border occasionally is present, and 20% to 40% of the time it occurs bilaterally. Safran et al. stated that MRI definitively shows that the dorsal defect does not involve the articular surface compared with osteochondritis dissecans (Figs. 4.37C and D and 4.38C and D). A bone scan also can help differentiate between the two. In osteochondritis dissecans of the patella, the bone scan is exceptionally "hot" (Fig. 4.37B) compared with dorsal defects in which it is "cold."

Treatment of osteochondritis dissecans of the patella, especially in young children whose physes are still open, is nonoperative if possible. Restriction of activities and immobilization for a time are recommended to avoid surgical excision. If conservative treatment fails, the lesion can be drilled, and if it is loose but still in the crater, the lesion can be internally fixed with a small-diameter Herbert screw. If a defect and an old loose body are present, the loose body should be removed and the crater debrided and drilled. If the loose body appears to have viable subchondral bone, the crater should be freshened and the loose body placed within the crater and internally fixed.

Peters et al. used arthroscopic chondroplasty, removal of loose bodies, and retinacular release in 37 patients with mechanical symptoms (24 patellar and 13 trochlear groove).

The average age of their patients was 15 years, and 54% had open physes. Most patients improved after surgery, but patients with articular cartilage loss had persistent patellofemoral crepitus and discomfort. In our experience, the results after chondroplasty of the patella have been unsatisfactory.

OSTEOCHONDRITIS DISSECANS OF THE HIP

Osteochondritis dissecans of the hip occurs most frequently after Legg-Calvé-Perthes disease, although it can occur as an isolated entity and may be related to FAI. In children, loose bodies secondary to Legg-Calvé-Perthes disease, osteonecrosis of sickle cell disease, and multiple epiphyseal dysplasia have to be ruled out before this can be established as an isolated diagnosis. In adults, idiopathic osteonecrosis, Gaucher disease, and occult trauma, such as a torn acetabular labrum, have to be considered in the differential diagnosis.

Unless the fragment interferes with hip mechanics, treatment of osteochondritis dissecans of the hip after Legg-Calvé-Perthes disease or idiopathic lesions should be conservative (Fig. 4.39). In an asymptomatic child with osteochondritis dissecans of the hip, restriction of activity and prolonged observation are indicated to allow healing and revascularization.

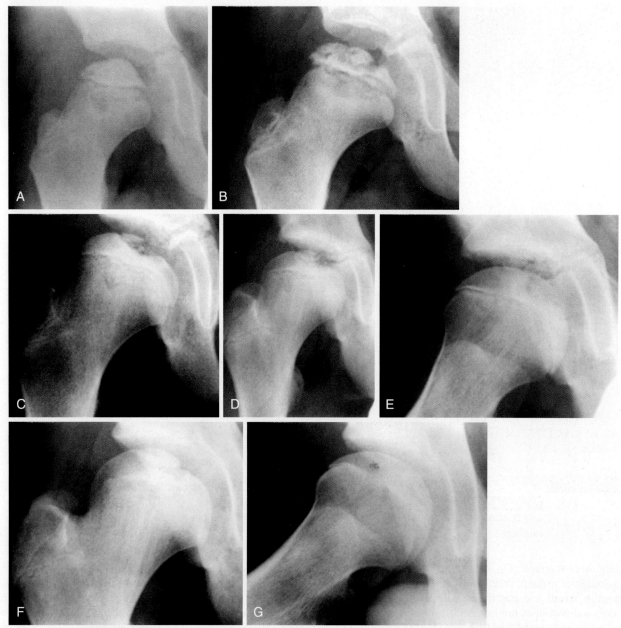

FIGURE 4.39 Osteochondritis dissecans of hip. **A,** Onset of Legg-Calvé-Perthes disease in 6-year-old patient. **B,** Fourteen months later, fragmentation and reossification stage. **C,** Persistent defect 5 years after onset. **D,** Osteochondritic lesion at 7 years with some evidence of healing. **E,** Lateral radiograph during same period shows osteochondritic lesion. Note air arthrogram with smooth cartilage surface. **F,** At 8 years defect is healing. **G,** Lateral radiograph at same time shows no evidence of defect.

Operative treatment is indicated for severe lesions with mechanical symptoms. The choice of operative procedure depends on the extent and location of the lesion, the age and activity expectations of the patient, and the presence of degenerative joint changes. Surgical dislocation of the hip as described by Ganz and others may be necessary. Good results have been reported in small series of patients who had open or arthroscopic excision of the fragment, internal fixation of the fragment, curettage or drilling, and arthroscopic removal of loose osteocartilaginous fragments. Osteochondral grafts have been used as well. None of these procedures is recommended if severe osteoarthritic changes are present.

OSTEOCHONDROSIS OF THE CAPITELLUM (OSTEOCHONDRITIS DISSECANS)

Little Leaguer's elbow is a term that has been used loosely to describe changes in the elbow secondary to baseball pitching and usually limited to the capitellum, radial head, or medial epicondyle. We have seen osteochondrosis of the capitellum (Panner disease) and osteochondritis dissecans of the capitellum. The cause of both is obscure and is not limited to throwing a baseball. A relationship may or may not exist between osteochondrosis and osteochondritis dissecans of the capitellum (Fig. 4.40).

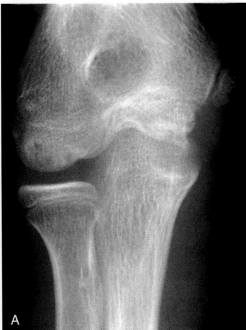

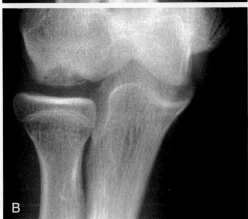

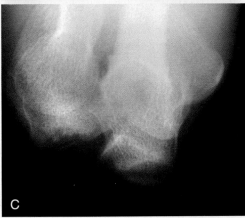

FIGURE 4.40 **A,** Osteochondrosis of capitellum. Anteroposterior **(B)** and Jones **(C)** views 1 year later show evidence of some consolidation, but osteochondritis dissecans appears to be forming.

presence of loose bodies within the joint. Anteroposterior and lateral radiographs should be obtained, and comparison views of the contralateral elbow are helpful to identify subtle changes in the capitellum, surrounded by subchondral sclerosis demarcated by a characteristic semilunar rarefied zone (crescent signs); older lesions may have a sclerotic border. Loose bodies may be seen in the joint. MRI often identifies early changes of marrow edema before changes are seen on plain radiographs. Recent studies revealed that MRI could reliably predict instability of an elbow lesion.

Classification systems for OCDs of the elbow have been developed based on radiographic, MRI, and arthroscopic findings. It can be broadly classified into the following groups:

- Ia: Intact/stable: Intact articular cartilage, no loss of subchondral stability
- Ib: Intact/unstable: Intact articular cartilage, unstable subchondral bone with impending collapse
- II: Open unstable: Cartilage fracture, collapse or partial displacement of subchondral bone
- III: Detached: Loose cartilaginous fragments within the joint

Also, lesions can be described as contained or uncontained. Contained lesions have intact articular cartilage, while uncontained lesions extend beyond the cartilaginous margin. Compared with elbows that have contained osteochondritis dissecans lesions, elbows with uncontained lesions are more broad and shallow, have greater flexion contractures, and higher rates of joint effusion. If a loose body is not present, nonsurgical treatment usually is satisfactory, especially if the lesion seems stable (type Ia). Resting the joint for 3 to 6 weeks with the use of a hinged elbow brace to eliminate excessive valgus stress usually allows return to activity in 3 to 6 months. This may be very difficult in a minimally symptomatic child playing year-round sports. Indications for operative treatment include persistent symptoms, symptomatic loose bodies, fracture of the articular cartilage, and displacement of the osteochondral lesion. Operative management may involve excision of loose bodies or partially attached lesions, chondroplasty with osteochondral autogenous graft (mosaicplasty) or subchondral drilling, or internal fixation of a loose fragment. Mixed results have been reported for all of these techniques, with rates of poor results up to 50%.

In more recent literature, the surgical results seem to be better, especially concerning motion, because of arthroscopic techniques. Arthroscopic procedures include partial synovectomy, excision of loose bodies, drilling the crater or the intact lesion, microfracture, internally fixing the unstable viable fragment with bioabsorbable pins or headless compression screws, and osteotomy of the capitellum. Although the arthroscopic results seem to be better than nonarthroscopic techniques, no procedure, as noted by Byrd and Jones, ensures return to a throwing sport, such as baseball, and the prognosis should be guarded especially if the lesion is large, widespread, or unstable. Arthroscopy and especially an elbow arthrogram or MRI may be indicated when a loose body is suspected but not seen on plain radiographs. Arthroscopy of the elbow is described in other chapter.

Most patients with osteochondritis dissecans of the capitellum report symptoms of elbow pain and stiffness that are aggravated by activity and relieved by rest. Reports of locking or catching of the joint suggest the

RECONSTRUCTION OF THE ARTICULAR SURFACE WITH OSTEOCHONDRAL PLUG GRAFTS FOR OSTEOCHONDROSIS OF THE CAPITELLUM

TECHNIQUE 4.14

(TAKAHARA ET AL.)

ARTHROSCOPIC FRAGMENT REMOVAL

- After administering general anesthesia, place the patient supine.
- Inject 10 to 20 mL of 1% lidocaine with epinephrine into the elbow joint. A tourniquet usually is not necessary.
- Flex the shoulder 90 degrees, and elevate the elbow until the upper arm is almost vertical. Maintain this position with skin traction applied from the forearm to the overhead bar.
- Confirm the suitable position and direction of the portals with a 23-gauge needle. Create posterior, posterolateral, anteromedial, and anterolateral portals with a sharp blade.
- Bluntly release the subcutaneous tissues avoiding the cutaneous nerves.
- Widen the portals with the use of step-up cannulas.
- Insert a 4-mm-diameter, 30-degree oblique arthroscope to remove the loose bodies.

OPEN APPROACH FOR FRAGMENT REMOVAL

- For a posterolateral approach, place the upper arm on the operative bed with the shoulder in abduction and the elbow fully flexed.
- Make a 4- to 6-cm posterolateral oblique skin incision on a line from the posterior edge of the lateral epicondyle to the posterior aspect of the radioulnar joint.
- After inflating the tourniquet, incise the skin and fascia. Develop the intermuscular plane between the extensor carpi ulnaris and anconeus muscles or muscle fibers.
- Incise the capsule over the capitellar lesion and elongate the incision from the posterior edge of the lateral epicondyle to the posterior aspect of the radioulnar joint.
- Perform a limited local synovectomy.

RECONSTRUCTION USING BONE PLUG GRAFTS

- After removal of loose fragments arthroscopically or through an open approach, harvest cylindrical osteochondral bone plugs from the lateral part of the lateral femoral condyle at the level of the patellofemoral joint, keeping the tube harvester at a 90-degree angle to the articular surface. One to three plugs may be necessary depending on the size of the defect.
- Prepare the recipient bed.
- Place the osteochondral plugs toward the center of the capitellum to obtain stable fixation. Take care not to damage the capitellar physis or the distal part of the femur in skeletally immature patients (Fig. 4.41). Because the thickness of hyaline cartilage and its surface curvature differ between the elbow and the knee, insert the plugs to match the spherical articular surface of the capitel-

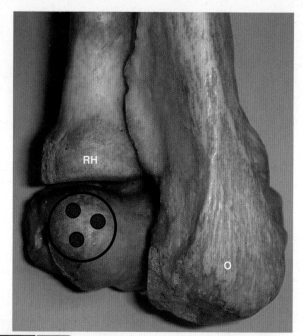

FIGURE 4.41 Reconstruction of the articular surface of the humeral capitellum using osteochondral plug grafts from the lateral femoral condyle. O, olecranon; RH, radial head. (From Takahara M, Mura N, Sasaki J, et al: Classification, treatment, and outcome of osteochondritis dissecans of the humeral capitellum, *J Bone Joint Surg* 90A:47–62, 2008.) **SEE TECHNIQUE 4.14**.

lum. The articular surface of the osteochondral plug graft should be slightly depressed rather than prominent relative to the capitellar surface, and the step-off should be less than 1 mm. Rarely is shaving the articular surface of the osteochondral plug graft necessary. Reconstructing the entire capitellar defect is not necessary.

POSTOPERATIVE CARE Immobilize the elbow for 1 to 2 weeks, and protect the knee from vigorous flexion for 3 weeks. Physical therapy should focus on reducing pain and swelling and regaining range of motion. Three months after the procedure, gentle elbow exercises against resistance are progressed to full resistance at 4 months. Throwing is allowed at 4 to 5 months if there is no pain and elbow range of motion has returned to preoperative levels. The patient is released for full sports activity at 6 to 8 months.

TIBIA VARA (BLOUNT DISEASE)

Erlacher is credited with the first description of tibia vara and internal tibial torsion (1922), but it was Blount's article in 1937 that prompted recognition of this disorder. Blount described tibia vara as "an osteochondrosis similar to coxa plana and Madelung deformity but located at the medial side of the proximal tibial epiphysis." Currently, tibia vara is considered an acquired disease of the proximal tibial metaphysis, however, rather than an epiphyseal dysplasia or osteochondrosis. The exact cause is unknown, but enchondral ossification seems to be altered. Suggested causative factors include infection, trauma, osteonecrosis, and a latent form of rickets, although none of these has been proved. A combination of hereditary and developmental factors is the most likely cause. Weight bearing must be necessary for its development because it does not occur in nonambulatory patients, and the relationship of early walking and obesity to Blount disease has been clearly documented. Because of the "obesity epidemic" and vitamin D deficiency in children in the United States, it has been speculated that the number of cases of Blount disease will rise.

Although the exact cause of tibia vara is controversial, the clinical and radiographic findings are consistent. The abnormality is characterized by varus and internal torsion of the tibia and genu procurvatum. Blount distinguished, according to age at onset, two types of tibia vara: infantile, which begins before 8 years of age, and adolescent, which begins after 8 years of age but before skeletal maturity. The infantile form is difficult to differentiate from physiologic bowing common in this age group, especially before the age of 2 years. Infantile tibia vara is bilateral and symmetric in approximately 60% of affected children; physiologic bowing is almost always bilateral. In Blount disease, the varus deformity increases progressively, whereas physiologic bowing tends to resolve with growth.

Although not as common as the infantile form, adolescent Blount disease has been divided into two types: (1) an adolescent form occurring between ages 8 and 13 years caused by partial closure of the physis after trauma or infection and (2) "late-onset" tibia vara that occurs in obese children, between ages 8 and 13, without a distinct cause. The marked similarity of histologic changes that occur in patients with late-onset tibia vara and in patients with infantile tibia vara and slipped capital femoral epiphysis suggests a common cause for these conditions.

In tibia vara, characteristically the medial half of the proximal tibial epiphysis as seen on radiographs is short, thin, and wedged; the physis is irregular in contour and slopes medially. The proximal metaphysis forms a projection medially that is often palpable, but this projection is not diagnostic of tibia vara. Medial metaphyseal fragmentation *is* pathognomonic for the development of a progressive tibia vara. The angular deformity occurs just distal to the projection. MRI studies reveal other soft-tissue abnormalities: (1) increased thickness of the chondroepiphysis of the proximal medial aspect of the tibia, (2) increased height and width of the medial meniscus, and (3) abnormal medial femoral epiphysis.

Langenskiöld noted progression of epiphyseal changes and the deformity through six stages with growth and development (Fig. 4.42). At stage VI, the medial portion of the epiphysis fuses at a 90-degree downward angle.

Normally, the tibiofemoral angle progresses from pronounced varus before the age of 1 year to valgus between ages 1.5 and 3 years. Several authors have suggested that deviation from normal tibiofemoral angle development indicates Blount disease, and the metaphyseal-diaphyseal angle is an early indicator of Blount disease. In one study, most children with metaphyseal-diaphyseal angles of 11 degrees or more developed Blount disease, whereas children with angles of less than 11 degrees had physiologic bowing that resolved with growth. This measurement is not an absolute prognosticator of Blount disease, but a metaphyseal-diaphyseal angle of more than 11 degrees warrants close observation (Fig. 4.43). Because of rotation, the Drennan angle is believed by some to be unreliable, although excellent interobserver reliability has been noted, and other angle

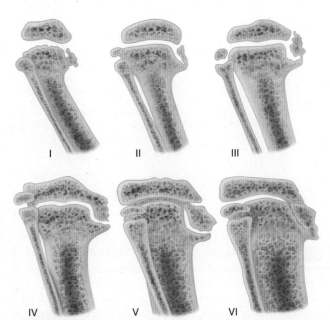

FIGURE 4.42 Diagram of radiographic changes seen in infantile type of tibia vara and their development with increasing age. (From Langenskiöld A, Riska EB: Tibia vara [osteochondrosis deformans tibiae]: a survey of seventy-one cases, *J Bone Joint Surg* 46A:1405–1420, 1964.)

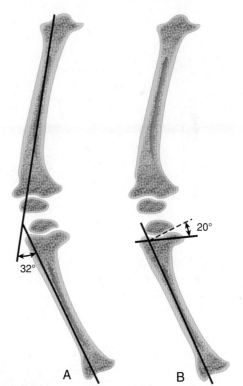

FIGURE 4.43 **A,** Tibiofemoral angle is formed by lines drawn along longitudinal axes of tibia and femur. **B,** Metaphyseal-diaphyseal angle is formed by line drawn perpendicular to longitudinal axis of the tibia and line drawn through two beaks of metaphysis to determine transverse axis of tibial metaphysis. (Redrawn from Levine A, Drennan J: Physiological bowing and tibia vara: the metaphyseal-diaphyseal angle in measurement of bowleg deformities, *J Bone Joint Surg* 64:1158–1163, 1982.)

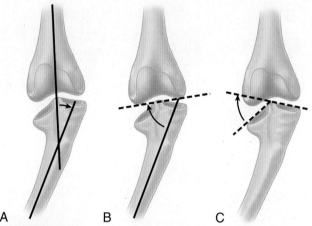

FIGURE 4.44 **A,** Angle formed by femoral shaft and tibial shaft. **B,** Angle formed by femoral condyle and tibial shaft. **C,** Depression of medial plateau of tibia. (From Schoenecker PL, Johnston R, Rich MM, et al: Elevation of the medial plateau of the tibia in the treatment of Blount disease, *J Bone Joint Surg* 74:351–358, 1992.)

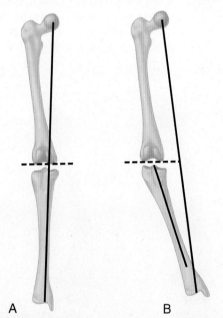

FIGURE 4.45 Mechanical axis of limb as it relates to angle formed by femoral condyle and tibial shaft. **A,** Normal alignment. Angle formed by femoral condyle and tibial shaft is approximately 90 degrees. **B,** Tibia vara. Angle formed by femoral condyle and tibial shaft is less than 90 degrees. (From Schoenecker PL, Johnston R, Rich MM, et al: Elevation of the medial plateau of the tibia in the treatment of Blount disease, *J Bone Joint Surg* 74:351–358, 1992.)

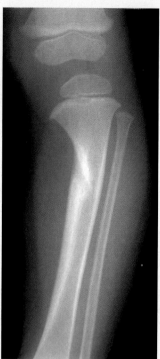

FIGURE 4.46 Fibrocartilaginous dysplasia in proximal tibia with resultant varus deformity simulating "bowlegs" of Blount disease.

measurements have been suggested: MRI to predict late resolution of tibial bowing, length of the fibula compared with the tibia, and the severity of proximal tibial angulation compared with distal femoral angulation. Although other angles of the femur and tibia at the knee can be determined (Fig. 4.44), when the deformity is present, most authors agree that the mechanical axis of the limb, as it relates to the tibiofemoral angle on radiographs, should be the most functional measurement of the amount of deformity present (Fig. 4.45).

Kline et al. described femoral varus as a significant deformity of late-onset Blount disease. They showed an average deformity of 10 degrees of femoral varus more than the calculated ideal femoral-tibial joint angle. This represented 34% to 76% of the genu varum deformity of the affected limbs. Gordon and Schoenecker recommended that calculations be made on standing long-film radiographs to determine the amount of excessive femoral varus and that this should be corrected by femoral osteotomy or epiphysiodesis at the time of tibial osteotomy to avoid a subsequent compensatory deformity.

Focal fibrocartilaginous dysplasia has been reported as a cause of tibia vara in a few patients. Bell described the characteristic radiographic appearance and unilateral nature of this lesion of the proximal medial metaphysis. Later reports suggest that this generally is a self-limiting condition that corrects spontaneously (Fig. 4.46) and that severe progression should be documented before valgus osteotomy is done. The proximal tibial physis has the potential to correct the deformity in the adjacent metaphysis, depending on the age of the patient and the severity of the deformity. Osteotomy is indicated only for significant deformity in an older child when spontaneous correction no longer can be expected. Infantile tibia vara resulting from slipping of the proximal tibial epiphysis has been described. It appears to be an atraumatic "slip" of the proximal tibial epiphysis on the metaphysis in severely obese children. Radiographically, the condition is characterized by a dome-shaped metaphysis, an open growth plate, and disruption of the continuity between the lateral borders of the epiphysis and metaphysis, with inferomedial translation of the proximal tibial epiphysis. It is important to recognize this entity because of the differences in treatment between it and conventional Blount disease.

The treatment of Blount disease depends on the age of the child and the severity of the varus deformity. Generally, observation or bracing with a knee-ankle-foot orthosis may be indicated for children between ages 2 and 3 years, but progressive deformity in children older than 3 years usually requires osteotomy. Recurrence of the deformity is not as frequent after osteotomy at an early age as after osteotomy when the child is older, with recurrence rates of about 80% reported in older children compared with less than 20% in younger children. Beaty et al. reported that early osteotomy (2 to 4 years old) produced the best results, with only one of their 10 patients having recurrence of the deformity. Conversely, of 12 patients in whom osteotomy was done after age 5 years, 10 (83%) had recurrence of the deformity necessitating repeated osteotomy. They recommended valgus osteotomies of the proximal tibia and fibula with mild overcorrection in young children.

Rab described a proximal tibial osteotomy for Blount disease in which a single-plane oblique cut allows simultaneous correction of varus and internal rotation and permits postoperative cast wedging if necessary to obtain appropriate position. More recently, Laurencin et al., in an effort to avoid neurovascular and physeal complications, described an oblique incomplete closing wedge osteotomy fixed with a lateral tension plate. Greene also described a chevron osteotomy in which opening and closing wedges can be made so that the limb-length deformity present in moderate to severe tibia vara is not increased. He prefers a crescent-shaped osteotomy, using a one-half lateral closing wedge and using the graft medially in an opening wedge to maintain length. Internal fixation of the graft often is necessary.

One cause of recurrence of the deformity after osteotomy is a physeal bar. Greene listed the following criteria for deciding if CT studies should be done preoperatively to determine if a bony bar is present: (1) age older than 5 years, (2) medial physeal slope of 50 to 70 degrees, (3) Langenskiöld grade IV radiographic changes, and (4) body weight greater than the 95th percentile. Alternatively, to decrease radiation exposure, MRI can be obtained to identify a physeal bar. Bony bridge resection should be considered in children with remaining growth potential and can be done in conjunction with tibial osteotomy if angulation is significant.

In children older than age 9 years with more severe involvement, osteotomy alone, with bony bar resection, or with epiphysiodesis of the lateral tibial and the fibular physes may be indicated. Medial physeal bar resection alone has been reported to be effective when premature closure of the physis is evident, but significant angular deformity would not be corrected by bar resection alone. Lateral tibial epiphysiodesis can be done, with or without osteotomy, after the age of 9 years but before skeletal maturity. In unilateral involvement, epiphysiodesis of the uninvolved leg may be indicated to correct leg-length discrepancy. Several early reports in the literature have described lateral guided growth correction (manipulation) with temporary epiphysiodesis for infantile Blount disease with tension band plates (eight-plate technique). The results have been satisfactory in selected patients but with the following observations: (1) recurrence of the deformity after plate removal is secondary to a slower growth rate of the medial physis; (2) mechanical failure of the tension band plate screws can occur in those who are obese, and, if in doubt, four screws or two eight-plates can be used; and (3) tension band plates are as effective as staple hemiepiphysiodesis for guided correction of growth with respect to rate of correction and complications.

For older patients in whom bracing and tibial osteotomy have failed to prevent progressive deformity, and when the risk of abnormal spontaneous medial epiphysiodesis is great, as evidenced by severe disorderly enchondral ossification, an intraepiphyseal osteotomy to correct severe joint instability and a valgus metaphyseal osteotomy to correct the varus angulation may be indicated.

An essential element of this procedure is reconstruction of the horizontal level of the medial tibial plateau. This method is for considerable depression of the medial femoral condyle within the defect of the tibial epiphyseal bone and when there is the possibility of a bony bridge between the metaphysis and epiphysis of the medial tibia. In addition to elevation of the depressed medial tibial plateau, metaphyseal valgus osteotomy may be needed to correct alignment of the tibia (Fig. 4.47).

Zayer described a hemicondylar tibial osteotomy through the epiphysis, but not through the physis, into the intercondylar notch (Fig. 4.48). This method corrects the medial slope of the tibial epiphysis while avoiding the physis. Because obesity, unequal limb lengths, and femoral deformity often are present in patients with Blount disease, external fixation, including the Taylor spatial frame, may be indicated to achieve stability after osteotomy and immediate correction and seems to be an excellent method of treating an extremely obese patient for whom

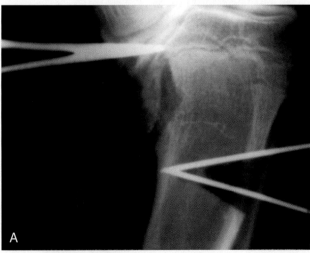
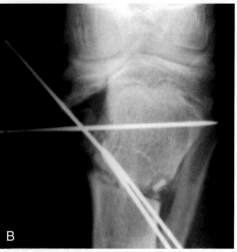

FIGURE 4.47 Severe Blount disease. **A,** Closing wedge metaphyseal osteotomy. **B,** Epiphyseal elevation. **SEE TECHNIQUE 4.15.**

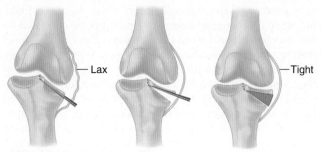

FIGURE 4.48 Hemicondylar osteotomy. (From Zayer M: Hemicondylar tibial osteotomy in Blount's disease: a report of two cases, *Acta Orthop Scand* 63:350–352, 1992.)

unilateral or especially bilateral casting is impractical. A uniplanar external fixator also can be used especially for isolated frontal one-plane deformities with satisfactory results. The advantages seem to be ease of application, adjustability, early weight bearing, the ability to lengthen the extremity, and avoiding a second operation to remove the implant (Fig. 4.49). The Ilizarov technique is effective for correction of deformity and lengthening if needed in adolescent patients. Various multiplanar external fixators allow computer-navigated correction of residual deformity after initial intraoperative correction and have been shown to be safe while providing excellent correction. This technique allows adjustment of limb alignment postoperatively, if necessary, to obtain a perfect mechanical axis.

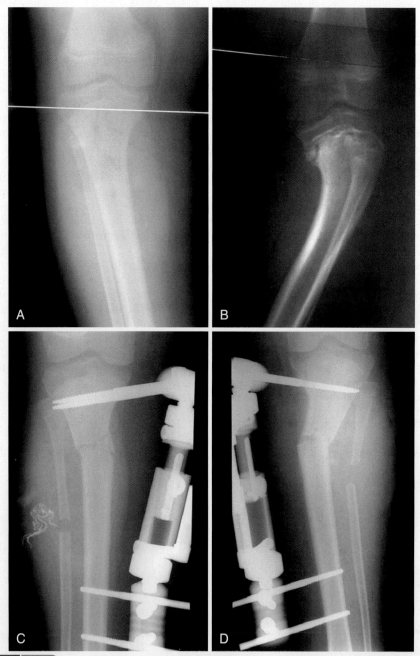

FIGURE 4.49 **A** and **B,** Anteroposterior radiographs of severe bilateral tibia vara in obese adolescent. **C** and **D,** Radiographs of unilateral frame external fixators after metaphyseal osteotomies.

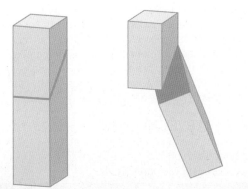

FIGURE 4.50 Principle of oblique osteotomy for tibia vara. Rotation around face of cut produces valgus and external rotation.

Fixation of the tibia is achieved through four proximal and four distal wires that are affixed to rings and tensioned. Half-pin modifications also can be used.

OSTEOTOMIES

The oblique osteotomy described by Rab begins at a point distal to the tibial tubercle, proximal to the posterior tibial metaphysis, and just distal to the physis and is done through a cosmetic transverse incision. Fasciotomy and fibular osteotomy are done through a separate incision. Because rigid internal fixation is not used, postoperative adjustments through cast wedging are possible.

Correction is obtained by rotating around the face of the oblique osteotomy and can be described best by considering the individual cuts in their anatomic planes (Fig. 4.50). Correction of a purely rotational deformity requires an osteotomy in the transverse plane, whereas purely varus or valgus correction requires osteotomy in the frontal (coronal) plane. An oblique osteotomy, directed from anterodistal to posteroproximal, splits the difference between the transverse and frontal planes. Rotation with its two faces in contact corrects varus and internal rotation. Osteotomy cuts that are more vertical (frontal) correct more varus than internal rotation. More horizontal (transverse) cuts do the opposite. According to Rab, patients with Blount disease have almost equal amounts of varus and internal rotation and in practice a 45-degree upward osteotomy provides adequate correction in most patients. He reported simultaneous correction of varus deformity of 44 degrees and internal rotation of 30 degrees. A quick estimate of the osteotomy angle when different degrees of external rotation and valgus correction are required is provided in Figure 4.51. A mathematic model of the osteotomy rotations is shown in Figure 4.52.

METAPHYSEAL OSTEOTOMY FOR TIBIA VARA

TECHNIQUE 4.15

(RAB)
- Prepare and drape the patient in the usual manner, and apply and inflate a tourniquet.

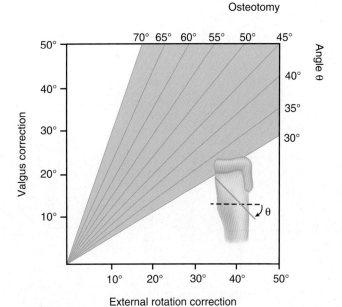

FIGURE 4.51 Nomogram for calculation of angle of oblique osteotomy for tibia vara. Desired valgus correction is found on vertical axis, and desired rotational correction is found on horizontal axis; intersection indicates osteotomy angle from horizontal as shown *(inset)*. (Redrawn from Rab GT: Oblique tibial osteotomy for Blount's disease [tibia vara], *J Pediatr Orthop* 8:715–720, 1988.)

- Make a transverse incision at the lower pole of the tibial tubercle (Fig. 4.53A). Make a Y-shaped incision in the periosteum and dissect periosteally (including the pes anserinus insertion medially) until malleable or Blount retractors can be placed behind the tibia (Fig. 4.53B). Elongate the periosteal incision distally, if necessary, to obtain subperiosteal protection posteriorly.
- Place a small Steinmann pin at a 45-degree angle 1 cm distal to the tibial tubercle, and advance it under image intensifier control until it passes just into the posterior cortex (Fig. 4.53C). Ensure the pin is distal to the physis at the posterior cortex on the image intensifier view. Measure the pin length, and use a marking pen or Steri-Strip to mark the same length on the osteotomes and sagittal saw blades (Fig. 4.53D). This serves as a reminder of the saw depth and can indicate if a lateral image intensifier exposure is appropriate.
- With the saw and osteotome, carefully make the osteotomy cut immediately distal to the Steinmann pin, checking frequently with image intensification (Fig. 4.53E). As the cut nears completion, it may be helpful to make some of the cut from the anteromedial side of the tibia where subperiosteal exposure is better.
- Make a second small incision over the midfibula, and excise a 1- to 2-cm subperiosteal segment of the fibula. Move the tibial osteotomy back and forth to free some of the posterior periosteum from the fragments.
- Drill a hole in the anteroposterior direction across the osteotomy cut lateral to the tibial tubercle. Rotate the osteotomy on its face by external rotation and valgus rotation (in Blount disease), overcorrecting if necessary. Through

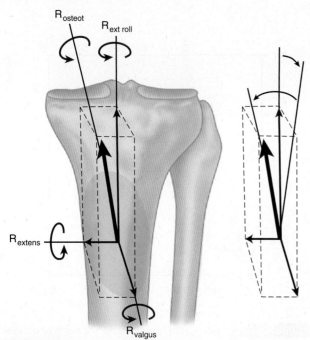

FIGURE 4.52 Mathematic description of osteotomy rotations. Vectors represent rotation in frontal, transverse, and sagittal planes, and R_{osteot} is actual rotation around face of osteotomy cut. Vectors describing rotation are normal to (at right angles to) plane of osteotomy cut.

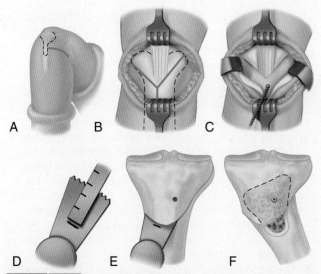

FIGURE 4.53 Oblique tibial osteotomy (see text) for tibia vara. **A,** Transverse incision at tibial tubercle. **B,** Y-shaped periosteal incision. **C,** Insertion of Steinmann pin after subperiosteal exposure. **D,** Marking of saw and osteotomies to avoid overpenetration. **E,** Oblique cut beneath pin. **F,** Rotation of osteotomy and fixation with single lag screw. **SEE TECHNIQUE 4.15**.

the drill hole, secure the osteotomy with a single 3.5-mm cortical or cancellous lag screw overdrilled anteriorly (Fig. 4.53F). Do not overtighten this screw.
- Perform a subcutaneous fasciotomy between the two incisions, and release the tourniquet. Check for return of

pulses, especially in the dorsalis pedis artery. Obtain hemostasis, and close the wound over suction drains with fine absorbable subcutaneous and subcuticular sutures. Check both extremities for correct clinical alignment, which is crucial at this stage. The single screw is loose enough to allow adjustment of the osteotomy position by cast wedging if necessary. Apply a long leg, bent-knee cast.

POSTOPERATIVE CARE The cast is changed at 4 weeks, and weight bearing is allowed as tolerated if callus is visible on radiograph. The cast is worn for 8 weeks or until union is evident radiographically.

Greene described an opening-closing chevron osteotomy that is a modification of the dome osteotomy and has the advantage of providing greater stability and minimal changes in leg length. Theoretical disadvantages are a slightly longer period of cast immobilization, which may be necessary to incorporate the wedge segment, and loss of correction caused by loss of fixation.

CHEVRON OSTEOTOMY FOR TIBIA VARA

TECHNIQUE 4.16

(GREENE)
- Before surgery, make a paper template that outlines the desired lateral wedge.
- Place the patient supine on the operating table with a sandbag under the ipsilateral hip to improve exposure of the fibula. Prepare the leg from the toes to the proximal thigh. Preparing the foot allows more accurate evaluation of the tibial torsion and allows evaluation of the dorsalis pedis and posterior tibial pulses when the tourniquet is deflated.

FIBULAR OSTEOTOMY
- Expose the middle third of the fibula through the interval between the lateral and posterior compartments. Sharply incise the periosteum of the fibula, and carefully elevate the periosteum circumferentially to prevent injury to the adjacent peroneal vessels.
- Remove a 1-cm segment of the fibula with a reciprocating saw. Cut the fibula obliquely, from superolateral to inferomedial. This allows the distal portion of the fibula to slide past the proximal fragment as the leg is brought from a varus to a valgus position.

TIBIAL OSTEOTOMY
- Make a hockey-stick incision 4 to 5 cm distal to the tibial tubercle staying medial and lateral to the anterior spine of the tibia. Extend the incision to the tibial tubercle and curve it laterally toward Gerdy's tubercle. Sharply incise the periosteum immediately adjacent to the anterior compartment muscles. Incise the periosteum transversely just distal to the tibial tubercle, and elevate it circumferentially so that curved retractors can be placed to protect the posterior

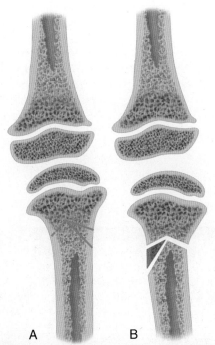

FIGURE 4.54   Opening-closing chevron osteotomy for tibia vara. **A,** Osteotomy cuts. **B,** Lateral wedge is inserted medially. (From Greene WB: Infantile tibia vara, *J Bone Joint Surg* 75A:130–143, 1993.) **SEE TECHNIQUE 4.16.**

soft tissues. Because of its triangular shape, more care is required at the posterolateral and posteromedial edges of the tibia to ensure that dissection remains subperiosteal.

■ Outline the osseous cuts on the anterior surface of the tibia with an osteotome or cautery (Fig. 4.54). The apex of the osteotomy should be just distal to the tibial tubercle. Drill a hole from anterior to posterior at this point to minimize the risk of extending the osteotomy beyond the desired location. Complete the osteotomy with an oscillating saw, and remove the lateral wedge.

■ Swing the distal tibia into the desired position of valgus and external rotation. Insert the lateral wedge medially in a position that maintains the correction.

■ Depending on the age of the child, the degree of obesity, and the stability of the osteotomy, a single pin or two crossed pins may be used for fixation if necessary. Use smooth or threaded pins, and predrill the diaphysis to make pin insertion easier and more accurate. Any pin used for fixation should cross the osteotomy and exit through the proximal cortex without crossing the physis.

■ Release the tourniquet, and check the circulation in the foot. If circulation is satisfactory and correction is adequate on radiographs, bury the ends of the pins beneath the skin to prevent pin track infection and skin ulceration. Perform subcutaneous fasciotomy in the anterolateral compartment.

■ Close the fibular and tibial incisions, leaving the fascia open, and close the skin with subcuticular sutures. Apply a long leg, bent-knee cast with the knee flexed 45 degrees and the ankle in the neutral position.

POSTOPERATIVE CARE No weight bearing is allowed for the first 4 weeks after surgery. The cast is changed at 4 weeks, and, if healing is satisfactory on radiographs, the pins are removed and weight bearing is begun. Usually 8 to 10 weeks of immobilization is necessary, depending on the age of the child. The osteotomy must be protected long enough to minimize the risk of fracture that accompanies a quick resumption of vigorous play activity.

EPIPHYSEAL AND METAPHYSEAL OSTEOTOMY FOR TIBIA VARA

TECHNIQUE 4.17

(INGRAM, CANALE, BEATY)

■ Determine preoperatively the amount of wedge to be removed from the epiphyseal and metaphyseal areas (Fig. 4.47) and whether a graft is to be taken from the fibula or tibia.

■ Prepare and drape the patient in the usual manner, and apply and inflate a tourniquet.

■ Expose the proximal tibia through a longitudinal incision approximately 10 cm long at the lateral border of the bone in the area of the physis. Carry the dissection through the soft tissue to expose the physis (Fig. 4.55B). Continue subperiosteal exposure distally and place reverse retractors in the metaphyseal area of the bone into the area of the tibial collateral ligament attachment on the tibia. Make a short incision in the proximal third of the lateral compartment, and carry soft-tissue dissection down to the fibula, avoiding the peroneal nerve.

■ Remove a segment of the fibula approximately 1.5 cm long. If a graft is to be used beneath the tibial plateau, a longer segment of fibula may be required.

■ Fasciotomy can be done through this incision or through the tibial incision. With an osteotome and mallet, make an osteotomy through the physis, resecting any bony bar (Fig. 4.55C). Complete the osteotomy from the periphery to the center of the knee anteriorly to posteriorly, avoiding vessels and nerves posteriorly. Place an elevator in the osteotomy site, and gently pry open and elevate the medial tibial plateau until it is as nearly parallel as possible to the lateral tibial plateau (Fig. 4.55D). If there is any offset of the osteotomy in the middle of the joint, arthrotomy can be done to inspect the joint; the abundant soft tissue and cartilage in the area of the tibial eminence act as a hinge, preventing any offset.

■ Cut the appropriate closing lateral wedge in the metaphysis and insert two parallel Steinmann pins. Place the wedge of bone (or bone graft from the fibula) beneath the elevated tibial plateau (Fig. 4.55E); apply compression if desired (Fig. 4.55E).

■ Insert crossed Steinmann pins through the epiphysis and proximal tibial graft.

■ Close the wound and apply a long leg, bent-knee cast incorporating the pins in the plaster (Fig. 4.55F) or in an external fixator apparatus.

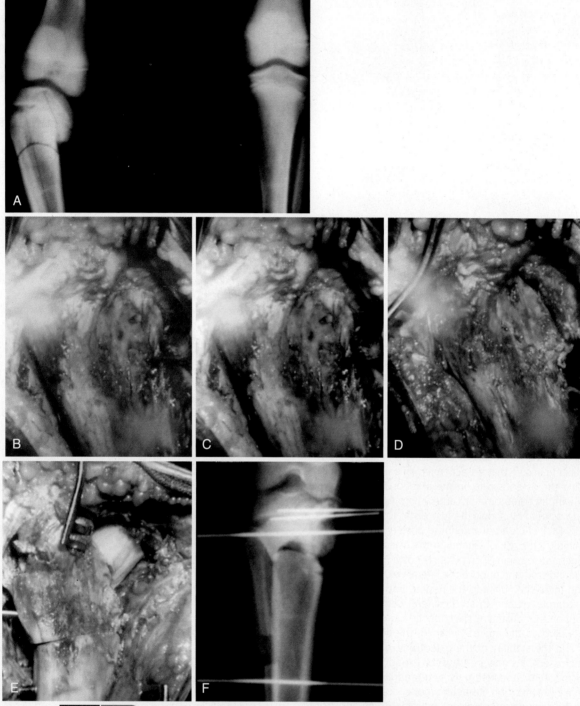

FIGURE 4.55 Epiphyseal and metaphyseal osteotomy for tibia vara. **A,** Severe Blount disease with physis slipped 90 degrees. **B,** Exposure of physis. **C,** Osteotomy. **D,** Elevation of medial tibial plateau. **E,** Placement of bone graft under compression. **F,** Cast incorporating pins in plaster. **SEE TECHNIQUE 4.17**.

POSTOPERATIVE CARE The pins in the osteotomy site are removed at 6 weeks, and the pins in the medial plateau are removed at 12 weeks. Cast immobilization is discontinued at 12 weeks, and range-of-motion exercises are begun.

INTRAEPIPHYSEAL OSTEOTOMY FOR TIBIA VARA

TECHNIQUE 4.18

(SIFFERT, STØREN, JOHNSON ET AL.)

- With the knee in extension, begin a medial longitudinal incision at the medial femoral epicondyle, extend it distally and anteriorly, and end it 2 cm medial and distal to the tibial tuberosity. (Siffert prefers a transverse incision along the medial joint line, curved distally to the tibial tuberosity.) Take care to preserve the infrapatellar branch of the saphenous nerve at the inferior aspect of the wound.
- Open the knee joint through a capsular incision anterior to the medial collateral ligament. The medial meniscus may be found hypertrophied; we try to preserve it. The capsular incision allows inspection of the articular surface of the tibia as the osteotomy is made.
- With a scalpel, make a circumferential incision through the epiphyseal cartilage down to the primary ossification center of the proximal tibial epiphysis, extending from the posteromedial corner of the tibia to the anteromedial corner; make the incision midway between the articular surface and the prominent vascular ring of vessels penetrating the epiphysis just proximal to the physis.
- Using a ¾-inch (18-mm), gently curved osteotome, make an osteotomy through the medial aspect of the primary ossification center of the epiphysis. Because of the abnormal slope of the medial tibial plateau, the osteotomy parallels the articular surface medially and should reach the subchondral bone in the intercondylar area adjacent to the anterior cruciate ligament (Fig. 4.56). Gently elevate this segment, bringing the medial tibial plateau congruent with the medial femoral condyle and level with the lateral tibial plateau. Siffert stated this should correct the genu recurvatum that is frequently present.
- Insert small cortical grafts from the medial proximal tibia (or bank bone) into the opened osteotomy. Because the articular depression usually is more posterior than anterior, grafts of different sizes and shapes are needed to maintain articular congruity and contact throughout a normal range of motion. It is important that the grafts be placed only in the opened wedge of the epiphyseal bone and not in the cartilage medially.

Andrade and Johnston described a more extensive operation using dental burrs and methyl methacrylate pin construct for fixation. They emphasized the importance of elevating the depression (Fig. 4.57). A medially based opening wedge osteotomy of the proximal tibia also may be required to correct varus of the tibia. A proximal fibular osteotomy is needed, and

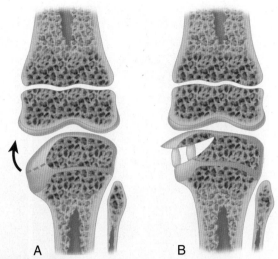

A   **B**

FIGURE 4.56 Correction of intraarticular component of Blount disease by osteotomy of epiphysis. **A,** Incision made into epiphyseal cartilage at its midportion medially. Curved osteotomy directed laterally and proximally to subchondral intercondylar region paralleling articular surface. **B,** Osteotomized tibial condyle elevated on its intercondylar cartilage hinge to position of congruity with femur; bone struts are placed into gap to maintain contact in all planes of motion and to tighten medial ligament. (From Siffert RS: Intraepiphyseal osteotomy for progressive tibia vara: case report and rationale of management, *J Pediatr Orthop* 2:81–85, 1982.) **SEE TECHNIQUE 4.18.**

through the lateral incision required for the fibular osteotomy we recommend a subcutaneous fasciotomy, taking care to protect the superficial peroneal nerve as it penetrates the deep investing fascia of the lower leg to become subcutaneous. We also insert a smooth Steinmann pin proximal and distal to the osteotomy of the proximal tibia, and with these incorporated in a long leg cast the position of the osteotomy is maintained without a graft. A cortical graft also can be used in an opening wedge and is held with crossed Steinmann pins. The technique of osteotomy of the proximal tibia is described in other chapter.

A lateral epiphysiodesis can be done with any of the osteotomies by extending the subperiosteal dissection proximally to expose the physis. A curet or dental burr can be used to excise the cartilaginous physis. The technique for epiphysiodesis is described in other chapter.

HEMIELEVATION OF THE EPIPHYSIS OSTEOTOMY WITH LEG LENGTHENING USING AN ILIZAROV FRAME FOR TIBIA VARA

TECHNIQUE 4.19

(JONES ET AL., HEFNY ET AL.)

STAGE 1

- Place the patient supine, and apply a tourniquet.
- Make a J-shaped skin incision on the medial side of the knee for subperiosteal exposure of the proximal tibia.

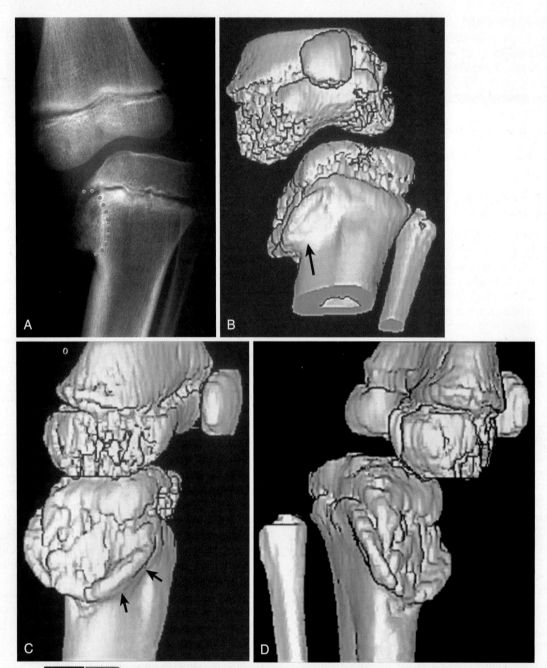

FIGURE 4.57 Medial epiphysiolysis for stage IV infantile tibia vara. **A,** Metaphyseal bone and Blount lesion to be excised is outlined. **B,** Three-dimensional reconstruction from CT showing extent of abnormally depressed epiphyseal bone anteriorly. *Arrow* indicates cleft on the anterior surface of the metaphysis where initial resection for epiphysiolysis begins. **C** and **D,** Lateral and posterolateral views of the metaphyseal beak. (From Andrade N, Johnston CE: Medial epiphysiolysis in severe infantile tibia vara, *J Pediatr Orthop* 26:652–658, 2006.)

- Place a ring-handled retractor subperiosteally behind the knee to protect the neurovascular structures.
- Determine the level of the proposed osteotomy using image intensification, and insert a Kirschner wire into the midline of the tibia anteriorly just below the tibial spine. Place a second Kirschner wire into the medial aspect of the proximal tibia (distal to the first wire) to mark the distal extent of the osteotomy (usually at the metaphyseal-diaphyseal junction). Predrill the osteotomy in line with

the Kirschner wires, verifying the position of the drill holes using image intensification.
- Close the skin temporarily.
- Insert three 4-mm or 5-mm half-pins, depending on the size of the patient, into the fragment of the medial tibial plateau, parallel to the medial joint line as determined by an intraoperative arthrogram and three-dimensional CT (Fig. 4.58). If there is a posterior slope, pins should be placed parallel to it from anterior to posterior. The skin

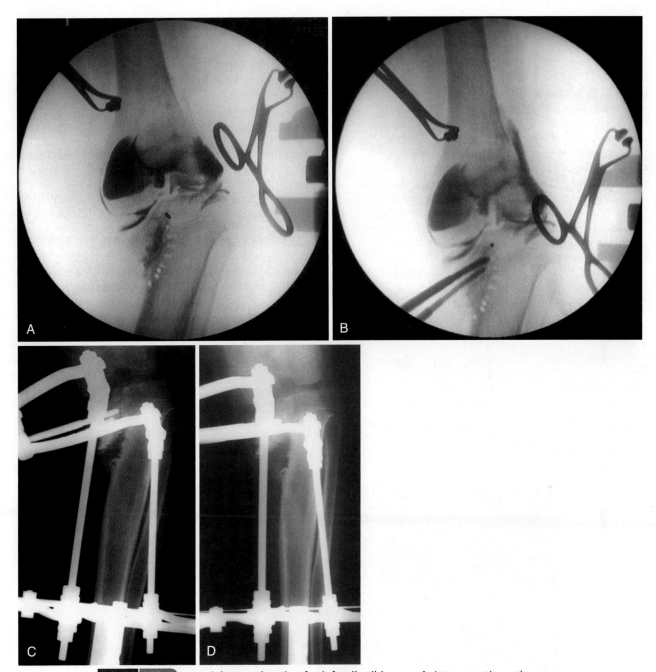

FIGURE 4.58 Hemiplateau elevation for infantile tibia vara. **A,** Intraoperative arthrogram using image intensifier showing drill holes marking proposed osteotomy site. **B,** Two half-pins inserted into fragment of medial tibial plateau parallel to true medial knee joint line. **C** and **D,** Completed osteotomy with elevation of hemiplateau under way using Ilizarov frame. (From Jones S, Hosalkar HS, Hill RA, et al: Relapsed infantile Blount's disease treated by hemiplateau elevation using the Ilizarov frame, *J Bone Joint Surg* 85:565–571, 2003. Copyright British Editorial Society of Bone and Joint Surgery.) **SEE TECHNIQUE 4.19.**

wound can be reopened and the osteotomy completed with Lambotte osteotomes, leaving the articular cartilage intact proximally. Examine the osteotomy clinically and radiographically.

■ Attach a half-ring of appropriate size to the three half-pins orientated parallel to the joint line in the anteroposterior and mediolateral planes. Apply a two-ring frame distally perpendicular to the long axis of the tibia and

attach to the half ring using anterior and posterior hinges. Place the hinges opposite the intact articular cartilage at the proximal end of the osteotomy. In the presence of a posterior slope, based on CT, the posterior hinge acts as a distraction hinge to elevate the posterior slope while the anterior hinge is fixed. Position the anterior hinge carefully in the midline over the tibial spine. The hinge must lie over the cartilage-bone junction because the osteotomy hinges here. Two threaded rods, mounted medially, act as motors. Use a 4-mm half-pin and an olive wire at each level for distal ring fixation.

STAGE 2

- The second stage is done after the medial plateau and the regenerate bone consolidates.
- Remove or adjust the Ilizarov frame for lengthening; if necessary, correct rotational deformities. Correct any residual varus.
- In patients with open physes, epiphysiodesis of the proximal fibular and lateral tibial physes should be done with the use of image intensification to prevent recurrence of deformity. The tibia should be lengthened by the amount equal to the anticipated shortening (using a Moseley graph) and the measured leg-length difference.
- Perform a fibular osteotomy at the level of the tibial osteotomy through a longitudinal skin incision using an oscillating saw.
- Using image intensification, mark the site of the proposed tibial osteotomy, and place a Gigli saw subperiosteally with two mini skin incisions.
- Add a half-ring to the existing half-ring over the medial plateau to convert it to a full ring. Attach the proximal tibial using olive wires. Attach the proximal ring block to the existing distal ring block by threaded rods for simple lengthening or derotation devices for correction of rotation if necessary.

- Complete the tibial osteotomy with the Gigli saw, and suture the skin incisions.

POSTOPERATIVE CARE The leg is kept elevated, and a radiograph of the tibia is obtained. Distraction is started 3 to 5 days later under the supervision of a physiotherapist. Weight bearing is allowed as tolerated.

Janoyer et al. used an Orthofix (Gentilly, France) external fixator prototype, which is composed of an upper epiphyseal articulating ring. This allows medial plateau elevation in the orthogonal slope with a posteromedial axis of 10 to 20 degrees. Early results were good with similar complications as other external fixation devices. Van Huyssteen reported a medial plateau elevating tibial osteotomy with lateral epiphysiodesis (performed delayed or concomitantly) for late presenting Blount disease (Fig. 4.59). The advantage of this procedure is that all deformities can be corrected in one operation.

NEUROVASCULAR COMPLICATIONS OF HIGH TIBIAL OSTEOTOMY

Neurovascular complications after an osteotomy for genu varum result most commonly from vascular occlusion or peroneal nerve palsy. Stretching of the anterior tibial artery occurs at the interosseous membrane with varus correction (as for genu valgum), and compression of the artery occurs with valgus correction (as for genu varum). Regardless of the cause, early recognition is mandatory. Immediate diagnosis with

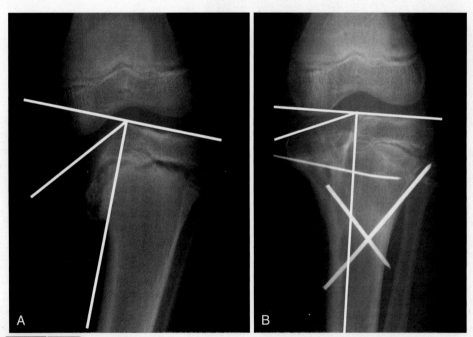

FIGURE 4.59 Anteroposterior radiographs of left knee in 12-year-old boy with stage V Blount disease. **A,** Preoperative radiograph showing angle of depression of medial tibial plateau of 50 degrees and tibial varus angle of 95 degrees. **B,** At 10 months after surgery note recurrent mechanical varus of 5 degrees; the angle of depression of the medial tibial plateau was maintained at 25 degrees but the tibial varus angle increased to 90 degrees because of fusion of the medial tibial physis with an open lateral physis. (From van Huyssteen AL, Olesak M, Hoffman EB: Double-elevating osteotomy for late-presenting infantile Blount's disease, *J Bone Joint Surg* 87:710–715, 2005. Copyright British Editorial Society of Bone and Joint Surgery.)

return of the extremity to the preoperative position of deformity is beneficial regardless of the cause, especially because the causative factors may not be clearly evident in each patient. Sensory loss on the dorsum of the foot and loss of active dorsiflexion of the foot without pain usually are caused by paralysis of the common peroneal nerve. Decrease in dorsiflexion and severe pain on plantar flexion of the toes are the most common clinical signs of occlusion of the artery or of an anterior compartment syndrome. Matsen and Staheli outlined appropriate treatment for each as follows:

1. For traction on the peroneal nerve (more common with varus correction), remove the cast and return the leg to the preoperative position. Remove all pressure on the peroneal nerve, loosen all dressings from the thigh to the toes, and observe closely.
2. For anterior compartment syndrome, remove the cast and return the leg to the preoperative position. Loosen all dressings from the thigh to the toes. If improvement does not occur immediately, fasciotomy without delay is mandatory.
3. For anterior tibial artery occlusion, remove the cast and return the leg to the preoperative position. Loosen all dressings from the thigh to the toes, and observe closely. If immediate improvement is not evident and vascular compromise is present, immediate vascular surgery is indicated.

RICKETS, OSTEOMALACIA, AND RENAL OSTEODYSTROPHY

Rickets is the bony manifestation of altered vitamin D, calcium, and phosphorus metabolism in a child; osteomalacia is the adult form. There are multiple causes of rickets and osteomalacia, but, regardless of the cause of the abnormal metabolism, children with rickets have similar long bone and trunk deformities.

Because vitamin D deficiency has become less common in the United States, rickets and osteomalacia are not often considered as differential diagnoses in patients who have extremity pain or deformity. According to Clarke et al., the children now at greatest risk for vitamin D deficiency are "white, breastfed, protected from the sun, and obese." Rickets can manifest as atypical muscle pain, bowed legs, a pathologic fracture, or slipped capital femoral epiphysis. The orthopaedist should remain familiar with the radiographic and laboratory findings that accompany these diseases. When treating patients with rickets, osteomalacia, or renal dystrophy, the orthopaedist always must be concerned about the effect treatment may have on impaired calcium homeostasis.

In very young children with deformity, treatment of the metabolic defect supplemented by corrective splinting or bracing may correct the deformity (Fig. 4.60). In prepubertal children or adolescents, medical management and bracing usually do not correct an established deformity, and early osteotomy or growth modulation is indicated to ensure that the joints are in a position of function if they became stiff.

Before surgery, management of the metabolic defect with vitamin D, phosphorus, and calcium or other appropriate measures should be done for several months. If the disease is not controlled metabolically, the deformity is likely to recur after corrective osteotomy. Treatment with large doses of

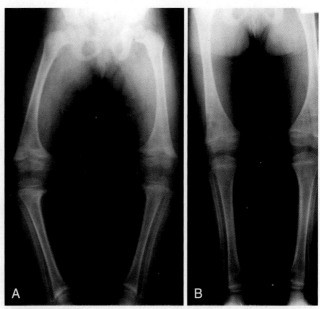

FIGURE 4.60 Vitamin D–deficient rickets. **A,** Standing radiograph of young child with nutritional rickets from vitamin D deficiency. **B,** Same child 18 months later after treatment with vitamin D and braces.

vitamin D should be discontinued for at least 3 weeks before surgery, however, because otherwise hypercalcemia is likely to occur with immobilization.

If a water-soluble preparation of vitamin D, such as dihydrotachysterol, is used instead of cholecalciferol that is stored in the liver, the period without medication before surgery can be shortened. In addition, in hypophosphatemic vitamin D–resistant rickets, if the disease is controlled by using inorganic phosphate plus 50,000 U or less of vitamin D per day, symptoms of hypercalcemia during the immediate postoperative period are less likely to occur, even if the preoperative vitamin D medication is not discontinued. We recommend stopping the administration of vitamin D 3 weeks before surgery, however, because hypercalcemia can cause severe symptoms of anorexia, nausea, vomiting, weight loss, confusion, and seizures. Mobilization of the patient as quickly as possible after surgery to allow early resumption of medical treatment would prevent delayed mineralization of the healing osteotomy and avoid recurrence of deformity with continued growth. When deformity is severe in older children, and there has been no previous medical treatment, after complete diagnostic studies are made, and if the patient does not have renal osteodystrophy, it may be better to proceed with the surgery with the patient in a less than homeostatic but compensated metabolic condition rather than to load the patient preoperatively with high doses of vitamin D, calcium, and phosphorus and run the risk of hypercalcemia and extraosseous calcification, especially in the kidney.

With renal osteodystrophy, expert preoperative and postoperative medical management is essential and ideally is done by a special team trained in the treatment of chronic renal failure. Correction of anemia, adequate hydration, uremia control, and electrolyte balance are required for safe administration of anesthesia. Peritoneal dialysis or hemodialysis may be required before surgery. If attention is given to detail, children with renal osteodystrophy can undergo orthopaedic surgery successfully. Requisites for surgery are a reasonable life

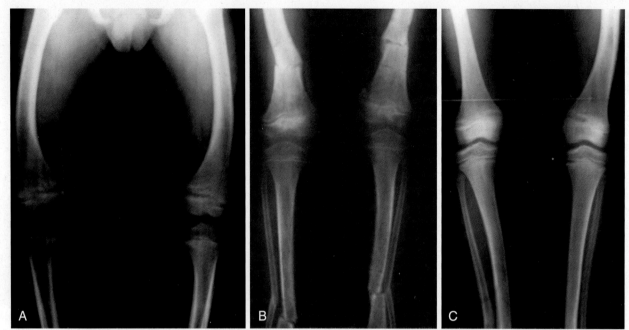

FIGURE 4.61 Vitamin D–resistant rickets. **A,** Child before treatment has deformities in distal femurs. Tibias are not shown in this film. **B,** Three months after valgus osteotomies of distal femurs and tibias using pins incorporated in plaster above and below osteotomy sites. **C,** Two years after osteotomies vitamin D–resistant rickets is well controlled with large doses of vitamin D, calcium, and phosphorus. No deformities have recurred.

expectancy, an intelligent and motivated patient and parents, demonstrated improvement of bone lesions on medical management, deformities that can be corrected with one or two orthopaedic procedures, and the likelihood that the surgery would significantly reduce the patient's disability. Surgery for children with renal osteodystrophy and knee deformities is feasible, but careful surgical planning and preoperative metabolic stabilization are essential. Use of an external fixator can allow precise correction of the deformities without interruption of medical management. Patients with resistant hypertension usually have short life expectancies and should not be considered as surgical candidates. In addition, when parathyroid autonomy is present and not controlled by parathyroidectomy and medical treatment, surgery is not indicated.

The deformities that require surgical correction most often are genu varum and genu valgum. In genu varum, usually the femur, tibia, and fibula all are deformed, often the latter two more severely; there is not only lateral bowing but also internal torsion. Osteotomy of the tibia and the fibula near the apex of the most severe bowing usually is required. Sometimes osteotomy of the femur also is necessary (Fig. 4.61). Osteotomies can be done bilaterally at one operation.

In genu valgum, most of the bowing usually is in the femur, and a severe deformity in older children and in adults can be corrected by supracondylar osteotomy of the femur. The goal of tibial and femoral osteotomies should be correction of deformity and alignment so that the plane of each knee joint is perfectly horizontal with the patient standing.

In addition to osteotomy, guided-growth modulation with hemiepiphysiodesis has had promising results, especially in X-linked hypophosphatemic rickets. Coronal plane correction with appropriate medical management can decrease the need for osteotomy; however, if appropriate medical management is not secured, recurrence is common after correction and removal of implants.

The techniques of osteotomy are described in other chapter.

HEMOPHILIA

Elective surgery for patients with classic hemophilia (factor VIII deficiency), hemophilia A and Christmas disease (factor IX deficiency), or hemophilia B has become possible and reasonable with the availability of factor VIII and factor IX concentrates. Previously, only lifesaving surgery was performed and mortality was high. Wound hematomas with massive sloughs and infection were common. Catastrophic complications can be minimized only by expert management and strict control of the clotting mechanism, and surgery in patients with hemophilia must not be undertaken casually. Bracing and casting techniques, such as the spring-loaded Dynasplint, can be used along with physical therapy to protect joints or to stretch soft-tissue contractures. These measures may be as important as hematologic management in avoiding surgery.

The current popularity of home therapy for hemophilic patients with self-administration of factor VIII or IX as soon as periarticular stiffness and pain occur may result in a lower incidence of degenerative arthritis and in fewer indications for major reconstructive procedures. Factor given prophylactically from age 1 or 2 years through adolescence (preventing the factor VIII concentration from decreasing to <1 of normal) seems to prevent hemophilic arthropathy, and only minor joint defects have been noted. The National Hemophiliac Foundation recommends prophylactic factor; however, prophylactic factor given daily has to be given intravenously, which increases the possibility of contamination and infection. Also, the use of ultrasound to determine early soft-tissue bleeds has been recommended to aid in the use of prophylactic factor.

Three changes have been noted regarding surgery in hemophiliacs: (1) a decrease in the need for surgery Tobase et al. showed a 5.6% decrease in need for invasive orthopaedic intervention in people with hemophilia over the previous 11 years, likely due to improved outpatient medical management, (2) an increase in the age of the patient, and (3) changes in types of operations. The indications for surgery include the following:

1. Chronic, progressive hypertrophic synovial enlargement from repeated hemarthrosis that cannot be controlled by adequate factor replacement; preferably, synovectomy is done before the cartilage becomes thin and at least some of the articular cartilage is preserved. Timely synovectomy also may decrease the incidence of hemorrhage into the joint. This can be done by intraarticular radioisotope injection, arthroscopically, or with an open procedure.
2. Severe soft-tissue contractures that have not responded to nonoperative measures (e.g., a knee flexion contracture that is so severe that serial casting or a turn-buckle casting technique causes subluxation of the knee joint); supracondylar osteotomy of the femur has been beneficial in this instance, provided that 70 to 80 degrees of knee motion remains and the contracture is not so severe that correction would result in excessive traction on the neurovascular bundle in the popliteal space. For correction of a knee flexion contracture of less than 45 degrees after conservative measures have failed, good results have been reported with hamstring release and posterior transverse capsulotomy. Correction by osteotomy of a contracture of more than 50 to 60 degrees probably should be done in stages and preferably after physeal closure.
3. A bony deformity severe enough to require osteotomy.
4. An expanding hematoma (pseudotumor) that continues to enlarge despite adequate factor replacement and possibly radiation therapy.
5. Useless or chronically infected extremities (amputation).
6. Severe arthritic changes with incapacitating pain and hemorrhage (total joint arthroplasty) (Fig. 4.62).

Successful surgery in hemophilia depends on a close working relationship between the orthopaedist and an experienced hematologist. All hematologic aspects of the patient's care must be the responsibility of the hematologist, including a hematologic team consisting of a hematologic nurse, surgeon, and physical therapist.

The hemorrhagic disorder must be diagnosed accurately before surgery is contemplated. Correct replacement of coagulation factors cannot be undertaken without precise identification and quantitation of the missing factor. Adequate reserve supplies of concentrate must be available in advance, and the supporting laboratory must be able to perform unlimited assays for the factor. It also is essential to determine within a few days of the operation whether the patient has developed an inhibitor against his or her deficient factor because the inhibitor hinders hematologic therapy and may eliminate the possibility of elective or semielective surgery. A bypass agent (described later) should be available at the time to counteract an inhibitor. In addition, a factor assay should be obtained at the time of surgery. The hematocrit should be measured for several days after surgery, especially in blood groups A, B, and AB, because a Coombs-positive hemolytic

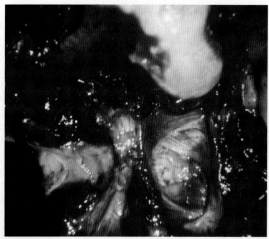

FIGURE 4.62 Damaged knee joint with hemophilia (factor VIII deficiency). *Upper right,* Marked destruction and erosion of articular surface of femoral condyle. *Center,* Anterior cruciate ligament and intercondylar notch. Tibial plateaus are grossly eroded, and articular surfaces and menisci are destroyed by invasion of synovium.

anemia may develop. The patient's HIV and hepatitis status should be known before surgery. In patients with HIV or hepatitis, the extent of involvement should be investigated. T lymphocyte counts and other parameters should be known to determine the ability to heal and the potential for infection. Fortunately, HIV and hepatitis that were prevalent in the 1990s have almost disappeared in the hemophiliac population because of the use of "clean" factor.

Post and Telfer emphasized meticulous surgical technique and detailed preoperative evaluation in this surgery. They recommended (1) as many procedures at one surgical session as the patient can tolerate—this reduces the times that the patient is at risk of bleeding complications and hepatitis and reduces the high cost of the concentrate and the possibility of inducing an inhibitor; (2) meticulous aseptic technique and pneumatic tourniquets whenever possible; (3) tight, careful wound closure to avoid dead space; (4) avoidance of electrocautery because of the tendency of the coagulated areas to slough after surgery; (5) wound suction in deep wounds for a minimum of 24 hours; (6) no aspirin or other medications postoperatively that inhibit platelet function; and (7) as far as possible, no intramuscular injections postoperatively for pain relief.

When coagulation is controlled with hematologic therapy, wound slough or infection usually does not occur. Pain relief and a substantial decrease in recurrent bleeding into joints usually result.

With the availability of factor, elective orthopaedic surgery can be safely performed utilizing a multidisciplinary team approach; however, an inhibitor is a life-threatening risk factor and a major risk factor for infection. Factor VII and IX "bypassing" agents have been used to counteract inhibitors and obtain hemostatic control after surgery. With the use of recombinant activated factor VII (RFVIIa) and plasma-activated prothrombin complex concentrates (pd-APCC), elective orthopaedic surgery is a viable option for hemophiliac patients with inhibitors. For minor surgery (100%) and for major surgery (85% to 100%) coagulation, a bolus of the RFVIIa usually is given with continuous infusion. This "inhibitor" surgery should not be taken lightly and should only be performed with an experienced hematologist team at a specialized hemophiliac center.

TOTAL JOINT ARTHROPLASTY

Synovectomy or total knee arthroplasty may be cost effective in that the cost of hematologic maintenance (concentrate) is markedly lower after surgery. Total knee arthroplasty should be considered only if hemophilic arthritis is advanced and range of motion is adequate because the arthroplasty is unlikely to increase motion. Careful examination of the quadriceps mechanism and correction of any flexion contracture of more than 30 degrees are recommended before surgery. We also suspect that late complications similar to those seen in rheumatoid arthritis would develop because of disuse osteopenia (Fig. 4.63). Because most candidates for total knee arthroplasty in hemophilic arthropathy are relatively young, all other means of relieving the symptoms should be attempted first, such as hyaluronic acid injection (viscosupplementation) in milder disease, radiosynovectomy, or arthroscopic synovectomy. Most often, both knees are involved, and bilateral arthroplasties are indicated, although arthrodesis of one knee and total knee arthroplasty of the other is a reasonable alternative to bilateral arthroplasty, provided that motion in the knee selected for arthroplasty is 80 to 90 degrees preoperatively.

Reports in the literature, although not conclusive, state that hemophiliac patients are less prone to venous thrombosis because of their disease than the normal population, and the same is true for those undergoing major orthopaedic surgery, including synovectomy and total joint replacement. Even so, a postoperative compression device, early ambulation, and joint mobilization with physical therapy are recommended. Routine use of antithrombotic agents prophylactically is controversial and not recommended in the face of an inhibitor. The exception is the hemophiliac patient undergoing major orthopaedic surgery with risk factors for venous thrombosis, such as a history of venous thromboembolism, obesity, malignancy, and varicose veins, or women with von Willebrand disease taking oral contraception. If prophylaxis is for venous thrombosis, enoxaparin has been used successfully.

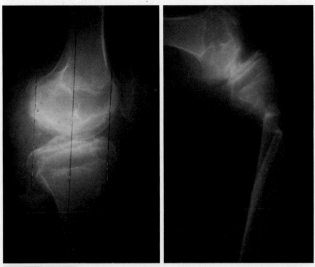

FIGURE **4.63** Late complications of hemophilic arthropathy. Note osteopenia and resulting fractures owing to manipulation.

Surgical infection in this patient population is related to lack of meticulous technique and the amount and length of time factor is given. Most series report an 8% infection rate if factor is given less than 2 weeks and much lower than 8% if given for 2 weeks with the patient 100% "covered." Continuous factor should be given for 2 weeks after total knee or total hip arthroplasty at 100%.

Total hip arthroplasty is an appropriate operation for disabling hemophilic hip arthropathy. In the shoulder or elbow, we have little or no experience with arthroplasty in these joints in hemophiliacs. In the ankle, there are several small series in the literature of total ankle arthroplasty being done in hemophiliacs with encouraging results.

SYNOVECTOMY

Although synovectomy of joints can decrease pain and the number of bleeding episodes in patients with hemophilia, it does not seem to alter the course of joint destruction. We performed 16 synovectomies of the knee in 14 children, adolescents, and young adults with hemophilia. Pain was eliminated or decreased in all patients, and the number of bleeding episodes dramatically decreased in all patients at 3-year follow-up. Some knee motion was lost in five patients. At long-term follow-up (average 9 years) of nine of these patients (11 knees), decreases in pain and frequency of bleeding episodes were sustained, but arthropathy had progressed in all 11 knees, and 8 knees had lost motion compared with short-term follow-up. A disturbing finding in this group of patients was that at long-term follow-up all nine were either HIV positive or had developed acquired immunodeficiency syndrome (AIDS). Fortunately, HIV-contaminated factor has virtually been eliminated.

Both open and arthroscopic synovectomies of the knee in patients with "classic" hemophilia can reduce hemarthrosis; however, the arthroscopic procedure seems to be less complete but have less morbidity. Although arthroscopy may require a longer operative time, it requires shorter hospitalization and less factor replacement.

The elbow is a frequent site (second only to the knee) of repeated hemorrhage followed by enlargement of the radial head and degenerative arthritis of the radiocapitellar and ulnar-trochlear articulations. The ankle is a common site as well and is a frequent cause of morbidity. We have been pleased with the pain relief resulting from synovectomy of the elbow joint and excision of the radial head. Improvement in flexion and extension of the elbow cannot be expected, but increased forearm rotation frequently results.

Synovectomy also has proven beneficial for hemophilic arthropathy of the ankle. Open synovectomy or arthroscopic synovectomy can be performed because removal of the posterior synovial tissue from the crypts of the malleoli is difficult and may injure the articular cartilage even with the use of the posterolateral portal and distraction of the joint arthroscopically may be difficult.

Ankle, knee, and elbow arthroscopic synovectomy are described in *Foot and Ankle Surgery*.

Radionuclide synovectomy, or radiosynovectomy (destruction of synovial tissue by intraarticular injection of a radioactive agent), has produced encouraging results. The procedure has little morbidity and can be done on an outpatient basis in the radiology department. The isotope appears to shrink the outer layer of synovium, decreasing pain, bleeding, and the recurrence rate.

Improved range of motion and decreased frequency of hemorrhage have been reported in nearly 80% of adult patients treated with radiosynovectomy of the elbow or knee using chromic phosphate P32 and 0.5 to 1 mCi of yttrium-90 silicate, depending on the joint involved. New isotopes using holmium-166-chitosan 186Re complex have been advocated. In situations where radioisotopes are not available, chemical synovectomy can be used with rifampicin. Two to three injections may be necessary (at 6-month intervals), and if not successful then a surgical synovectomy should be performed. Radiosynovectomy appears to be most effective when done early, before the synovium enlarges. Because most recurrent joint hemorrhages begin in early childhood, this procedure would be useful in the prevention of bony joint damage in children with hemophilia who have developed chronic hemarthrosis or synovitis. The long-term effects on joints in children, such as premature physeal closure or irritation, are not known. Most of the literature recommends radioisotope synovectomy at age 12 or older using yttrium-90 at a dose of 90 mBq in children, viscosupplementation with stearic acid and joint lavage, or holmium-16-chitosan complex. If not effective, chemical synovectomy with rifampicin can be used. If needed earlier than 12 years, a surgical synovectomy should be performed. The long-term effects on joints in children, such as premature physeal closure or tumor formation, are unknown, however. Two patients with hemophilia who developed acute lymphoblastic leukemia after radionuclide synovectomy have been reported.

In our experience, short-term results of radionuclide synovectomy of the ankle and knee in children and adults have been encouraging because the nuclide seems to be able to penetrate posteriorly; however, the recurrence rate (need for a second radiosynovectomy) seems to be higher than for open or arthroscopic synovectomy.

SYNOVECTOMY OF THE KNEE IN HEMOPHILIA

TECHNIQUE 4.20

- Inflate a pneumatic tourniquet around the thigh.
- Through a medial parapatellar incision (see Technique 1.48), remove as much synovium from the knee capsule as possible. Removal of all synovium from the lateral gutter is extremely difficult, and considerable hemorrhage usually occurs in this area.
- Remove synovium from the medial joint space, including over and around the medial meniscus and collateral ligament. Remove synovium from the intercondylar notch and anterior cruciate ligament and finally from the lateral joint space.
- Release the tourniquet, and obtain meticulous hemostasis with electrocautery; this may require more time than the removal of the synovium.
- Tightly close the capsule and soft tissues in layers to obliterate any dead space; insert a closed suction drainage tube.
- If the medial capsule is redundant, oversew it to prevent recurrent dislocation of the patella.

POSTOPERATIVE CARE The knee is immobilized for 24 hours, then motion is initiated with the aid of the physical therapist and a continuous passive motion machine, if available. The drain is removed at 48 hours under adequate clotting factor replacement. Physical therapy is continued for 6 weeks; the continuous passive motion machine can be used at home.

■ ARTHROSCOPIC SYNOVECTOMY

Arthroscopic synovectomy is described in other chapter.

SYNOVIORTHESIS FOR TREATMENT OF HEMOPHILIC ARTHROPATHY

TECHNIQUE 4.21

- Replacement therapy for hemostasis at the time of the synoviorthesis is the same as that used for minor operations. For patients in whom an inhibitor is present, synoviorthesis is sometimes done without preparation for hemostasis.
- Using aseptic technique, anesthetize the skin with 2% procaine (without epinephrine) with a 23-gauge needle. Note free flow of procaine indicating the introduction of the needle into the intraarticular space.
- Withdraw synovial fluid when possible.
- Inject 2 to 5 mL of contrast medium, and with radiography ensure there is no obvious leak from the synovial space. Inject colloidal chromic phosphate P32 (Phosphocol P32) intraarticularly.
- Use 1 mCi for knees and 0.5 mCi for other joints.
- Flush the needle with 2% lidocaine and remove.
- Apply a sterile plastic bandage and an appropriate immobilizer.

POSTOPERATIVE CARE The patient can bear weight immediately, but activity should be decreased for 48 hours.

■ OPEN ANKLE SYNOVECTOMY

Transfusion of the missing clotting factor (factor VIII or IX) is based on the previously described protocol. Approximately 2 hours before the operation, the patient is given a transfusion to increase the level of the deficient clotting factor to close to 100%. Open synovectomy of the ankle is done through anteromedial, anterolateral, and posterior incisions.

OPEN ANKLE SYNOVECTOMY IN HEMOPHILIA

TECHNIQUE 4.22

(GREENE)
- Place a sandbag underneath the ipsilateral buttock to facilitate positioning of the ankle for the anterior portion of the synovectomy.

- Make an anteromedial incision 3 cm long just medial to the anterior tibial tendon.
- Retract the anterior tibial tendon laterally, and retract the branches of the saphenous vein medially.
- Make a longitudinal incision in the joint capsule. Preserve the capsule even though it is stretched and attenuated by the underlying hypertrophic synovial tissue because its presence may facilitate postoperative rehabilitation. Free the joint capsule from the adherent synovial tissue by sharp dissection.
- Remove all visible synovial tissue. Use small pituitary rongeurs to remove folds of synovial tissue that extend into the crypts between the talus and the medial malleolus.
- Make a 3-cm long anterolateral incision centered just lateral to the peroneus tertius tendon, and retract this tendon medially.
- Open the joint capsule longitudinally, and excise the synovial tissue in the same manner described for the anteromedial incision.
- Resect the folds of synovial tissue interposed between the talus and the lateral malleolus.
- Remove the sandbag beneath the ipsilateral buttock, and place it beneath the contralateral buttock before making the posterior incision. Make a posterior incision approximately twice as long as the anterior incision, and center it between the medial malleolus and the Achilles tendon. Open the sheath of the posterior tibial tendon so that it can be retracted adequately. Dissect the other posterior tendons and the neurovascular structures away from the posterior portion of the capsule of the ankle joint.
- Place a retractor lateral to the flexor hallucis muscle and medial to the posterior tibial tendon, permitting retraction of the soft-tissue structures located posterior to the ankle joint. This provides full exposure of the posterior portion of the capsule. Incise the capsule horizontally from the medial malleolus to the distal end of the fibula.
- Dissect the insertion of synovial tissue on the talus and the distal end of the tibia. Use pituitary rongeurs to remove any residual folds of synovial tissue lying in the crypts of the malleoli. If the synovium cannot be removed from the capsule, or the capsule appears intimately involved, removal of large sections of the capsule may be necessary. According to Greene, postoperative rehabilitation may be impeded by extensive scar reaction in the posterior capsule.
- When the synovectomy has been completed, deflate the pneumatic tourniquet and secure hemostasis meticulously.
- Repair the anterior portion of the capsule, but leave the posterior portion open and place a drain. Close the wounds in a standard fashion and immobilize the ankle joint in a neutral position with a bulky dressing augmented by a plaster of Paris splint.

POSTOPERATIVE CARE Patients who have factor VIII deficiency should receive continuous transfusion therapy, and patients with factor IX deficiency should be given a bolus of factor IX every 12 hours. Transfusion should be continued throughout the hospital stay (7 to 10 days). After discharge, transfusion is given three times a week for 4 weeks. This regimen keeps the deficient clotting factor level sufficiently elevated to minimize the risk of a spontaneous hemarthrosis during the immediate postoperative period while the soft-tissue reaction is resolving. The drain is removed on the first postoperative day, and active range-of-motion exercises with the aid of hydrotherapy are begun on postoperative day 2. Initially, weight bearing is not permitted. Also, the ankle is intermittently splinted in a neutral position until range of motion of the ankle from neutral dorsiflexion to 25 degrees of plantar flexion is obtained. The hematologist and the surgeon determine discharge from the hospital. Walking with crutches with touch-down weight bearing is continued for approximately 5 weeks after discharge from the hospital.

ARTHRODESIS
Arthrodesis of the ankle, shoulder, and knee has been satisfactory in small series of patients with hemophilia. The use of internal fixation rather than external fixators that require transcutaneous pins is recommended to reduce bleeding and infection around the pins (Fig. 4.64). Fixed flexion contractures can be corrected by removing appropriate bone wedges at the time of arthrodesis.

OSTEOTOMY
For hemophilic patients with symptomatic bony deformities, osteotomies may be necessary. In patients with symptomatic genu varum deformities, proximal valgus closing wedge osteotomies may be done.

COMPLICATIONS OF HEMOPHILIA
A rare, yet disabling and frequently life-threatening complication, iliac hemophilic pseudotumor occurs in 1% to 2% of patients with factor VIII deficiency. Two types of pseudotumors have been identified: one occurs primarily in the femur or pelvis in adults and has an exceptionally poor prognosis, and one occurs more distally in the extremities in children and has a better prognosis. Recommended treatment includes factor replacement, immobilization, close observation, and avoidance of cyst aspiration. Operative resection for the adult-type pseudotumor may be life threatening, and amputation should be considered. Preoperative consideration of the tumor size and degree of infiltration is crucial in operative management. Early excision eliminates the possibility of endogenous infection. Partial resection of huge tumors that leave the lateral wall intact for compression and recovery of function may be preferable to excision of the entire wall, leaving a huge dead space that allows massive hematoma and sepsis. Several studies have shown early promising results using radiation for pseudotumors that are inaccessible or inappropriate for resection.

In addition to involvement of various joints, nerve lesions are common in patients with hemophilia. Katz et al. described 81 such peripheral nerve lesions. The femoral nerve was the most commonly involved, followed by the median nerve and the ulnar nerve. In 49% of the lesions, the nerves had full motor and sensory recovery after significant bleeds. In 34%, a residual sensory deficit (normal motor) was present, and in 16% persistent motor and sensory deficits were present. Patients who had inhibitors to factor VIII were significantly less likely to recover full motor or sensory function than patients who did not have antibodies, and time to full motor recovery in these patients was significantly longer.

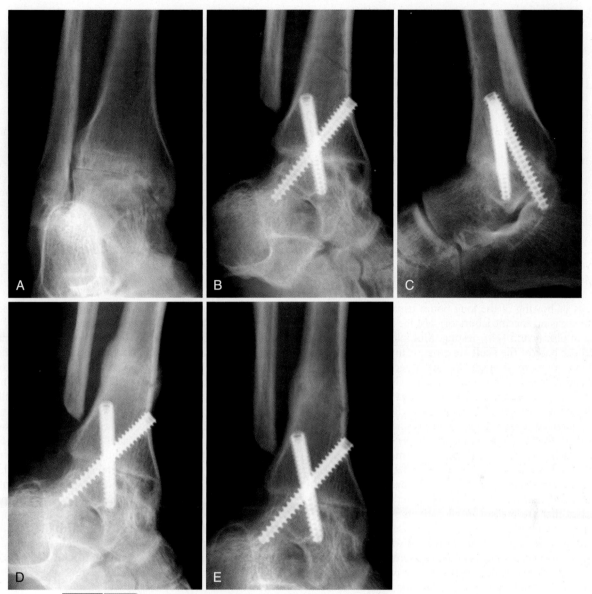

FIGURE 4.64   **A,** Preoperative radiograph of severe hemophilic arthropathy and painful swollen ankle. **B** and **C,** Postoperative radiographs of cross-threaded screw fixation. At 6 months, distal tibial pain and stress fracture are noted. **D,** At 12 months, stress fracture callus is noted but no pain. **E,** At 24 months, there is solid fusion. Stress fracture has resolved.

Hemophilia-related AIDS was first reported in the United States in 1981. Current estimates of the percentage of hemophilic patients with HIV antibodies range from 30% to 90%. Before 1985, it was estimated that 90% of patients seen in hemophiliac clinics were HIV positive, and a large percentage of patients also had laboratory evidence of hepatitis. The Centers for Disease Control and Prevention estimated that 9000 hemophiliacs, or 45% of the hemophiliac population, contracted AIDS and that 1900 patients died as the result of AIDS. The screening for the presence of HIV in blood and blood products for transfusion since 1985 and the development of monoclonal antibodies to factor VIII and of synthetically derived blood products have decreased the rate of transmission markedly. Because of this increased risk of HIV infection in hemophilic patients, albeit now small, orthopaedic surgeons treating these patients should observe not only the universal precautions recommended by the Centers for

Disease Control and Prevention but also the recommendations of the American Academy of Orthopaedic Surgeons Task Force on AIDS and Orthopaedic Surgery.

CONGENITAL AFFECTIONS

Most affections of bone seemingly of congenital origin may respond favorably to surgery. The surgical treatment of enchondromatosis (Ollier disease) and of hereditary multiple exostoses is described in other chapter.

OSTEOGENESIS IMPERFECTA

Osteogenesis imperfecta is a disease apparently of the mesodermal tissues with abnormal or deficient collagen that has been shown in bone, skin, sclerae, and dentin. The so-called diagnostic triad of blue sclerae, dentinogenesis imperfecta, and generalized osteoporosis in a patient with multiple

TABLE 4.7			
Sillence Classification of Osteogenesis Imperfecta (Simplified)			
TYPE	**INHERITANCE**	**SCLERAE**	**FEATURES**
Type I	Autosomal dominant	Blue	Mildest form. Presents at preschool age (tarda). Hearing deficit in 50%. Divided into type A and B based on tooth involvement
Type II	Autosomal recessive	Blue	Lethal in perinatal period
Type III	Autosomal recessive	Normal	Fractures at birth. Progressively short stature. Most severe survivable form
Type IV	Autosomal dominant	Normal	Moderate severity. Bowing bones and vertebral fractures are common. Hearing normal. Divided into type A and B based on tooth involvement
Type V			Hypertrophic callus after fracture. Ossification of IOM between radius and ulna and tibia and fibula
Type VI			Moderate severity. Similar to type IV
Type VII			Associated with rhizomelia and coxa vara

Type V, VI, VII have been added to the original classification system (these have no type I collagen mutation but have abnormal bone on microscopy and a similar phenotype). IOM, interosseous membrane.

fractures or bowing of the long bones usually is used clinically. There is no specific laboratory test for this disease other than skin biopsy and DNA testing. Multiple wormian bones around the base of the skull are a major finding only in the congenital type of osteogenesis imperfecta. Osteogenesis imperfecta congenita is characterized at birth by multiple fractures, bowing of the long bones, short extremities, and generalized osteoporosis. The most used classification noted in the literature is by Sillence, who originally classified the disease into four types, although it is likely that osteogenesis imperfecta is a continuum (Table 4.7). Since Sillence's classification, additional types have been added. Ninety percent of patients are type I or IV. Although many children with osteogenesis imperfecta have blue sclerae, the only two characteristics that are present in all patients with osteogenesis imperfecta are fractures and generalized osteoporosis.

Orthopaedic surgery is most involved with the bowing of the long bones in osteogenesis imperfecta tarda type 1, in which progressively increasing deformities may cause deterioration in activity of these children from walkers to sitters and from braceable to unbraceable. Healing of fractures and osteotomies usually is satisfactory, although the healed bone may be no stronger than the original. Hyperplastic callus occasionally is seen after fractures and osteotomies, although difficult and persistent nonunions have been noted. Because of frequently frail and disabling bone and joint deformities and fractures that preclude ambulation, a comprehensive rehabilitation program with long leg bracing has been suggested to result in a high level of functional activity with an acceptable level of risk of fracture in children with osteogenesis imperfecta. Results of surgery in these patients have been inconsistent, with frequent complications reported. Patients should be examined for scoliosis before surgical procedures are undertaken because thoracic scoliosis of greater than 60 degrees has severe adverse effects on pulmonary function in patients with osteogenesis imperfecta, which may partly explain the increased pulmonary morbidity in adult patients with osteogenesis imperfecta and scoliosis compared with that in the general population. Besides pulmonary problems other anesthetic complications can occur such as difficulty in positioning the patient, malignant hyperthermia, basilar invagination, cardiac abnormalities, or bleeding from platelet dysfunction. Although a transfusion rate of 14% was noted in one series of patients with

osteogenesis imperfecta treated with intramedullary rods, the blood loss was described as low and manageable.

The use of bisphosphonates has been shown to reduce osteoclast-mediated bone resorption. Intravenous administration of bisphosphonates, such as pamidronate, zoledronate, and risedronate, has been shown to decrease bone pain and incidence of fracture and to increase bone density and level of ambulation with minimal side effects. Increase in size of vertebral bodies and thickening of cortical bone also have been reported. There are no standardized guidelines for initiating bisphosphonate treatment in children. A Cochrane review showed that both intravenous or oral bisphosphonates are effective at increasing bone density, but which medication and dosing regimens are optimal and how long patients should be treated have not been established. Furthermore, no regimen was found that consistently reduced the fracture rate, although multiple independent studies did show a reduction in fracture rate. Furthermore, no study showed an increased rate of fractures given the well-studied topic of atypical femoral fractures with bisphosphonate use. Finally, there was no clear improvement in pain or functional mobility. The authors of the review concluded that the optimal type, duration, and safety of bisphosphonate use require further study. Besides fracture procedures (e.g., intramedullary rods) elective procedures, such as total joint arthroplasty and, spine surgery, including scoliosis surgery, are being reported with increasing frequency.

■ MULTIPLE OSTEOTOMIES, REALIGNMENT, AND MEDULLARY NAIL FIXATION

The most successful surgical method of treating the deformities of osteogenesis imperfecta is based on the work of Sofield and Millar who used a method of multiple osteotomies, realignment of fragments, and medullary nail fixation for long bones (Fig. 4.65).

Complications reported with the telescoping rod include fracture at the tip of the rod, proximal migration secondary to angular deformity, and eccentric rod positioning at the distal physis, and rod cut out (Fig. 4.66). Even so, the telescoping rod appears to be superior to the nontelescoping rod. In one study, the 3-year survival rate of the telescoping rod was 92.9% compared with 7.2% of the nontelescoping rod, and the reoperation rate was 7.2% compared with 31.6%, respectively.

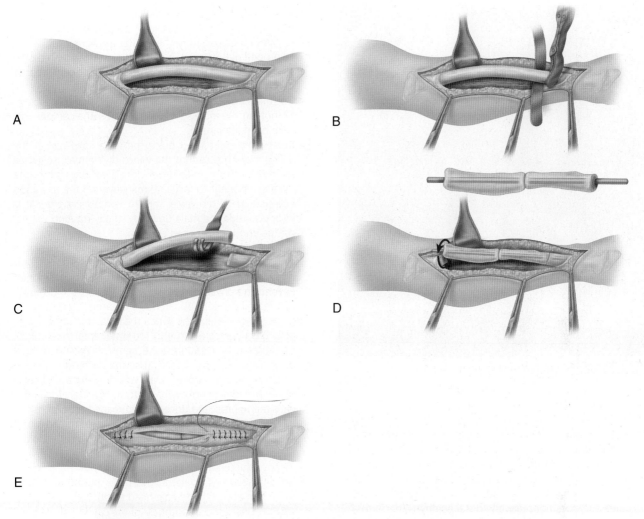

FIGURE 4.65 **A to E,** Technique for fragmentation and realignment of bone and insertion of medullary nail. **A-C,** Exposure and removal of shaft. **D,** Osteotomies. **E,** Closure. (From Sofield HA, Millar EA: Fragmentation, realignment, and intramedullary rod fixation of deformities of the long bones in children: a 10-year appraisal, *J Bone Joint Surg* 41:1371–1391, 1959.)

A more recent study compared survival of Fassier-Duval rods to static implants and found that the risk of failure of static implants was 13 times that of the risk with Fassier-Duval rods. For these reasons, we have been using the Fassier-Duval elongating intramedullary rod system.

For the tibia, to allow use of the longest possible medullary rod, Williams reported a technique in which an extension is screwed onto the distal end of the rod and is pushed through the distal tibia and out the sole of the foot. After the fragments of the tibia are realigned, the nail is reinserted in a retrograde fashion until the distal end lies just proximal to the surface of the ankle joint. The extension is unscrewed, leaving the rod extending only into the distal tibial epiphysis.

■ FASSIER-DUVAL TELESCOPING ROD (PEGA MEDICAL, INC., LAVAL, QUEBEC, CANADA)

Fassier-Duval and other intramedullary devices have been used for humeral and forearm deformities, with reported improvements in functional scores (Fig. 4.67).

This expandable rod is designed for children with osteogenesis imperfecta to prevent or stabilize fractures or correct deformity of the long bones during growth. It is indicated for children 18 months of age or older. It has been designed for use in the femur, tibia, and humerus. The main advantage is its easy placement and better fixation in the physis of long bones. As compared with other expandable rods, an open or percutaneous osteotomy technique can be employed for the femur. For patients with large bones and thin cortices, a percutaneous technique is recommended. For the tibia an open osteotomy technique is recommended.

FASSIER-DUVAL TELESCOPING ROD, FEMUR

TECHNIQUE 4.23

OPEN OSTEOTOMY
■ Through a posterolateral approach, expose the femur subperiosteally.

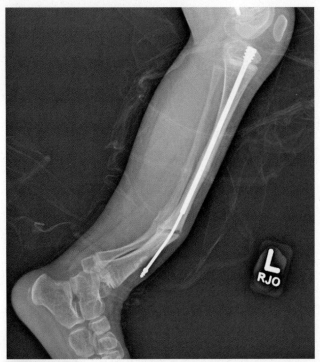

Cut-out of telescoping rod.

- Perform an osteotomy under C-arm guidance (Fig. 4.68A and B).
- With a cannulated reamer, ream the proximal fragment or drill up to the greater trochanter over a small-diameter guidewire. The diameter of the reamer should be 0.25 to 0.35 mm larger than the diameter of the nail implant size chosen. Prepare the distal fragment in same fashion. If the guidewire does not reach the distal epiphysis, perform a second osteotomy after reaming the intermediate fragment (Fig. 4.68C).
- Insert a male-size Kirschner wire retrograde from the direction of the osteotomy through the proximal fragment (Fig. 4.68D).
- Make a second incision at the buttock to allow the extremity of the Kirschner wire to exit proximally (Fig. 4.68E).

PERCUTANEOUS OSTEOTOMY

- If a percutaneous technique for osteotomy is chosen, insert a small-diameter guidewire through the greater trochanter into the apex of the deformity. Ream the femur to the appropriate size with a cannulated reamer (Fig. 4.68F).
- Through a 0.5-cm incision perform the first osteotomy in the convexity of the deformity just distal to the reamer (Fig. 4.68G).
- Apply counterpressure at the osteotomy site, and with gentle manipulation progressively correct the deformity. When the bone is straightened, push the guidewire distally and advance the reamer accordingly (Fig. 4.68H).
- Push the guidewire distally to the apex of the second deformity, then perform a second osteotomy as described for the first osteotomy until the length of the medullary canal has been reamed to just before the physis (Fig. 4.68I).

TELESCOPING ROD INSERTION

- After a corrective osteotomy is completed, estimate the length of the bone from the greater trochanter to the distal growth plate. Based on the height of the distal epiphysis as measured on an anteroposterior radiograph, choose a long (L) or short (S) nail.
- Cut the length of the female hollow component to size. Do not cut the male solid nail until after the components have been implanted.
- Remove the wire, and place the male solid nail in the driver, making sure that the wings of the male solid nail are fitted into the male driver slot. These drivers lock the male component to facilitate maneuvering the nail upon insertion. Lock the male implant component after it is inserted inside the male driver by simply rotating the eccentric ring to the locked position.
- Push the male solid nail distally after reduction of the osteotomy(ies), and screw it into the distal epiphysis. Verify with fluoroscopy that the distal thread is positioned beyond the physis (Fig. 4.68J to L). Center the distal tip of the nail on anteroposterior and lateral views on the distal femoral epiphysis. Once the male implant component has been screwed into the distal epiphysis, unlock the implant by rotating the eccentric ring and remove the male driver (Fig. 4.68M). Use the pushrod to reduce stress to the nail fixation while withdrawing the driver.
- Screw the female hollow nail into the greater trochanter with the appropriate driver. The threaded portion of the nail is inserted into bone (at least one or two threads), and the nonthreaded part of the female head is inserted in the nonossified part of the greater trochanter (Fig. 4.68N).
- Remove the female driver.
- Cut the solid nail (male) at this time, leaving a stub 10 to 15 mm above the female head for future growth (Fig. 4.68O). Check the smoothness of the cut end of the male nail with an appropriately sized probe.
- Close the incisions.

POSTOPERATIVE CARE The limb is immobilized until the osteotomies heal.

■ OSTEOTOMY AND MEDULLARY NAILING WITH LOCKED NAIL

In an older child in whom disturbance of the physis would not cause a significant growth problem, a small-diameter medullary nail can be used, with or without proximal or distal locking. There are several locked nails that come in sizes as small as 7 mm, and we have used this successfully in several older children with osteogenesis imperfecta. The guidewire is passed, in a closed manner, proximally to the point of angulation (Fig. 4.69A). Through a small incision, an osteotomy is made at this site where the guidewire is impeded (Fig. 4.69B). The medullary nail is inserted in a closed manner and locked proximally and distally. The nail should extend as far distally as possible to prevent fracture distal to it. The technique for insertion of an interlocking medullary rod is described in other chapter.

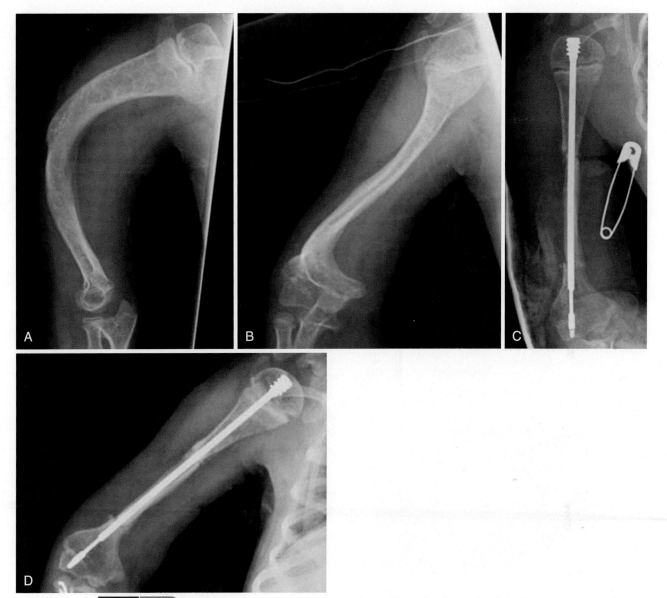

FIGURE 4.67 **A** and **B,** Preoperative anteroposterior and lateral radiographs of the humerus showing an angular deformity of more than 90 degrees. **C** and **D,** Postoperative radiographs showing correction of angular deformity and stabilization with an expandable Fassier-Duval rod. (From Ashby E, Montpetit K, Hamdy R, et al: Functional outcome of humeral rodding in children with osteogenesis imperfecta, *J Pediatr Orthop* 38:49–53, 2018.)

DWARFISM (SHORT STATURE)

Dwarfism with disproportionate shortness of the trunk or extremities has many different causes and is commonly difficult to classify, but certain orthopaedic problems are common to many of these patients. The main areas of concern to orthopaedic surgeons are atlantoaxial instability, hip dysplasia, and malalignment of the lower extremities.

Cervical myelopathy and anomalies of the cervical spine are especially common in dwarfs with a disproportionately short trunk and are rare in achondroplasia. Dwarfs with a short trunk may exhibit a rudimentary or absent odontoid process with ligamentous laxity and resultant atlantoaxial instability.

The first symptoms of myelopathy are a decrease in physical endurance and an early fatigue without neurologic deficit. Neurologic signs may develop later. Cord compression occurs because of bony displacement, ligamentous instability, and hypertrophy of the posterior longitudinal ligament. Often the spinal cord shifts laterally within the canal and accounts for the unilateral neurologic signs and symptoms. Cord compression also can occur at the foramen magnum (achondroplastic dwarfs) or secondary to severe cervical kyphosis from ligamentous laxity. The diagnosis of atlantoaxial instability can be made from lateral flexion and extension radiographic views or with cineradiography. Cervical fusion generally is indicated only when (1) there are obvious clinical signs of compression myelopathy or (2) there is obliteration of the subarachnoid space around the cord in flexion or extension as seen on gas myelography. Atlantoaxial instability shown on radiographs or cineradiography is not in itself an indication for surgery, and prophylactic bracing is not indicated.

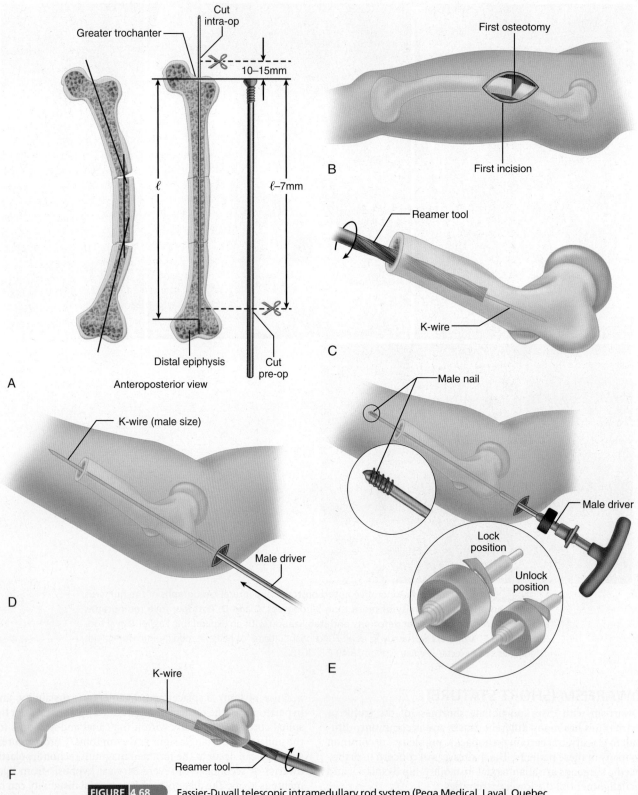

FIGURE 4.68 Fassier-Duvall telescopic intramedullary rod system (Pega Medical, Laval, Quebec, Canada). **SEE TECHNIQUE 4.23.**

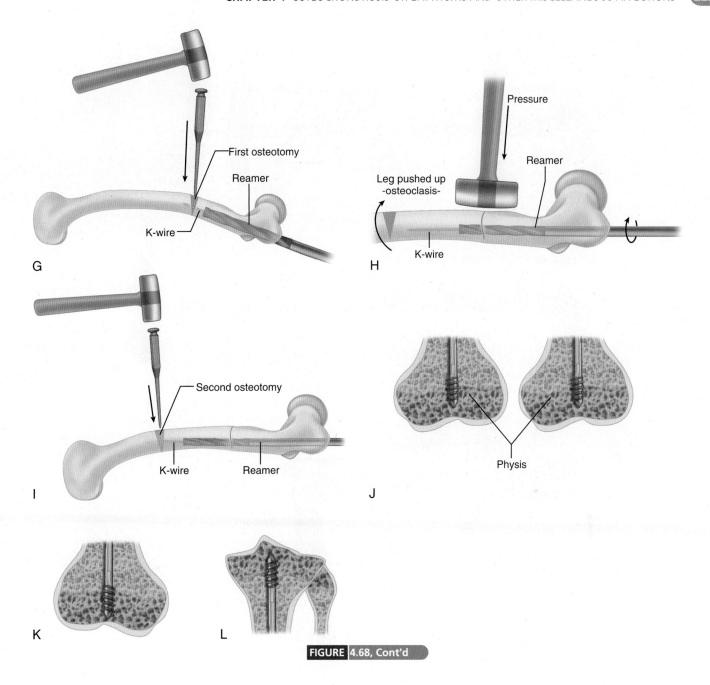

FIGURE 4.68, Cont'd

Kyphosis or scoliosis occurs commonly in short-trunk dwarfs, but with the exception of diastrophic dwarfs, the scoliosis usually is mild and does not require surgery. Severe scoliosis is common in diastrophic dwarfs, and surgical correction and fusion seem to be the only reasonably effective treatment. With profound hypotonia, ligamentous laxity, and a collapsing spine, fusion may be necessary for stability while sitting.

Ligamentous laxity can cause kyphosis in achondroplasia. Severe progressive kyphoscoliosis with a posteriorly displaced vertebral body occasionally occurs in achondroplasia and in a variety of dwarfs. For neurologic deficit, anterior decompression and fusion are best and are followed by posterior fusion when the deformity is greater than 60 degrees.

In the *lumbar spine,* profound lordosis, bulging intervertebral discs, and a narrowed spinal canal are characteristic of achondroplasia. By the third decade of life, many of these patients complain of low back pain, have nerve root signs, and occasionally have a cauda equina syndrome and claudication. Laminectomy, cord and nerve root decompression, disc excision, and spinal fusion ultimately may be needed to relieve symptoms in some patients.

The *hip joint* in many dwarfing syndromes is spared compared with the remainder of the lower extremity. Multiple epiphyseal dysplasia and spondyloepiphyseal dysplasia involve the epiphysis and may cause severe, early crippling arthritis. Hip fusion usually is not indicated in dwarfs for three reasons: (1) with extremely short stature, mobility is crucial for activities of daily living such as dressing and stepping up stairs; (2) hip fusion may increase low back pain that already may be present from lumbar lordosis; and (3) hip fusion would shorten further a patient of already short stature. We have performed total hip

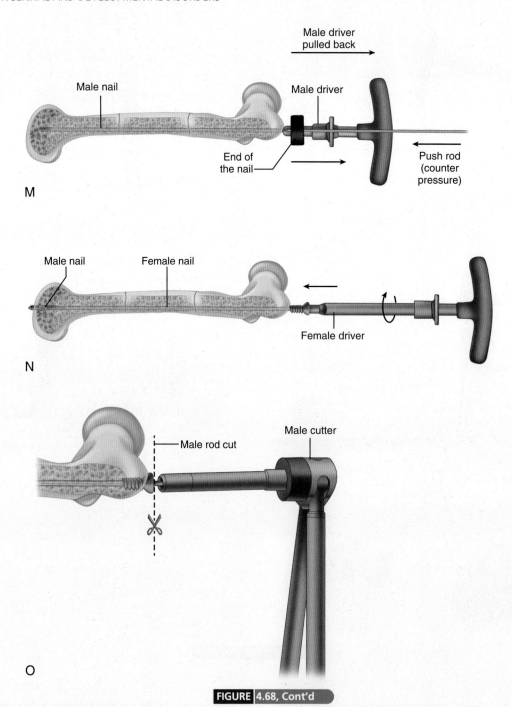

FIGURE 4.68, Cont'd

arthroplasty in dwarfs with severe arthritis. Careful planning is necessary because nonstandard size femoral and acetabular components almost always are necessary. Bilateral dislocation of the hips is commonly seen in Morquio syndrome and usually is not vigorously treated (Fig. 4.70).

Two other conditions, *coxa vara* and *coxa valga,* occur in a substantial percentage of dwarfs. Coxa valga is commonly seen with Morquio syndrome, and coxa vara is commonly seen with spondyloepiphyseal dysplasia (Fig. 4.71). Varus and valgus osteotomies of the hips of patients with bone dysplasias should be done only rarely and after much study because of probable instability. Intertrochanteric osteotomies for

severe coxa valga should be reserved for proven hip instability resulting from the valgus deformity, and for severe coxa vara they should be reserved for a waddling gait and cartilaginous defects. Varus and valgus osteotomies of the hip are described in other chapters.

A substantial percentage of dwarfs have *genu varum* or *genu valgum.* In general, dwarfs with disproportionately short trunks have genu valgum, whereas dwarfs with disproportionately short extremities have genu varum. Angulation may be the result of ligamentous laxity, bowing of the proximal tibia and distal femur, or, as is characteristic of achondroplastic dwarfs, bowing of the distal tibia.

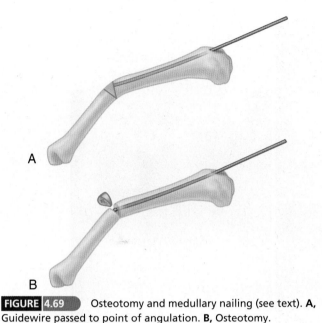

FIGURE 4.69 Osteotomy and medullary nailing (see text). **A,** Guidewire passed to point of angulation. **B,** Osteotomy.

The deformity usually is progressive with an ultimate length discrepancy between the fibula and the tibia. Foot placement is in a forced varus or valgus position depending on the direction of angulation at the knees. Osteotomy at or near the site of the deformity is our preferred treatment. When operating on recurrent genu valgum, such as in Ellis-van Creveld syndrome, the surgeon should be prepared to release the lateral structures such as the iliotibial band and tighten the medial structures by reefing the vastus medialis. We have tried to control the deformity in young children with ambulatory "knock-knee" or "bowleg" braces. These braces are heavy and cumbersome and may promote ligamentous laxity, but in several patients we have been able to stop the progression or improve the deformity (Fig. 4.72). At a later age, we have performed an osteotomy without recurrence of the angulation.

Because of the disproportionate length of the extremities, especially the lower, limb lengthening has been attempted by several methods. Formerly, the most often used method in the United States was that popularized by Wagner, which combines osteotomy with slow distraction (see chapter 1). The Ilizarov and DeBastiani techniques have

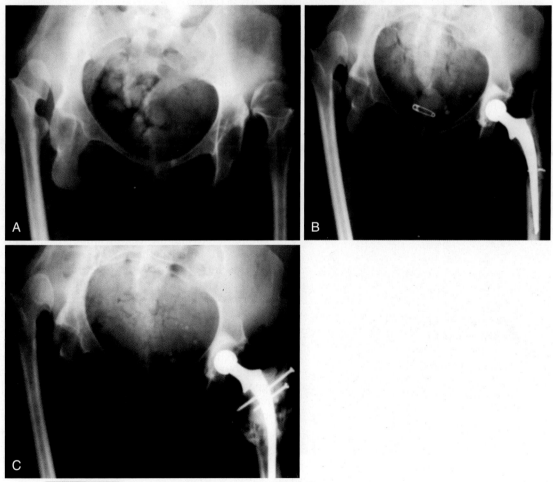

FIGURE 4.70 **A,** Adult patient with Morquio disease with bilateral dislocated hips. Left hip was painful and disabling. **B,** Appearance after total hip arthroplasty using custom-designed femoral component with small stem. Despite this, femoral shaft proximally was fractured during insertion. **C,** Appearance after revision of total hip arthroplasty with second custom-designed long-stem femoral component and anchoring screws in methylmethacrylate. Result was satisfactory.

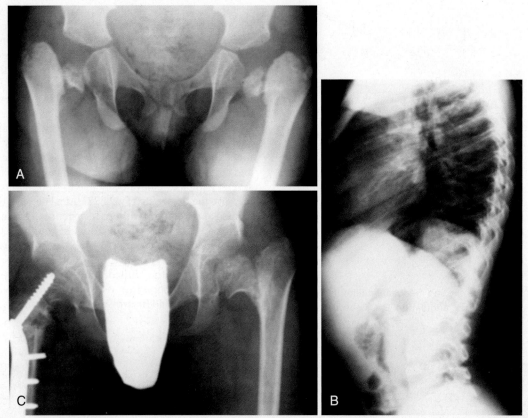

FIGURE 4.71   Spondyloepiphyseal dysplasia. **A,** Severe bilateral coxa vara deformity. **B,** Platyspondyly in same patient. **C,** After valgus osteotomy of right hip using Coventry lag screw. Cartilaginous defect is now more horizontal and under compression rather than shear.

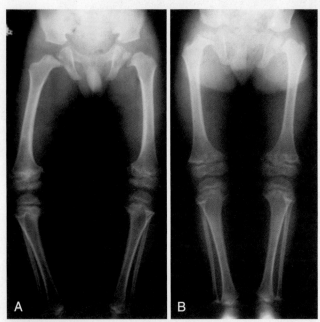

FIGURE 4.72   Multiple epiphyseal dysplasia. **A,** Radiograph obtained while weight bearing in 4-year-old boy showing delayed ossification of capital femoral epiphyses, coxa vara, and femoral and tibial bowing. **B,** Appearance 1 year after treatment in ambulatory bowleg braces. Femoral and tibial bowing is markedly improved.

been reported to achieve greater lengthening with fewer complications. More recently, tibial lengthening over an intramedullary nail with the use of an external fixator has shown to result in new bone formation equal to the conventional Ilizarov technique, however, with fewer complications and less time required for internal fixation. The frequency of complications and the lengthy immobilization period associated with limb lengthening by any method caused some authors in the past to discourage its use, however, especially in dwarfs. Limb lengthening should be attempted only in informed, cooperative patients committed to the lengthy procedure and with realistic expectations of the result. As the lengthening procedures have been better perfected and the complications fewer, disproportionate extremity dwarfs are commonly having lower extremity lengthenings done. In the recent literature, large series have been described with good results with the following observations: (1) lengthening should be started in children early but not before the age of 9 years, (2) premature physeal arrest (closure) of the distal femur and proximal tibia in extensive lengthening should be included in the preoperative calculations and counseling, and (3) humeral lengthenings compared with femoral lengthenings seem to have fewer complications, and callus forms at a higher rate. Humeral hybrid monolateral fixators can be used that are less bulky and allow patients to perform activities of daily living.

TIBIAL LENGTHENING OVER AN INTRAMEDULLARY NAIL WITH EXTERNAL FIXATION IN DWARFISM

TECHNIQUE 4.24

(PARK ET AL.)

- To be treated with lengthening over an intramedullary nail, the tibial medullary diameter must be at least 8 mm.
- Insert an AO tibial nail with a diameter 1 mm smaller than that of the tibial isthmus. To make passage less traumatic, remove irregularities on the endosteal surface with a single pass of a reamer.
- Insert two proximal interlocking screws in a mediolateral direction.
- Parallel to the nail, apply a preconstructed Ilizarov frame with two rings connected with telescoping rods.
- Insert two proximal tensioned wires posterior to the nail. At least one wire at each ring should pass the fibular head or the distal part of the fibula to prevent migration of a fibular segment during lengthening.
- Perform a tibial corticotomy at the metaphyseal-diaphyseal junction with a technique utilizing multiple drill holes.
- Initiate lengthening 7 to 10 days postoperatively at a rate of 0.25 mm four times daily at each distraction site. Obtain radiographs every week during the distraction phase and every 4 weeks during the consolidation phase. Callus formation is determined to have occurred when new bone formation is seen in the distraction gap on lateral radiographs.

- When the desired length has been achieved, insert two distal interlocking screws and one distal tibiofibular transfixing screw after consolidation of the fibula.

POSTOPERATIVE CARE Patients are allowed to bear weight with the use of two crutches (Fig. 4.73).

TRAUMATIC PHYSEAL ARREST FROM BRIDGE OF BONE

Physeal arrest after fracture in young children can produce significant limb shortening and angulatory deformity. Angulation osteotomies, epiphysiodesis of the involved epiphysis, and epiphysiodesis of the contralateral epiphysis are worthwhile and time-honored procedures to reduce angular deformity and limb-length discrepancy.

Bright and Langenskiöld described resection of small, localized bony bridges (after fracture across a physis) that produced angular deformity or limb-length discrepancy. They recommended this procedure for a young child with a significant deformity caused by a bony bridge across less than one half of the physis of a bone that is peripheral and accessible. Tomograms, CT, and MRI are helpful in determining the extent of the bony bridge. Three-dimensional reconstruction to produce a three-dimensional model has been described to show the extent and to help in preoperative "mapping" of the bar.

After resection, Langenskiöld filled the space with fat and Bright used Silastic 382. Although the physis apparently does not regenerate in the area where the bony bridge was resected, the remaining normal physeal cartilage cells surrounding this area can produce bone in a more linear and orderly fashion than before. In a rabbit model, Lee et al. compared the results

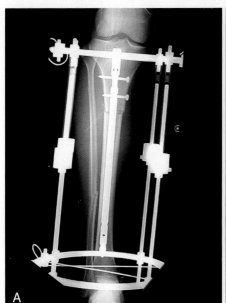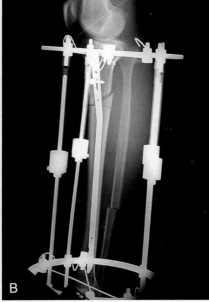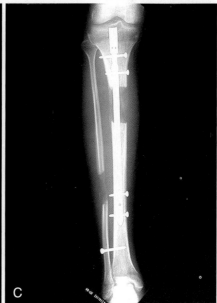

FIGURE 4.73 **A** and **B,** Immediate postoperative anteroposterior and lateral radiographs demonstrating tibial lengthening over an intramedullary nail. **C,** After gradual lengthening, two distal interlocking screws and one distal tibiofibular transfixing screw are inserted. The external fixator is removed. (From Park HW, et al: Tibial lengthening over an intramedullary nail with use of the Ilizarov external fixator for idiopathic short stature, *J Bone Joint Surg* 90:1970–1978, 2008.) **SEE TECHNIQUE 4.24.**

of interposition with physeal grafts, free fat, and Silastic after epiphysiodesis for correction of partial growth arrest. Clinical, radiographic, and histologic studies showed physeal grafts (from the iliac crest) to be superior to Silastic in correcting angular deformity and contributing to the longitudinal growth of the tibia after resection of a large, peripherally situated bony bridge. Interposition of fat produced the worst results. We have resected a bony bridge in conjunction with an angulation osteotomy and used fat or silicone to fill the resected area.

Depending on the location of the physis and the amount of the deformity, we agree with MacEwen (personal communication) that bony bridge resection usually does not correct a significant angular deformity but that the resection may decrease the number of osteotomies necessary during the growth of a young child by decreasing the rate of recurrence of the angular deformity.

Ingram at this clinic described a technique for osteotomy at the level of the bony bridge adjacent and parallel to the physis. With this technique, the bridge does not have to be peripheral. When the osteotomy is opened, the white, sclerotic bridge of bone can be differentiated easily from the normal cancellous metaphyseal bone with or without a magnifying optical loupe or microscope. The bridge is resected with a dental burr, leaving only the normal physis and cancellous bone of the epiphysis and the metaphysis. A free graft of fat or a piece of silicone is placed in the defect, and the osteotomy is secured after insertion of a wedge of bone to correct deformity.

BONY BRIDGE RESECTION FOR PHYSEAL ARREST

TECHNIQUE 4.25

(LANGENSKIÖLD)
- Before the operation, exact localization and estimation of the size of the bony bridge by MRI, CT, and tomography in at least two planes are essential (Fig. 4.74A and B). More than half of the physis should be normal, and the bony bridge should be peripheral, causing a progressive angular deformity or progressive discrepancy of leg length or both.
- Expose the periphery of the physis by a suitable approach near the bony bridge. Use a tourniquet for a bloodless field for localization of the cartilaginous plate, which may be thin when close to the bridge. Use of a microscope or binocular loupe makes the procedure easier.
- Define the most peripheral part of the bony bridge, and remove the overlying periosteum. Remove the bony bridge until the normal periphery of the physis is reached on both sides of the bridge and until the cartilaginous plate can be seen around the whole cavity. It is essential that no part of the bridge be left and that normal physeal cartilage not be removed unnecessarily.
- Release the tourniquet, and while hemostasis is occurring, secure a piece of fat from the subcutaneous tissue, preferably from the gluteal fold, to fill the cavity. After cessation

of bleeding, fill the cavity with the autogenous fat. When the resected cavity is irregular, divide the fat transplant into several pieces to ensure complete filling.
- To keep the autogenous fat in place, suture ligament, muscle, or subcutaneous tissue over the defect. Close the wound in layers without drainage.

BONY BRIDGE RESECTION AND ANGULATION OSTEOTOMY FOR PHYSEAL ARREST

TECHNIQUE 4.26

(INGRAM)
- Accompanying a bony bridge there is usually not only angular deformity but also shortening, and an opening wedge osteotomy usually is indicated to gain length.
- Perform the osteotomy on the same side of the bone as the bony bridge causing the angular deformity (Fig. 4.74A and B). Expose the metaphyseal area of the bone without damaging the periphery of the physis on the side of the bone where the bridge is located.
- After subperiosteal exposure, place a guide pin in the metaphysis parallel to the physis and just adjacent to it, using either radiographic control or image intensifier fluoroscopy. The guide pin should penetrate or lie just adjacent to the bony bridge (Fig. 4.74C).
- Perform an osteotomy at the level of the guide pin, and open the osteotomy site wide with a laminar spreader. Using a small dental burr, resect completely the white sclerotic bony bridge, using an operating microscope or a magnifying loupe for improved vision (Fig. 4.74D). Carry the resection through the physis, ensuring that all of the bony bridge is resected and that normal physeal cartilage appears on all sides of the cavity. This can be facilitated with the use of a dental mirror.
- After adequate resection, obtain hemostasis and fill the area with autogenous fat obtained from the subcutaneous tissue at the incision or with a silicone implant. Correct the angular deformity appropriately by inserting a wedge of autogenous bone into the osteotomy and secure the osteotomy with smooth pins (Fig. 4.74E).
- Close the wound in layers, and apply a sterile dressing and a plaster splint.

POSTOPERATIVE CARE Weight bearing and activities should be limited until the osteotomy has completely healed and the pins are removed.

Peripheral and linear bars are more easily approached and identified than are central bars. The normal perichondral ring at the perimeter of the healthy physis is replaced by periosteum over the bar and is easily stripped. Peripheral bar resection involves scooping out the bar but leaving the residual healthy physis intact. This requires knowing where the bar meets the physis at the perimeter of the bone and the depth that the bar reaches into the physis.

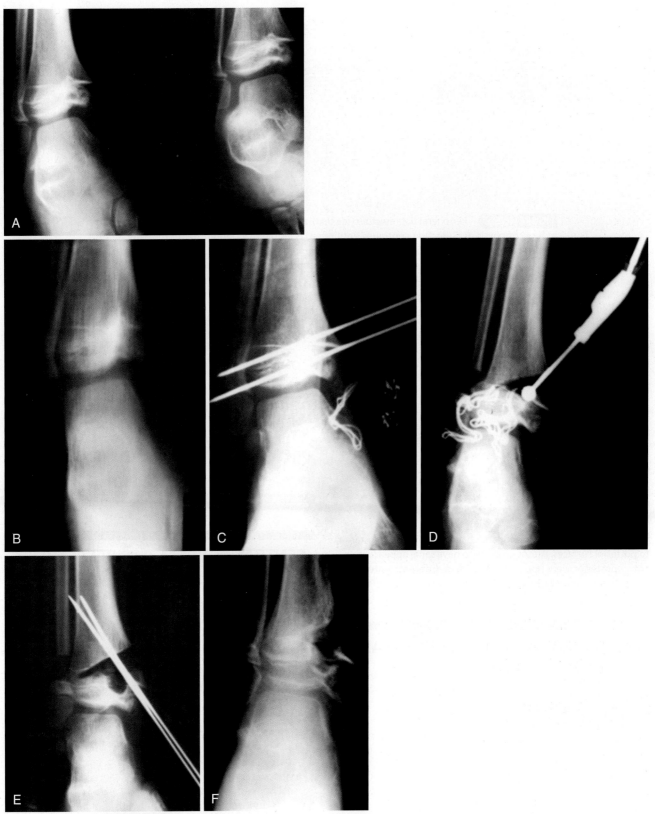

FIGURE 4.74 Traumatic epiphyseal arrest from bridge of bone. **A** and **B,** Anteroposterior radiographs and tomogram of lesion resulting from trauma to medial aspect of the distal tibial epiphysis. **C-E,** Steps in operative technique of Ingram for excision of bony bar and wedge osteotomy of distal tibia (see text). **F,** Radiograph showing correction of deformity and defect at bony bridge site. (**C** to **F** from Canale ST, Harper MC: Biotrigonometric analysis and practical applications of osteotomies of tibia in children, *Instr Course Lect* 30:85–101, 1981.) **SEE TECHNIQUES 4.25 AND 4.26.**

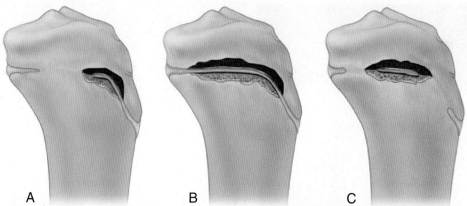

FIGURE 4.75   Peripheral bar resection (see text). **A,** Fluoroscopy ensures that resection remains at level of physis. **B,** Resection continues until physis is visible throughout depth of cavity. **C,** An alternative method for exposure is periosteal stripping with fluoroscopic guidance. (Redrawn from Birch JG: Technique of partial physeal bar resection, *Op Tech Orthop* 3:166–173, 1993.) **SEE TECHNIQUES 4.27 AND 4.28**.

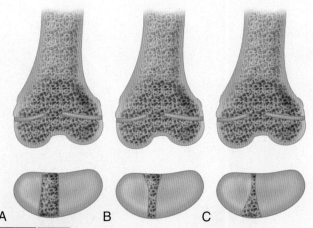

FIGURE 4.76   **A** to **C,** Elongated bar extending from anterior to posterior surfaces. Although all three have same appearance on anteroposterior view *(top row),* they have different contours on transverse sections *(bottom row)* (see text).

PERIPHERAL AND LINEAR PHYSEAL BAR RESECTION FOR PHYSEAL ARREST

TECHNIQUE 4.27

(BIRCH ET AL.)
- Carefully expose the peripheral junction of the bar and the healthy perichondral ring at one, or preferably both, edges of the bar. This junction serves as an excellent starting point for removing the bar. Use fluoroscopy to ensure that the resection remains at the level of the physis and does not drift into the metaphysis or epiphysis (Fig. 4.75A).
- Continue resection until the physis is visible from each edge of healthy perichondrium and throughout the depth of the cavity (Fig. 4.75B). As an alternative, identify the

bar with periosteal stripping and fluoroscopic guidance and develop a cavity directed toward the physis until it is identified (Fig. 4.75C). Extend this cavity peripherally until healthy perichondrium is identified at either end of the bar.
- Fill the defect with autogenous fat from the area or from a small incision in the buttocks or groin.
  Central bars can be approached from the metaphyseal marrow cavity through a metaphyseal cortical window or an osteotomy. Arthroscopically assisted central bar resection has been described using the scope to identify the normal cartilage after dental burr resection in the defect.

CENTRAL PHYSEAL BAR RESECTION FOR PHYSEAL ARREST

TECHNIQUE 4.28

(PETERSON)
- For bars extending completely across the physis, evaluate tomographic maps to determine surgical approach, and ensure complete removal (Fig. 4.76). Approach centrally located bars (Fig. 4.77A) through the metaphysis or epiphysis. Because the bar is not readily accessible through the transepiphyseal approach, and because it usually requires traversing the joint, the transmetaphyseal approach is preferable, although it requires removal of a window of cortical bone and some cancellous metaphyseal bone to reach the bony bar (Fig. 4.77B).
- After removal of the entire bar with a high-speed burr, inspect the normal physis with a small dental mirror (Fig. 4.77C). The sides of the cavity should be flat and smooth (Fig. 4.78).
- Place metal markers, such as surgical clips, in the metaphysis and epiphysis to aid in accurate measurement of subsequent growth of the involved physis. Place these

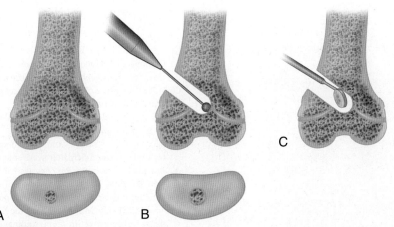

FIGURE 4.77 **A,** Central bar with peripheral growth results in "tenting" or "cupping" of physis (see text). **B,** Excision of central bar through window in metaphysis (see text). **C,** Examination of entire physis with dental mirror (see text). **SEE TECHNIQUE 4.37.**

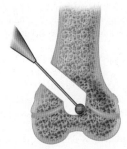

FIGURE 4.78 Smoothing metaphyseal bone surface (see text). **SEE TECHNIQUE 4.37.**

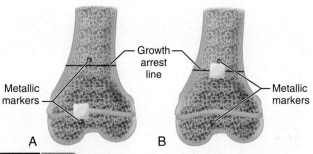

FIGURE 4.80 **A,** Plug growing away from proximal marker and growth arrest line (see text). **B,** Plug remaining with metaphysis as epiphysis grows (see text). **SEE TECHNIQUE 4.37.**

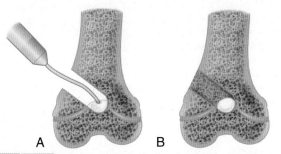

FIGURE 4.79 **A,** Insertion of Cranioplast with syringe (see text). **B,** Bone graft filling remainder of defect (see text). **SEE TECHNIQUE 4.37.**

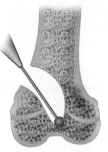

FIGURE 4.81 Undermining of epiphysis (see text). **SEE TECHNIQUE 4.37.**

markers in cancellous bone, not in contact with the cavity, and in the same longitudinal plane proximally and distally to the defect.
- In a large cavity that is gravity dependent, pour liquid Cranioplast into the defect. If the cavity is not gravity dependent, place the Cranioplast in a syringe and push it into the defect through a short polyethylene tube (Fig. 4.79A) or allow the Cranioplast to set partially and push it like putty into the defect. Allow as little Cranioplast as possible to

remain in the metaphysis. After the Cranioplast has set, fill the remainder of the metaphyseal cavity with cancellous bone (Fig. 4.79B). The contour of the cavity also is important. Bar formation is less likely when the interposition material remains in the epiphysis (Fig. 4.80A) than when the epiphysis grows away from it (Fig. 4.80B).
- Methods of keeping the plug in the epiphysis include drilling holes in the cavity (undermining) (Fig. 4.81) and enlarging the cavity (Fig. 4.82).

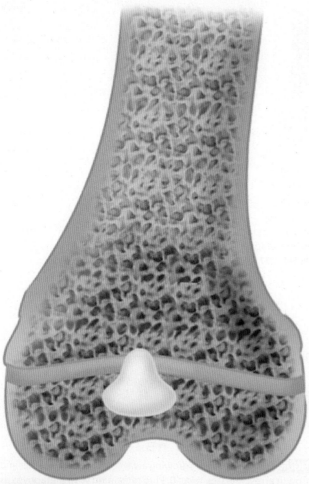

Camp CL, Krych AJ, Stuart MJ: Arthroscopic preparation and internal fixation of an unstable osteochondritis dissecans lesion of the knee, *Arthrosc Tech* 2:3461, 2013.

Chambers HG, Shea KG, Anderson AF, et al.: American Academy of Orthopaedic Surgeons clinical practice guideline on: the diagnosis and treatment of osteochondritis dissecans, *J Bone Joint Surg* 94A:1322, 2012.

Chan JY, Young JL: Köhler disease: avascular necrosis in the child, *Foot Ankle Clin* 24:83, 2019.

Czyrny Z: Osgood-Schlatter disease in ultrasound diagnostics—a pictorial essay, *Med Ultrason* 12:323, 2010.

De Lucena GL, dos Santos Gomes C, Guerra RO: Prevalence and associated factors of Osgood-Schlatter syndrome in a population-based sample of Brazilian adolescents, *Am J Sports Med* 39:415, 2011.

Duncan B, Hurst D: Osteochondrosis of the tarsal navicular and medial cuneiform in a child, *Proc (Bayl Univ Med Cent)* 31:539, 2018.

Heywood CS, Benke MT, Brindle K, Fine KM: Correlation of magnetic resonance imaging to arthroscopic findings of stability in juvenile osteochondritis dissecans, *Arthroscopy* 27:194, 2011.

Itsubo T, Murakami N, Uemura K, et al.: Magnetic resonance imaging staging to evaluate the stability of capitellar osteochondritis dissecans lesions, *Am J Sports Med* 42:1972–1977, 2014.

Iwasaki N, Kamishima T, Kato H, et al.: A retrospective evaluation of magnetic resonance imaging effectiveness on capitellar osteochondritis dissecans among overhead athletes, *Am J Sports Med* 40:624, 2012.

Jans LB, Ditchfield M, Anna G, et al.: MR imaging findings and MR criteria for instability in osteochondritis dissecans of the elbow in children, *Eur J Radiol* 81:1306, 2012.

Jones KJ, Wiesel BB, Sankar WN, Ganley TJ: Arthroscopic management of osteochondritis dissecans of the capitellum: mid-term results in adolescent athletes, *J Pediatr Orthop* 30:8, 2010.

Kessler JI, Weiss JM, Nikizad H, et al.: Osteochondritis dissecans of the ankle in children and adolescents: demographics and epidemiology, *Am J Sports Med* 42:2165–2167, 2014.

Kida Y, Morihara T, Kotoura Y, et al.: Prevalence and clinical characteristics of osteochondritis dissecans of the humeral capitellum among adolescent baseball players, *Am J Sports Med* 42:1963–1971, 2014.

Kosaka M, Nakase J, Takahashi R, et al.: Outcomes and failure factors in surgical treatment for osteochondritis dissecans of the capitellum, *J Pediatr Orthop* 33:719, 2013.

Krause M, Hapfelmeier A, Möller M, et al.: Healing predictors of stable juvenile osteochondritis disecans knee lesions after 6 and 12 months of nonoperative treatment, *Am J Sports Med* 41:2384, 2013.

Lam KY, Siow HM: Conservative treatment for juvenile osteochondritis dissecans of the talus, *J Orthop Surg (Hong Kong)* 20:176, 2012.

Lykissas MG, Wall EJ, Nathan S: Retro-articular drilling and bone grafting of juvenile knee osteochondritis dissecans: a technical description, *Knee Surg Sports Traumatol Arthrosc* 22:274, 2014.

Maier GS, Lazovic D, Maus U, et al.: Vitamin D deficiency: the missing etiological factor in the development of juvenile osteochondrosis dissecans? *J Pediatr Orthop* 39:51, 2019.

Murphy RT, Pennock AT, Bugbee WD: Osteochondral allograft transplantation of the knee in the pediatric and adolescent population, *Am J Sports Med* 42:635, 2014.

Nierenberg G, Falah M, Keren Y, Eidelman M: Surgical treatment of residual Osgood-Schlatter disease in young adults: role of the mobile osseous fragment, *Orthopedics* 34:176, 2011.

Olstad K, Shea KG, Cannamela PC, et al.: Juvenile osteochondritis dissecans of the knee is a results of failure of the blood supply to growth cartilage and osteochondrosis, *Osteoarthritis Cartilage* 26:1691, 2018.

Pengas IP, Assiotis A, Kokkinakis M, et al.: Knee osteochondritis dissecans treated by the AO hook fixation system: a four year follow-up of an alternative technique, *Open Orthop J* 8:209, 2014.

Pennock AT, Bomar JD, Chambers HG: Extra-articular, intraepiphyseal drilling for osteochondritis dissecans of the knee, *Arthrosc Tech* 2:e231, 2013.

Pihlajamäki HK: Visuri TI: Long-term outcome after surgical treatment of unresolved Osgood-Schlatter disease in young men. Surgical Technique, *J Bone Joint Surg* 92(Suppl 1):258, 2010.

FIGURE **4.82**   "Collar button" contour of plug to act as anchor (see text). **SEE TECHNIQUE 4.37.**

POSTOPERATIVE CARE Joint motion is begun immediately. If osteotomy has not been done, no cast or other immobilization is necessary. Weight bearing is encouraged on the day of surgery or as soon as comfort permits. Follow-up with scanograms continues until maturity.

REFERENCES

FREIBERG DISEASE; OSTEOCHONDROSIS OF THE ANKLE, KNEE, AND ELBOW; AND OSGOOD-SCHLATTER DISEASE

Abouassaly M, Peterson D, Salci L, et al.: Surgical management of osteochondritis dissecans of the knee in the paediatric population: a systematic review addressing surgical techniques, *Knee Surg Sports Traumatol Arthrosc* 22:1216, 2014.

Achar S, Yamanaka J: Apophysitis and osteochondrosis: common causes of pain in growing bones, *Am Fam Physician* 99:610, 2019.

Adachi N, Deie M, Nakamae A, et al.: Functional and radiographic outcomes of unstable juvenile osteochondritis dissecans of the knee treated with lesion fixation using bioabsorbable pins, *J Pediatr Orthop* 35:82–88, 2015.

Al-Ashhab MEA, Kandel WA, Rizk AS: A simple surgical technique for treatment of Freiberg's disease, *The Foot* 23:29, 2013.

Boughanem J, Riaz R, Patel RM, Sarwark JF: Functional and radiographic outcomes of juvenile osteochondritis dissecans of the knee treated with extra-articular retrograde drilling, *Am J Sports Med* 39:2212, 2011.

Sabo MT, McDonald CP, Ferreira LM, et al.: Osteochondral lesions of the capitellum do not affect elbow kinematics and stability with intact collateral ligaments: an in vitro biomechanical study, *J Hand Surg [Am]* 36:74, 2011.

Salci L, Ayeni O, Abouassaly M, et al.: Indications for surgical management of osteochondritis dissecans of the knee in the pediatric population: a systematic review, *J Knee Surg* 27:147, 2014.

Samora WP, Chevillet J, Adler B, et al.: Juvenile osteochondritis dissecans of the knee: predictors of lesion stability, *J Pediatr Orthop* 32:1, 2012.

Satake H, Takahara M, Harada M, Maruyama M: Preoperative imaging criteria for unstable osteochondritis dissecans of the capitellum, *Clin Orthop Relat Res* 471:1137, 2013.

Shane A, Reeves C, Wobst G, Thurston P: Second metatarsophalangeal joint pathology and Freiberg disease, *Clin Podiatr Med Surg* 30:313, 2013.

Shi LL, Bae DS, Kocher MS, et al.: Contained versus uncontained lesions in juvenile elbow osteochondritis dissecans, *J Pediatr Orthop* 32:221, 2012.

Shimada K, Tanaka H, Matsumoto T, et al.: Cylindrical costal osteochondral autograft for reconstruction of large defects of the capitellum due to osteochondritis dissecans, *J Bone Joint Surg* 94A:992, 2012.

Siegall E, Faust JR, Herzog MM, et al.: Age predicts disruption of the articular surface of the femoral condyles in knee OCD: Can we reduce usage of arthroscopy and MRI? *J Pediatr Orthop* 38:176, 2018.

Tabaddor RR, Banffy MB, Andersen JS, et al.: Fixation of juvenile osteochondritis dissecans lesions of knee using poly 96L/4D-lactide copolymer bioabsorbable implants, *J Pediatr Orthop* 30:14, 2010.

Takeba J, Takahashi T, Hino K, et al.: Arthroscopic technique for fragment fixation using absorbable pins for osteochondritis dissecans of the humeral capitellum: a report of 4 cases, *Knee Surg Sports Traumatol Arthrosc* 18:831, 2010.

Tatebe M, Hirata H, Shinohara T, et al.: Pathomechanical significance of radial head subluxation in the onset of osteochondritis dissecans of the radial head, *J Orthop Trauma* 26:e4, 2012.

Thacker MM, Dabney KW, Mackenzie WG: Osteochondritis dissecans of the talar head: natural history and review of the literature, *J Pediatric Orthop* 21:373, 2012.

Tis JE, Edmonds EW, Bastrom T, Chambers HG: Short-term results of arthroscopic treatment of osteochondritis dissecans in skeletally immature patients, *J Pediatr Orthop* 32:226, 2012.

Van den Ende KI, McIntosh AL, Adams JE, Steinmann SP: Osteochondritis dissecans of the capitellum: a review of the literature and a distal ulnar portal, *Arthroscopy* 27:122, 2011.

Viladot A, Sodano L, Marcellini L: Joint debridement and microfracture for treatment of late-stage Freiberg-Kohler's disease: long-term follow-up study, *Foot Ankle Surg*, 2018 Feb 17, [Epub ahead of print].

Wax A, Leland R: Freiberg disease and avascular necrosis of the metatarsal heads, *Foot Ankle Clin* 24:69, 2019.

Webb JE, Lewallen LW, Christophersen C, et al.: Clinical outcome of internal fixation of unstable juvenile osteochondritis dissecans lesions of the knee, *Orthopedics* 36:31444, 2013.

Wulf CA, Stone RM, Giveans MR, Lervick GN: Magnetic resonance imaging after arthroscopic microfracture of capitellar osteochondritis dissecans, *Am J Sports Med* 40:2549, 2012.

Yonetani Y, Tanaka Y, Shiozaki Y, et al.: Transarticular drilling for stable juvenile osteochondritis dissecans of the medial femoral condyle, *Knee Surg Sports Traumatol Arthrosc* 20:1528, 2012.

LEGG-CALVÉ-PERTHES DISEASE

Albers CE, Steppacher SD, Ganz R, et al.: Joint-preserving surgery improves pain, range of motion, and abductor strength after Legg-Calvé-Perthes disease, *Clin Orthop Relat Res* 470:2450, 2012.

Anderson LA, Erickson JA, Severson EP, Peters CL: Sequelae of Perthes disease: treatment with surgical hip dislocation and relative femoral neck lengthening, *J Pediatr Orthop* 30:758, 2010.

Baunin C, Sanmartin-Viron D, Accadbled F, et al.: Prognosis value of early diffusion MRI in Legg-Calvé-Perthes disease, *Orthop Traumatol Surg Res* 100:317, 2014.

Boutault JR, Baunin C, Bérard E, et al.: Diffusion MRI of the neck of the femur in Legg-Calvé-Perthes disease: a preliminary study, *Diagn Interv Imaging* 94:78, 2013.

Bowen JR, Guille JT, Jeong C, et al.: Labral support shelf arthroplasty for containment in early stages of Legg-Calvé-Perthes disease, *J Pediatr Orthop* 31(Suppl 2):S206, 2011.

Bulut M, Demirts A, Ucar BY, et al.: Salter pelvic osteotomy in the treatment of Legg-Calvé-Perthes disease: the medium-term results, *Acta Orthop Belg* 80:56, 2014.

Carsi B, Judd J, Clarke NM: Shelf acetabuloplasty for containment in the early stages of Legg-Calvé-Perthes disease, *J Pediatr Orthop* 35:151–156, 2015.

Chang JH, Kuo KN, Huang SC: Outcomes in advanced Legg-Calvé-Perthes disease treated with the Staheli procedure, *J Surg Res* 168:237, 2011.

Chiarapattanakom P, Thanacharoenpanich S, Pakpianpairoj C, Liupolvanish P: The remodeling of the neck-shaft angle after proximal femoral varus osteotomy for the treatment of Legg-Calvé-Perthes syndrome, *J Med Assoc Thai* 95(Suppl 10):S135, 2012.

Citlak A, Kerimoglu S, Baki C, Aydin H: Comparison between conservative and surgical treatment in Perthes disease, *Arch Orthop Trauma Surg* 132:87, 2012.

Clohisy JC, Ross JR, North JD, et al.: What are the factors associated with acetabular correction in Perthes-like hip deformities, *Clin Orthop Relat Res* 470:3439, 2012.

Conroy E, Sheehan E, O'Connor P, et al.: Triple pelvic osteotomy in Legg-Calvé-Perthes disease using a single anterolateral incision: a 4-year review, *J Pediatr Orthop B* 19:323, 2010.

Du J, Lu A, Dempsey M, et al.: MR perfusion index as a quantitative method of evaluation epiphyseal perfusion in Legg-Calvé-Perthes disease and correlation with short-term radiographic outcome: a preliminary study, *J Pediatr Orthop* 33:707, 2013.

Eamsobhana P, Kaewporsawan K: Combined osteotomy in patients with severe Legg-Calvé-Perthes disease, *J Med Assoc Thai* 95(Suppl 10):S128, 2012.

Edmonds EW, Heyworth BE: Osteochondritis dissecans of the shoulder and hip, *Clin Sports Med* 33:285, 2014.

Freeman CR, Jones K, Byrd JWT: Hip arthroscopy for Legg-Calvé-Perthes disease: minimum 2-year follow-up, *Arthroscopy* 29:666, 2013.

Ghanem I, Haddad E, Haidar R, et al.: Lateral shelf acetabuloplasty in the treatment of Legg-Calvé-Perthes disease: improving mid-term outcome in severely deformed hips, *J Child Orthop* 4:13, 2010.

Grigoryan G, Korcek L, Eidelman M, et al.: Direct lateral approach for triple pelvic osteotomy, *J Am Acad Orthop Surg* 2019. [Epub ahead of print].

Grzegorzewski A, Synder M, Kmiec K, et al.: Shelf acetabuloplasty in the treatment of severe Legg-Calvé-Perthes disease: good outcomes at mid-term follow-up, *Biomed Res Int* 2013: 859483, 2013; 2013:859483.

Hailer YD, Haag AC, Nilsson O: Legg-Calvé Perthes disease: quality of life, physical activity, and behavior pattern, *J Pediatr Orthop* 34:514, 2014.

Hailer YD, Montgomery SM, Ekbom A, et al.: Legg-Calvé-Perthes disease and risks for cardiovascular diseases and blood diseases, *Pediatrics* 125:e1308, 2010.

Hailer YD, Penno E: Agreement of radiographic measurements and patient-reported outcome in 61 patients with Legg-Calvé-Perthes disease at mean follow-up of 28 years, *J Pediatr Orthop* 28:100, 2019.

Hardesty CK, Liu RW, Thompson GH: The role of bracing in Legg-Calvé-Perthes disease, *J Pediatr Orthop* 31(Suppl 2):S178, 2011.

Hosalkar H, Munhoz da Cunha AL, Baldwin K, et al.: Triple innominate osteotomy for Legg-Calvé-Perthes disease in children: does the lateral coverage change with time? *Clin Orthop Relat Res* 470:2402, 2012.

Hyman JE, Trupia EP, Wright ML, et al.: Interobserver and intraobserver reliability of the modified Waldenström classification system for staging of Legg-Calvé-Perthes disease, *J Bone Joint Surg Am* 987:643, 2015.

Kim HK, Burgess J, Thoveson Am, et al.: Assessment of femoral head revascularization in Legg-Calvé-Perthes disease using serial perfusion MRI, *J Bone Joint Surg Am* 98:1897, 2016.

Kim HK, da Cunha AM, Browne R, et al.: How much varus is optimal with proximal femoral osteotomy to preserve the femoral head in Legg-Calvé-Perthes disease? *J Bone Joint Surg* 93A:341, 2011.

Kim HK, Kaste S, Dempsey M, Wilkes D: A comparison of non-contrast and contrast-enhanced MRI in the initial stage of Legg-Calvé-Perthes disease, *Pediatr Radiol* 43:1166, 2013.

Kim HT, Gu JK, Bae SH, et al.: Does valgus femoral osteotomy improve femoral head roundness in severe Legg-Calvé-Perthes disease? *Clin Orthop Relat Res* 471:1021, 2013.

Kim HT, Oh MH, Lee JS: MR imaging as a supplement to traditional decision-making in the treatment of LCP disease, *J Pediatr Orthop* 31:246, 2011.

Kitoh H, Kaneko H, Mishima K, et al.: Prognostic factors for trochanteric overgrowth after containment treatment in Legg-Calvé-Perthes disease, *J Pediatr Orthop B* 22:432, 2013.

Kosashvili Y, Raz G, Backstein D, et al.: Fresh-stored osteochondral allografts for the treatment of femoral head defects: surgical technique and preliminary results, *Int Orthop* 37:1001, 2013.

Laklouk MA, Hosny GA: Hinged distraction of the hip joint in the treatment of Perthes disease: evaluation at skeletal maturity, *J Pediatr Orthop B* 21:386, 2012.

Larson AN, Sucato DJ, Herring JA, et al.: A prospective multicenter study of Legg-Calvé-Perthes disease: functional and radiographic outcomes of nonoperative treatment at a mean follow-up of twenty years, *J Bone Joint Surg* 94:584, 2012.

Leunig M, Ganz R: Relative neck lengthening and intracapital osteotomy for severe Perthes and Perthes-like deformities, *Bull NYU Hosp Joint Dis* 69:S62, 2011.

Moya-Angeler J, Abril JC, Rodriguez IV: Legg-Calvé-Perthes disease: role of isolated adductor tenotomy? *Eur J Orthop Surg Traumatol* 8:921, 2013.

Mundluru SN, Feldman D: Varus derotational osteotomy, *Bull Hosp Jt Dis* 77(2013):53, 2019.

Nakamura J, Kamegaya M, Saisu T, et al.: Outcome of patients with Legg-Calvé-Perthes onset before 6 years of age, *J Pediatr Orthop* 35:144–150, 2015.

Nguyen NA, Klein G, Dogbey G, et al.: Operative versus nonoperative treatments for Legg-Calvé-Perthes disease: a meta-analysis, *J Pediatr Orthop* 32:697, 2012.

Novais EN: Application of the surgical dislocation approach to residual hip deformity secondary to Legg-Calvé-Perthes disease, *J Pediatr Orthop* 33:S62, 2013.

Oh CW, Rodriguez A, Guille JT, Bowen JR: Labral support shelf arthroplasty for the early stages of severe Legg-Calvé-Perthes disease, *Am J Orthop* 39:26, 2010.

Onishi E, Ikeda N, Ueo T: Degenerative osteoarthritis after Perthes' disease: a 36-year follow-up, *Arch Orthop Trauma Surg* 131:701, 2011.

Pailhé R, Cavaignac E, Murgier J, et al.: Triple osteotomy of the pelvic for Legg-Calvé-Perthes disease: a mean fifteen year follow-up, *Int Orthop* 40:115, 2016.

Park MS, Chung CY, Lee KM, et al.: Reliability and stability of three common classifications for Legg-Calvé-Perthes disease, *Clin Orthop Relat Res* 470:2376, 2012.

Rich MM, Schoenecker PL: Management of Legg-Calvé-Perthes disease using an A-frame orthosis and hip range of motion: a 25-year experience, *J Pediatr Orthop* 33:112, 2013.

Ross JR, Nepple JJ, Baca G, et al.: Intraarticular abnormalities in residual Perthes and Perthes-like hip deformities, *Clin Orthop Relat Res* 470:2968, 2012.

Sankar WN, Castaneda TS, Hont T, et al.: Feasibility and safety of perfusion MRI for Legg-Calvé-Perthes disease, *J Pediatr Orthop* 2014. [Epub ahead of print].

Sankar WN, Thomas S, Castaneda P, et al.: Feasibility and safety of perfusion MRI for Legg-Calvé-Perthes disease, *J Pediatr Orthop* 34:679–682, 2014.

Shohat N, Copeliovitch L, Smorgick Y, et al.: The long-term outcome after varus derotational osteotomy for Legg-Calvé-Perthes disease: a mean follow-up of 42 years, *J Bone Joint Surg Am* 98:1277, 2016.

Schoenecker PL: Do we need another gold standard to assess acute Legg-Calvé-Perthes disease? *J Bone Joint Surg* 96A(1):e125, 2014.

Shore BJ, Millis MB, Kim YJ: Vascular safe zones for surgical dislocation in children with healed Legg-Calvé-Perthes disease, *J Bone Joint Surg* 94A:721, 2012.

Shore BJ, Novais EN, Millis MB, Kim Y-J: Low early failure rates using a surgical dislocation approach in healed Legg-Calvé-Perthes disease, *Clin Orthop Relat Res* 470:2441, 2012.

Siebenrock KA, Pwell JN, Ganz R: Osteochondritis dissecans of the femoral head, *Hip Int* 20:489, 2010.

Sink E, Zaltz I, Session Participants: Report of break-out session: management of sequelae of Legg-Calvé-Perthes disease, *Clin Orthop Relat Res* 470:3462, 2012.

Tannast M, Hanke M, Ecker TM, et al.: LCPD: reduced range of motion resulting from extra- and intraarticular impingement, *Clin Orthop Relat Res* 470:2431, 2012.

Terjesen T, Wiig O, Svenningsen S: Varus femoral improves sphericity of the femoral head in older children with severe form of Legg-Calvé-Perthes disease, *Clin Orthop Relat Res* 470:2394, 2012.

Thompson GH: Salter osteotomy in Legg-Calvé-Perthes disease, *J Pediatr Orthop* 31(Suppl 2):S192, 2011.

Volpon JB: Comparison between innominate osteotomy and arthrodistraction as a primary treatment for Legg-Calvé-Perthes disease: a prospective controlled trial, *Int Orthop* 36:1899, 2012.

Yoo W, Choi IH, Moon HJ, et al.: Valgus femoral osteotomy for noncontainable Perthes hips: prognostic factors of remodeling, *J Pediatr Orthop* 33:650, 2013.

Wright DM, Perry DC, Bruce CE: Shelf acetabuloplasty for Perthes disease in patients older than eight years of age: an observational cohort study, *J Pediatr Orthop B* 22:96, 2013.

HEMOPHILIA

Bai Z, Zhang E, He Y, et al.: Arthroscopic ankle arthrodesis in hemophilic arthropathy, *Foot Ankle Int* 34:1147, 2013.

Barg A, Elsner A, Hefti D, Hintermann B: Haemophilic arthropathy of the ankle treated by total ankle replacement: a case series, *Haemophilia* 16:647, 2010.

Bluth BE, Fong YJ, Houman JJ, et al.: Ankle fusion in patients with haemophilia, *Haemophilia* 19:432, 2013.

Carulli C, Matassi F, Civinini R, et al.: Intra-articular injections of hyaluronic acid induce positive clinical effects in knees of patients affected by haemophilic arthropathy, *Knee* 20:36, 2013.

Caviglia H, Candela M, Galatro G, et al.: Elective orthopaedic surgery for haemophilia patients with inhibitors: single centre experience of 40 procedures and review of the literature, *Haemophilia* 17:910, 2011.

Chevalier Y, Dargaud Y, Lienhart A, et al.: Seventy-two total knee arthroplasties performed in patients with haemophilia using continuous infusion, *Vox Sang* 104:135, 2013.

Cho YJ, Kim KI, Chun YS, et al.: Radioisotope synoviorthesis with Holmium-166-chitosan complex in haemophilic arthropathy, *Haemophilia* 16:640, 2010.

De Almeida AM, de Rezende MU, Cordeiro FG, et al.: Arthroscopic partial anterior synovectomy of the knee on patients with haemophilia, *Knee Surg Sports Traumatol Arthrosc* 23:785–791, 2015.

Feng B, Xiao K, Gao P, et al.: Comparison of 90-day complication rates and cost between single and multiple joint procedures for end-stage arthropathy in patients with hemophilia, *JB JS Open Access* 3:e0026, 2018.

Goddard NJ, Mann HA, Lee CA: Total knee replacement in patients with end-stage haemophilic arthropathy: 25-year results, *J Bone Joint Surg* 92B:1085, 2010.

Hirose J, Takedani H, Koibuchi T: The risk of elective orthopaedic surgery for haemophilia patients: Japanese single-centre experience, *Haemophilia* 19:951, 2013.

Kuijlaars IAR, Timmer MA, de Kleijn P, et al.: Monitoring joint health in haemophilia: factors associated with deterioration, *Haemophilia* 23:934, 2017.

Lambert T, Auerswald G, Benson G, et al.: Joint disease, the hallmark of haemophilia: what issues and challenges remain despite the development of effective therapies? *Thromb Res* 133:967, 2014.

Melchiorre D, Linari S, Innocenti M, et al.: Ultrasound detects joint damage and bleeding in haemophilic arthropathy: a proposal of a score, *Haemophilia* 17:112, 2011.

Ozelo MC: Surgery in patients with hemophilia: is thromboprophylaxis mandatory? *Thromb Res* 130(Suppl 1):S23, 2012.

Poenaru DV, Patrascu JM, Andor BC, Popa I: Orthopaedic and surgical features in the management of patients with haemophilia, *Eur J Orthop Surg Traumatol* 24:685, 2014.

Rangarajan S, Austin S, Goddard NJ, et al.: Consensus recommendations for the use of FEIBA(*) in haemophilia A patients with inhibitors undergoing elective orthopaedic and non-orthopaedic surgery, *Haemophilia* 19:294, 2013.

Raza S, Kale G, Kim D, et al.: Thromboprophylaxis and incidence of venous thromboembolism in patients with hemophilia A or B who underwent high-risk orthopedic surgeries, *Clin Appl Thromb Hemost* 2014. [Epub ahead of print].

Rezazadeh S, Haghighat A, Mahmoodi M, et al.: Synviorthesis induced by rifampicin in hemophilic arthropathy: a report of 24 treated joints, *Ann Hematol* 90:963, 2011.

Rodriguez-Merchan EC: Hemophilic synovitis of the knee: radiosynovectomy or arthroscopic synovectomy? *Expert Rev Hematol* 7:507, 2014.

Rodriguez-Merchan EC: Haemophilic synovitis of the elbow: radiosynovectomy, open synovectomy or arthroscopic synovectomy? *Thromb Res* 132:15, 2013.

Rodriguez-Merchan EC: Intra-articular injections of hyaluronic acid (viscosupplementation) in the haemophilic knee, *Blood Coagul Fibrinolysis* 23:580, 2012.

Rodriguez-Merchan EC, De La Corte-Rodriguez H, Jiminez-Yuste V: Is radiosynovectomy (RS) effective for joints damaged by haemophilia with articular degeneration in simple radiography (ADSR)? *Expert Rev Hematol* 7:507, 2014.

Rodriguez-Merchan EC: Orthopaedic problems about the ankle in hemophilia, *J Foot Ankle Surg* 51:772, 2012.

Rodriguez-Merchan EC: Special features of total knee replacement in hemophilia, *Epert Rev Hematol* 6:337, 2013.

Siboni SM, Biguzzi E, Solimeno LP, et al.: Orthopaedic surgery in patients with von Willebrand disease, *Haemophilia* 20:133, 2014.

Takedani H, Kawahara H, Kajiwara M: Major orthopaedic surgeries for haemophilia with inhibitors using rFVIIa, *Haemophilia* 16:290, 2010.

Tobase P, Lane H, Siddiqi AE, et al.: Declining trends in invasive orthopedic interventions for people with hemophilia enrolled in the Universal Data Collection program (2000-2010), *Haemophilia* 22:604, 2016.

Tsukamoto S, Tanaka Y, Matsuda T, et al.: Arthroscopic ankle arthrodesis for hemophilic arthropathy: two case reports, *Foot (Edinb)* 21:103, 2011.

Westberg M, Paus AC, Holme PA, Tjonnfjord GE: Haemophilic arthropathy: long-term outcomes in 107 primary total knee arthroplasties, *Knee* 21:147, 2014.

Wong JM, Mann HA, Goddard NJ: Perioperative clotting factor replacement and infection in total knee arthroplasty, *Haemophilia* 18:607, 2012.

Zhai J, Weng X, Zhang B, et al.: Management of knee flexion contracture in haemophilia with the Ilizarov technique, *Knee* 26:201, 2019.

RICKETS, OSTEOMALACIA, AND RENAL OSTEODYSTROPHY

Bitzan M, Goodyer PR: Hypophosphatemic rickets, *Pediatr Clin North Am* 66:179, 2019.

Clarke NM, Page JE: Vitamin D deficiency: a paediatric orthopaedic perspective, *Curr Opin Pediatr* 24:46, 2012.

Eralp L, Kocaoglu M, Toker B, et al.: Comparison of fixator-assisted nailing versus circular external fixator for bone realignment of lower extremity angular deformity in rickets disease, *Arch Orthop Trauma Surg* 131:581, 2011.

Gizard A, Rothenbuhler A, Pejin Z, et al.: Outcomes of orthopedic surgery in a cohort of 49 patients with X-linked hypophosphatemic rickets (XLHR), *Endocr Connect* 6:566, 2017.

Horn A, Wright J, Bockenhauer D, et al.: The orthopaedic management of lower limb deformity in hypophosphataemic rickets, *J Child Orthop* 11:298, 2017.

Larson AN, Trousdale RT, Pagnano MW, et al.: Hip and knee arthroplasty in hypophosphatemic rickets, *J Arthroplast* 25:1099, 2010.

Veilleux LN, Cheung M, Ben Amor M, Rauch F: Abnormalities in muscle density and muscle function in hypophosphatemic rickets, *J Clin Endocrinol Metab* 97:E1492, 2012.

Veilleux LN, Cheung MS, Glorieux FH, Rauch F: The muscle-bone relationship in X-linked hypophosphatemic rickets, *J Clin Endocrinol* 98:E990, 2013.

Wirth T: The orthopaedic management of long bone deformities in genetically and acquired generalized bone weakening conditions, *J Child Orthop* 13:12, 2019.

TIBIA VARA

Abraham E, Toby D, Welborn MC, et al.: New single-stage double osteotomy for late-presenting infantile tibia vara: a comprehensive approach, *J Pediatr Orthop* 39:247, 2019.

Burghardt RD, Specht SC, Herzenberg JE: Mechanical failures of eight-plate guided growth system for temporary hemiepiphysiodesis, *J Pediatr Orthop* 30:594, 2010.

Gkiokas A, Brilakis E: Management of neglected Blount disease using double corrective tibia osteotomy and medial plateau elevation, *J Child Orthop* 6:411, 2012.

Ho-Fung V, James C, Delgado J, et al.: MRI evaluation of the knee in children with infantile Blount disease: tibial and extra-tibial findings, *Pediatr Radiol* 43:1316, 2013.

Jain MJ, Inneh IA, Zhu H, et al.: Tension band plate (TBP)-guided hemiepiphysiodesis in Blount disease: 10-year single-center experience with a systematic review of the literature, *J Pediatr Orthop* 2019. [Epub ahead of print].

Khanfour AA: Does Langenskiold staging have a good prognostic value in late onset tibia vara? *J Orthop Surg Res* 7:23, 2012.

Laville JM, Wiart Y, Salmeron F: Can Blount's disease heal spontaneously? *Orthop Traumatol Surg Res* 96:531, 2010.

Li Y, Spencer SA, Hedequist D: Proximal tibial osteotomy and Taylor Spatial Frame application for correction of tibia vara in morbidly obese adolescents, *J Pediatr Orthop* 33:276, 2013.

Masrouha KZ, Sraj S, Lakkis S, Saghieh S: High tibial osteotomy in young adults with constitutional tibial vara, *Knee Surg Sports Traumatol Arthrosc* 19:89, 2011.

Mayer SW, Hubbad EW, Sun D, et al.: Gradual deformity correction in Blount disease, *J Pediatr Orthop* 39:257, 2019.

Montgomery CO, Young KL, Austen M, et al.: Increased risk of Blount disease in obese children and adolescents with vitamin D deficiency, *J Pediatr Orthop* 30:879, 2010.

Oh CW, Kim SJ, Park SK, et al.: Hemicallotasis for correction of varus deformity of the proximal tibia using a unilateral external fixator, *J Orthop Sci* 16:44, 2011.

Sabharwal S, Wenokor C, Mehta A, Zhao C: Intra-articular morphology of the knee joint in children with Blount disease: a case-control study using MRI, *J Bone Joint Surg* 94A:883, 2012.

Sabharwal S, Zhao C, Sakamoto SM, McClemens E: Do children with Blount disease have lower body mass index after lower limb realignment? *J Pediatr Orthop* 34:213, 2014.

Sanghrajka AP, Hill RA, Murnaghan CF, et al.: Slipped upper tibial epiphysis in infantile tibial vara. Three cases, *J Bone Joint Surg* 94B:1288, 2012.

Scott AC: Treatment of infantile Blount disease with lateral tension band plating, *J Pediatr Orthop* 32:29, 2012.

OSTEOGENESIS IMPERFECTA

Aglan MS, Hosny L, El-Houssini R, et al.: A scoring system for the assessment of clinical severity in osteogenesis imperfecta, *J Child Orthop* 6:29, 2012.

Anissipour AK, Hammerberg KW, Caudill A, et al.: Behavior of scoliosis during growth in children with osteogenesis imperfecta, *J Bone Joint Surg* 96A:237, 2014.

Ashby E, Montpetit K, Hamdy RC, et al.: Functional outcome of forearm rodding in children with osteogenesis imperfecta, *J Pediatr Orthop* 38:54, 2018.

Ashby E, Montpetit K, Hamdy RC, et al.: Functional outcome of humeral rodding in children with osteogenesis imperfecta, *J Pediatr Orthop* 38:49, 2018.

Azzam KA, Rush ET, Burke BR, et al.: Mid-term results of femoral and tibial osteotomies and Fassier-Duval nailing in children with osteogenesis imperfecta, *J Pediatr Orthop* 38:331, 2018.

Biggin A, Briody JN, Ormshaw E, et al.: Fracture during intravenous bisphosphonate treatment in a child with osteogenesis imperfecta: an argument for a more frequent, low-dose treatment regimen, *Horm Res Paediatr* 81:204, 2014.

Cho TJ, Kim JB, Lee JW, et al.: Fracture in long bones stabilised by telescopic intramedullary rods in patients with osteogenesis imperfecta, *J Bone Joint Surg* 93B:634, 2011.

Chow W, Negandhi R, Kuong E, To M: Management pitfalls of fractured neck of femur in osteogenesis imperfecta, *J Child Orthop* 7:195, 2013.

Dwan K, Phillipi CA, Steiner RD, et al.: Bisphosphonate therapy for osteogenesis imperfecta, *Cochrane Database Syst Rev* 7:CD005088, 2014.

Dwan K, Phillipi CA, Steiner RD, et al.: Bisphosphonate therapy for osteogenesis imperfecta, *Cochrane Database Syst Rev* 10:CD005088, 2016.

Franzone JM, Shah SA, Wallace MJ, et al.: Osteogenesis imperfecta: a pediatric orthopedic perspective, *Orthop Clin North Am* 50:193, 2019.

Grossman LS, Price AL, Rush ET, et al.: Initial experience with percutaneous IM rodding of the humeri in children with osteogenesis imperfecta, *J Pediatr Orthop* 38:484, 2018.

Hatz D, Esposito PW, Schroeder B, et al.: The incidence of spondylolysis and spondylolisthesis in children with osteogenesis imperfecta, *J Pediatr Orthop* 31:655, 2011.

Kim RH, Scuderi GR, Dennis DA, Nakano SW: Technical challenges of total knee arthroplasty in skeletal dysplasia, *Clin Orthop Relat Res* 469:69, 2011.

Kocher S, Dichtel L: Osteogenesis imperfecta misdiagnosed as child abuse, *J Pediatr Orthop B* 20:440, 2011.

Krishnan H, Patel NK, Skinner JA, et al.: Primary and revision total hip arthroplasty in osteogenesis imperfecta, *Hip Int* 23:303, 2013.

Lafage-Proust MH, Courtois I: The management of osteogenesis imperfecta in adults: state of the art, *Joint Bone Spin* 2019. [Epub ahead of print].

Lee K, Park MS, Yoo WJ, et al.: Proximal migration of femoral telescopic rod in children with osteogenesis imperfecta, *J Pediatr Orthop* 35:178–184, 2015.

Mesfin A, Nesterenko SO, Al-Hourani KG, et al.: Management of hangman's fractures and a subaxial compression fracture in two children with osteogenesis imperfecta, *J Surg Orthop Adv* 22:326, 2013.

Nicolaou N, Agrawal Y, Padman M, et al.: Changing pattern of femoral fractures in osteogenesis imperfecta with prolonged use of bisphosphonates, *J Child Orthop* 6:21, 2012.

Nijhuis WH, Eastwood DM, Allgrove J, et al.: Current concepts in osteogenesis imperfecta: bone structure, biomechanics, and medical management, *J Child Orthop* 13:1, 2019.

Oakley I, Reece LP: Anesthetic implications for the patient with osteogenesis imperfecta, *AANA J* 78:47, 2010.

Persiani P, Martini L, Ranaldi FM, et al.: Elastic intramedullary nailing of the femur fracture in patients affected by osteogenesis imperfecta type 3: indications, limits and pitfalls, *Injury* 2019. [Epub ahead of print].

Persiani P, Ranaldi FM, Martini L, et al.: Treatment of tibial deformities with the Fassier-Duval telescopic nail and minimally invasive percutaneous osteotomies in patients with osteogenesis imperfecta type III, *J Pediatr Orthop B* 28:179, 2019.

Popkov D, Popkov A, Mingazov E: Use of sliding transphyseal flexible intramedullary nailing in pediatric osteogenesis imperfect patients, *Acta Orthop Belg* 85:1, 2019.

Ruck J, Dahan-Oliel N, Montpetit K, et al.: Fassier-Duval femoral rodding in children with osteogenesis imperfecta receiving bisphosphonates: functional outcomes at one year, *J Child Orthop* 5:217, 2011.

Spahn KM, Mickel T, Carry PM, et al.: Fassier-Duval rods are associated with superior probability of survival compared with static implants in a cohort of children with osteogenesis imperfecta deformities, *J Pediatr Orthop* 39:e396, 2019.

Wagner R, Luedke C: Total knee arthroplasty with concurrent femoral and tibial osteotomies in osteogenesis imperfecta, *Am J Orthop* 43:37, 2014.

Yilmaz G, Hwang S, Oto M, et al.: Surgical treatment of scoliosis in osteogenesis imperfecta with cement-augmented pedicle screw instrumentation, *J Spinal Disord Tech* 27:174, 2014.

DWARFISM

Kim SJ, Agashe V, Song SH, et al.: Comparison between upper and lower limb lengthening in patients with achondroplasia: a retrospective study, *J Bone Joint Surg* 94B:128, 2012.

Kim SJ, Balce GC, Agashe MV, et al.: Is bilateral lower limb lengthening appropriate for achondroplasia? Midterm analysis of the complications and quality of life, *Clin Orthop Relat Res* 470:616, 2012.

Launay F, Younsi R, Pithioux M, et al.: Fracture following lower limb lengthening in children: a series of 58 patients, *Orthop Traumatol Surg Res* 99:72, 2013.

Malot R, Park KW, Song SH, et al.: Role of hybrid monolateral fixators in managing humeral length and deformity correction, *BMJ Case Rep* 2013. pii:bcr2013008793.

Song SH, Agashe MV, Huh YJ, et al.: Physeal growth arrest after tibial lengthening in achrondroplasia: 23 children followed to skeletal maturity, *Acta Orthop* 83:282, 2012.

Song SH, Kim SE, Agashe MV, et al.: Growth disturbance after lengthening of the lower limb and quantitative assessment of physeal closure in skeletally immature patients with achondroplasia, *J Bone Joint Surg* 94B:556, 2012.

Weiner DS, Jonah D, Leighley B, et al.: Orthopaedic manifestations of chondroectodermal dysplasia: the Ellis-van Creveld syndrome, *J Child Orthop* 7:465, 2013.

TRAUMATIC EPIPHYSEAL ARREST FROM BRIDGE OF BONE

Kang HG, Yoon SJ, Kim JR: Resection of a physeal bar under computer-assisted guidance, *J Bone Joint Surg* 92B:1452–1455, 2010.

Miyamura S, Tanaka H, Oka K, et al.: Physeal bar resection using a patient-specific guide with intramedullary endoscopic assistance for partial physeal arrest of the distal radius, *Arch Orthop Trauma Surg* 138:1179, 2018.

Pharr ZK, Roaten JD, Moisan A, et al.: Use of a core reamer for the resection of a central distal femoral physeal bone bridge: a novel technique with 3-year follow-up, *Am J Orthop (Belle Mead NJ)* 47:5, 2018.

The complete list of references is available online at Expert Consult.com

PART II

NERVOUS SYSTEM DISORDERS IN CHILDREN

CHAPTER 5

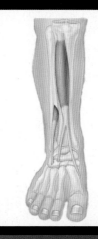

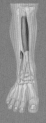

CEREBRAL PALSY

David D. Spence, Benjamin W. Sheffer

ETIOLOGY

Cerebral palsy is a heterogeneous disorder of movement and posture that has a wide variety of presentations, ranging from mild motor disturbance to severe total body involvement. Because of this variability in clinical presentation and the absence of a definitive diagnostic test, defining exactly what cerebral palsy is has been difficult and controversial. It is generally agreed that there are three distinctive features common to all patients with cerebral palsy: (1) some degree of motor impairment, which distinguishes it from other conditions, such as global developmental delay or autism; (2) an insult to the developing brain, making it different from conditions that affect the mature brain in older children and adults; and (3) a neurologic deficit that is nonprogressive, which distinguishes it from other motor diseases of childhood, such as the muscular dystrophies. In 2004 the International Executive Committee for the Definition of Cerebral Palsy revised the definition of cerebral palsy to state: Cerebral palsy (CP) describes a group of permanent disorders of the development of movement and posture, causing activity limitation, that are attributed to nonprogressive disturbances that occurred in the developing fetal or infant brain. The motor disorders of cerebral palsy often are accompanied by disturbances of sensation, perception, cognition, communication, behavior, epilepsy, and secondary musculoskeletal problems.

The insult to the brain is believed to occur between the time of conception and age 2 years, at which time a significant amount of motor development has already occurred. A similar injury to the brain after age 2 years can have a similar effect, however, and often is called cerebral palsy. By 8 years of age, most of the development of the immature brain is complete, as is gait development, and an insult to the brain results in a more adult-type clinical picture and outcome.

Although the neurologic deficit is permanent and nonprogressive, the effect it can have on the patient is dynamic, and the orthopaedic aspects of cerebral palsy can change dramatically with growth and development. Growth, along with altered muscle forces across joints, can lead to progressive loss of motion, contracture, and eventually joint subluxation or dislocation, resulting in degeneration that may require orthopaedic intervention.

Children with cerebral palsy constitute the largest group of pediatric patients with neuromuscular disorders in the United States. The prevalence of cerebral palsy varies around the world according to the amount and quality of prenatal care, the socioeconomic condition of the parents, the environment, and the type of obstetric and pediatric care the mother and child receive. The determination of the true prevalence also is difficult because many children are not diagnosed until age 2 or 3 years; this most often occurs in socioeconomic groups that have decreased access to medical care. In the United States, the occurrence is approximately two per 1000 live births; there are approximately 25,000 new patients with cerebral palsy each year, and approximately 400,000 children with cerebral palsy at any given time. The United States experienced an initial decrease in the number of affected children in the 1950s and 1960s as a result of better understanding and treatment of maternal-fetal Rh incompatibility and improvements in obstetric techniques. More recently, the prevalence of cerebral palsy was thought to be increasing because of the increased survival of premature and low-birth-weight infants; however, two large population-based studies showed that the improved survival of these infants has not contributed to the increase in prevalence of cerebral palsy in the United States. Worldwide, the prevalence ranges from 0.6 to 7.0 cases per 1000 live births. The cost of operative treatment in children with cerebral palsy is substantial. In 1997, there were an estimated 37,000 operative procedures performed, with the most common being gastrostomy tube placements, soft-tissue releases, fundoplications, spinal fusions, and hip osteotomies. These procedures accounted for 50,000 hospital days and $150 million in charges.

Injury to the developing brain can occur at any time from gestation to early childhood and typically is categorized as prenatal, perinatal, or postnatal. Contrary to popular belief, fewer than 10% of injuries that result in cerebral palsy occur during the birth process, with most occurring in the prenatal period. A wide variety of risk factors for cerebral palsy have been identified in the prenatal period, including risk factors inherent to the fetus (most commonly genetic disorders), factors inherent to the mother (seizure disorders, mental retardation, and previous pregnancy loss), and factors inherent to the pregnancy itself (Rh incompatibility, polyhydramnios, placental rupture, and drug or alcohol exposure). External factors, such as TORCH syndrome (toxoplasmosis, other agents, rubella, cytomegalovirus, herpes simplex), also can lead to cerebral palsy in the prenatal period. Occurrences in the absence of any known risk factors may be caused by some yet unknown factor during this critical time in brain development. Several more recent studies have suggested a possible role of chorioamnionitis as one of these factors.

Cerebral palsy in the perinatal period, from birth until a few days after birth, typically is associated with asphyxia or trauma that occurs during labor. Oxytocin augmentation, umbilical cord prolapse, and breech presentation all have been associated with an increased occurrence of cerebral palsy. Only 10% of cases of cerebral palsy occur during this time period, and most patients with cerebral palsy have no history of asphyxia. Although cerebral palsy is often associated with low Apgar scores during this period, many neonates have low scores because of other conditions, such as genetic disorders, that are completely unrelated to asphyxia.

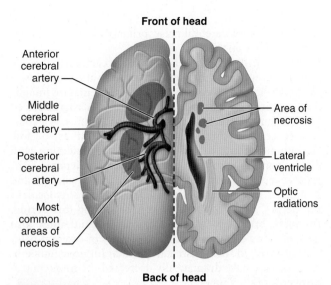

Front of head

Anterior cerebral artery

Middle cerebral artery

Posterior cerebral artery

Most common areas of necrosis

Area of necrosis

Lateral ventricle

Optic radiations

Back of head

FIGURE 5.1   Periventricular leukomalacia. Cross-sectional view shows blood vessels that supply brain with blood *(left)* and brain structures *(right)*. Area surrounding ventricles contains "white matter" that includes descending neuronal pathways of motor control system. This area, especially farther forward in brain, is susceptible to damage in premature infants because of relative paucity of blood vessels. Fluctuations in blood flow, blood oxygen, or blood glucose levels can cause damage in this area, resulting in disturbance of motor control system and subsequent (usually spastic) cerebral palsy.

TABLE 5.1

Grading of Periventricular Lesions	
I	Bleeding confined to germinal matrix
II	Bleeding extends into ventricles
III	Bleeding into ventricles with dilation
IV	Bleeding into brain substance

Adapted from Pellegrino L, Dormans JP: Definitions, etiology, and epidemiology of cerebral palsy. In Pellegrino L, Dormans JP, editors: *Caring for children with cerebral palsy: a team-based approach*, Baltimore, 1998, Paul Brookes.

Low-birth-weight infants (<1500 g) are at dramatically increased risk of cerebral palsy, with an incidence of 60 per 1000 births compared with two per 1000 births in infants of normal weight. This increased incidence is believed to be caused by the fragility of the periventricular blood vessels, which are highly susceptible to physiologic fluctuations during pregnancy (Fig. 5.1). These fluctuations, which include hypoxic episodes, placental pathology, maternal diabetes, and infection, can injure these vessels and lead to subsequent intraventricular hemorrhages. These injuries are graded on a scale from I to IV (Table 5.1), with an increased incidence of neurologic consequences such as hydrocephalus and cerebral palsy in grade III (bleeding into ventricles with dilation) and grade IV (bleeding into brain substance). In addition, the periventricular area, which is important for motor control, is especially susceptible from the 26th to the 32nd week of pregnancy. If this area is injured, diplegia usually results. Often, a synergistic combination of events leads to brain injury and the subsequent development of cerebral palsy. Pregnancies involving multiple births also are at increased risk for cerebral palsy, primarily because of their association with premature delivery.

Although most children born with cerebral palsy are delivered at full term, full-term infants are at a much lower risk of developing cerebral palsy than are premature infants. Hypoxic-ischemic encephalopathy, which is characterized by hypotonia, decreased movement, and seizures, is a common cause of cerebral palsy during the postnatal period. Meconium aspiration and persistent fetal circulation with true ischemia are the most common causes of hypoxic-ischemic encephalopathy. Infections such as encephalitis and meningitis, most commonly caused by group B *Streptococcus* and herpes, can lead to cerebral palsy during this period. Traumatic brain injury from accidents or child abuse also accounts for a significant number of cases of cerebral palsy that develop in the postnatal period. Improvements in obstetric care have dramatically decreased the frequency of iatrogenic brain injury.

CLASSIFICATION

Because of the wide variability in presentation and types of cerebral palsy, various classification schemes have been described. Traditionally, cerebral palsy has been classified by the clinical physiologic picture, the region of the body affected, or the neuroanatomic region of the brain that was injured. More recently, the Gross Motor Function Classification System (GMFCS) has been adopted as the most widely used classification scheme; this system stratifies children based on function at various ages.

GEOGRAPHIC CLASSIFICATION

The anatomic region of the body affected with the movement disorder should be identified as shown in Table 5.2. Often, it is difficult to classify completely the pattern of involvement geographically because some extremities may be only subtly involved and a patient's pattern of involvement can change over time. This classification is useful, however, in describing general patterns of involvement.

■ MONOPLEGIA

Monoplegia is very rare and usually occurs after meningitis. Most patients diagnosed with monoplegia actually have hemiplegia with one extremity only very mildly affected.

■ HEMIPLEGIA

In hemiplegia, one side of the body is involved, with the upper extremity usually more affected than the lower extremity. Patients with hemiplegia, approximately 30% of patients with cerebral palsy, typically have sensory changes in the affected extremities as well. Severe sensory changes, especially in the upper extremity, are a predictor of poor functional outcome after reconstructive surgery. Hemiplegic patients also may have a leg-length discrepancy, with shortening on the affected side, which can be treated with contralateral epiphysiodesis or leg lengthening.

■ DIPLEGIA

Diplegia is the most common anatomic type of cerebral palsy, constituting approximately 50% of all cases. Patients with

TABLE 5.2

Geographic Classification of Cerebral Palsy

TYPE	DESCRIPTION/INVOLVEMENT
Monoplegia	One extremity involved, usually lower
Hemiplegia	Both extremities on same side involved Usually upper extremity involved more than lower extremity
Paraplegia	Both lower extremities equally involved
Diplegia	Lower extremities more involved than upper extremities Fine-motor/sensory abnormalities in upper extremity
Quadriplegia	All extremities involved equally Normal head/neck control
Double hemiplegia	All extremities involved, upper more than lower
Total body	All extremities severely involved No head/neck control

diplegia have motor abnormalities in all four extremities, with the lower extremities more affected than the upper. The close proximity of the lower extremity tracts to the ventricles most likely explains the more frequent involvement of the lower extremities with periventricular lesions (Fig. 5.1). This type of cerebral palsy is most common in premature infants; intelligence usually is normal. Most children with diplegia walk eventually, although walking is delayed usually until around age 4 years.

■ QUADRIPLEGIA

In quadriplegia, all four extremities are equally involved and many patients have significant cognitive deficiencies that make care more difficult. Head and neck control usually is present, which helps with communication, education, and seating. Treatment goals for patients with quadriplegia include a straight spine and level pelvis, located mobile hips with 90 degrees of flexion for sitting and 30 degrees of extension for pivoting, plantigrade feet that can fit in shoes, and an appropriate wheelchair.

■ TOTAL BODY

Patients with total body involvement typically have profound cognitive deficits in addition to loss of head and neck control. These patients usually require full-time assistance for activities of daily living and specialized seating systems to assist with head positioning. Drooling, dysarthria, and dysphagia also are common and complicate care.

■ OTHER TYPES

Some patients have a double hemiplegia pattern as a result of bleeding in both hemispheres of the brain. It often is difficult to differentiate this from diplegia or quadriplegia; however, in double hemiplegia, the upper extremities typically are more involved than the lower.

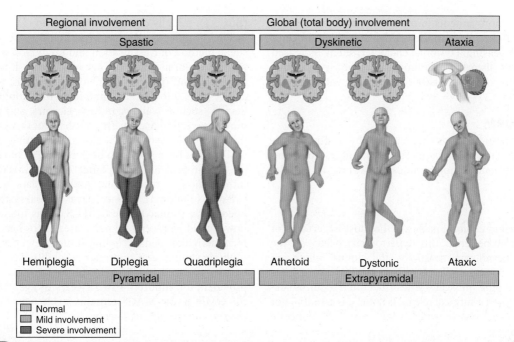

Regional involvement	Global (total body) involvement	
Spastic	Dyskinetic	Ataxia

Hemiplegia	Diplegia	Quadriplegia	Athetoid	Dystonic	Ataxic
Pyramidal			Extrapyramidal		

☐ Normal
☐ Mild involvement
■ Severe involvement

FIGURE 5.2   Classification of cerebral palsy. Although overlaps in terminology exist, cerebral palsy can be classified according to distribution (regional versus global involvement, hemiplegic, diplegic, quadriplegic), physiologic type (spastic, dyskinetic/dystonic, dyskinetic/athetoid, ataxic), or presumed neurologic substrate (pyramidal, extrapyramidal). (Redrawn from Pellegrino L: Cerebral palsy. In Batshaw ML, editor: *Children with disabilities*, ed 4, Baltimore, 1997, Paul H. Brookes.)

Paraplegia is very rare and is characterized by bilateral lower extremity involvement with (in contrast to diplegia) completely normal gross and fine motor skills in the upper extremity. Many patients diagnosed with paraplegia actually are diplegic with very mildly involved upper extremities. Although occasionally mentioned, triplegia, the involvement of three extremities, probably does not exist. With careful examination, most patients believed to have triplegia actually have subtle motor deficits of the least involved limb.

PHYSIOLOGIC CLASSIFICATION

Most patients with cerebral palsy have recognizable patterns of movement that also can be classified. A basic understanding of normal brain development is important to understanding the various types. During the first trimester, the immature brain separates into the gross structures, including the cerebrum, cerebellum, and medulla. Neurons begin to form in the second trimester, and the total number of neurons an individual eventually has are present at the end of this time frame. Any neurons lost from this point forward are irreplaceable. Synaptic connections and myelination begin during the third trimester and continue through adolescence in a highly organized fashion. As these synapses develop and myelinization continues, primitive reflexes disappear and more mature motor patterns arise. Because of this continued development after birth, many injuries to the newborn nervous system go unrecognized until the absence of expected patterns can be detected. Different pathways of the brain are myelinated at different times; therefore spastic diplegia usually is not detected until 8 to 10 months of age; hemiplegia, 20 months of age; and athetoid cerebral palsy, after 24 months of age. This should be kept in mind because a child's pattern may change over time.

Physiologically, cerebral palsy can be divided into a spastic type, which affects the corticospinal (pyramidal) tracts, and an extrapyramidal type, which affects the other regions of the developing brain. The extrapyramidal types of cerebral palsy include athetoid, choreiform, ataxic, rigid, and hypotonic (Fig. 5.2).

■ SPASTIC

Spastic is the most common form of cerebral palsy, constituting approximately 80% of cases, and usually is associated with injury to the pyramidal tracts in the immature brain. Spasticity, or the velocity-dependent increase in muscle tone with passive stretch, is caused by an exaggeration of the normal muscle passive stretch reflex. Booth showed histologically that this altered muscle function leads to the deposition of type I collagen in the endomysium of the affected muscle, leading to thickening and fibrosis, the degree of which correlated to the severity of the spasticity. Often, patients have simultaneous cocontraction of normally antagonistic muscle groups leading to fatigue, loss of dexterity and coordination, and balance difficulties. Joint contractures, subluxation, and degeneration are common in patients with spastic cerebral palsy.

■ ATHETOID

Athetoid cerebral palsy is caused by an injury to the extrapyramidal tracts and is characterized by dyskinetic, purposeless movements that may be exacerbated by environmental stimulation. The clinical picture varies based on the level of excitement of the patient. In pure athetoid cerebral palsy, joint contractures are uncommon; the results of soft-tissue releases, in contrast to those seen in spastic cerebral palsy, are unpredictable, and the procedures have a high complication rate. With the improvements in prevention of Rh incompatibility leading to kernicterus, the incidence of athetoid cerebral palsy is decreasing. Dystonia, characterized by increased overall tone and distorted positioning in response to voluntary movements, or hypotonia also can occur with athetoid cerebral palsy.

■ CHOREIFORM

Choreiform cerebral palsy is characterized by continual purposeless movements of the patient's wrists, fingers, toes, and ankles. This continuous movement can make bracing and sitting difficult.

■ RIGID

Patients with rigid cerebral palsy are the most hypertonic of all cerebral palsy patients. This hypertonicity occurs in the absence of hyperreflexia, spasticity, and clonus, which are common in spastic cerebral palsy. These patients have a "cogwheel" or "lead pipe" muscle stiffness that often requires surgical release. When a surgical release is done, it is essential not to overweaken the muscle, which would cause the opposite deformity to occur.

■ ATAXIC

Ataxic cerebral palsy is very rare and probably is the most often misdiagnosed type. It is characterized by the disturbance of coordinated movement, most commonly walking, as a result of an injury to the developing cerebellum. It is important to distinguish true ataxia from spasticity because with treatment many children with ataxia are able to improve their gait function without surgery. Overaggressive tendon lengthening in patients with ataxia can lead to iatrogenic weakness, which further interferes with gait function.

■ HYPOTONIC

Hypotonic cerebral palsy is characterized by weakness in conjunction with low muscle tone and normal deep tendon reflexes. Many children who ultimately develop spastic or ataxic cerebral palsy pass through a hypotonic stage lasting 1 or 2 years before the true nature of their brain injury becomes apparent. Persistent hypotonia can lead to difficulties with sitting balance, head positioning, and communication.

■ MIXED

Many patients with cerebral palsy have features of more than one type and are referred to as having mixed cerebral palsy. Patients with mixed cerebral palsy usually show signs of pyramidal and extrapyramidal deficits. The final clinical appearance is determined by the relative components of spasticity, athetosis, and ataxia. Surgical releases in this group can be less predictable, especially when a large athetoid or ataxic component is present.

FUNCTIONAL CLASSIFICATION

In recent years, newer classification systems have been developed based on function. Functional classification systems are able to grade individuals based on their abilities instead of their deficiencies and promote the concepts of the World Health Organization's International Classification of Functioning, Disability, and Health, which focuses on activity and participation. The first widely accepted functional classification was the Gross Motor Function Classification System (GMFCS)

(Box 5.1). Initially described by Palisano et al., this five-level ordinal grading system has been found to be a reliable and stable method of classification and prediction of motor function for children under the age of 12 years. It has since been expanded and revised to include children 12 to 18 years of age. It takes into account functional limitations for assistive devices, such as walkers and wheelchairs, and the quality of movement based on age. The emphasis of this scale is on self-initiated movement and walking and sitting function. The GMFCS has been shown to be predictive of hip dislocation.

The impact and acceptance of the GMFCS led to the introduction of the Manual Abilities Classification System (MACS) (Table 5.3). This five-level ordinal system was developed to be similar to the GMFCS but is intended to assess how a child with cerebral palsy uses his or her hands to perform activities of daily living. It also has been validated by multiple studies, and interrater reliability has been found to be good to excellent among health care professionals and care providers for children 4 to 18 years of age. Also similar to the GMFCS, the MACS remains stable over time with little change after the age of 4 years.

DIAGNOSIS

History and physical examination are the primary tools in making the diagnosis of cerebral palsy. The history should include a thorough investigation of the pregnancy and delivery. With the exception of several rare conditions, such as familial spastic paraparesis and congenital ataxia, there is no known genetic component to cerebral palsy. Ancillary studies, such as radiographs, hematologic studies, chromosomal analysis, computed tomography (CT), magnetic resonance imaging, and positron emission tomography, rarely are needed to make the diagnosis but may be helpful in determining the type and extent of cerebral palsy present. Diagnosis of cerebral palsy before 2 years of age can be difficult. One study found that 55% of children diagnosed with cerebral palsy by 1 year of age did not meet the criteria by 7 years of age. Transient dystonia of prematurity is a condition characterized by increased tone in the lower extremities between 4 and 14 months old and often is confused with cerebral palsy. This is a self-limiting condition and resolves without treatment. In addition, African-American children tend to have higher muscle tone than other ethnic groups, which also can lead to a misdiagnosis of cerebral palsy.

Knowledge of normal motor developmental milestones and primitive reflexes allows identification of children who are delayed in their motor development. Motor development usually occurs in a cephalad-to-caudal pattern, starting with swallowing and sucking, which are present at birth, and proceeding to sphincter control, which occurs at 24 to 36 months of age (Table 5.4). Primitive reflex patterns of motor activity that are outgrown as part of the normal maturation process persist longer than normal and in some cases permanently in children with cerebral palsy. Other, more mature motor patterns, which are essential for normal ambulation, may be significantly delayed or never appear. By determining which reflexes are present or absent, the child's neurologic age can be determined. By comparing the neurologic age with the chronologic age, a neurologic quotient can be determined, which is useful in determining prognosis and treatment. The presence of these primitive reflexes also can contribute to further deformity.

BOX 5.1

Gross Motor Functional Classification System

Level I
- **Up to 2 Years of Age:** Infants start to learn to sit on the floor and use both hands to play with and manipulate objects. Infants are also capable of crawling and pulling themselves up, and by 18 months, can walk.
- **Ages 2 to 4:** Children can successfully sit on the floor with no assistance. They may also begin to stand without adult assistance and walk. Walking is typically preferred over crawling.
- **Ages 4 to 6:** Children can sit in a chair and get up from a chair without assistance. They can also move to the floor from a chair without assistance, walk freely without assistance, and begin to run and jump.
- **Ages 6 to 12:** Children can run, walk, jump, and climb stairs without assistance; balance and coordination may be lacking still.

Level II
- **Up to 2 Years of Age:** Infants may begin to sit on the floor but only with adult assistance or by relying on their hands for support. They may begin to crawl on hands and knees or "creep" on their belly.
- **Ages 2 to 4:** Children can sit on the floor but require assistance, especially if they're using their hands to manipulate and grab objects. Reciprocal patterns are used when crawling on hands and knees, and children can walk either with assistive devices or by holding onto furniture or other sturdy objects.
- **Ages 4 to 6:** Children can now sit in a chair without assistance but need assistance from standing to moving to the floor, such as a sturdy table or surface. Additionally, they can walk for short distances without support and can climb stairs as long as they are holding the rails for support. However, they cannot skip, run, or jump.
- **Ages 6 to 12:** Children can walk both indoors and outdoors with little to no assistance but will need help with walking in crowds, in unfamiliar settings, and on inclined surfaces. They still need rails when climbing steps and only possess minimal abilities for gross motor skills, such as running, jumping, and skipping.

Level III
- **Up to 2 Years of Age:** Infants can roll and creep in a forward position while on their stomachs but will need assistance with sitting via lower back support.
- **Ages 2 to 4:** Children can sit on the floor unsupported but typically in the "W" position: rotated hips and knees. They also can crawl on their hands and knees, usually without moving the legs. Crawling tends to be the preferred method of moving around.

- **Ages 4 to 6:** Children can sit upright on a chair but require trunk support if using their hands. Additionally, they can lift themselves from the chair with the assistance of sturdy furniture, such as a table, and can climb stairs with adult help. They can also walk while using a mobility device for assistance.
- **Ages 6 to 12:** With a mobility device for assistance, children walk both outdoors and indoors. They may be able to climb stairs without adult assistance but with the use of handrails. If they are traveling long distances or walking on uneven or inclined distances, they will either need to be carried or use a wheelchair.

Level IV
- **Up to 2 Years of Age:** Infants can roll from back to stomach and vice versa but can only sit upright with trunk assistance.
- **Ages 2 to 4:** When placed on the floor, children can sit up, but will need to use their hands and arms for support. In most instances, they will need adaptive equipment for both sitting and standing, but crawling on their hands and knees, stomach creeping, and/or rolling are the preferred methods of moving.
- **Ages 4 to 6:** Children can sit on a chair with trunk support and can move from the chair by holding onto a sturdy surface. They can walk short distances, but adult supervision is highly recommended as they may have problems turning and keeping their balance.
- **Ages 6 to 12:** Children will maintain the same mobility from age 6, but they may rely more on wheelchairs and walk-assisting devices, especially at school or in the community.

Level V
- **Up to 2 Years of Age:** Voluntary control of movements are physically impaired and, in turn, the infant cannot hold his or her head and trunk without support. They also need assistance in rolling over.
- **Ages 2 to 4:** All areas of motor function are still limited, rendering it difficult for the child to sit without assistance, to crawl, or achieve any type of independent mobility at all.
- **Ages 4 to 6:** Children can now sit on a chair but will need adaptive equipment to hold them in place. In addition, they will need to be transported, even for daily activities, as they still have no independent mobility.
- **Ages 6 to 12:** Some children may be able to achieve mobility on their own via an electronic wheelchair, but mobility will still be limited to the point where they cannot move on their own, including the inability to support their trunks and bodies. Additional expansive adaptation equipment is used in some instances.

PROGNOSTIC FACTORS

Considerable work has been done investigating prognostic factors for function, including ambulation, in patients with cerebral palsy. The presence of tonic neck reflexes usually is incompatible with independent standing balance and the ability to perform alternating movements of the lower extremities necessary for walking. Sitting independently by 2 years of age is a good predictor of independent ambulation. If a child cannot sit independently by 4 years, it is unlikely he or she will ever walk without assistance. If a child has not learned to walk by 8 years of age, and he or she is not limited by severe contractures, it is unlikely he or she will ever walk at all.

Poor prognostic signs for walking reported by Bleck included (1) an imposable asymmetric tonic neck reflex, (2) persistent Moro reflex, (3) strong extensor thrust on vertical suspension, (4) persistent neck-righting reflex, and (5) absence of normal parachute reaction after 11 months.

TABLE 5.3

Manual Ability Classification System (MACS) Levels

LEVEL	DESCRIPTION	COMMENTS
1	Handles objects easily and successfully	At most, limitations in the ease of performing manual tasks requiring speed and accuracy; however, any limitations in manual abilities do not restrict independence in daily activities
2	Handles most objects but with somewhat reduced quality and/or speed	Certain activities may be avoided or be achieved with some difficulty; alternative ways of performance might be used, but manual abilities do not usually restrict independence in daily activities
3	Handles objects with difficulty; needs help to prepare and/or modify activities	Performance is slow and is achieved with limited success regarding quality and quantity; activities are performed independently if they have been set up or adapted
4	Handles a limited selection of easily managed objects in adapted situations	Performs parts of activities with effort and with limited success; requires continuous support and assistance and/or adapted equipment for even partial achievement of the activity
5	Does not handle objects and has severely limited ability to perform even simple actions	Requires total assistance

TABLE 5.4

Early Motor Developmental Milestones

MILESTONE	AVERAGE AGE (MO)	95TH PERCENTILE
Head control	3	6
Independent sitting	6	9
Crawling	8	Variable, some never do
Pull to stand	8	12
Independent walking	12	17

The persistence of these primitive reflexes is associated with extensive and severe brain damage and a poor prognosis for independent ambulation, self-care, and activities of daily living.

GAIT ANALYSIS

Before the development of computer-based gait analysis systems, careful clinical observation was the primary method of diagnosing gait disturbances in children with cerebral palsy. It is still an essential component in making the diagnosis. This clinical observation is done by repeatedly watching the child walk from the front, sides, and back, studying one component of gait at a time. Attention should be paid to the pelvis, hip, knee, ankle, and foot and to stride length, cadence, rotational alignment, trunk position, and side-to-side differences.

Modern quantitative gait analysis uses high-speed motion picture cameras from different angles, retroreflective markers on the surface of the skin aligned with palpable skeletal landmarks, and force platforms to measure the various components of gait. Kinematic data are obtained and presented in a waveform that represents the three-dimensional motion of the joints during the gait cycle. Electromyographic (EMG) testing, which documents the activation of various muscles during the gait cycle, also is used to determine which muscles are firing in a normal pattern and which are firing out of phase. Other components of quantitative gait analysis include pedobarography (foot pressure) and oxygen consumption measurement. Combined, these give the trained observer an accurate representation of the complex interaction of all of the components of gait. Gait analysis frequently is used in preoperative planning before lower extremity surgery to delineate a patient's specific gait deviations and plan the appropriate intervention. One study found that when experienced observers were given quantitative gait analysis for patients after surgical recommendations had already been made based on clinical observation, the surgical recommendation changed 52% of the time.

Although quantitative gait analysis provides objective data, interpretation of that data seems to be subjective. Only slight-to-moderate agreement has been noted among physicians in identification of soft-tissue and bony problems and in recommendations for treatment. Significant institutional differences in diagnosis and treatment recommendations also have been found. Clinical examination combined with gait analysis has been reported to improve surgical outcome. As noted, postoperative gait analysis may be useful not only in assessing outcomes but also in making further treatment recommendations, including recommendations for bracing, specific physical therapy protocols, and further surgical intervention.

Although quantitative gait analysis techniques continue to improve, their role in the evaluation and treatment of children with cerebral palsy remains controversial. Although gait analysis has been shown to alter decision-making, studies are necessary to determine if these changes lead to improved clinical outcomes. Davids et al. proposed a five-step paradigm for clinical decision making to optimize the walking ability of children with cerebral palsy. The five points are clinical history, physical examination, diagnostic imaging, quantitative gait analysis, and examination under anesthesia. We believe that this type of approach is better than relying on quantitative gait analysis alone in the diagnosis and treatment of children with cerebral palsy.

ASSOCIATED CONDITIONS

Most patients with cerebral palsy have associated impairments that interfere with their daily function, independence, mobility, and overall health. These issues may be more important to the patient, the patient's family, and their caregivers than the child's ambulatory status. These conditions must be taken into account when considering any type of therapeutic intervention. In one study, adults with cerebral palsy ranked what was most important to them, and education and communication were most important, followed by activities of daily living and mobility. Ambulation was ranked fourth. Because of the complex nature of these conditions, a multidisciplinary team approach to patients with cerebral palsy is essential.

The most common associated conditions in patients with cerebral palsy are mental impairment or learning disability (40%); seizures (30%); complex movement disorders (20%); visual impairment (16%); malnutrition and related conditions, such as gastroesophageal reflux, obesity, and undernutrition (15%); and hydrocephalus (14%). Mental impairment and learning disability can range from very mild deficits to severe impairment and inability to live independently. Mental retardation, as defined as an IQ less than 50, occurs in 30% to 65% of children with cerebral palsy, most commonly in quadriplegics. Learning disabilities are worsened by seizure disorders, various medications with central nervous system side effects, and communication difficulties. Bulbar involvement can lead to drooling, dysphagia, and speech difficulties, which can limit cognitive and social development further.

Many children with cerebral palsy (50% in some series) have significant visual difficulties, with 7% having a severe visual defect. Common visual disturbances include myopia, amblyopia, strabismus, visual field defects, and cortical blindness. Visual screening is indicated in all children with cerebral palsy. Hearing loss has been reported to occur in 10% to 25% of children with cerebral palsy, which can exacerbate communication and learning difficulties further. Hearing screenings, similar to visual screenings, should be part of the routine evaluation of patients with cerebral palsy.

Approximately 30% of patients with cerebral palsy also have seizures, most commonly patients with hemiplegia, quadriplegia, or postnatally acquired syndromes. Seizures and the medications used in their management can have profound effects on learning, communication, and ambulation. This has led to renewed interest in alternative medication delivery systems, such as intrathecal baclofen and intramuscular botulinum toxin injections.

Osteopenia with increased risk of fracture also is common in children with cerebral palsy, especially children who are more severely affected. Fractures often can be difficult to diagnose, especially in nonverbal patients. The use of whole-body technetium bone scanning can be helpful to identify occult fractures in these patients. The nonoperative and operative treatment of these fractures has a high complication rate and usually interferes with the child's social and school activities and can make it difficult for caretakers. Significant femoral osteopenia (bone mineral density Z-score of <−2) has been identified in nearly 80% of children with cerebral palsy and 97% of nonstanders. Femoral fractures can occur especially in nonambulatory patients with severe involvement. Although these can be treated nonoperatively, there is a high rate of malunion requiring surgery and increased cast-related complications. Bisphosphonates and growth hormone have been shown in small studies to be safe and effective in increasing bone mineral density in children with cerebral palsy, but large multicenter trials are lacking. Severe medical problems, such as aspiration pneumonia and profound feeding problems, can lead to malnutrition, immune suppression, and metabolic abnormalities. Gastroesophageal reflux often can be managed medically and with positioning, but fundoplication may be necessary. Enteral feeding augmentation often is necessary because of swallowing dysfunction and the risk of aspiration pneumonia. This can be done with a gastrostomy or jejunostomy tube. Patients with protein malnutrition have been shown to be at increased risk of postoperative infection.

Emotional problems add to these associated conditions. The child's self-image plays an important role, especially in adolescence, when the differences between the affected child and peers become more apparent. Communication difficulties also may affect self-image at this stage. The attitudes of the parents, siblings, treatment team, and community are important to help the child or young adult maximize his or her independence and function. As young adulthood is reached, concerns about employment, self-care, sexual function, marriage, childbearing, and caring for aging parents may become emotional stressors.

TREATMENT

Because of the heterogeneous nature of cerebral palsy, it is difficult to make generalized statements regarding treatment, and it is best to have an individualized approach to each patient and his or her needs. In some centers, a multidisciplinary team approach (including physical, occupational, and speech therapy; orthotics; nutrition; social work; orthopaedics; and general pediatrics) has been successful. Four basic treatment principles exist. The first is that although the central nervous system injury, by definition, is nonprogressive, the deformities caused by abnormal muscle forces and contractures are progressive. The second, which can be a source of frustration, is that the treatments currently available correct the secondary deformities only and not the primary problem, which is the brain injury. The third is that the deformities typically become worse during times of rapid growth. For some patients, it may be beneficial to delay surgery until after a significant growth spurt to decrease the risk of recurrence. When determining the timing of surgery, consider the fact that most children with cerebral palsy have an advanced skeletal age compared with chronologic age by approximately 2 years and a significantly advanced age compared with normal controls of both sexes. The highest correlation between advanced bone age was found in quadriplegics and in boys with GMFCS level III and girls with a body mass index of less than 15. The fourth is that treatment should be done to minimize the negative effect that cerebral palsy has on the patient's socialization and education. It is important to be aware of these timing issues when considering any form of treatment in this patient population. For most patients a combined approach using nonoperative and operative methods is more beneficial than one form of treatment alone.

NONOPERATIVE TREATMENT

Nonoperative modalities, such as medication, splinting and bracing, and physical therapy, commonly are used as primary treatment or in conjunction with other forms of treatment such as surgery. A wide variety of medications have been used to treat cerebral palsy. The three most common agents are diazepam and baclofen, which act centrally, and dantrolene, which acts at the level of skeletal muscle. Baclofen mimics the action of γ-aminobutyric acid, a powerful inhibitory neurotransmitter centrally and peripherally, whereas diazepam potentiates the activity of γ-aminobutyric acid. These medications can be difficult to use because of wide variability in effectiveness among children and a narrow therapeutic window. Because these drugs increase inhibitory neurotransmitter activity, common systemic side effects include sedation, balance difficulties, and cognitive dysfunction, which can have a dramatic detrimental effect on ambulation, education, and communication.

Dantrolene acts at the level of skeletal muscle and decreases muscle calcium ion release. It has an affinity for fast twitch muscle fibers and selectively decreases abnormal muscle stretch reflexes and tone. Dantrolene is used less frequently than other medications because some patients taking it develop profound weakness, and there is a risk of hepatotoxicity with long-term use. Because of the systemic side effects of these medications, there is a renewed interest in alternative drug delivery systems, such as intrathecal baclofen and intramuscular botulinum toxin injections.

Baclofen, in addition to inhibiting abnormal monosynaptic extensor activity and polysynaptic flexor activity, has been shown to decrease substance P levels, which limits nociception. Baclofen has been shown to penetrate the blood-brain barrier poorly, and it has a short half-life (3 to 4 hours). This requires gradual titration of medication and the use of extremely high systemic levels to obtain a central effect of spasticity reduction. Intrathecal injection of baclofen requires 1/30 the dose of oral baclofen to achieve a similar or better response. Injecting baclofen intrathecally with an implantable programmable pump dramatically decreases the dose required to affect spasticity and decreases some of the side effects such as sedation. This pump typically is implanted subcutaneously in the abdominal wall and requires refilling approximately every 2 to 3 months (Fig. 5.3). A meta-analysis of 14 studies of intrathecal baclofen management found that it reduced lower extremity spasticity, seemed to improve function and ease of care, and had manageable complications. Baclofen also works at the level of the spinal cord to slow abnormal spinal reflexes and decrease motor neuron drive, which can reduce spasticity further. Careful monitoring is required to prevent overdosage, which can cause a decrease in trunk tone, weakness, and sedation. Complications from intrathecal baclofen include catheter and pump infection or malfunction, spinal fluid leak, respiratory depression, drug reactions, and oversedation. Ten to 20 percent of patients require further surgery or pump removal. There also have been concerns about the progression of scoliosis in patients who receive intrathecal baclofen therapy. One study, however, comparing curve magnitude progression in patients with and without the use of intrathecal baclofen showed no differences in curve progression between the groups. Until longer-term studies can be done, this treatment method is

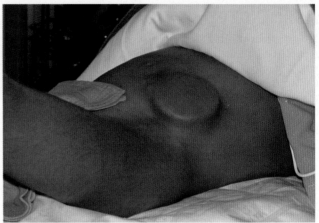

FIGURE 5.3 Continuous intrathecal baclofen infusion. Baclofen is injected through skin to reservoir, which is located within surgically placed pump beneath skin of abdomen. The pump, which is about the size of a hockey puck, is programmable using a device placed against skin and over the pump. Medication is continuously infused through catheter that tunnels under skin and is inserted directly into spinal canal; baclofen mixes with spinal fluid, directly affecting spinal cord and decreasing spasticity.

indicated for patients whose spasticity significantly interferes with self-care and quality of life and in whom other modalities have failed.

Botulinum toxin is a potent neurotoxin, of which there are seven serotypes, produced by *Clostridium botulinum*. Botulinum toxin type A (BTX-A) (Botox, Dysport) has been used to weaken muscles selectively in patients with cerebral palsy. BTX-A injected directly into the muscle acts at the level of the motor end plate, blocking the release of the neurotransmitter acetylcholine and inhibiting muscle contraction. Because it can diffuse 2 to 3 cm in the tissues, it is easier to achieve the desired effect with BTX-A than with other agents, such as phenol or alcohol, which require more accurate injection. It also is safer than these other agents because it binds selectively to the neuromuscular junction and not to other surrounding tissues. This effect begins approximately 24 hours after injection and lasts 2 to 6 months. Care must be taken to prevent systemic injection of this toxin, which in large enough doses can cause respiratory depression and death. The maximal safe dose of BTX-A based on primate data is 36 to 50 units/kg of body weight; however, most studies report doses of less than 20 units/kg. BTX-A has been shown to be effective when used in conjunction with other modalities, such as physical therapy or serial casting. The most common side effects are local pain and irritation from the injection. The most common use of BTX-A is as an adjuvant to a bracing, casting, or physical therapy treatment program over a finite period. It is beneficial in young patients before the onset of fixed contractures. It also has been used to predict the results of tendon-lengthening surgery; however, this is controversial. BTX-A also has been shown to improve energy expenditure with walking and has been reported to improve upper extremity function and self-care, but the results are highly variable. With long-term use, efficacy may decrease because of the production of antibodies to the toxin; it is recommended that injections be done 3 to 4 months apart and only when other methods have failed. Contraindications to BTX-A therapy include known resistance or antibodies, fixed deformity or contracture, concurrent use of aminoglycoside antibiotics, failure of previous response, and certain neurologic conditions such as myasthenia gravis.

Physical therapy is an essential component in the treatment of patients with cerebral palsy. Physical therapy typically is used as a primary treatment modality and in conjunction with other modalities, such as casting, bracing, BTX-A, and surgery. The therapist plays a crucial role in all aspects of care, including identifying children who may have cerebral palsy, treating their spasticity and contractures, fabricating splints and simple braces, providing family education and follow-up, acting as a liaison with the school and other health care providers, and implementing home stretching and exercise programs with the patients and their families. Because of the variability in patients with cerebral palsy, an individualized approach to therapy is necessary. Goals for ambulatory patients include strengthening of weakened muscles, contracture prevention, and gait and balance training; for severely affected individuals, goals are improvements in sitting balance, hygiene, and ease of care for caregivers. The parents should be encouraged from the beginning to take an active role in the child's therapy program.

Objective data in the literature supporting or disputing the use of physical therapy in patients with cerebral palsy are few because most studies involve small groups of heterogeneous patients who are not randomized. Unanswered questions include what types of therapeutic modalities should be used, by whom, and for how long. There are no clear data to support lifelong physical therapy, although many parents request this. Lifelong physical therapy may be detrimental to the child and the family financially, developmentally, socially, and emotionally.

Bracing, as with physical therapy and medication, typically is used in conjunction with other modalities. Bracing in patients with cerebral palsy most commonly is used to prevent or slow progression of deformity. The most commonly used braces for the treatment of cerebral palsy include ankle-foot orthoses, hip abduction braces, hand and wrist splints, and spinal braces or jackets. A patient-centered approach should be used. The goals of bracing for an ambulatory child differ from the goals for a child with severe involvement. Bracing of the lower extremities, most commonly with ankle-foot orthoses, is common in patients with cerebral palsy. These have been shown to improve gait function and decrease crouch during walking, even in the absence of surgery in ambulatory children. The goals of bracing in a severely affected child include facilitating shoe wear, preventing further progression of contractures, improving wheelchair positioning, and assisting standing programs. The use of floor-reaction ankle-foot orthoses, which use a plantar flexion–knee extension couple to help eliminate crouched-knee gait and improve stance phase knee extension, has dramatically decreased the need for bracing above the knee with knee-ankle-foot orthoses.

OPERATIVE TREATMENT

Operative treatment typically is indicated when contractures or deformities decrease function, cause pain, or interfere with activities of daily living. Because many patients with cerebral palsy have significant comorbidities, operative treatment carries with it an increased risk of complications compared with the general population. Preoperative consultation with the patient's pediatrician, pulmonologist, and other members of the care team can help optimize the patient's condition before surgery. Surgical procedures should be scheduled to minimize the number of hospitalizations and interference with school and social activities. "Birthday surgery," or multiple procedures performed at different times, as described by Rang, should be avoided whenever possible. Although comparison studies of staged and single-event multilevel surgery are lacking, the use of single-event multilevel surgery has become the most common method to minimize a patient's exposure to repeated hospitalizations and rehabilitation. Newer techniques, such as percutaneous muscle lengthening and osteotomies, show promise in terms of decreased blood loss, operative time, and return to mobilization, but further research is necessary.

Up to 30% of patients with cerebral palsy have been shown to be malnourished, which increases the risk of postoperative wound healing problems and infection. In a study of 1746 patients with cerebral palsy, Minas et al. found underweight to be an independent predictor of increased complications after osteotomies and spine surgery, with no independent increased risk in overweight or obese patients. A serum albumin level less than 35 g/L and a blood lymphocyte count of less than 1.5 g/L have been associated with a significant increase in the risk of postoperative infection. Determination of a patient's nutritional status and improving it before surgery may decrease the overall complication rate.

It is essential to ensure that parental and patient concerns and expectations are discussed before operative intervention. Parents of younger children and children with more severe manifestations show higher levels of concern about surgery. The top preoperative concerns are the duration of rehabilitation, immediate postoperative pain, general anesthesia, and cost. Postoperative parental satisfaction has been shown to be correlated with a higher GMFCS level (level I), unilateral involvement, and younger age at the time of surgery.

Operative treatment of deformities related to cerebral palsy can be divided into several groups, including procedures to (1) correct static or dynamic deformity, (2) balance muscle power across a joint, (3) reduce spasticity (neurectomy), and (4) stabilize uncontrollable joints. Often, procedures can be combined; for example, an adductor tendon release can be done at the time of pelvic osteotomy for hip subluxation.

Flexible static and dynamic deformities typically are corrected with a muscle-tendon lengthening procedure; capsulotomies and osteotomies are reserved for more severe or rigid deformities. Over time, spasticity causes a relative shortening of the musculotendinous unit because the skeleton grows at a faster pace than the musculotendinous unit can lengthen, leading to abnormal joint motion and loading and, if left untreated, degenerative changes. Operative lengthening of the musculotendinous unit causes a relative weakening of the muscle with restoration of more normal forces and motion across the joint. Lengthening can be done using a recession or release of the muscular aponeurosis at the musculotendinous junction, a Z-plasty within the substance of the tendon itself, or a complete tenotomy depending on the circumstances. Recessions tend to avoid complications that can occur with overlengthening and subsequent weakness that can occur with tenotomy or Z-plasty. More severe deformities usually cannot be corrected with soft-tissue release alone and typically require osteotomy.

Balancing muscle forces across any joint can be difficult and is even more difficult in patients with cerebral palsy because of the decreased control of voluntary muscle function, lowered threshold of stretch reflexes, increased frequency of cocontraction of antagonistic muscle groups, and inability to learn to use the transferred muscle in an altered location or function. In addition, muscles that are spastic throughout the gait cycle typically remain spastic after transfer. Often, the goal of tendon transfer in this patient population is either to remove a deforming or out-of-phase muscle force away from a joint or to act as a passive tendon sling.

Neurectomy, by a variety of mechanical and chemical methods, has been proposed as a way to decrease the muscle forces acting across a joint. A primary concern about neurectomy is the overweakening of the affected muscle, leading to uncontrolled antagonistic function and development of a secondary opposite deformity. Because of these concerns, neurectomy is not commonly performed. If neurectomy is considered, a trial can be conducted by temporarily disrupting nerve function using a local anesthetic such as lidocaine or a longer-acting agent to determine if neurectomy will have the desired effect.

With continued abnormal muscle forces applied across a joint, pathologic changes to the joint can occur, including subluxation, dislocation, and cartilaginous degeneration. Joint stabilization procedures, such as osteotomies, usually combined with soft-tissue releases, have produced good long-term results. For severe joint destruction, procedures such as arthrodesis, especially in the foot, and resection arthroplasty, especially in the hip, have been shown to be beneficial. Joint replacement, which was initially contraindicated in patients with neuromuscular diseases such as cerebral palsy, also has been used in this population with end-stage arthritis with good functional improvement and pain relief. Joint replacement should be done only in carefully selected patients and in a center with experience with this type of procedure.

NEUROSURGICAL INTERVENTION

Selective dorsal root rhizotomy is a technique to reduce spasticity and balance muscle tone in carefully selected patients. In patients with cerebral palsy, the normal central nervous system inhibitory control of the gamma efferent system is deficient, leading to the exaggerated stretch reflex response. In addition, the ability to coordinate movement, mediated by the alpha motor neurons, is abnormal. Stimulatory afferent input from the muscle spindle travels to the spinal cord through the dorsal rootlets. The goal of selective dorsal rhizotomy is to identify the rootlets carrying excessive stimulatory information and section them to reduce the stimulatory input from the dorsal sensory fibers.

The indications for rhizotomy are variable, and further work is necessary to develop more uniform consensus guidelines. Three randomized trials of rhizotomy, with and without physical therapy, compared with physical therapy alone showed improvement in both groups, but slightly more in the rhizotomy group. There also is some limited evidence to show that rhizotomy decreases the need for orthopaedic procedures as well. The ideal patient for this procedure is a child 3 to 8 years old with a history of preterm birth, GMFCS II or III, with spastic diplegia, fair voluntary motor and trunk control, primary spastic tone, and no fixed contractures. Children who were born preterm or with low birth weight tend to have better results than children who were born full term because they tend to have pure spasticity, whereas children born full term are more likely to have rigidity plus spasticity. In addition, the patient and family should exhibit intelligence and a high level of motivation because this procedure requires extensive physical therapy postoperatively. In the early postoperative period, patients have significant weakness, but when rehabilitation is complete, most patients show significant improvement in lower extremity function, including decreased spasticity in the ankle dorsiflexors, increased strength in the knee flexors/extensors and foot dorsiflexors and plantarflexors, and more efficient ambulation. If surgery is performed in the appropriate patient, gross function can be expected to improve one GMFCS level. Improvements also can occur in upper extremity function, swallowing and speech, bladder function, pain control, and overall happiness, but these are less predictable. In addition, patients have been shown to have a decreased need for adjunct orthopaedic surgical procedures or botulinum toxin injections after rhizotomy. The role of selective dorsal rhizotomy is less clear in patients with spastic quadriplegia and hemiplegia, and usually it is not recommended. A 10-year follow-up study showed that peak joint range of motion and ambulatory status occurred 3 years after rhizotomy and then declined gradually. In this cohort, 16 of 19 patients (84%) had a mean of three orthopaedic procedures, indicating that contracture development in cerebral palsy is not mediated entirely by spasticity. Although there is some decline in results with time after rhizotomy, it appears that patients still show statistical improvement in terms of gait mechanics from their preoperative measurements, and the majority of adults who had rhizotomy would recommend the procedure to others.

Complications of selective dorsal root rhizotomy include hip subluxation and dislocation in patients with increased GMFCS level, lumbar hyperlordosis (especially in patients with > 60 degrees of lordosis preoperatively), scoliosis, spondylolysis, and spondylolisthesis. It is difficult to determine to what extent these complications are related to the rhizotomy or to the disease progression itself. Progression of coronal and sagittal plane abnormalities has been documented in 25% of patients with scoliosis, 32% of patients with kyphosis, and 36% of patients with hyperlordosis. Approximately half of patients also develop planovalgus foot deformities. One of the most difficult postoperative complications to manage is weakness, either iatrogenic or unrecognized preoperative weakness that becomes apparent after surgery.

HIP

Deformities of the hip in patients with cerebral palsy range from mild painless dysplasia or subluxation to complete dislocation with joint destruction, pain, and impaired mobility. When a hip begins to dislocate, it rarely improves without treatment. Hip pain is one of the main complaints of young adults with cerebral palsy, affecting up to 47% of patients. Most studies show that the risk of hip dislocation is correlated with the GMFCS score (Fig. 5.4). Ninety-two percent of patients with spastic cerebral palsy were found in one study to have some degree of hip deformity, and another study found hip subluxation and dislocation in 60% of dependent sitters.

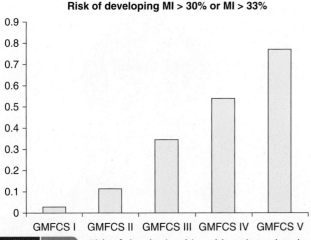

Risk of developing MI > 30% or MI > 33%

FIGURE 5.4 Risk of developing hip subluxation related to GMFCS (1=100% risk of subluxation). *GMFCS*, Gross Motor Function Classification System; *MI*, migration index. (From Pruszczynski B, Sees J, Miller F: Risk factors for hip displacement in children with cerebral palsy: systematic review, *J Pediatr Orthop* 36:829, 2016.)

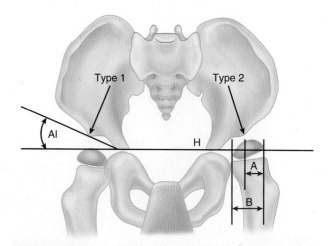

FIGURE 5.5 Subluxated hip joint *(left side of image)*. Migration index (MI) is calculated by dividing width of uncovered femoral head *A* by total width of femoral head *B*. Acetabulum is dysplastic (type 2 sourcil) with lateral corner of acetabulum above weight-bearing dome. Normal hip (left side) with acetabular index (AI) indicated. Acetabulum is normal (type 1 sourcil); lateral corner is sharp and below weight-bearing dome. *H*, Horizontal axis.

In most patients, the hip is normal at birth and radiographic changes typically become apparent between 2 and 4 years of age. The cause of this progressive deformity is multifactorial and includes muscle imbalance, retained primitive reflexes, abnormal positioning, and pelvic obliquity. These altered forces across the hip along with decreased weight bearing lead to bony deformities, including acetabular dysplasia, excessive femoral anteversion, increased neck-shaft angle, and osteopenia. Prolonged spasticity of the adductor muscles leads to a relative overpowering of the abductor muscles, causing a growth inhibition of the greater trochanter and producing a relative valgus overgrowth of the proximal femur. In many patients, the apparent increase in neck-shaft angle observed may be caused, however, more by the appearance of increased anteversion on the radiograph than to an actual increase in the neck-shaft angle.

The neck-shaft angle in children with cerebral palsy has been shown to increase with age, and anteversion, which normally decreases with age, often does not change in children with cerebral palsy. Increased anteversion is more common in ambulators than nonambulators and does not change significantly after age 6 years.

In a study of the incidence and pathogenesis of structural changes around the hip in patients with cerebral palsy, only 21% were considered normal. Hip subluxation in patients with cerebral palsy can be difficult to detect clinically because of the presence of abnormal muscle forces and contractures, and because early hip subluxation typically is painless. This has led to the development of hip surveillance programs for children with cerebral palsy in which routine clinical and radiographic examinations are performed at intervals based on severity of their cerebral palsy and GMFCS level until skeletal maturity. The primary goal of such programs is to ensure that progressive hip displacement is detected early enough to allow timely referral for orthopaedic evaluation and treatment. Hip surveillance programs were begun in Australia, and, based on the growing evidence supporting hip surveillance for children with cerebral palsy, a number of developed countries have adopted national hip surveillance programs; however, no such national program exists in the United States. Many pediatric orthopaedic centers, however, use their own internal hip radiographic schedule parameters, which, in large part, are based on established formal international hip surveillance programs. The American Academy for Cerebral Palsy and Developmental Medicine (AACPDM) has developed clinical pathways to help guide physicians in a variety of clinical care areas, one of which is a hip surveillance pathway.

These programs have been effective in reducing the rate of hip dislocation in these screened populations. A practical radiographic method for quantifying the amount of hip subluxation present was described by Reimers as the "migration percentage." Careful patient positioning, with the patient supine, the hips together, and the patellae facing forward, increases the accuracy of the measurement. If a hip flexion contracture or excessive lumbar lordosis is present, then the knees should be elevated with a bump to maintain the pelvis in an appropriate position. The measurement error for an experienced observer using this method is approximately 5 degrees. The migration percentage (Fig. 5.5) is determined by drawing the Hilgenreiner line connecting the two triradiate cartilages and then perpendicular lines at the lateral margins of the bony acetabula. The width of the femoral head uncovered (lateral to the perpendicular line) is divided by the total width of the femoral head and multiplied by 100 to give the migration percentage (Fig. 5.5). The measurement error for an experienced observer using this method is approximately 5 degrees. This index typically is 0 until age 4 years and less than 5% from 4 years until skeletal maturity. A migration of greater than 33% is considered subluxation and greater than 100% as dislocation. Hip subluxation, as measured by the migration percentage, is related to the GMFCS score and has been shown to increase approximately 12% per year in nonambulators as compared with 2% per year in ambulators, with the highest risk being in quadriplegic nonambulators who are

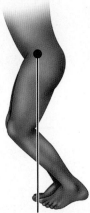

FIGURE 5.6   Typical crouch posture caused by flexion deformities of hips or fixed flexion deformities of knees.

younger than 5 years old. More important than the absolute value is the change observed within a given patient.

FLEXION DEFORMITIES

Crouched gait, or flexion of the hip, with or without flexion contractures around the hip, knee, and ankle, has been well described. Excessive hip flexion brings the center of gravity anteriorly and is compensated for by increased lumbar lordosis, knee flexion, and ankle dorsiflexion (Fig. 5.6). It is important to determine whether the increased hip flexion is the primary deformity or is secondary to other deformities around the lower extremities, such as knee or ankle contractures. If an unrecognized knee flexion contracture is present, hip flexor release can weaken the hip further and increase hip flexion. Careful physical examination is helpful in making this determination. One source of confusion is differentiating flexion-internal rotation deformity of the hip, or "pseudoadduction," from isolated adduction deformity, although often both coexist in the same patient. Children with flexion-internal rotation deformity sit with a wide base of support in the W position: hips flexed 90 degrees and maximally internally rotated, knees maximally flexed, and feet externally rotated (Fig. 5.7). With flexion-internal rotation deformity, femoral anteversion and external tibial torsion are increased, and planovalgus feet are present. With a true adduction contracture, these secondary deformities in the femoral neck, tibia, and feet are absent.

At the time of hip surgery, contractures around the knees and ankles also should be corrected. Single-stage multilevel procedures are preferable to staged single-level procedures. Hip flexion contractures from 15 to 30 degrees usually are treated with psoas lengthening through an intramuscular recession over the pelvic brim, especially in ambulatory children in whom complete iliopsoas release at its insertion may lead to excessive hip flexion weakness and difficulties with clearance of the foot during the swing phase of gait. Contractures of more than 30 degrees may require more extensive releases of the rectus femoris, sartorius, and tensor fasciae latae and the anterior fibers of the gluteus minimus and medius, in addition to the iliopsoas. Release of these muscles, because of its extensive nature, is used only for large deformities, and isolated iliopsoas lengthening is better suited for smaller ones.

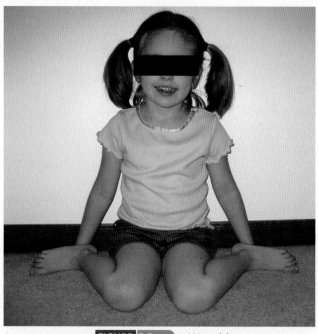

FIGURE 5.7   W position.

ADDUCTION DEFORMITIES

Adduction is the most common deformity of the hip in children with cerebral palsy. Adduction contractures can cause various difficulties, including scissoring of the legs during gait, hip subluxation, and, in severely affected children, difficulty with perineal hygiene. For mild contractures, an adductor tenotomy usually is sufficient; more severe contractures often require release of the gracilis and the anterior half of the adductor brevis. Adductor tenotomies usually are done bilaterally to prevent a "windswept" pelvis. Immediately after surgery, a program of physical therapy and abduction bracing is begun.

ADDUCTOR TENOTOMY AND RELEASE

Adductor tenotomy is indicated for a patient with a mild adduction contracture, as indicated by a scissoring gait or early hip subluxation. This procedure should be done early because damage to the developing acetabulum from abnormal hip muscle forces is greatest before 4 years of age. The ideal candidate for soft-tissue lengthening is an ambulatory child younger than 8 years, and preferably younger than 4 years, who has hip abduction of less than 30 degrees and a migration index of less than 50%. Neurectomy of the anterior branch of the obturator nerve should be avoided to prevent iatrogenic hip abduction contracture. Miller et al. reported the results of adductor release in 147 hips (74 children) with hip abduction of less than 30 degrees or migration index of more than 25%. At an average follow-up of 39 months, 54% of hips were classified as good, 34% as fair, and 12% as poor based on the migration index. A longer-term study with an 8-year average follow-up showed that 58% of patients required a second surgical procedure, indicating that, although still beneficial, early soft-tissue release alone may be insufficient to prevent long-term hip subluxation and dislocation. While adductor lengthening is effective in the short term, its long-term success, as defined by no additional surgery and a migration percentage under 50%, is highly correlated with the patient's GMFCS level. Shore et al. demonstrated a success rate of only 14% in children with a GMFCS level of V compared to 94% in children with a GMFCS level of II. It may delay major bony surgery, however, until the risk of recurrence is decreased.

TECHNIQUE 5.1

- Place the patient supine on the operating table and prepare the area from the toes to the inferior costal margin, isolating the perineum (Fig. 5.8A).
- Identify the adductor longus by palpation and make a 2- to 3-cm transverse incision over the adductor longus tendon approximately 1 cm distal from its origin.
- Dissect through the subcutaneous tissue and identify the adductor longus fascia (Fig. 5.8B).
- Make a longitudinal incision in the adductor fascia, identify the tendinous portion of the adductor longus, and resect it with electrocautery.
- Release with electrocautery any remaining muscle fibers of the adductor longus as necessary. Avoid injury to the anterior branch of the obturator nerve, which is in the interval between the adductor longus and brevis (Fig. 5.8C).
- Gradually abduct the hip and determine the amount of correction obtained. If further correction is required, slowly release the anterior half of the adductor brevis using electrocautery and avoiding injury to the branches of the obturator nerve. Do not release an excessive amount of the adductor brevis and protect the posterior branch of the obturator nerve to prevent an abduction contracture.
- If the gracilis muscle is found to be tight, release it with electrocautery (Fig. 5.8D).
- When the final correction is obtained, close the wound in layers. Take care to close the adductor fascia to help prevent skin dimpling postoperatively (Fig. 5.8E).

POSTOPERATIVE CARE Postoperatively, the patient is placed in the abducted position. Depending on the patient's functional status, quality of caregivers, and other procedures done, the patient can be immobilized in bilateral long leg casts with an abduction bar or abduction pillow for 1 month. A removable abduction pillow can be used, which allows physical therapy to be started immediately after surgery to help maintain and increase optimally hip range of motion.

ILIOPSOAS RECESSION

Bleck recommended iliopsoas recession when the hip internally rotates during walking or when passive external rotation is absent with the hip in full extension and present when the joint is passively flexed to 90 degrees. This procedure usually is done in conjunction with other soft-tissue releases of the lower extremities. Iliopsoas recession is used more commonly than complete tenotomy at the level of the lesser trochanter to avoid causing excessive hip flexion weakness.

TECHNIQUE 5.2   *Figure 5.9*

- Place the patient supine with a roll under the buttock of the operative side.
- Palpate the course of the femoral artery and mark it on the skin, keeping in mind that the femoral nerve is lateral to it.
- For an isolated iliopsoas recession, make a 5-cm "bikini" incision. This incision can be modified as needed if other procedures are going to be done at the same time. Center the incision medial to and 2 cm below the anterior superior iliac spine.
- Identify and develop the interval between the tensor fasciae latae and sartorius to expose the direct head of the rectus femoris with its origin at the anterior inferior iliac spine. It is not necessary to identify the femoral neurovascular structures.
- Palpate the pelvic brim just medial and inferior to the rectus femoris origin to locate the iliopsoas tendon in a shallow groove.
- Slightly flex the hip to relax the soft-tissue structures around the hip.
- Place a right-angle retractor on the lateral aspect of the iliopsoas muscle and pull the retractor medially and anteriorly, exposing the posteromedial aspect of the muscle and the psoas tendon (Fig. 5.9). The retractor is protecting the femoral nerve, which is medial to it.
- Dissect the surrounding muscle fascia and isolate the tendon from the muscle with a right-angle clamp. Verify that there is enough muscle remaining at that level so that continuity is maintained after tendon release.
- Under direct vision, carefully internally and externally rotate the hip to see the tendon loosen and tighten. If there is any doubt as to the identification of the tendon, use an elevator to dissect around the tendon proximally until its muscle fibers are identified. An electrical nerve stimulator or careful brief stimulation with electrocautery also can be used to help confirm that the tendon has been found and that the femoral nerve has not been mistakenly identified.
- Release the tendinous portion, leaving the muscle fibers in continuity. Extend and internally rotate the hip to separate the tendon ends.
- Close the wound in layers and apply sterile dressings.

POSTOPERATIVE CARE Patients with an isolated iliopsoas release are started immediately in a physical therapy program emphasizing hip extension and external rotation. Patients, especially those who are unable to cooperate with physical therapy, are placed prone at bed rest to help improve hip extension. This can be modified as needed if other procedures are done at the same time.

ILIOPSOAS RELEASE AT THE LESSER TROCHANTER

Iliopsoas release at its insertion on the lesser trochanter is better for nonambulatory patients than for ambulatory patients because of the risk of causing excessive hip flexion

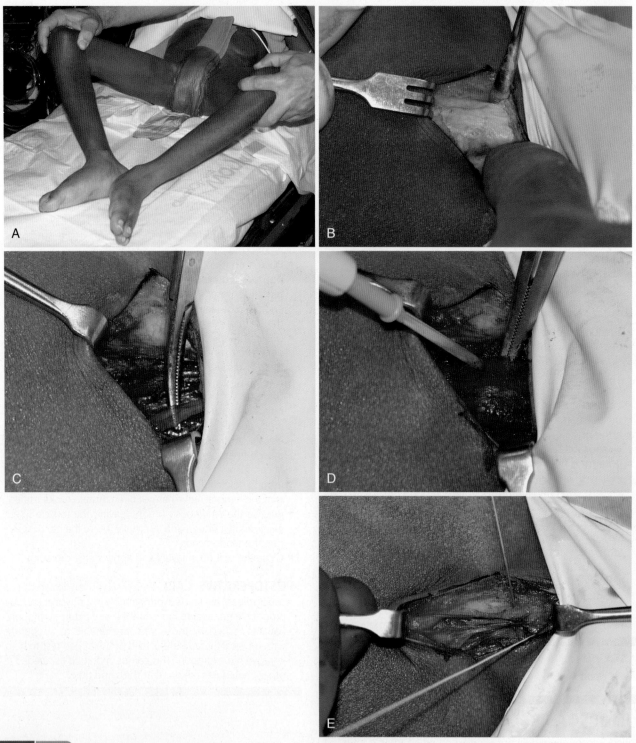

FIGURE 5.8 Adductor tenotomy. **A,** Patient positioning. **B,** Skin incision and subcutaneous dissection to identify adductor longus fascia. **C,** Hemostat placed under anterior branch of obturator nerve. **D,** Release of tight gracilis muscle with electrocautery. **E,** Closure of adductor fascia. **SEE TECHNIQUE 5.1.**

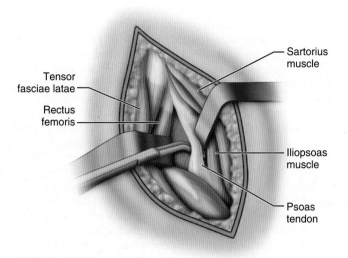

Tensor fasciae latae

Rectus femoris

Sartorius muscle

Iliopsoas muscle

Psoas tendon

FIGURE 5.9   Skaggs et al. surgical approach for iliopsoas recession. When procedure is done alone, much smaller incision is adequate. **SEE TECHNIQUE 5.2.**

weakness, which can severely affect an ambulatory patient. It often is done at the same time as another procedure, such as an adductor release or varus derotational osteotomy.

Additional release of the secondary hip flexors including the sartorius and rectus femoris also may be used for severe deformities.

TECHNIQUE 5.3

- Make a transverse incision 1 to 3 cm distal to the inguinal crease. If an adductor release is to be done at the same time, make a longitudinal incision in the adductor longus fascia and transect the adductor longus with electrocautery; perform a myotomy of the gracilis if necessary.
- Resect as much of the adductor brevis as necessary to obtain 45 degrees of abduction.
- Develop the interval between the residual adductor brevis and the pectineus or between the pectineus and the neurovascular bundle until the femur is identified.
- Open the bursa over the iliopsoas and its sheath.
- Place a retractor into the tendon sheath and retract the tendon medially.
- Pass a right-angle clamp under the tendon of the iliopsoas, which can be completely released with electrocautery in a nonambulatory child.
- Release the iliopsoas as far proximally as possible in an ambulatory child to preserve the iliacus muscle attachment to the iliopsoas tendon.

POSTOPERATIVE CARE Physical therapy is started 2 days after surgery, emphasizing range-of-motion exercises of the hips and knees. Leg-knee immobilizers are used 8 to 12 hours a day for 1 month. Parents are encouraged to have the child sleep prone as much as possible.

SUBLUXATION AND DISLOCATION

Hip dislocation occurs on a continuum from mild subluxation to true dislocation with significant degenerative changes. Because early intervention can be very effective in preventing or delaying the development of dislocation, considerable work has been done to identify hips at risk. Children with risk factors for subluxation or dislocation should be examined and radiographs obtained at 6-month intervals until it can be established that the hips are stable, and then follow-up can be less frequent. Of hip dislocations, 70% to 90% occur in patients with quadriplegia, which necessitates screening for all patients in this high-risk group. Clinically, a hip at risk has contractures of the adductors and flexors. Hips with flexion contractures of more than 20 degrees and abduction of less than 30 degrees are at increased risk of progressive subluxation. Radiographically, a hip at risk has an increased neck-shaft angle and increased femoral anteversion. Acetabular dysplasia and an abnormal migration index also may be present. When a hip at risk is identified, a program of aggressive physical therapy and abduction splinting typically is started, although there are no well-controlled long-term studies to support this. If further progression continues, early operative treatment consisting of soft-tissue release of contracted tendons is indicated. The goal of adductor release is restoration of more than 60 degrees of abduction with the hips flexed and 45 degrees with the hips extended. The release begins sequentially with the complete release of the adductor longus, the anterior half of the adductor brevis, and occasionally the gracilis until the desired range of motion is achieved. Care must be taken not to perform too extensive a release, which can cause an abduction contracture that is extremely difficult to manage. For this reason, neurectomy of the anterior branch of the obturator nerve should not be done. Immediately after adductor release or transfer, a program of physical therapy is begun, emphasizing hip abduction and night splinting for 6 months.

Hip subluxation occurs when more than one third of the femoral head is uncovered and there is a break in the Shenton line. Nonoperative treatment alone at this point is ineffective. In younger children, soft-tissue releases alone may be sufficient, but most patients with hip subluxation require osteotomy in addition to soft-tissue release. Operative correction of femoral valgus and anteversion and acetabular dysplasia is necessary at this stage to prevent further subluxation and dislocation. Plain radiographs are necessary and, if available, CT or MRI three-dimensional reconstructions can help evaluate the proximal femoral and acetabular deformities. Rotational studies using CT can be helpful in quantifying the amount of femoral anteversion and any tibial rotation.

A femoral varus and derotation (external rotation) osteotomy, often combined with femoral shortening, generally is used to reduce the neck-shaft angle to 115 degrees in ambulatory patients and often less in nonambulatory patients. A wide variety of acetabular osteotomies have been used in the treatment of acetabular dysplasia in patients with cerebral palsy, including osteotomies described by Salter, Pemberton, Dega, Ganz, and Steel and salvage-type osteotomies such as the Chiari and shelf. Careful matching of the procedure to the deformity is essential to prevent inadvertent iatrogenic worsening of the deformity. For example, a Salter osteotomy, which redirects the acetabulum posteriorly and laterally, if done in a patient with posterior acetabular deficiency would uncover the femoral head further. Often patients with cerebral palsy have a posterosuperior deficiency for which a Dega osteotomy, San

Diego type osteotomy, or shelf procedure is effective. The Dega osteotomy has been shown by CT morphometry to increase anterosuperior, superolateral, and posterosuperior coverage. Although typically done before the time of triradiate cartilage closure, it has been done in patients with cerebral palsy after triradiate closure with good improvement in subluxation and dislocation radiographically. Postoperatively, patients can be immobilized for a brief time in a spica cast, followed by a period of aggressive rehabilitation that includes physical therapy, bracing, and progressive weight bearing. Because of concerns about skin breakdown, difficulty with transfers, and lack of mobility, we now avoid casting when possible and use early physical therapy to increase range of motion.

Hip dislocation is common in patients with cerebral palsy, especially in severely affected children. Radiographic abnormalities, such as increased femoral neck-shaft angle and increased internal femoral rotation, have been shown to be correlated with increased GMFCS level (see Fig. 5.4). Similar acetabular changes also are seen in patients with dislocated hips having global acetabular defects and smaller acetabular volume than in those with subluxed hips having more posterior acetabular defects and greater acetabular volume. The patient's risk of hip dislocation is related to GMFCS level, with a 0% incidence for patients with grade I and 90% for patients with grade V. The head-shaft angle, which measures the amount of proximal femoral valgus, has been shown to be predictive of hip dislocation: for every 10-degree increase in head-shaft angle, the risk of dislocation increases 1.6-fold. The natural history of the untreated hip in these patients is progressive subluxation associated with bony deformity of the proximal femur and acetabulum. The spastic adductors and hip flexors compress the femoral head against the posterolateral acetabulum and labrum. The capsule and superior rim of the acetabulum cause focal deformation of the femoral head. The indented femoral head locks on the acetabular rim, causing significant cartilage loss and pain. Mathematic models have predicted that a child with spastic hip disease has a sixfold increase in forces across the hip. The acetabulum in affected children usually is normal until about 30 months of age, when a change in the acetabular index is seen. With continued abnormal muscle forces, the hip typically dislocates superolaterally, which has been confirmed by CT studies. Late findings include dislocation of the hip and degenerative changes. Most authors agree that hip subluxation and dislocation should be prevented in all patients who are medically able to tolerate treatment. The treatment of an established dislocation is more controversial. A patient with a long-standing dislocation is not a good candidate for a relocation procedure because of the deformities of the proximal femur and acetabulum, which also may be associated with degenerative changes. Treatment options for hip dislocations in patients with cerebral palsy include observation; relocation procedures on the femur, acetabulum, or both; proximal femoral resection; hip arthrodesis; and, in carefully selected patients, total hip arthroplasty.

The heterogeneous literature concerning surgical treatment of dislocated hips in patients with cerebral palsy makes it difficult to compare outcomes across studies. Because of the variable nature of cerebral palsy, most studies include a wide spectrum of severity of neurologic involvement and a wide variety of procedures used. Varus femoral osteotomy was found in one study to be effective in preventing redislocation and surgery in 84%. The amount of bony deformity present preoperatively, as measured by center-edge angle and migration index, was a predictor of final outcome. Worse results were reported in quadriplegics than in diplegics and hemiplegics.

Good results were reported in 95% of patients at mean 7-year follow-up after a one-stage combined approach that included soft-tissue lengthenings, open reduction with capsulorrhaphy (open if migration index was more than 70 degrees), varus derotational osteotomy, and pericapsular acetabuloplasty. A recent report of 168 hip reconstructions in children with cerebral palsy showed statistically significant improvement in pain relief and function (GMFCS level) with a 10% complication rate. Preoperative migration percentage was correlated with increasing pain and worse outcome while femoral head shape was not. Although most centers favor a one-stage approach, good results have been obtained with femoral osteotomy and later acetabular osteotomy if needed; however, this approach requires a second hospitalization and rehabilitation. Despite these good outcomes, complications following hip osteotomy are common. In one large series, 65% of children with cerebral palsy who had hip osteotomy had at least one postoperative complication, most (83%) of which were medical rather than orthopaedic. Redislocations also can occur, especially in GMFCS IV and V patients in whom the migration percentage was found to increase 2% per year and 3.5% per year in GMFCS IV and V patients, respectively. Long-term follow-up monitoring is necessary.

In a series of patients treated with Chiari osteotomies, 79% of 23 hips were reportedly painless at an average follow-up of 7 years; however, 29% of the hips had a migration index of 30% or greater; resubluxation typically occurred in the first year after surgery.

Recently, there has been study in the area of proximal femoral medial hemiepiphysiodesis to prevent hip migration. One study showed significant improvements in head-shaft angle, migration percentage, and acetabular index at final follow-up. Progression of deformity occurred in three (5%) of 56 hips, to the point of needing reconstructive surgery such as proximal femoral or pelvic osteotomies.

■ VARUS DEROTATIONAL OSTEOTOMY

Varus derotational osteotomy, usually combined with soft-tissue releases, is indicated for patients with hip subluxation or dislocation and excessive anteversion and valgus deformity of the proximal femur. Computer models have shown that to normalize the muscle forces across a spastic hip, the psoas, iliacus, gracilis, and adductor longus and brevis must be released. The benefit of a varus derotational osteotomy comes primarily through the bony shortening that acts biomechanically similar to a soft-tissue lengthening. Decreasing the neck-shaft angle and anteversion has little effect on the hip forces. An isolated varus derotational osteotomy, often with femoral shortening, is indicated only when there is mild or no acetabular dysplasia present because, although there is some remodeling potential of the acetabulum, it is variable in patients with cerebral palsy. Acetabular remodeling is better in GMFCS I–III patients and is correlated with the amount of varus produced. Varus derotational osteotomy can be combined with an acetabular osteotomy if significant subluxation and acetabular dysplasia are present. In a prospective gait study of 37 patients, varus derotational osteotomy improved hip external rotation and extension, knee extension strength, and cosmetic appearance and decreased anterior pelvic tilt. Patients who are nonambulatory and patients with a gastrostomy or tracheostomy are at increased risk of postoperative complications, including decubitus ulcers and fractures. The risk of recurrent dislocation is higher in patients with higher GMFCS levels or insufficient correction of valgus and acetabular dysplasia, and the risk of osteonecrosis is proportional to the patient's age and degree of preoperative subluxation.

The technique of varus derotational osteotomy is described in other chapter (see Technique 30.6).

COMBINED ONE-STAGE CORRECTION OF SPASTIC DISLOCATED HIP

TECHNIQUE 5.4

MEDIAL APPROACH (SOFT-TISSUE RELEASE)
- With the patient on a radiolucent table, prepare and drape the hip from the toes to the costal margin.
- Use electrocautery to release the adductor longus and gracilis.
- Release the psoas in the interval between the neurovascular bundle and the pectineus. After the sciatic nerve is carefully identified, release the proximal hamstrings posterior to the adductor magnus. Avoid the sciatic nerve.

ANTERIOR APPROACH (OPEN REDUCTION)
- Make the second incision parallel to the iliac crest using a Salter incision (see Technique 30.3).
- Divide the iliac crest apophysis and strip the iliac wing subperiosteally down to the sciatic notch medially and laterally. Alternatively, the iliac crest apophysis can be elevated instead of split by placing a Freer elevator underneath the apophysis and lifting it gently.
- Resect the direct and indirect heads of the rectus femoris and retract them distally to expose the underlying capsule.
- If an open reduction is needed, make a T-capsulotomy, and identify the ligamentum teres.
- Remove the ligamentum teres, cut the contracted transverse acetabular ligament, and clear the acetabulum of any remaining soft tissue.
- Inspect the femoral head to assess deformity and cartilage loss. If more than 50% of the cartilage is lost, reduction may be unsuccessful and other options (e.g., valgus osteotomy or resection of the femoral head) should be considered.

LATERAL APPROACH (FEMORAL OSTEOTOMY)
- Make an incision on the lateral aspect of the proximal femur and perform a lateral exposure.
- Split the tensor fasciae latae and dissect to the lateral aspect of the femur.
- Perform a varus derotational shortening femoral osteotomy at the lesser trochanter. Remove 1 to 2 cm of bone (Fig. 5.10).
- The neck-shaft angle should be decreased to approximately 110 degrees, and anteversion should be corrected to 10 to 20 degrees.
- Fix the femoral osteotomy with an AO blade plate of the appropriate size for the child. Several implant systems have been developed to accommodate infantile, pediatric, and adolescent anatomic variations. Alternatively, a size-appropriate proximal femoral locking plate can be used.

ANTERIOR APPROACH (PERICAPSULAR PELVIC OSTEOTOMY)
- The type of pericapsular pelvic osteotomy is patient-specific. Here, a San Diego type osteotomy is described. Other osteotomies use a similar approach, but differ in the location of the bone cuts. See other chapter for other pelvic osteotomy techniques.
- Return to the anterior incision and place five nonabsorbable No. 1 sutures into the capsulotomy for later closure.
- With a straight osteotome, make an osteotomy 0.5 to 1.0 cm above the edge of the acetabulum, on a line drawn between the anterior inferior iliac spine and the sciatic notch. Extend this through the lateral wall of the pelvis, but not through the medial wall (Fig. 5.11). To allow proper bending, both corners should be cut at the anterior and posterior ends of the osteotomy (anterior superior iliac spine and sciatic notch). This is most easily done by using a regular rongeur anteriorly and a large Kerrison rongeur posteriorly in the sciatic notch.
- Use a curved osteotome 1.0 to 2.5 cm wide and an image intensifier to perform the second part of the osteotomy. Direct the osteotome halfway between the articular surface and the medial cortex. Extend the cut medially and distally to the level of the triradiate cartilage. Use gentle downward pressure on the osteotome to open the osteotomy site 1.0 to 1.5 cm (Fig. 5.12).
- Remove a bicortical graft from the iliac crest and shape it into three or four triangular grafts measuring approximately 1 cm at the base. Insert the grafts into the osteotomy, using the largest one for the area of most desired coverage. The portion of the proximal femur removed earlier also can be used as autograft.
- Alternatively, tricortical allograft bone can be used, which gives good structural support to the osteotomy.
- When a stable reduction is obtained, repair the capsule using the sutures placed earlier.
- Close all three wounds in standard fashion and check a radiograph to ensure proper reduction before application of a hip spica cast with the hip in 45 degrees of flexion and 30 degrees of abduction.

POSTOPERATIVE CARE The patient is placed in an abduction pillow or a well-padded spica cast, which typically is removed at 6 weeks postoperatively with the patient anesthetized. Physical therapy for range of motion and progressive weight bearing are started after cast removal, but vigorous physical therapy and attempted weight bearing are not advised until 10 weeks after surgery.

Resection arthroplasty, arthrodesis, and total hip arthroplasty have been proposed for the treatment of a painful dislocated hip when a relocation procedure is impossible. Because of the heterogeneous nature of the patients and procedures performed, as well as the lack of large long-term comparison studies, the optimal treatment for the painful

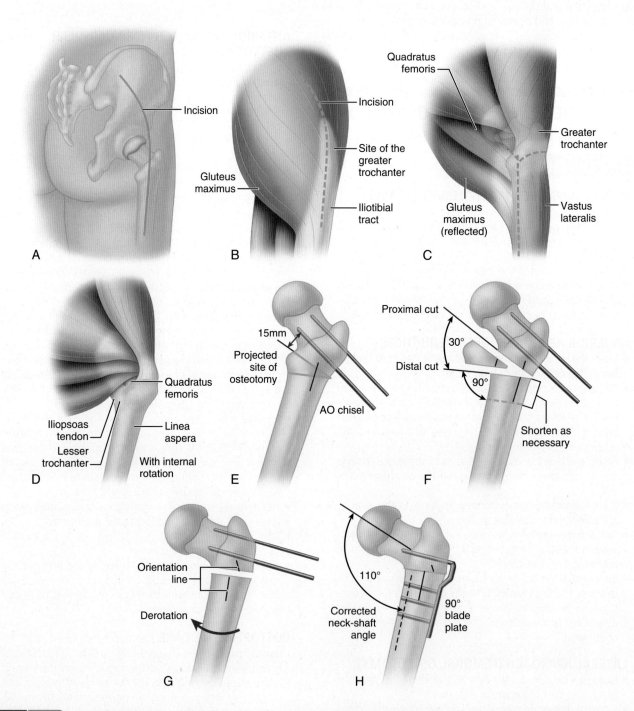

FIGURE 5.10 Root and Siegal varus derotational osteotomy of hip. **A,** Skin incision. **B,** Incision through gluteus maximus and fascia lata (iliotibial tract). **C,** Greater trochanter, quadratus femoris, origin of vastus lateralis, tendinous attachment of gluteus maximus, and linea aspera are identified. **D,** Osteotomy site is exposed in area of lesser trochanter; psoas tendon can be released if necessary. **E,** Guidewire and chisel are inserted in parallel position. *Shaded area* represents wedge to be excised; *scored line* is for reference for later rotation. **F,** Location of osteotomy planes; proximal osteotomy is 15 mm distal to chisel. **G,** Rotation is accomplished by external rotation of femur. **H,** Osteotomy is fixed with AO blade plate, or proximal femoral locking plate. **SEE TECHNIQUE 5.4.**

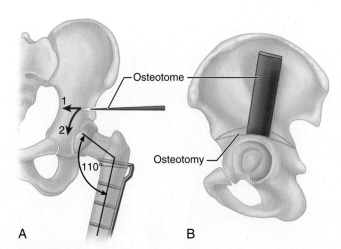

FIGURE 5.11 Mubarak et al. one-stage correction of spastic dislocated hip. **A,** Pericapsular acetabuloplasty is begun approximately 1 cm above lateral margin of acetabulum. **B,** Osteotomy proceeds in line between anterior inferior iliac spine and sciatic notch, penetrating outer wall of ilium only. Bicortical cuts are made at anterior inferior iliac spine and sciatic notch. Straight or slightly curved osteotome extends osteotomy toward triradiate cartilage, avoiding penetration of joint or inner pelvic wall. **SEE TECHNIQUE 5.4.**

dislocated nonreconstructable hip is unclear. The goals of these procedures are pain relief, improved function, and increased ease of care for caregivers. Hip resection arthroplasty, most commonly a Girdlestone intertrochanteric resection, has been used for the treatment of end-stage hip degeneration caused by other conditions, such as osteoarthritis, osteonecrosis, septic arthritis, and slipped capital femoral epiphysis. In patients with cerebral palsy, the use of this type of resection arthroplasty has been modified because of the high rate of postoperative pain from femoral-iliac impingement. Proximal femoral resection, combined with capsular interposition, has been effective. The advantage of this type of resection is that it is technically straightforward, requires less postoperative immobilization and operating room time, and requires no permanent implants, in contrast to other techniques such as relocation procedures and arthrodesis. The use of capsular interposition (Castle and Schneider) has been shown to have a lower complication rate than the interposition of capsule and iliopsoas and gluteal muscles (McCarthy). In a study of 34 severely affected institutionalized patients who had proximal femoral resections (56 hips), 33 were able to sit comfortably and have painless perineal care at 2-year follow-up; 79% of patients developed heterotopic ossification postoperatively, but this

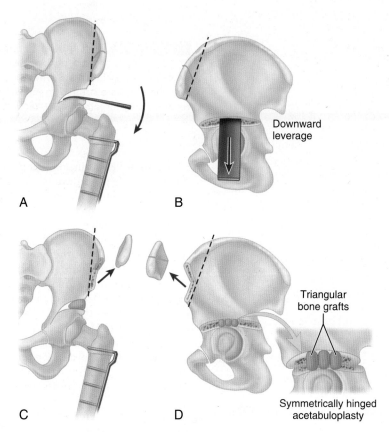

FIGURE 5.12 Mubarak et al. one-stage correction of spastic dislocated hip. Osteotomy stops several millimeters from triradiate cartilage and is hinged open laterally to correct dysplasia. **A,** Tricortical segment of iliac wing is harvested for bone graft. **B,** Trapezoidal segments are fashioned to fit into osteotomy site. **C** and **D,** Three trapezoidal segments of tricortical bone graft are impacted into place to hold osteotomy site open. Elasticity of intact medial cortex holds bone grafts in place; fixation is not required. **SEE TECHNIQUE 5.4.**

had little to no effect on overall function. Although initially recommended, the use of postoperative traction following proximal femoral resection has become less common and may not improve outcome.

PROXIMAL FEMORAL RESECTION

TECHNIQUE 5.5

- Preoperatively, determine the level of the osteotomy by drawing a line on the preoperative anteroposterior radiograph from the ischium to the femur, parallel to the inferior border of the ischium.
- After administration of general anesthesia, place the patient supine with a sandbag elevating the affected hip.
- Make a straight lateral incision along the proximal femur beginning superior to the greater trochanter and ending inferior to the level of the lesser trochanter.
- Split the fascia of the tensor fasciae latae and femoris and extraperiosteally detach the insertions of the vastus lateralis and gluteus medius and minimus from the proximal femur.
- Detach the psoas tendon from the lesser trochanter and complete the exposure of the proximal femur extraperiosteally.
- Incise the periosteum circumferentially around the femur just distal to the insertion of the gluteus maximus or at the proposed level of femoral resection.
- Divide the short external rotators.
- Incise the capsule circumferentially and free it from the base of the femoral neck.
- Divide the ligamentum teres and remove the proximal femur, using an oscillating saw to make the osteotomy (Fig. 5.13A).
- Test the range of motion of the hip at this point and, if necessary for motion, tenotomize the proximal hamstrings through the same incision after identifying the sciatic nerve. If necessary, also release the adductors.
- Seal the acetabular cavity by oversewing the capsular edges. Alternatively, the iliopsoas can be sutured to the lateral part of the capsule and the abductors to the medial part of the capsule.
- Bring the vastus lateralis lateral to medial over the femoral stump, sewing it into the rectus femoris muscle.
- To decrease the risk of heterotopic ossification, handle tissue carefully, completely excise the periosteum, and irrigate thoroughly. Consider the use of nonsteroidal anti-inflammatories perioperatively.
- Secure meticulous hemostasis and close the wound over a suction drain.

POSTOPERATIVE CARE Postoperatively, the patient uses an abduction pillow for 2 weeks and then is progressed in therapy with gentle range of motion.

▌REDIRECTIONAL OSTEOTOMY

Redirectional osteotomy also has been proposed as an alternative to resection arthroplasty. This proximal femoral valgus osteotomy places the legs in a more abducted position,

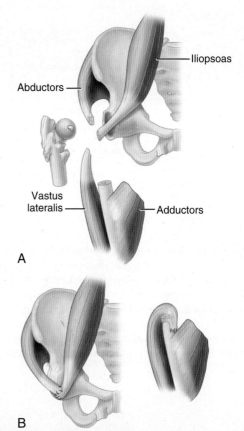

FIGURE 5.13 McCarthy et al. proximal femoral resection. **A,** Extraperiosteal approach, periosteal excision, and release of musculotendinous attachments. **B,** Interpositional arthroplasty-iliopsoas and abductors are sutured to hip capsule, and femoral stump is covered by vastus lateralis. **SEE TECHNIQUE 5.5.**

which improves perineal hygiene and sitting. The ideal candidate for this procedure is a child with severe hip adduction with minimal or no pain. The osteotomy directs the lesser trochanter into the acetabulum and the femoral head away from the pelvis.

The procedure described by McHale et al. in 1990 involves resection of the femoral head and neck, valgus-producing subtrochanteric osteotomy to reposition the leg relative to the trunk, and advancement of the lesser trochanter into the acetabulum by attaching the ligamentum teres to the intact iliopsoas. The technique was modified by Godfrey et al., who placed the patient in the lateral position rather than supine, released the short external rotators to easily expose the femoral head, and did not attach the iliopsoas to the ligamentum teres. They reported that these modifications resulted in shorter surgical time, less blood loss, and shorter hospital stays. This has become a preferred technique at many centers, but we have little experience with it. In a later comparison of Schanz, Girdlestone, Castle, and McHale procedures in 69 hips, these authors determined that, while all four procedures provided pain relief, bone resorption and revision surgery were more frequent after the McHale procedure.

REDIRECTIONAL OSTEOTOMY (MCHALE PROCEDURE FOR NEGLECTED HIP DISLOCATION)

TECHNIQUE 5.6

(MCHALE ET AL.)

- Place a "bump" underneath the sacrum to improve access to the affected hip, and make an anterolateral Watson-Jones approach (see chapter 1).
- Resect the femoral head, preserving the ligamentum teres for further attachment to the iliopsoas tendon (Fig. 5.14A).
- Make an opening wedge valgus osteotomy distal to the lesser trochanter, taking into account that 3 holes of the LCP plate should be proximal to the osteotomy (Fig. 5.14B).
- After attachment of the ligamentum teres to the iliopsoas tendon, pre-bend and contour a 4.5-mm LCP plate to accommodate to the shape of the femur after the osteotomy (Fig. 5.14C).
- Fix the plate to the femur with locking screws.

POSTOPERATIVE CARE The patient uses an abduction pillow for the first 2 weeks after surgery. Gentle passive range of motion and sitting in a wheelchair are allowed immediately after surgery.

HIP ARTHRODESIS

Hip arthrodesis also can be effective in relieving pain and improving function in carefully selected patients. The ideal candidate is a patient with unilateral disease and no spinal involvement. Hip arthrodesis may be preferable in ambulatory patients because it allows weight bearing, in contrast to proximal femoral resections. In two studies of arthrodesis in patients with cerebral palsy and painful hip dislocation, fusions were obtained in 6 of 8 patients and 11 of 14 hips after the first attempt, resulting in pain relief and improvement in posture. The remainder required repeat arthrodesis. One negative aspect of hip arthrodesis is the need for postoperative casting for 2 months and the complications associated with it.

TECHNIQUE 5.7

- Place the patient supine with a soft pad under the gluteal region.
- Perform an adductor tenotomy as described in Technique 5.1.
- Through a longitudinal lateral incision to the hip, split the gluteal muscles.
- Extend the exposure of the hip joint to allow an iliopsoas tenotomy.
- Resect the pulvinar and ligamentum teres, remove any remaining cartilage from the femoral head and acetabulum, and deepen the dysplastic acetabulum.
- Position the hip in 40 degrees of flexion, 15 degrees of abduction, and neutral rotation. The fixation device used depends on the local bone width and quality, the size of the femoral head and neck, and the desirable degree of hip flexion. Appropriate implants include a 4.5-mm AO-D cerebral palsy plate, AO-Cobra plate, and 6.5-mm cannulated screws.

POSTOPERATIVE CARE A hip spica cast is worn for 2 months postoperatively. Patients are then started in a progressive range-of-motion and weight-bearing program.

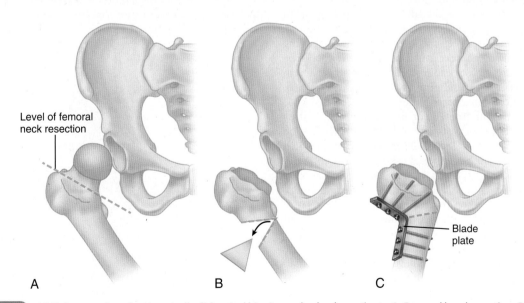

Level of femoral neck resection

A   B   C

Blade plate

FIGURE 5.14 McHale procedure for chronically dislocated hips in cerebral palsy patients. **A,** Femoral head resection. **B,** Lateral wedge varus osteotomy. **C,** Fixation with hand-contoured plate. (Redrawn from McHale KA, Bagg M, Nason SS: Treatment of the chronically dislocated hip in adolescents with cerebral palsy with femoral resection and subtrochanteric valgus osteotomy, *J Pediatr Orthop* 10:504, 1990.)

Total hip arthroplasty is an option for patients with cerebral palsy with end-stage hip degeneration. The ideal candidate is an intelligent, independent ambulator with mild soft-tissue contractures. Good midterm results (10 years) have been reported after hip arthroplasty. Another study reported return to preoperative function in all patients, return to prepain function in 88%, and implant survivorship in 95% at 2 years and 85% at 10 years. Increasing the anteversion and inclination of the acetabular component may help increase stability. Although the results of total hip replacement are best in GMFCS I and II patients, surface replacement has been shown to be effective for pain relief in a small series of GMFCS III-V patients.

KNEE
HIP AND KNEE RELATIONSHIPS

Deformities of the knee in patients with cerebral palsy are difficult to evaluate and treat and rarely occur in isolation. Pelvic, hip, knee, ankle, and foot deformities are interrelated. The hip and the knee are tightly coupled because of the muscles that cross both joints, the "two-joint muscles." These muscles include the rectus femoris anteriorly, gracilis medially, and semimembranosus, semitendinosus, and biceps femoris posteriorly. Pathologic conditions that affect these muscles, such as spasticity or contracture, and surgical changes affect the function of both joints. A similar relationship exists between the knee and ankle with the gastrocnemius muscle, which crosses both joints. A patient with cerebral palsy who ambulates with his or her knees flexed may not have hamstrings that are tight or spastic. A patient with a hip flexion contracture ambulates with increased knee flexion to help maintain sagittal balance. Likewise, surgical correction of a knee flexion contracture may lead to spontaneous improvement in hip flexion. Because of these relationships, a careful physical examination of the entire lower extremity is essential when evaluating the knee in patients with cerebral palsy.

FLEXION DEFORMITY

Flexion is the most common knee deformity in patients with cerebral palsy and frequently occurs in ambulatory children. Knee flexion deformities keep the knee from fully extending at the end of the swing phase of gait. This causes the knee to be flexed during stance phase, leading to decreased stride length and increased energy expenditure. Spastic hamstrings, weak quadriceps, or a combination of both can cause isolated knee flexion. It also can result from hip or ankle pathology. Patients with spastic hip flexors or weak hip extensors or both develop compensatory knee flexion that results in crouch gait in which the hips, knees, and ankles are flexed (Fig. 5.15). Patients with weakened gastrocnemius-soleus muscles, from cerebral palsy or more commonly from Achilles tendon overlengthenings, ambulate with knee flexion to accommodate for the relative overpull of the ankle dorsiflexors. Prolonged spasticity and crouched knee gait can lead to true contracture of the knee itself. This is a difficult problem to deal with and has led to the increased use of single-event multilevel surgery rather than staged procedures. A wide variety of procedures has been proposed for this, including femoral shortening or distal femoral extension osteotomy with patellar tendon advancement or both. Patellar advancement has been shown to improve gait mechanics better than extension osteotomy alone.

To find the source of the knee flexion, the muscles must be assessed to determine if the deformity is caused by spasticity or contracture or both. Strength testing should be done, although this can be difficult in patients with cerebral palsy. In patients with cerebral palsy, if the hamstrings are affected, most likely the quadriceps are affected to some degree as well. Quadriceps strength, spasticity, and firing pattern should be evaluated throughout the gait cycle. Lengthening, and essentially weakening, the hamstrings in the presence of a spastic rectus femoris can lead to hyperextension deformity of the knee and significant gait disturbance.

Hamstring strength, spasticity, and knee contracture are assessed with the patient prone and supine. With the patient prone, the examiner extends the hips as much as possible and exerts gentle pressure on the calves. The angle that the femur and the tibia make after spasticity has been overcome is the degree of contracture of the soft tissues behind the knee. Next, the patient is placed supine to test hamstring spasticity. The examiner stabilizes the opposite knee in as much extension as possible and raises the leg being examined with the knee straight. If knee extension is limited as the hip is flexed, either medial or lateral hamstring tightness is present (Fig. 5.16). The patient can be examined for medial hamstring spasticity in the supine position with the knees flexed and feet off the table. This relaxes the hamstrings proximally and allows the hip to be abducted if there is no contracture of the adductor muscles. If extension is not possible unless the hip is adducted, there is tightness in the medial hamstrings and gracilis (Fig. 5.17). The amount of equinus in the ankle should be measured with the knee flexed and fully extended (Fig. 5.18). If ankle dorsiflexion improves with knee flexion, there is gastrocnemius spasticity or contracture.

As previously mentioned, quadriceps strength, contracture, and function should be evaluated when examining a patient with knee flexion deformity. Quadriceps strength is best assessed with the patient supine and the feet off the end of the table. The examiner extends the hips and allows the knees to flex passively (Fig. 5.19A) and then asks the patient to extend the knees voluntarily against resistance (Fig. 5.19B). To determine if the rectus femoris is spastic, the examiner turns the patient prone and performs the prone rectus (Ely) test (Fig. 5.20A). With the patient prone and the knees extended,

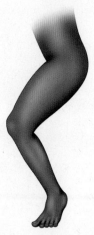

FIGURE **5.15** Typical crouch posture caused by plantar flexion deformities of ankles, which require flexion of knees, hip, and lumbar spine to place center of gravity over weight-bearing surface.

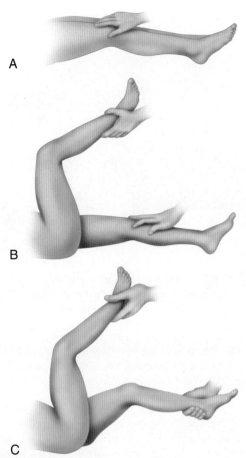

FIGURE 5.16 Testing for hamstring spasticity and contracture. **A,** Patient is supine with hips extended. Pressure is exerted over knees, forcing them into extension. Flexion remaining in knees is absolute knee flexion contracture. **B,** Knee on side to be tested is flexed while opposite knee is stabilized in extension. **C,** Attempted flexion of hip results in more flexion of knee.

the examiner flexes the knees. If the rectus is spastic, the hips flex and the buttocks rise off the table when the rectus is stretched. It is best to do this one side at a time to determine the relative spasticity of each rectus femoris muscle.

Physical therapy and bracing can be used for milder deformities. Serial stretch casting has been shown to be effective as well, but care is necessary to prevent soft-tissue complications or breakdown and neurapraxia. The indications for hamstring lengthening are a straight-leg raise of less than 70 degrees or a popliteal angle of less than 135 degrees in the absence of significant bony deformity. In an ambulatory patient, knee contracture of more than 10 degrees can lead to excessive compensatory hip flexion and ankle dorsiflexion. Care must be taken not to overlengthen the hamstrings because it can lead to excessive weakness and knee hyperextension gait. In hyperextension gait, the femur moves forward over a fixed tibia, which is prevented from moving forward either by a spastic gastrocnemius-soleus or a limited ankle dorsiflexion. Rectus femoris spasticity, which is common in patients with cerebral palsy, also can exacerbate this condition. For this reason, most surgeons begin with lengthening the medial hamstrings by a Z-plasty of the gracilis and semitendinosus tendons and a fractional lengthening of the semimembranosus. If further correction is desired, the biceps femoris laterally can be lengthened using fractional lengthening.

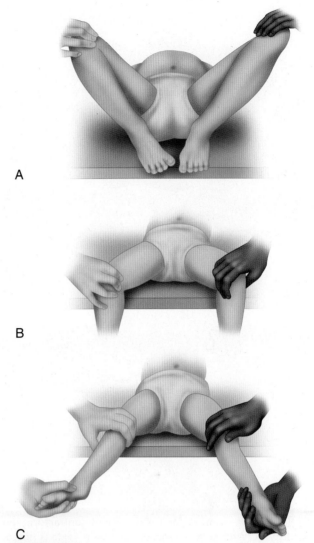

FIGURE 5.17 Testing for adductor and medial hamstring tightness. **A,** Thighs abduct well with hips and knees flexed, indicating no adductor contracture. **B,** With hips extended and knees flexed, hips abduct well. **C,** With hips extended, bringing knees into extension causes thighs to adduct, indicating medial hamstring spasticity.

Identify the proximal aponeurosis of the semimembranosus anteriorly as it arises from the tendon of the proximal attachment. It is separate and proximal from the distal aponeurosis and should be released at the time of surgery as well.

FRACTIONAL LENGTHENING OF HAMSTRING TENDONS

Although knee extension in stance phase has been shown to improve dramatically after hamstring lengthening, velocity, stride length, and cadence have not been shown to improve. With spastic hamstrings and quadriceps, knee flexion during swing phase markedly diminishes. In addition, the results of surgery have been reported to deteriorate with time, with reoperation being necessary in up to 17%. Because very little change can be expected from repeat hamstring lengthen-

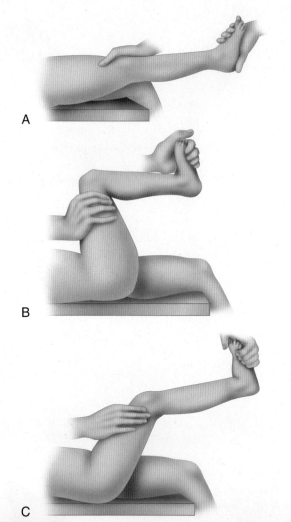

FIGURE 5.18 Testing for gastrocnemius contracture and spasticity. **A,** With knee extended, equinus in ankle is noted. **B,** With knee flexed, ankle is easily dorsiflexed, indicating no soleus contracture. **C,** As knee is extended, ankle dorsiflexion is resisted by tight or spastic gastrocnemius muscles.

ing in patients with recurrent knee flexion after hamstring lengthening, alternative surgical interventions may be more beneficial. Some improvement in the popliteal angle and knee extension has been noted in patients with combined medial and lateral hamstring lengthenings, however, with greater risk of knee hyperextension and hamstring weakness.

TECHNIQUE 5.8

- Place the patient prone and inflate the thigh tourniquet.
- Make medial and lateral posterior incisions just above the popliteal crease extending 4 to 6 cm proximally. Alternatively, a single midline incision can be used (Fig. 5.21A).
- Divide the subcutaneous tissue and deep fascia in line with the skin incision, protecting the posterior femoral cutaneous nerve in the proximal portion of the wound.
- Expose the semitendinosus tendon, which is the most superficial posteromedial structure and is tendinous at this level. Incise the tendon transversely or, alternatively, perform a Z-plasty.

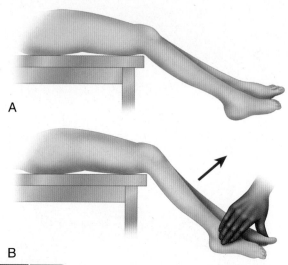

FIGURE 5.19 Testing for quadriceps strength. **A,** With hips extended, knees are allowed to flex off end of table. **B,** Patient voluntarily extends knees from flexed position against resistance.

- Identify and isolate the semimembranosus and incise its tendon sheath longitudinally. Divide its aponeurosis sharply at two levels, leaving the underlying muscle intact (Fig. 5.21B,C).
- Extend the knee with the hip in extension and the tendinous portion of the semimembranosus slides on the muscle. If further correction is required, identify the biceps femoris tendon laterally and isolate it from the peroneal nerve lying along its medial side. Pass a blunt instrument deep to the biceps femoris tendon, incise its tendinous portion transversely at two levels 3 cm apart, and leave the muscle fibers intact (Fig. 5.21D).
- Perform a similar lengthening maneuver by extending the knee with the hip in extension. Do not forcefully extend the knee with the hip flexed because this may cause a traction injury to the sciatic nerve and risk injury to the peroneal injury.
- Close all tendon sheaths, but do not close the deep fascia (Fig. 5.21E).
- After deflating the tourniquet, obtain hemostasis and close the subcutaneous tissues and skin.
- Apply a long leg cast with the knee in maximal extension.

POSTOPERATIVE CARE Straight-leg raises are begun immediately postoperatively with the cast on to help stretch the hamstring tendons. The patient may walk with crutches and bear weight as tolerated. After 3 to 4 weeks, the casts are removed and the patient is started on a physical therapy program to maintain, and in some cases improve, range of motion. Nighttime extension splints or knee immobilizers are used for 8 to 12 weeks postoperatively.

▇ COMBINED HAMSTRING LENGTHENING, POSTERIOR CAPSULAR RELEASE

If hamstring lengthening alone is ineffective in achieving the desired range of motion, a posterior capsular release can be used. This most commonly occurs in older children with

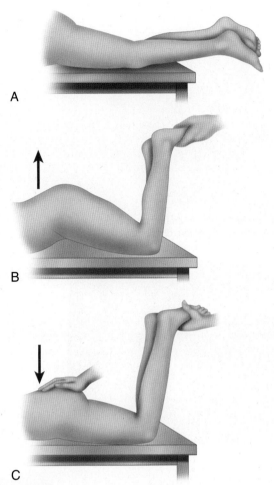

FIGURE 5.20 Prone rectus test. **A,** Patient is prone, and knees are extended. **B,** Flexing knees causes buttocks to rise from table. **C,** Spasticity in rectus is overcome by downward pressure on buttocks.

significant fixed knee flexion contractures. This technique also can be combined with quadriceps shortening to help correct elongation of the infrapatellar tendon caused by chronic quadriceps weakening to obtain improved range of motion.

DISTAL FEMORAL EXTENSION OSTEOTOMY AND PATELLAR TENDON ADVANCEMENT

Because the results of revision hamstring lengthening are poor, the use of a distal femoral extension osteotomy has increased, especially for severe or recurrent knee flexion contractures after hamstring release. Stout et al. described a distal femoral extension osteotomy and patellar tendon advancement for treatment of crouch gait in cerebral palsy and obtained improved function and level of community ambulation. The osteotomy is most commonly fixed with distal femoral plates, but external fixation has also been used. Recurrence of deformity is less likely in patients in whom growth is complete. This procedure is most commonly done for patients who stand or ambulate. Patients

should be followed closely after surgery because up to 10% of children have a postoperative nerve palsy that is unrelated to the degree of correction. To avoid these complications of acute correction, anterior distal femoral hemiepiphysiodesis has been used in small series to correct fixed knee flexion contractures (Fig. 5.22). This technique requires that patients have significant growth remaining to allow for correction. Immature patients (age < 11 years) should be followed for premature closure of the proximal tibial physis leading to decreased posterior slope.

TECHNIQUE 5.9

(STOUT ET AL.)

- Approach the distal part of the femur posterior to the vastus lateralis.
- Insert a chisel for a 90-degree blade plate just proximal to a guidewire placed at a 90-degree angle to the femoral shaft and just proximal to the physis (or physeal scar) with the angle guide of the chisel parallel to the tibia. This placement avoids varus or valgus displacement of the osteotomy. Alternatively, a distal femoral locking plate can be used with an estimate for correction based on the guide being in line with the tibia.
- Remove an anterior triangular wedge of bone that matches the degree of contracture. Also, remove any bone protruding posteriorly from the distal fragment (Fig. 5.23). Coronal and transverse plane abnormalities can be corrected simultaneously.
- The type of patellar tendon advancement depends on the skeletal maturity of the patient. If the physis is open, sharply divide the patellar tendon from the tibial tubercle to avoid physeal injury and advance it under a periosteal flap. If the physis is closed, transpose the tibial tubercle with the attached patellar tendon distally and secure it with a compression screw.
- Alternatively, the redundant patellar tendon can be oversewn onto itself with satisfactory results.
- Insert a 16-gauge wire or tension-band wire transversely through the patella and the proximal part of the tibia to protect the repair.

■ DISTAL TRANSFER OF RECTUS FEMORIS

Stiff knee gait is common in patients with cerebral palsy and is caused by co-contracture of the quadriceps and hamstring muscles or weakness caused by previous hamstring lengthening, or both. Co-spasticity of the hamstrings and quadriceps causes a loss of knee flexion that leads to decreased power and difficulties with foot clearance during the swing phase of gait. Patients with rectus femoris spasticity also have difficulty transitioning from standing to sitting. Dynamic EMG analysis often reveals a rectus femoris muscle that also is abnormally active during swing phase. To help achieve balanced knee function during swing phase, transfer of the distal rectus femoral tendon to the semitendinosus medially or iliotibial band laterally can be done, depending on the presence of malrotation. No functional differences in knee flexion are seen between the transfer sites, and this should then be determined by surgeon preference and concomitant procedures. Ten degrees of

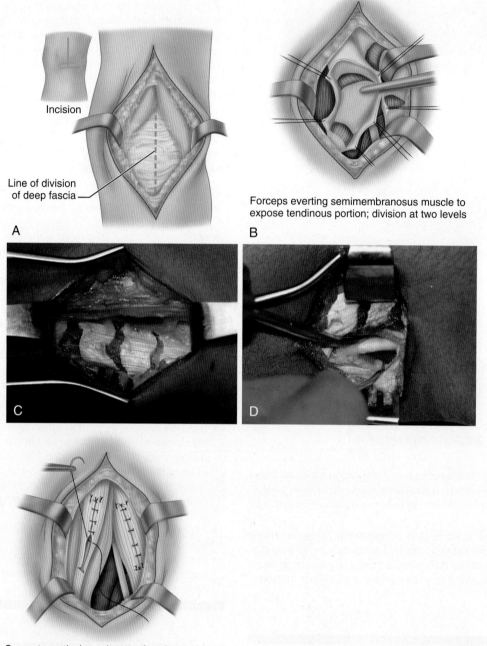

Incision

Line of division
of deep fascia

A

Forceps everting semimembranosus muscle to
expose tendinous portion; division at two levels

B

C

D

Separate meticulous closure of each
tendon sheath; deep fascia is not sutured

E

FIGURE 5.21 Fractional lengthening of hamstrings. **A,** Skin incision and incision in deep fascia over back of knee. **B** and **C,** Incisions in semimembranosus. **D,** Incisions in biceps femoris; note hemostat anterior to peroneal nerve. **E,** Tendon sheaths of biceps femoris and semimembranosus are sutured before wound closure. **SEE TECHNIQUE 5.8.**

malrotation can be corrected depending on the direction of transfer, but larger degrees of malrotation require rotational osteotomy of the affected bone. Gage et al. found significant improvement in swing-phase knee motion and foot clearance when the following criteria were met: (1) hamstring contractures corrected so that the knee can extend fully in midstance, (2) foot plantigrade and stable in stance, and (3) foot in line of progression to generate a moment of sufficient magnitude to maintain knee extension in midstance and terminal stance. In

comparison studies of hamstring lengthening with and without rectus femoris transfer, patients with rectus femoris transfer had significantly improved foot clearance and gait efficiency, most markedly in GMFCS I and II patients. In patients who are GMFCS III or IV, rectus transfer can lead to a persistent crouch gait and should be avoided because of the importance of an upright posture for the patients and their caregivers. More improvements than deterioration of results have been reported in ambulatory children at long-term follow-up.

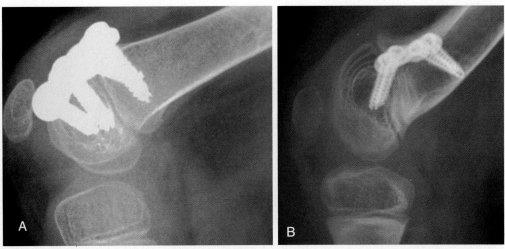

FIGURE 5.22 **A,** Patient with cerebral palsy and fixed knee flexion contracture treated with anterior distal femoral epiphysiodesis using 8-plates. **B,** 20 months after surgery. (From Al-aubaidi Z, Lundgaard B, Pedersen NW: Anterior distal femoral hemi-epiphysiodesis in the treatment of fixed knee flexion contracture in neuromuscular patients, *J Chil Orthop* 6:313, 2012.) **SEE TECHNIQUE 5.8.**

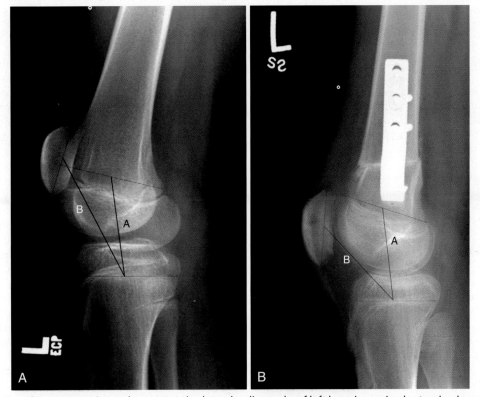

FIGURE 5.23 **A** and **B,** Preoperative and postoperative lateral radiographs of left knee in maximal extension in patient treated with distal femoral extension osteotomy. **SEE TECHNIQUE 5.9.** (From Stout JL, Gage JR, Schwartz MH, Novacheck TF: Distal femoral extension osteotomy and patellar tendon advancement to treat persistent crouch gait in cerebral palsy, *J Bone Joint Surg* 90A:2470, 2008.)

RECTUS FEMORIS TRANSFER

TECHNIQUE 5.10   *Figure 5.24*

(GAGE ET AL.)
- With the patient anesthetized and supine, make a longitudinal incision in the anterior thigh, 5 to 6 cm proximal to the superior pole of the patella.

- Identify the rectus femoris tendon proximally as it lies between the vastus medialis and vastus lateralis. Separate the rectus tendon from the remainder of the quadriceps tendon; avoid entering the knee joint. Dissect it free to approximately 3 cm proximal to the patella. Divide the tendon and separate it from the vastus intermedius tendon posteriorly.
- Transfer the freed tendon stump to either the distal stump of the semitendinosus or the iliotibial band depending on whether the desired rotatory effect is lateral rotation

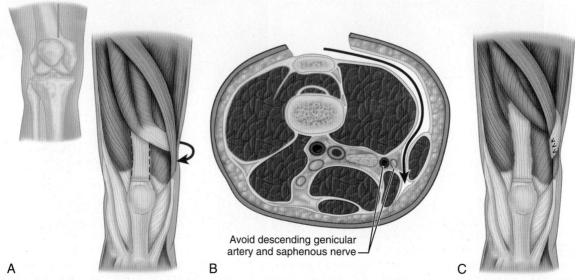

FIGURE 5.24 Distal release or transfer of rectus femoris. **A,** Rectus femoris is separated from vastus medialis, vastus lateralis, and vastus intermedius. *Inset,* Longitudinal incision along medial side of distal third of rectus femoris. **B,** Rectus femoris may be transferred through medial intermuscular septum to sartorius if desired. **C,** Rectus femoris is sutured to sartorius. **SEE TECHNIQUE 5.10.**

Avoid descending genicular artery and saphenous nerve

(to the iliotibial band) or medial (to the semitendinosus stump).

- For medial transfer to the semitendinosus, divide the semitendinosus 2 to 3 cm proximal to its musculotendinous junction and dissect the distal stump to its insertion at the pes anserinus. Transfer the tendon through the medial intermuscular septum and suture it to the distal end of the rectus femoris tendon.
- For a lateral transfer to the iliotibial band, resect the fibers of the iliotibial band until the remaining fibers are posterior to the knee joint axis. Pass the distal end of the rectus femoris around the iliotibial band and suture it onto itself.

POSTOPERATIVE CARE If hamstring lengthening also has been done, patients are placed in long leg casts for 3 to 4 weeks. If hamstring lengthening has not been done, cast immobilization is unnecessary; instead, a knee immobilizer is used. The patient is allowed to sit in a reclining wheelchair and is gradually moved to the upright sitting position with the knee fully flexed. Standing with support is allowed on the third day, and the knee immobilizer is removed for passive and active range of motion of the knee. At 4 weeks, the patient is instructed by the physical therapist to begin vigorous exercises to encourage muscle strengthening and gait training. Improvements in gait function typically are seen for 12 months postoperatively.

RECURVATUM OF THE KNEE

Recurvatum of the knee is caused by a relative imbalance between the quadriceps and the hamstrings owing to several factors, including (1) co-spasticity of the quadriceps and hamstrings in which the quadriceps is stronger; (2) weakened hamstrings secondary to previous surgery, overlengthening, or transfer; (3) gastrocnemius-soleus weakness secondary to proximal head recession; and (4) ankle equinus. For a patient

with an ankle equinus contracture, the only way to put the feet flat is to compensate with knee recurvatum.

The prone rectus test can be used to test for quadriceps spasticity. If the rectus femoris is tight, it can be lengthened or released in nonambulatory patients and transferred posteriorly in ambulatory children. Recurvatum of the knee caused by excessive hamstring weakness is difficult to treat. Replantation of transferred tendons or shortening of overlengthened tendons would not improve functional strength because the muscles have been permanently weakened by the previous surgery.

To determine if recurvatum of the knee is caused by ankle equinus, a short leg cast or ankle orthosis is applied with the ankle in the neutral position. If the knee goes into recurvatum with the foot plantigrade, the recurvatum is not caused by ankle equinus. If ankle equinus does exist, correction of this operatively or nonoperatively is indicated. Significant recurvatum should be treated with bilateral long leg braces with a pelvic band with the knees locked in 20 degrees of flexion and ankle stops at 5 degrees of dorsiflexion. When hip control is achieved, the pelvic band can be removed, but long leg braces often are used for years until a stable knee is obtained. Flexion osteotomy for this condition is not advised.

KNEE VALGUS

Knee valgus in patients with cerebral palsy usually is caused by a hip adduction deformity and rarely occurs independently. It is usually associated with hip internal rotation and flexion of the knees, which can accentuate the appearance of valgus. In most patients, correction of the hip adduction and internal rotation improves the position and appearance of the knee. In these patients, surgery on the knee itself is rarely indicated.

A tight iliotibial band also can cause a knee valgus deformity. The presence of iliotibial band tightness can be determined by having the patient lie on the contralateral side and flex the knee nearest the table to the chest. With the knee flexed, the hip being tested is flexed and abducted, moved

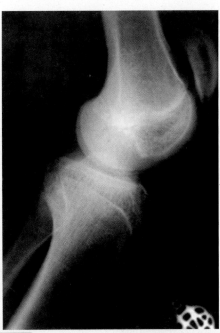

FIGURE 5.25 Patella alta in patient with cerebral palsy.

from the position of flexion to extension, and then adducted. If the hip does not adduct without flexing, the iliotibial band is tight and usually can be palpated subcutaneously along the distal third of the thigh. The tight band should be resected.

PATELLA ALTA

Patella alta is common in patients with cerebral palsy (93% in one study) and usually is associated with crouched gait and a knee flexion contracture (Fig. 5.25). Despite this frequent occurrence, the prevalence of anterior knee pain in these patients is approximately 10% to 20%, being more common in older children, females, and possibly those with larger flexion contractures. Patellar subluxation and dislocation are rare; they can be caused by quadriceps spasticity or long-standing knee flexion deformity. Patella alta leads to a decrease in the moment arm of terminal knee extension, which further weakens an already weakened extensor mechanism. This increased tension can lead to repetitive microtrauma to the patellar and quadriceps tendons, causing elongation of these structures and fragmentation and stress fractures of the patella and tibial tubercle; it is thought to be one of the causes of knee pain in patients with cerebral palsy. Because these changes are almost universal in ambulatory patients with cerebral palsy and most patients are pain free, operative treatment rarely is indicated. Often, correction of the flexion deformity of the knee with hamstring lengthening and other associated procedures causes improvement in not only the patella alta but also knee function in general. Operative treatment to correct the underlying pathologic process, which usually is patellar subluxation and dislocation, is helpful in patients in whom conservative treatment has failed.

ROTATIONAL ABNORMALITIES

Rotational abnormalities, either internal or external, can cause significant gait dysfunction in patients with cerebral palsy. These deformities usually occur at multiple levels including the hip or femur, tibia or ankle, and foot. There is no role for bracing in correction of these deformities in patients with cerebral palsy. A thorough rotational evaluation is essential before any operative intervention. A large gait analysis study of 412 children found that the most common cause of internal rotation gait was internal hip rotation, followed by internal tibial torsion, and multiple abnormalities were found in almost 50% of affected limbs. Differences were noted between hemiplegic and diplegic patients, with the most common site of internal rotation deformity in diplegics being the hip (57%), tibia (52%), and pelvis (19%) compared with hemiplegics, in whom foot deformities included pes varus (42%) and metatarsus adductus (24%).

These deformities should be corrected at the time of soft-tissue procedures. Minimally invasive percutaneous osteotomies of the femur and supramalleolar tibia have been described.

FOOT AND ANKLE

Foot deformities in children with cerebral palsy can be difficult to fully understand. The goals of treatment in ambulatory children differ from those in non-ambulatory children, but generally a braceable plantigrade foot should be the desired outcome. Foot deformities caused by altered or abnormal muscle forces are common in patients with cerebral palsy, with 70% to 90% of children affected. The most common deformity is ankle equinus, with equinovarus and equinovalgus deformities being equally common. In a series of 306 children with cerebral palsy, approximately 50% had normal "side-to-side" balance, 25% had valgus deformities, and 23% had varus deformities. The presence of a bilateral as opposed to a unilateral foot deformity, regardless of the type, has been shown to have a significant effect on overall level of ambulation. A patient's deformity may change over time, especially in young children. For example, in a very young child with a valgus foot deformity, persistent tonic reflexes and abnormal muscle forces may over time cause a varus foot position to develop. Digital deformity is caused by an imbalance between the intrinsic muscles of the foot and extrinsic muscles of the leg (intrinsic plus foot) and can cause hallux valgus, claw toes, and forefoot adduction. Spasticity of the smaller muscles of the foot can lead to other deformities, such as hallux valgus, claw toes, and forefoot adduction. These can occur in isolation but more often occur in association with other deformities related to abnormal extrinsic foot musculature.

EQUINUS DEFORMITY

Equinus deformity is the most common foot and ankle deformity in patients with cerebral palsy, affecting 70% of children, of whom approximately 25% develop a deformity severe enough to require operative treatment. Conservative treatment consisting of stretching, bracing, BTX-A, and, occasionally, casting remains the primary form of treatment or means of delaying operative intervention. Ankle-foot orthoses, in addition to preventing or delaying surgical treatment, often improve gait parameters and decrease energy expenditure in children with cerebral palsy by positioning joints in the proper position and reducing pathologic reflex or spasticity. As equinus is caused by spasticity of the gastrocnemius-soleus muscle, it often worsens during periods of rapid growth because of overgrowth of the tibia relative to the gastrocnemius-soleus. Animal models have shown that muscles in mice with hereditary spasticity grow at a slower rate than normal muscle. Ultrasound evaluation of the musculotendinous junction showed that patients with cerebral palsy have longer Achilles tendons and shorter muscle bellies than normal controls. Whereas ankle dorsiflexion increases in operatively treated patients, the muscle-tendon architecture remains abnormal. Bracing, especially at night, to prevent the foot from going into the equinus position is essential. The exact indications for surgery for equinus-related conditions are unclear given the variable nature of cerebral palsy; however, surgery typically is indicated when the ankle cannot be brought into the neutral position in an ambulatory child because ankle kinematics change dramatically with the ankle fixed in more than 10 degrees of dorsiflexion. Other indications include difficulties with hygiene, foot wear, and standing programs in a nonambulatory child.

■ SURGICAL CORRECTION OF EQUINUS DEFORMITY

Because of the variable nature of cerebral palsy and the fact that numerous procedures and postoperative regimens have been used in the treatment of equinus contracture, it is difficult to compare studies and success rates. In addition, many recurrences are more than 5 years after the initial operation and may not be included in short-term studies. The recurrence rate in the literature ranges from 0% to 50%, depending on the type of patient and the length of follow-up. Younger patients, especially those younger than 3 years, and hemiplegics are most likely to have recurrence. Recurrence in patients older than 6 years is uncommon. A study of 243 children with cerebral palsy (mean age, 7.8 years) who had Achilles tendon lengthening showed a recurrence rate of 11% at 10 years. A large meta-analysis showed that age is the most important determinant of recurrence and that overcorrection leading to a calcaneal deformity and crouch gait was more common in diplegics (15%) compared with hemiplegics (1%). Despite numerous techniques used, there did not seem to be a significant difference in outcomes between techniques, although the majority of the studies were level IV evidence.

The gastrocnemius-soleus can be lengthened at either the musculotendinous junction with an aponeurotic recession or at the level of the Achilles tendon through an open or percutaneous approach. For mild to moderate contractures, it is recommended that lengthening be done at the level of the musculotendinous junction; the higher rate of overlengthening seen with the use of open Z-plasty techniques leads to residual weakness. The use of the percutaneous approach has been shown in a small (28 feet) randomized, blinded study to provide rapid healing as demonstrated on ultrasound evaluation of the tendon, shorter operative and hospitalization times, postoperative dorsiflexion, and higher parental satisfaction. Larger studies are necessary to further evaluate this. Overlengthening of the gastrocnemius-soleus should be avoided, especially in an ambulatory child, because it can cause weakness in push-off and crouch gait. Because overlengthening is less common with an aponeurosis recession, this is the most commonly used procedure in ambulatory children, with open Achilles lengthening reserved for patients with severe deformities and for nonambulatory patients. It is important to evaluate patients after release for toe flexion

contractures that have been unmasked after Achilles tendon lengthening, because this can lead to abnormal weight bearing on the tips of the toes. This can be treated with simultaneous Z-lengthenings of the flexor digitorum longus and flexor hallucis longus.

Z-PLASTY LENGTHENING OF THE ACHILLES TENDON

Rattey et al. reported recurrence of contractures in 18% and 41% of diplegic and hemiplegic patients 10 years after 77 open Z-plasty lengthenings of the Achilles tendon. Children 6 years old or older at the time of lengthening did not have recurrence. Diplegic patients who were operated on before age 4 years and patients who had longitudinal incisions had statistically significantly higher recurrence rates.

TECHNIQUE 5.11

- Make a posteromedial incision midway between the Achilles tendon and the posterior aspect of the medial malleolus. The lower extent of the incision is at the superior border of the calcaneus, and it continues cephalad for 4 to 5 cm (Fig. 5.26A).
- Expose the Achilles tendon with sharp dissection directed posteriorly toward it.
- Incise the sheath of the Achilles tendon longitudinally from the superior to the inferior extent of the incision. Free the tendon from the surrounding tissues.
- Make a longitudinal incision in the center of the Achilles tendon from proximal to distal (Fig. 5.26A).
- Turn the scalpel either medially or laterally distally and divide that half of the tendon transversely. Make the distal cut toward the medial side for a varus deformity and toward the lateral for a valgus deformity.
- Hold this cut portion of the tendon with forceps and bring the scalpel to the proximal portion of the longitudinal incision in the tendon.
- Turn the scalpel opposite the distal cut and divide that half of the tendon transversely to free the Achilles tendon completely.
- Divide the plantaris tendon on the medial aspect of the Achilles tendon transversely.
- Evaluate the passive excursion of the triceps surae muscle using a Kocher clamp to pull the proximal stump of the tendon to its maximally stretched length.
- Allow the tendon to retract halfway back to its resting length and suture it to the distal tendon end at that point (Fig. 5.26B).
- Control tension further by adjusting the foot position: neutral for mild spasticity, 10 degrees of dorsiflexion for moderate involvement, and 20 degrees of dorsiflexion for severe deformity.
- Perform the repair in a side-to-side or if needed, end-to-end, manner with heavy absorbable sutures.
- Close the wound with absorbable sutures or subcuticular sutures and skin strips and apply a long leg cast.

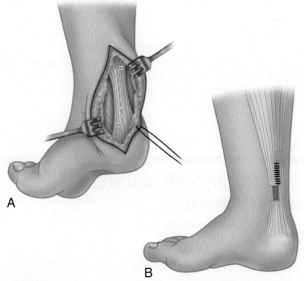

FIGURE 5.26 Z-plasty lengthening of Achilles tendon. **A,** Longitudinal incision, halfway between posterior aspect of medial malleolus and tendon. Longitudinal cut in tendon is brought out proximally in one direction and distally in opposite direction. **B,** Ends are sutured to repair tendon. **SEE TECHNIQUE 5.12.**

POSTOPERATIVE CARE The patient is allowed to bear full weight on the leg postoperatively. The cast is left on for approximately 4 weeks. During this time, knee extension is encouraged to maintain the lengthening of the gastrocnemius-soleus complex. The cast is removed, and an ankle-foot orthosis is fitted with the ankle in maximal dorsiflexion. Alternatively, a mold for a custom ankle-foot orthosis can be made at the time of the initial procedure so that it is ready at the time of cast removal. This is especially helpful if patient compliance and follow-up are questionable. The patient begins with full-time brace wear, and this is modified depending on the patient's growth remaining and progress in physical therapy.

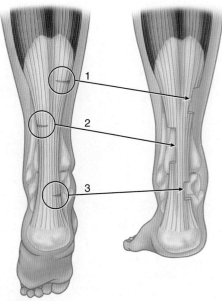

FIGURE 5.27 Incisions for percutaneous Achilles tendon lengthening. Cut ends slide on themselves with forceful dorsiflexion of foot. **SEE TECHNIQUE 5.13.**

- Make three partial tenotomies in the Achilles tendon (Fig. 5.27). Make the first medial cut, just at the insertion of the tendon onto the calcaneus, through one half of the width of the tendon. Make the second tenotomy proximally and medially, just below the musculotendinous junction. Make the third laterally through half the width of the tendon midway between the two medial cuts.
- Place the two incisions on the medial side if the heel is in varus as it usually is and on the lateral side if the heel is in valgus.
- Dorsiflex the ankle to the desired angle.
- The incisions do not require closure, only a sterile dressing and a long leg cast with the knee in full extension.

POSTOPERATIVE CARE The postoperative care is the same as that described for Technique 5.11.

PERCUTANEOUS LENGTHENING OF THE ACHILLES TENDON

Moreau and Lake found that when done as an outpatient procedure, percutaneous lengthening of the Achilles tendon was quick, inexpensive, and free of complications. Of the 90 legs treated in this fashion, 97% showed improvement in gait function.

TECHNIQUE 5.12

- With the patient prone and the leg prepared to the midthigh to include the toes, extend the knee and dorsiflex the ankle to tense the Achilles tendon so that it is subcutaneous, easily outlined, and away from the neurovascular structures anteriorly.

■ LENGTHENING OF THE GASTROCNEMIUS-SOLEUS MUSCLE COMPLEX

Surgical lengthening of the gastrocnemius-soleus complex is commonly performed to treat equinus deformity, either as an isolated procedure or as part of other reconstructive surgery. A variety of surgical procedures have been described to accomplish this lengthening, varying in terms of selectivity, stability, and amount of correction. In a systematic review by Shore et al., 10 different procedures were summarized and grouped by anatomic zone (Fig. 5.28). They concluded that cerebral palsy subtype (hemiplegia or diplegia) and age at index surgery were more important in determining outcomes of surgery than the choice of surgical procedure. In a biomechanical cadaver study, Firth et al. tested six procedures in the three zones and determined that zone 1 procedures were very stable but obtained limited lengthening, zone 2 procedures were stable and obtained more lengthening, and zone 3 procedures were not stable but obtained the most lengthening

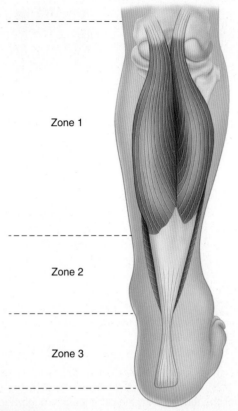

FIGURE 5.28 Three discrete anatomical zones of the gastroc-soleus complex. (Redrawn from Shore BJ, White N, Graham HK: Surgical correction of equinus deformity in children with cerebral palsy: a systematic review, *J Child Orthop* 4:277, 2010.)

(Fig. 5.29). The clinical implications of these findings are unclear. In a later clinical study of 40 children with spastic diplegia, Firth et al. found that equinus gait usually could be corrected by conservative procedures in zone 1; severe crouch gait was abolished, calcaneal deformity was infrequent, and the rate of overcorrection was low (2.5%). The procedure chosen should be based on the surgeon's experience and the unique clinical presentation of the patient.

GASTROCNEMIUS-SOLEUS LENGTHENING

TECHNIQUE 5.13

- Make a posteromedial longitudinal incision at the level of the musculotendinous junction, expose the aponeurosis of the gastrocnemius, and make an inverted V or transverse incision through it (Fig. 5.30A). Release this in a lateral-to-medial fashion to ensure complete release.
- Release the raphes of the gastrocnemius-soleus and the plantaris tendon (Fig. 5.30B) completely.
- Bring the ankle into slight dorsiflexion, which separates the ends of the tendon (Fig. 5.30C).
- If the aponeurosis of the soleus tendon is contracted and further correction is desired, divide it, but do not disturb the soleus muscle itself.

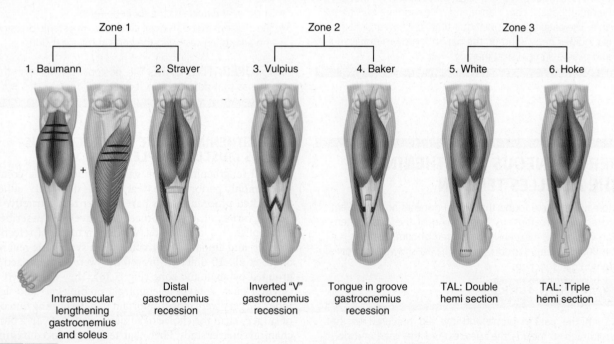

FIGURE 5.29 Six procedures for gastrocnemius-soleus lengthening according to zone. *TAL,* Tendo Achilles lengthening. (Redrawn from Firth BM, McMullean M, Chin T, et al: Lengthening of the gastrocnemius-soleus complex: an anatomical and biomechanical study in human cadavers, *J Bone Joint Surg* 95:1489, 2013.)

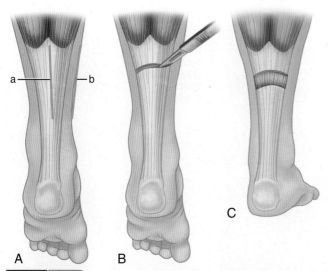

FIGURE 5.30 Gastrocnemius lengthening. **A,** Incision over posterior aspect of calf. **B,** Transverse cut through tendon. **C,** Foot is placed in dorsiflexion to neutral to separate tendon ends. **SEE TECHNIQUE 5.14.**

- Baker modified the Vulpius technique by lengthening the aponeurotic tendon of the gastrocnemius in a tongue-in-groove fashion. We prefer a simple transverse incision, through a slightly posteromedial approach, releasing the plantaris tendon as well.

POSTOPERATIVE CARE Postoperative care is the same as after Technique 5.11.

VARUS OR VALGUS DEFORMITY

Varus and valgus deformities can occur in patients with cerebral palsy, most commonly in association with an equinus deformity. The direction of deformity depends on the type and severity of cerebral palsy and the overall biomechanics of the affected limb. Computer motion analysis and dynamic EMG have shown that anterior tibial muscle dysfunction alone or in combination with dysfunction of the posterior tibial muscle is more commonly the cause of varus deformity than isolated posterior tibial dysfunction. In hemiplegia the foot deformity has been found to be either equinus or equinovarus, and in diplegia and quadriplegia it was valgus in 64% or varus in 36% of affected children. Although less common, varus deformities are more functionally disabling, more difficult to manage nonoperatively, and easier to correct operatively. Consequently, surgery is done more often and more successfully for varus than for valgus deformities.

The biomechanics of the hip and knee also influence whether a varus or valgus deformity is present. Diplegic patients typically have internally rotated and adducted hips, flexed knees, and external rotation deformity of the tibia. This combination of deformities causes the foot to assume a valgus position. In hemiplegic patients, the internally rotated thigh with the knee coming to full extension in stance phase causes the foot to internally rotate and produce a varus deformity.

■ EQUINOVARUS DEFORMITY

Varus deformity, which usually is accompanied by equinus, is caused most commonly by an abnormal posterior tibial muscle that is overactive or firing out of phase. The normal posterior tibial muscle is active during stance phase to stabilize the foot and inactive during swing phase. In many children with cerebral palsy, the posterior tibial muscle contracts during swing phase, leading to the varus position of the foot at heel strike. This also may be associated with anterior tibial muscle dysfunction; however, isolated anterior tibial muscle function is less likely to cause a varus deformity of the foot. Gait studies using EMG are helpful in determining which muscles are overactive or out of phase. It is essential to determine which muscles are responsible for the deformity before any attempt at surgical correction. The gastrocnemius-soleus contracture that usually accompanies the varus contracture also contributes to the overall varus deformity of the foot. It also is important to determine whether the deformity is flexible and correctable or rigid because patients with flexible deformities are more likely to be successfully treated nonoperatively with orthotics and shoe modifications and operatively with soft-tissue procedures such as tendon lengthenings, releases, or transfers (usually of the abnormally active muscle). Patients with rigid varus deformities generally require bone procedures, such as calcaneal osteotomy.

LENGTHENING OF THE POSTERIOR TIBIAL TENDON

The posterior tibial tendon can be lengthened in a variety of ways, including open Z-plasty of the tendon itself and various recession procedures, such as step-cut lengthening and intramuscular lengthening. The type of procedure used depends on the severity of the deformity and other procedures being done. A Z-plasty lengthening of the tendon, although it gives a large amount of correction, can cause scarring and tethering of the tendon in its sheath, leading to recurrence of deformity. Recession procedures such as lengthening at the musculotendinous junction have a lower risk of overlengthening and scarring of the tendon sheath. Recession procedures, because the muscle itself is spared, are good for patients at high risk of recurrence or in whom a posterior tibial transfer may be needed in the future.

MUSCULOTENDINOUS RECESSION OF THE POSTERIOR TIBIAL TENDON

TECHNIQUE 5.14

- This technique is commonly done in conjunction with other soft-tissue procedures such as a gastrocnemius recession.
- Place the patient supine and make a 3-cm longitudinal incision over the posteromedial aspect of the tibia, at the junction between the middle and distal thirds.
- Incise the deep fascia and identify the flexor digitorum longus and retract it posteriorly.

- Identify the posterior tibial musculotendinous junction by placing a hemostat beneath it and observing its action when inverting the foot without flexing the toes.
- Pass a hemostat around the tendinous portion of the musculotendinous junction to isolate it from the surrounding muscle, protecting the neurovascular bundle.
- Divide the tendinous portion of the posterior tibial musculotendinous unit, leaving its muscular fibers intact (Fig. 5.31A).
- Manipulate the foot into an overcorrected position (Fig. 5.31B).
- Close the wound and apply a short leg walking cast.

POSTOPERATIVE CARE The postoperative care is the same as for Technique 5.11.

■ SPLIT TENDON TRANSFERS

Depending on the muscles that are out of phase, split tendon transfers of the posterior or anterior tendon can be done. Full tendon transfers should be avoided because of the higher risk of complications and overcorrection of the deformity. Full posterior tibial tendon transfer to the dorsum of the foot has fallen out of favor for these reasons. Seventy-eight percent poor results were reported in one study with full tendon transfer because of unrecognized rigid varus deformity, simultaneous Achilles tendon lengthening leading to calcaneus deformity, lateral transplant of the tendon leading to valgus deformity, and detachment of the transferred tendon at the bone-tendon interface. Preoperatively, it is essential to ensure that the deformity is flexible and to identify the correct tendon to be transferred. A tendon transfer alone is insufficient to correct a rigid deformity. The split transfer not only improves active muscle function during gait but also acts as a dynamic sling, balancing the abnormal forces evenly across the foot.

SPLIT POSTERIOR TIBIAL TENDON TRANSFER

A study of 37 split posterior tibial tendon transfers in 30 children with cerebral palsy showed that in an average follow-up of 8 years there were 30 excellent, 4 good, and 3 poor results. Results did not deteriorate with time, and most patients were able to ambulate without braces.

TECHNIQUE 5.15 Figure 5.32

- Begin the first of two incisions 5 cm proximal and medial to the medial malleolus and extend the incision distally, ending over the navicular.
- Identify the posterior tibial muscle and tendon and the Achilles tendon, which can be lengthened as necessary.
- Identify and protect the neurovascular bundle with a vessel loop throughout the entire procedure.
- Open the anterior aspect of the posterior tibial tendon sheath from the navicular to the musculotendinous junc-

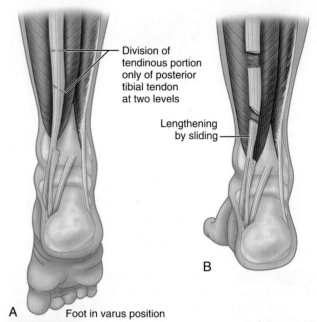

Division of tendinous portion only of posterior tibial tendon at two levels

Lengthening by sliding

B

A Foot in varus position

FIGURE 5.31 Sliding lengthening of posterior tibial tendon. **A,** Position of cuts in tendon. **B,** Lengthening by sliding. **SEE TECHNIQUE 5.14.**

tion, preserving the posterior tunnel to prevent dislocation of the tendon.
- Dissect the plantar portion of the posterior tibial tendon from its insertion on the navicular, preserving as much length for transfer as possible.
- Deliver this portion of the tendon into the proximal aspect of the wound and place a nonabsorbable suture in the free end of the tendon.
- Make a second incision over the lateral side of the ankle 2 cm proximal to the lateral malleolus and extend it to the insertion of the peroneus brevis tendon at the base of the fifth metatarsal.
- Open the sheath of the peroneus brevis tendon.
- Through the medial incision, create a tunnel posterior to the tibia and anterior to the neurovascular bundle, directed laterally toward the fibula.
- Pass the free end of the tendon through the tunnel, ensuring that the transferred tendon is posterior to the tibia and fibula and anterior to the neurovascular bundle and toe-flexor tendons to prevent neurovascular and flexor tendon compression during muscle contraction.
- Weave the end of the tendon through the peroneus brevis tendon and suture it to the tendon.
- Adjust tension on the transferred tendon so that the hindfoot is in neutral with the ankle in neutral dorsiflexion.
- If the Achilles tendon was lengthened with a Z-plasty, repair it at this time.
- Close the wounds in routine fashion and apply a long leg cast with the knee slightly flexed and the foot in neutral.

POSTOPERATIVE CARE Weight bearing is allowed immediately. The long leg cast is worn for 6 weeks, and then a short leg cast is worn for 2 weeks. An ankle-foot orthosis is prescribed only if patients have weak or absent anterior tibial muscle function preoperatively.

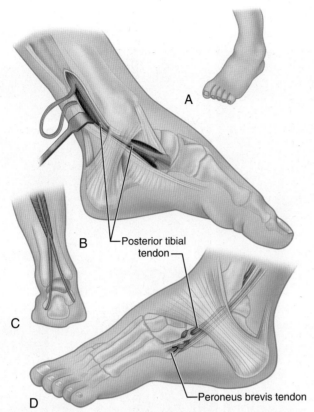

FIGURE 5.32 Kaufer split transfer of posterior tibial tendon for varus deformity. **A,** Foot is in varus position. **B,** Posterior tibial tendon has been split, one half is freed distally, and flexor tendons of toes and neurovascular bundle are retracted posteriorly. **C** and **D,** Freed half of tendon is passed from medial to lateral behind tibia and sutured to peroneus brevis tendon near its insertion. **SEE TECHNIQUE 5.15.**

SPLIT ANTERIOR TIBIAL TENDON TRANSFER

A 10-year follow-up of 21 patients who had split anterior tibial tendon transfers found that 19 were community ambulators with improved gait without the use of orthotics. Posterior tibial intramuscular lengthening and Achilles tendon lengthening combined with split anterior tibial tendon transfer was reported to produce excellent or good results in 18 of 20 children. The poor results were in patients with fixed hindfoot deformities and weak anterior tibial tendons preoperatively. A biomechanical study found that for a split tendon transfer the ideal insertion site, biomechanically, is the fourth metatarsal, and for whole tendon transfers it is the third metatarsal.

TECHNIQUE 5.16

(HOFFER ET AL.)
- Three incisions are used for the split anterior tibial tendon transfer.
- With the patient supine, make the first incision medially over the anterior tibial insertion on the medial cuneiform and first metatarsal.

- Identify the anterior tibial tendon, protecting the dorsalis pedis artery, and split the tendon with an umbilical tape (Fig. 5.33B).
- Make a second incision over the anterior aspect of the leg at the musculotendinous junction and identify the anterior tibial tendon; pass the umbilical tape into the second incision (Fig. 5.33C).
- Identify the lateral half of the tendon, release it from its insertion, and secure it with a locking stitch (Fig. 5.33D), preserving as much length as possible, and then pass it into the second incision as well.
- Make the third incision on the foot over the dorsal aspect of the cuboid. Pass the lateral half of the tendon subcutaneously into the third incision and close the first two incisions (Fig. 5.33E).
- Drill a hole into the cuboid, preserving a roof of bone. Pass the lateral slip of tendon through the drill hole and suture it to itself with nonabsorbable suture with the ankle in slight dorsiflexion and hindfoot eversion.
- If this is combined with lengthening of the Achilles tendon or posterior tibial tendon recession, these procedures should be done before the anterior tibial tendon transfer.
- Carefully hold the foot in the corrected position during wound closure and application of a short leg cast (Fig. 5.33F).

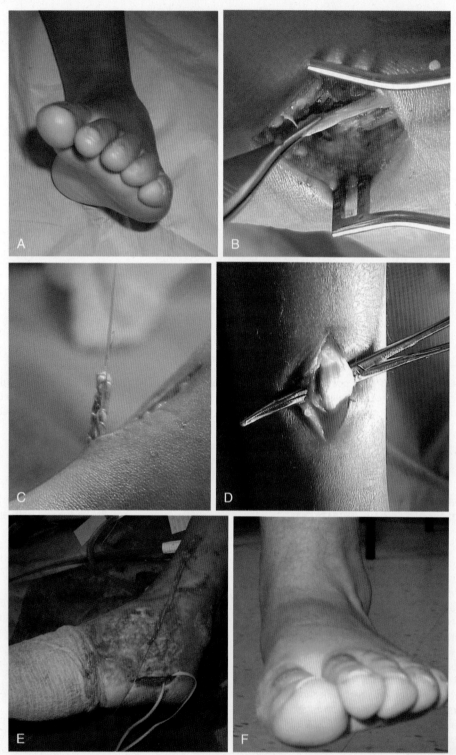

FIGURE 5.33 Transfer of anterior tibial tendon. **A,** Preoperative appearance of foot; note flexible forefoot supination. **B,** Lateral half of anterior tibial tendon is released from insertion, with care to resect as distally as possible to maximize graft length. **C,** Anterior tibial tendon is identified in anterior compartment, and graft is brought into anterior incision. **D,** Tendon is secured with locked nonabsorbable suture. **E,** Lateral slip of tendon is passed subcutaneously into third incision on lateral border of foot. **F,** Corrected position of foot postoperatively; note improved forefoot position and position of transferred tendon. **SEE TECHNIQUE 5.16.**

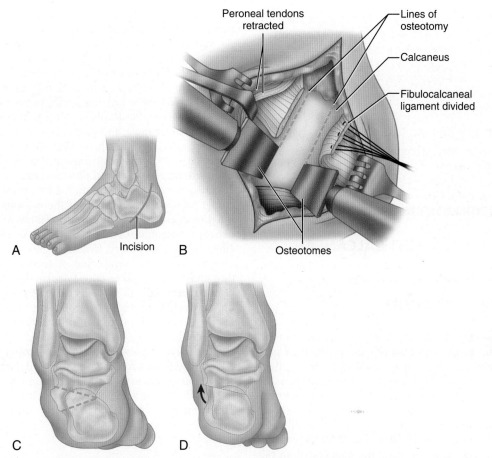

Peroneal tendons
retracted

Lines of
osteotomy

Calcaneus

Fibulocalcaneal
ligament divided

A   Incision   B   Osteotomes

C   D

FIGURE 5.34 Dwyer closing wedge osteotomy of calcaneus for varus heel. **A,** Lateral skin incision is made inferior and parallel to peroneal tendons. **B,** Wedge of bone is resected with its base laterally. **C,** Wedge of bone is tapered medially. **D,** Calcaneus is closed after bone has been removed, and varus deformity is corrected to slight valgus. **SEE TECHNIQUE 5.17.**

POSTOPERATIVE CARE A short leg cast is worn for 6 weeks, and weight bearing is allowed immediately. An ankle-foot orthosis is worn for 6 months to prevent recurrence.

■ OSTEOTOMY OF THE CALCANEUS

When the heel becomes fixed in varus, a corrective procedure on the bone is required, combined with a muscle balancing soft-tissue procedure. Osteotomy of the calcaneus as advocated by Dwyer corrects the varus of the heel and, in contrast to a triple arthrodesis, does not impair mobility in the subtalar or midtarsal joints. For varus deformities, the incision is lateral and the base of the wedge of bone removed is lateral. Alternatively, a lateral displacement osteotomy can be used to correct hindfoot varus. Although widely discussed as a treatment option, there are no good long-term outcome studies of this technique or comparisons with Dwyer osteotomy.

Good long-term results have been reported after a modified Dwyer calcaneal osteotomy (Fig. 5.34). A minimum age of 3 years is recommended for this osteotomy. Triple arthrodesis is recommended in children 9 years old or older.

LATERAL CLOSING-WEDGE CALCANEAL OSTEOTOMY

TECHNIQUE 5.17

(DWYER)

- Expose the lateral aspect of the foot through a curved incision parallel and about 1 cm posterior and inferior to the peroneus longus tendon (Fig. 5.34A).
- Retract the superior wound edge until the tendon sheath of the peroneus longus is exposed.
- Strip the periosteum from the superior, lateral, and inferior surfaces of the calcaneus posterior to this tendon.
- Remove a wedge of bone from the calcaneus just inferior and posterior to the tendon and parallel with it (Fig. 5.34B). Make the base of the wedge 8 to 12 mm wide as needed for correction of the deformity and taper the wedge medially to, but not through, the medial cortex of the calcaneus (Fig. 5.34C).
- Manually break the medial cortex and close the gap in the bone. Bring the bony surfaces snugly together by pressing the foot into dorsiflexion against the pull of the Achilles

tendon (Fig. 5.34D). Failure to close the gap in the calcaneus indicates that a small piece of bone has been left behind at the apex of the wedge and should be removed. Ensure that the varus deformity has been corrected and that the heel is in the neutral or a slightly varus position. Close the wound and apply a cast from the toes to the tibial tuberosity.

POSTOPERATIVE CARE The patient is placed in a short leg cast and weight bearing is protected for 4 weeks when possible. Weight bearing is progressed at that time, and cast immobilization is continued until the osteotomy is solid, usually no longer than 8 weeks.

LATERAL DISPLACEMENT CALCANEAL OSTEOTOMY

This technique is described in other chapter.

■ PLANOVALGUS DEFORMITY

Planovalgus is a common foot deformity in children with diplegia and quadriplegia, which, in contrast to equinovarus, rarely causes pain or gait dysfunction. Spasticity of the gastrocnemius-soleus usually is accompanied by overpull of the peroneal muscles or weakness of the foot inverters or both. The gastrocnemius-soleus acts as the primary deforming force. The contracted Achilles tendon acts as a bowstring, preventing dorsiflexion of the ankle. The dorsiflexion observed during gait occurs at the midtarsal joints, causing the calcaneus to evert and removing the sustentaculum tali from its normal supporting position underneath the talus. This, along with abduction of the midtarsal joint, causes the talus to move into a more medial and vertical position. External rotation deformity of the tibia, which is common in patients with diplegia and quadriplegia, also plays a role in this deformity. This altered talar position may cause pain with weight bearing and callus formation over the uncovered talar head. For this reason, gastrocnemius-soleus lengthening should accompany any procedure intended to correct planovalgus.

Most patients can be treated conservatively with shoe modifications or an orthosis to help control the hindfoot eversion. Operative treatment is indicated for patients in whom conservative treatment fails and who have significant deformity that is either painful or limits function. Soft-tissue procedures alone, such as lengthening or transfer of the peroneal tendons, usually are insufficient to correct this deformity. Perry and Hoffer transferred the peroneus longus or brevis into the posterior tibial tendon if either or both were active during stance phase only. Subtalar joint arthroereisis has fallen out of favor because of the unpredictable results and approximately 50% failure rate. Surgical treatment usually consists of calcaneal osteotomy, especially for milder deformities and GMFCS I and II patients, and subtalar arthrodesis for more severe deformities most commonly in GMFCS III to V patients. A 10-year follow-up study of cerebral palsy patients who had either calcaneal lengthening or subtalar fusion showed improvement in both groups; however, patients with poor functional abilities and those who had fusion had less foot pain. Regardless of the procedure, a recent gait study showed that correction of a planovalgus foot

deformity led to improvements in knee flexion, especially in patients with milder deformities.

Calcaneal osteotomy, consisting of lateral column lengthening, is effective in the treatment of mild-to-moderate deformities and is more effective in normalizing foot contact pressures than subtalar arthrodesis. It has been shown that preoperative weight bearing lateral radiographs with a less than 35-degree talocalcaneal angle, less than 25-degree talo–first metatarsal angle, and greater than 5 degrees of calcaneal pitch are associated with good outcomes. Although graft failure is rare (5%), it is less common with tricortical allografts than with patellar allografts. Postoperative subluxation of the calcaneocuboid joint is common after lateral column lengthening; however, stabilization of the calcaneocuboid joint at the time of correction has been shown not to reduce the incidence or magnitude of this. It also has been shown to be more effective in ambulatory children; nonambulatory children have a higher recurrence rate. A medial column stabilization consisting of either talonavicular stapling or fusion can be used, especially in GMFCS III to V patients. Medial column arthrodesis has also been shown to be effective in treating recurrent planovalgus deformity following lateral column lengthening.

A review of lateral column lengthening in 31 feet in 20 children with severe hindfoot valgus deformities in whom conservative treatment had failed found satisfactory results in 29 of the 31 feet with good preservation of subtalar motion. This technique is described in other chapter.

MEDIAL DISPLACEMENT CALCANEAL OSTEOTOMY

For more severe deformities, a translational osteotomy of the calcaneus can be used. Excellent results were reported in 17 of 18 patients at an average of 42 months after medial displacement calcaneal osteotomy to correct hindfoot valgus. A combined procedure of medial displacement osteotomy, opening wedge cuboid osteotomy, and pronation plantar flexion osteotomy of the medial cuneiform also has shown good restoration of foot position.

TECHNIQUE 5.18

- Place the patient supine and apply a midthigh tourniquet.
- Expose the lateral surface of the calcaneus through an incision beginning near the lateral tuberosity of the Achilles tendon attachment and extending distally and parallel but inferior to the sural nerve.
- By blunt dissection, expose the lateral surface of the calcaneus, reflecting the peroneal tendons and sural nerve superiorly.
- Using the plantar surface of the foot as a guide, place a Kirschner wire along the lateral side of the calcaneus and with a fluoroscopic image determine the appropriate placement of the osteotomy. It should not extend forward into the subtalar or calcaneocuboid joint.
- Make the osteotomy transverse and parallel to the sole of the foot, beginning just posterior to the subtalar joint,

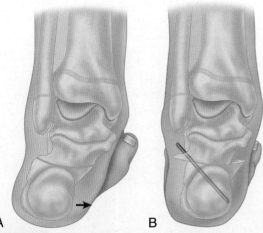

FIGURE 5.35 Medial displacement of calcaneus for hindfoot valgus. **A,** Transverse osteotomy of calcaneus. **B,** Fixation with Kirschner wire after distal fragment has been shifted medially to place calcaneus in weight-bearing line of tibia. **SEE TECHNIQUE 5.18.**

and direct it plantarward toward the attachment of the plantar fascia to the calcaneus (Fig. 5.35A). In making the osteotomy, protect the Achilles tendon superiorly and the plantar muscles, nerves, and vessels inferiorly. Do not penetrate the medial periosteum.

- When the osteotomy is complete, slide the inferior fragment medially to align the calcaneus with the tibia.
- Insert a threaded Kirschner wire, directed downward and medially, through the two fragments of calcaneus (Fig. 5.35B).
- Close the wound over suction drainage and apply a short leg cast.

POSTOPERATIVE CARE The cast is changed at 4 weeks, and the wire is removed. A new short leg cast is placed, and weight bearing is progressed over the next 4 weeks.

HINDFOOT ARTHRODESIS

Arthrodesis also has been used in the treatment of calcaneovalgus feet, with the classic procedure being the Grice extraarticular subtalar arthrodesis. It should be noted that although hindfoot alignment is improved this does not treat residual forefoot supination and ankle equinus. Because of high graft failure and pseudarthrosis rates of the initial procedure, a variety of modifications have been proposed. The modifications have been aimed at better retention of the calcaneus beneath the talus with internal fixation and decreased rates of pseudarthrosis. Good results have been reported in 70% of patients at an average follow-up of 5.6 years after Dennyson-Fulford modification of the extraarticular arthrodesis according to Hadley et al. The pseudarthrosis rate has been reported to be 6.4%. A report of 46 children who had bilateral subtalar fusion using an Ollier incision and precut corticocancellous graft found that at mean follow-up of 55 months functional mobility scores

improved in all patients, especially GMFS III patients, with no wound complications and fusion in 45. Alternatively, tibiotalocalcaneal arthrodesis has been reported in a small series of patients with severe calcaneovalgus deformity as a salvage procedure.

Triple arthrodesis can be performed for the severe planovalgus or cavovarus deformity that is rigid and painful. Techniques for triple arthrodesis are discussed in further detail in other chapter. One study reported fusion in 96% of feet at an average follow-up of 22-years; radiographic tibiotalar arthritis was found in only 11.5% of feet, and 95% of patients reported a good outcome.

TECHNIQUE 5.19

- See subtalar arthrodesis in other chapter.
- Obliquely incise the skin over the sinus tarsi beginning anteriorly at the middle of the ankle and proceeding laterally to the peroneal tendons (Fig. 5.36A).
- Incise and reflect as one flap the subcutaneous fat and origins of the extensor digitorum brevis muscles.
- By sharp dissection, excise the fat from the sinus tarsi down to bone proximally and distally.
- With a small gouge or burr, remove cortical bone from the apex of the sinus tarsi to expose cancellous bone on the talar neck and the superior surface of the calcaneus. Do not remove the cortical bone from the outer part of the sinus tarsi where a transfixion screw is to pass.
- Dorsally expose the small depression just behind the neck of the talus through a small separate skin incision and by blunt dissection between the neurovascular bundle and the tendons of the extensor digitorum longus.
- Hold the calcaneus in the corrected position and pass an awl posteriorly, inferiorly, and slightly laterally so that it passes through the cortical bone of the talus above and below and through the cortical bone of the calcaneus above and inferolaterally. Use the awl to determine the desired length of a screw needed for fixation into the hole and insert the screw in the hole.
- Alternatively, a cannulated screw can be placed using fluoroscopy (Fig. 5.36B).
- Remove chips of cancellous bone from the iliac crest and pack them into the sinus tarsi and above the bone that has been denuded on the talus and calcaneus.
- Replace the extensor digitorum brevis and close the skin.

POSTOPERATIVE CARE A short leg cast is applied with careful padding and molding around the heel. This cast is worn for 6 to 8 weeks with the patient kept non–weight bearing. The cast is changed to a short leg walking cast, and gradual weight bearing is begun.

Triple arthrodesis also has been used in the treatment of equinovalgus foot deformities. The addition of a lateral column lengthening as proposed by Horton allows better correction of the flatfoot deformity while offering good pain relief. A long-term study of 21 patients (26 feet) with cerebral palsy and a mean follow-up of 19 years after triple arthrodesis showed that although residual deformity was present in 39% of feet, 62% of patients were pain free and 95% were happy

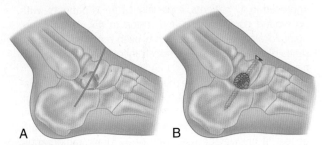

FIGURE 5.36 Dennyson and Fulford technique of extraarticular subtalar arthrodesis using screw and cancellous bone chips. **A,** Skin incision and bone area curetted from lateral side of talus and calcaneus. **B,** Placement of iliac bone chips in side of talus and calcaneus after screw has been inserted across subtalar joint with heel in corrected position. **SEE TECHNIQUE 5.19.**

with the operation. The rate of adjacent joint arthritis was 12% tibiotalar and 4% midfoot. After skeletal maturity, all residual deformities in the ankle, hindfoot, and midfoot can be corrected by a triple arthrodesis with appropriate wedge resections. Before undertaking a triple arthrodesis in a child with cerebral palsy, the surgeon always should obtain standing anteroposterior radiographs of the ankle. What often appears to be a valgus of the heel may be valgus of the ankle mortise, which should be corrected by a supramalleolar osteotomy and realignment of the ankle, rather than by creation of a secondary compensatory deformity in the subtalar joint (Fig. 5.37). Any external tibial torsion should be recognized before a triple arthrodesis is done because if the ankle joint is externally rotated, the foot will still appear to be in valgus and abduction after the triple arthrodesis.

■ CALCANEUS DEFORMITY

Pure calcaneus deformity is rare in patients with cerebral palsy and usually is associated with calcaneovalgus. It is most commonly caused by overlengthening or repeated lengthenings of the Achilles tendon. It can develop as a primary deformity when the dorsiflexors of the foot are spastic and the gastrocnemius-soleus is weak. This condition tends to be progressive and unresponsive to bracing. A variety of soft-tissue transfers have been proposed to help correct the deformity, including transfer of the anterior tibial or the peroneal tendons to the calcaneus, with limited success. The best treatment of this condition is prevention of excessive lengthening or denervation of the gastrocnemius-soleus complex.

■ CAVUS DEFORMITY

Cavus deformity is rare in children with cerebral palsy and is typically caused by an imbalance between the extrinsic and intrinsic musculature of the foot. In a review of 33 children in whom 38 osteotomies were done for cavus deformity, only one child (two feet) had cerebral palsy. Cavus deformity can be caused by hindfoot deformity in which the calcaneus is in a dorsiflexed position, or by midfoot deformity, in which the angulation of the foot occurs at the level of the midfoot. Conservative treatment alone rarely is successful in the treatment of this condition. Mild forefoot cavus may respond to plantar fascia release and casting; however, most such deformities require osteotomies as described in other chapter. Severe cavus deformities can be treated with triple arthrodesis. One must ensure that the patient does not have significant

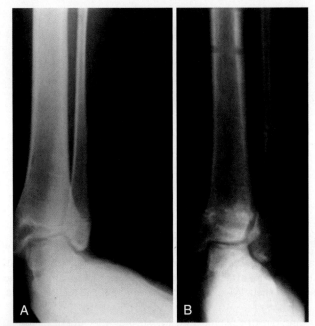

FIGURE 5.37 **A,** Standing anteroposterior view of ankle shows valgus deformity of ankle joint. **B,** Alignment of ankle achieved by supramalleolar osteotomy.

ankle valgus or external tibial deformity before performing triple arthrodesis.

■ FOREFOOT ADDUCTION DEFORMITY

Adduction deformity of the forefoot can occur in patients with cerebral palsy as an isolated deformity or in association with other deformities, such as in an incompletely corrected or recurrent clubfoot. In patients with an isolated abductor hallucis contracture, the tight tendon usually can be palpated when the great toe is adducted. Patients with isolated abductor hallucis spasticity have a passively correctable forefoot with the heel and ankle stabilized.

❚ CORRECTION OF FLEXIBLE FOREFOOT ADDUCTUS

If the forefoot is passively correctable, resecting a segment of the muscle and its tendon can be done. In a report of 18 feet treated with this procedure, 16 had no increase in the adduction deformity and 2 developed hallux valgus deformities.

In older children, forefoot adduction that interferes with shoe wear or is painful should be corrected by osteotomy of the metatarsals, realignment, and Kirschner wire fixation as described in other chapter. Medial column opening wedge (medial cuneiform) and lateral column closing wedge (cuboid) osteotomies also have been used to treat this condition.

■ HALLUX VALGUS DEFORMITY

Hallux valgus deformity in patients with cerebral palsy usually is associated with other deformities, such as equinovalgus foot, heel valgus, and external rotation of the tibia. These conditions cause the foot to pronate, forcing the first metatarsophalangeal joint into abduction and creating a hallux valgus deformity. The extensor hallucis tendon may sublux into the first web space and become an abductor of the hallux, leading to further deformity.

Any other underlying deformities, such as heel valgus or external rotation of the tibia, should be corrected before surgical correction of the hallux valgus. If the causative deformities are not corrected, recurrence is almost certain, especially if fusion of the first metatarsophalangeal joint is not done. Isolated soft-tissue procedures for hallux valgus in patients with cerebral palsy, because of altered muscle forces, rarely are successful and have a high recurrence rate, and great toe metatarsophalangeal joint fusion is recommended.

First metatarsophalangeal joint fusion has been shown to provide the best overall outcome with functional gains and anatomic correction of the deformity being maintained. Surgical procedures for the correction of hallux valgus are discussed in other chapter.

■ CLAW TOES

Claw toe deformities are common in adolescents and adults with cerebral palsy, although most require only observation and foot wear modifications, such as high toe box shoes. Operative treatment is recommended if the claw toe deformity becomes painful, interferes with foot wear, or interferes with walking. Although neurectomy of the lateral plantar nerve has been proposed, the method most commonly used to treat claw toes is metatarsophalangeal joint capsulotomies and tenotomy of the long toe extensors to the lesser toes, with proximal interphalangeal joint resections or fusions using Kirschner wire fixation until bony fusion occurs. Surgical procedures for claw toes are discussed in other chapter.

SPINE-PELVIC OBLIQUITY AND SCOLIOSIS

The combination of hip dislocation, pelvic obliquity, and scoliosis is common in wheelchair-bound patients with cerebral palsy and can cause significant difficulties with pain, sitting balance, and overall independence (Fig. 5.38). In an ambulatory child, spinal deformity and imbalance can make standing erect difficult if not impossible. In a nonambulatory child, scoliosis can lead to abnormal skin pressure areas and decubitus ulcers, seating/positioning difficulties, and, in severe cases, cardiopulmonary compromise. The scoliosis in patients with cerebral palsy is different from that of idiopathic adolescent scoliosis in that the curves tend to be long thoracolumbar C-shaped curves, with or without accompanying pelvic obliquity. The optimal treatment of scoliosis associated with hip dislocation and pelvic obliquity is controversial.

Although pelvic obliquity and scoliosis are common and related to disease severity in patients with cerebral palsy, the relationship between the two is not well established. A review of 500 children with cerebral palsy found no correlation between the frequency of dislocated hips, either bilateral or unilateral, and pelvic obliquity. All degrees of pelvic obliquity were found in children in whom both hips were dislocated. The frequency of hip dislocation on the same side as the elevated hemipelvis had no direct correlation with the degree of pelvic obliquity. In "windswept" hips there was no correlation between the direction of the windswept hips and the direction of the pelvic obliquity. This and other studies have shown that hip pathology is a result of muscle imbalance around the

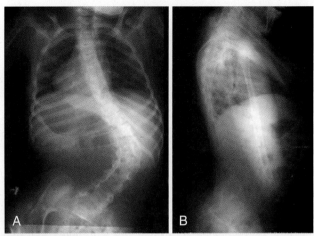

FIGURE 5.38 A, Posteroanterior view of spine of patient with spastic quadriplegic cerebral palsy with 73-degree thoracolumbar scoliosis and pelvic obliquity. B, Lateral view of spine of same patient shows progressive lumbar lordosis. This deformity was believed to contribute to increased skin pressures and seating difficulties. (From McCarthy JJ, D'Andrea LP, Betz RR, et al: Scoliosis in the child with cerebral palsy, J Am Acad Orthop Surg 14:367, 2006.)

hip and that pelvic obliquity and scoliosis are related to muscle imbalance of the trunk and independent of the position of the hips.

Scoliosis associated with cerebral palsy is related to the severity of motor involvement, with 50% to 75% of quadriplegics affected compared with fewer than 5% of hemiplegics. Compared with curves in idiopathic scoliosis, curves in patients with cerebral palsy tend to occur at a younger age and be more progressive and usually require operative treatment. Orthotic management has been shown to be ineffective in preventing progression of scoliosis but is occasionally used to help improve sitting balance or in efforts to delay surgery in immature patients to allow for further thoracic development. For nonambulatory patients with poor trunk control, chair modifications are necessary. Risk factors for curve progression include GMFCS level, younger age, poor sitting balance, and multiple curves. A study of 182 cerebral palsy patients with scoliosis showed that for GMFCS IV and V patients mean progression of the coronal Cobb angle was 3.4 degrees, thoracic kyphosis was 2.2 degrees, and apical translation was 5.4 mm per year. Curves of more than 30 degrees tend to progress, even after skeletal maturity.

Patients with cerebral palsy also have sagittal plane abnormalities. Hyperkyphosis is the most common deformity, especially in young children with weak spinal extensor muscles. This can significantly interfere with sitting balance and communication and usually is treated with wheelchair modifications, such as adding chest supports or reclining the seat. A soft body orthosis can be used as well. Hyperlordosis occurs less commonly and usually is associated with hip flexion contractures or a rigid thoracic kyphosis. Treatment of the primary deformity usually improves or corrects hyperlordosis.

Operative treatment should be considered for patients in whom scoliosis or pelvic obliquity interferes with overall function, rather than based on the absolute magnitude of the curve. The goals of treatment should be functionally oriented and related to loss of sitting balance, pelvic obliquity, and presence of pain rather than to the degree of curvature.

Improvement in pain is one of the most important factors in the improvement in quality of life after spinal surgery. The goals of surgery are to prevent further deformity, provide a well-balanced spine in the coronal and sagittal planes, correct any underlying pelvic obliquity, and improve pulmonary function. Complication rates after scoliosis surgery in patients with cerebral palsy are markedly higher, up to 25% to 50% in some series, than for adolescent idiopathic scoliosis and are often related to comorbidities such as aspiration, poor nutritional status, cardiopulmonary compromise, and increased risk of infection. The incidence of deep wound infection after scoliosis surgery in patients with cerebral palsy may be as high as 10%. Patients with wound breakdown and greater residual curves, greater preoperative white blood cell count, and fusion using unit rods may be at higher risk. *Escherichia coli* and *Pseudomonas aeruginosa* are commonly cultured organisms and, therefore, gram-negative prophylaxis should be considered. Surgical stabilization usually consists of posterior spinal instrumentation with segmental fixation, using screws, hooks, or wires. The use of pedicle screw fixation has become more common and has been shown to be effective in correcting coronal and sagittal deformity and pelvic obliquity. Osteotomies can be used in selected patients with severe focal deformities. Growth-sparing techniques, both rib-based and spine-based, have been shown in small series to be effective in controlling scoliosis while maintaining growth in patients with cerebral palsy; however, complications, especially infection, are frequent. The use of antibiotic-impregnated bone graft may decrease the rate of postoperative infection, and it is becoming more widely used.

Although parental and caretaker satisfaction after spinal fusion in patients with cerebral palsy remains high, it is difficult to find objective criteria that correlate with this. A review of 50 patients with scoliosis and cerebral palsy treated with posterior spinal fusion showed statistically significant improvement in the health-related quality of life (HRQL) scores postoperatively. However, only a weak correlation was found between the magnitude of curve correction and HRQL scores, and no correlation was found between complications and extension of the fusion to the pelvis. Another large study of 84 patients found that although functional improvement postoperatively was limited, satisfaction was high and was thought to be related to sitting balance and cosmesis. Factors in this study associated with less satisfaction included a higher complication rate, greater residual major curve magnitude, and hyperlordosis, which may relate to poorer overall sitting balance. Further study of factors leading to parental and caregiver satisfaction after spinal fusion in patients with cerebral palsy is necessary. A comparison of patients with cerebral palsy who had spinal fusion with patients who did not have fusion found no significant differences in pain, need for pulmonary medication or therapy, the presence of decubitus ulcers, patient function, or time required for daily care. Subjectively, however, most health care workers believed that patients who had undergone fusion were more comfortable.

UPPER EXTREMITY

Many patients with cerebral palsy have involvement of the upper extremities, especially patients with hemiplegia and quadriplegia. A review of 100 cerebral palsy patients found that 83% had upper limb involvement and 69% had reduced hand control. The most common contracture patterns were thumb in palm/clasped hand and shoulder adduction/internal rotation and wrist flexion/pronation. Functionally, 70% of children have limitation of forearm supination, and 63% have limitation of wrist and finger extension in the affected limb(s). The degree of upper extremity deformity is significantly related to GMFCS function in hemiplegic, but not diplegic patients. Most patients can be treated nonoperatively with physical therapy, splinting, and BTX-A. Selective dorsal rhizotomy, usually done to reduce lower extremity tone, has been shown to decrease upper extremity tone as well. Despite this high prevalence of deformity and functional limitations, only approximately 5% are surgical candidates. This may be related to the fact that in patients with cerebral palsy the upper extremity movement disorder often is associated with sensory deficits, particularly in proprioception, stereognosis, barognosis, and light touch, and there is seldom normal sensation in the affected hand. This alteration in sensation can cause a complete neglect of the affected extremity. Children who are likely to benefit from upper extremity surgery are highly functioning and have difficulties with activities of daily living, such as dressing and hygiene, or have severe contractures and deformities leading to pain and skin breakdown. Other positive predictors for a good outcome after upper extremity surgery include high motivation, reasonable intelligence, emotional stability, no neglect, good voluntary control, strength, and normal sensation. A randomized study of 39 children with cerebral palsy undergoing upper extremity surgery found that a combination of flexor carpi ulnaris to extensor carpi radialis brevis transfer, pronator teres release, and extensor pollicis brevis rerouting produced more improvement, although modest, than treatment with BTX-A injections or physical therapy. Children with severe spasticity, athetosis, and neglect still may benefit from surgery, which consists of static joint stabilizing procedures such as arthrodesis. The family should be considered so that they have realistic expectations regarding the goals of upper extremity surgery to prevent disappointment with the surgical outcome. Ancillary studies, such as kinetic EMG studies, are useful in evaluating the upper extremity before surgery.

The function of the upper extremity is to position the hand in space to perform a specific activity. If the hand is functional, procedures to correct these deformities may be useful in improving overall function. A review of the results of surgery in 84 upper limbs of 64 patients with cerebral palsy found a statistically significant improvement in functional status, hygiene, and appearance in carefully selected patients at an average follow-up of 4 years.

SHOULDER

Contracture of the shoulder or spasticity of the muscles that control it usually is not sufficiently disabling to justify surgery. The deformity usually is adduction and internal rotation. When surgery is indicated, useful procedures include procedures similar to those performed for brachial plexus palsy (see chapter 6) and rotational osteotomy of the humerus done at the level of the deltoid tubercle. The use of pectoralis major release alone and combined with latissimus dorsi release for severe deformities may be beneficial in patients with severe cerebral palsy to improve axillary hygiene, bathing, and dressing.

ELBOW

The two groups of patients who have been shown to benefit from surgical procedures around the elbow are highly functioning patients with useful hand function and severely involved patients with significant contractures leading to antecubital fossa skin breakdown. When releasing a flexion contracture around the elbow, acutely extending the elbow fully should be avoided to prevent stretch injury to the brachial artery and median nerve, which have shortened as well. The addition of partial biceps tendon lengthening has been shown to increase elbow extension better than brachialis fractional lengthening, lacertus fibrosis division, and pretendinous adventitia debridement alone. The improvements gained are maintained in long-term outcome studies. Note that biceps lengthening will weaken it, which is important in patients with underlying supination weakness.

RELEASE OF ELBOW FLEXION CONTRACTURE

A report of 32 anterior elbow releases in patients with cerebral palsy showed no neurovascular injuries and no recurrence of deformity. The indications for this operation are fixed elbow contracture of 45 degrees or more that interferes with the ability to reach forward with a functional forearm and hand. Other procedures that improve forearm supination and hand function by releasing the flexor-pronator muscle origins from the medial capsule result in a mild gain in elbow flexion as well.

TECHNIQUE 5.20

- With the patient supine and the arm fully draped and with or without a tourniquet, approach the antecubital space with a gently curving S-shaped incision over the flexor crease. If necessary, ligate the veins that cross the region.
- Dissect the soft tissue and deep fascia to the muscle belly of the biceps proximally and follow the muscle distally to its tendon and the lacertus fibrosus. Isolate the lacertus fibrosus and resect it (Fig. 5.39A).
- Identify and protect the lateral antebrachial cutaneous nerve as it enters the area between the biceps and the brachialis laterally.
- Retract the nerve laterally and then flex the elbow partially and free the biceps tendon down to its insertion on the tuberosity of the proximal radius.
- Divide the biceps tendon for a Z-plasty lengthening (Fig. 5.39B). The musculofascial surface of the brachialis muscle can be seen under it. The radial nerve lies lateral to the bra-

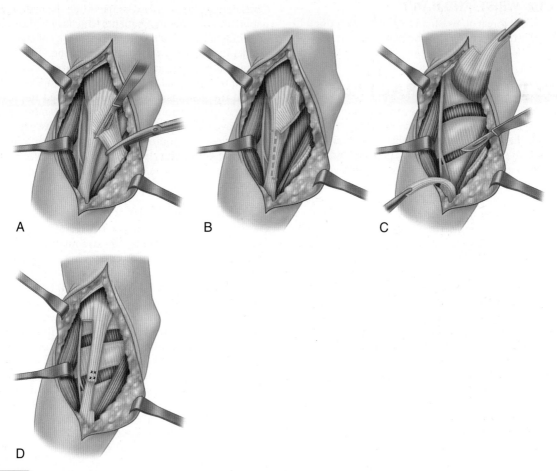

A   B   C

D

FIGURE 5.39   Mital elbow flexion release. **A,** Lacertus fibrosus is severed through incision in antecubital space. **B,** Tendon of insertion of biceps muscle is lengthened by Z-plasty. **C,** Fascia covering brachialis muscle anteriorly is cut at two levels. **D,** Z-plasty in biceps tendon is sutured after elbow is extended.

chialis muscle, and the brachial artery and median nerve lie medial to it. Identify and protect these structures.

- Extend the elbow maximally and circumferentially incise the aponeurotic tendinous fibers of the brachialis muscle at its distal end at one or two levels (Fig. 5.39C).
- Maximally extend the elbow and, if necessary, perform an anterior elbow capsulotomy. Allow the tourniquet to deflate and secure hemostasis.
- Extend the elbow and repair the previously divided biceps tendon (Fig. 5.39D).
- Ensure the integrity of the median nerve and brachial artery.
- Close only the subcutaneous tissue and skin and immobilize the arm in a well-padded cast with the elbow maximally, but not forcefully, extended and the forearm fully supinated. Bivalve the cast.

POSTOPERATIVE CARE The arm is elevated for 48 hours, and finger motion is encouraged. At 5 days, flexion and extension exercises out of the cast are begun. For 6 weeks after surgery, the arm is replaced in the cast when the exercise period has been completed. Nighttime splinting is continued for 6 months. Maximal elbow extension usually is obtained 3 to 5 months postoperatively.

■ FOREARM, WRIST, AND HAND

Deformities of the forearm, wrist, and hand are described in other chapter in the discussion of the hand in patients with cerebral palsy.

ADULTS WITH CEREBRAL PALSY

Because of the tremendous advances in the care given to patients with cerebral palsy, a generation of children who in the past would have been institutionalized now have been integrated into the family and society. These advances have been relatively recent, and more is becoming known about adults with cerebral palsy and the long-term outcomes of treatment. Population-based studies have shown that adults with cerebral palsy can live independently and maintain a high level of function. Long-term outcome studies of adults with cerebral palsy have found that for individuals who are mobile as young adults there is a marked decline in ambulation with age, with fatigue and falls having a negative impact on quality of life. Approximately 25% of ambulatory adults with cerebral palsy will experience a gait decline sooner than their nondisabled peers, especially older patients with bilateral motor impairment, with more frequent use of assistive devices and higher levels of pain and/or fatigue. The exact cause of this decline is unknown but likely is multifactorial. Skills such as feeding, speech, and ability to order meals in public are well preserved. In one long-term study, 18% of 60-year-olds lived independently and 41% resided in facilities providing higher-level medical care. Long-term survival rates were moderately worse than the general population, especially in nonambulatory patients. In a review of 819 adults with cerebral palsy, 33% of patients (77% controls) had education beyond secondary school, 29% (82% controls) were competitively employed, and 5% had specially created jobs. Social outcome studies have found a higher rate

of unemployment in patients with other comorbidities, such as seizures, self-care limitations, and cognitive and communication impairments, with no substantial impact of severity of motor involvement on employment rate. Although more likely to be single and living with parents, 14% to 28% of patients with cerebral palsy without intellectual impairment were in a long-term partnership or had established their own families.

Many patients with cerebral palsy return for orthopaedic care in their thirties and forties when compensatory mechanisms they have relied on in the past begin to fail. This transition from care in the pediatric setting to the adult setting can be challenging for patients and physicians because of a lack of communication between the two systems, fear of the new system, and different treatment styles for adults and children. Common orthopaedic problems for adults with cerebral palsy include fatigue, knee instability that arises from long-standing ankle equinus, degenerative hip disease, flatfoot deformity, and scoliosis. Osteopenia also is frequently present in adults with cerebral palsy, which can predispose them to fractures. A patient-centered approach, just as with children, should be used in treating an adult with cerebral palsy. Not all deformities require treatment, and attention should be focused on the deformities that cause pain or interfere with independent function.

ADULT STROKE PATIENTS

Considerable literature exists regarding the orthopaedic evaluation and treatment of patients who have had cerebrovascular accidents, especially with the incidence of cerebrovascular accidents and the survival rate increasing. The development a multidisciplinary team approach incorporating early physical and occupational therapy, bracing, standing, use of BTX-A, and the gait analysis has led to marked improvement in the treatment of adult stroke patients. Randomized clinical trials have shown benefits of BTX-A in post-stroke hemiparesis patients by improving walking speed and likelihood of achieving community ambulation. BTX-A use continues to be explored to improve functionality of both upper and lower extremities after stroke in adult patients.

LOWER EXTREMITY

Of patients who have had a stroke, 65% to 75% recover enough function in their lower extremities to permit ambulation. This is because the lower extremity does not depend as much on sensation for its function as does the upper extremity and the activities necessary for walking are gross motor functions that are enhanced by primitive postural reflexes. Most patients with residual hemiparesis require the use of an external support and a brace to ambulate independently.

Orthotic positioning and range-of-motion exercises of the lower extremity begin in the early phases of recovery when the primary goal is prevention of fixed contractures. This treatment extends through the period of motor recovery and gait training to the time when the neurologic deficit becomes stationary and a definitive brace to aid in ambulation is required. In the early phase, the paralysis usually is flaccid and deformities occur as a result of poor positioning. Passive range-of-motion exercises help prevent undesirable patterning of movements, which often occurs in the recovery phase. Equinus deformity should be prevented by appropriate splinting and frequent range-of-motion exercises. Preventing deformity of the lower extremity is greatly assisted by having the patient stand and walk as soon as his or her medical condition permits. The use of BTX-A has become more common and has been shown to improve range of motion, lower extremity function, and ability to perform activities of daily living. Electrical stimulation can be used to help maintain strength and keep joints mobilized, and as a sensorimotor educational tool to increase the awareness of the sensation of muscle contractions, especially in the anterior tibial and peroneal muscles. In the early phase, this can be done with cutaneous stimulation; later in recovery, electrodes can be placed directly on a motor nerve with stimulation controlled through an externally placed transmitter. Various pharmacologic agents have been used in the treatment of spasticity, including baclofen, oral muscle relaxants, anticonvulsants, and cannabis, with limited success because of the variable nature of stroke patients, side effects, and the fact that these are systemic treatments for targeted dysfunctional muscle groups.

Motor recovery occurs during the first 3 to 4 months, and the quality of gait can change dramatically during that time. To become a functional ambulator, the patient must obtain adequate spontaneous improvement to allow voluntary control of the hip and knee. Bracing may be necessary to help achieve this goal; however, many of the braces used to stabilize the knee can be difficult to apply and manage and can negatively affect the ability to ambulate. When maximal motor recovery has been obtained and the gait function has stabilized, definitive bracing can be done.

Neurophysiologic studies have shown that there are seven neurologic sources of motion, two of which are sophisticated components of normal function (selective control and habitual control) and five are primitive forms of control. These primitive forms, which are present and suppressed in the normal state, become expressed as overt sources of motion (locomotor pattern, verticality, limb synergy, fast stretch, slow stretch) following a stroke.

Selected control is the normal ability to move one joint independently of another, to contract an isolated muscle, or to select a desired combination of motions. *Habitual control* is the normal automatic performance of a learned skill, such as walking.

Primitive *locomotor patterns* are mass movements of flexion and extension. The patient can initiate or terminate the movements but cannot otherwise modify them. If the knee is extended, the ankle also is automatically plantar flexed and the hip is extended. The opposite movements occur in knee flexion. This voluntary motion is preserved after a loss of cortical control and presumably is controlled by the midbrain. *Control of verticality* is a vestibular function and is an antigravity mechanism. When the body is erect, the extensor muscles have more tone than when the body is supine; additionally, standing creates a more intense stimulus than does sitting. In the upper extremity, the flexor muscles respond in this manner. Primitive *limb synergy* is the result of a multisegmental spinal cord reflex, tying the action of the extensor muscles to the posture of the limb. When the knee is extended, the tone of the soleus and the gastrocnemius is greatly increased, making both muscles much more sensitive to stretch than when the knee is flexed. Similarly, the tone in the antagonistic muscles may be inhibited. This activity confuses the results in the Silfverskiöld test used to differentiate contracture of the gastrocnemius from that of the soleus. The *fast stretch reflex,* characterized by the familiar clonic

response, is caused by an intermittent burst of muscle activity. It is initiated by the velocity sensors in the muscle spindles. The *slow stretch reflex* is characterized by rigidity, a clinical term for continuous muscle reaction to stretch and often misinterpreted as contracture. This reflex disappears under anesthesia when length-change sensors in the muscle spindles are inactive. Primitive locomotor patterns and control of verticality, and stretch reflex activity, are especially troublesome to stroke patients.

In addition to motor problems, stroke patients frequently have impaired sensation. Impaired proprioception is especially important because it causes a delay or hesitancy in making a voluntary motor response. The duration of this delay indicates the time it takes to process the central nervous signals, and if the delay is too great, walking may not be a reasonable goal.

Gait analysis and various standing tests, including double limb support, hemiparetic single limb stance, and hemiparetic limb flexion, are useful in determining whether or not the patient can walk and if orthopaedic surgery is necessary.

Surgery should be deferred until at least 6 months after the stroke. Most patients make a rapid spontaneous recovery during the first 6 to 8 weeks. They subsequently strengthen these gains and learn to live with their disability. Progress in control of the limb occurs, and this typically is the result of extensive therapy. Patients with better early functional scores maintain better function at 6 months than those with lower scores. By 6 to 9 months after a stroke, patients have obtained maximal spontaneous improvement and must come to realize the permanence of their residual deficits. Surgical intervention, which usually is soft-tissue release, is indicated if it is likely to improve function or hygiene or decrease pain, and occasionally, improve cosmesis. The goals of surgery must be clearly explained to prevent unrealistic expectations. Although improvement in a single deficit may be expected, restoration of normal function in the extremity is almost impossible.

HIP

Scissoring gait secondary to adductor spasticity can be corrected by soft-tissue release. To determine whether or not the hip adductors are necessary for hip flexion in a patient, a diagnostic block of the obturator nerve before surgery is performed. If the effect of the nerve block is prolonged, it can be repeated once or twice, and occasionally the results are permanent.

Surgical release of a hip flexion contracture rarely is indicated in stroke patients because the decrease in hip flexion power may make the patient unable to walk. When gait EMG shows continuous activity of the hip flexors and medial hamstrings, releasing the iliopsoas and adductor longus and medial hamstring transfer to the femur sometimes allow the limb to assume an upright position.

KNEE

Flexion contractures of the knee can be treated operatively if the patient has adequate power in the gluteus maximus and quadriceps muscles to extend the hip when the hamstrings are lengthened. One study reported that 43% of 30 patients obtained ambulation ability after hamstring release, and 17% gained the ability to transfer. Caution was recommended in patients with severe peripheral vascular disease because of an increased risk of complications as a result of poor wound healing and risk of neurovascular injury.

Stiff knee gait, caused by increased activity of the rectus femoris during the swing phase of gait, can cause difficulties with foot clearance for stroke patients. A meta-analysis of the effect of chemodenervation of the rectus femoris on stiff knee gait showed that it does lead to improved peak knee flexion during swing phase. Release of the rectus femoris from the patella by excision of its distal segment can improve knee flexion by 15 to 20 degrees.

FOOT

Talipes equinovarus is the most common foot deformity in a stroke patient. Other deformities can occur, such as equinus without varus, varus of the forefoot, footdrop, planovalgus foot, and in-curling of the toes. Early physical therapy, use of ankle foot orthoses, and BTX-A have been shown to be effective in preventing equinus deformity and improving gait function in some patients.

▥ TALIPES EQUINUS

The goal of surgery is to correct talipes equinus in the mid-swing and midstance phases while preserving heel lift support in the terminal stance phase and accepting a flat-footed contact with the floor. This goal can be accomplished with a closed subcutaneous triple hemisection of the Achilles tendon. The distal cut is made medially, proximal to the insertion of the tendon; the next is made 2.5 cm proximal to the first through the lateral half of the tendon; and the final one is made 2.5 cm proximal to the second through the medial half of the tendon. After surgery, the foot is immobilized in a cast in a slight equinus position so that walking does not overstretch the tendon. Patients can bear weight on the cast for 4 weeks before cast removal.

▥ TALIPES EQUINOVARUS

Talipes equinovarus is common in stroke patients because of weakness in the foot dorsiflexors and evertors or spasticity of their antagonists. The goal of surgery is either to provide a plantigrade foot that can be braced in a nonambulatory patient or to rid an ambulator of braces. In the presence of moderate action of the anterior tibial muscle without the assistance of the toe extensors, the equinus deformity is corrected by rebalancing the foot to eliminate the varus deformity. The anterior and posterior tibial, soleus, flexor hallucis longus, and flexor digitorum longus, despite their swing phase and stance phase action, can be active well into the other phase and often are active continuously. They also can be inactive. A varus deformity in either swing or stance phase can be caused by any one or a combination of these muscles being abnormal, in contrast to varus deformity in patients with cerebral palsy. The posterior tibial muscle-tendon unit rarely is the deforming force in a stroke patient.

CORRECTION OF TALIPES EQUINOVARUS

Soft-tissue releases and tendon transfers can be used in adults to help balance the muscle forces across the foot. Historically, this has been done by transferring three fourths of the anterior tibial tendon to the third cuneiform, the flexor

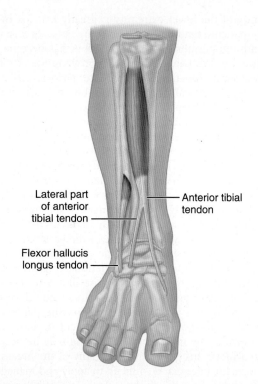

Lateral part of anterior tibial tendon

Anterior tibial tendon

Flexor hallucis longus tendon

FIGURE **5.40** Technique of Perry et al. to correct equinovarus deformity in stroke patients. Lateral three fourths of anterior tibial tendon and flexor hallucis longus tendon are transferred to third cuneiform. Flexor digitorum longus is released (see text).

hallucis longus tendon to the same area, with the flexor digitorum longus tendon released and the posterior tibial tendon undisturbed (Fig. 5.40). Significant improvement in patient autonomy, ability to ambulate independently, and increased ability to wear normal shoes have been reported after this procedure. Similar results have been reported with the use of a split anterior tendon transfer alone in 132 feet in which improvements were made in walking distance and shoewear.

TECHNIQUE 5.21

- Make a 2-cm incision on the medial border of the foot over the navicular.
- Identify and expose the insertion of the anterior tibial tendon.
- Separate and detach the lateral three fourths of the tendon from the medial one fourth.
- Bring the detached part out through an incision made 2 cm proximal to the ankle and route it subcutaneously to the dorsal surface of the third cuneiform.
- Expose the cuneiform, drill converging holes in the bone, and use a curet to construct a tunnel. Loop the free part of the tendon through this tunnel to be anchored later.
- Through a separate 4-cm incision in the arch of the foot, use electrocautery to release the plantar flexors of the toes.
- Through a posterior incision at the level of the ankle, identify the flexor hallucis longus tendon at its tunnel, detach it, and pass it anteriorly through a large window made in the interosseous membrane.

- Insert this tendon through the tunnel in the third cuneiform opposite to the direction of the anterior tibial tendon.
- Lengthen the Achilles tendon as described in Technique 5.11.
- With the ankle in the neutral position and the foot slightly everted, sew the two tendons to themselves as loops and to each other.
- The flexor digitorum longus can be transferred instead of the flexor hallucis longus if the toe flexors are active in the swing phase of gait.

POSTOPERATIVE CARE Because the Achilles tendon has been lengthened, a cast is applied with the foot in slight plantar flexion. At 6 weeks, the cast is removed and the foot is protected with a locked ankle brace for an additional 6 months. Because the muscles in a hemiplegic patient pull strongly or not at all, several months are necessary for the scar to mature enough not to yield under tension.

Satisfactory results have been reported in adult hemiplegics with talipes equinovarus using a procedure that consists of triple sectioning of the Achilles tendon, open Z-plasty lengthening and suturing of the posterior tibial tendon just proximal to the medial malleolus, transfer of one half of the anterior tibial tendon to the third cuneiform, and transverse division of the flexor digitorum brevis and the flexor digitorum longus tendons at the base of each toe.

■ VARUS FOOT

The anterior tibial muscle usually is the deforming force in a patient with forefoot varus. A split anterior tibial tendon transfer (see Technique 5.15) is the procedure of choice for this condition as long as a fixed hindfoot varus is not present. A short leg walking cast is worn for 6 weeks. An ankle-foot orthosis is used when walking to protect the muscle transfer for an additional 6 months.

■ PLANOVALGUS

If pes planus preceded the stroke, in rare cases a planovalgus deformity can occur after the stroke. Spasticity of the triceps surae pulls the calcaneus laterally, and the peroneals may be hyperactive with no opposing posterior tibial muscle function during stance phase. If walking is impeded by pain, surgical correction is indicated. As in equinus deformity, the treatment involves lengthening of the Achilles tendon with a triple-level hemitenotomy. The distal hemisection in the Achilles tendon is performed in the lateral half of the tendon to reduce the valgus placement or thrust of the tendon on the calcaneus.

If the peroneals are hyperactive during stance phase, the peroneus brevis can be transferred medially into the posterior tibial tendon to support the medial border of the foot or the peroneus longus and brevis can be lengthened. A triple arthrodesis ultimately is required if an ankle-foot orthosis does not control the deformity.

■ TOE FLEXION

Toe flexion occurs at the metatarsophalangeal joint and is different from the claw toe deformity in most neurologic disorders in which the extensors are hyperactive. Toe curling or toe flexion in a stroke patient occurs from overactivity of the long toe flexors. These can be released by tenotomies of the toe flexor tendons at the level of the metatarsophalangeal joint.

UPPER EXTREMITY

The prognosis for recovering normal function in the upper extremity in stroke patients is poor, and approximately one third are left with a permanently functionless limb. The most important reason for this is that the patterns of neuromuscular activity in the normally functioning upper extremity are highly sophisticated and complex and are modified by multiple sophisticated somatosensory impulses. Permanent impairment in motor and sensory function in the upper extremity is incurable, and permanent impairment of function is to be expected. Upper limb recovery after stroke is adaptive and consists of training the individual to accomplish activities of daily living as a one-handed person. For patients who show sufficient neurologic recovery, additional training for development of assistive function is indicated.

The orthopaedic surgeon may release contractures, weaken spastic muscles that cause imbalance and deformity, and transfer functioning muscle units to attempt to restore some balance to the affected extremity. These operations also can relieve persistent pain, which causes further immobility and lack of participation in other areas of rehabilitation.

■ SHOULDER

Some stroke patients report pain localized precisely to the shoulder and specifically to the adductor and internal rotator groups. In others, a hemicorporeal type of diffuse discomfort is present and is untreatable by present methods. Patients with the first type of pain develop progressively decreasing ranges of motion despite intensive conservative treatment. They also have an exaggerated stretch reflex on rapid external rotation of the shoulder, abduction of less than 45 degrees, and internal rotation of less than 15 degrees. Modalities such as suprascapular nerve blocks, joint injection, use of BTX-A, and therapy/taping programs are of minimal benefit. Surgery is recommended only for patients who have a reasonable potential for rehabilitation. A review of 34 adults with spastic hemiparesis who had fractional lengthening of the pectoralis major, latissimus dorsi, and teres major had improvements in their spasticity scores, shoulder range of motion, especially external rotation, as well as pain relief and a high degree of satisfaction with the outcome.

RELEASE OF INTERNAL ROTATION CONTRACTURE OF THE SHOULDER

In a comparison study, patients who had internal rotation contracture release showed significant improvement in motion in 10 of 13 patients. Of 12 control patients with similar symptoms not treated by surgery, none had a spontaneous resolution of the painful joint contracture.

TECHNIQUE 5.22

- Make an anterior deltopectoral approach to the shoulder.
- Identify the subscapularis tendon and cauterize the vascular bundle at its distal edge. Excise this tendon, but preserve the anterior capsule of the shoulder joint.
- Palpate the tendon of the pectoralis major and, with scissors passed distally along the humerus, cut its tendinous insertion.

POSTOPERATIVE CARE A sling is worn on the arm, and a program of assisted range-of-motion exercises is begun within the first few days of surgery. Reciprocal pulley exercises are begun within the first 5 days. It is important to supervise the patient's participation in the exercises.

FRACTIONAL LENGTHENING OF PECTORALIS MAJOR, LATISSIMUS DORSI, TERES MAJOR

TECHNIQUE 5.23

- With the patient in the beach chair position with a bolster between the scapula, make a deltopectoral approach (see Technique 1.87) to expose the pectoralis major tendon.
- Divide the tendon as it overlaps the muscle belly on the undersurface.
- Identify the brachial plexus and retract it medially.
- Identify the insertions of the latissimus dorsi and teres major in the interval between the short head of the biceps and the deltoid.
- Lengthen the tendons at the musculotendinous junction.
- The long head of the triceps can be lengthened if further correction of elbow extension is desired.
- Place a drain and close in layers.

POSTOPERATIVE CARE A sling is worn on the arm for comfort, and a program of assisted range-of-motion exercises is begun within the first few days of surgery.

▓ ELBOW

Fixed flexion of the elbow seriously impairs function of the upper extremity. Some patients with mild spasticity may benefit from the early use of BTX-A in conjunction with physical therapy. For those who do not respond to nonoperative measures and who have reasonable functional goals, surgical release of the elbow can be considered. A review of 42 patients with elbow flexion deformities showed improvements in active and passive range of motion with a low rate of superficial wound problems at a mean of 6 years after anterior release and fractional myotendinous elbow flexor lengthening.

▌ PHENOL NERVE BLOCK

Phenol injection into motor nerves in adults and children with spastic hemiplegia produced early improvement in 17 of 18 patients. Unfortunately, the results deteriorated over 6 months, with 2 patients having recurrence of the deformity within 1 year. The 6-month window allows time to begin treatment programs aimed at decreasing contractures and to train weakened muscles before the spasticity returns. In addition, patients who receive nerve ablation can have sensory loss that can lead to painful dysesthesia. For these reasons, as well as the reversible nature of BTX-A, the use of phenol nerve block is decreasing.

▌ FUNCTIONAL ELECTRICAL NERVE STIMULATION

Functional electrical stimulation allows restoration of function in paralyzed muscles by electrical stimulation. The aim is to have functional muscle control occur during stimulation, but occasionally a carryover occurs, and the muscle comes under voluntary control. Functional electrical stimulation theoretically depends on a single stimulation, such as heel lift, being transferred through an antenna to an electrical implant, which fires another signal to the nerve supply to the muscles, such as the peroneal nerve, to perform a function, such as dorsiflexion to the foot. The device needs to be small and cosmetically acceptable, and the activity should be under some degree of voluntary control; otherwise too much stimulation may occur. Functional electrical stimulation is used in the upper and lower extremities, around the foot and ankle to suppress spasticity, to correct scoliosis, for electrophrenic respiration, and for bladder control. There remains a need for external control of motor unit gradation, for synergistic activity in other muscles, and for some proprioceptive kinesthetic feedback.

REFERENCES

GENERAL

Akerstedt A, Risto O, Odman P, et al.: Evaluation of single event multilevel surgery and rehabilitation in children and youth with cerebral palsy—a 2-year follow-up study, *Disabil Rehabil* 32:530, 2010.

Akpinar P, Tezel CG, Eliasson AC, et al.: Reliability and cross-cultural validation of the Turkish version of Manual Ability Classification System (MACS) for children with cerebral palsy, *Disabil Rehabil* 32:1910, 2010.

Brandenburg JE, Fogarty MJ, Sieck GC: A critical evaluation of current concepts in cerebral palsy, *Physiology (Bethesda)* 34:216, 2019.

Gannotti ME, Gorton 3rd GE, Nahorniak MT, et al.: Walking abilities of young adults with cerebral palsy: changes after multilevel surgery and adolescence, *Gait Posture* 32:46, 2010.

Imms C, Carlin J, Eliasson AC: Stability of caregiver-reported manual ability and gross motor function classifications of cerebral palsy, *Dev Med Child Neurol* 52:153, 2010.

Minhas SV, Chow I, Otsuka NY: The effect of body mass index on postoperative morbidity after orthopaedic surgery in children with cerebral palsy, *J Pediatr Orthop* 36:505, 2016.

Park MS, Chung CY, Lee KM, et al.: Issues of concern before single event multilevel surgery in patients with cerebral palsy, *J Pediatr Orthop* 30:489, 2010.

Svehlik M, Steinwender G, Kraus T, et al.: The influence of age at single-event multilevel surgery on outcome in children with cerebral palsy who walk with flexed knee gait, *Dev Med Child Neurol* 53:730, 2011.

te Velde A, Morgan C, Novak I, et al.: Early diagnosis and classification of cerebral palsy: an historical perspective and barriers to an early diagnosis, *J Clin Med* 8(ppi):E1599, 2019.

Thompson N, Stebbins J, Seniorou M, et al.: The use of minimally invasive techniques in multi-level surgery for children with cerebral palsy: preliminary results, *J Bone Joint Surg* 92B:1442, 2010.

Westbomb L, Bergsrand L, Wagner P, et al.: Survival at 19 years of age in a total population of children and young people with cerebral palsy, *Dev Med Child Neurol* 53:808, 2011.

NEUROSURGICAL TREATMENT

Blumetti FC, Belloti JC, Tamaoki MJ, et al.: Botulinum toxin type A in the treatment of lower limb spasticity in children with cerebral palsy, *Cochrane Database Syst Rev*, 2019, [Epub ahead of print].

Carraro E, Zeme S, Ticcinelli V, et al.: Multidimensional outcome measure of selective dorsal rhizotomy in spastic cerebral palsy, *Eur J Paediatr Neurol* 18:704, 2014.

D'Aquino D, Moussa AA, Ammar A, et al.: Selective dorsal rhizotomy for the treatment of severe spastic cerebral palsy: efficacy and therapeutic durability in GMFCS grade IV and V children, *Acta Neurochir (Wien)* 160:811, 2018.

Dudley RW, Parolin M, Gagnon B, et al.: Long-term functional benefits of selective dorsal rhizotomy for spastic cerebral palsy, *J Neurosurg Pediatr* 12:142, 2013.

Grunt S, Fieggen AG, Vermeulen RJ, et al.: Selection criteria for selective dorsal rhizotomy in children with spastic cerebral palsy: a systematic review of the literature, *Dev Med Child Neurol* 56:302, 2014.

Hurvitz EA, Marciniak CM, Daunter AK, et al.: Functional outcomes of childhood dorsal rhizotomy in adults and adolescents with cerebral palsy, *J Neurosurg Pediatr* 11:380, 2013.

Jeffrey SMT, Markia B, Pople IK, et al.: Surgical outcomes of single-level bilateral selective dorsal rhizotomy for spastic diplegia in 150 consecutive patients, *World Neurosurg* 125:e60, 2019.

Park TS, Dobbs MB, Cho J: Evidence supporting selective dorsal rhizotomy for treatment of spastic cerebral palsy, *Cureus* 10:e3466, 2018.

Tedroff K, Löwing K, Jacobson DN, et al.: Does loss of spasticity matter? A 10-year follow-up after selective dorsal rhizotomy in cerebral palsy, *Dev Med Child Neurol* 53:724, 2011.

HIP

Bayusentono S, Choi Y, Chung CY, et al.: Recurrence of hip instability after reconstructive surgery in patients with cerebral palsy, *J Bone Joint Surg* 96:1527, 2014.

Boldingh EJ, Bouwhuis CB, van der Heijden-Maessen HC, et al.: Palliative hip surgery in severe cerebral palsy: a systematic review, *J Pediatr Orthop B* 23:86, 2014.

Braatz F, Staude D, Klotz MC, et al.: Hip-joint congruity after Dega osteotomy in patients with cerebral palsy: long-term results, *Int Orthop* 40:1663, 2016.

Chan P, Hsu A, Godfrey J, et al.: Outcomes of salvage hip surgery in children with cerebral palsy, *J Pediatr Orthop B* 28:314, 2019.

Chang CH, Chen YY, Wang CJ, et al.: Dynamic displacement of the femoral head by hamstring stretching in children with cerebral palsy, *J Pediatr Orthop* 30:475, 2010.

Chang FM, Ma J, Pan Z, et al.: Acetabular remodeling after a varus derotational osteotomy in children with cerebral palsy, *J Pediatr Orthop* 36(2):198–204, 2016.

Cobanoglu M, Cullu E, Omurlu I: The effect of hip reconstruction on gross motor function levels in children with cerebral palsy, *Acat Orthop Traumatol Turc* 52:44, 2018.

Cottrill EJ, Johnson DC, Silberstein CE: A single-center retrospective review of factors influencing success in patients with cerebral palsy undergoing corrective hip surgery, *J Pediatr Rehabil Med* 12:263, 2019.

Dartnell J, Gough M, Paterson JM, et al.: Proximal femoral resection without post-operative traction for the painful dislocated hip in patients with cerebral palsy: a review of 79 cases, *Bone Joint J* 96B:701, 2014.

DiFazio R, Vessey JA, Miller P, et al.: Postoperative complications after hip surgery in patients with cerebral palsy: a retrospective matched cohort study, *J Pediatr Orthop* 36:56, 2016.

El Hage S, Rachkidi R, Noun Z, et al.: Is percutaneous adductor tenotomy as effective and safe as the open procedure, *J Pediatr Orthop* 30:485, 2010.

Fucs PM, Yamada HH: Hip fusion as hip salvage procedure in cerebral palsy, *J Pediatr Orthop* 34(Suppl 1):S32, 2014.

Hachache B, Eid T, Ghosn E, et al.: Is percutaneous proximal gracilis tenotomy as effective and safe as the open procedure? *J Child Orthop* 9(6):477–481, 2015.

Hägglund G, Alriksson-Schmidt A, Lauge-Pedersen H, et al.: Prevention of dislocation of the hip in children with cerebral palsy: 20-year results of a population-based prevention programme, *Bone Joint J* 96B:1546, 2014.

Hermanson M, Hägglund G, Riad J, et al.: Head-shaft angle is a risk factor for hip displacement in children with cerebral palsy, *Acta Orthop* 86:229, 2015.

Hsieh HC, Wang TM, Kuo KN, et al.: Guided growth improves coxa valga and hip subluxation in children with cerebral palsy, *Clin Orthop Relat Res* 477:2568, 2019.

Huh K, Rethlefsen SA, Wren TA, Kay RM: Surgical management of hip subluxation and dislocation in children with cerebral palsy: isolated VDRO or combined surgery? *J Pediatr Orthop* 31:858, 2011.

Khalife R, Ghanem I, El Hage S, et al.: Risk of recurrent dislocation and avascular necrosis after proximal femoral varus osteotomy in children with cerebral palsy, *J Pediatr Orthop* 19:32, 2010.

Koi PS, Jameson 2nd PG, Chang TL, et al.: Transverse-plane pelvic asymmetry in patients with cerebral palsy and scoliosis, *J Pediatr Orthop* 31:277, 2011.

Lanert P, Risto O, Hägglund G, et al.: Hip displacement in relation to age and gross motor function in children with cerebral palsy, *J Child Orthop* 8:129, 2014.

Miller SD, Shore BJ, Mulpuri K: Hip surveillance is important to children with cerebral palsy: stop waiting, start now, *J Am Acad Orthop Surg Glob Res Rev* 3:e021, 2019.

Portinaro N, Turati M, Cometto M, et al.: Guided growth of the proximal femur for the management of hip dysplasia in children with cerebral palsy, *J Pediatr Orthop* 39:e622, 2019.

Pruszczynaki B, Sees J, Miller F: Risk factors for hip displacement in children with cerebral palsy: systematic review, *Pediatr Orthop* 36:829, 2016.

Raphael BS, Dines JS, Akerman M, et al.: Long-term followup of total hip arthroplasty in patients with cerebral palsy, *Clin Orthop Relat Res* 468:1845, 2010.

Riccio AI, Carney CD, Hammell LC, et al.: Three-dimensional computed tomography for determination of femoral anteversion in a cerebral palsy model, *J Pediatr Orthop* 35:167, 2015.

Rutz E, Gaston MS, Tirosh O, et al.: Hip flexion deformity improves without psoas-lengthening after surgical correction of fixed knee flexion deformity in spastic diplegia, *Hip Int* 22:379, 2012.

Rutz E, Vavken P, Camathias C, et al.: Long-term results and outcome predictors in one-stage hip reconstruction in children with cerebral palsy, *J Bone Joint Surg* 97:500, 2015.

Ruzbarsky JJ, Beck NA, Baldwin KD, et al.: Risk factors and complications in hip reconstruction for nonambulatory patients with cerebral palsy, *J Child Orthop* 7:487, 2013.

Shaw KA, Hire JM, Cearley DM: Salvage treatment options for painful hip dislocations in nonambulatory cerebral palsy patients, *J Am Acad Orthop Surg*, 2019, [Epub ahead of print].

Shore B, Spence D, Graham H: The role for hip surveillance in children with cerebral palsy, *Curr Rev Musculoskelet Med* 5:126, 2012.

Shore BJ, Yu X, Desai S, et al.: Adductor surgery to prevent hip displacement in children with cerebral palsy: the predictive role of the Gross Motor Function Classification System, *J Bone Joint Surg Am* 94:326, 2012.

Shrader MW, Wimberly L, Thompson R: Hip surveillance in children with cerebral palsy, *J Am Acad Orthop Surg* 27:760, 2019.

Terjesen T: Femoral and pelvic osteotomies for severe hip displacement in nonambulatory children with cerebral palsy: a prospective population-based study of 31 patients with 7 years' follow-up, *Acta Orthop* 90:614, 2019.

Zhang S, Wilson NC, Mackey AH, et al.: Radiological outcome of reconstructive hip surgery in children with gross motor function classification system IV and V cerebral palsy, *J Pediatr Orthop B* 23:430, 2014.

KNEE

Al-Aubaidi Z, Lundgaard B, Pedersen NW: Anterior distal femoral hemiepiphysiodesis in the treatment of fixed knee flexion contracture in neuromuscular patients, *J Child Orthop* 6:313, 2012.

Blumetti FC, Morais Filho MC, Kawamura CM, et al.: Does the GMFCS level influence the improvement in knee range of motion after rectus femoris transfer in cerebral palsy? *J Pediatr Orthop B* 24:433, 2015.

Brunner R, Camathias C, Gaston M, et al.: Supracondylar osteotomy of the paediatric femur using the locking compression plate: a refined surgical technique, *J Child Orthop* 7:571, 2013.

Choi Y, Lee SH, Chung CY, et al.: Anterior knee pain in patients with cerebral palsy, *Clin Orthop Surg* 6:426, 2014.

Inan M, Sarikaya IA, Yildirim E, et al.: Neurological complications after supracondylar femoral osteotomy in cerebral palsy, *J Pediatr Orthop* 35:290, 2015.

Lee SY, Kwon SS, Chung CY, et al.: Rectus femoris transfer in cerebral palsy patients with stiff knee gait, *Gait Posture* 40:76, 2014.

McMulkin ML, Gordon AB, Caskey PM, et al.: Outcomes of orthopaedic surgery with and without an external femoral derotational osteotomy in children with cerebral palsy, *J Pediatr Orthop* 36:382, 2016.

O'Sullivan R, Leonard J, Quinn A, et al.: The short-term effects of selective dorsal rhizotomy on gait compared to matched cerebral palsy control groups, *PLoS One* 14:e0220119, 2019.

Patthanacharoenphon C, Maples DL, Saad C, et al.: The effects of patellar tendon advancement on the immature proximal tibia, *J Child Orthop* 7:139, 2013.

Rethlefsen SA, Nguyen DT, Wren TA, et al.: Knee pain and patellofemoral symptoms in patients with cerebral palsy, *J Pediatr Orthop* 35:519, 2015.

Rethlefsen SA, Yasmeh S, Wren TA, et al.: Repeat hamstring lengthening for crouch gait in children with cerebral palsy, *J Pediat Orthop* 33:501, 2013.

Scully WF, McMulkin ML, Baird GO, et al.: Outcomes of rectus femoris transfer in children with cerebral palsy: effect of transfer site, *J Pediatr Orthop* 33:303, 2013.

Skiak E, Karakasli A, Basci O, et al.: Distal femoral derotational osteotomy with external fixation for correction of excessive femoral anteversion in patients with cerebral palsy, *J Pediatr Orthop B* 24:425, 2015.

Sousa TC, Nazareth A, Rethlefsen SA, et al.: Rectus femoris transfer surgery worsens crouch gait in children with cerebral palsy at GMFCS levels III and IV, *J Pediatr Orthop* 39:466, 2019.

Stiel N, Babin K, Bettorazzi E, et al.: Anterior distal femoral hemiepiphysiodesis can reduce fixed flexion deformity of the knee: a retrospective study of 83 knees, *Acta Orthop* 89:555, 2018.

FOOT AND ANKLE

Aleksic M, Bascarevic Z, Stevanovic V, et al.: Modified split tendon transfer of posterior tibialis muscle in the treatment of spastic equinovarus foot deformity: long-term results and comparison with the standard procedure, *Int Orthop* 44:155, 2020.

Boffeli TJ, Collier RC: Surgical treatment guidelines for digital deformity associated with intrinsic muscle spasticity (intrinsic plus foot) in adults with cerebral palsy, *J Foot Ankle Surg* 54:985, 2015.

Costici PF, Donati F, Russo R, et al.: Double hindfoot arthrodesis technique for the treatment of severe equino-plano-valgus foot deformity in cerebral palsy: long-term results and radiological evaluation, *J Pediatr Orthop B* 28:235, 2019.

Danino B, Erel S, Kfir M, et al.: Are gait indices sensitive enough to reflect the effect of ankle foot orthosis on gait impairment in cerebral palsy diplegic patients? *J Pediatr Orthop* 36:294, 2016.

Firouzeh P, Sonnenberg LK, Morris C, et al.: Ankle foot orthoses for young children with cerebral palsy: a scoping review, *Disabil Rehabil*, 2019, [Epub ahead of print].

Firth GB, McMullan M, Chin T, et al.: Lengthening of the gastrocnemius-soleus complex: an anatomical and biomechanical study in human cadavers, *J Bone Joint Surg* 95:1489, 2013.

Firth BG, Passmore E, Sangeux M, et al.: Multilevel surgery for equinus gait in children with spastic diplegic cerebral palsy. Medium-term follow-up with gait analysis, *J Bone Joint Surg* 95:931, 2013.

Houx L, Lempereur M, Rémy-Néris O, et al.: Threshold of equinus which alters biomechanical gait parameters in children, *Gait Posture* 38:582, 2013.

Huang CN, Wu KW, Hunag SC, et al.: Medial column stabilization improves the early result of calcaneal lengthening in children with cerebral palsy, *J Pediatr Orthop B* 22:233, 2013.

Jaddue DA, Abbas MA, Sayed-Noor AS: Open versus percutaneous tendo-achilles lengthening in spastic cerebral palsy with equinus deformity of the foot in children, *J Surg Orthop Adv* 19:196, 2010.

Kadhim M, Holmes Jr L, Church C, et al.: Pes planovalgus deformity surgical correction in ambulatory children with cerebral palsy, *J Child Orthop* 6:217, 2012.

Kadhim M, Holmes Jr L, Miller F: Long-term ourcome of planovalgus foot surgical correction in children with cerebral palsy, *J Foot Ankle Surg* 52:697, 2013.

Kadhim M, Miller F: Crouch gait changes after planovalgus foot deformity correction in ambulatory children with cerebral palsy, *Gait Posture* 39:793, 2014.

Kadhim M, Miller F: Pes planovalgus deformity in children with cerebral palsy: review article, *J Pediatr Orthop B* 23:400, 2014.

Lee IH, Chung CY, Lee KM, et al.: Incidence and risk factors of allograft bone failure after calcaneal lengthening, *Clin Orthop Relat Res* 473:1765, 2015.

Nahm NJ, Sohrweide SS, Wervey RA, et al.: Surgical treatment of pes planovalgus in ambulatory children with cerebral palsy: static and dynamic changes as characterized by multi-segment foot modeling, physical examination, and radiographs, *Gait Posture*, 2019, [Epub ahead of print].

Ries AJ, Novacheck TF, Schwartz MH: The efficacy of ankle-foot orthoses on improving the gait of children with diplegic cerebral palsy: a multiple outcome analysis, *PM R* 7:922, 2015.

Shore BJ, Smith KR, Riazi A, et al.: Subtalar fusion for pes valgus in cerebral palsy: results of a modified technique in the setting of single event multilevel surgery, *J Pediatr Orthop* 33:431, 2013.

Shore BJ, White N, Kerr Graham H: Surgical correction of equinus deformity in children with cerebral palsy: a systematic review, *J Child Orthop* 4:277, 2010.

Trehan SK, Ihekweazu UN, Root L: Long-term outcomes of triple arthrodesis in cerebral palsy patients, *J Pediatr Orthop* 35:751, 2015.

Wren TA, Chatwood AP, Rethlefsen SA, et al.: Achilles tendon length and medial gastrocnemius architecture in children with cerebral palsy and equinus gait, *J Pediatr Orthop* 30:479, 2010.

SPINE

Abol Oyoun N, Stuecker R: Bilateral rib-to-pelvis Eiffel Tower VEPTR construct for children with neuromuscular scoliosis: a preliminary report, *Spine J* 14:1183, 2014.

Bohtz C, Meyer-Heim A, Min K: Changes in health-related quality of life after spinal fusion and scoliosis correction in patients with cerebral palsy, *J Pediatr Orthop* 31:668, 2011.

Hasler CC: Operative treatment for spinal deformities in cerebral palsy, *J Child Orthop* 7:419, 2013.

Brooks JT, Yaszay B, Bartley CE, et al.: Do all patients with cerebral palsy require postoperative intensive care admission after spinal fusion? *Spine Deform* 7:112, 2019.

Demura S, Kato S, Shinmura K, et al.: *More than 10-year follow-up after laminoplasty and pedicle screw fixation for cervical myelopathy associated with athetoid cerebral palsy*, Spine (Phila Pa 1976), 20202020, [Epub ahead of print].

Jackson T, Yaszay B, Sponseller PD, et al.: Factors associated with surgical approach and outcomes in cerebral palsy scoliosis, *Eur Spine J* 28:567, 2019.

Lee SY, Chung CY, Lee KM, et al.: Annual changes in radiographic indices of the spine in cerebral palsy patients, *Eur Spine J* 25:679, 2016.

Lins LAB, Nechyporenko AV, Halanski MA, et al.: Does an intrathecal pump impact scoliosis progression and complicate posterior spine fusion in patients with cerebral palsy? *Spine Deform*, 2020, [Epub ahead of print].

Lonstein JE, Koop SE, Novachek TF, et al.: Results and complications after spinal fusion for neuromuscular scoliosis in cerebral palsy and static encephalopathy using Luque Galveston instrumentation: experience in 93 patients, *Spine* 37:583, 2012.

McElroy MJ, Sponseller PD, Dattilo JR, et al.: Growing rods for the treatment of scoliosis in children with cerebral palsy: a critical assessment, *Spine* 37:E1504, 2012.

Mohamed A, Koutharawu DN, Miller F, et al.: Operative and clinical markers of deep wound infection after spine fusion in children with cerebral palsy, *J Pediatr Orthop* 30:851, 2010.

Sewell MD, Malagelada F, Wallace C, et al.: A preliminary study to assess whether spinal fusion for scoliosis improves carer-assessed quality of life for children with GMFCS level IV or V cerebral palsy, *J Pediatr Orthop* 36:299, 2016.

Sponseller PD, Jain A, Shah SA, et al.: Deep wound infections after fusion in children with cerebral palsy: a prospective cohort study, *Spine* 38:2023, 2013.

Sponseller PD, Shah SA, Abel MF, et al.: Infection rate of spine surgery in cerebral palsy is high and impairs results: multicenter analysis of risk factors and treatment, *Clin Orthop Relat Res* 468:711, 2010.

Tsirikos AI, Mains E: Surgical correction of spinal deformity in patients with cerebral palsy using pedicle screw instrumentation, *J Spinal Disord Tech* 25:401, 2012.

UPPER EXTREMITY

Gigante P, McDowell MM, Bruce SS, et al.: Reduction in upper-extremity tone after lumbar selective dorsal rhizotomy in children with spastic cerebral palsy, *J Neurosurg Pediatr* 12:588, 2013.

Gong HS, Cho HE, Chung CY, et al.: Early results of anterior elbow release with and without biceps lengthening in patients with cerebral palsy, *J Hand Surg [Am]* 39:902, 2014.

Koman LA, Smith BP, Williams R, et al.: Upper extremity spasticity in children with cerebral palsy: a randomized, double-blind, placebo-controlled study of the short-term outcomes of treatment with botulinum A toxin, *J Hand Surg [Am]* 38:435, 2013.

Leafblad ND, Van Heest AE: Management of the spastic wrist and hand in cerebral palsy, *J Hand Surg [Am]* 40:1035, 2015.

Louwers A, Warnink-Kavelaars J, Objeijn M, et al.: Effects of upper-extremity surgery on manual performance of children and adolescents with cerebral palsy: a multidisciplinary approach using shared decision-making, *J Bone Joint Surg Am* 100:1416, 2018.

Makki D, Duodu J, Nixon M: Prevalence and pattern of upper limb involvement in cerebral palsy, *J Child Orthop* 8:215, 2014.

Marigi EM, Statz JM, Sperling JW, et al.: Shoulder arthroplasty in patients with cerebral palsy: a matched cohort study to patients with osteoarthritis, *J Shoulder Elbow Surg*, 2019, [Epub ahead of print].

Park ES, Sim EG, Rha DW: Effect of upper limb deformities on gross motor and upper limb functions in children with spastic cerebral palsy, *Res Dev Disabil* 32:2389, 2011.

Pontén E, von Walden F, Lenk-Ekholm C, et al.: Outcome of hand surgery in children with spasticity—a 9-year follow-up study, *J Pediatr Orthop B* 28:301, 2019.

Smitherman JA, Davids JR, Tanner S, et al.: Functional outcomes following single-event multilevel surgery of the upper extremity for children with hemiplegic cerebral palsy, *J Bone Joint Surg* 93A:655, 2011.

Tranchida GV, Van Heest A: Preferred options and evidence for upper limb surgery for spasticity in cerebral palsy, stroke, and brain injury, *J Hand Surg Eur* 45:34, 2020.

Van Heest AE, Bagley A, Molitor F, et al.: Tendon transfer surgery in upper-extremity cerebral palsy is more effective than botulinum toxin injections or regular ongoing therapy, *J Bone Joint Surg* 97:529, 2015.

ADULTS WITH CEREBRAL PALSY

Flanigan M, Gaebler-Spira D, Kocherginsky M, et al.: Spasticity and pain in adults with cerebral palsy, *Dev Med Child Neurol*, 2019, [Epub head of print].

French ZP, Torres RV, Whitney DG: Elevated prevalence of osteoarthritis among adults with cerebral palsy, *J Rehabil Med* 51:575, 2019.

Frisch D, Msall ME: Health, functioning, and participation of adolescents and adults with cerebral palsy: a review of outcomes research, *Dev Disabil Res Rev* 18:84, 2013.

Jacobson DN, Löwing K, Tedroff K: Health-related quality of life, pain, and fatigue in young adults with cerebral palsy, *Dev Med Child Neurol*, 2019, [Epub ahead of print].

Kim JH, Jung NY, Chang WS, et al.: Intrathecal baclofen pump versus globus pallidus interna deep brain stimulation in adult patients with severe cerebral palsy, *World Neurosurg* 126:e550, 2019.

Lariviere-Bastien D, Bell E, Majnemer A, et al.: Perspectives of young adults with cerebral palsy on transitioning from pediatric to adult healthcare systems, *Semin Pediatr Neurol* 20:154, 2013.

Lomax MR, Shrader MW: Orthopedic conditions in adults with cerebral palsy, *Phys Med Rehabil Clin N Am* 31:171, 2020.

Morgan P, McGinley J: Gait function and decline in adults with cerebral palsy: a systematic review, *Disabil Rehabil* 36:1, 2014.

Morgan PE, Soh SE, McGinley JL: Health-related quality of life of ambulant adults with cerebral palsy and its association with falls and mobility decline: a preliminary cross sectional study, *Health Qual Life Outcomes* 12:132, 2014.

Oetgen ME, Ayyala H, Martin BD: Treatment of hip subluxation in skeletally mature patients with cerebral palsy, *Orthopedics* 38:e248, 2015.

Opheim A, McGinley JL, Olsson E, et al.: Walking deterioration and gait analysis in adults with spastic bilateral cerebral palsy, *Gait Posture* 37:165, 2013.

Putz C, Blessing AK, Erhard S, et al.: Long-term results of multilevel surgery in adults with cerebral palsy, *Int Orthop* 43:255, 2019.

Reddihough DS, Jiang B, Lanigan A, et al.: Social outcomes of young adults with cerebral palsy, *J Intellect Dev Disabil* 38:215, 2013.

Vogtle LK, Malone LA, Azuero A: Outcomes of an exercise program for pain and fatigue management in adults with cerebral palsy, *Disabil Rehabil* 36:818, 2014.

Whitney DG, Kamdar NS, Ng S, et al.: Prevalence of high-burden medical conditions and health care resource utilization and costs among adults with cerebral palsy, *Clin Epidemiol* 11:469, 2019.

ADULT STROKE PATIENTS

Anakwenze OA, Namdari S, Hsu JE, et al.: Myotendinous lengthening of the elbow flexor muscles to improve active motion in patients with elbow spasticity following brain injury, *J Shoulder Elbow Surg* 22:318, 2013.

Appel C, Perry L, Jones F: Shoulder strapping for stroke-related upper limb dysfunction and shoulder impairments: systematic review, *Neurorehabilitation* 35:191, 2014.

Bakheit AM: The pharmacological management of post-stroke muscle spasticity, *Drugs Aging* 29:941, 2012.

Carda S, Invernizzi M, Baricich A, et al.: Casting, taping or stretching after botulinum toxin type A for spastic equinus foot: a single-blind randomized trial on adult stroke patients, *Clin Rehabil* 25:1119, 2011.

Gracies JM, Esquenazi A, Brashear A, et al.: Efficacy and safety of abobotulinumtoxinA in spastic lower limb: randomized trial and extension, *Neurology* 89:2245, 2017.

Hugues A, Di Marco J, Ribault S, et al.: Limited evidence of physical therapy on balance after stroke: a systematic review and meta-analysis, *PLoS One* 14:e0221700, 2019.

Jeon WH, Park GW, Jeong HJ, et al.: The comparison of effects of suprascapular nerve block, intra-articular steroid injection, and a combination therapy on hemiplegic shoulder pain: pilot study, *Ann Rehabil Med* 38:167, 2014.

Lee J, Stone AJ: Combined aerobic and resistance training for cardiorespiratory fitness, muscle strength, and walking capacity after stroke: a systematic review and meta-analysis, *J Stroke Cerebrovasc Dis* 29:104498, 2020.

Marciniak CM, Harvey RL, Gagnon CM, et al.: Does botulinum toxin type A decrease pain and lessen disability in hemiplegic survivors of stroke with shoulder pain and spasticity? A randomized, double-blind, placebo-controlled trial, *Am J Phys Med Rehabil* 91:1007, 2012.

Mercer VS, Freburger JK, Yin Z, et al.: Recovery of paretic lower extremity loading ability and physical function in the first six months after stroke, *Arch Phys Med Rehabil* 95:1547, 2014.

Namdari S, Alosh H, Baldwin K, et al.: Outcomes of tendon fractional lengthenings to improve shoulder function in patients with spastic hemiparesis, *J Shoulder Elbow Surg* 21:691, 2012.

Otom AH, Al-Khawaja IM, Al-Quliti KW: Botulinum toxin type-A in the management of spastic equinovarus deformity after stroke. Comparison of 2 injection techniques, *Neurosciences (Riyadh)* 19:199, 2014.

Rosales RL, Kong KH, Goh KJ, et al.: Botulinum toxin injection for hypertonicity of the upper extremity within 12 weeks after stroke: a randomized controlled trial, *Neurorehabil Neural Repair* 26:812, 2012.

Rousseaux M, Daveluy W, Kozlowski O, et al.: Onabotulinumtoxin-A injection for disabling lower limb flexion in hemiplegic patients, *Neurorehabilitation* 35:25, 2014.

Tenniglo MJ, Nederhand MJ, Prinsen EC, et al.: Effect of chemodenervation of the rectus femoris muscle in adults with a stiff knee gait due to spastic paresis: a systematic review with a meta-analysis in patients with stroke, *Arch Phys Med Rehabil* 95:576, 2014.

Vogt JC, Bach G, Cantini B, et al.: Split anterior tibial tendon transfer for varus equinus spastic foot deformity. Initial clinical findings correlate with functional results: a series of 132 operated feet, *Foot Ankle Surg* 17:178, 2011.

The complete list of references is available online at Expert Consult.com.

CHAPTER 6

PARALYTIC DISORDERS

William C. Warner Jr., James H. Beaty

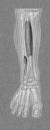

POLIOMYELITIS

Acute anterior poliomyelitis is a viral infection localized in the anterior horn cells of the spinal cord and certain brainstem motor nuclei. One of three types of poliomyelitis viruses is usually the cause of infection, but other members of the enteroviral group can cause a condition clinically and pathologically indistinguishable from poliomyelitis. Viral transmission is primarily fecal-oral, and initial invasion by the virus occurs through the gastrointestinal and respiratory tracts and spreads to the central nervous system through a hematogenous route. Although most individuals in an endemic area are infected with poliovirus, only 0.5% of infected individuals develop paralytic poliomyelitis.

Since the introduction and extensive use of the poliomyelitis vaccine, the incidence of acute anterior poliomyelitis has decreased dramatically. In 1988, there were an estimated 350,000 cases; in 2013, fewer than 400 cases were reported. In 2017, there were 22 reported cases and in 2018, 29 cases. Currently, it most often affects children younger than 5 years old in developing tropical and subtropical countries and unimmunized individuals. In 2014, only three countries

(Afghanistan, Nigeria, and Pakistan) were classified as polio-endemic by the WHO. Isolated outbreaks of poliomyelitis occurred in North America and Europe in the 1990s.

Administration of three doses of the Sabin oral polio vaccine, containing all three types of attenuated virus, can prevent the disease. The use of the live attenuated virus vaccine remains controversial. Live oral poliovirus vaccine (OPV) may immunize contacts who have not been vaccinated; however, this carries a risk of developing vaccine-associated paralytic polio, which has been estimated at 1 case per 2.5 million doses. Outbreaks of paralytic poliomyelitis in the United States have been associated with the use of live poliovirus vaccine. The implementation of an all-inactive polio vaccine (IPV) schedule in the United States in 2000 has eliminated indigenous acquired vaccine-associated poliomyelitis. Despite the safety and efficacy of the IPV, OPV remains the vaccine of choice for global eradication in many parts of the world where logistical issues and the higher cost of IPV prohibit its use and in places where inadequate sanitation necessitates an optimal mucosal barrier to wild-type poliovirus circulation. Challenges to the complete eradication of polio include the transmission of wild-type viruses in endemic areas, outbreaks related to vaccine-related polioviruses, and excretion of vaccine-related viruses in vaccines with B-cell immunodeficiencies.

In August of 2018, the Centers for Disease Control and Prevention (CDC) noted an increased number of reports of patients having symptoms clinically compatible with acute flaccid myelitis, a polio-like condition characterized by rapid onset of flaccid weakness in one or more limbs and spinal cord gray matter lesions. First described in 2014, the disease appears to have established a biennial pattern of recurrence, usually in the summer and fall and often following a viral respiratory infection. Of 106 patients identified with acute flaccid myelitis in 2018, 80 were classified as confirmed, six as probable, and 20 as noncases, a threefold increase in confirmed cases compared with 2017. The pattern of spinal cord involvement, similar to poliomyelitis, is suggestive of a viral infection, but a definitive connection with a particular virus has yet to be established. The most frequently cited causative agent is enterovirus D68, but the absence of direct virus isolation from affected tissues, infrequent detection in cerebrospinal fluid, and the limited number of animal studies has left the causal nature of the relationship unproven. A number of treatments have been tried, including immunoglobulin, corticosteroids, plasma exchange, and antiviral therapy. To date, however, no systematic studies have identified an effective medical treatment of acute flaccid myelitis, and supportive care is the mainstay of treatment. Most patients have some residual weakness a year or more after onset.

PATHOLOGIC FINDINGS

When the poliomyelitis virus invades the body through the oropharyngeal route, it multiplies in the alimentary tract lymph nodes and spreads through the blood, acutely attacking the anterior horn ganglion cells of the spinal cord, especially in the lumbar and cervical enlargements. How the virus penetrates the blood-brain barrier and why the virus has a predilection for the anterior horn cell is under investigation. The incubation period is 6 to 20 days. The anterior horn motor cells may be damaged directly by viral multiplication or toxic by-products of the virus or indirectly by ischemia, edema, and hemorrhage in the glial tissues surrounding them.

Destruction of the spinal cord occurs focally and randomly, and within 3 days, Wallerian degeneration is evident throughout the length of the individual nerve fiber. Macrophages and neutrophils surround and partially remove necrotic ganglion cells, and the inflammatory response gradually subsides. Within the muscle, axonal "sprouting" occurs when nerve cells from surviving motor units develop new axons, which innervate muscle cells that have lost their lower motor neuron, thus expanding the size of the motor unit. After 4 months, residual areas of gliosis and lymphocytic cells fill the area of destroyed motor cells in the spine. Reparative neuroglial cells proliferate. Continuous disease activity has been reported in spinal cord segments 20 years after disease onset.

The number of individual muscles affected by the resultant flaccid paralysis and the severity of paralysis vary; the clinical weakness is proportional to the number of lost motor units. Weakness is clinically detectable only when more than 60% of the nerve cells supplying the muscle have been destroyed. Muscles innervated by the cervical and lumbar spinal segments are most often affected, and paralysis occurs twice as often in the lower extremity muscles as in upper extremity muscles. In the lower extremity, the most commonly affected muscles are the quadriceps, glutei, anterior tibial, medial hamstrings, and hip flexors; in the upper extremity, the deltoid, triceps, and pectoralis major are most often affected.

The potential for recovery of muscle function depends on the recovery of damaged, but not destroyed, anterior horn cells. Most clinical recovery occurs during the first month after the acute illness and is almost complete within 6 months, although limited recovery may occur for about 2 years. A muscle paralyzed at 6 months remains paralyzed.

CLINICAL COURSE AND TREATMENT

Approximately 95% of patients infected with poliovirus remain asymptomatic. Nonspecific findings such as fever and sore throat occur in 4% to 8% of people infected. Between 0.5% and 2% of patients will progress to poliomyelitis. The course of poliomyelitis can be divided into three stages: acute, convalescent, and chronic. General guidelines for treatment are described here. Specific indications and techniques for operative procedures are discussed in specific sections.

■ ACUTE STAGE

The acute stage generally lasts 7 to 10 days, and up to 95% of all anterior horn cells may be infected. Symptoms range from mild malaise to generalized encephalomyelitis with widespread paralysis. With upper spinal cord involvement, diaphragmatic dysfunction and respiratory compromise can be life threatening. A high index of suspicion of this is necessary, especially in patients with shoulder involvement, given the close proximity of their respective anterior horn cells. In younger children, systemic symptoms include listlessness, sore throat, and a slight temperature elevation; these may resolve, but recurrent symptoms, including hyperesthesia or paresthesia in the extremities, severe headache, sore throat, vomiting, nuchal rigidity, back pain, and limitation of straight-leg raising, culminate in characteristically asymmetric paralysis. In older children and adults, symptoms include slight temperature elevation, marked flushing of the skin, and apprehension; muscular pain is common. Muscles are tender even to gentle palpation. Superficial reflexes usually are absent first, and deep tendon reflexes disappear when the muscle group is paralyzed. Differential diagnoses include Guillain-Barré syndrome and other forms of encephalomyelitis. In rare cases, transverse myelitis can follow receipt of OPV.

Treatment of poliomyelitis in the acute stage generally consists of bed rest, analgesics, and anatomic positioning of the limbs to prevent contractures. Gentle, passive range-of-motion exercises of all joints should be performed several times daily.

■ CONVALESCENT STAGE

The convalescent stage begins 2 days after the temperature returns to normal and continues for 2 years. It has been estimated that approximately half of the infected anterior horn cells survive the initial infection, and muscle power improves spontaneously during this stage, especially during the first 4 months and more gradually thereafter. Treatment during this stage is similar to that during the acute stage. Muscle strength should be assessed monthly for 6 months and then every 3 months. Physical therapy should emphasize muscle activity in normal patterns and development of maximal capability of individual muscles. Muscles with more than 80% return of strength recover spontaneously without specific therapy. According to Johnson, an individual muscle with less than 30% of normal strength at 3 months should be considered permanently paralyzed.

Vigorous passive stretching exercises and wedging casts can be used for mild or moderate contractures. Surgical release of tight fascia and muscle aponeuroses and lengthening of tendons may be necessary for contractures persisting longer than 6 months. Orthoses should be used until no further recovery is anticipated.

■ CHRONIC STAGE

The chronic stage of poliomyelitis usually begins 24 months after the acute illness. During this time, the orthopaedist attempts to help the patient achieve maximal functional activity by management of the long-term consequences of muscle imbalance. Goals of treatment include correcting any significant muscle imbalances and preventing or correcting soft-tissue or bony deformities. Static joint instability usually can be controlled indefinitely by orthoses. Dynamic joint instability eventually results in a fixed deformity that cannot be controlled with orthoses. Young children are more prone than adults to develop bony deformity because of their growth potential. Soft-tissue surgery, such as tendon transfers, should be done in young children before the development of any fixed bony changes; bony procedures for correcting a deformity usually can be delayed until skeletal growth is near completion.

TENDON TRANSFERS

Tendon transfers are indicated when dynamic muscle imbalance results in a deformity that interferes with ambulation or function of the upper extremities. Surgery should be delayed until the maximal return of expected muscle strength in the involved muscle has been achieved. The objectives of a tendon transfer are (1) to provide active motor power to replace function of a paralyzed muscle or muscles, (2) to eliminate the deforming effect of a muscle when its antagonist is paralyzed, and (3) to improve stability by improving muscle balance.

Tendon transfer shifts a tendinous insertion from its normal attachment to another location so that its muscle can be substituted for a paralyzed muscle in the same region. In selecting a tendon for transfer, the following factors must be carefully considered:

1. *Strength.* The muscle to be transferred must be strong enough to accomplish what the paralyzed muscle did or to supplement the power of a partially paralyzed muscle. A muscle to be transferred should have a rating of *good* or *better* because a transferred muscle loses at least one grade in power after transfer.
2. *Efficiency.* The transferred tendon should be attached as close to the insertion of the paralyzed tendon as possible and should be routed in as direct a line as possible between the muscle's origin and its new insertion.
3. *Excursion.* The tendon to be transferred should have a range of excursion similar to the one it is reinforcing or replacing. It should be retained in its own sheath or placed into the sheath of another tendon, or it should be passed through tissues, such as subcutaneous fat, that would allow it to glide. Routing a tendon through fascial or osseous tunnels can lead to scarring and decreased excursion.
4. *Neurovascular.* The nerve and blood supply to the transferred muscle must not be impaired or traumatized in making the transfer.
5. *Articular.* The joint on which the muscle is to act must be in a satisfactory position; any contractures must be released before the tendon transfer. A transferred muscle cannot be expected to correct a fixed deformity.
6. *Tension.* The transferred tendon must be securely attached under tension slightly greater than normal. If tension is insufficient, excursion is used in removing slack in the musculotendinous unit, rather than in producing the desired function.

Muscle transfers, whenever possible, should occur between agonistic muscles that are phasic, or active at the same time in the gait cycle. The anterior muscles of the leg are predominantly swing-phase muscles, and the posterior muscles, or flexors, are stance-phase muscles; in the thigh, the quadriceps is characteristically a stance-phase muscle, and the hamstrings are swing-phase muscles. In general, phasic transfers retain their preoperative phasic activities and regain their preoperative duration of contraction and electrical intensity. In contrast, nonphasic muscle transfers often retain their preoperative phasic activity and fail to assume the action of the muscles for which they are substituted and are not recommended. Some nonphasic transfers are capable of phasic conversion; however, phasic conversion is somewhat unpredictable and requires extensive postoperative physical therapy. Phasic conversion is not related to the use of splints and/or braces or time between disease onset and muscle transfer.

The ideal muscle for tendon transfer would have the same phasic activity as the paralyzed muscle, would be of about the same size in cross section and of equal strength, and could be placed in proper relationship to the axis of the joint to allow maximal mechanical effectiveness. Not all of these criteria can be met in every instance.

Paralytic deformities from muscle paralysis can be dynamic or static, and often both types are present. The extent to which the paralytic deformity is dynamic or static should be determined because a static deformity can be controlled with a brace in a growing child or with arthrodesis in an adult. A dynamic deformity is more likely to be appropriate for tendon transfer in children and adults. In a growing child with dynamic deformity, recurrence is possible with arthrodesis alone; in a child with static deformity, however, recurrence after arthrodesis is rare. In a growing child with dynamic deformity, an appropriate tendon transfer with minimal external support redistributes muscle power, preventing permanent deformity until the patient is old enough for an arthrodesis.

ARTHRODESIS

A relaxed or flail joint is stabilized by restricting its range of motion. Although a properly constructed brace may control a flail joint, a reconstructive operation that would not only eliminate the need for a brace but also improve function may be more effective. Arthrodesis is the most efficient method of permanent stabilization of a joint. Tenodeses that use flexor or extensor tendons to stabilize joints of the fingers are notable exceptions, as are tenodeses of the peroneus longus or Achilles tendon in paralytic calcaneal deformity; results are satisfactory here because the pull of gravity and body weight usually are not enough to overstretch the tendons.

Because the lower extremities are designed primarily to support the weight of the body, it is important that their joints are stable and their muscles have sufficient power. When the control of one or more joints of the foot and ankle is lost because of paralysis, stabilization may be required. In the upper extremity, reach, grasp, pinch, and release require more mobility than stability and more dexterity than power. An operation to limit or obliterate motion in a joint of an upper extremity should be performed only after careful study of its advantages and disadvantages and of its general effect on the patient, especially in normal daily activity. Because of the high prevalence of lower extremity weakness in patients with poliomyelitis and because many patients use ambulatory assistive devices, any surgical treatment that affects the upper extremity can have a dramatic impact on ambulation as well. Arthrodesis of the shoulder is useful for some patients but has certain cosmetic and functional disadvantages that must be weighed. Arthrodesis of the elbow is rarely indicated in poliomyelitis. Arthrodesis of the wrist, although useful for some patients, may increase the disability of other patients. A patient who must use a wheelchair or crutches and has a wrist that is fused in the "optimal" position (for grasp and pinch) may be unable to rise from a chair or to manipulate crutches because he or she cannot shift the body weight to the palm of the hand with the wrist extended.

FOOT AND ANKLE

Because the foot and ankle are the most dependent parts of the body and are subjected to significant amounts of stress, they are especially susceptible to deformity from paralysis. The most common deformities of the foot and ankle include claw toes, cavovarus foot, dorsal bunion, talipes equinus, talipes equinovarus, talipes cavovarus, talipes equinovalgus, and talipes calcaneus. When the paralysis is of short duration, these dynamic deformities are not fixed and may be evident only on contraction of unopposed muscles or on weight bearing; later, as a result of muscle imbalance, habitual posturing, growth, and abnormal weight-bearing alignment, a permanent deformity can occur from contracture of the soft tissues and eventual osseous changes.

Ambulation requires a stable plantigrade foot with even weight distribution between the heel and forefoot and no significant fixed deformity. In the foot, muscle transfer is

performed to prevent contracture formation, balance the muscles responsible for dorsiflexion and plantarflexion and for inversion and eversion, and reestablish as normal a gait as possible. Arthrodesis to correct deformity or stabilize the joints usually should be delayed until about age 10 to 12 years to allow for adequate growth of the foot.

■ TENDON TRANSFERS

Tendon transfers around the foot and ankle after 10 years of age can be supplemented by arthrodesis to correct fixed deformities, to establish enough lateral stability for weight bearing, and to compensate in part for the loss of function in the evertor and invertor muscles of the foot. When tendon transfers and arthrodesis are combined in the same operation, the arthrodesis should be performed first.

Transfer of a tendon usually is preferable to excision, not only to preserve function but also to prevent further atrophy of the leg. When the paralysis is severe enough to require arthrodesis, there usually is some weakness of the dorsiflexor or plantar flexor muscles. In this case, the invertor or evertor muscles can be transferred to the midline of the foot anteriorly or posteriorly into the calcaneus and Achilles tendon. In the rare instance when a muscle function is discarded, 7 to 10 cm of its tendon should be excised to prevent scarring of the tendon ends by fibrous tissue. In addition to arthrodesis and tendon transfers, any deformities of the leg, such as excessive tibial torsion, genu varum, or genu valgum (bowlegs), should be corrected because otherwise they might cause recurrence of the foot deformity.

▌PARALYSIS OF SPECIFIC MUSCLES

Isolated muscles may be paralyzed in patients with poliomyelitis, but more often combinations of muscles are affected. The specific muscle or muscles involved and the resulting muscle imbalance should be determined before treatment is started. Common deformities caused by muscle imbalance in the foot and ankle are described, according to the muscles involved. The exact pattern of muscle paralysis and the specific deformity that occurs must be carefully determined before any surgical intervention is undertaken.

▌ANTERIOR TIBIAL MUSCLE

Severe weakness or paralysis of the anterior tibial muscle results in loss of dorsiflexion and inversion power and produces a slowly progressive deformity (equinus and cavus or varying degrees of planovalgus) that is first evident in the swing phase of gait. The extensors of the long toe, which usually assist dorsiflexion, become overactive in an attempt to replace the paralyzed anterior tibial muscle, causing hyperextension of the proximal phalanges and depression of the metatarsal heads. A cavovarus deformity occasionally results from unopposed activity of the peroneus longus combined with an active posterior tibial muscle.

Passive stretching and serial casting can be tried before surgery to correct the equinus contracture. Posterior ankle capsulotomy and Achilles tendon lengthening occasionally are required and are combined with anterior transfer of the peroneus longus to the base of the second metatarsal. The peroneus brevis is sutured to the stump of the peroneus longus to prevent a dorsal bunion. As an alternative, the extensor digitorum longus can be recessed to the dorsum of the midfoot to supply active dorsiflexion. Claw toe deformity is managed by transfer of the long toe extensors into the metatarsal necks.

Plantar fasciotomy and release of intrinsic muscles may be necessary before tendon surgery for a fixed cavovarus deformity. In this situation, the peroneus longus is transferred to the base of the second metatarsal and the extensor hallucis longus is transferred to the neck of the first metatarsal. The claw toe deformity frequently recurs because of reattachment of the extensor hallucis longus; this can be prevented by suturing its distal stump to the extensor hallucis brevis.

ANTERIOR AND POSTERIOR TIBIAL MUSCLES

If the anterior tibial and the posterior tibial muscles are paralyzed, development of hindfoot and forefoot equinovalgus is more rapid and the deformity becomes fixed as the Achilles tendon and peroneal muscles shorten. This deformity may be similar to congenital vertical talus on a standing lateral radiograph, but the apparent vertical talus is not confirmed when a plantarflexion lateral view is obtained. Serial casting is used before surgery to stretch the tight Achilles tendon and to avoid weakening the gastrocnemius-soleus. If the peroneal muscles are normal, and both tibial muscles are paralyzed, one of the peroneal muscles must be transferred. Because of its greater excursion, the peroneus longus is transferred to the base of the second metatarsal to replace the anterior tibial and one of the long toe flexors replaces the posterior tibial. The peroneus brevis is sutured to the distal stump of the peroneus longus tendon.

POSTERIOR TIBIAL MUSCLE

Isolated paralysis of the posterior tibial muscle is rare but can result in hindfoot and forefoot eversion. The flexor hallucis longus and the flexor digitorum longus have been used for tendon transfers in this situation. Through a posteromedial incision, the intrinsic plantar muscles are dissected sharply from their calcaneal origin, and one of the long toe flexors is exposed and divided. If the flexor digitorum longus is used, it is dissected from its tendon sheath posterior and proximal to the medial malleolus, rerouted through the posterior tibial sheath, and attached to the navicular. In rare cases, as an alternative, the extensor hallucis longus can be transferred posteriorly through the interosseous membrane and then through the posterior tibial tunnel.

For children 3 to 6 years old, Axer recommended bringing the conjoined extensor digitorum longus and peroneus tertius tendons through a transverse tunnel in the talar neck and suturing the tendon back onto itself. For fixed equinus deformity, lengthening of the Achilles tendon may be required before tendon transfer. For severe valgus, Axer recommended transfer of the peroneus longus into the medial side of the talar neck and transfer of the peroneus brevis into the lateral side. Isolated transfer of the peroneus brevis should not be done because it can cause a forefoot inversion deformity. After surgery, cast immobilization is continued for 6 weeks, followed by 6 months of orthosis wear.

ANTERIOR TIBIAL, TOE EXTENSOR, AND PERONEAL MUSCLES

Progressively severe equinovarus deformity develops when the posterior tibial and gastrocnemius-soleus are unopposed. The posterior tibial muscle increases forefoot equinus and cavus deformity by depressing the metatarsal head

and shortening the medial arch of the foot. Further equinus and varus deformity result from contracture of the gastrocnemius-soleus, which acts as a fixed point toward which the plantar intrinsic muscles pull and increase forefoot adduction.

Stretching by serial casting may be attempted, but lengthening of the Achilles tendon usually is required. Radical soft-tissue release of the forefoot cavus deformity also may be necessary. Anterior transfer of the posterior tibial to the base of the third metatarsal or middle cuneiform can be supplemented by anterior transfer of the long toe flexors. Arthrodesis usually is not required; the deformity can be controlled by physical therapy and orthoses. A bony tunnel can be made through the base of the third metatarsal or the middle cuneiform, with suture of the transfer to a button over a felt pad placed on the non–weight bearing area of the plantar surface of the foot.

PERONEAL MUSCLES

Isolated paralysis of the peroneal muscles is rare in patients with poliomyelitis but can cause severe hindfoot varus deformity because of the unopposed activity of the posterior tibial muscle. The calcaneus becomes inverted, the forefoot is adducted, and the varus deformity is increased by the action of the invertor muscles during gait. The unopposed anterior tibial activity can cause a dorsal bunion. In this situation, the anterior tibial muscle can be transferred laterally to the base of the second metatarsal; however, isolated transfer of the anterior tibial muscle can result in overactivity of the extensor hallucis longus, causing hyperextension of the hallux and development of a painful callus under the first metatarsal head. In children younger than 5 years of age, lengthening of the extensor hallucis longus tendon may be required. In children older than 5 years, the extensor hallucis longus should be transferred to the first metatarsal neck before the bony deformity becomes fixed.

PERONEAL AND LONG TOE EXTENSOR MUSCLES

Paralysis of the peroneal muscles and long toe extensors causes a less severe equinovarus deformity that can be treated by transfer of the anterior tibial tendon to the base of the third metatarsal or the middle cuneiform.

GASTROCNEMIUS-SOLEUS MUSCLES

The gastrocnemius-soleus is a strong muscle group in the body, lifting the entire body weight with each step. Paralysis of the gastrocnemius-soleus, leaving the dorsiflexors unopposed, causes a rapidly progressive calcaneal deformity. Adequate tension of the Achilles tendon is important to the normal function of the long toe flexors and extensors and to the intrinsic foot muscles. If the gastrocnemius-soleus is weak, the posterior tibial, the peroneal muscles, and the long toe flexors cannot effectively plantarflex the hindfoot; however, they can depress the metatarsal heads and cause an equinus deformity. Shortening of the intrinsics and plantar fascia draws the metatarsal heads and the calcaneus together, similar to a bowstring. The long axes of the tibia and the calcaneus coincide, negating any residual power in the gastrocnemius-soleus.

Keeping the foot in slight equinus during the acute stage of poliomyelitis helps prevent overstretching of the gastrocnemius-soleus, and the position is maintained in the convalescent stage. If the gastrocnemius-soleus is weak, early walking is discouraged. Serial standing radiographs should be obtained frequently, especially in children younger than 5 years old, because of the rapid development of the deformity.

Surgical correction is indicated to prevent development of calcaneal deformity and to restore hindfoot plantarflexion. In the acute stage, the only absolute indication for tendon transfer in children younger than 5 years old is a progressive calcaneal deformity.

The combination of muscles transferred posteriorly depends on the residual strength of the gastrocnemius-soleus and the pattern of remaining muscle function. If the motor strength of the gastrocnemius-soleus is fair, posterior transfer of two or three muscles may be sufficient for normal gait. If the gastrocnemius-soleus is completely paralyzed, as many muscles as are available should be transferred. Plantar fasciotomy and intrinsic muscle release are required before tendon transfer in fixed forefoot cavus deformity.

The anterior tibial muscle can be transferred posteriorly 18 months after the acute stage of poliomyelitis. This can be done as an isolated procedure if the lateral stabilizers are balanced and the strong toe extensors can be used for dorsiflexion. In more severe deformity, transfer of the toe extensors to the metatarsal heads and fusion of the interphalangeal joints may be required to prevent claw toe deformity.

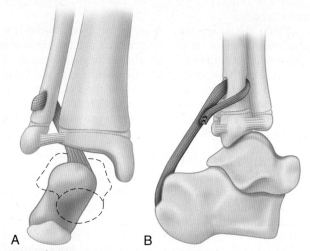

FIGURE 6.1   Anterior **(A)** and lateral **(B)** views of tenodesis of Achilles tendon to fibula.

POSTERIOR TRANSFER OF ANTERIOR TIBIAL TENDON

TECHNIQUE 6.1

(DRENNAN)
- Take care to obtain maximal length of the anterior tibial tendon, which may have shortened because of the calcaneal deformity of the interosseous membrane.
- Split the insertion of the Achilles tendon longitudinally and develop osteoperiosteal flaps on the calcaneal tuberosity.
- Place the foot in maximal plantarflexion to ensure that the transfer is attached under appropriate tension. If necessary to obtain adequate plantarflexion, release other dorsal soft structures, including the ankle joint capsule, or lengthen the long toe extensors. If the attenuated Achilles tendon requires shortening, use a Z-plasty technique, resecting the redundant tendon from the proximal part.
- Attach the transferred anterior tibial tendon to the tuberosity of the calcaneus and to the distal stump of the Achilles tendon, which has retained its normal attachment to the calcaneal tuberosity.
- Close the wound in normal fashion and apply a long leg cast with the foot in the plantarflexed position. The cast is worn for 5 weeks, and a brace is worn for an additional 4 months.

If the invertors and evertors are balanced, a pure calcaneocavus deformity develops. Posterior transfer of only one set of these muscles causes instability and deformity. If the gastrocnemius-soleus strength is fair, transfer of the peroneus brevis and posterior tibial to the heel is sufficient to control the calcaneal deformity and allow normal gait. Lateral imbalance requires transposition of the acting invertor or evertor to the heel. Both peroneals are transferred to the heel for calcaneovalgus deformity, and the posterior tibial and flexor hallucis longus can be transferred for cavovarus deformity.

Westin and Defiore recommended tenodesis of the Achilles tendon to the fibula for paralytic calcaneovalgus deformity (Fig. 6.1). They used a T-shaped incision in the periosteum instead of a drill hole, with imbrication of the distal segment of the sectioned tendon below the periosteum. For mobile calcaneal deformities, Makin recommended transfer of the peroneus longus into a groove cut in the posterior calcaneus, without disturbance of the origin or insertion of the tendon. The tendon is freed proximal to the lateral malleolus and at the cuboid groove, and the foot is maximally plantarflexed, allowing the peroneus longus to displace posteriorly into the calcaneal groove, where it eventually unites with the bone. Extraarticular subtalar arthrodesis may be required as a second procedure.

In rare cases, if no invertors or evertors are present for transfer, the hamstrings can be used to replace the gastrocnemius-soleus. Prerequisites for this procedure include complete paralysis of the gastrocnemius-soleus, strong medial hamstrings or biceps femoris muscles, and strong ankle dorsiflexors and quadriceps muscles. The insertions of the semitendinosus and gracilis and occasionally the semimembranosus are mobilized, passed subcutaneously, and attached to the sagittally incised Achilles tendon. A mattress suture at the proximal end of the Achilles tendon prevents this incision from extending proximally. The tendons are sutured with the knee flexed to 25 degrees and the foot in plantarflexion.

FLAIL FOOT

When all muscles distal to the knee are paralyzed, equinus deformity results because of passive plantarflexion. The intrinsic muscles may retain some function, leading to forefoot equinus or cavoequinus deformity. Radical plantar release, sometimes combined with plantar neurectomy, usually controls this deformity. Midfoot wedge resection may be required for the forefoot equinus deformity in older patients.

DORSAL BUNION

In a dorsal bunion deformity, the shaft of the first metatarsal is dorsiflexed and the great toe is plantarflexed; it usually results from muscle imbalance, although occasionally there may be other causes. In its early stages, the deformity is not fixed but is present only on weight bearing, especially walking. If the muscle imbalance is not corrected, the deformity becomes fixed, although it remains more pronounced on weight bearing.

Usually, only the metatarsophalangeal joint of the great toe is flexed, and on weight bearing the first metatarsal head is displaced upward; the longitudinal axis of the metatarsal shaft can be horizontal, or its distal end can even be directed slightly upward. The first cuneiform also can be tilted upward. A small exostosis can form on the dorsum of the metatarsal head. When flexion of the great toe is severe enough, the metatarsophalangeal joint can subluxate and the dorsal part of the cartilage of the metatarsal head eventually can degenerate. The plantar part of the joint capsule and the flexor hallucis brevis muscle can become contracted.

Two types of muscle imbalance can cause a dorsal bunion. The more common dorsiflexes the first metatarsal, and the plantarflexion of the great toe is secondary. The less common plantarflexes the great toe, and dorsiflexion of the first metatarsal is secondary.

The most common imbalance is between the anterior tibial and peroneus longus muscles; normally, the anterior tibial muscle raises the first cuneiform and the base of the first metatarsal, and the peroneus longus opposes this action. When the peroneus longus is weak or paralyzed or has been transferred elsewhere, the first metatarsal can be dorsiflexed by a strong anterior tibial muscle or by a muscle substituting for it. When the first metatarsal is dorsiflexed, the great toe becomes actively plantarflexed to establish a weight-bearing point for the medial side of the forefoot and to assist push-off in walking. Weakness of the dorsiflexor muscles of the great toe also may favor the development of this position of the toe. Many dorsal bunions develop after ill-advised tendon transfers for residual poliomyelitis. In such patients, the opposing actions of the peroneus longus and anterior tibial muscles on the first metatarsal were considered in the transfers. Before any transfer of the peroneus longus tendon, the effect of its loss on the first metatarsal must be carefully considered. When the anterior tibial is paralyzed and tendon transfer is feasible, the peroneus longus tendon or the tendons of the peroneus longus and peroneus brevis should be transferred to the third cuneiform, rather than to the insertion of the anterior tibial; as an alternative, the peroneus brevis tendon can be transferred to the insertion of the anterior tibial, leaving the peroneus longus tendon undisturbed. We believe that when the peroneus longus tendon is transferred, the proximal end of its distal segment should be securely fixed to bone at the level of division. When the gastrocnemius-soleus group is weak or paralyzed, and the anterior tibial and peroneus longus muscles are strong, the peroneus longus should not be transferred to the calcaneus unless the anterior tibial is transferred to the midline of the foot. A dorsal bunion does not always follow ill-advised tendon transfers, however, because the muscle imbalance may not be severe enough to cause it. When the deformity is progressive, surgery may simply consist of transferring the anterior tibial (or the previously transferred peroneus longus) to the third cuneiform; correcting the deformity itself may be unnecessary. When the deformity is fixed, however, surgery must correct not only the muscle imbalance but also the deformity.

The second and less common muscle imbalance that can cause a dorsal bunion results from paralysis of all muscles controlling the foot except the gastrocnemius-soleus group, which may be of variable strength, and the long toe flexors, which are strong. These strong toe flexors help steady the foot in weight bearing and sustain the push-off in walking. The flexor hallucis longus assumes a large share of this added function and with active use, the great toe may be almost constantly plantarflexed; the first metatarsal head is displaced upward to accommodate it. A strong flexor hallucis brevis muscle also may help produce the deformity.

There are other, less common causes for the deformity. It can develop in conjunction with a hallux rigidus in which dorsiflexion of the first metatarsophalangeal joint is painful. The articular surfaces become irregular, and the plantar part of the joint capsule gradually contracts; proliferation of bone on the dorsum of the first metatarsal head often becomes pronounced and blocks dorsiflexion of the joint. When walking, the patient may unconsciously supinate the foot and plantarflex the great toe to protect the weight-bearing pad of the great toe. A dorsal bunion also is sometimes seen in a severe congenital flatfoot with a rocker-bottom deformity (see chapter 1). Transfer of the flexor hallucis longus to the neck of the first metatarsal, combined with bony correction by plantar closing wedge osteotomy of the first metatarsal when necessary, currently is our preferred technique for correction of dorsal bunions (Chapter 1, Technique 1.19). A strong unopposed anterior tibial tendon that contributes to forefoot supination is an indication for addition of a split anterior tibial tendon transfer.

BONY PROCEDURES (OSTEOTOMY AND ARTHRODESIS)

The object of arthrodesis in patients with poliomyelitis is to reduce the number of joints the weakened or paralyzed muscles must control. The structural bony deformity must be corrected before a tendon transfer is performed. Stabilizing procedures for the foot and ankle are traditionally of five types: (1) calcaneal osteotomy, (2) extraarticular subtalar arthrodesis, (3) triple arthrodesis, (4) ankle arthrodesis, and (5) bone blocks to limit motion at the ankle joint. These procedures can be performed singly or in combination with other procedures. The choice of operations depends on the age of the patient and the particular deformity that must be corrected.

CALCANEAL OSTEOTOMY

Calcaneal osteotomy can be performed for correction of hindfoot varus or valgus deformity in growing children. For cavovarus deformity, it can be combined with release of the intrinsic muscles and the plantar fascia, and for calcaneovarus deformity, with posterior displacement calcaneal osteotomy. Fixed valgus deformity may require medial displacement osteotomy in a plane parallel to the peroneal tendons.

DILLWYN EVANS OSTEOTOMY

The Dillwyn Evans osteotomy can be used for talipes calcaneovalgus deformity as an alternative to triple arthrodesis in children 8 to 12 years old. This osteotomy, the reverse of the original technique used in clubfeet, lengthens the calcaneus by a transverse osteotomy of the calcaneus and the insertion

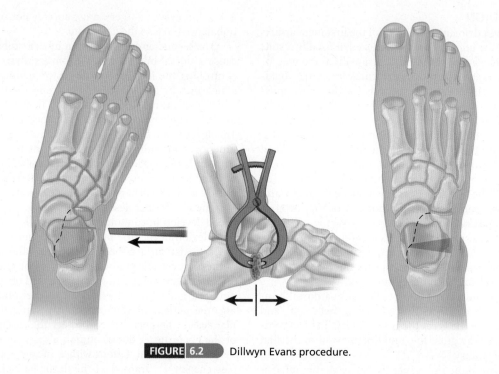

FIGURE 6.2 Dillwyn Evans procedure.

of a bone graft to open a wedge and lengthen the lateral border of the foot (Fig. 6.2).

SUBTALAR ARTHRODESIS

Paralytic equinovalgus deformity results from paralysis of the anterior tibial and posterior tibial and the unopposed action of the peroneals and gastrocnemius-soleus. The calcaneus is everted and displaced laterally and posteriorly. The sustentaculum tali no longer functions as the calcaneal buttress for the talar head, which shifts medially and into equinus. Hindfoot and forefoot equinovalgus deformities develop rapidly and, with growth, become fixed and require bony correction.

Grice and Green developed an extraarticular subtalar fusion to restore the height of the medial longitudinal arch in patients 3 to 8 years old. Ideally, this procedure is performed when the valgus deformity is localized to the subtalar joint and when the calcaneus can be manipulated into its normal position beneath the talus. Careful clinical and radiographic examinations should determine whether the valgus deformity is located primarily in the subtalar joint or the ankle joint. If the forefoot is not mobile enough to be made plantigrade when the hindfoot is corrected, the procedure is contraindicated. The most common complications of the Grice and Green arthrodesis are varus deformity and increased ankle joint valgus because of overcorrection. Bone infection, pseudarthrosis, graft resorption, and degenerative arthritis of the metatarsal joints also have been reported.

Dennyson and Fulford described a technique for subtalar arthrodesis in which a screw is inserted across the subtalar joint for internal fixation and an iliac crest graft is placed in the sinus tarsi. Because the screw provides internal fixation, maintenance of the correct position does not depend on the bone graft.

SUBTALAR ARTHRODESIS

TECHNIQUE 6.2

(GRICE AND GREEN)

- Make a short curvilinear incision on the lateral aspect of the foot directly over the subtalar joint.
- Carry the incision down through the soft tissues to expose the cruciate ligament overlying the joint. Split this ligament in the direction of its fibers, and dissect the fatty and ligamentous tissues from the sinus tarsi.
- Dissect the short toe extensors from the calcaneus, and reflect them distally. The relationship of the calcaneus to the talus now can be determined, and the mechanism of the deformity can be demonstrated.
- Place the foot in equinus, and then invert it to position the calcaneus beneath the talus. A severe, long-standing deformity may require division of the posterior subtalar joint capsule or removal of a small piece of bone laterally from beneath the anterosuperior calcaneal articular surface.
- Insert an osteotome or broad periosteal elevator into the sinus tarsi, and block the subtalar joint to evaluate the stability of the graft and its proper size and position.
- Prepare the graft beds by removing a thin layer of cortical bone from the inferior surface of the talus and the superior surface of the calcaneus (Fig. 6.3).
- Now make a linear incision over the anteromedial surface of the proximal tibial metaphysis, incise the periosteum, and take a block of bone large enough for two grafts (usually 3.5 to 4.5 cm long and 1.5 cm wide). As alternatives

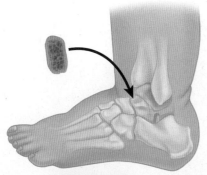 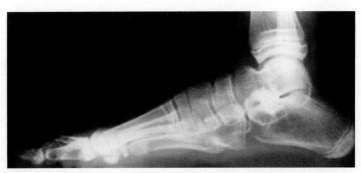

FIGURE 6.3 Grice-Green subtalar fusion. Preparation of graft bed and placement of graft in lateral aspect of subtalar joint. **SEE TECHNIQUE 6.2.**

to tibial bone, take a short segment of the distal fibula or a circular segment of the iliac crest.

- Cut the grafts to fit the prepared beds. Use a rongeur to shape the grafts so that they can be countersunk into the cancellous bone to prevent lateral displacement.
- With the foot held in a slightly overcorrected position, place the grafts in the sinus tarsi. Evert the foot to lock the grafts in place.
- If a segment of the fibula or iliac crest is used, a smooth Kirschner wire can be used to hold the graft in place for 12 weeks. A screw can be inserted anteriorly from the talar neck into the calcaneus for rigid fixation.
- Apply a long leg cast with the knee flexed, the ankle in maximal dorsiflexion, and the foot in the corrected position.

POSTOPERATIVE CARE After 12 weeks of non–weight bearing, the long leg cast is removed and a short leg walking cast is applied and worn for an additional 4 weeks.

SUBTALAR ARTHRODESIS

TECHNIQUE 6.3

(DENNYSON AND FULFORD)

- Make an oblique incision in the line of the skin creases, centered over the sinus tarsi and extending from the middle of the front of the ankle proximally and laterally to the peroneal tendons (Fig. 6.4A).
- Raise the origin of the extensor digitorum brevis, along with a pad of subcutaneous fat, proximally and reflect it distally to expose the sinus tarsi.
- Remove the fat from the sinus tarsi by sharp dissection close to the bone and, with a narrow gouge, remove cortical bone from the apex of the sinus tarsi to expose cancellous bone on the undersurface of the talar neck and on the nonarticular area in the upper calcaneal surface (Fig. 6.4B). Do not remove cortical bone from the outer part of the sinus tarsi in the area through which the screw will pass.
- Expose the depression on the superior surface of the talar neck by blunt dissection between the tendon of the extensor digitorum longus and the neurovascular bundle.

- Hold the calcaneus in its correct position, and pass a bone awl from this depression through the neck of the talus and across the sinus tarsi to enter the upper surface of the calcaneus toward the lateral side until it pierces the cortex of the calcaneus at its inferolateral border (Fig. 6.4C). The awl must pass through cortical bone on both the superior and inferior surfaces of the talar neck and on the superior and inferolateral surfaces of the calcaneus.
- Determine the length of the awl that is within the bones, and insert a minifragment cancellous screw of the same length. Tighten the screw until its head is seated into the superior surface of the talus.
- Pack chips of cancellous bone from the iliac crest into the apex of the sinus tarsi (Fig. 6.4D).
- Replace the extensor digitorum brevis, and close the wound.
- Apply a long leg, non–weight bearing cast.

POSTOPERATIVE CARE The long leg cast is removed at 6 to 8 weeks, and a short leg walking cast is applied and worn for an additional 4 to 6 weeks.

▌TRIPLE ARTHRODESIS

The most effective stabilizing procedure in the foot is triple arthrodesis (Fig. 6.5): fusion of the subtalar, calcaneocuboid, and talonavicular joints. Triple arthrodesis limits motion of the foot and ankle to plantarflexion and dorsiflexion. It is indicated when most of the weakness and deformity are at the subtalar and midtarsal joints. Triple arthrodesis is performed (1) to obtain stable and static realignment of the foot, (2) to remove deforming forces, (3) to arrest progression of deformity, (4) to eliminate pain, (5) to eliminate the use of a short leg brace or to provide sufficient correction to allow fitting of a long leg brace to control the knee joint, and (6) to obtain a more normal-appearing foot. Generally, triple arthrodesis is reserved for severe deformity in children 12 years old and older; occasionally, it may be required in children 8 to 12 years old with progressive, uncontrollable deformity.

The exact technique of triple arthrodesis depends on the type of deformity, and this should be determined before surgery. A paper tracing can be made from a lateral radiograph of the ankle, and the components of the subtalar joint are divided into three sections: the tibiotalar and calcaneal components and another component comprising all the bones of the foot

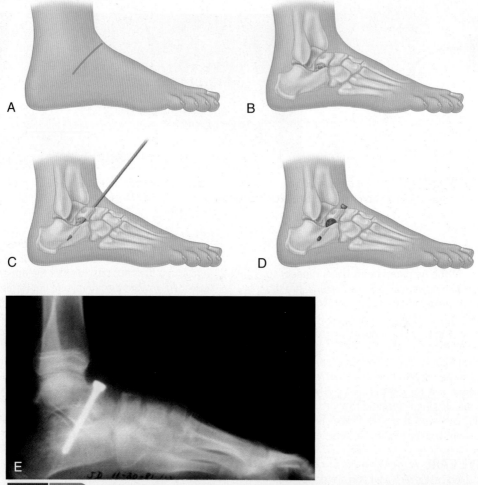

FIGURE 6.4 Subtalar arthrodesis with internal fixation. **A,** Oblique incision over sinus tarsi. **B,** Exposure of sinus tarsi, cancellous bone of calcaneus, and talus. **C,** Steinmann pin is placed across subtalar joint entering talus as far distal as possible with foot held in corrected position. **D,** Screw is placed across subtalar joint from talar neck into calcaneus; sinus tarsi is filled with iliac crest bone graft. **E,** Radiograph of corrected foot with screw in place. **SEE TECHNIQUE 6.3.**

distal to the midtarsal joint. These are reassembled with the foot in the corrected position so that the size and shape of the wedges to be removed can be measured accurately.

In talipes equinovalgus, the medial longitudinal arch of the foot is depressed, the talar head is enlarged and plantarflexed, and the forefoot is abducted. Raising the talar head and shifting the sustentaculum tali medially beneath the talar head and neck restores the arch. A medially based wedge consisting of a portion of the talar head and neck is excised (Fig. 6.5C). When the hindfoot valgus deformity is corrected, the forefoot tends to supinate; this is controlled by midtarsal joint resection with a medially based wedge. An additional medial incision may be required for resection of the talonavicular joint.

In talipes equinovarus, the enlarged talar head lies lateral to the midline axis of the foot and blocks dorsiflexion. A laterally based subtalar wedge, combined with midtarsal joint resection, places the talar head slightly medial to the midline axis of the foot (Fig. 6.5D).

In talipes calcaneocavus, the arthrodesis should allow posterior displacement of the foot at the subtalar joint. After stripping of the plantar fascia, a wedge-shaped or cuneiform

section of bone is removed to allow correction of the cavus deformity, and a wedge of bone is removed from the subtalar joint to correct the rotation of the calcaneus (Fig. 6.5D).

The muscle balance of the foot and ankle determines how much the foot should be displaced posteriorly. Posterior displacement of the foot transfers its fulcrum (the ankle) anteriorly to a position near its center and lengthens its posterior lever arm; this is especially important when the gastrocnemius-soleus group is weak.

TRIPLE ARTHRODESIS

TECHNIQUE 6.4

- Make an oblique incision centered over the sinus tarsi in line with the skin creases on the lateral side of the foot, beginning dorsolaterally at the lateral border of the tendons of the long toe extensors at the level of the talonavicular joint (Fig. 6.5A). Continue the incision posteriorly,

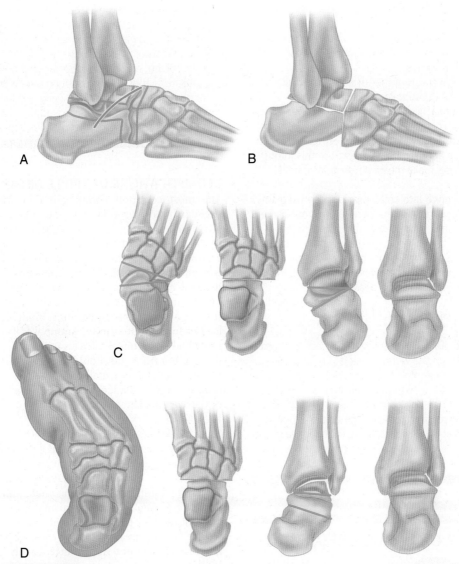

FIGURE 6.5 Triple arthrodesis. **A,** Oblique incision in sinus tarsi to expose subtalar, talonavicular, and calcaneocuboid joints. **B,** Cartilage and cortical bone removed from all joint surfaces; appropriate wedges are removed if necessary. **C,** Wedges necessary for correction of valgus deformity. **D,** Wedges necessary for correction of varus deformity. **SEE TECHNIQUES 6.4 AND 6.5.**

angling plantarward and ending at the level of the peroneal tendons. Carefully protect the extensor and peroneal tendons, and carry the incision sharply down through the sinus tarsi to the extensor digitorum brevis muscle.

- Reflect the origin of this muscle distally along with the fat in the sinus tarsi.
- Clean the remainder of the sinus tarsi of all tissue to expose the subtalar and calcaneocuboid joints and the lateral portion of the talonavicular joint.
- Incise the capsules of the talonavicular, calcaneocuboid, and subtalar joints circumferentially to obtain as much mobility as possible. If this release allows the foot to be placed in a normal position, removal of large bony wedges is not required. If correction is impossible after soft-tissue release, appropriate bone wedges are removed (Fig. 6.5C and D).

- Identify the anterior articular process of the calcaneus and excise it at the level of the floor of the sinus tarsi for better exposure of all joints.
- To make this osteotomy, use an osteotome placed parallel to the plantar surface of the foot; preserve the bone for grafting.
- With an osteotome, remove the articular surfaces of the calcaneocuboid joint to expose cancellous bone.
- Remove an equal amount from both bones unless wedge correction of a bone deformity is required (Fig. 6.5B).
- Remove the distal portion of the head of the talus with ¼-inch and ½-inch straight and curved osteotomes. Remove only enough bone to expose the cancellous bone of the talar head unless a medial wedge is required to correct a fixed deformity. A small lamina spreader can be inserted for better exposure. A second medial incision

may be necessary to expose the most medial portion of the talonavicular joint.

- Remove the proximal articular surface and subchondral bone of the navicular and shape and roughen the surfaces for a snug fit with the talus.
- Excise the articular surfaces of the sustentaculum tali and the anterior facet of the subtalar joint.
- Approach the subtalar joint and completely remove its articular surfaces. For better exposure of the posterior portion, use the small lamina spreader to expose the subtalar joint. Remove appropriate wedges from this joint if necessary; otherwise, make the joint resections parallel to the articular surfaces.
- Cut the removed bone into small pieces to be used for bone grafting. Place most of the bone graft around the talonavicular joint and in the depth of the sinus tarsi.
- Correction is maintained with internal fixation, usually smooth Steinmann pins or Kirschner wires.
- Close the muscle pedicle of the extensor digitorum brevis over the sinus tarsi to reduce the dead space.
- Close the wound over a suction drain and apply a well-padded, short leg cast.

POSTOPERATIVE CARE Considerable bleeding from the drain and through the wound itself can be expected. The foot should be elevated to minimize swelling. The drain is removed at 24 to 48 hours. Walking with crutches or a walker, with touch-down weight bearing on the operated foot, is allowed as tolerated. The cast and pins or wires are removed at 6 to 8 weeks, and a short leg walking cast is applied and worn until union is complete, usually 4 weeks more.

CORRECTION OF CAVUS DEFORMITY

TECHNIQUE 6.5

- Perform a medial radical plantar release to correct the contracted soft tissues bridging the longitudinal arch. Then forcibly correct the cavus deformity as much as possible.
- Expose the calcaneocuboid, talonavicular, and subtalar joints through the incision described earlier.
- With an osteotome, remove from the talonavicular and calcaneocuboid joints a wedge-shaped or cuneiform section of bone with its base anterior and large enough to correct the cavus deformity that remains after the plantar fascial stripping.
- Dorsiflex the forefoot and appose the raw surfaces to see if the cavus is corrected; if so, expose the subtalar joint and remove from it a wedge of bone with its base posterior to correct the deformity or rotation of the calcaneus (see Fig. 6.5D). Be sure that all bone surfaces fit together well and that the foot is in satisfactory position before closing the wound.

POSTOPERATIVE CARE Correction usually is maintained with Steinmann pins or Kirschner wires. A cast is applied, and firm pressure is exerted on the sole of the foot while the plaster is setting to stretch the plantar structures as much as possible. When internal fixation is not used, the cast and sutures are removed at 10 to 14 days, the foot is inspected, and radiographs are made. If the position is not satisfactory, the foot is manipulated with the patient under general anesthesia. A new cast, snug but properly padded, is then applied and is molded to the contour of the foot; this cast is removed at 12 weeks.

COMPLICATIONS OF TRIPLE ARTHRODESIS

The most common complication of triple arthrodesis is pseudarthrosis, especially of the talonavicular joint. The additional stress on the ankle joint caused by loss of mobility of the hindfoot can lead to the development of degenerative arthritis. Excessive resection of the talus can cause osteonecrosis, especially in adolescents; this usually is evident on radiographs 8 to 12 weeks after triple arthrodesis. Ligamentous laxity around the ankle joint may require ankle fusion. Muscle imbalance after hindfoot stabilization can lead to forefoot deformity; unopposed function of the anterior tibial or peroneal muscles is the most common cause of this complication and should be corrected by tendon transfer. Residual deformity usually is caused by insufficient correction at surgery, inadequate immobilization, pseudarthrosis, or muscle imbalance.

TALECTOMY

Talectomy provides stability and posterior displacement of the foot and generally is recommended for children 5 to 12 years old when the deformity is not correctable by arthrodesis. Talectomy limits motion of the ankle joint, especially dorsiflexion, and creates a tibiotarsal ankylosis. Posterior displacement of the foot places the distal tibia over the center of the weight-bearing area, producing even weight distribution and good lateral stability. Appearance usually is satisfactory, pain is relieved, and special shoes or orthoses are not required.

The most common cause of failure of talectomy is muscle imbalance, usually the presence of a strong anterior or posterior tibial muscle. Intrinsic muscle activity can cause contracture of the plantar fascia, resulting in a forefoot equinus deformity. In children younger than 5 years old, recurrence of the deformity is frequent, and pain is common in individuals older than 15 years, especially with inadequate excision of the entire talus. Tibiocalcaneal arthrodesis can be performed for failed talectomy and most commonly is indicated because of persistent pain. The technique of talectomy is described in other chapter.

LAMBRINUDI ARTHRODESIS

The Lambrinudi arthrodesis is recommended for correction of isolated fixed equinus deformity in patients older than 10 years. Retained activity in the gastrocnemius-soleus, combined with inactive dorsiflexors and peroneals, causes the footdrop deformity. The posterior talus abuts the undersurface of the tibia, and the posterior ankle joint capsule contracts to create a fixed equinus deformity. In the Lambrinudi procedure, a wedge of bone is removed from the plantar distal part of the talus so that the talus remains in complete equinus at the ankle joint while the remainder of the foot is repositioned to the desired degree of plantarflexion. Tendon resection or transfer may be necessary to prevent varus or valgus deformity if active muscle power remains. The Lambrinudi arthrodesis is not recommended for a flail foot or when hip or knee instability requires a brace. A good result depends on the strength of the dorsal ankle ligaments. If anterior subluxation of the talus is noted on a weight-bearing lateral radiograph, a two-stage pantalar arthrodesis is recommended. Complications of the Lambrinudi arthrodesis include ankle instability, residual varus or valgus deformities caused by muscle imbalance, and pseudarthrosis of the talonavicular joint.

TECHNIQUE 6.6

(LAMBRINUDI)

- With the foot and ankle in extreme plantarflexion, make a lateral radiograph and trace the film. Cut the tracing into three pieces along the outlines of the subtalar and midtarsal joints; from these pieces the exact amount of bone to be removed from the talus can be determined with accuracy before surgery. In the tracing, the line representing the articulation of the talus with the tibia is left undisturbed but that corresponding to its plantar and distal parts is to be cut so that when the navicular and the calcaneocuboid joint are later fitted to it, the foot will be in 5 to 10 degrees of equinus relative to the tibia (Fig. 6.6) unless the extremity has shortened; more equinus may then be desirable.
- Expose the sinus tarsi through a long, lateral curved incision.
- Section the peroneal tendons by a Z-shaped cut, open the talonavicular and calcaneocuboid joints, and divide the interosseous and lateral collateral ligaments of the ankle to permit complete medial dislocation of the tarsus at the subtalar joint.
- With a small power saw (more accurate than a chisel or osteotome), remove the predetermined wedge of bone from the plantar and distal parts of the neck and body of the talus. Remove the cartilage and bone from the superior surface of the calcaneus to form a plane parallel with the longitudinal axis of the foot.
- Next make a V-shaped trough transversely in the inferior part of the proximal navicular and denude the calcaneocuboid joint of enough bone to correct any lateral deformity.
- Firmly wedge the sharp distal margin of the remaining part of the talus into the prepared trough in the navicular and appose the calcaneus and talus. Take care to place the distal margin of the talus well medially in the trough; otherwise, the position of the foot will not be satisfactory. The talus is now locked in the ankle joint in complete equinus, and the foot cannot be further plantarflexed.
- Insert smooth Kirschner wires for fixation of the talonavicular and calcaneocuboid joints.
- Suture the peroneal tendons, close the wound in the routine manner, and apply a cast with the ankle in neutral or slight dorsiflexion.

POSTOPERATIVE CARE The cast and sutures are removed at 10 to 14 days, and the position of the foot is

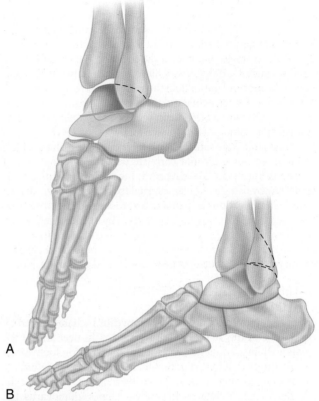

A

B

FIGURE 6.6 Lambrinudi operation for talipes equinus. **A,** *Colored area* indicates part of talus to be resected. **B,** Sharp distal margin of remaining part of talus has been wedged into prepared trough in navicular, and raw osseous surfaces of talus, calcaneus, and cuboid have been apposed. **SEE TECHNIQUE 6.6.**

evaluated by radiographs. If the position is satisfactory, a short leg cast is applied, but weight bearing is not allowed for another 6 weeks, after which a short leg walking cast is applied and is worn until fusion is complete, usually at 3 months.

ANKLE ARTHRODESIS

Ankle fusion may be indicated for a flail foot or for recurrence of deformity after triple arthrodesis. Compression arthrodesis generally is recommended for older children and adolescents. Subcutaneous plantar fasciotomy and lengthening of the Achilles tendon can be performed initially, followed by ankle arthrodesis.

PANTALAR ARTHRODESIS

Pantalar arthrodesis is fusion of the tibiotalar, talonavicular, subtalar, and calcaneocuboid joints. For flail feet with paralyzed quadriceps, pantalar arthrodesis may be indicated to eliminate the need for long leg braces. The ideal patient for this operation is one with a flail foot and ankle and normal muscles around the hip and knee. Absolute prerequisites for this procedure include a strong gluteus maximus to initiate toe-off during gait and a normally aligned knee with full extension or a few degrees of hyperextension.

The ankle should be fused in 5 to 10 degrees of plantarflexion to produce the backward thrust on the knee joint necessary for stable weight bearing. Excessive plantarflexion of the ankle results in pain and increased pressure under the metatarsal heads; acceptable plantarflexion should be confirmed with a lateral radiograph during surgery. Pantalar arthrodesis can be done in two stages: the first in the foot and the second in the ankle because it is difficult to achieve and maintain proper position of the foot and the ankle at the same time. Provelengios et al. described one-stage pantalar arthrodesis in 24 patients (average age, 20 years) with a Steinmann pin used to stabilize the ankle and subtalar joints. At an average follow-up of 37 years, 22 of the 24 patients were satisfied with their outcomes. The position of the fused ankle did not correlate with the development of ipsilateral knee pain. More recently, the authors modified their technique by using a circular external fixator to stabilize all four joints. Complications of pantalar arthrodesis include pseudarthrosis, painful plantar callosities caused by unequal weight distribution, and excessive heel equinus, which causes increased pressure on the forefoot. Provelengios et al. reported a complication rate of 46%, but all were minor wound or skin problems.

■ TENDON TRANSFER TECHNIQUES
▌ TALIPES EQUINOVARUS

Talipes equinovarus caused by poliomyelitis is characterized by equinus deformity of the ankle, inversion of the heel, and, at the midtarsal joints, adduction and supination of the forefoot. When the deformity is of long duration there also is a cavus deformity of the foot; clawing of the toes may develop secondary to substitution of motor patterns. In paralytic talipes equinovarus, the peroneal muscles are paralyzed or severely weakened but the posterior tibial muscle usually is normal; the anterior tibial may be weakened or normal. The gastrocnemius-soleus is comparatively strong but becomes contracted by a combination of motor imbalance, growth, gravity, and posture. Treatment depends on the age of the patient, the forces causing the deformity, the severity of the deformity, and its rate of increase.

Anterior transfer of the posterior tibial tendon removes a dynamic deforming force and aids active dorsiflexion of the foot; however, transfer alone rarely restores active dorsiflexion. Rerouting of the tendon anterior to the medial malleolus diminishes its plantarflexion power and lengthens the posterior tibial muscle; the deformity may not be corrected, however, because the muscle retains its varus pull. The entire tendon can be transferred through the interosseous membrane to the middle cuneiform, or the tendon can be split, with the lateral half transferred to the cuboid.

ANTERIOR TRANSFER OF POSTERIOR TIBIAL TENDON

TECHNIQUE 6.7

(BARR)
- Make a skin incision on the medial side of the ankle, beginning distally at the insertion of the posterior tibial tendon and extending proximally over the tendon just posterior to the malleolus and from there proximally along the medial border of the tibia for 5.0 to 7.5 cm.
- Free the tendon from its insertion, preserving as much of its length as possible.

- Split its sheath, and free it in a proximal direction until the distal 5.0 cm of the muscle has been mobilized. Carefully preserve the nerves and vessels supplying the muscle.
- Make a second skin incision anteriorly; begin it distally at the level of the ankle joint and extend it proximally for 7.5 cm just lateral to the anterior tibial tendon. Carry the dissection deep between the tendons of the anterior tibial muscle and the extensor hallucis longus, carefully preserving the dorsalis pedis artery; expose the interosseous membrane just proximal to the malleoli.
- Cut a generous window in the interosseous membrane but avoid stripping the periosteum from the tibia or fibula.
- Pass the posterior tibial tendon through the window between the bones, taking care that it is not kinked, twisted, or constricted and that the vessels and nerves to the muscle are not damaged. Pass the tendon beneath the cruciate ligament, which can be divided if necessary to relieve pressure on the tendon.
- Expose the third cuneiform or the base of the third metatarsal through a transverse incision 2.5 cm long.
- Retract the extensor tendons, sharply incise the periosteum over the bone in a cruciate fashion, and fold back osteoperiosteal flaps.
- Drill a hole through the bone in line with the tendon and large enough to receive it; anchor it in the bone with a pull-out wire. Be sure that the button on the plantar surface of the foot is well padded.
- Suture the osteoperiosteal flaps to the tendon with two figure-of-eight nonabsorbable sutures.
- Close the incision and apply a plaster cast to hold the foot in calcaneovalgus position.

Instead of the long medial incision used by Barr, we make a short longitudinal one to free the posterior tibial tendon at its insertion and withdraw it through another incision 5 cm long at the musculotendinous junction just posterior to the subcutaneous border of the tibia (Fig. 6.7). The tendon also can be anchored to bone by passing it through a hole drilled in the bone, looping it back, and suturing it to itself with nonabsorbable sutures.

POSTOPERATIVE CARE The cast is removed at 3 weeks, the wounds are inspected, the sutures are removed, and a short leg walking cast is applied with the foot in the neutral position and the ankle in slight dorsiflexion. Six weeks after surgery the cast is removed, and a program of rehabilitative exercises is started that is continued under supervision until a full range of active resisted function is obtained. The transfer is protected for 6 months by a double-bar foot-drop brace with an outside T-strap.

ANTERIOR TRANSFER OF POSTERIOR TIBIAL TENDON

TECHNIQUE 6.8

(OBER)
- Through a medial longitudinal incision 7.5 cm long, free the posterior tibial tendon from its attachment to the navicular (Fig. 6.7A).

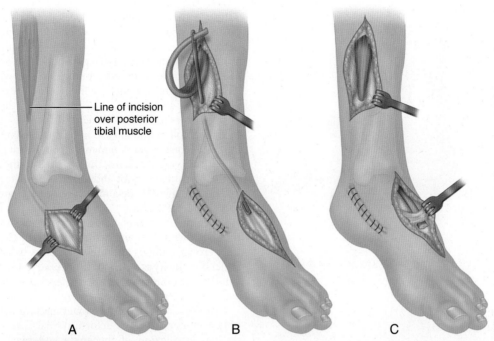

FIGURE 6.7 Ober anterior transfer of posterior tibial tendon. **A,** Insertion of posterior tibial tendon has been exposed. Note line of skin incision over muscle. **B,** Tendon has been freed from its insertion, and muscle has been dissected from tibia. **C,** Tendon and muscle have been passed through anterior tibial compartment to dorsum of foot, and tendon has been anchored in third metatarsal. **SEE TECHNIQUES 6.7 AND 6.8.**

- Make a second longitudinal medial incision 10 cm long centered over the musculotendinous junction of the posterior tibial tendon and muscle.
- Withdraw the tendon from the proximal wound and free the muscle belly well up on the tibia (Fig. 6.7B).
- Strip the periosteum obliquely on the medial surface of the tibia so that when the tendon is moved into the anterior tibial compartment only the belly of the muscle will come in contact with denuded bone. The tendon must not be in contact with the tibia.
- Make a third incision over the base of the third metatarsal, draw the posterior tibial tendon from the second into the third incision, and anchor its distal end in the base of the third metatarsal (Fig. 6.7C).

POSTOPERATIVE CARE Postoperative care is the same as after Technique 6.7.

SPLIT TRANSFER OF ANTERIOR TIBIAL TENDON

TECHNIQUE 6.9

- Make a 2- to 3-cm longitudinal incision dorsomedially over the medial cuneiform (Fig. 6.8A).
- Identify the anterior tibial tendon and split it longitudinally in the midportion. Detach the lateral half of the

tendon from its insertion, preserving as much length as possible, and continue the split proximally to the extent of the incision.
- Make a second 2- to 3-cm incision anteriorly over the distal tibia, identify the tibialis anterior tendon sheath, and split it longitudinally.
- Continue the split in the anterior tibial tendon proximally into this incision and up to the musculotendinous junction. Umbilical tape can be used to continue the split in the tendon. Place the tape into the split and bring its two ends into the proximal incision. Before the lateral half of the tendon is detached, continue the split to the musculotendinous junction by pulling on the tape.
- Once the split in the tendon is complete, detach the lateral half and bring it into the proximal wound.
- Make a third 2- to 3-cm longitudinal incision over the cuboid on the dorsolateral aspect of the foot.
- Drill two holes in the cuboid, placing them as far away from each other as possible so that they meet well within the body of the cuboid (Fig. 6.8B). Enlarge the holes with a curet if necessary, but be certain to leave a bridge of bone between the two holes.
- Pass the split lateral portion of the anterior tibial tendon distally through the subcutaneous tunnel from the proximal incision to the dorsolateral incision over the cuboid.
- Attach a nonabsorbable suture to the end of the tendon, and pass it into one hole in the cuboid and out the other (Fig. 6.8C).
- Hold the foot in dorsiflexion, pull the tendon tight, and suture the free end to the proximal portion of the tendon under moderate tension (Fig. 6.8D).

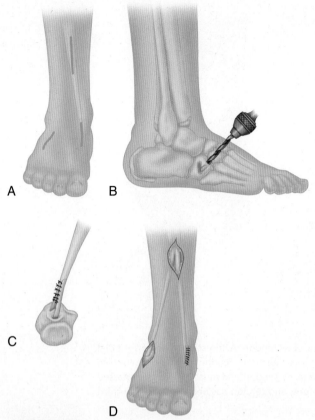

FIGURE 6.8 Split transfer of anterior tibial tendon. **A,** Three incisions: longitudinal over insertion of anterior tibial tendon and longitudinally over distal leg and over cuboid. **B,** Two holes are drilled in cuboid. **C,** Split portion of anterior tibial tendon is pulled into one hole and out the other and sutured to itself. **D,** New split portion of tendon in its redirected position. **SEE TECHNIQUE 6.9.**

- As an alternative, drill a hole in the cuneiform through the plantar cortex, pass the tendon through this hole, and anchor it on the plantar aspect of the foot with a suture over felt and a button.

POSTOPERATIVE CARE A short leg cast is worn for 6 weeks. An ankle-foot orthosis may be needed for 6 months.

SPLIT TRANSFER OF THE POSTERIOR TIBIAL TENDON

The split transfer of the posterior tibial tendon technique is used more often for patients with cerebral palsy and is described in other chapter.

TALIPES CAVOVARUS

Paralytic talipes cavovarus can be caused by an imbalance of the extrinsic muscles or by persistent function of the short toe flexors and other intrinsic muscles when the foot is otherwise flail. Treatment of the cavus foot is discussed in other chapter.

TALIPES EQUINOVALGUS

Talipes equinovalgus usually develops when the anterior and posterior tibial muscles are weak, the peroneus longus and peroneus brevis are strong, and the gastrocnemius-soleus is strong and contracted. The gastrocnemius-soleus pulls the foot into equinus and the peroneals into valgus position; when the extensor digitorum longus and the peroneus tertius muscles are also strong, they help to pull the foot into valgus position on walking. Structural changes in the bones and ligaments follow the muscle imbalance; eventually, the plantar calcaneonavicular ligament becomes stretched and attenuated, the weight-bearing thrust shifts to the medial border of the foot, the forefoot abducts and pronates, and the head and neck of the talus become depressed and prominent on the medial side of the foot.

Treatment of this deformity in a skeletally immature foot is difficult. Subtalar arthrodesis and anterior transfer of the peroneus longus and brevis tendons usually suffice until skeletal maturity is reached; if necessary, a triple arthrodesis can then be done. Failure to transfer the tendons is the usual cause of recurrence.

Paralysis of the anterior tibial muscle alone usually causes only a moderate valgus deformity that is more pronounced during dorsiflexion of the ankle and may disappear during plantarflexion. Treatment of this deformity may require transfer of the peroneus longus to the first cuneiform, transfer of the extensor digitorum longus, or the Jones procedure. Paralysis of the posterior tibial alone can cause a planovalgus deformity. Normally, this muscle inverts the foot during plantarflexion; when it is paralyzed, a valgus deformity develops. Because most of the functions of the foot are performed during plantarflexion, loss of the posterior tibial is a severe impairment. Treatment of this deformity may involve transfer of the peroneus longus tendon, the flexor digitorum longus, the flexor hallucis longus, or the extensor hallucis longus. Paralysis of the anterior tibial and the posterior tibial muscles results in an extreme deformity similar to rocker-bottom flatfoot. For this deformity, a transfer to replace the posterior tibial is necessary, followed by another to replace the anterior tibial if necessary. Extraarticular subtalar arthrodesis may be indicated for equinovalgus deformity in children 4 to 10 years old. The equinus must be corrected by Achilles tendon lengthening at surgery to allow the calcaneus to be brought far enough distally beneath the talus to correct the deformity. The technique of Grice and Green (see Technique 6.2) or preferably of Dennyson and Fulford (see Technique 6.3) can be used. Talipes equinovalgus in skeletally mature patients usually requires triple arthrodesis (see Technique 6.4) and lengthening of the Achilles tendon, followed in 4 to 6 weeks by appropriate tendon transfers.

PERONEAL TENDON TRANSFER

TECHNIQUE 6.10

- Expose the tendons of the peroneus longus and peroneus brevis through an oblique incision paralleling the skin creases at a point midway between the distal tip of the lateral malleolus and the base of the fifth metatarsal.

- Divide the tendons as far distally as possible, securely suture the distal end of the peroneus longus to its sheath to prevent the development of a dorsal bunion, and free the tendons proximally to the posterior border of the lateral malleolus. (When they are to be transferred at the time of arthrodesis, they can be divided through a short extension of the routine incision, as shown in Fig. 6.5.)
- Make a second incision 5 cm long at the junction of the middle and distal thirds of the leg overlying the tendons. Gently withdraw the tendons from their sheaths, taking care not to disrupt the origin of the peroneus brevis muscle.
- The new site of insertion of the peroneal tendons is determined by the severity of the deformity and the existing muscle power. When the extensor hallucis longus is functioning and is to be transferred to the neck of the first metatarsal, the peroneal tendons should be transferred to the lateral cuneiform; when no other functioning dorsiflexor is available, they should be transferred to the middle cuneiform anteriorly.
- Expose the new site of insertion of the tendons through a short longitudinal incision.
- Retract the tendons of the extensor digitorum longus, and make a cruciate or H-shaped cut in the periosteum of the recipient bone.
- Raise and fold back osteoperiosteal flaps and drill a hole in the bone large enough to receive the tendons. Then bring the tendons out beneath the cruciate crural ligament into this incision and anchor them side by side and under equal tension through a hole drilled in the bone, either by suturing them back on themselves or by securely fixing them to bone using a platform staple.
- As an alternative, drill a hole through the middle cuneiform and pull the tendons through the hole and then through a button on the plantar aspect of the foot.
- When there is significant clawing of the great toe, the extensor hallucis longus tendon should be transferred to the neck of the first metatarsal and then the interphalangeal joint is fused (Jones procedure).
- Residual clawing of the lateral four toes usually is of little or no significance after transfer of the peroneal and extensor hallucis longus tendons.

PERONEUS LONGUS, FLEXOR DIGITORUM LONGUS, OR FLEXOR OR EXTENSOR HALLUCIS LONGUS TENDON TRANSFER

TECHNIQUE 6.11

(FRIED AND HENDEL)
- In this operation the tendon of the peroneus longus, flexor digitorum longus, flexor hallucis longus, or extensor hallucis longus can be transferred to replace a paralyzed posterior tibial muscle.
- When the peroneus longus tendon is to be transferred, make a longitudinal incision 5 to 8 cm long laterally over the shaft of the fibula.

- After incising the fascia of the peroneal muscles, inspect them; if their color does not confirm their preoperative grading, the transfer will fail.
- Now make a second incision along the lateral border of the foot over the cuboid and the peroneus longus tendon.
- Free the tendon, divide it as far distally in the sole of the foot as possible, suture its distal end in its sheath, and withdraw the tendon through the first incision.
- By blunt dissection create a space between the gastrocnemius-soleus and the deep layer of leg muscles; from here make a wide tunnel posterior to the fibula and to the deep muscles and directed to a point proximal and posterior to the medial malleolus.
- Now make a small incision at this point, and draw the peroneus longus tendon through the tunnel; it now emerges where the posterior tibial tendon enters its sheath.
- Make a fourth incision 5 cm long over the middle of the medial side of the foot centered below the tuberosity of the navicular.
- Free and retract plantarward the anterior border of the abductor hallucis muscle, and expose the tuberosity of the navicular and the insertion of the posterior tibial tendon; proximal to the medial malleolus, open the sheath of this tendon, and into it introduce and advance a curved probe until it emerges with the tendon at the sole of the foot.
- Using the probe, pull the peroneus longus tendon through the same sheath, which is large enough to contain this second tendon.
- Drill a narrow tunnel through the navicular, beginning on its plantar surface lateral to the tuberosity and emerging through its anterior surface.
- Pull the peroneus longus tendon through the tunnel in an anterior direction and anchor it with a Bunnell pull-out suture. Also, suture it to the posterior tibial tendon close to its insertion.
- Close the wounds, and apply a short leg cast with the foot in slight equinus and varus position.
- When the flexor digitorum longus tendon is to be transferred, make the incision near the medial malleolus as just described but extend it for about 7 cm.
- Free the three deep muscles and observe their color; if it is satisfactory, make the incision on the medial side of the foot as just described.
- Free and retract the short plantar muscles and expose the flexor digitorum longus tendon as it emerges from behind the medial malleolus.
- Free the tendon as far distally as possible, divide it, and withdraw it through the first incision; now pass it through the sheath of the posterior tibial tendon and anchor it in the navicular as just described.
- When the flexor hallucis longus tendon is to be transferred, use the same procedure as described for the flexor digitorum longus.
- When the extensor hallucis longus tendon is to be transferred, cut it near the metatarsophalangeal joint of the great toe.
- Suture its distal end to the long extensor tendon of the second toe.
- Withdraw the proximal end through an anterolateral longitudinal incision over the distal part of the leg.

- Open the interosseous membrane widely, make the incision near the medial malleolus as previously described, and with a broad probe draw the tendon through the interosseous space and through the sheath of the posterior tibial tendon to the insertion of that tendon.
- Then continue with the operation as described for transfer of the peroneus longus tendon.

POSTOPERATIVE CARE A short leg walking cast is applied. At 6 weeks the walking cast is removed, a splint is used at night, and muscle reeducation is started.

▌TALIPES CALCANEUS

Talipes calcaneus is a rapidly progressive paralytic deformity that results when the gastrocnemius-soleus is paralyzed and the other extrinsic foot muscles, especially the muscles that dorsiflex the ankle, remain functional. Mild deformity in skeletally immature patients should be treated conservatively with braces or orthoses until the rate of progression of the deformity can be determined. For rapidly progressing deformities, especially in young children, early tendon transfers are recommended. The goal of surgery in the skeletally immature foot is to stop progression of the deformity or to correct severe deformity without damaging skeletal growth; arthrodesis may be necessary after skeletal maturity. If muscles of adequate power are available, tendons should be transferred early to improve function and avoid progressive deformity. If adequate muscles are unavailable, tenodesis of the Achilles tendon to the fibula may be appropriate.

The calcaneotibial angle (Fig. 6.9) is formed by the intersection of the axis of the tibia with a line drawn along the plantar aspect of the calcaneus. Normally, this angle measures between 70 and 80 degrees; in equinus deformity it is greater than 80 degrees, and in calcaneal deformity it is less than 70

degrees. When the tenodesis is fixed at 70 degrees or more at the time of surgery, a tendency to develop a progressive equinus deformity with growth has been noted. Progressive equinus also is directly related to the patient's age at surgery: the younger the patient, the greater the calcaneotibial angle and the more likely the development of progressive equinus deformity with subsequent growth.

In skeletally mature feet, initial surgery for talipes calcaneus consists of plantar fasciotomy and triple arthrodesis that corrects the calcaneus and the cavus deformities; the arthrodesis should displace the foot as far posteriorly as possible to lengthen its posterior lever arm (the calcaneus) and reduce the muscle power required to lift the heel. Six weeks after arthrodesis, the tendons of the peroneus longus and peroneus brevis and the posterior tibial tendon are transferred to the calcaneus; and when the extensor digitorum longus is functional, it can be transferred to a cuneiform and then the anterior tibial tendon can be transferred to the calcaneus.

TENODESIS OF THE ACHILLES TENDON

TECHNIQUE 6.12

(WESTIN)
- With the patient supine and tilted toward the nonoperative side, apply and inflate a pneumatic tourniquet.
- Make a posterolateral longitudinal incision just behind the posterior border of the fibula beginning 7 to 10 cm above the tip of the lateral malleolus and extending distally to the insertion of the Achilles tendon on the calcaneus.
- Expose the tendon and section it transversely at the musculotendinous junction, usually 6 cm from its insertion. Stevens advised that the tendon be split eccentrically, leaving the lateral one fifth to prevent retraction. Transect the medial four fifths proximally.
- Expose the peroneus brevis and longus tendons, and if they are completely paralyzed or spastic, excise them. Expose the distal fibula, taking care not to damage the distal fibular physis.
- About 4 cm proximal to the distal physis, use a fine drill bit to make a transverse hole in an anteroposterior direction. Make the hole large enough for the Achilles tendon to pass through it easily (Fig. 6.10A).
- If the tendon is too large, trim it longitudinally for about 2.5 cm. Bring the tendon through the hole, and suture it to itself under enough tension to limit ankle dorsiflexion to 0 degrees (Fig. 6.10B). Do not suture the tendon with the foot in too much equinus because of the possibility of causing a fixed equinus deformity.
- In patients with active anterior tibial tendons, simultaneous transfer of this tendon through the interosseous membrane to the calcaneus is indicated to avoid stretching of the Achilles tendon after surgery (Fig. 6.10C).

POSTOPERATIVE CARE Weight bearing is allowed in a short leg cast with the ankle in 5 to 10 degrees of equinus.

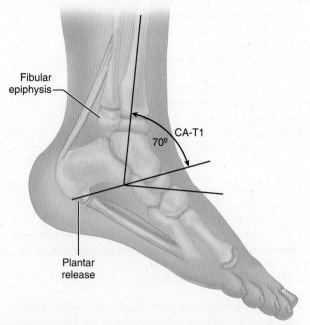

Fibular epiphysis

CA-T1

70°

Plantar release

FIGURE 6.9 Measurement of calcaneotibial angle (see text).

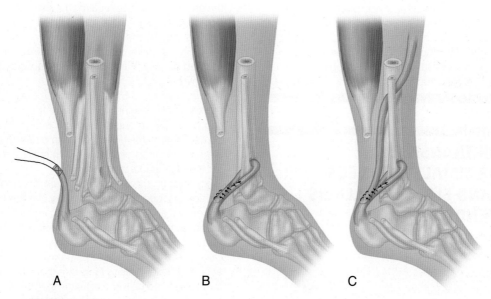

FIGURE 6.10 Calcaneal tenodesis. **A,** After division of Achilles tendon, tenotomy of peroneus brevis and longus, and detachment of anterior tibial tendon from its insertion, transverse hole is made in fibula 2 cm proximal to epiphysis. **B,** Achilles tendon is passed through hole in fibula and sutured to itself. **C,** If necessary, anterior tibial tendon can be passed through interosseous membrane and attached to calcaneus. **SEE TECHNIQUE 6.12.**

The cast is removed at 6 weeks, and an ankle-foot orthosis is fitted with the ankle in neutral position. Any residual cavus deformity is corrected by plantar release 3 to 6 months after tenodesis.

In skeletally mature feet, initial surgery for talipes calcaneus consists of plantar fasciotomy and triple arthrodesis that corrects both the calcaneus and cavus deformities; the arthrodesis should displace the foot as far posteriorly as possible to lengthen its posterior lever arm (the calcaneus) and reduce the muscle power required to lift the heel. Six weeks after arthrodesis, the tendons of the peroneus longus and peroneus brevis and the posterior tibial muscles are transferred to the calcaneus, and when the extensor digitorum longus is functional, it can be transferred to a cuneiform and then the anterior tibial muscle can be transferred to the calcaneus.

POSTERIOR TRANSFER OF PERONEUS LONGUS, PERONEUS BREVIS, AND POSTERIOR TIBIAL TENDONS

TECHNIQUE 6.13

- Expose the peroneus longus and peroneus brevis tendons through an oblique incision 2.5 cm long midway between the tip of the lateral malleolus and the base of the fifth metatarsal.
- Divide the tendons as far distally as possible and securely suture the distal end of the peroneus longus tendon to its sheath.
- Bring the tendons out through a second incision overlying the peroneal sheath at the junction of the middle and distal thirds of the leg.
- If desired, suture the peroneus brevis at its musculotendinous junction to the peroneus longus tendon and discard the distal end of the peroneus brevis tendon.
- Expose the posterior tibial tendon through a short incision over its insertion; free its distal end, and gently bring it out through a second incision 2.5 cm long at its musculotendinous junction 5 cm proximal to the medial malleolus.
- Reroute all three tendons subcutaneously to and out of a separate incision lateral and anterior to the insertion of the Achilles tendon.
- Drill a hole in the superior surface of the posterior part of the calcaneus just lateral to the midline of the bone and enlarge it enough to receive the tendons; anchor the tendons in the hole with a large pull-out suture while holding the foot in equinus and the heel in the corrected position. An axial pin also can be inserted into the calcaneus and left in place for 6 weeks.
- With interrupted figure-of-eight sutures, fix the tendons to the Achilles tendon near its insertion; then close the wounds.

POSTOPERATIVE CARE The foot is immobilized in a long leg cast with the ankle in plantarflexion and the knee at 20 degrees. The pull-out sutures and cast (and axial pin, if used) are removed at 6 weeks, and physical therapy is started. Weight bearing is not allowed until active plantar flexion is possible and dorsiflexion to the neutral position has been regained. The foot is protected for at least 6 more months by a reverse 90-degree ankle stop brace and an appropriate heel elevation.

POSTERIOR TRANSFER OF POSTERIOR TIBIAL, PERONEUS LONGUS, AND FLEXOR HALLUCIS LONGUS TENDONS

TECHNIQUE 6.14

(GREEN AND GRICE)

- Place the patient prone for easier access to the heel.
- First, expose the posterior tibial tendon through an oblique incision 3 or 4 cm long from just inferior to the medial malleolus to the plantar aspect of the talonavicular joint; open its sheath, and divide it as close to bone as possible for maximal length.
- Remove the epitenon from its distal 3 or 4 cm, scarify it, and insert a 1-0 or 2-0 braided nonabsorbable suture into its distal end.
- When the flexor hallucis longus tendon also is to be transferred, expose it through this same incision where it lies posterior and lateral to the flexor digitorum longus tendon.
- At the proper level for the desired tendon length, place two braided nonabsorbable sutures in the flexor hallucis longus tendon and divide it between them; suture the distal end of this tendon to the flexor digitorum longus tendon.
- Second, make a longitudinal medial incision, usually about 10 cm long, over the posterior tibial muscle, extending distally from the junction of the middle and distal thirds of the leg.
- Open the medial compartment of the leg, and identify the posterior tibial and flexor hallucis longus muscle bellies.
- Using moist sponges, deliver the tendons of these two muscles into this wound.
- Third, make an incision parallel to the bottom of the foot from about a fingerbreadth distal to the lateral malleolus to the base of the fifth metatarsal.
- Expose the peroneus longus and peroneus brevis tendons throughout the length of the incision and divide that of the peroneus longus between sutures as far distally as possible in the sole of the foot and free its proximal end to behind the lateral malleolus.
- Place a suture in the peroneus brevis tendon, detach it from its insertion on the fifth metatarsal, and suture it to the distal end of the peroneus longus tendon.
- Make a lateral longitudinal incision over the posterior aspect of the fibula at the same level as the medial incision and deliver the peroneus longus tendon into it.
- Make a posterolateral transverse incision 6 cm long over the calcaneus in the part of the heel that neither strikes

the ground nor presses against the shoe. Deepen the incision, reflect the skin flaps subcutaneously, and expose the Achilles tendon and calcaneus.
- Beginning laterally, partially divide the Achilles tendon at its insertion and reflect it medially, exposing the calcaneal apophysis.
- With a 9/64-inch (3.57-mm) drill bit, make a hole through the calcaneus beginning in the center of its apophysis and emerging through its plantar aspect near its lateral border. Enlarge the hole enough to receive the three tendons and ream its posterior end to make a shallow facet for their easier insertion.
- Next, through the medial wound on the leg (the second incision), incise widely the intermuscular septum between the medial and posterior compartments; insert a tendon passer through the wound and along the anterior side of the Achilles tendon to the transverse incision over the calcaneus. Thread the sutures in the ends of the posterior tibial and flexor hallucis longus tendons through the tendon passer and deliver the tendons at the heel.
- Through the lateral wound on the leg (the fourth incision), open widely the intermuscular septum between the medial and posterior compartments in this area and pass the peroneus longus tendon to the heel.
- Pass all tendons through smooth tissues in a straight line from as far proximally as possible to avoid angulation.
- With a twisted wire probe, bring the tendons through the hole in the calcaneus; suture them to the periosteum and ligamentous attachments where they emerge.
- When the dorsiflexors are weak, suture them under enough tension to hold the foot in 10 to 15 degrees of equinus, and when they are strong, suture them in about 30 degrees of equinus. Also, suture the tendons to the apophysis at the proximal end of the tunnel and to each other with 2-0 or 3-0 sutures.
- Replace the Achilles tendon posterior to the transferred tendons and suture it in its original position.
- Close the wounds, and apply a long leg cast with the foot in equinus.

POSTOPERATIVE CARE At 3 weeks, the cast is bivalved and exercises are started with the leg in the anterior half of the cast; the bivalved cast is reapplied between exercise periods. At first, dorsiflexion exercises are not permitted, but, later, guided reciprocal motion is allowed. The exercises are gradually increased, and at 6 weeks the patient is allowed to stand but not to bear full weight on the foot. The periods of partial weight bearing on crutches are increased, depending on the effectiveness of the transfer, the cooperation of the patient, and the ability to control his or her motions. Usually at 6 to 8 weeks a single step is allowed, using crutches and an elevated heel; later more steps are allowed, using crutches and a plantarflexion spring brace with an elastic strap posteriorly. Crutches are used for 6 to 12 months.

KNEE

The disabilities caused by paralysis of the muscles acting across the knee joint include (1) flexion contracture of the knee, (2) quadriceps paralysis, (3) genu recurvatum, and (4) flail knee.

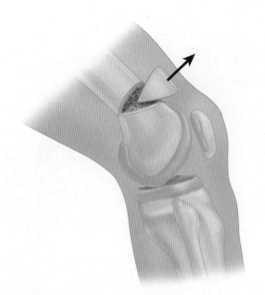

FIGURE 6.11 Supracondylar extension osteotomy of femur for fixed knee flexion deformity in older child.

■ FLEXION CONTRACTURE OF THE KNEE

Flexion contracture of the knee can be caused by a contracture of the iliotibial band; contracture of this band can cause not only flexion contracture but also genu valgum and an external rotation deformity of the tibia on the femur. Flexion contracture also can be caused by paralysis of the quadriceps muscle when the hamstrings are normal or only partially paralyzed. When the biceps femoris is stronger than the medial hamstrings, there may be genu valgum and an external rotation deformity of the tibia on the femur; often the tibia subluxates posteriorly on the femur.

Contractures of 15 to 20 degrees or less in young children can be treated with posterior hamstring lengthening and capsulotomy. More severe contractures usually require a supracondylar extension osteotomy of the femur (Fig. 6.11).

Flexion contractures of more than 70 degrees result in deformity of the articular surfaces of the knee. In a growing child with poliomyelitis, a decrease in pressure and a tendency toward posterior subluxation cause increased growth on the anterior surface of the proximal tibia and distal femur. The quadriceps expansion adheres to the femoral condyles, and the collateral ligaments are unable to glide easily. Severe knee flexion contractures in growing children can be treated by division of the iliotibial band and hamstring tendons, combined with posterior capsulotomy. Skeletal traction after surgery is maintained through a pin in the distal tibia; a second pin in the proximal tibia pulls anteriorly to avoid posterior subluxation of the tibia. Long-term use of a long leg brace may be required to allow the joint to remodel. Supracondylar osteotomy may be required as a second-stage procedure in older patients near skeletal maturity.

■ QUADRICEPS PARALYSIS

Disability from paralysis of the quadriceps muscle is severe because the knee may be extremely unstable, especially if there is even a mild fixed flexion contracture. When there is slight recurvatum, the knee may be stable if the gastrocnemius-soleus is active.

Tendons usually are transferred around the knee joint to reinforce a weak or paralyzed quadriceps muscle; transfers are unnecessary for paralysis of the hamstring muscles because, in walking, gravity flexes the knee as the hip is flexed. Several muscles are available for transfer to the quadriceps tendon and patella: the biceps femoris, semitendinosus, sartorius, and tensor fasciae latae. When the power of certain other muscles is satisfactory, transfer of the biceps femoris has been the most successful. Transfer of one or more of the hamstring tendons is contraindicated unless one other flexor in the thigh and the gastrocnemius-soleus, which also acts as a knee flexor, are functioning. If a satisfactory result is to be expected after hamstring transfer, the power not only of the hamstrings but also of the hip flexors, the gluteus maximus, and the gastrocnemius-soleus must be fair or better; when the power of the hip flexor muscles are less than fair, clearing the extremity from the floor may be difficult after surgery. Transfer of the tensor fasciae latae and sartorius muscles, although theoretically more satisfactory, is insufficient because these muscles are not strong enough to replace the quadriceps.

Ease in ascending or descending steps depends on the strength of the hip flexors and extensors. Strong hamstrings are necessary for active extension of the knee against gravity after the transfer; however, a weak medial hamstring can be transferred to serve as a checkrein on the patella to prevent it from dislocating laterally. A normal gastrocnemius-soleus is desirable because it aids in preventing genu recurvatum and remains as an active knee flexor after surgery; it may not always prevent genu recurvatum, however, which can result from other factors. Recurvatum after hamstring transfers can be kept to a minimum if (1) strength in the gastrocnemius-soleus is fair or better; (2) the knee is not immobilized in hyperextension after surgery; (3) talipes equinus, when present, is corrected before weight bearing is resumed; (4) postoperative bracing is used to prevent knee hyperextension; and (5) physical therapy is begun to promote active knee extension.

TRANSFER OF BICEPS FEMORIS AND SEMITENDINOSUS TENDONS

TECHNIQUE 6.15

- Make an incision along the anteromedial aspect of the knee to conform to the medial border of the quadriceps tendon, the patella, and the patellar tendon.
- Retract the lateral edge of the incision, and expose the patella and the quadriceps tendon.
- Incise longitudinally the lateral side of the thigh and leg from a point 7.5 cm distal to the head of the fibula to the junction of the proximal and middle thirds of the thigh.
- Isolate and retract the common peroneal nerve, which is near the medial side of the biceps tendon.
- With an osteotome, free the biceps tendon, along with a thin piece of bone, from the head of the fibula. Do not divide the lateral collateral ligament, which lies firmly adherent to the biceps tendon at its point of insertion.
- Free the tendon and its muscle belly proximally as far as the incision will permit; free the origin of the short head

of the biceps proximally to where its nerve and blood supplies enter so that the new line of pull of the muscle may be as oblique as possible.

- Create a subcutaneous tunnel from the first incision to the lateral thigh incision, and make it wide enough for the transferred muscle belly to glide freely.
- To further increase the obliquity of pull of the transferred muscle, divide the iliotibial band, the fascia of the vastus lateralis, and the lateral intermuscular septum at a point distal to where the muscle will pass.
- Beginning distally over the insertion of the medial hamstring tendons into the tibia, make a third incision longitudinally along the posteromedial aspect of the knee and extend it to the middle of the thigh.
- Locate the semitendinosus tendon; it inserts on the medial side of the tibia as far anteriorly as its crest and lies posterior to the tendon of the sartorius and distal to that of the gracilis. Divide the insertion of the semitendinosus tendon and free the muscle to the middle third of the thigh.
- Reroute this muscle and tendon subcutaneously to emerge in the first incision over the knee.
- Make an I-shaped incision through the fascia, quadriceps tendon, and periosteum over the anterior surface of the patella, and strip these tissues medially and laterally. With an 11/64-inch (4.36-mm) drill bit, make a hole transversely through the patella at the junction of its middle and proximal thirds; if necessary, enlarge the tunnel with a small curet.
- Place the biceps tendon in line with and anterior to the quadriceps tendon, the patella, and the patellar tendon.
- Suture the biceps tendon to the patella with the knee in extension or hyperextension.
- When only the biceps tendon is transferred, close the soft tissues over the anterior aspect of the patella and the transferred tendon. With interrupted sutures, fix the biceps tendon to the medial side of the quadriceps tendon.
- When the semitendinosus also is transferred, place it over the biceps and suture the two together with interrupted sutures; place additional sutures proximally and distally through the semitendinosus, quadriceps, and patellar tendons.
- Alternatively, detach the insertion of the semitendinosus from the tibia through an incision 2.5 cm long and bring it out through a posteromedial incision 7.5 cm long over its musculotendinous junction (Fig. 6.12). Incise the enveloping fascia to prevent acute angulation of the muscle, and pass the tendon subcutaneously in a straight line to the patellar incision.

POSTOPERATIVE CARE With the knee in the neutral position, a long leg cast is applied. To prevent swelling, the extremity is elevated by raising the foot of the bed rather than by using pillows; otherwise, flexion of the hip may put too much tension on the transferred tendons. At 3 weeks, physical therapy and active and passive exercises are started. Knee flexion is gradually developed, and the hamstring muscles are reeducated. At 8 weeks, weight bearing is started, with the extremity supported by a controlled dial knee brace locked in extension. Knee motion is gradually allowed in the brace when the muscles of the transferred tendons are strong enough to extend the knee

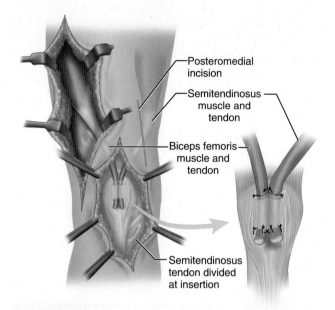

FIGURE 6.12 Transfer of semitendinosus and biceps femoris tendons to patella for quadriceps paralysis. **SEE TECHNIQUE 6.15.**

actively against considerable force. To prevent overstretching or strain of the muscles, a night splint is worn for at least 6 weeks and the brace for at least 12 weeks.

GENU RECURVATUM

In genu recurvatum the deformity is the opposite of that in a flexion contracture and the knee is hyperextended. Mild genu recurvatum can cause some disability, but when the quadriceps is severely weakened or paralyzed, such a deformity is desirable because it stabilizes the knee in walking. Severe genu recurvatum is significantly disabling, however.

Genu recurvatum from poliomyelitis is of two types: that caused by structural articular and bone changes stemming from lack of power in the quadriceps and that caused by relaxation of the soft tissues around the posterior aspect of the knee. In the first type, the quadriceps lacks the power to lock the knee in extension; the hamstrings and gastrocnemius-soleus usually are normal. The pressures of weight bearing and gravity cause changes in the tibial condyles and in the proximal third of the tibial shaft. The condyles become elongated posteriorly; their anterior margins are depressed compared with their posterior margins; and the angle of their articular surfaces to the long axis of the tibia, which is normally 90 degrees, becomes more acute. The proximal third of the tibial shaft usually bows posteriorly, and partial subluxation of the tibia may gradually occur. In the second type, the hamstrings and the gastrocnemius-soleus muscles are weak. Hyperextension of the knee results from stretching of these muscles, often followed by stretching of the posterior capsular ligament.

The prognosis after correction of the first type of recurvatum is excellent. The skeletal deformity is corrected first, and then one or more hamstrings can be transferred to the patella. Irwin described an osteotomy of the proximal tibia to correct the first type of genu recurvatum caused by structural bone changes. Storen modified the Campbell osteotomy by immobilizing the fragments of the tibia with a Charnley clamp.

OSTEOTOMY OF THE TIBIA FOR GENU RECURVATUM

TECHNIQUE 6.16

(IRWIN)

- Through a short longitudinal incision, remove a section of the shaft of the fibula about 2.5 cm long from just distal to the neck.
- Pack the defect with chips from the sectioned piece of bone.
- Close the periosteum and overlying soft tissues.
- Through an anteromedial incision, expose and, without entering the joint, osteotomize the proximal fourth of the tibia as follows: With a thin osteotome or a power saw, outline a tongue of bone but leave it attached to the anterior cortex of the distal fragment. At a right angle to the longitudinal axis of the knee joint and parallel to its lateral plane, pass a Kirschner wire through the distal end of the proposed proximal fragment before the tibial shaft is divided. Complete the osteotomy with a Gigli saw, an osteotome, or a power saw.
- Lift the proximal end of the distal fragment from its periosteal bed, and remove from it a wedge of bone of predetermined size, its base being the posterior cortex.
- Replace the tongue of bone in its recess in the proximal fragment, and push the fragments firmly together.
- Suture the periosteum, which is quite thick in this area, firmly over the tongue of bone; this is enough fixation to keep the fragments in position until a cast can be applied.

The osteotomy can be fixed with percutaneous Kirschner wires, an external fixator, or, in adults, rigid plate fixation. Figure 6.13 shows correction of genu recurvatum by the Campbell technique.

SOFT-TISSUE OPERATIONS FOR GENU RECURVATUM

Another type of genu recurvatum results from stretching of the posterior soft tissues. The prognosis is less certain after correction of this type of deformity; no muscles are available for transfer, the underlying cause cannot be corrected, and the deformity can recur. An operation on the soft tissues, triple tenodesis of the knee, has been described for correcting paralytic genu recurvatum. If the deformity is 30 degrees or less, prolonged bracing of the knee in flexion usually prevents an increase in deformity. When the deformity is severe, however, bracing is ineffective, the knee becomes unstable and weak, the gait is inefficient, and, in adults, pain is marked. The three following principles must be considered if operations on the soft tissues for genu recurvatum are to be successful:

1. The fibrous tissue mass used for tenodesis must be sufficient to withstand the stretching forces generated by walking; all available tendons must be used.
2. Healing tissues must be protected until they are fully mature. The operation should not be undertaken unless the surgeon is sure that the patient will conscientiously use a brace that limits extension to 15 degrees of flexion for 1 year.
3. The alignment and stability of the ankle must meet the basic requirements of gait. Any equinus deformity must be corrected to at least neutral. If the strength of the soleus is less than good on the standing test, this defect must be corrected by tendon transfer, tenodesis, or arthrodesis of the ankle in the neutral position.

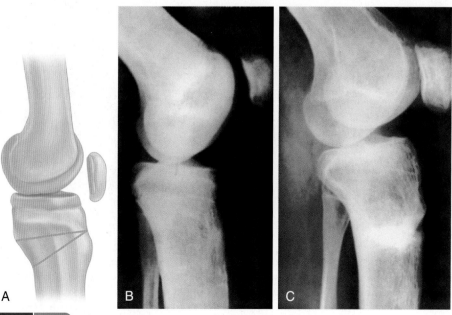

FIGURE 6.13   Closing wedge osteotomy for genu recurvatum. **A,** Wedge of bone removed from tibia. **B,** Recurvatum secondary to anterior tilt of tibial plateau. **C,** Five months after operation. **SEE TECHNIQUE 6.16.**

TRIPLE TENODESIS FOR GENU RECURVATUM

The operation for triple tenodesis for genu recurvatum consists of three parts: proximal advancement of the posterior capsule of the knee with the joint flexed 20 degrees, construction of a checkrein in the midline posteriorly using the tendons of the semitendinosus and gracilis, and creation of two diagonal straps posteriorly using the biceps tendon and the anterior half of the iliotibial band.

TECHNIQUE 6.17

(PERRY, O'BRIEN, AND HODGSON)
- Place the patient prone, apply a tourniquet high on the thigh, and place a large sandbag beneath the ankle to flex the knee about 20 degrees.
- Make an S-shaped incision beginning laterally parallel to and 1 cm anterior to the biceps tendon; extend it distally 4 cm to the transverse flexion crease of the knee, carry it medially across the popliteal fossa, and extend it distally for 4 or 5 cm overlying or just medial to the semitendinosus tendon.
- Identify the sural nerve and retract it laterally. Then identify the tibial nerve and the popliteal artery and vein, and protect them with a soft rubber tape. Next, identify and free the peroneal nerve and protect it in a similar manner. Retract the neurovascular bundle laterally and identify the posterior part of the joint capsule.
- Detach the medial head of the gastrocnemius muscle in a step-cut fashion, preserving a long, strong proximal strap of the Z to be used in the tenodesis (Fig. 6.14A).
- Next, use a knife to detach the joint capsule from its attachment to the femur just proximal to the condyles and the intercondylar notch.

- Detach the tendons of the gracilis and semitendinosus at their musculotendinous junctions, and suture their proximal ends to the sartorius. Be sure to divide these tendons as far proximally as possible because all available length will be needed.
- Next, drill a hole in the tibia, beginning at a point in the midline posteriorly inferior to the physis and emerging near the insertion of the pes anserinus; take care to avoid the physis.
- Drill a hole in the femur, beginning in the midline posteriorly proximal to the femoral physis and emerging on the lateral aspect of the distal femur (Fig. 6.14B).
- Draw the tendons of the gracilis and semitendinosus through the hole in the tibia, pass them posterior to the detached part of the capsule, and pull them through the hole in the femur to emerge on the lateral aspect of the distal femur; suture the tendons to the periosteum here under moderate tension with heavy nonabsorbable sutures with the knee flexed 20 degrees.
- Advance the free edge of the joint capsule proximally on the femur until all slack has disappeared and suture it to the periosteum in its new position using nonabsorbable sutures.
- Detach the biceps tendon from its muscle, rotate it on its fibular insertion, pass it across the posterior aspect of the joint deep to the neurovascular structures, and anchor it to the femoral origin of the medial head of the gastrocnemius under moderate tension (Fig. 6.14C).
- Detach the anterior half of the iliotibial band from its insertion on the tibia, pass it deep to the intact part of the band, the biceps tendon, and the neurovascular structures, and suture it to the semimembranosus insertion on the tibia under moderate tension.

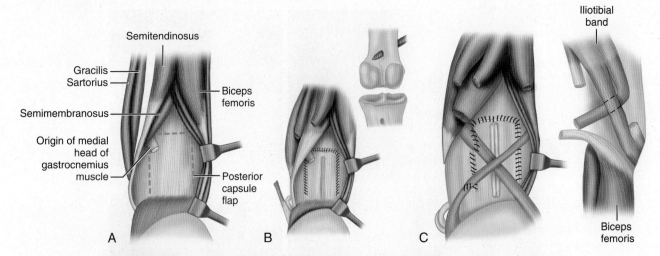

FIGURE 6.14 Perry, O'Brien, and Hodgson operation for genu recurvatum. **A,** Origin of medial head of gastrocnemius has been released, leaving proximal strap. Broad flap of posterior capsule is released for future advancement. **B,** Semitendinosus and gracilis tendons are divided at musculotendinous junctions. Each is passed through tunnel in tibia, then across exterior of joint, and then through tunnel in femur. Flap of posterior capsule is advanced and sutured snugly with knee flexed 20 degrees. **C,** Cross straps are made with biceps femoris and iliotibial band. **SEE TECHNIQUE 6.17.**

- If one of the tendons being used is of an active muscle, split that tendon and use only half of it in the tenodesis, leaving the other half attached at its insertion.
- Close the wound in layers, and use suction drainage for 48 hours. Apply a well-padded cast from groin to toes with the knee flexed 30 degrees to prevent tension on the sutures.

POSTOPERATIVE CARE The cast is removed at 6 weeks, and a long leg brace that was fitted before surgery is applied. The brace is designed to limit extension of the knee to 15 degrees of flexion. Full weight bearing is allowed in the brace, and at night a plaster shell is used to hold the knee flexed 15 degrees. Twelve months after surgery the patient is readmitted to the hospital and the flexion contracture of the knee is corrected gradually to neutral by serial plaster casts; unprotected weight bearing is then permitted. It is important that the soft tissues are completely healed before being subjected to excessive stretching caused by unprotected weight bearing or by wedging plaster casts.

■ FLAIL KNEE

When the knee is unstable in all directions, and muscle power sufficient to overcome this instability is unavailable for tendon transfer, either a long leg brace with a locking knee joint must be worn or the knee must be fused. Fusion of the knee in a good position not only permits a satisfactory gait but also improves it by eliminating the weight of the brace; fusion of the knee causes inconvenience while sitting. One option is to defer fusion until the patient is old enough to weigh its advantages and disadvantages before a final decision is made. For patients who are heavy laborers and would have trouble maintaining a brace, the advantages of being free of a brace outweigh the advantages of being able to sit with the knee flexed in a brace; in these patients, an arthrodesis is indicated. Others who sit much of the time may prefer to use a brace permanently. When both legs are badly paralyzed, one knee can be fused and the other stabilized with a brace.

Before an arthrodesis is performed, a cylinder cast can be applied on a trial basis, immobilizing the knee in the position in which it would be fused; this allows the patient to make an informed decision concerning the advantages and disadvantages of arthrodesis of the knee. The techniques of knee fusion are described in other chapter.

TIBIA AND FEMUR

Angular and torsional deformities of the tibia and femur are more often caused by conditions other than poliomyelitis, such as congenital abnormalities, metabolic disorders, or trauma, and the various osteotomies used for their treatment are discussed in chapters 1 and 8.

HIP

Paralysis of the muscles around the hip can cause severe impairment. This impairment may include flexion and abduction contractures of the hip, hip instability and limping caused by paralysis of the gluteus maximus and medius muscles, and paralytic hip dislocation.

■ FLEXION AND ABDUCTION CONTRACTURES OF THE HIP

An abduction contracture is the most common deformity associated with paralysis of the muscles around the hip; it usually occurs in conjunction with flexion and external rotation contractures of varying degrees. Less often, a contracture of the hip may occur that consists of adduction with flexion and internal rotation. When contractures of the hip are severe and bilateral, locomotion is possible only as a quadruped; the upright position is possible after the contractures have been released.

Spasm of the hamstrings, hip flexors, tensor fasciae latae, and hip abductors is common during the acute and convalescent stages of poliomyelitis. Straight-leg raising usually is limited. The patient assumes the frog position, with the knees and hips flexed and the extremities completely externally rotated. When this position is maintained for even a few weeks, secondary soft-tissue contractures occur; a permanent deformity develops, especially when the gluteal muscles have been weakened. The deformity puts the gluteus maximus at a disadvantage and prevents its return to normal strength. If the faulty position is not corrected, growth of the contracted soft tissues would fail to keep pace with bone growth and the deformity would progressively increase. If positioning in bed is correct while muscle spasm is present, and if the joints are carried through a full range of motion at regular intervals after the muscle spasm disappears, contractures can be prevented and soft tissues can be kept sufficiently long and elastic to meet normal functional demands.

The large expanse of the tensor fasciae latae must be recognized before the deforming possibilities of the iliotibial band can be appreciated. Proximally, the fascia lata arises from the coccyx, the sacrum, the crest of the ilium, the inguinal ligament, and the pubic arch and invests the muscles of the thigh and buttock. Either the superficial or the deep layer is attached to most of the gluteus maximus muscle and to all of the tensor fasciae latae muscle. All of the attachments of the fascia converge to form the iliotibial band on the lateral side of the thigh.

Contracture of the iliotibial band can contribute to the following deformities:

1. *Flexion, abduction, and external rotation contracture of the hip.* The iliotibial band lies lateral and anterior to the hip joint, and its contracture can cause flexion and abduction deformity. The hip is externally rotated for comfort and, if not corrected, the external rotators of the hip contract and contribute to a fixed deformity.
2. *Genu valgum and flexion contracture of the knee.* With growth, the contracted iliotibial band acts as a taut bowstring across the knee joint and gradually abducts and flexes the tibia.
3. *Limb-length discrepancy.* Although the exact mechanism has not been clearly defined and may be related more to the loss of neurologic and muscle function, a contracted iliotibial band on one side may be associated with considerable shortening of that extremity after years of growth.
4. *External tibial torsion, with or without knee joint subluxation.* Because of its lateral attachment distally, the iliotibial band gradually rotates the tibia and fibula externally on the femur; this rotation may be increased if the short head of the biceps is strong. When the deformity becomes extreme, the lateral tibial condyle subluxates on the lateral femoral condyle and the head of the fibula lies in the popliteal space.
5. *Secondary ankle and foot deformities.* With external torsion of the tibia, the axes of the ankle and knee

joints are malaligned, causing structural changes that may require surgical correction.

6. *Pelvic obliquity.* When the iliotibial band is contracted, and the patient is supine with the hip in abduction and flexion, the pelvis may remain at a right angle to the long axis of the spine (see Fig. 6.18). When the patient stands, however, and the affected extremity is brought into the weight-bearing position (parallel to the vertical axis of the trunk), the pelvis assumes an oblique position: The iliac crest is low on the contracted side and high on the opposite side. The lateral thrust forces the pelvis toward the unaffected side. The trunk muscles on the affected side lengthen, and the muscles on the opposite side contract. An associated lumbar scoliosis can develop. If not corrected, the two contralateral contractures (i.e., the band on the affected side and the trunk muscles on the unaffected side) hold the pelvis in this oblique position until skeletal changes fix the deformity (see Fig. 6.19).

7. *Increased lumbar lordosis.* Bilateral flexion contractures of the hip pull the proximal part of the pelvis anteriorly; for the trunk to assume an upright position, a compensatory increase in lumbar lordosis must develop.

A flexion and abduction contracture of the hip can be minimized or prevented in the early convalescent stage of poliomyelitis. The patient should be placed in bed with the hips in neutral rotation, slight abduction, and no flexion. All joints must be carried through a full range of passive motion several times daily; the hips must be stretched in extension, adduction, and internal rotation. To prevent rotation, a bar similar to a Denis Browne splint is useful, especially when a knee roll is used to prevent a genu recurvatum deformity; the bar is clamped to the shoe soles to hold the feet in slight internal rotation. The contracture is carefully watched for in the acute and early convalescent stages; if found, it must be corrected before ambulation is allowed.

Secondary adaptive changes occur soon after the iliotibial band contracts, and the resulting deformity, regardless of its duration or of the patient's age, cannot be corrected by conservative measures; on the contrary, attempts at correction with traction only increase the obliquity and hyperextension of the pelvis and cannot exert any helpful corrective force on the deformity.

Simple fasciotomies around the hip and knee may correct a minor contracture, but recurrence is common; they do not correct a severe contracture. For abduction and external rotation contractures, a complete release of the hip muscles (Ober-Yount procedure) is indicated. For severe deformities, complete release of all muscles from the iliac wing with transfer of the crest of the ilium (Campbell technique) is indicated.

COMPLETE RELEASE OF HIP FLEXION, ABDUCTION, AND EXTERNAL ROTATION CONTRACTURE

TECHNIQUE 6.18

(OBER; YOUNT)
- With the patient in a lateral position, make a transverse incision medial and distal to the anterior superior iliac spine, extending it laterally above the greater trochanter.

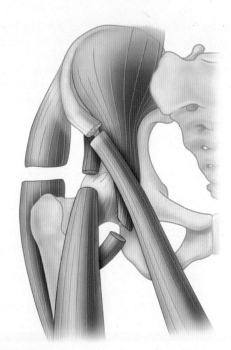

FIGURE 6.15 Complete release of flexion-abduction–external rotation contracture of hip. **SEE TECHNIQUE 6.18.**

- Divide the iliopsoas tendon distally, and excise 1 cm of it.
- Detach the sartorius from its origin in the anterior superior iliac spine, detach the rectus from the anterior inferior iliac spine, and divide the tensor fasciae latae from its anterior border completely posteriorly (Fig. 6.15).
- Detach the gluteus medius and minimus and the short external rotators from their insertions on the trochanter.
- Retract the sciatic nerve posteriorly and then open the hip capsule from anterior to posterior, parallel with the acetabular labrum.
- Close the wound over a suction drain, and apply a hip spica cast with the hip in full extension, 10 degrees of abduction, and, if possible, internal rotation.
- For the Yount procedure, expose the fascia lata through a lateral longitudinal incision just proximal to the femoral condyle.
- Divide the iliotibial band and fascia lata posteriorly to the biceps tendon and anteriorly to the midline of the thigh at a level 2.5 cm proximal to the patella.
- At this level, excise a segment of the iliotibial band and lateral intermuscular septum 5 to 8 cm long.
- Before closing the wound, determine by palpation that all tight bands have been divided.

POSTOPERATIVE CARE The cast is removed at 2 weeks, and a long leg brace with a pelvic band is fitted with the hip in the same position.

COMPLETE RELEASE OF MUSCLES FROM ILIAC WING AND TRANSFER OF CREST OF ILIUM

TECHNIQUE 6.19

(CAMPBELL)

- Incise the skin along the anterior one half or two thirds of the iliac crest to the anterior superior spine and then distally for 5 to 10 cm on the anterior surface of the thigh.
- Divide the superficial and deep fasciae to the crest of the ilium.
- Strip the origins of the tensor fasciae latae and gluteus medius and minimus muscles subperiosteally from the wing of the ilium down to the acetabulum (Fig. 6.16A).
- Free the proximal part of the sartorius from the tensor fasciae latae.
- With an osteotome, resect the anterior superior iliac spine along with the origin of the sartorius muscle and allow both to retract distally and posteriorly.
- Denude the anterior border of the ilium down to the anterior inferior iliac spine. Free subperiosteally the attachments of the abdominal muscles from the iliac crest (or resect a narrow strip of bone with the attachments). Strip the iliacus muscle subperiosteally from the inner table.
- Free the straight tendon of the rectus femoris muscle from the anterior inferior iliac spine and the reflected tendon from the anterior margin of the acetabulum, or simply divide the conjoined tendon of the muscle. Releasing these contracted structures often will allow the hip to be hyperextended without increasing the lumbar lordosis; this is a most important point because, in this situation, correction may be more apparent than real.
- If the hip cannot be hyperextended, other contracted structures must be divided. If necessary, divide the capsule of the hip obliquely from proximally to distally and, as a last resort, free the iliopsoas muscle from the lesser trochanter by tenotomy.
- After the deformity has been completely corrected, resect the redundant part of the denuded ilium with an osteotome (Fig. 6.16B).
- Suture the abdominal muscles to the edge of the gluteal muscles and tensor fasciae latae over the remaining rim of the ilium with interrupted sutures. Suture the superficial fascia on the medial side of the incision to the deep fascia on the lateral side to bring the skin incision 2.5 cm posterior to the rim of the ilium.
- To preserve the iliac physis in a young child, modify the procedure as follows. Free the muscles subperiosteally from the lateral surface of the ilium.
- Detach the sartorius and rectus femoris as just described and, if necessary, release the capsule and iliopsoas muscle. Stripping the muscles from the medial surface of the ilium is unnecessary.
- Now with an osteotome, remove a wedge of bone from the crest of the ilium distal to the physis from anterior to posterior; its apex should be as far posterior as the end of the incision and its base anterior and 2.5 cm or more in width, as necessary to correct the deformity.

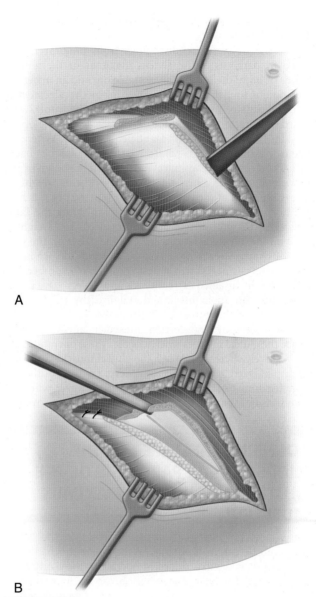

A

B

FIGURE 6.16 Campbell transfer of crest of ilium for flexion contracture of hip. **A,** Origins of sartorius, tensor fasciae latae, and gluteus medius muscles are detached from ilium. **B,** Redundant part of ilium is resected. **SEE TECHNIQUE 6.19.**

- Then displace the crest of the ilium distally to contact the main part of the ilium, and fix it in place with sutures through the soft tissues.

POSTOPERATIVE CARE When the deformity is mild, the hip is placed in hyperextension and about 10 degrees of abduction, and a spica cast is applied on the affected side and to above the knee on the opposite side. After 3 or 4 weeks, the cast is removed, and the hip is mobilized. Support may be unnecessary during the day when the patient is on crutches; however, Buck extension or an appropriate splint should be used at night.

■ PARALYSIS OF THE GLUTEUS MAXIMUS AND MEDIUS MUSCLES

One of the most severe disabilities from poliomyelitis is caused by paralysis of the gluteus maximus or the gluteus medius or both; the result is an unstable hip and an unsightly and fatiguing limp. During weight bearing on the affected side when the gluteus medius alone is paralyzed, the trunk sways toward the affected side and the pelvis elevates on the opposite side (the "compensated" Trendelenburg gait). When the gluteus maximus alone is paralyzed, the body lurches backward. The strength of the gluteal muscles can be shown by the Trendelenburg test. When a normal person bears weight on one extremity and flexes the other at the hip, the pelvis is held on a horizontal plane and the gluteal folds are on the same level; when the gluteal muscles are impaired, and weight is borne on the affected side, the level of the pelvis on the normal side drops lower than that on the affected side; when the gluteal paralysis is severe, the test cannot be made because balance on the disabled extremity is impossible.

Because no apparatus would stabilize the pelvis when one or both of these muscles is paralyzed, function can be improved only by transferring muscular attachments to replace the gluteal muscles when feasible. These operations are only relatively successful. When the gluteal muscles are completely paralyzed, normal balance is never restored. Although the gluteal limp can be lessened, it remains; however, when the paralysis is only partial, the gait can be markedly improved.

POSTERIOR TRANSFER OF THE ILIOPSOAS FOR PARALYSIS OF THE GLUTEUS MEDIUS AND MAXIMUS MUSCLES

For weakness of the hip abductors the tendon of the iliopsoas muscle can be transferred to the greater trochanter. Although it is a more extensive operation, the iliopsoas tendon and the entire iliacus muscle can be transferred posteriorly when the gluteus maximus and gluteus medius are paralyzed. Open adductor tenotomy should always precede iliopsoas transfer.

TECHNIQUE 6.20

(SHARRARD)
- Place the patient on the operating table, slightly tilted toward the nonoperative side. Through a transverse incision overlying the adductor longus, expose and divide the adductor muscles.
- Expose the lesser trochanter and detach it from the femur (Fig. 6.17A). Then clear the psoas muscle as far proximally as possible.
- Make a second incision just below and parallel to the iliac crest.
- Detach the crest with the muscles of the abdominal wall and open the psoas muscle sheath. Locate the insertion of the muscle with a fingertip.
- Through the first incision, grasp the lesser trochanter with a Kocher forceps and pull it upward, within the psoas sheath and into the upper operative area (Fig. 6.17B).

- Next, expose the sartorius muscle and divide it in its proximal half. Allow the muscle to remain in the cartilaginous portion of the anterior superior iliac spine, which is retracted medially.
- Identify the direct head of the rectus femoris muscle and divide it at its origin in the anterior inferior iliac spine. Identify the reflected head of the rectus femoris muscle, dissect it free from the hip capsule, and elevate it posteriorly.
- If the hip is dislocated, open the capsule anteriorly and laterally, parallel to the labrum, excise the ligamentum teres, and remove any hypertrophic pulvinar.
- Reduce the hip joint.
- Make a hole through the iliac wing just lateral to the sacroiliac joint. Make an oval with its long axis longitudinal, its width slightly more than one third of that of the iliac wing, and its length 1½ times as long as its width.
- Pass the iliopsoas tendon and the entire iliacus muscle through the hole (Fig. 6.17C). Pass a finger from the gluteal region distally and posteriorly into the bursa deep to the gluteus maximus tendon and identify by touch the posterolateral aspect of the greater trochanter. By referring to this point, expose the corresponding anterior aspect of the greater trochanter by dissecting through the fascia.
- With awls and burs and from anteriorly to posteriorly, make a hole through the greater trochanter until it is big enough to receive the tendon.
- While the hip is held in abduction, extension, and neutral rotation, pass the end of the tendon through the buttock and from posteriorly to anteriorly through the tunnel in the greater trochanter (Fig. 6.17C).
- Secure the psoas and lesser trochanter to the greater trochanter with sutures or a screw (Fig. 6.17D).
- Suture the origin of the iliacus muscle to the ilium inferior to the crest.
- For severe coxa valga or anteversion that requires more than 20 to 30 degrees of abduction for stability, a varus derotation osteotomy with internal fixation can be performed before insertion and suturing of the iliopsoas tendon in the greater trochanter.
- As an alternative, cut a "gutter," or notch, into the posterior lateral iliac crest rather than a window in the ilium. The muscle and its tendon can be redirected laterally through the notch and inserted into the greater trochanter (Fig. 6.17E and F). This is technically simpler because the iliacus muscle is not transferred to the outside of the pelvis.

POSTOPERATIVE CARE The hip is immobilized for 6 weeks in an abduction spica cast.

■ PARALYTIC DISLOCATION OF THE HIP

If a child contracts poliomyelitis before age 2 years, and the gluteal muscles become paralyzed but the flexors and adductors of the hip do not, the child may develop a paralytic dislocation of the hip before he or she is grown. That the combination of imbalance in muscle power, habitually faulty postures, and growth is important in producing deformity is illustrated nowhere better than in this situation. Generally, children with paralytic dislocation of the hip have normal strength of the flexors and adductors but paralysis of the gluteal muscles. Unless this muscle imbalance is corrected, dislocation is likely

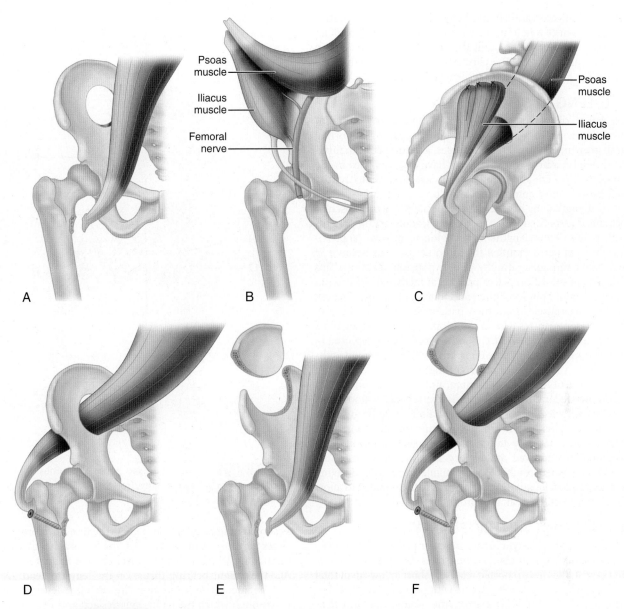

Psoas muscle

Iliacus muscle

Femoral nerve

Psoas muscle

Iliacus muscle

A   B   C

D   E   F

FIGURE 6.17   Sharrard transfer of iliopsoas muscle. **A,** Iliopsoas tendon is released from lesser trochanter. **B,** Tendon and lesser trochanter are detached, iliacus and psoas muscles are elevated, origin of iliacus is freed, and hole is made in ilium. **C,** Iliopsoas tendon is passed from posterior to anterior through hole in greater trochanter. **D,** Iliopsoas muscle and lesser trochanter are secured to greater trochanter with screw. **E** and **F,** Modification of technique in which muscle and tendon are redirected laterally through notch in ilium and inserted into greater trochanter, as described by Weisinger et al. **SEE TECHNIQUE 6.20.**

to recur regardless of other treatment. Dislocation also can develop because of fixed pelvic obliquity, in which the contralateral hip is held in marked abduction, usually by a tight iliotibial band or a structural scoliosis. If the pelvic obliquity is not corrected, the hip gradually subluxates and eventually dislocates. Weakness of the abductor musculature retards the growth of the greater trochanteric apophysis. The proximal femoral capital epiphysis continues to grow away from the greater trochanter and increases the valgus deformity of the femoral neck; femoral anteversion also may be increased; and the hip becomes mechanically unstable and gradually subluxates. The uneven pressure in the acetabulum causes an increased obliquity in the acetabular roof.

The goals of treatment of paralytic hip dislocations are reduction of the femoral head into the acetabulum and restoration of muscle balance. The bony deformity should be corrected before or at the time of any muscle-balancing procedures. Reduction of the hip in young children can often be achieved by simple abduction, sometimes aided by open adductor tenotomy and traction. Traction can be used to bring the femoral head opposite the acetabulum before closed reduction is attempted. If the hip cannot be reduced by traction, open reduction and adductor tenotomy may be required, in combination with primary femoral shortening, varus derotation osteotomy of the femur, and appropriate acetabular reconstructions (see chapter 2). Hip arthrodesis rarely is indicated and should be used as the last alternative for treatment of a flail hip that requires stabilization or of an arthritic hip in a young adult that cannot be corrected with total hip arthroplasty. The Girdlestone procedure is the final option for failed correction of the dislocation.

LEG-LENGTH DISCREPANCY

Leg-length discrepancies are common in patients with poliomyelitis owing to a variety of factors, including abnormal limb growth, abnormal muscle forces, and joint contractures. At skeletal maturity, most patients have discrepancies in the range of 4 to 7 cm and many have associated lower extremity deformities, most commonly of the foot.

Leg lengthening in general and especially in neuromuscular patients is associated with a high complication rate. In patients with poliomyelitis, lengthening is a longer process (approximately 1 cm per 2 months) than in other patients because of associated muscular atrophy and hypoplasia of bone. This delayed consolidation places patients at increased risks of pin track infection, pin loosening, and joint contracture. Because of abnormal muscle forces, these patients also are at greater risk for joint contractures. Use of an intramedullary nail for tibial lengthening in patients with poliomyelitis has been reported to decrease mean healing time compared with lengthening without a nail. A high rate of recurrent foot deformity was found with the use of Ilizarov lengthening, and triple arthrodesis was recommended rather than contracture release. Poliomyelitis patients with leg-length discrepancy alone have been found not have a higher level of ambulatory function than those with leg-length discrepancy and associated angular deformity. Leg lengthening improved ambulatory function at various distances only when combined with angular correction. Leaving a small residual length discrepancy was recommended to allow for clearance of the weak limb from the ground.

TOTAL JOINT ARTHROPLASTY

Total joint arthroplasty in neuromuscular patients also is associated with increased complication rates. Several small series and case studies have reported relatively short follow-up of total joint arthroplasty in adult patients with poliomyelitis sequelae. Chichos et al., using data from the Nationwide Inpatient Sample, determined that neuromuscular patients had increased risks of total surgical complications, medical complications, and overall complications after total joint arthroplasty; nearly half of their patient cohort, however, were older than 70 years of age and had multiple comorbidities. Poliomyelitis was not associated with increased odds of any type of complications except periprosthetic fracture and wound dehiscence. Improvements in knee range of motion, pain, and function have been reported after total knee arthroplasty, but further study and longer follow-up are necessary to fully establish the efficacy and safety of total joint arthroplasty in patients with poliomyelitis.

TRUNK

To understand the deformities and disabilities that may occur when the muscles of the trunk and hips are affected by poliomyelitis requires knowledge of the normal actions and interactions of these muscles. Irwin described the actions of the hip abductors and of the lateral trunk muscles during weight bearing as follows.

The different muscle groups, bone levers, and weight-bearing thrusts have a symmetric and triangular relationship,

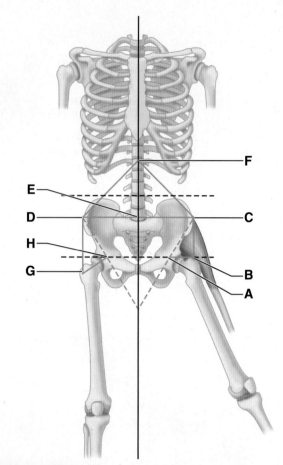

FIGURE 6.18 Most true fixed pelvic obliquities are initiated by contractures below iliac crest (see text).

as shown in Figures 6.18 and 6.19. The line *BC* represents the abductor muscles of the hip; *AB*, the femoral head, neck, and trochanter, which provide a lever for the abductor muscles; *AC*, the weight-bearing thrust on the femoral head; *DF* and *CF*, the lateral trunk muscles; *CE*, the bone lever of the pelvis through which the trunk muscles act; and *FE*, the weight-bearing thrust through the midline of the pelvis from above. When the body is balanced, the triangles above and below the pelvis are symmetric.

During normal walking, the abductors of the hip on the weight-bearing side pull downward on the pelvis and the lateral trunk muscles on the opposite side pull upward; these two sets of muscles hold the pelvis at a right angle to the longitudinal axis of the trunk. The femoral head on the weight-bearing side serves as the fulcrum. The point of fixation of the trunk muscles (the ribs and spine) is less stable than that of the abductor muscles. When *DF* elevates the pelvis, *CF* must provide counterfixation; *CF* depends on the abductors of the hip, *BC*, for counterfixation. With each step, the femur on the weight-bearing side is the central point of action for this coordinated system of fixation and counterfixation. Each part of the system depends on the others for proper pelvic balance during walking.

■ PELVIC OBLIQUITY

When there is an abduction contracture of the hip, line *BC* is shortened; as the affected extremity is placed in the

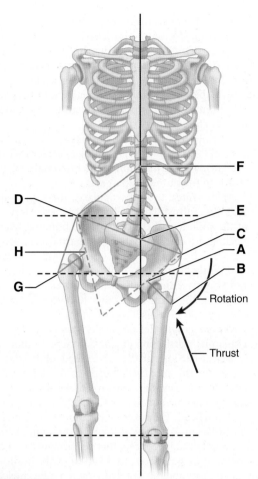

FIGURE 6.19   Abnormal mechanical relationships are created when contracted hip is brought down into weight-bearing position (see text).

weight-bearing position, the femur, acting through the contracted abductor group, *BC*, depresses the pelvis on that side. During this motion, the affected extremity and the pelvis act as a unit; the pelvis is displaced by the lateral thrust toward the opposite side, and the normal symmetry of the pelvis in relation to the weight-bearing thrust from above is altered. This thrust from above, *FE*, now closely approaches the affected hip, and the pelvis is tilted obliquely. The adducted position of the unaffected hip elongates the abductor muscles, *DG*, to about the same extent that the abductors on the affected side, *BC*, have been shortened, so even when the abductors, *DG*, are normal, their contractility and efficiency are diminished. The demand on these weakened muscles is increased by the increase in the length of line *DE*.

The trunk muscles also are affected by this asymmetry. The lateral trunk muscles, *CF*, become elongated, and their efficiency is impaired. The elongation of the abductors, *DG*, alters their interrelation with the lateral trunk muscles, *DF*, in providing a fixed point for contraction of the lateral trunk muscles, *CF*. The lateral trunk muscles, *CF*, normally elevate the pelvis on that side, but their position now prevents efficient function. Shortening of the lever, *EC*, places the trunk muscles, *CF*, at a further disadvantage. All these alterations in function and structure disrupt the mechanics of walking.

When the contracted lateral trunk muscles, *DF*, and contracted hip abductors, *BC*, hold the pelvis in this position long enough, its obliquity becomes fixed through adaptive changes in the spine.

When pelvic obliquity is associated with paralysis of the legs severe enough to require two long leg braces, walking is even more difficult. When the quadriceps is strong on the side of the abduction contracture (the apparently long extremity), the brace can be unlocked to allow knee flexion, and walking becomes possible, although with a marked limp. When the brace on the affected side cannot be unlocked, and the heel on the opposite side (the apparently short extremity) is not elevated, the affected extremity must be widely abducted in walking; otherwise, weight is borne only on the affected extremity and the opposite one becomes almost useless.

▌TREATMENT

Most pelvic obliquities arise from contractures distal to the iliac crest, and a few arise from unilateral weakness of the abdominal and lateral trunk muscles. When contractures are absent distal to the iliac crest, a pelvic obliquity should not be considered a true one but one secondary to scoliosis.

The early origin of a true pelvic obliquity from contracture of the iliotibial band has already been discussed. Before starting treatment, the degree of fixation of the lumbar scoliosis should be determined by radiographs. When the deformity is mild and the lumbar scoliosis is not fixed, the pelvic obliquity is corrected by treating the flexion and abduction contracture of the hip (see Technique 6.18). When the pelvic obliquity is moderately severe and the lumbar scoliosis is fixed, the scoliosis is corrected first by instrumentation, as described in other chapter. After this treatment has been completed, the contractures around the hip are released.

For adults with arthritic changes in the lumbar spine that make correction impossible, the weight borne on the adducted extremity (the apparently short one) can be shifted nearer the midline by valgus osteotomy; a severe unilateral weakness of the gluteus medius also can be treated in this way. This procedure may enable a patient to walk who could not do so before. When the pelvic obliquity is extreme and the femoral head of the abducted extremity (the apparently long one) is almost within the center of gravity, varus osteotomy of the femur is indicated. The osteotomy usually is made at the level of the lesser trochanter, and the fragments are immobilized by appropriate internal fixation.

▌SERRATUS ANTERIOR PARALYSIS

The following procedures were devised to treat serratus anterior paralysis:

1. Fascial transplant to anchor the inferior angle of the scapula to the inferior border of the pectoralis major
2. Multiple fascial transplants extending from the vertebral border of the scapula to the fourth, fifth, sixth, and seventh thoracic spinous processes
3. Transfer of the teres major tendon from the humerus to the fifth and sixth ribs
4. Transfer of the coracoid insertion of the pectoralis minor muscle to the vertebral border of the scapula
5. Transfer of the coracoid insertion of the pectoralis minor to the inferior angle of the scapula
6. Transfer of the pectoralis minor to distal third of the scapula

TRAPEZIUS AND LEVATOR SCAPULAE PARALYSIS

The following procedures are used to treat trapezius and levator scapulae paralysis:

1. Fascial transplants extending from the spine of the scapula to the cervical muscles and to the first thoracic spinous process; also, anchoring of the inferior angle of the scapula to the adjacent paraspinal muscles for stability

2. Transplant of two fascial strips, one extending from the vertebral border of the scapula just proximal to its spine to the sixth cervical spinous process and the other from a point 6 cm distal to the first transplant to the third thoracic spinous process

3. Fascial transplant extending from the middle of the vertebral border of the scapula to the spinous process of the second and third thoracic vertebrae and transfer of the insertion of the levator scapulae muscle lateralward on the spine of the scapula to a point adjacent to the acromion

PARALYTIC SCOLIOSIS

The treatment of paralytic scoliosis is discussed in *Spine Surgery*.

SHOULDER

The disability caused by paralysis of the muscles around the shoulder can be diminished to some extent by tendon and muscle transfers or by arthrodesis of the joint; the pattern and severity of the paralysis determine which method is most appropriate. Neither procedure is indicated, however, unless the hand, forearm, and elbow have remained functional or have already been made so by reconstructive surgery.

Tendons and muscles are transferred to substitute for a paralyzed deltoid muscle or to reinforce a weak one. For these operations to be successful, power must be fair or better in the serratus anterior, the trapezius, and the short external rotators of the shoulder (for the trapezius transfer, power must be fair or better in the pectoralis major, the rhomboids, and the levator scapulae). When the short external rotators are below functional level, the latissimus dorsi or teres major can be transferred to the lateral aspect of the humerus to reinforce them (Harmon). When the supraspinatus is below functional level, the levator scapulae (preferred), sternocleidomastoid, scalenus anterior, scalenus medius, or scalenus capitis can be transferred to the greater tuberosity. When the subscapularis is below functional level, the pectoralis minor or the superior two digitations of the serratus anterior or the latissimus dorsi or teres major posteriorly can be transferred to the lesser tuberosity to a point exactly opposite the insertion of the subscapularis (here the action is backward, although identical to that of the subscapularis after elevation >90 degrees). Arthrodesis of the shoulder may be indicated when the paralysis around the joint is extensive, provided that power in at least the serratus anterior and the trapezius is fair or better.

■ TENDON AND MUSCLE TRANSFERS FOR PARALYSIS OF THE DELTOID

Transfer of the insertion of the trapezius is the most satisfactory operation for complete paralysis of the deltoid. Resecting a part of the spine of the scapula and including it in the transfer permits fixation of the transfer with screws after the muscle is pulled like a hood over the head of the humerus (Fig. 6.20). In a technique modification, the superior and middle trapezius is completely mobilized laterally from its origin and the transfer is made 5 cm longer without endangering its nerve or blood supply; this added length greatly increases leverage of the transfer on the humerus. The entire insertion of the trapezius is freed by resecting the lateral clavicle, the acromion, and the adjoining part of the scapular spine; these are anchored to the humerus by screws (Fig. 6.21).

Saha developed a functional classification of the muscles around the joint and recommended careful assessment of their strength before surgery.

1. *Prime movers:* the deltoid and clavicular head of the pectoralis major, which in lifting exert forces in three directions at the junction of the proximal and middle thirds of the humeral shaft axis.

2. *Steering group:* the subscapularis, the supraspinatus, and the infraspinatus. These muscles exert forces at the junction of the axes of the humeral head and neck and humeral shaft. As the arm is elevated, the humeral head, by rolling and gliding movements, constantly changes its point of contact with the glenoid cavity. Although these muscles exert a little force in lifting the arm, their chief function is stabilizing the humeral head as it moves in the glenoid.

3. *Depressor group:* the pectoralis major (sternal head), latissimus dorsi, teres major, and teres minor. These muscles are intermediately located and exert their forces on the proximal fourth of the humeral shaft axis. During elevation, they rotate the shaft, and in the last few degrees of this movement, they depress the humeral head. They exert only minimal steering action on the head. Absence of their power would cause no apparent disability except that performance of the limb in lifting weights above the head would be diminished.

The classic methods of transferring a single muscle (or even several muscles to a common attachment) to restore abduction of the shoulder do not consider the functions of the steering muscles. When the steering muscles are paralyzed and a single muscle has been transferred to restore functions only of the deltoid, the arm cannot be elevated more than 90 degrees and scapulohumeral motion is significantly disturbed. For paralysis of the deltoid, the entire insertion of the trapezius can be transferred to the humerus to replace the anterior and middle parts of the muscle; however, the subscapularis, the supraspinatus, and the infraspinatus must be carefully evaluated. When any two are paralyzed, their functions also must be restored because otherwise the effectiveness of the transferred trapezius as an elevator of the shoulder would be greatly reduced. As already mentioned, for paralysis of the subscapularis, either the pectoralis minor or the superior two digitations of the serratus anterior can be transferred because either can be rerouted and anchored to the lesser tuberosity; as an alternative procedure, the latissimus dorsi or the teres major can be transferred posteriorly to a point exactly opposite the lesser tuberosity. For paralysis of the supraspinatus, the levator scapulae, sternocleidomastoid, scalenus anterior, scalenus medius, or scalenus capitis can be transferred to the greater tuberosity; of these, the levator scapulae is the best because of the direction and length of its fibers. When suitable transfers are unavailable, the insertion of the trapezius can be anchored more anteriorly or posteriorly on the humerus to restore internal or external rotation. Contractures of unopposed muscles around the shoulder rarely are severe enough to cause extreme disability; most can be corrected at the time of transfer or arthrodesis.

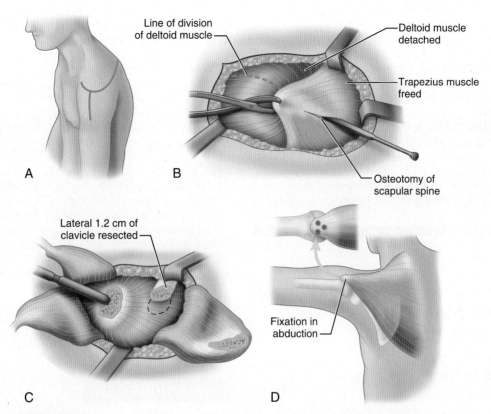

FIGURE 6.20   Bateman trapezius transfer for paralysis of deltoid. **A,** Skin incision. **B,** Spine of scapula is osteotomized near its base in obliquely distal and lateral plane. *Broken line* indicates division of deltoid. **C,** Atrophic deltoid has been split, deep surface of acromion and spine and corresponding area on lateral aspect of humerus have been roughened, and lateral end of clavicle has been resected. **D,** Acromion has been anchored to humerus as far distally as possible with two or three screws. **SEE TECHNIQUE 6.21.**

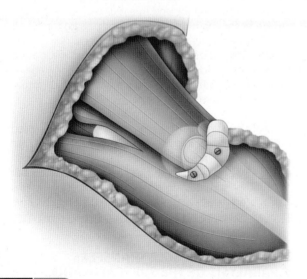

FIGURE 6.21   Saha trapezius transfer for paralysis of deltoid. Entire insertion of trapezius along with attached lateral end of clavicle, acromioclavicular joint, and acromion and adjoining part of scapular spine have been anchored to lateral aspect of humerus distal to tuberosities by two screws. **SEE TECHNIQUE 6.22.**

TRAPEZIUS TRANSFER FOR PARALYSIS OF DELTOID

TECHNIQUE 6.21

(BATEMAN)

- With the patient prone, approach the shoulder through a T-shaped incision (Fig. 6.20A); extend the transverse part around the shoulder over the spine of the scapula and the acromion and end it just above the coracoid process; extend the longitudinal limb distally over the lateral aspect of the shoulder and upper arm for 6 cm.
- Mobilize the flaps, split the atrophic deltoid muscle, and expose the joint.
- Free the undersurface of the acromion and spine of the scapula of soft tissue and osteotomize the spine of the scapula near its base in an obliquely distal and lateral plane; thus, a broad cuff of the trapezius is freed but still attached to the spine and the acromion.
- Resect the lateral 2 cm of the clavicle, taking care to avoid damaging the coracoclavicular ligament.
- Roughen the deep surface of the acromion and spine, abduct the arm to 90 degrees, and at the appropriate

level on the lateral aspect of the humerus roughen a corresponding area.

- With firm traction, bring the muscular cuff laterally over the humeral head and anchor the acromion to the humerus as far distally as possible with two or three screws (Fig. 6.20D). Immobilize the arm in a shoulder spica cast with the shoulder abducted to 90 degrees.

POSTOPERATIVE CARE Immobilization is continued for 8 weeks, but at 4 to 6 weeks the arm and shoulder part of the spica is bivalved to allow some movement. When the transplanted acromion has united with the humerus, the arm is placed on an abduction humeral splint and is gradually lowered to the side and the muscle is reeducated by exercises.

TRAPEZIUS TRANSFER FOR PARALYSIS OF DELTOID

TECHNIQUE 6.22

(SAHA)
- Make a saber-cut incision convex medially; begin it anteriorly a little superior to the inferior margin of the anterior axillary fold at about its middle, extend it superiorly, then posteriorly, and finally inferiorly, and end it slightly inferior to the base of the scapular spine and 2.5 cm lateral to the vertebral border of the scapula.
- Mobilize the skin flaps, and expose the trapezius medially to 2.5 cm medial to the vertebral border of the scapula; expose the acromion, the capsule of the acromioclavicular joint, the lateral third of the clavicle, and the entire origin of the paralyzed deltoid muscle.
- Detach and reflect laterally the origin of the deltoid, and locate the anterior border of the trapezius.
- Identify the coronoid ligament, and divide the clavicle just lateral to it.
- Palpate the scapular notch, identify the acromion and the adjoining part of the scapular spine, and with a Gigli saw and beveling posteriorly, resect the spine.
- Elevate the insertion of the trapezius along with the attached lateral end of the clavicle, the acromioclavicular joint, and the acromion and adjoining part of the scapular spine. Then free the trapezius from the superior border of the remaining part of the scapular spine medially to the base of the spine where the inferior fibers of the muscle glide over the triangular area of the scapula. Next free from the investing layer of deep cervical fascia the anterior border of the trapezius, and raise the muscle from its bed for rerouting.
- Denude the inferior surfaces of the bones attached to the freed trapezius insertion; with forceps, break these bones in several places but leave intact the periosteum on their superior surfaces. Denude also the area on the lateral aspect of the proximal humerus selected for attachment of the transfer.

- With the shoulder in neutral rotation and 45 degrees of abduction, anchor the transfer by two screws passed through fragments of bone and into the proximal humerus (Fig. 6.21).
- When suitable transfers are unavailable to replace any paralyzed external or internal rotators, anchor the muscle a little more anteriorly or posteriorly. Transfers for paralysis of the subscapularis, supraspinatus, or infraspinatus are discussed later; when indicated, they should be performed at the time of trapezius transfer.

POSTOPERATIVE CARE A spica cast is applied with the shoulder abducted 45 degrees, neutrally rotated, and flexed in the plane of the scapula. At 10 days, the sutures are removed and radiographs are made to be sure that the humeral head has not become dislocated inferiorly. At 6 to 8 weeks, the cast is removed and active exercises are started.

TRANSFER OF DELTOID ORIGIN FOR PARTIAL PARALYSIS

TECHNIQUE 6.23

(HARMON)
- Make a U-shaped incision 20 cm long extending from the middle third of the clavicle laterally and posteriorly around the shoulder just distal to the acromion to the middle of the spine of the scapula.
- Raise flaps of skin and subcutaneous tissue proximally and distally.
- Detach subperiosteally from its origin the active posterior part of the deltoid, and free it distally from the deep structures for about one half its length, being careful not to injure the axillary nerve and its branches.
- Expose subperiosteally the lateral third of the clavicle, transfer the muscle flap anteriorly, and anchor it against the clavicle with interrupted nonabsorbable sutures through the adjacent soft tissues (Fig. 6.22).

POSTOPERATIVE CARE A shoulder spica cast is applied, holding the arm abducted 75 degrees. At 3 weeks, part of the cast is removed for massage and active exercise. At 6 weeks, the entire cast is removed and an abduction humeral splint is fitted to be worn for at least 4 months; supervised active exercises are continued during this time.

▤ TENDON AND MUSCLE TRANSFERS FOR PARALYSIS OF THE SUBSCAPULARIS, SUPRASCAPULARIS, SUPRASPINATUS, OR INFRASPINATUS

When two of these three muscles are paralyzed, their functions must be restored by suitable transfers; this is just as necessary as the trapezius transfer for paralysis of the deltoid. Without the function of these muscles or their substitutes the effectiveness of the transferred trapezius in elevating the

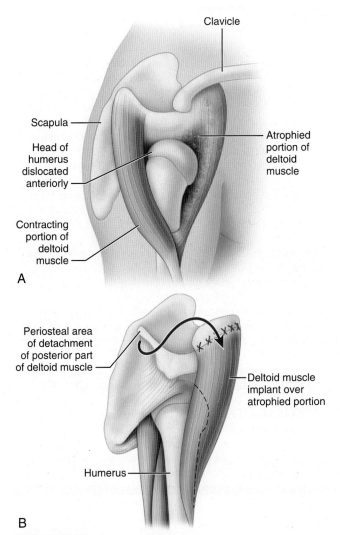

Clavicle

Scapula

Head of humerus dislocated anteriorly

Atrophied portion of deltoid muscle

Contracting portion of deltoid muscle

A

Periosteal area of detachment of posterior part of deltoid muscle

Deltoid muscle implant over atrophied portion

Humerus

B

FIGURE 6.22 Harmon transfer of origin of deltoid for partial paralysis. **A,** Posterior part of deltoid is functioning; middle and anterior parts are paralyzed. **B,** Transferred posterior part of deltoid is overlying atrophic anterior part. When transfer contracts, it prevents anterior dislocation of shoulder and exerts more direct abduction force than in its previous posterior location. **SEE TECHNIQUE 6.23.**

shoulder would be markedly reduced. Muscles suitable for transfer are muscles whose distal ends can be carried to the tuberosities of the humerus and whose general directions of pull correspond to those of the muscles they are to replace. The transfers should be rerouted close to the end of the axis of the humeral head and neck, or the desired functions will not be restored. The nerve and blood supply to any transferred muscle must be protected. Currently, the most commonly performed transfers are transfer of the latissimus dorsi or teres major or both and posterior transfer of the pectoralis minor to the scapula. These transfers, when indicated, are done at the same time as the Saha trapezius transfer for paralysis of the deltoid. Consequently, in each instance, the saber-cut incision would have been made, the lateral end of the clavicle and the acromion and adjoining part of the scapular spine would have been elevated, and the superior and middle trapezius would have been mobilized as already described.

TRANSFER OF LATISSIMUS DORSI OR TERES MAJOR OR BOTH FOR PARALYSIS OF SUBSCAPULARIS OR INFRASPINATUS

TECHNIQUE 6.24

(SAHA)

- Elevate the arm about 130 degrees. Then make an incision in the posterior axillary fold beginning in the upper arm about 6.5 cm inferior to the crease of the axilla and extending to the inferior angle of the scapula, crossing the crease in a zigzag manner.
- Expose and free the insertion of the latissimus dorsi, and raise the muscle from its bed, taking care to preserve its nerve and blood supply.
- If the transfer is to be reinforced by the teres major, free and raise both muscles.
- Fold the freed insertion on itself and close its margins by interrupted sutures; place in its end a strong mattress suture.
- With a blunt instrument, open the interval between the deltoid and long head of the triceps.
- Identify the tubercle at the inferior end of the greater tuberosity, carry the end of the transfer to this tubercle, and while holding the limb in neutral rotation, anchor the transfer there by interrupted sutures.

■ ARTHRODESIS

When paralysis around the shoulder is extensive, arthrodesis may be the procedure of choice, especially when there is a paralytic dislocation, the muscles of the forearm and hand are functional, and the serratus anterior and trapezius are strong. Motion of the scapula compensates for lack of motion in the joint. Normal function of the forearm and hand is a prerequisite.

The position of the shoulder for arthrodesis is similar to that recommended for any shoulder fusion. The angle of abduction should be determined on the basis of the clinical presentation of the arm's position in relation to the body. This angle traditionally is obtained by measuring the angle between the vertebral border of the scapula and the humerus; however, this frequently is difficult to determine on radiographs. The position of the arm in shoulder arthrodesis should be established with the arm at the side of the body, with enough abduction of the arm clinically determined from the side of the body to clear the axilla (15 to 20 degrees) and enough forward flexion (25 to 30 degrees) and internal rotation (40 to 50 degrees) to bring the hand to the midline of the body. An additional 10 degrees of abduction should be obtained in children with poliomyelitis when no internal fixation is used. When both shoulders must be fused, their positions should allow the patient to bring the hands together. A weak or flail shoulder should be fused in only slight abduction. A study of 11 patients (average age, 15 years) with 13 shoulder arthrodesis reported great variability in the position of fusion, but improved function in all patients. The authors concluded that the position of arthrodesis and the resulting arc of motion were less important than stability of the glenohumeral joint. Care must be taken to preserve the proximal humeral physis in skeletally immature patients. The techniques for shoulder arthrodesis are described in other chapter.

ELBOW

Most operations for paralysis of the muscles acting across the elbow are designed to restore active flexion or extension of the joint. Operations to correct deformity or operations to stabilize the joint, such as posterior bone block or arthrodesis, rarely are necessary.

■ MUSCLE AND TENDON TRANSFERS TO RESTORE ELBOW FLEXION

Several methods of restoring active elbow flexion are available. Here, as elsewhere, the actual and the relative power of the remaining muscles must be accurately determined before a transfer procedure is chosen. Also, because the function of the hand is more important than flexion of the elbow, these operations should not be done when the muscles controlling the fingers are paralyzed, unless their function has been or can be restored by tendon transfers. Several methods of restoring elbow flexion have been described: (1) flexorplasty (Steindler), (2) anterior transfer of the triceps tendon (Bunnell and Carroll), (3) transfer of part of the pectoralis major muscle (Clark), (4) transfer of the sternocleidomastoid muscle (Bunnell), (5) transfer of the pectoralis minor muscle (Spira), (6) transfer of the pectoralis major tendon (Brooks and Seddon), and (7) transfer of the latissimus dorsi muscle (Hovnanian).

FLEXORPLASTY

Flexorplasty consists of transferring the common origin of the pronator teres, the flexor carpi radialis, the palmaris longus, the flexor digitorum sublimis, and the flexor carpi ulnaris muscles from the medial epicondylar region of the humerus proximally about 5 cm. Its chief disadvantage is the frequent development of a pronation deformity of the forearm.

Flexorplasty is indicated when the biceps brachii and brachialis are paralyzed, and the group of muscles arising from the medial epicondyle are fair or better in strength. The best results are obtained when the elbow flexors are only partially paralyzed and the finger and wrist flexors are normal. The strength in active flexion and the range of motion of the elbow after surgery do not compare favorably with that of the normal elbow, but the usefulness of the arm is nonetheless increased. When only the flexor digitorum sublimis is active, the elbow can be flexed only if the fingers are strongly flexed; this interferes with the function of the hand, and another method should be used to restore elbow flexion. Unsuccessful results from this procedure usually are caused by overestimating the strength of the muscles to be transferred. A practical way to test them is to hold the patient's arm at a right angle to the body, rotate it to eliminate the influence of gravity, and determine whether the muscles to be transferred can flex the elbow in this position; if not, this type of transfer would fail and another should be used.

TECHNIQUE 6.25

(BUNNELL)

- Make a curved longitudinal incision over the medial side of the elbow, beginning 7.5 cm proximal to the medial epicondyle and extending distally posterior to the medial condyle and thence anteriorly on the volar surface of the forearm along the course of the pronator teres muscle.
- Locate the ulnar nerve posterior to the medial epicondyle, and retract it posteriorly.
- Detach en bloc the common origin of the pronator teres, flexor carpi radialis, palmaris longus, flexor digitorum sublimis, and flexor carpi ulnaris from the medial epicondyle close to the periosteum. Free these muscles distally for 4 cm and prolong the common muscle origin with a free graft of fascia lata.
- Advance this origin 5 cm up the lateral side rather than the medial side of the humerus (Fig. 6.23); this results in a moderate, although not complete, correction of the tendency of the transfer to pronate the forearm.
- Should a pronation deformity persist after this procedure, it can be corrected by transferring the tendon of the flexor carpi ulnaris around the ulnar margin of the forearm into the distal radius.
- Apply a cast with the elbow in acute flexion and the forearm midway between pronation and supination.

POSTOPERATIVE CARE At 2 weeks the cast is replaced by a splint that holds the arm in this same position for at least 6 weeks; physical therapy and active exercises are then started and are gradually increased to strengthen the transferred muscles.

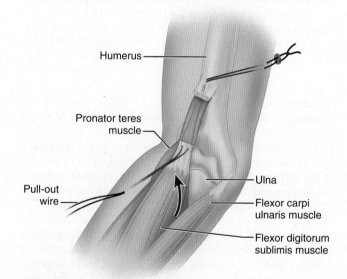

FIGURE 6.23 Bunnell modification of Steindler flexorplasty. Common muscle origin is transferred laterally on humerus by means of fascial transplant. **SEE TECHNIQUE 6.25.**

ANTERIOR TRANSFER OF THE TRICEPS

Anterior transfer of the triceps tendon can be done to regain active elbow flexion. One disadvantage of this transfer is that the triceps tendon would not reach the tuberosity of the radius; a short graft of fascia or a tendon graft must be used to complete the transfer.

TECHNIQUE 6.26

(BUNNELL)

- Through a posterolateral incision expose the triceps tendon, and divide it at its insertion.
- Dissect it from the posterior aspect of the distal fourth of the humerus, and transfer it around the lateral aspect.
- Make an anterolateral curvilinear incision, and retract the brachioradialis and pronator teres muscles to expose the tuberosity of the radius.
- Prolong the triceps tendon by a graft of fascia lata that is 4 cm long and wide enough to make a tube.
- Attach it to the roughened tuberosity of the radius with a steel pull-out suture passed to the dorsum of the forearm via a hole drilled through the tuberosity and the neck of the radius (Fig. 6.24).
- Flex the elbow, gently pull the suture taut to snug the tendon against the bone, and tie the suture over a padded button.
- Apply a cast with the elbow in acute flexion and the forearm midway between pronation and supination.
- Carroll described a similar method of triceps transfer in which the tendon is passed superficial to the radial nerve and through a longitudinal slit in the biceps tendon and is sutured under tension with the elbow in flexion.

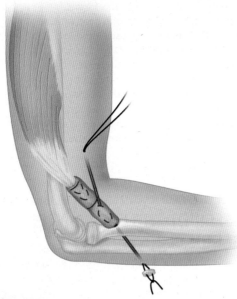

FIGURE 6.24 Bunnell anterior transfer of triceps for paralysis of biceps. Triceps tendon elongated by short graft of fascia or tendon, routed laterally, and inserted into tuberosity of radius by pull-out suture. **SEE TECHNIQUE 6.26.**

POSTOPERATIVE CARE At 2 weeks the cast is replaced by a splint that holds the arm in the same position for at least 6 weeks. The pull-out wire is removed at 4 weeks. Physical therapy and active exercises are begun at 6 weeks and are gradually increased.

TRANSFER OF THE PECTORALIS MAJOR TENDON

Brooks and Seddon described an operation to restore elbow flexion in which the entire pectoralis major muscle is used as the motor and its tendon is prolonged distally by means of the long head of the biceps brachii. This transfer is contraindicated unless the biceps is completely paralyzed; they recommended it when flexorplasty is not applicable, when the distal part of the pectoralis major is weak but the proximal part is strong, or when both parts of the muscle are so weak that the entire muscle is needed for transfer. To avoid undesirable movements of the shoulder during elbow flexion after this procedure, muscular control of the shoulder and scapula must be good, or an arthrodesis of the shoulder should be performed.

TECHNIQUE 6.27

(BROOKS AND SEDDON)

- Make an incision from the distal end of the deltopectoral groove distally to the junction of the proximal and middle thirds of the arm.
- Detach the tendon of insertion of the pectoralis major as close to bone as possible and by blunt dissection mobilize the muscle from the chest wall proximally toward the clavicle (Fig. 6.25A).
- Retract the deltoid laterally and superiorly, and expose the tendon of the long head of the biceps as it runs proximally into the shoulder joint; sever this tendon at the proximal end of the bicipital groove and withdraw it into the wound.
- By blunt and sharp dissection, free the belly of the long head of the biceps from that of the short head and ligate and divide all vessels entering it.
- Make an L-shaped incision at the elbow with its transverse limb in the flexor crease and its longitudinal limb extending proximally along the medial border of the biceps muscle.
- Mobilize the long head of the biceps by dividing its remaining neurovascular bundles so that the tendon and muscle are completely freed distally to the tuberosity of the radius; withdraw the tendon and muscle through the distal incision (Fig. 6.25B and C). (When the muscle belly is adherent to the overlying fascia, free it by sharp dissection.)
- Replace the long head of the biceps in its original position, and through the proximal incision pass its tendon and muscle belly through two slits in the tendon of the pectoralis major; loop the long head of the biceps on itself so that its proximal tendon is brought into the distal incision.
- Then, using nonabsorbable sutures, suture the end of the proximal tendon through a slit in the distal tendon

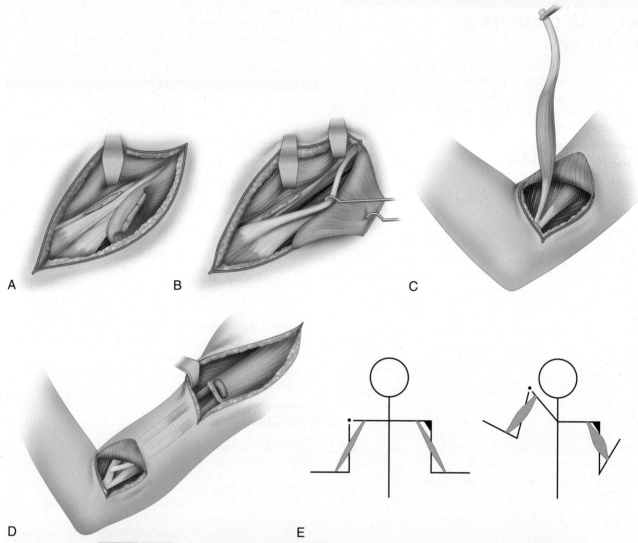

A   B   C

D   E

FIGURE **6.25**   Brooks-Seddon transfer of pectoralis major tendon for paralysis of elbow flexors. **A,** Insertion of pectoralis major is detached as close to bone as possible. **B,** Tendon of long head of biceps is exposed and divided at proximal end of bicipital groove. **C,** Tendon and muscle of long head of biceps are completely mobilized distally to tuberosity of radius by dividing all vessels and nerves that enter muscle proximal to elbow. **D,** Long head of biceps is passed through two slits in pectoralis major, is looped on itself so that its proximal tendon is brought into distal incision, and is sutured through slit in its distal tendon. **E,** To avoid undesirable movements of shoulder during elbow flexion after this transfer, muscular control of shoulder and scapula must be good, or shoulder must be fused. Left shoulder shown is flail; right has been fused. When transfer on left contracts, some of its force is wasted because of lack of control of shoulder, but, on right, transfer moves only elbow. **SEE TECHNIQUE 6.27.**

(Fig. 6.25D) and suture the tendon of the pectoralis major to the long head of the biceps at their junction.

- Close the incisions, and apply a posterior plaster splint with the elbow in flexion.

POSTOPERATIVE CARE At 3 weeks, the splint is removed and muscle reeducation is started. Care must be taken to extend the elbow gradually so that active flexion of more than 90 degrees is preserved. It may be 2 or 3 months before full extension is possible.

TRANSFER OF THE LATISSIMUS DORSI MUSCLE

Hovnanian described a method of restoring active elbow flexion by transferring the origin and belly of the latissimus dorsi to the arm and anchoring the origin near the radial tuberosity. This transfer is possible because the neurovascular bundle of the muscle is long and easily mobilized (Fig. 6.26A); a similar transfer in which the origin is anchored to the olecranon to restore active extension also is possible.

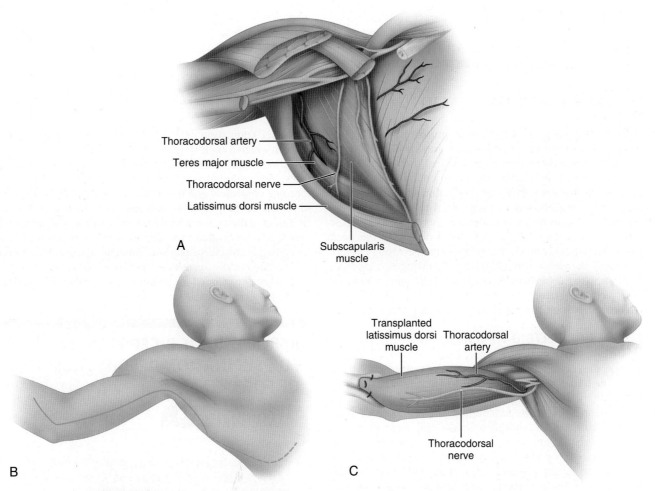

Thoracodorsal artery

Teres major muscle

Thoracodorsal nerve

Latissimus dorsi muscle

A

Subscapularis muscle

B

Transplanted latissimus dorsi muscle   Thoracodorsal artery

Thoracodorsal nerve

C

FIGURE 6.26   Hovnanian transfer of latissimus dorsi muscle for paralysis of biceps and brachialis muscles. **A,** Normal anatomy of axilla; note that thoracodorsal nerve and artery are long and can be easily mobilized. **B,** Skin incision. **C,** Origin and belly of latissimus dorsi have been transferred to arm, and origin has been sutured to biceps tendon and to other structures distal to elbow joint. **SEE TECHNIQUE 6.28.**

TECHNIQUE 6.28

(HOVNANIAN)

- Place the patient on his or her side with the affected extremity upward. Start the skin incision over the loin, and extend it superiorly along the lateral border of the latissimus dorsi to the posterior axillary fold, distally along the medial aspect of the arm, and finally laterally to end in the antecubital fossa (Fig. 6.26B). Carefully expose the dorsal and lateral aspects of the latissimus dorsi, leaving its investing fascia intact.
- Free the origin of the muscle by cutting across its musculofascial junction inferiorly and its muscle fibers superiorly. Then gradually free the muscle from the underlying abdominal and flank muscles.
- Divide the four slips of the muscle that arise from the inferior four ribs and the few arising from the angle of the scapula.
- Carefully protect the neurovascular bundle that enters the superior third of the muscle. To prevent injury of the

vessels to the latissimus dorsi, ligate their branches that anastomose with the lateral thoracic vessels. Identify and gently free the thoracodorsal nerve that supplies the muscle; its trunk is about 15 cm long and runs from the apex of the axilla along the deep surface of the muscle belly.
- Next prepare a bed in the anteromedial aspect of the arm to receive the transfer.
- Carefully swing the transfer into this bed without twisting its vessels or nerve. To prevent kinking of the vessels, divide the intercostobrachial nerve and the lateral cutaneous branches of the third and fourth intercostal nerves; also free as necessary any fascial bands.
- Now suture the aponeurotic origin of the muscle to the biceps tendon and the periosteal tissues about the radial tuberosity and then suture the remaining origin to the sheaths of the forearm muscles and to the lacertus fibrosus (Fig. 6.26C).
- Close the wound in layers and bandage the arm against the thorax with the elbow flexed and the forearm pronated.

POSTOPERATIVE CARE Exercises of the fingers are encouraged early. At 3 or 4 weeks, the bandage is removed and passive and active exercises of the elbow are started.

■ MUSCLE TRANSFERS FOR PARALYSIS OF THE TRICEPS

Weakness or paralysis of the triceps muscle usually is considered of little importance because gravity would extend the elbow passively in most positions that the arm assumes. A good triceps is essential, however, to crutch walking or to shifting the body weight to the hands during such activities as moving from a bed to a wheelchair. A functioning triceps allows the patient to perform these activities by locking the elbow in extension. To place the hand on top of the head when the patient is erect, the triceps must be strong enough to extend the elbow against gravity; thrusting and pushing motions with the forearm also require a functional triceps. In other activities, strong active extension of the elbow is relatively unimportant compared with strong active flexion.

▮ POSTERIOR DELTOID TRANSFER (MOBERG PROCEDURE)

Moberg described an operation to transfer the posterior third of the deltoid muscle to the triceps to restore active elbow extension in the quadriplegic patient. Patients with complete quadriplegia at the functioning level of C5 or C6 have active elbow flexion, shoulder flexion and abduction, and possibly wrist extension. Elbow extension is by gravity only, without triceps function (C7). Active extension is impossible. Ambulation is not a realistic goal in such patients. Rather, improved strength, mobility, and function and improved ability to reach overhead, to perform personal hygiene and grooming, to relieve ischial pressure from the wheelchair, to achieve driving ability and wheelchair use, and to eat and control eating utensils are sought.

The Moberg procedure has been modified by the construction of tendinoperiosteal tongues proximally and distally instead of using the free tendon grafts from the foot. The posterior belly of the deltoid muscle is freed, along with the most distal insertion of the muscle and including a strip of periosteum 1.0 × 3.0 cm, continuous with the muscle and its insertion. A tongue of the triceps tendon 1.5 to 2.0 cm wide is developed by parallel incisions and including a continuous strip of periosteum similar to that for the deltoid, if possible.

The length of the tendinoperiosteal tongues should be such that with the elbow extended and the arm adducted their deep surfaces should appose when the triceps tendon is folded over 180 degrees. The angle of tendinous reflection is reinforced by a narrow sheet of Dacron wrapped around the grafts and sutured to the tongues and to itself.

FOREARM

Operations on the forearm after poliomyelitis consist of tenotomy, fasciotomy, and osteotomy to correct deformities and tendon transfers to restore function.

■ PRONATION CONTRACTURE

Deformities of the forearm seldom are disabling enough in themselves to warrant surgery; the most common exception is a fixed pronation contracture from imbalance between the supinators and pronators. When the pronator teres is not strong enough to transfer to replace the paralyzed supinators, correcting the contracture alone is indicated, provided that there is active flexion of the elbow. When the pronators of the forearm and the flexors of the wrist are active, however, function can be improved not only by correcting the pronation contracture but also by transferring the flexor carpi ulnaris.

Fixed supination deformity develops from muscle imbalance in which usually the pronators and finger flexors are weak and the biceps and wrist extensors are strong. The soft tissues, such as the interosseous membrane, contract; the bones become deformed, and eventually the radioulnar joints may dislocate. A fixed supination deformity combined with weak shoulder abduction markedly limits an otherwise functional hand. Recommended procedures for this deformity include rerouting of the biceps tendon (Zancolli) and manual osteoclasis of the middle thirds of the radius and ulna (Blount). The latter is recommended for children younger than 12 years old with insufficient muscle power for tendon transfer.

REROUTING OF BICEPS TENDON FOR SUPINATION DEFORMITIES OF FOREARM

TECHNIQUE 6.29

(ZANCOLLI)

- If full passive pronation is already possible before surgery, omit the first part of the operation. Otherwise, make a longitudinal incision on the dorsum of the forearm over the radial shaft (Fig. 6.27A, *1*).
- By blunt dissection, expose the interosseous membrane and retract the dorsal muscles radialward to protect the posterior interosseous nerve (Fig. 6.27B).
- Divide the interosseous membrane throughout its length close to the ulna. If the dorsal ligaments of the distal radioulnar joint are contracted, extend the incision distally and perform a capsulotomy of this joint.
- If necessary, release the supinator muscle after identifying and protecting the posterior interosseous nerve in the proximal part of the incision. At this point in the operation full passive pronation of the forearm should be possible.
- Now make a second incision; begin it on the medial aspect of the arm proximal to the elbow and extend it distally to the flexion crease of the joint, then laterally across the joint in the crease, and then distally over the anterior aspect of the radial head (Fig. 6.27A, *2*).
- Identify and retract the median nerve and brachial artery.
- Divide the lacertus fibrosus and expose the insertion of the biceps tendon on the radial tuberosity.
- Now divide the biceps tendon by a long Z-plasty (Fig. 6.27C).
- Reroute the distal segment of the tendon around the radial neck medially, then posteriorly, and then laterally so that traction on it will pronate the forearm (Fig. 6.27D).
- Place the ends of the biceps tendon side-by-side and suture them together under tension that will maintain full pronation and yet allow extension of the elbow.

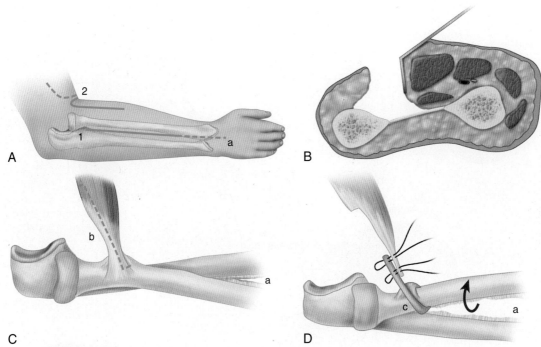

FIGURE 6.27   Zancolli rerouting of biceps tendon for supination deformity of forearm. **A,** *1,* Dorsal skin incision *(dotted line)* is extended distally to *a* when distal radioulnar joint requires capsulotomy. *2,* Anterior incision to expose biceps tendon and radial head. **B,** Exposure of interosseous membrane by retracting dorsal muscles radially (see text). **C,** Line at *b* shows Z-plasty incision to be made in biceps tendon. Interosseous membrane has been divided at *a*. **D,** At *c*, biceps tendon has been divided by Z-plasty, distal segment has been rerouted around radial neck medially, and ends of tendon are being sutured together. Traction on tendon will now pronate forearm as indicated by *arrow*. **SEE TECHNIQUE 6.29.**

- If the radial head is subluxated or is dislocated, reduce it if possible and hold it in place by capsulorrhaphy of the radiohumeral joint; if the radial head cannot be reduced, excise it and transfer the proximal segment of the biceps tendon to the brachialis tendon.
- Close the incisions and apply a cast with the elbow flexed 90 degrees and the forearm moderately pronated.

POSTOPERATIVE CARE   At about 3 weeks, the cast and sutures are removed and passive and active exercises are begun.

WRIST AND HAND

The treatment of disabilities of the wrist and hand caused by paralysis is discussed in *Hand Surgery*.

MYELOMENINGOCELE
EPIDEMIOLOGY

Myelomeningocele is a complex congenital malformation of the central nervous system. Advances in medicine, surgery, and allied health services have reduced the mortality rates in patients born with severe defects of the central nervous system. The challenge for orthopaedic surgeons is to assist these patients in attaining the best possible function within their anatomic and physiologic limitations. With advances in technology such as gait analysis, as well as the use of evidence-based medicine and multispecialty care models, significant changes in the management of patients with myelomeningocele are occurring.

Myelomeningocele is the most common of the spectrum of conditions described as spina bifida. Myelomeningocele is a severe form of spinal dysraphism that also includes meningocele, lipomeningocele, and caudal regression syndrome. *Neural tube defect* is a broader term that includes myelomeningocele, anencephaly, and encephalocele. A myelomeningocele is a sac-like structure containing cerebrospinal fluid and neural tissue (Fig. 6.28A). The herniation of the spinal cord and its meninges through a defect in the vertebral canal results in variable neurologic defects depending on the location and severity of the lesion. A meningocele is a cystic distention of the meninges through unfused vertebral arches, but the spinal cord remains in the vertebral canal. Most lesions are posterior, but rarely an anterior or lateral meningocele may occur. Neurologic deficits are not as common as in myelomeningocele. *Spina bifida occulta* is a term that refers to a defect in the posterior vertebral elements that includes the spinous process and often part of the lamina, most commonly of the fifth lumbar and first sacral vertebrae. Spina bifida occulta occurs in approximately 10% of asymptomatic adult spines and is often an incidental finding on plain radiographs that is rarely associated with neurologic involvement.

The nervous system develops by the formation of a tubular structure (neurulation). Closure of this tube is completed

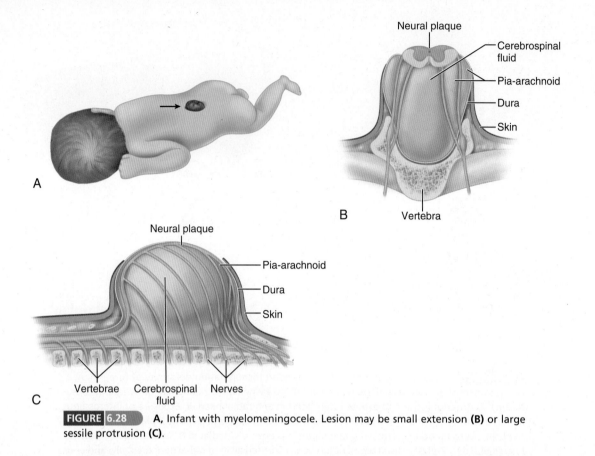

Neural plaque
Cerebrospinal fluid
Pia-arachnoid
Dura
Skin
B Vertebra
Neural plaque
Pia-arachnoid
Dura
Skin
C Vertebrae Cerebrospinal Nerves fluid
A

FIGURE 6.28   **A,** Infant with myelomeningocele. Lesion may be small extension **(B)** or large sessile protrusion **(C)**.

by closure of the cranial and caudal neuropores between day 26 to 28 of gestation. Myelomeningocele and anencephaly occur because of abnormalities during this phase of closure of the neural tube. Conditions such as meningocele, lipomeningocele, and diastematomyelia occur from abnormalities during the canalization phase from day 28 to 48 of gestation and are referred to as *postneurulation defects*.

The myelomeningocele is formed by the protrusion of dura and arachnoid through the defect in the vertebral arches. The spinal cord and nerve roots are carried out through this defect (Fig. 6.28B and C). These lesions can occur at any level along the spinal column but occur most commonly in the lower thoracic and lumbosacral regions. The skin over a myelomeningocele is almost always absent. The neural placode is covered by a thin membrane (arachnoid) that breaks down in a couple of days, leaving an ulcerated granulating surface. The superficial surface of the neural placode represents the everted interior of the neural tube. The ventral surface represents what should have been the outside of a closed neural tube. Because of this pathologic anatomy, the nerve roots arise from the ventral part of the neural placode. The pedicles are everted and lie almost horizontal in the coronal plane. The affected laminae are hypoplastic and everted, and the paraspinal muscles are everted with the pedicles and lie in an anterior position. These muscles act as flexors of the spine instead of functioning normally as extensors because of their anterior position.

The incidence of myelomeningocele in the United States is 2.5 to 1.1 per 1000 births. The overall incidence of infants born with neural tube defects is decreasing, which is most likely related to better prenatal screening and the use of folic

acid supplementation before conception and during the first month of pregnancy; an estimated 23% of pregnancies with myelomeningocele are terminated. Testing for elevated levels of maternal serum α-fetoprotein between 16 and 18 weeks of gestation can detect 75% to 80% of affected pregnancies. If the maternal serum α-fetoprotein is found to be elevated, ultrasound examination, ultrafast MRI, and amniocentesis for α-fetoprotein and acetylcholinesterase may be needed to confirm a possible neural tube defect. Ultrasound is a sensitive and efficient test to determine the presence and location of a neural tube defect. If no abnormalities are found on ultrasound examination, an amniocentesis is recommended to evaluate for α-fetoprotein and acetylcholinesterase. With this prenatal screening program, there has been a reported decrease in birth prevalence of anencephaly from 100% to 80% and birth prevalence of myelomeningocele from 80% to 60%. Other studies have shown a 60% to 100% reduction in the risk of neural tube defects when adequate levels of folate are taken by pregnant women. The U.S. Food and Drug Administration recommends that all women of childbearing age receive 0.4 mg folate before conception and during early pregnancy. The CDC also recommends that women who are at high risk (i.e., women who have given birth to a prior affected child or who have a first-degree relative with a neural tube defect) receive 4 mg of folate daily.

Genetic factors also play a role in myelomeningocele. There is a greater incidence of neural tube defects, including myelomeningocele, in siblings of affected children, in the range of 2% to 7%. There also is a higher frequency in twins than in single births. For a couple who has a child with myelomeningocele the chance that a subsequent child will be affected by a major malformation of the central nervous system is approximately 1 in 14. With over 100 known genes that affect neurulation and the low frequency of occurrence in the population, the determination of the exact molecular defect(s) remains difficult.

ASSOCIATED CONDITIONS

The natural history of myelomeningocele has changed over the past several decades because of advances in medical treatment. Patients born with myelomeningocele often died of urinary tract infection, renal failure, meningitis, and sepsis. With early neurosurgical and urologic intervention, patients born with myelomeningocele are surviving into adult life, with about 65% having normal intelligence. Myelomeningocele was believed to be nonprogressive, but studies have shown progressive neurologic deterioration can occur, manifested by increasing levels of paralysis and decreasing upper extremity function. Hydrocephalus and associated hydrosyringomyelia, Arnold-Chiari malformation, and tethered cord syndrome have been associated with progressive neurologic deterioration.

■ HYDROCEPHALUS

Hydrocephalus is a dilation of the ventricles of the brain from excessive cerebrospinal fluid. Before closure of the myelomeningocele defect, the ventricles are decompressed by their direct communication to the persistently open central canal of the cord. Of children with myelomeningocele, 80% to 90% have hydrocephalus that requires cerebrospinal shunting. Chakarborty et al. described new protocols aimed at reducing shunt placement rates in myelomeningocele patients. Using these protocols, the shunt rate in infants with myelomeningocele was decreased to 60%.

The incidence of hydrocephalus is related to the neurologic level of the lesion, with patients with thoracic and upper lumbar lesions having a higher incidence than those with lower lumbar and sacral level lesions. Early treatment of hydrocephalus has improved the early mortality rate and, more importantly, improved the long-term intellectual development of these children. If the hydrocephalus is not treated, the increased fluid pressure results in atrophy of the brain, hydromyelia, and syringomyelia. Children who do not require shunting have a better prognosis for upper extremity function and trunk balance than children who require shunting. Shunt malfunctions, manifested by signs of acute hydrocephaly such as nausea, vomiting, and severe headaches, do occur. In older children, the diagnosis may be more difficult because the shunt malfunction may be associated with increased irritability, decreased perceptual motor function, short attention span, intermittent headaches, increasing scoliosis, and increased level of paralysis.

■ HYDROSYRINGOMYELIA

Hydrosyringomyelia is an accumulation of fluid in the enlarged central canal of the spinal cord. This usually is the result of hydrocephalus or an alteration in the normal cerebrospinal fluid dynamics. Hydrosyringomyelia can cause three problems in patients with myelomeningocele: (1) an increasing level of paralysis of the lower extremities, often associated with an increase in spasticity of the lower extremity, (2) progressive scoliosis, and (3) weakness in the hands and upper extremities. This condition can be diagnosed with MRI; early treatment may reverse some of the neurologic loss and scoliosis.

■ ARNOLD-CHIARI MALFORMATION

Arnold-Chiari malformation (caudal displacement of the posterior lobe of the cerebellum) is a consistent finding in patients with myelomeningocele. Type II Arnold-Chiari malformation is seen most often in children with myelomeningocele and is characterized by displacement of the medulla oblongata into the cervical neural canal through the foramen magnum. This malformation causes dysfunction of the lower cranial nerves, resulting in weakness or paralysis of vocal cords and difficulty in feeding, crying, and breathing. Sometimes, these symptoms are episodic, which makes diagnosis difficult. In childhood, symptoms may consist of nystagmus, stridor, swallowing difficulties, and a depressed cough reflex. Spastic weakness of the upper extremities also may be present. Placement of a ventriculoperitoneal shunt to control hydrocephalus often resolves brainstem symptoms, and surgical decompression of the Arnold-Chiari malformation is unnecessary unless the neurologic symptoms are not relieved by shunting. In these rare cases, the posterior fossa and upper cervical spine require surgical decompression.

■ TETHERED SPINAL CORD

MRI shows signs of tethering of the spinal cord in most children with myelomeningocele, but only 20% to 30% have clinical manifestations. Clinical signs vary, but the most consistent are (1) loss of motor function, (2) development of spasticity in the lower extremities, primarily the medial hamstrings and ankle dorsiflexors and evertors, (3) development of scoliosis before age 6 years in the absence of congenital anomalies of the vertebral bodies, (4) back pain and increased lumbar lordosis in an older child, and (5) changes in urologic function. Deterioration in somatosensory evoked potentials of the posterior tibial nerve has been used to document deterioration of lower extremity function and a clinically significant tethered cord. MRI evaluation should be performed in any child suspected of having a tethered cord syndrome. Because dermal elements are left attached during initial closure, a dermal cyst often is seen in association with a tethered cord. If clinical signs are documented, surgical treatment is indicated to prevent further deterioration of the motor function and to diminish the progress of spasticity and scoliosis. It is important to make an early diagnosis and start treatment because surgical release of the tethered cord rarely provides complete return of lost function.

■ OTHER SPINAL ABNORMALITIES

Vertebral bone anomalies, such as a defect in segmentation and failure of formation of vertebral bodies, may cause congenital scoliosis, kyphosis, and kyphoscoliosis. Other spinal anomalies the treating physician should be aware of are duplication of the spinal cord and diastematomyelia. Diastematomyelia may cause progressive loss of neurologic function.

■ UROLOGIC DYSFUNCTION

Almost all children with myelomeningocele have some form of bladder dysfunction, with most having bladder paralysis. Chronic renal failure and sepsis from urinary tract infections were the most common causes of delayed mortality in patients with myelomeningocele before modern urologic treatment methods. The goal of urologic management is to achieve continence at an appropriate age, decompress the upper urinary tract to prevent renal failure, and prevent urinary tract infections. The mainstay of treatment is clean intermittent catheterization to prevent hydronephrosis and maintain bladder compliance and capacity. Antibiotic prophylaxis and anticholinergic medication to reduce infection and vesicoureteral reflux may be beneficial. Screening examinations, consisting of voiding cystometrograms and renal sonograms, are routinely done every 6 to 12 months. Surgical options for patients in whom medical treatment is unsuccessful include vesicostomy, a diversion of the bladder to the lower abdominal wall to facilitate catheterization, and bladder augmentation in which a segment of the ileum is added to the bladder to increase capacity and reduce bladder pressure. The orthopaedist must be aware of the effects any orthopaedic surgery may have on the need for self-catheterization and any possible urinary diversion procedures.

■ BOWEL DYSFUNCTION

Most patients with myelomeningocele have innervation of the bowel and anus that results in dysmotility, poor sphincter control, and often fecal incontinence. Constipation and fecal impaction resulting from decreased bowel motility can cause increased intraabdominal pressure that leads to ventriculo-peritoneal shunt malfunction. Oral laxatives, suppositories, or enemas can be used to achieve continence and avoid fecal impaction by promoting regular fecal elimination. If these are unsuccessful, the Malone antegrade continence enema (MACE) procedure is an option: the appendix and cecum are used to create a stoma through which the colon can be irrigated. In one study evaluating the results of the MACE procedure in 108 patients with myelomeningocele, approximately 85% achieved continence.

■ LATEX HYPERSENSITIVITY

Latex hypersensitivity has been noted in children with myelomeningocele, with a reported incidence of 3.8% to 38%. The hypersensitivity is a type 1 IgE-mediated response to residual free protein found in latex products. Tosi et al. reported a serologic prevalence of hypersensitivity in 38% of at-risk patients but a clinical prevalence of 10%. A detailed history is the most sensitive way to detect individuals at risk for latex reaction. It is recommended that all patients with myelomeningocele be treated "latex free" during surgery with avoidance of latex gloves and latex-containing accessories (catheters, adhesives, tourniquets, and anesthesia equipment) (Box 6.1). High-risk patients or those with known hypersensitivity reactions can be treated prophylactically with corticosteroids and/or antihistamines before medical procedures.

■ MISCELLANEOUS MEDICAL ISSUES

Depending on the severity of involvement, children with myelomeningocele are at risk for depression, as well as cognitive dysfunction and learning difficulties. Obesity also is a problem for children with myelomeningocele both medically and functionally. This is especially true in nonambulatory children in whom it may be difficult to increase caloric expenditure. Small changes in body weight can have a dramatic impact on ambulation because of the increased demands placed on already weak muscles by the additional body weight. It is exceptionally rare for an obese nonambulatory child to lose weight and regain ambulation.

CLASSIFICATION

The most commonly used classification of myelomeningocele is based on the neurologic level of the lesion (Fig. 6.29);

BOX 6.1

Steps to Ensure a Latex-Safe Office Visit or Surgical Procedure

Prior to the Visit/Surgery

- Assess the examination room or surgical suite for latex-containing products.
- Find suitable nonlatex alternatives for use during the procedure, or prepare for modifications that can make the products safe for use with latex-allergic patients. Be sure to include proper latex-free resuscitation equipment in the preparation for surgery for a latex-sensitive patient.
- Schedule latex-sensitive patients for the first procedure of the day, which will decrease the risk of contamination from powdered latex surgical gloves used in other procedures.
- Inform all staff of the patient's allergy and the precautions that must be taken.
- Label the room that will be used as a "Latex-Free Room."
- Label the patient's chart with information on his or her latex allergy.
- Sterilize equipment for the procedure in a latex-free load.

During the Visit/Surgery

- Closely assess the patient before surgery, noting any skin rashes and documenting lung examination and blood pressure.
- Place only nonlatex products (e.g., bouffant, mask) on the patient.
- Monitor the patient closely during the procedure for changes in respiratory function, blood pressure, or new skin findings.

From Accetta D, Kelly KH: Recognition and management of the latex-allergic patient in the ambulatory plastic surgical suite, *Anesth Surg J* 31:560, 2011.

---

however, there are several difficulties with this classification system, including performing isolated muscle testing in young children, differences in classification systems, and differences in the affected neurologic level compared with the anatomic defect. In addition, not all patients have these distinct levels of paralysis. Some patients may not have symmetric levels for each extremity, and some may be flaccid, whereas others may have some associated spasticity in the involved lower extremities.

Despite these limitations, patients with myelomeningocele can be grouped into four distinct levels: thoracic level, upper lumbar level, lower lumbar level, and sacral level. This classification assists in predicting the patient's natural history and expected deformities that may need intervention. Patients can be placed into one of four groups according to the level of the lesion and resultant muscle function. Patients with thoracic level lesions have no active hip flexion and no voluntary muscle control in the lower extremities. Patients with upper lumbar level lesions have variable power with hip flexion and adduction (L1-2) and quadriceps function (L3). Patients with lower lumbar level lesions have active knee flexion against gravity (hamstring power), anterior tibial function (L4), and extensor hallucis longus function (L5). Patients with sacral level lesions have weakness of the peroneals and intrinsic muscles of the foot but have some active toe flexor function and hip extensor and abductor power.

The sensory level has been suggested to be a better way to define the level of paralysis because muscles that can

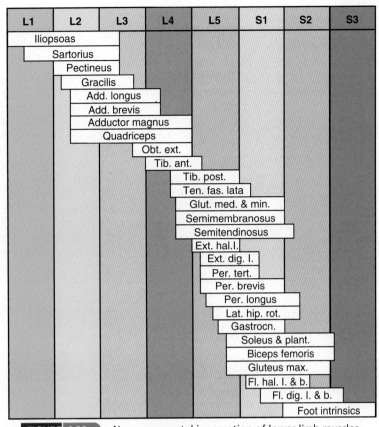

L1	L2	L3	L4	L5	S1	S2	S3

Iliopsoas
Sartorius
Pectineus
Gracilis
Add. longus
Add. brevis
Adductor magnus
Quadriceps
Obt. ext.
Tib. ant.
Tib. post.
Ten. fas. lata
Glut. med. & min.
Semimembranosus
Semitendinosus
Ext. hal.l.
Ext. dig. l.
Per. tert.
Per. brevis
Per. longus
Lat. hip. rot.
Gastrocn.
Soleus & plant.
Biceps femoris
Gluteus max.
Fl. hal. l. & b.
Fl. dig. l. & b.
Foot intrinsics

FIGURE 6.29 Neurosegmental innervation of lower limb muscles.

communicate with the brain through sensory feedback are functional but muscles that cannot become flaccid or spastic, functioning only by reflex. A sensory level classification also may be more reproducible between different observers.

The functional classification described by Swaroop and Dias is useful in determining a child's prognosis for ambulation and bracing. Patients are divided into four groups based on lesion level and accompanying functional and ambulatory capacity (Table 6.1).

The Functional Mobility Scale (FMS) also has been used to evaluate the functional ability of children with neuromuscular disorders. This scale is simple and fast, rating the child's mobility on a scale of 1 to 6 (1 = wheelchair, 2 = walker, 3 = two crutches, 4 = one crutch, 5 = independent on level surfaces, 6 = independent on all surfaces) over three different distances: home (5 m), school (50 m), and community (500 m). Additional advantages of the FMS include the ability to systematically compare children affected with different neuromuscular diseases and the fact that this is more a true measure of the child's functional abilities than isolated motor or sensory testing.

Hoffer et al. also described a functional five-category classification of patients with myelomeningocele: normal ambulator, community ambulator, household ambulator, therapy ambulatory, and wheelchair ambulator.

ORTHOPAEDIC EVALUATION

Orthopaedic evaluation of children with myelomeningocele should include the following:

1. *Serial sensory and motor examinations:* Evaluate the neurologic level of function; this may be difficult before 4 years of age.

2. *Sitting balance:* Indicates central nervous system function; if significant support is required for sitting, the probability of ambulation is significantly decreased.

3. *Upper extremity function:* Assesses ability to use assistive devices; decreased grip strength and atrophy of the thenar musculature are indications of hydromyelia.

4. *Spine evaluation:* Clinical evaluation and yearly radiographs are needed to detect development of scoliosis and/or kyphosis and lumbar hyperlordosis.

5. *Hip evaluation:* Range of motion, stability, contractures, pelvic obliquity

6. *Knee evaluation:* Range of motion, alignment, contractures, and spasticity

7. *Rotational evaluation:* Including internal/external tibial torsion and femoral anteversion and retroversion

8. *Ankle evaluation:* Range of motion, valgus deformity

9. *Foot evaluation:* Foot deformities, skin breakdown

10. *Mobility and bracing evaluation:* Changes in mobility that have remained stable; braces fitting properly and in good condition

11. *Miscellaneous:* Depression, obesity, school performance

GAIT EVALUATION

Advances in the quality and use of gait analysis have produced useful information about gait function and energy expenditure in patients with myelomeningocele. Most patients with myelomeningocele, especially those with higher level involvement, have multilevel three-dimensional deformities. These deformities can be difficult to assess on isolated clinical examination. Gait analysis allows assessment of the patient in real time during ambulation, which can be helpful diagnostically

TABLE 6.1

TABLE 6.1

Functional Classification of Myelomeningocele

GROUP	NEUROLOGIC LEVEL OF LESION	PREVALENCE (%)	FUNCTIONAL CAPACITY	AMBULATORY CAPABILITY	FUNCTIONAL MOBILITY SCALE
Thoracic/high lumbar	L3 or above	30	No functional quadriceps (≤grade 2)	During childhood, require bracing to level of pelvis for ambulation (RGO, HKAFO) 70%-99% require wheelchair for mobility in adulthood	1,1,1
Low lumbar	L3-L5	30	Quadriceps, medial hamstring ≥grade 3 No functional activity (≤grade 2) of gluteus medius and maximus, gastrocsoleus	Require AFOs and crutches for ambulation 80%-95% maintain community ambulation in adulthood	3,3,1
High sacral	S1-S3	30	Quadriceps, gluteus medius ≥grade 3 No functional activity (≤grade 2) of gastrocsoleus	Require AFOs for ambulation 94%-100% maintain community ambulation in adulthood	6,6,6
Low sacral	S3-S5	5-10	Quadriceps, gluteus medius, gastrocsoleus ≥grade 3	Ambulate without braces or support 94%-100% maintain community ambulation in adulthood	6,6,6

AFO, Ankle-foot orthosis; *HKAFO*, hip-knee-ankle-foot orthosis; *RGO*, reciprocal gait orthosis.
From Swaroop VT, Dias L: Myelomeningocele. In Weinstein SL, Flynn JM, editors: *Lovell and winter's pediatric orthopaedics*, ed 7, Philadelphia, 2014, Wolters Kluwer.

and in planning treatment strategies. Gait analysis has shown that hip abductor strength is one of the most important determinants of ambulatory kinematics and ability; that pelvic obliquity, determined by hip abductor strength, has the strongest correlation to oxygen cost during gait; and that children tend to self-select both velocity and dynamics to maintain a comfortable level of exertion. Gait studies also have shown increased dynamic knee flexion in patients with myelomeningocele compared with static examination. Patients with low lumbar level lesions have a walking velocity that is 60% of normal, and patients with high sacral level lesions have a walking velocity approximately 70% of normal.

PRINCIPLES OF ORTHOPAEDIC MANAGEMENT

Orthopaedic management should be tailored to meet specific goals during childhood, taking into account the expected function in adulthood. The goal for a child with myelomeningocele is to establish a pattern of development for the child that is as near normal as possible. Ambulation is not the goal for every child. Despite the best medical and surgical care, about 40% of children with myelomeningocele are unable to walk as adults. An evidence-based review found that neurosegmental level is the primary determinant of walking ability and physical function. Other factors believed to play a lesser role in the ability to ambulate in children with myelomeningocele include cognitive ability, physical therapy, compliant parents, clubfoot deformity, scoliosis, increased age, back pain, and lack of motivation. Often, the goal of orthopaedic treatment is a stable posture in braces or in a wheelchair. Surgery may be more detrimental than helpful, causing long-term disability. Before aggressive orthopaedic treatment is instituted, the

lifetime prognosis for the patient should be considered. Only 30% of all patients with myelomeningocele are functionally independent, and only 30% of adults with myelomeningocele are employed full time or part time. Almost all patients with L2 or higher-level lesions use a wheelchair, and more than two thirds of patients with lower-level lesions (L3-5) use a wheelchair at least part of the time.

Most children achieve their maximal level of ambulation around age 4 to 6 years. If a child with myelomeningocele is not standing independently by about age 6 years, walking is unlikely. Prerequisites for walking include a spine balanced over the pelvis; absence of hip and knee contractures (or only mild contractures); and plantigrade, supple, braceable feet with the center of gravity centered over them. An extension posture at the hip and knee can be maintained with minimal support from leg and arm muscles, whereas a flexion posture tends to be a collapsing posture (Fig. 6.30). At least 80% of children with myelomeningocele have some impairment of their upper extremities; effective ambulation with low energy consumption and minimal bracing is possible in only about 50% of adult patients. If a child has functioning quadriceps and medial hamstring muscles, good sitting balance, and upper extremity function, all efforts should be made to achieve ambulation.

■ NONOPERATIVE MANAGEMENT

Almost all children with myelomeningocele except those with low sacral level lesions will require some type of orthotic device. Orthotic treatment goals include maintenance of motion, prevention of deformity, assistance with ambulation/mobility, and the protection of insensate skin. Bracing and splinting vary with the degree of motor deficit and trunk balance, and each child should be carefully evaluated using

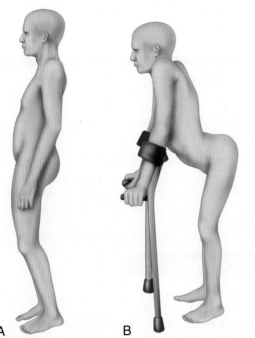

A

B

FIGURE 6.30 **A,** Extension posture with hips and knees extended, feet plantigrade; posture aimed for regardless of bracing necessary. **B,** Flexion posture at the hips imposes lumbar lordosis and patient uses both arms for weight bearing and loses other, more valuable function.

a team approach. Children 12 to 18 months old may benefit from the use of a standing frame for upright positioning, and for children older than 2 years, a parapodium that supports the spine and allows a swing-to or swing-through gait with crutches or a walker may be beneficial. An ankle-foot orthosis is used in children with low lumbar or sacral level lesions and fair quadriceps muscle function. The ankle-foot orthosis should be rigid enough to provide ankle and foot stabilization and to maintain the ankle at 90 degrees. A knee-ankle-foot orthosis (KAFO) may be indicated for a child with a lumbar level lesion and weak quadriceps function to prevent abnormal valgus of the knee during the stance phase of gait. Children with high-level lesions often have excessive anterior pelvic tilt and lumbar lordosis and require a pelvic band, either a conventional HKAFO or a reciprocating gait orthosis. The reciprocating gait orthosis also can be used in patients with upper lumbar lesions, allowing them to be upright and assisting them in attempts at ambulation. This brace is started around the age of 2 and provides the ability to walk in a reciprocal fashion by dynamically coupling the flexion of one hip to the simultaneous extension of the contralateral hip. For the reciprocating orthosis to be effective, the patient should have good upper extremity strength, sitting (trunk) balance, and active hip flexion. Energy expenditure for children in reciprocal gait orthoses and traditional HKAFO are similar; however, children with HKAFO have a faster gait velocity. A child can be tapered from a reciprocal gait orthosis to a HKAFO if he or she develops enough upper body strength to use crutches safely.

The use of materials such as carbon fiber may provide an alternative to patients who do not benefit from current braces.

Carbon fiber ankle-foot orthoses have been shown to increase energy return and ankle plantarflexion motion, positive work, and stride length compared with standard materials.

■ OPERATIVE MANAGEMENT

Orthopaedic deformities in children with myelomeningocele are caused by (1) muscle imbalance resulting from the neurologic abnormality, (2) habitually assumed posture, and (3) associated congenital malformations. Surgical correction of deformities may be indicated. Most surgical procedures in patients with myelomeningocele are performed during the first 15 years of life. When surgical correction is indicated, the deformity should be completely and permanently corrected.

Principles of orthopaedic management include:
1. Multiple procedures should be done simultaneously to minimize repeated anesthetic exposures.
2. Cast immobilization, especially in recumbency, should be minimized owing to the risk of osteopenia and pathologic fracture.
3. The orthopaedic treatment program must be integrated with the total treatment program.
4. The absence of sensation, osteopenia, and the increased risk of infection secondary to urinary tract problems must be constantly considered.
5. Hospitalization must be kept at a minimum.
6. The demands on the family in terms of time, effort, expense, and separation must be minimized.

FOOT

Approximately 75% of children with myelomeningocele have foot deformities that can seriously limit function. These deformities can take many forms including clubfoot, acquired equinovarus, varus, metatarsus adductus, equinus, equinovalgus, vertical talus, talipes calcaneus, calcaneovalgus, calcaneovarus, calcaneocavus, cavus, cavovarus, supination, pes planovalgus, and toe deformities.

The goal of orthopaedic treatment of foot deformities is a plantigrade, painless, mobile, braceable foot. Muscle-balancing procedures that remove deforming muscular forces are more reliable than tendon transfer procedures. Often tendon excision is more reliable than tendon lengthening or transfer. Bone deformities should be corrected by appropriate osteotomies that preserve joint motion. Arthrodesis should be avoided if possible because most feet in patients with myelomeningocele are insensate, which can lead to neuropathic problems including joint destruction and pressure sores.

Manipulation and casting should be used with caution in these patients to avoid pressure sores and iatrogenic fractures. Most foot deformities may eventually require surgical correction if correction of the deformity is needed to improve function. Despite surgical correction, there is a relatively high recurrence rate of the deformity because of the deforming neurologic forces present.

■ EQUINUS DEFORMITY

Equinus usually is an acquired deformity that may be prevented or delayed by bracing and splinting. Depending on the ambulatory function of the patient, an Achilles tendon lengthening, tenotomy, or resection can be performed. Equinus is seen more frequently in children with high lumbar or thoracic level lesions. For mild deformities, excision of 2 cm of the Achilles tendon through a vertical incision usually is sufficient. Alternatively, a percutaneous Achilles tendon lengthening or tenotomy may be performed. Often the long toe flexors must be released to prevent persistent toe flexion deformities that can result in pressure sores. For more severe deformity, radical posterior release is required, including excision of all the tendons contributing to the equinus and extensive capsulotomies of the ankle and subtalar joints. In rare cases, salvage procedures such as osteotomy or talectomy may be required for a symptomatic deformity.

■ CLUBFOOT

Clubfoot is present at birth in approximately 30% to 50% of children with myelomeningocele. The deformity usually is rigid and resembles that of arthrogryposis multiplex congenita and differs markedly from idiopathic clubfoot. It is characterized by severe rigidity, supination-varus deformity, rotational malalignment of the calcaneus and talus, subluxation of the calcaneocuboid and talonavicular joints, and often a cavus component. Internal tibial torsion often is present. With the increased use of the Ponseti clubfoot casting technique, infants with myelomeningocele are being treated with this method. Patients can be successfully treated with this technique, but the complication and recurrence rates are much higher than in idiopathic clubfoot. A 68% early relapse rate and a 33% surgical release rate have been reported in children with myelomeningocele treated with this method. In a series of 24 infants (48 feet), however, only 5 feet (10%) failed to show improvement. Even with adequate surgical correction, recurrence of the clubfoot deformity is frequent.

Surgery can be done between 10 and 12 months of age. Radical posteromedial-lateral release through the Cincinnati incision (see chapter 1) is recommended. If there is significant equinus, a variety of techniques have been described to help prevent posterior soft-tissue and incision breakdown including the use of medial and posterior incisions (Carroll), a modification of the Cincinnati incision that includes a complete circumferential skin release (Noonan et al.), and a modified V-Y plasty (Lubicky and Altiok) (Fig. 6.31). Another method to avoid undue tension on the incision posteriorly is to immobilize the foot postoperatively in an undercorrected position until the wound is healed. Two weeks later, when the incision has healed, the cast can be changed and the foot can be placed in a corrected position safely.

Tenotomies instead of tendon lengthening should be done to minimize any recurrence with growth. If the anterior tibial tendon is active, simple tenotomy should be performed to prevent recurrent supination deformity. In older children, the imbalance between the medial and lateral columns of the foot may be so severe that it cannot be corrected by soft-tissue release alone. Closing wedge osteotomy of the cuboid (see chapter 1), lateral wedge resection of the distal calcaneus (Lichtblau procedure; see chapter 1), or calcaneocuboid arthrodesis (Dillwyn Evans procedure; Fig. 6.2) may be required to shorten the lateral column. Talectomy (see chapter 1) is indicated as a salvage procedure for a severely deformed rigid clubfoot in an older child. The talus should be completely removed because any fragment left behind would resume its growth and cause recurrence of the deformity. The Achilles tendon may need to be resected after talectomy to prevent further equinus. Talectomy would correct the hindfoot deformity, but any adduction deformity should be corrected by shortening of the lateral column through the same

incision. Severe forefoot deformities require midtarsal or metatarsal osteotomies (see chapter 1).

V-O PROCEDURE

Verebelyi and Ogston described a decancellation procedure to correct residual clubfoot deformity in patients with myelomeningocele. This procedure consists of removing as much cancellous bone as possible from the talus and the cuboid. This leaves a hollow shell of bone and more space for correction. The foot is manipulated into calcaneus and valgus, which, because of collapse of the talus and cuboid bone, would lead to correction of the residual deformity. In selected patients, this procedure may be preferable to talectomy for correction of severe rigid clubfoot deformity.

TECHNIQUE 6.30

- Make an oblique incision on the dorsolateral aspect of the foot to expose the cuboid and the talus.
- Retract the peroneal tendons and sural nerve plantarly, and protect them while retracting the extensor digitorum brevis dorsally.
- Cut a square window in the cuboid with a ¼-inch osteotome and remove all cancellous bone with a curet.
- Along the lateral talus, cut a rectangular window with the longer dimension parallel to the long axis of the talus and curet the cancellous contents of the body, neck, and head.
- Confirm the removal of all cancellous bone, with fluoroscopy or radiography, especially at the posterior aspect of the talus.
- Obtain correction by collapsing the empty cartilaginous shells of the cuboid and talus. If satisfactory correction is not obtained, remove lateral wedges from the cuboid or the talar neck.
- If necessary, perform a percutaneous heel cord lengthening.
- Close the wounds routinely, and apply a short leg cast, monovalved for swelling.

POSTOPERATIVE CARE After the swelling has subsided, the cast is reinforced and initially changed at 10 days, maintaining the foot in a neutral or slightly overcorrected position. At 4 weeks after surgery, at the time of the second cast change, a mold is made of the foot in a slightly overcorrected position for an ankle-foot orthosis. When the cast is removed at 6 weeks, the orthosis is worn usually until skeletal maturity.

■ VARUS DEFORMITY

Isolated varus deformity of the hindfoot is rare; it is usually associated with adduction deformity of the forefoot, cavus deformity, or supination deformity. Imbalance between the invertors and evertors should be evaluated carefully. For isolated, rigid hindfoot varus deformity, a closing wedge osteotomy is indicated. After removal of the lateral wedge (Fig. 6.32), the calcaneus should be translated laterally, if needed to increase correction.

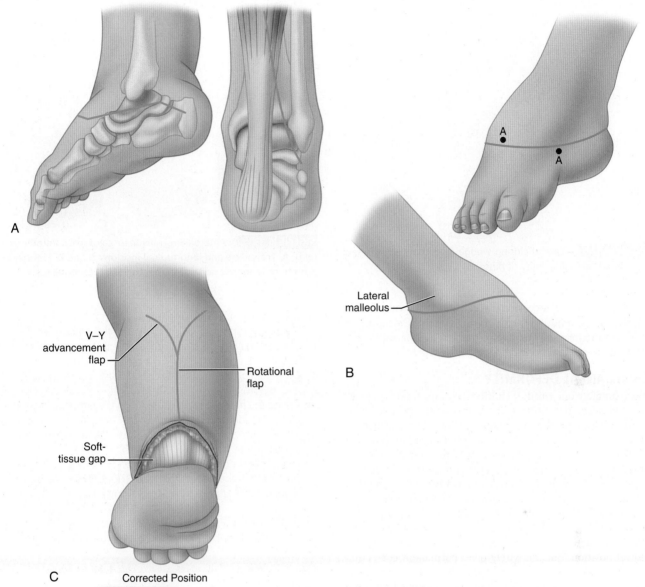

FIGURE 6.31 Incisions used for clubfoot correction. **A,** Carroll two-incision technique. **B,** Modification of the Cincinnati incision by Noonan et al. **C,** V–Y advancement flap technique of Lubicky and Altiok.

■ CAVOVARUS DEFORMITY

Cavovarus deformities occur mainly in children with sacral level lesions. The cavus is the primary deformity that causes the hindfoot varus. The Coleman test (see chapter 7) helps to determine the rigidity of the varus deformity. For a supple deformity, radical plantar release (see chapter 7) is indicated to correct the cavus deformity, without hindfoot bone surgery. If the varus deformity is rigid despite plantar release with or without midtarsal osteotomy, a closing wedge osteotomy is indicated. Any muscle balance must be corrected before the bony procedures or at the same time. Triple arthrodesis (see Technique 6.4) rarely is indicated as a salvage procedure and should be used with caution in myelomeningocele patients.

■ SUPINATION DEFORMITY

Supination deformity of the forefoot occurs most frequently in children with L5 to S1 level lesions and is caused by the unopposed action of the anterior tibial muscle when the peroneus brevis and peroneus longus are inactive. Adduction deformity also can be present. If the muscle imbalance is not corrected, the deformity becomes fixed. If the deformity is supple, simple tenotomy of the anterior tibial tendon is adequate. Simple tenotomy usually is the preferred treatment method for patients with myelomeningocele, but a tendon transfer may be indicated in selective situations. If there is some gastrocnemius-soleus activity and no spasticity, the anterior tibial tendon can be transferred to the midfoot in line with the third metatarsal. Split anterior tibial tendon transfer

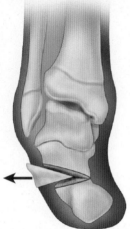

FIGURE 6.32 Lateral closing wedge osteotomy of calcaneus for isolated varus deformity of hindfoot.

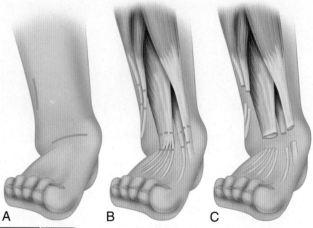

FIGURE 6.33 Anterolateral release for calcaneal deformity (see text). **A,** Transverse and longitudinal incisions. **B** and **C,** Excision of portion of tendons and tendon sheaths. **SEE TECHNIQUE 6.31.**

(see Technique 6.9) occasionally can be used, with the lateral half of the tendon inserted in the cuboid. Osteotomy of the first cuneiform or the base of the first metatarsal may be required for residual bone deformity.

■ CALCANEAL DEFORMITY
Approximately one third of children with myelomeningocele have calcaneal deformities, most frequently children with L4 and L5 lesions. The most common form is a calcaneovalgus deformity caused by the active anterior leg muscles and inactive posterior muscles. Spasticity of the evertors and dorsiflexors may cause calcaneal deformity in children with high-level lesions. Untreated calcaneal deformity produces a bulky, prominent heel that is prone to pressure sores and makes shoe wear difficult. Patients also lose toe-off power and develop an increased crouched gait. If the deformity is supple, as usually is the case, manipulation and splinting can bring the foot to a neutral position, but this rarely gives permanent correction. Muscle imbalance can be corrected early by simple tenotomy of all ankle dorsiflexors, as well as the peroneus brevis and peroneus longus. After anterolateral release in some patients, spasticity develops in the gastrocnemius-soleus muscle, causing an equinus deformity that requires tenotomy of the Achilles tendon or posterior release. Posterior transfer of the anterior tibial tendon has been reported to give good results. This often is combined with other soft-tissue and bony procedures to balance the foot. In older children with severe structural deformities, tendon transfers or tenotomies seldom achieve correction, and bone procedures are indicated.

ANTEROLATERAL RELEASE

TECHNIQUE 6.31

- With the patient supine, apply and inflate a pneumatic tourniquet.
- Make a transverse incision about 2.5 cm long 2.0 to 3.0 cm above the ankle joint (Fig. 6.33A). Alternatively, an an-

terior lazy-S incision may be made. With sharp dissection, divide the superficial fascia to expose the tendons of the extensor hallucis longus, extensor digitorum communis, and tibialis anterior.
- Divide each tendon, and excise at least 2.0 cm of each (Fig. 6.33B).
- Locate the peroneus tertius tendon in the lateralmost part of the wound, and divide it.
- Make a second longitudinal incision above the ankle joint lateral and posterior to the fibula (Fig. 6.33A).
- Identify and divide the peroneus brevis and longus tendons, and excise a section of each (Fig. 6.33C). Close the wounds, and apply a short leg walking cast.

POSTOPERATIVE CARE The cast is worn for 10 days, and then an ankle-foot orthosis is fabricated for night wear.

TRANSFER OF THE ANTERIOR TIBIAL TENDON TO THE CALCANEUS

TECHNIQUE 6.32

- With the patient supine, make an incision in the dorsal aspect of the foot at the level of the insertion of the anterior tibial tendon at the base of the first metatarsal.
- Carefully detach the tendon from its insertion and free it as far proximally as possible.
- Make a second incision on the anterolateral aspect of the leg, just lateral to the tibial crest and 3 to 5 cm above the ankle joint.
- Free the tendon as far distally as possible and bring it up into the proximal wound (Fig. 6.34A).
- Expose the interosseous membrane and make a wide opening in it (Fig. 6.34B).

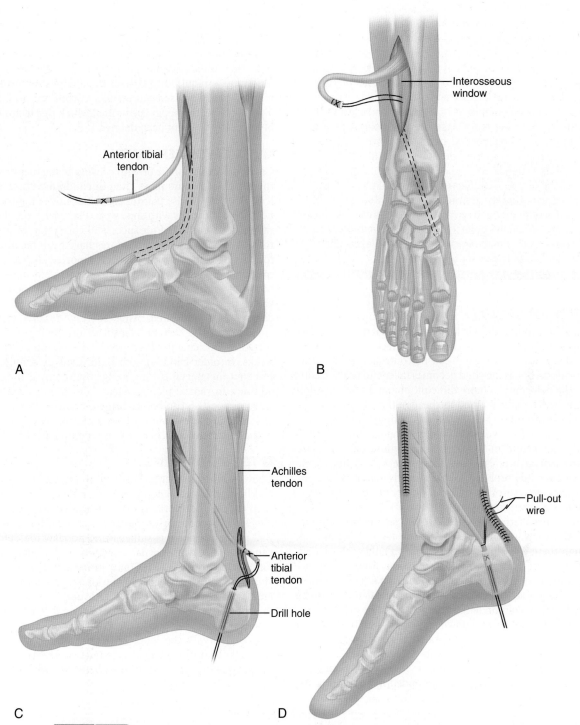

FIGURE 6.34 **A,** Anterior tibial tendon is divided distally and passed subcutaneously to the proximal incision. **B,** A 4 × 1.5 cm window is created in the interosseous membrane. **C,** The anterior tibial tendon is transferred posteriorly through the interosseous membrane. **D,** The transferred tendon is fixed to the calcaneus with a Bunnell suture or suture anchor. (Redrawn from Georgiadis GM, Aronson DD: Posterior transfer of the anterior tibial tendon in children who have a myelomeningocele, *J Bone Joint Surg* 72A:392, 1990.) **SEE TECHNIQUE 6.32.**

- Make a third transverse incision posteriorly at the level of the insertion of the Achilles tendon into the calcaneus.
- Using a tendon passer, bring the anterior tibial tendon through the interosseous membrane, from anterior to posterior, down to the level of this incision (Fig. 6.34C).
- Drill a large hole in the calcaneus, starting posteriorly and medially and exiting laterally and plantarward.
- Pass a Bunnell suture through the tendon, and use a Keith needle to draw the tendon through the hole. A button suture is not recommended because of pressure sores. Suture the tendon to the surrounding soft tissues to the level of its entrance into the calcaneus and to the Achilles tendon (Fig. 6.34D). Alternatively, a suture anchor can be used to secure the transferred tendon. The length of tendon is often not enough to secure the transfer to the calcaneus. When this occurs, the transferred anterior tibial tendon can be sutured directly into the Achilles tendon.
- Close the wounds and apply a short leg cast.

■ HINDFOOT VALGUS

Valgus deformity at the ankle joint and external rotation deformity of the tibia and fibula frequently can exacerbate a hindfoot valgus deformity. Initially, this can be controlled with a well-fitted orthosis, but as the child becomes taller and heavier, control of the deformity is more difficult, pressure sores develop over the medial malleolus and the head of the talus, and surgical treatment is indicated. Clinical and radiographic measurements of the hindfoot valgus should be obtained; more than 10 mm of "lateral shift" of the calcaneus is significant. The Grice extraarticular arthrodesis (see Technique 6.2) is the classic treatment for this problem, but frequently reported complications include resorption of the graft, nonunion, varus overcorrection, and residual valgus. A 19-year follow-up of 35 feet treated with the Grice arthrodesis found significant improvement in visual analog scale (VAS) satisfaction scores and, although there was some mild increase in ankle valgus, 83% of patients were satisfied with their outcome. Medial displacement osteotomy has been recommended for correction of hindfoot valgus so that arthrodesis of the subtalar joint can be avoided. Lateral column lengthening also can be done if there is significant midfoot breakdown associated with the hindfoot valgus. The combination of hindfoot and ankle valgus should be considered; if the ankle deformity is more than 10 to 15 degrees, closing wedge osteotomy or hemiepiphysiodesis of the distal tibial epiphysis is recommended in addition to the calcaneal osteotomy.

■ VERTICAL TALUS

Vertical talus deformities occur in approximately 10% of children with myelomeningocele. The deformity is characterized by malalignment of the hindfoot and midfoot. The talus is almost vertical, the calcaneus is in equinus and valgus, the navicular is dislocated dorsally on the talus, and the cuboid may be subluxated dorsally in relation to the calcaneus. In congenital vertical talus, manipulation and serial casting may partially correct the soft-tissue contractures in preparation for a complete posteromedial-lateral release (see chapter 1), which should be performed when the child is ready to stand in braces, usually between 12 and 18 months old. The anterior tibial tendon can be resected or transferred into the neck of

the talus. Occasionally, an extraarticular subtalar arthrodesis is needed to stabilize the subtalar joint. Dobbs et al. described a technique for correction of vertical talus in which serial manipulation and casting are followed by closed or open reduction of the talus and pin fixation. Percutaneous Achilles tenotomy is required to correct the equinus deformity. This method has been used successfully in children from birth to 4 years of age; the upper age limit at which this technique can be successful has not been defined.

■ PES CAVUS DEFORMITY

Cavus deformity, alone or with clawing of the toes or varus of the hindfoot, occurs most often in children with sacral level lesions. It may cause painful callosities under the metatarsal heads and difficulty with shoe wear. Plantarflexion of the first ray must be corrected for successful correction of the deformity. Although several procedures have been recommended for this deformity, few have been reported in patients with myelomeningocele. For an isolated cavus deformity with no hindfoot varus, radical plantar release is indicated. When varus deformity is present, medial subtalar release (see chapter 1) is indicated. After surgery, a short leg cast is applied, and 1 to 2 weeks later the deformity is gradually corrected by cast changes every week or every other week for 6 weeks. In older children with rigid cavus deformities, anterior first metatarsal closing wedge osteotomy is indicated in addition to radical plantar release. Opening wedge midfoot osteotomies also can be performed to correct the cavus. For residual varus deformity, a Dwyer closing wedge osteotomy of the calcaneus (see chapter 5) is recommended.

■ TOE DEFORMITIES

Claw toe or hammer toe deformities occur more often in children with sacral level lesions and can cause problems with shoe and orthotic fitting. For flexible claw toe deformities, simple tenotomy of the flexors at the level of the proximal phalanx usually is sufficient. Rigid claw toe deformities can be treated with partial resection of the interphalangeal joint or arthrodesis. The Jones procedure (tendon suspension) is indicated when clawing of the great toe is associated with a cavus deformity. Arthrodesis of the proximal interphalangeal joint or tenodesis of the distal stump of the extensor pollicis longus to the extensor pollicis brevis is recommended with the Jones procedure, although arthrodesis would hold up better than a tenodesis. The Hibbs transfer (see chapter 7) can be performed to treat clawing of the lesser toes.

ANKLE

Progressive valgus deformity at the ankle or in combination with hindfoot valgus occurs most frequently in children with low lumbar level lesions. The strength of the gastrocnemius-soleus muscle is diminished or absent, and excessive laxity of the Achilles tendon allows marked passive ankle dorsiflexion. The medial malleolus is bulky, the head of the talus is shifted medially, and pressure ulcerations in these areas are common. The calcaneovalgus deformity usually appears early, but problems with orthotic fitting do not arise until the child is about 6 years old. Fibular shortening is common in children with L4, L5, or higher-level lesions. In the paralytic limb, abnormal shortening of the fibula and lateral malleolus causes a valgus tilt of the talus, with subsequent valgus deformity at the ankle (Fig. 6.35). Shortening of the fibula alters the normal distribution of forces on the distal tibial articular surface and increases compression forces on the lateral portion of the tibial epiphysis, further inhibiting growth, whereas decreased compression on the medial portion of the tibial epiphysis accelerates growth. This imbalance causes the lateral wedging that produces a valgus inclination of the talus. The degree of lateral wedging of the tibial epiphysis correlates with the degree of fibular shortening.

To evaluate valgus ankle deformity in children with myelomeningocele accurately, three factors must be determined: (1) the degree of fibular shortening, (2) the degree of valgus tilt of the talus in the ankle mortise, and (3) the amount of "lateral shift" of the calcaneus in relation to the weight-bearing axis of the tibia. Fibular shortening can be evaluated by measuring the distance between the distal fibular physis and the dome of the talus. In the normal ankle joint, the distal fibular physis is 2 to 3 mm proximal to the dome of the talus in children 4 years old (Fig. 6.36A). Between ages 4 and 8 years, the physis is at the same level as the talar dome (Fig. 6.36B), and in children older than 8 years, it is

2 to 3 mm distal to the talar dome (Fig. 6.36C). Differences of more than 10 mm from these values are considered significant. The valgus tilt of the talus can be measured accurately on anteroposterior, weight-bearing radiographs. The lateral shift of the calcaneus is more difficult to determine, and radiographic techniques have been developed for evaluating ankle valgus and hindfoot alignment. If the talar tilt exceeds 10 degrees, the x-ray tube should be tilted appropriately to obtain a true lateral weight-bearing view of the foot. On this view, the weight-bearing axis of the tibia is drawn and the distance from this line to the center of the calcaneus is measured. On an anteroposterior weight-bearing view, the beam should be directed horizontally to preserve the coronal relationship in both dimensions. The foot is positioned in slight dorsiflexion by placing a hard foam wedge under the plantar surface, but not under the calcaneus, and by positioning the cassette behind the foot and ankle. The normal lateral shift of the calcaneus is 5 to 10 mm (Fig. 6.37A); if the center of the calcaneus is more than 10 mm lateral to the weight-bearing line, excessive valgus is present (Fig. 6.37B). This technique is useful to determine before surgery if the valgus deformity is at the ankle or subtalar level.

Operative treatment is indicated when the ankle valgus deformity causes problems with orthotic fitting and cannot be relieved with orthoses. Achilles tenodesis is indicated for valgus talar tilt between 10 and 25 degrees in patients 6 to 10 years old (Fig. 6.1). Other procedures to correct ankle valgus caused by bone deformities include hemiepiphysiodesis in children with remaining growth and supramalleolar derotation osteotomy for severe angular deformity. Medial sliding osteotomy of the calcaneus may be indicated if the valgus deformity is in the subtalar joint and calcaneus.

HEMIEPIPHYSIODESIS OF THE DISTAL TIBIAL EPIPHYSIS

Hemiepiphysiodesis of the distal tibial epiphysis is indicated in young children with valgus deformities of less than 20 degrees and mild fibular shortening. Through a medial incision at the ankle, the medial aspect of the epiphysis is exposed and epiphysiodesis is performed by a percutaneous or an

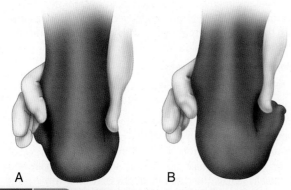

FIGURE 6.35 **A,** Posterior view of right foot of normal child with correct alignment of malleoli and hindfoot. **B,** In child with myelomeningocele, medial malleolus is prominent and lateral malleolus is shortened, causing valgus deformity of ankle.

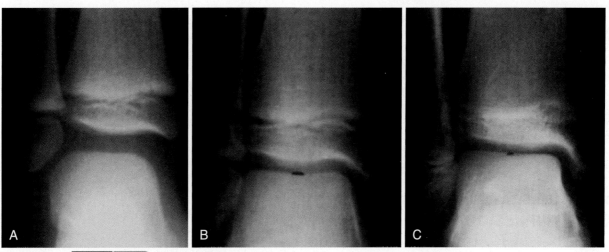

FIGURE 6.36 Normal position of distal fibular physis. **A,** Proximal to dome of talus in children up to 4 years of age. **B,** Level with dome of talus in children between 4 and 8 years of age. **C,** Distal to dome of talus in children older than 8 years of age.

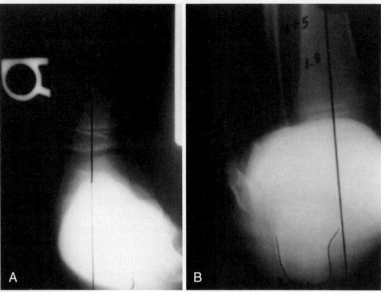

FIGURE 6.37 Radiographic technique for evaluation of ankle valgus. **A,** Normal shift of calcaneus is 5 to 10 mm. **B,** Lateral shift of 15 to 18 mm indicates excessive valgus.

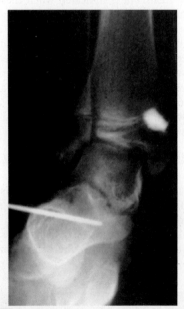

FIGURE 6.38 Radiopaque dye shows extent of medial hemiepiphysiodesis of distal tibial epiphysis.

open method (Fig. 6.38). The growth arrest of the medial physis combined with continued growth of the lateral side gradually corrects the lateral wedging of the tibial epiphysis. If overcorrection occurs, the epiphysiodesis should be completed laterally. This procedure does not correct any rotational component of the deformity, and derotation osteotomy of the distal tibia and fibula may be required.

SCREW EPIPHYSIODESIS

Good results have been obtained with screw epiphysiodesis for correction of ankle valgus, which involves placing a vertical 4.5-mm screw across the medial malleolar physis to slow medial growth, allowing gradual correction of

ankle valgus (median rate of correction of 0.59 degree per month). If the single screw is removed, growth can resume and the deformity may recur. This procedure is recommended in children older than 6 years (Fig. 6.39).

TECHNIQUE 6.33

- Place the patient supine.
- Make a 3-mm stab wound over the medial malleolus. Use image intensification to properly position the incision.
- Insert a guide pin from the 4.5-mm cannulated screw set into the medial malleolus and advance it proximally and medially across the distal tibial physis. Confirm the position of the guide pin by image intensification. The guide pin should be as vertical as possible in the medial one fourth of the medial distal tibial physis in the anteroposterior plane. In the sagittal plane the guide pin should cross the physis through its middle third.
- Place a tap over the guide pin and tap the bone across the physis. Insert a fully threaded, cannulated screw over the guide pin until it is completely seated

SUPRAMALLEOLAR VARUS DEROTATION OSTEOTOMY

Supramalleolar osteotomy is recommended for children older than 10 years of age with low lumbar level lesions, severe fibular shortening (>10 to 20 mm), valgus tilt of more than 20 degrees, and external tibial torsion.

TECHNIQUE 6.34

- With the patient supine, make an anterior longitudinal incision at the distal third of the leg. Expose the distal tibia and identify the epiphysis.

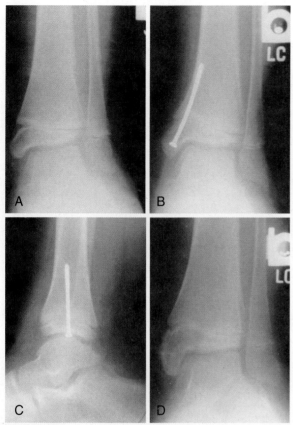

FIGURE 6.39 **A,** Preoperative standing anteroposterior radiographs of ankle in an 8-year, 6-month-old boy with symptomatic flexible pes planus. Note valgus alignment of tibiotalar axis (11 degrees valgus), increased fibular station (station 1), and distal tibial epiphyseal wedging (index 0.55). Standing anteroposterior **(B)** and lateral **(C)** radiographs 1 year, 3 months after placement of transphyseal medial malleolar screw. Tibiotalar axis is improved (3 degrees varus), whereas fibular station and epiphyseal wedging are unchanged. Note position of screw in both planes, subtle distal tibial metaphyseal deformity, and obliquity of physis created by screw. **D,** Standing anteroposterior radiograph of ankle 1 year, 4 months after screw removal. With release of medial tether and resumption of complete physeal growth, ankle valgus recurred (6 degrees valgus). (From Davids JR, Valadie AL, Ferguson RL, et al: Surgical management of ankle valgus in children: use of a transphyseal medial malleolar screw, *J Pediatr Orthop* 17:3, 1997.) **SEE TECHNIQUE 6.33.**

- Make a second incision over the distal third of the fibula and perform an oblique osteotomy beginning laterally and extending distally and medially, depending on the degree of valgus to be corrected.
- Make the medial-based wedge osteotomy as distal on the tibia as possible (Fig. 6.40A).
- At the time of correction of the valgus, rotate the distal fragment internally to correct external tibial torsion.
- Use two Kirschner wires to temporarily hold the fragments in place, and obtain radiographs to evaluate correction of the valgus deformity. The talus should be horizontal and the lateral malleolus lower than the medial malleolus.

- Staples or Kirschner wires (Fig. 6.40C) or, in patients nearing skeletal maturity, a plate and screws (Fig. 6.40B) can be used for internal fixation.
- Close the wounds, and apply a long leg cast with the ankle and foot in neutral.

POSTOPERATIVE CARE Partial weight bearing with crutches is allowed immediately. At 3 weeks, the cast is changed to a below-knee cast and full weight-bearing is allowed. The Kirschner wires can be removed at 8 to 12 weeks.

Rotational deformities of the lower extremity can cause functional problems in patients with myelomeningocele. Out-toeing can result either from an external rotation deformity of the hip or from external tibial torsion and can lead to abnormal knee stress, primarily valgus, as well as difficulties with brace fitting. Internal rotation osteotomies should be considered in children with 20 degrees or more of tibial torsion that interferes with gait. In-toeing can cause difficulties with foot clearance during swing phase of gait. In-toeing frequently occurs in patients with L4 or L5 lesions because of an imbalance between the medial and lateral hamstrings. The hamstrings tend to remain active during the stance phase of gait and, when the biceps femoris is paralyzed, the muscle imbalance produces an in-toeing gait. Another cause for in-toeing is residual internal tibial torsion.

Rotation deformity of the hip and external and internal tibial torsion can be corrected by derotation osteotomies. Dynamic in-toeing gait can be corrected by transferring the semitendinosus laterally to the biceps tendon.

KNEE
Knee deformities are common in patients with myelomeningocele and can cause significant difficulties in maintaining ambulatory function. Deformities of the knee in patients with myelomeningocele are of four types: (1) flexion contracture, (2) extension contracture, (3) valgus deformity, and (4) varus deformity.

▓ FLEXION CONTRACTURE
Flexion contractures are more common than extension contractures. About half of children with thoracic or lumbar level lesions have knee flexion contractures. Contractures of 20 degrees are common at birth, but most correct spontaneously. Knee flexion contractures may become fixed because of (1) the typical position assumed when supine—hips in abduction, flexion, and external rotation; knees in flexion; and feet in equinus; (2) gradual contracture of the hamstring and biceps muscles, with contracture of the posterior knee capsule from quadriceps weakness and prolonged sitting; (3) spasticity of the hamstrings that may occur with the tethered cord syndrome; and (4) hip flexion contracture or calcaneal deformity in the ambulatory patient. Knee flexion contractures of more than 20 degrees can interfere with an effective bracing and standing program and ambulation in an ambulatory patient. Patients who are nonambulatory may tolerate larger degrees of flexion contractures as long as it does not interfere with transfers and sitting balance. Radical flexor release usually is required for contractures of 20 to 30 degrees, especially in children who walk with below-knee orthoses.

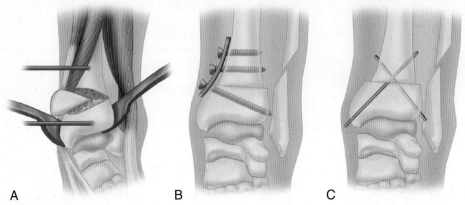

FIGURE 6.40 Supramalleolar varus derotation osteotomy for severe ankle valgus deformity in adolescents. **A,** Removal of medial bone wedge from distal tibial metaphysis. **B,** Fixation of osteotomy with plate and screws. **C,** Fixation with crossed wires. **SEE TECHNIQUE 6.34.**

Supracondylar extension osteotomy of the femur (Fig. 6.11) generally is required for contractures of more than 30 to 45 degrees in older children who are community ambulators and in whom radical flexor release was unsuccessful. If a hip flexion contracture is present, hip and knee contractures should be corrected at the same time. Spiro et al. reported that anterior femoral epiphysiodesis by stapling is an effective and safe method for the treatment of fixed knee flexion deformity in growing children and adolescents with spina bifida. Guided growth with plate and screws also can be used to correct fixed flexion deformities. No surgical treatment is indicated in older children who are not community ambulators if the contracture does not interfere with mobility and sitting balance.

RADICAL FLEXOR RELEASE

TECHNIQUE 6.35

- Make a medial and a lateral vertical incision just above the flexor crease. Alternatively, a vertical midline incision just above the flexor crease can be used. Z- or S-shaped incisions that cross the flexor crease should be avoided because of difficulty with skin closure after a radical flexor release.
- In a child with a high-level lesion, identify and divide the medial hamstring tendons (semitendinosus, semimembranosus, gracilis, and sartorius).
- Resect part of each tendon (Fig. 6.41A).
- Laterally, identify, divide, and resect the biceps tendon and the iliotibial band.
- In a child with a low lumbar level lesion, intramuscularly lengthen the biceps and semimembranosus to preserve some flexor power.
- Free the origin of the gastrocnemius from the medial and lateral condyles, exposing the posterior knee capsule, and perform an extensive capsulectomy (Fig. 6.41B).
- If full extension is not obtained, divide the medial and lateral collateral ligaments and the posterior cruciate ligament (Fig. 6.41C).

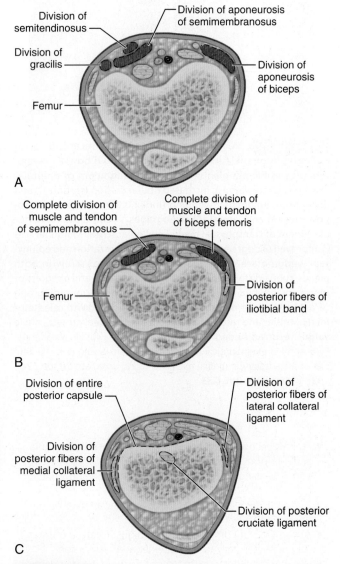

FIGURE 6.41 Release of flexor tendons for flexion contracture of knee. **A,** Minimal procedure. **B,** Additional optional procedures above joint level. **C,** Additional optional procedures at joint level. **SEE TECHNIQUE 6.35.**

- Close the wound over a suction drain and apply a long leg cast or brace with the knee in full extension. If the flexion contracture is greater than 45 degrees, because of the possibility of vascular problems the first cast should be applied with the knee in 20 to 30 degrees of flexion and gradually brought to full extension through serial cast changes.

POSTOPERATIVE CARE The cast is removed at 14 days, and a long leg splint is used at night. For children with low lumbar level lesions, intensive physical therapy for strengthening of the quadriceps mechanism is imperative after cast removal.

■ EXTENSION CONTRACTURE

Knee extension contractures can occur in patients with myelomeningocele. Approximately two thirds have no useful muscle function in the lower extremities, one third of which are caused by unopposed quadriceps function from paralytic hamstring muscles. Extension contractures usually are bilateral and frequently are associated with other congenital anomalies, such as dislocation of the ipsilateral hip, external rotation contracture of the hip, equinovarus deformity of the foot, and occasionally valgus deformity of the knee. Knee extension contracture can impair ambulation and make wheelchair sitting and transfers difficult. Serial casting, attempting to flex the knee to at least 90 degrees, is successful in some patients. If this does not correct the contracture, lengthening of the quadriceps mechanism is indicated. The most common procedure to correct this deformity is a V-Y quadriceps lengthening, capsular release, and posterior displacement of the hamstring muscles (Fig. 6.42). This usually is done by 1 year of age. Other methods of lengthening have been described, including "anterior circumcision," in which all of the structures in front and at the side of the knee are divided by subcutaneous tenotomy, subcutaneous release of quadriceps tendon, Z-plasty of the extensor mechanism combined with anterior capsulotomy, and subcutaneous release of the patellar ligament.

■ VARUS OR VALGUS DEFORMITY

Varus or valgus deformity of the knee can occur in patients with myelomeningocele and can result from abnormal trunk mechanics that lead to abnormal knee mechanics or from malunion of a supracondylar fracture of the femur or proximal metaphyseal fracture of the tibia. In ambulatory patients, valgus knee instability is more common. This is caused by several reasons in ambulatory patients. Weak quadriceps, gastrocnemius-soleus muscles, and hip abductors cause the knee to go into valgus as the patient displaces the hemipelvis laterally during stance phase. The amount of knee valgus is proportional to the degree of neurologic impairment. This deformity also can be associated with excessive femoral anteversion or excessive external tibial torsion. Both increase the valgus or adductor stresses at the knee during the stance phase of gait (Fig. 6.43). This eventually leads to increased joint laxity and degenerative changes around the knee. Nonoperative treatment consists of the use of forearm crutches to decrease the Trendelenburg gait. A KAFO can be used to stabilize the knee, but often they are too bulky and not well accepted by an ambulatory patient. Deformities that

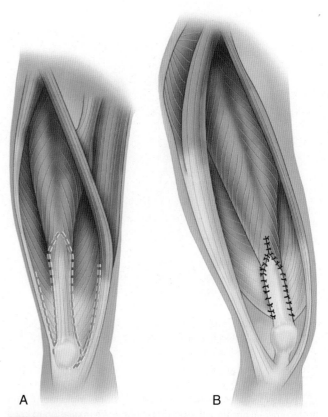

FIGURE 6.42 V-Y quadricepsplasty for hyperextension contracture of the knee. **A,** Detachment of rectus femoris tendon from muscle of rectus femoris, vastus medialis, and vastus lateralis muscles; vastus medialis and lateralis muscles are separated from iliotibial band, lateral hamstrings, medial hamstrings, and sartorius muscles. **B,** When knee is flexed, hamstring muscles and tensor fascia lata slip posterior to knee axis, restoring normal function. Quadriceps muscles are repaired in lengthened position.

interfere with bracing and mobility require supracondylar or tibial osteotomy with internal fixation to correct the deformity. Hemiepiphysiodesis, stapling, or guided growth with plate and screws also can be used for correction if the angular deformity is recognized early.

HIP

Treatment recommendations for deformities and instability around the hip in children with myelomeningocele have changed owing, in part, to the use of gait analysis. Deformities or instability of the hip in children with myelomeningocele can be caused by muscle imbalance, congenital dysplasia, habitual posture, or a combination of these three. Nearly half of children with myelomeningocele have hip subluxation or dislocation, which correlates poorly with overall hip function and ambulatory potential. Many authors found that the presence of a concentric reduction did not lead to improvements in hip range of motion, ability to ambulate, and decreased pain. The goal of current treatment protocols is to maintain hip range of motion through contracture prevention and release rather than obtaining anatomic concentric reduction.

Abduction or adduction contractures of the hip can cause infrapelvic obliquity that can interfere with ambulation and bracing. Hip flexion contractures with associated lumbar

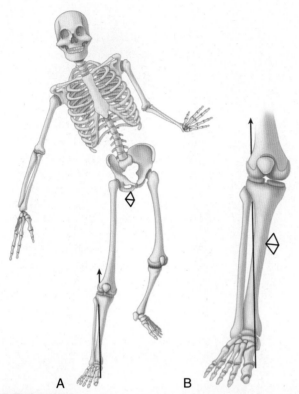

FIGURE 6.43 **A,** Maximal coronal plane movement and posteromedial position of ground reaction force in relation to knee joint center. **B,** Close-up of ground reaction force during maximal coronal plane displacement of trunk. (From Gupta RT, Vankoski S, Novak RA, Dias LS: Trunk kinematics and the influence on valgus knee stress in persons with high sacral level myelomeningocele, *J Pediatr Orthop* 25:89, 2005.)

lordosis and knee flexion contracture may cause more disability than mobile dislocated hips. Because of the different levels of paralysis and the combination of mixed and flaccid paralysis, treatment must be individualized for each patient. An evidence-based review of hip surgery in patients with myelomeningocele found that there was no benefit to surgical treatment of dislocated hips and that walking ability was related to the degree of contracture present. The only subgroup that might benefit from surgery is children with myelomeningocele below L4 with a unilateral hip dislocation. Children in this group may have a worsened Trendelenburg gait secondary to leg-length discrepancy; however, this remains controversial. Gait analysis has shown that walking speed is unaffected by the presence of a hip dislocation in patients with low-level myelomeningocele, and gait symmetry more closely correlates to the absence of joint contractures or the presence of symmetric contractures rather than the status of the hip itself.

In addition, the complication rate for surgical reduction of the hip in patients with myelomeningocele can be very high, ranging from 30% to 45%. Complications include loss of motion, pathologic fractures, worsening ambulatory function, and worsening neurologic deficits.

◼ FLEXION CONTRACTURE

Flexion deformity of the hip occurs most frequently in children with high lumbar or thoracic level lesions. The proposed causes for a hip flexion contracture are unopposed action of the hip flexors (iliopsoas, sartorius, and rectus femoris), habitual posture from long periods of lying supine or sitting, and spasticity of the hip flexors. Hip flexion contractures must be distinguished from the physiologic flexion position, and the amount of hip flexion should be determined by the Thomas test. Because of a tendency to improve, hip flexion deformities rarely should be surgically treated before 24 months of age. A hip flexion contracture of 20 to 30 degrees usually can be accommodated. Increased lumbar lordosis and knee flexion often are associated with hip flexion contractures and may make a stable upright posture difficult. Surgical release is indicated for contractures that interfere with bracing, walking, or obtaining an upright posture when hip flexion contractures are greater than 30 degrees. Knee flexion contractures, which commonly occur with the hip contractures, should be corrected at the same time as the hip contracture.

Anterior hip release involves release of the sartorius, rectus femoris, iliopsoas, and tensor fasciae latae muscles; the anterior hip capsule; and the iliopsoas tendon. This procedure should adequately correct flexion contractures of 60 degrees. If deformity remains after release, subtrochanteric extension osteotomy is indicated.

ANTERIOR HIP RELEASE

TECHNIQUE 6.36

- Make a "bikini-line" skin incision slightly distal and parallel to the iliac crest, extending it obliquely along the inguinal crease.
- Identify and protect the neurovascular bundle medially.
- Identify the iliopsoas tendon as far distally as possible and divide it transversely.
- Detach the sartorius muscle from its origin on the superior iliac crest.
- Identify the rectus insertion in the anterior inferior iliac crest and detach it.
- Laterally, identify the tensor fasciae latae muscle, and, after carefully separating it from the fascia, divide the fascia transversely completely posterior to the anterior border of the gluteal muscles to expose the anterior hip capsule.
- If any residual flexion contracture remains, open the joint capsule transversely about 2 cm from the acetabular labrum.
- Place a suction drain in the wound, suture the subcutaneous tissue with interrupted sutures, and approximate the skin edges with subcuticular nylon sutures.
- Apply a hip spica cast or a total body splint with the hip in full extension, 10 degrees of abduction, and neutral rotation.
- In children with low lumbar level lesions this release greatly reduces hip flexor power and may impair mobility. A free tendon graft, using part of the tensor fasciae latae, can be used to reattach the sartorius to the anterior superior iliac crest, and the rectus tendon can be sutured distal to the sartorius muscle in the hip capsule.

POSTOPERATIVE CARE Early weight bearing for 2 to 3 hours a day is encouraged. The spica cast is removed at 4 to 6 weeks. If a splint is used, it can be removed for range-of-motion exercises after the wounds are healed.

■ FLEXION-ABDUCTION–EXTERNAL ROTATION CONTRACTURE

Flexion-abduction–external rotation contractures are common in children with thoracic level lesions and complete paralysis of the muscles of the lower extremity. Continuous external rotation of the hip in the supine position causes contractures of the posterior hip capsule and short external rotator muscles; this occurrence may be decreased by the use of night splints (total body splints) and range-of-motion exercises. Complete hip release (see Technique 6.18) is indicated only when the deformity interferes with bracing. If both hips are contracted, as is often the case, both should be corrected at the same time.

■ EXTERNAL ROTATION CONTRACTURE

Isolated external rotation contracture of the hip occasionally occurs in children with low lumbar level lesions. Initially, bracing and physical therapy help improve the external rotation contracture. If the external hip rotation persists after the child is 5 or 6 years old, a subtrochanteric medial rotation osteotomy is indicated.

■ ABDUCTION CONTRACTURE

Isolated unilateral abduction contracture is a common cause of pelvic obliquity, scoliosis, and difficulty in sitting and ambulation. It generally is caused by contracture of the tensor fasciae latae, but it may occur after iliopsoas transfer. It is common in children with high-level lesions, and early splinting and physical therapy may decrease the risk of its occurrence. Fascial release is indicated when the abduction contracture causes pelvic obliquity and scoliosis and interferes with function or bracing.

FASCIAL RELEASE

TECHNIQUE 6.37

- Incise the skin along the anterior one half or two thirds of the iliac crest to the anterior superior iliac spine.
- Divide all thigh fascial and tendinous structures around the anterolateral aspect of the hip: fascia lata, fascia over the gluteus medius and gluteus minimus, and tensor fasciae latae.
- Do not divide the muscle tissue, only the enveloping fascial structures.
- Fasciotomy of the fascia lata distally, as described by Yount (see Technique 6.18), also may be required.
- Close the wound over a suction drain, and apply a hip spica cast with the operated hip in neutral abduction and the opposite hip in 20 degrees of abduction, enough to permit perineal care.

POSTOPERATIVE CARE The cast is removed at 2 weeks, and a total body splint is fitted.

■ ADDUCTION CONTRACTURE

Adduction contractures are common with dislocation or subluxation of the hip in children with high-level lesions because of spasticity and contracture of the adductor muscles. Surgery is indicated when the contracture causes pelvic obliquity and interferes with sitting or walking. Adductor release may be combined with operative treatment of hip subluxation or dislocation.

ADDUCTOR RELEASE

TECHNIQUE 6.38

- Make a transverse inguinal incision 2 to 3 cm long just distal to the inguinal crease over the adductor longus tendon.
- Open the superficial fascia to expose the adductor longus tendon.
- Using electrocautery, divide the tendon close to its insertion on the pubic ramus.
- If necessary, divide the muscle fibers of the gracilis proximally and completely divide the adductor brevis muscle fibers, taking care to protect the anterior branch of the obturator nerve. At least 45 degrees of abduction should be possible.
- Close the wound over a suction drain.

POSTOPERATIVE CARE A brace or cast that holds the hip in 25 to 30 degrees of abduction can be used postoperatively. If a cast is used, it is removed at 2 weeks, and a splint is fitted with the hip in 25 degrees of abduction.

■ HIP SUBLUXATION AND DISLOCATION

True developmental hip dislocation is rare in patients with myelomeningocele and occurs in children with sacral level lesions without significant muscle imbalance. Treatment should follow standard conservative methods (Pavlik harness, closed reduction, and spica cast immobilization). Teratologic dislocations usually occur in children with high-level lesions. Initial radiographs show a dysplastic acetabulum, with the head of the femur displaced proximally; these dislocations should not be treated initially.

Paralytic subluxation or dislocation is the most common type, occurring in 50% to 70% of children with low-level (L3 or L4) lesions. Dislocation occurs most frequently during the first 3 years of life because of an imbalance between abduction and adduction forces. Dislocations in older children usually are caused by contractures or spasticity of the unopposed adductors and flexors associated with a tethered cord syndrome or hydromyelia.

Reduction of hip dislocations in children with myelomeningocele is generally not recommended. Maintaining a level pelvis and flexible hips seems more important than reduction of the hip dislocation. The goal of treatment should be maximal function, rather than radiographic reduction. Soft-tissue release alone is indicated in patients without functional quadriceps muscles because only occasionally do they remain community ambulators as adults. Open reduction is appropriate only for rare children with sacral level involvement who have strong quadriceps muscles bilaterally, normal trunk balance, and normal upper extremity function. Bilateral or unilateral hip dislocation or subluxation in children with high-level lesions does not require extensive surgical treatment, but soft-tissue contractures should be corrected.

If treatment is undertaken for hip subluxation or dislocation in the rare patient who may benefit from it, the principles of paralytic hip surgery should be adhered to as follows: (1) obtain reduction of the hip into the acetabulum, (2) correct any residual bony deformity, and (3) balance the deforming muscle forces to prevent recurrence. The two most common procedures to balance the deforming muscle forces in an unstable hip in patients with myelomeningocele have been transfer of the iliopsoas muscle (Sharrad or Mustard procedure) and transfer of the external oblique muscle. Iliopsoas transfer with adductor release, capsulorrhaphy, and acetabuloplasty can be done in addition to open reduction. The Sharrad iliopsoas transfer through the posterolateral ilium (see Technique 6.21) is most often used. Iliopsoas transfer is controversial and is not routinely recommended; it has reported success rates ranging from 20% to 95%. Alternative procedures include transfer of the external oblique muscle to the greater trochanter (see Technique 6.19) in conjunction with femoral osteotomy and posterolateral transfer of the tensor fasciae latae with transfer of the adductor and external oblique muscles. This procedure also is controversial. Yildram et al. found no difference in functional improvement with external oblique transfer compared with surgery with internal oblique transfer.

TRANSFER OF ADDUCTORS, EXTERNAL OBLIQUE, AND TENSOR FASCIAE LATAE

TECHNIQUE 6.39

(PHILLIPS AND LINDSETH)
- Place the patient supine and expose the adductor muscles through a transverse incision beginning just anterior to the tendon of the adductor longus and extending posteriorly to the ischium.
- Incise the fascia longitudinally and detach the tendons of the gracilis, adductor longus and brevis, and the anterior third of the magnus from the pubis.
- Carry the dissection posteriorly to the ischial tuberosity and suture the detached origins of the adductor muscles to the ischium with nonabsorbable sutures. Take care not to disrupt the anterior branch of the obturator nerve that supplies the adductor muscles.
- Transfer the external abdominal oblique muscle to the gluteus medius tendon or preferably to the greater trochanter, as described by Thomas, Thompson, and Straub.
- Make an oblique skin incision extending from the posterior third of the iliac crest to the anterior superior iliac spine (Fig. 6.44A).
- Curve the incision distally and posteriorly to the junction of the proximal and middle third of the femur.
- With sharp and blunt dissection, raise skin flaps to expose the fascia of the leg from the lateral border of the sartorius to the level of the greater trochanter.
- Expose the external oblique similarly from the iliac crest to the posterior superior iliac spine and from its costal origin to the pubis (Fig. 6.44B).

- Make two incisions approximately 1 cm apart in the aponeurosis of the external oblique parallel to the Poupart ligament and join them close to the pubis at the external ring.
- Extend the superior incision proximally along the medial border of the muscle belly until the costal margin is reached.
- Free the muscle from the underlying internal oblique by blunt dissection until the posterior aspect is reached in the Petit triangle.
- Elevate the muscle fibers from the iliac crest by cutting from posterior to anterior along the crest.
- Close the defect that remains in the aponeurosis of the external oblique beginning at the pubis and extending as far laterally as possible.
- Fold the cut edges of the muscle and aponeurosis over and suture with a single suture at the muscle-tendinous junction.
- Weave a heavy, nonabsorbable suture through the aponeurosis in preparation for transfer (Fig. 6.44C).
- Attention is then directed to the tensor fasciae latae.
- Detach the origin of the tensor fasciae latae from the ilium.
- Separate the muscle along its anterior border from the sartorius down to its insertion into the iliotibial band.
- Divide the iliotibial band transversely to the posterior part of the thigh.
- Carry the incision in the iliotibial band proximally to the insertion of the oblique fibers of the tensor fasciae latae and the tendon of the gluteus maximus. Take care to preserve the superior gluteal nerve and arteries beneath the gluteus medius muscle approximately 1 cm distal and posterior to the anterior superior iliac spine (Fig. 6.44D).
- Abduct the hip and fold the origin of the tensor fasciae latae back on itself to the limit allowed by the neurovascular bundle and then suture it to the ilium with nonabsorbable sutures so that its origin overlies the gluteus medius muscle. Do not attach the distal end to the gluteus maximus tendon until the end of the procedure.
- The hip, proximal femur, and ilium are now easily accessible for indicated corrective procedures such as open reduction of the hip, capsular plication, proximal femoral osteotomy, and acetabular augmentation. The origins of the rectus femoris and the psoas tendon are not routinely divided, although they can be released at this time if there is a hip flexion contracture.
- With the patient maximally relaxed or paralyzed, transfer the tendon of the external oblique to the greater trochanter.
- Drill a hole in the greater trochanter and pass the tendon of the external oblique from posterior to anterior and suture it back on itself. The muscle should reach the greater trochanter and should follow a straight line from the rib cage to the trochanter; if it does not, the borders of the muscle should be inspected to ensure that they are free from all attachments (Fig. 6.44D).
- Weave the distal end of the tensor fasciae latae through the tendon of the gluteus maximus while the hip is abducted approximately 20 degrees.

POSTOPERATIVE CARE A hip spica cast is applied postoperatively with the hips in extension and abducted 20 degrees. The child is encouraged to stand in the cast to

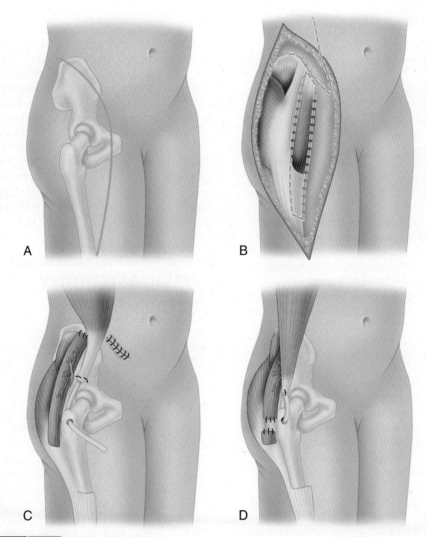

FIGURE 6.44   Transfer of adductors, external oblique, and tensor fasciae latae. **A,** Skin incision. **B,** Skin flaps are elevated to expose fascia of leg and external oblique muscle. **C,** Cut edges of external oblique muscle and aponeurosis are folded over and sutured. Defect in aponeurosis is sutured. Origin of tensor fasciae latae on ilium is detached, with care being taken to preserve neurovascular bundle. Remainder of muscle is prepared for transfer. **D,** Tendon of external oblique is transferred to greater trochanter from posterior to anterior. Distal end of tensor fasciae latae is woven through tendon of gluteus maximus. **SEE TECHNIQUE 6.39.**

prevent osteopenia. The cast is removed 1 month after surgery, and physical therapy is started. The patient is returned to the braces used before the operation. Any modification in bracing is made as indicated on follow-up.

For severe acetabular dysplasia, a shelf procedure or Chiari pelvic osteotomy can be done at the same time as the transfer. If more than 20 to 30 degrees of abduction is necessary to maintain concentric reduction of the hip, a varus femoral osteotomy is indicated. Even with these procedures to correct acetabular dysplasia there is a high failure rate if muscle-balancing procedures are not included as part of the procedure.

PROXIMAL FEMORAL RESECTION AND INTERPOSITION ARTHROPLASTY

Severe joint stiffness is one of the most disabling results of hip surgery in patients with myelomeningocele. If the hip is stiff in extension, the child cannot sit; if it is stiff in flexion, the child cannot stand; if it is stiff "in between," the child can neither sit nor stand. Resection of the femoral head and neck often is not effective. Proximal femoral resection and interposition arthroplasty are recommended in severely involved multiply handicapped children with dislocated hips and severe adduction contractures of the lower extremity.

TECHNIQUE 6.40

(BAXTER AND D'ASTOUS)
- Position the patient with a sandbag beneath the affected hip.
- Make a straight lateral approach beginning 10 cm proximal to the greater trochanter and extending down to the proximal femur.
- Split the fascia lata.
- Detach the vastus lateralis and gluteus maximus from their insertions, and detach them from the greater trochanter.
- Identify the psoas tendon, and detach its distal insertion on the lesser trochanter to expose extraperiosteally the proximal femur.
- Incise the periosteum circumferentially just distal to the gluteus maximus insertion, and transect the bone at this level.
- Divide the short external rotators. Incise the capsule circumferentially at the level of the basal neck.
- Cut the ligamentous teres, remove the proximal femur, and test the range of motion of the hip. If necessary, perform a proximal hamstring tenotomy through the same incision after identifying the sciatic nerve.
- Adductor release also can be performed through a separate groin incision.
- Seal the acetabular cavity by oversewing the capsular edges.
- Cover the proximal end of the femur with the vastus lateralis and rectus femoris muscles.
- Interpose the gluteal muscles between the closed acetabulum and the covered end of the proximal femur to act as a further soft-tissue cushion.
- Close the wound in layers over a suction drain.

POSTOPERATIVE CARE The operated lower extremity is placed in Russell traction in abduction until the soft tissues have healed, and then gentle range-of-motion exercises are begun. If traction is not tolerated, the patient can be placed in a cast or brace until the soft tissues have healed.

▓ PELVIC OBLIQUITY

Pelvic obliquity is common in patients with myelomeningocele. In addition to predisposing the hip to dislocation, it interferes with sitting, standing, and walking, and it can lead to ulceration under the prominent ischial tuberosity. Pelvic obliquity is an important determinant of ambulatory function, second only to neurologic level of involvement. Gait analysis has shown that pelvic obliquity has the strongest correlation with oxygen cost in ambulatory patients with myelomeningocele and that patients may self-select their walking speed to minimize the pelvic shift in the sagittal and coronal planes during gait. Mayer described three types of pelvic obliquity: (1) infrapelvic, caused by contracture of the abductor and tensor fasciae latae muscles of one hip and contracture of the adductors of the opposite hip; (2) suprapelvic, caused by uncompensated scoliosis resulting from bony deformity of the lumbosacral spine or severe paralytic scoliosis; and (3) pelvic, caused by bony deformity of the sacrum and sacroiliac joint, such as partial sacral agenesis, causing asymmetry of the pelvis. Incidence of infrapelvic obliquity can be decreased by splinting, range-of-motion exercises,

and positioning, but when hip contractures are well established, soft-tissue release is required. Occasionally, more severe deformities require proximal femoral osteotomy. Suprapelvic obliquity can be corrected by control of the scoliosis by orthoses or spinal fusion. If severe scoliosis cannot be completely corrected, bony pelvic obliquity becomes fixed.

Obliquity of 20 degrees is sufficient to interfere with walking and to produce ischial decubitus ulcerations; Mayer recommended pelvic osteotomy in this instance. Before osteotomy, hip contractures should be released and the scoliosis should be corrected by spinal fusion. The degree of correction of pelvic obliquity is determined preoperatively from appropriate radiographs of the pelvis and spine (Fig. 6.45A). The maximal correction obtainable with bilateral iliac osteotomies is 40 degrees.

PELVIC OSTEOTOMY

TECHNIQUE 6.41

(LINDSETH)
- The approach is similar to that described by O'Phelan for iliac osteotomy to correct exstrophy of the bladder.
- With the child prone, make bilateral, inverted, L-shaped incisions beginning above the iliac crest, proceeding medially to the posterior superior iliac spine, and then curving downward along each side of the sacrum to the sciatic notch.
- Detach the iliac apophysis by splitting it longitudinally starting at the anterior superior iliac spine and proceeding posteriorly.
- Retract the paraspinal muscles, the quadratus lumborum muscle, and the iliac muscles medially along the inner half of the epiphysis and the inner periosteum of the ilium.
- After the sacral origin of the gluteus maximus has been detached from the sacrum, divide the outer periosteum of the ilium longitudinally just lateral to the posteromedial iliac border, extending from the posterior superior iliac spine down to the sciatic notch.
- Strip the outer periosteum along the gluteus muscles and the outer half of the epiphysis from the outer table of the ilium, taking care to avoid damaging the superior and inferior gluteal vessels and nerves. Retract the soft tissues down to the sciatic notch, and protect them by inserting malleable retractors. Next, make bilateral osteotomies approximately 2 cm lateral to each sacroiliac joint. The size of the wedge is determined by the amount of the correction desired and is limited to no more than one third of the iliac crest; the base of the wedge usually is about 2.5 cm long (Fig. 6.45B).
- After the wedge of bone has been removed, correct the deformity by pulling on the limb on the short side and pushing up on the limb on the long side (Fig. 6.45C). Usually this closes the osteotomy on the long side. If upper migration of the ilium onto the sacrum is severe, trim the excess iliac crest.
- Close the wedge osteotomy with two threaded pins or sutures through drill holes.

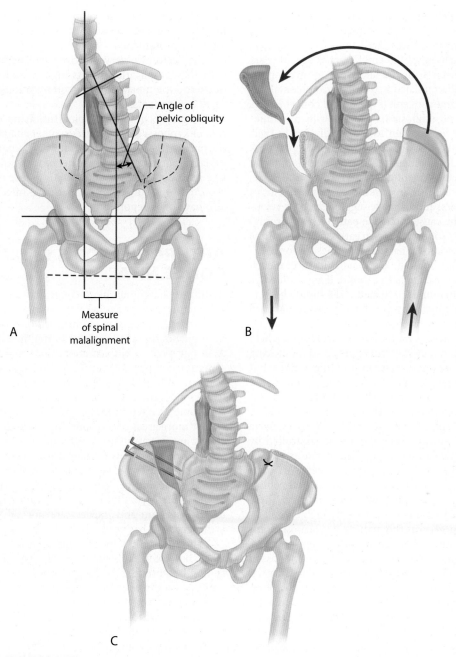

FIGURE 6.45 Pelvic osteotomy for pelvic obliquity, as described by Lindseth. **A,** Preoperative determination of size of iliac wedge to be removed and transferred. **B,** After bilateral osteotomies and removal of wedge from low side, deformity is corrected. **C,** Transferred iliac wedge is fixed with two Kirschner wires. **SEE TECHNIQUE 6.41.**

- Then use a spreader to open the osteotomy on the opposite (short) side sufficiently to receive the graft.
- Use two Kirschner wires to hold the graft in place (Fig. 6.45C).
- Close the wound over suction-irrigation drains, and apply a double full-hip spica cast.

POSTOPERATIVE CARE The cast is worn for 2 weeks. The Kirschner wires are removed when radiographs show sufficient healing of the osteotomy.

SPINE
■ SCOLIOSIS

Paralytic spinal deformities have been reported in 90% of patients with myelomeningocele. Scoliosis is the most common deformity and usually is progressive. The incidence of scoliosis is related to the level of the bone defect and the level of paralysis: 100% with T12 lesions, 80% with L2 lesions, 70% with L3 lesions, 60% with L4 lesions, 25% with L5 lesions, and 5% with S1 lesions. Glard expanded on this concept by dividing patients into four neurosegmental groups based on the spinal deformities that occur within each group. Group 1 (L5 or below) had no spinal deformity, group 2 (L3-L4) had variable deformities, group 3 (L1-L2) was predictive of spinal deformity, and group 4 (T12 and above) was predictive of kyphosis. The curves develop gradually until the child reaches age 10 years and may increase rapidly with the adolescent growth spurt. Raycroft and Curtis differentiated between developmental (no vertebral anomalies) and congenital (structural abnormalities of the vertebral bodies) scoliosis in patients with myelomeningocele. The two types were almost evenly divided in their patients. They suggested muscle imbalance and habitual posturing as causes of developmental scoliosis. Developmental curves occur later than congenital curves, are more flexible, and usually are in the lumbar area with compensatory curves above and below. Several authors have suggested that developmental scoliosis can be caused in some patients by hydromyelia or a tethered cord syndrome, and an early onset of scoliosis (<6 years) frequently occurs in patients with these lesions.

Spinal radiographs should be obtained at least once each year, beginning when the child is 5 years old. If any scoliosis is detected, further evaluation is indicated. MRI should be performed to determine if hydromyelia or a tethered spinal cord is present. The use of a thoracolumbosacral orthosis for daytime wear when the curve is more than 30 degrees may help with sitting balance and may slow curve progression. Bracing slows curve progression and delays surgical intervention but does not halt the progress of most curves. The use of a brace may be challenging because of poor skin and the risk of pressure sores, as well as interference with bowel and bladder care.

Indications for spinal fusion include a progressive increase in angular deformity that cannot be controlled by bracing and unacceptable deformities that create problems with sitting balance. The goals of surgery are to achieve a solid fusion with maximal safe correction, minimize pelvic obliquity, and increase sitting tolerance and independence. These goals must be weighed against the extremely high complication rate of spinal surgery in this patient population; complications include nonunion in up to 40%, deep infection, hardware irritation and resultant skin breakdown, and loss of ambulatory function. In 49 patients who had spinal surgery, sitting balance was improved in 70%, but the ability to ambulate was negatively affected in 67% of patients who had anterior and posterior surgery. Another study found that sitting was the only outcome measure to be improved by spinal surgery, and an evidence-based review concluded that the benefits of spine surgery in this patient population were uncertain. Anterior and posterior surgery was found to provide greater correction with lower pseudarthrosis rates (Fig. 6.46).

■ KYPHOSIS

The most severe spinal deformity in patients with myelomeningocele is congenital kyphosis; it occurs in approximately 10% of patients. The kyphosis usually is present at birth and may make sac closure difficult. The curve generally extends from the lower thoracic level to the sacral spine, with its apex in the midlumbar region. The deformity usually is progressive.

❚ KYPHECTOMY

Congenital kyphosis is unresponsive to bracing and usually requires surgery for correction. The goal of treatment of kyphosis is not to obtain a normal spine but to provide sitting balance without the use of the arms and hands for support. Other goals are to increase the lumbar height to allow

room for abdominal contents and provide better mechanics for breathing and to prevent pressure sores by reducing the kyphotic prominence.

Kyphectomy is very effective in correcting kyphosis; however, the complication rate is high. Wound and skin breakdown are the most common complications, occurring in up to 50% of patients.

Surgical techniques for spinal fusion in scoliosis and correction of kyphosis are described in other chapter. Complications of spinal surgery in patients with myelomeningocele are significantly greater than in patients with idiopathic scoliosis. The most common complication is failure of fusion, which is reported to occur in 40% of patients. Infection rates of 43% also have been reported.

ARTHROGRYPOSIS MULTIPLEX CONGENITA

Arthrogryposis multiplex congenita (multiple congenital contractures) is a physical finding, not a diagnosis, and the term represents a group of unrelated disorders with the common phenotypic characteristic of multiple joint contractures. Arthrogryposis multiplex congenita should be considered a symptom complex that results in this characteristic phenotype that can occur in 400 different disorders that have been linked to over 350 genes. Arthrogryposis usually is a nonprogressive syndrome characterized by deformed, rigid joints that affect two or more areas of the body. The involved muscles or muscle groups are atrophied or absent. The involved extremities appear cylindrical, fusiform, or cone-shaped and have diminished skin creases and subcutaneous tissue. Contracture of the joint capsule and periarticular tissues is present. Dislocation of the joints is common, especially of the hip and knee (Fig. 6.47). Sensation and intellect are normal. The incidence of arthrogryposis has been reported to be 1 in 3000 live births.

More than 400 specific entities can be associated with what has been known as arthrogryposis multiplex congenita; because it is no longer considered a discrete clinical entity, the term *multiple congenital contractures* is preferred. Determining whether a child has normal neurologic function is essential to establish a differential diagnosis. In a child with a normal neurologic examination, arthrogryposis is most likely caused by amyoplasia, distal arthrogryposis, generalized connective tissue disorder, or fetal crowding. An abnormal neurologic examination indicates that movement in utero was diminished as a result of an abnormality of the central or peripheral nervous system, the motor endplate, or muscle (Fig. 6.48). The deformities may result from neurogenic, myogenic, skeletal, or environmental factors. Genetic evaluation is recommended for patients with arthrogryposis. Limited intrauterine movement is common to all types of arthrogryposis. Histologic analysis shows a small muscle mass with fibrosis and fat between the muscle fibers. Myopathic and neuropathic features often are found in the muscle. The periarticular soft-tissue structures are fibrotic and create a fibrous ankylosis.

Clinical examination is the best modality for establishing the diagnosis of arthrogryposis multiplex congenita. Neurologic assessment, electromyography and nerve conduction studies, serum enzyme tests, DNA testing, and muscle biopsy can help to determine the underlying diagnosis. Radiographic examination assesses the integrity of the skeletal system, especially the

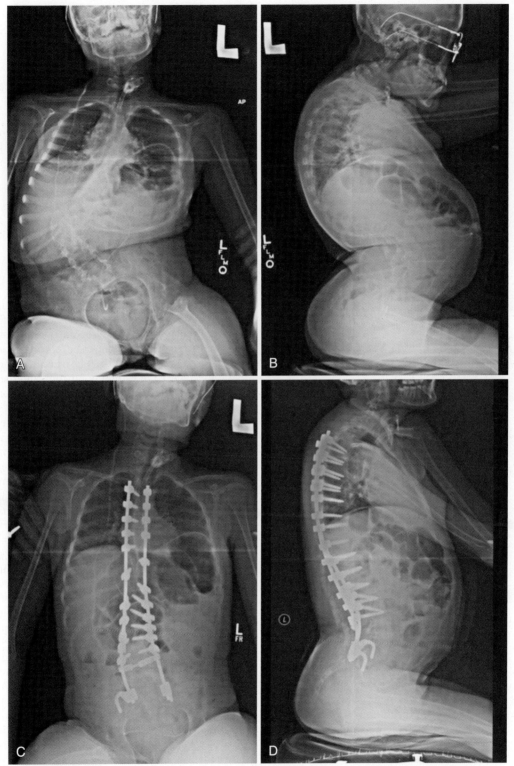

FIGURE 6.46 Anteroposterior (**A**) and lateral (**B**) radiographs of scoliosis in child with myelomeningocele. **C** and **D,** After correction with anteroposterior fusion.

presence or absence of dislocated hips or knees, scoliosis, and other skeletal anomalies. The most common lower extremity deformities are rigid clubfoot and fixed extension or flexion contractures of the knees. Major problems in the upper extremity usually are immobile, adducted, and internally rotated shoulders; elbow contractures; severe, fixed palmar flexion and ulnar-deviated deformities of the wrist; and contractures of the metacarpophalangeal and interphalangeal joints. Involvement usually is bilateral but not always symmetric. All four limbs are involved in 56% of patients with arthrogryposis, three limbs in 5%, legs only in 16%, and arms only in 17%. Scoliosis has been reported to occur in 10% to 30% of patients.

Classic arthrogryposis or amyoplasia usually involves all four extremities. The shoulders are internally rotated and

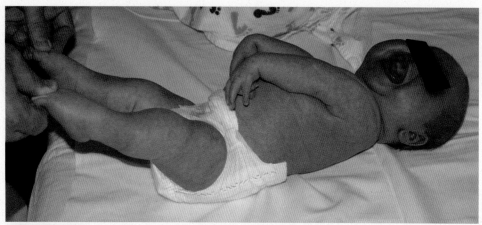

FIGURE 6.47 Newborn with multiple congenital contractures (arthrogryposis) Note orthopaedic conditions: congenital dislocation of knees, teratologic clubfeet, internal rotation contractures of shoulder, extension contractures of elbow, and flexion contractures of wrist.

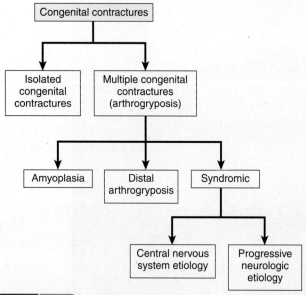

FIGURE 6.48 Types of congenital contractures. (From Bamshad M, Van Heest AE, Pleasure D: Arthrogryposis: a review and update. *J Bone Joint Surg* 91A[Suppl 4]:40, 2009.)

adducted. The elbow usually has an extension contracture, and the wrists are palmar flexed and ulnarly deviated. The fingers often are rigidly flexed with the thumbs adducted. There often is a midline cutaneous hemangioma on the forehead. Patients with distal arthrogryposis have fixed hand and foot contractures, but the major large joints of the arms and legs are spared. Distal arthrogryposis is divided into type I and type II based on the absence or presence of facial abnormalities. In contrast to amyoplasia, which occurs sporadically, distal arthrogryposis is inherited in an autosomal dominant fashion. Genetic analysis has identified 10 distinct types of distal arthrogryposis (Table 6.2).

TREATMENT
Most children with arthrogryposis have a relatively good prognosis; treatment should be focused on obtaining maximal

function. Some contractures may seem to worsen with age, but no new joints become involved. At least 25% of affected patients are nonambulatory. An early program of passive stretching exercises for each contracted joint, to be followed by serial splinting with custom thermoplastic splints, is recommended. Although gains are achieved in extremity function and the need for corrective surgery is reduced, recurrence of the deformity is likely.

The primary long-term goals of treatment are increased joint mobility and muscle strength and the development of adaptive use patterns that allow walking and independence with activities of daily living. To achieve these goals, correcting lower extremity alignment to make plantigrade standing and walking possible is necessary. Existing joint motion should be preserved and placed in the most functional location. Treatment should also focus on active motion, and tendon-muscle transfers should be done when necessary. In addition, stiff joints should be positioned for functional advantage. Surgical intervention can be divided into early and late treatment. Early treatment should accomplish as much functional improvement as possible in the involved extremities by 6 to 7 years of age. Knee and hip surgery should be done by 6 to 9 months of age. Treatment of foot deformities has shifted from surgery to more of an emphasis on deformity correction by casting and limited surgery. If foot surgery is required, it should be done close to the time the patient normally begins to stand, to decrease the likelihood of recurrence.

■ LOWER EXTREMITY
The rigid foot deformity in multiple congenital contractures usually is a clubfoot or congenital vertical talus. The goal of treatment is conversion of the rigid deformed foot into a plantigrade foot. If the valgus foot is plantigrade, treatment usually is not required. The most common foot deformity is clubfoot. The Ponseti method of clubfoot casting has been used successfully in patients with arthrogryposis and clubfeet, but a greater number of casts were required than for idiopathic clubfeet, and the relapse rate was 27% at 2-year follow-up. Matar et al. reported satisfactory outcomes at 6-year follow-up in 11 of 17 arthrogrypotic clubfeet treated with Ponseti casting. Three patients with bilateral severe deformities required operative treatment. If casting fails, an extensive posteromedial and posterolateral release

TABLE 6.2

Common Causes of Arthrogryposis

DISEASE	GENETIC INFLUENCE	ADDITIONAL FACTORS/FINDINGS
Amyoplasia	Sporadic	Usually quadrimelic involvement
Myelomeningocele	Multifactorial	Folic acid deficiency
Larsen syndrome	AD	Joint dislocations, spatulate thumbs, flattened nasal bridge
Distal arthrogryposis type I	AD	Hand, foot involvement
Multiple pterygium syndrome (Escobar syndrome)	AR	Pterygium of upper and lower extremities, neck
Freeman-Sheldon syndrome (whistling face syndrome)	AD	Whistling appearance of face, ulnar deviation of hands, club-foot, congenital vertical talus
Beal contractural arachnodactyly	AD	Slender limbs with knee, elbow, and hand contractures
Sacral agenesis	Sporadic	Maternal diabetes, exposure to organic solvents, retinoic acid
Diastrophic dysplasia	AR	Clubfoot, hitchhiker's thumb, short stature, scoliosis, hypertrophic pinnae
Metatropic dysplasia	AD, AR	Platyspondylia, kyphosis, scoliosis
Thrombocytopenia–absent radii (TAR) syndrome	AR	Absent radii with thumbs present, knee involvement, thrombocytopenia
Steinert myotonic dystrophy	AD	Myotonia, typical facies
Spinal muscular atrophy	AR	Anterior horn cell degeneration
Congenital muscular dystrophy	AR	Heterogeneous group of diseases, some with central nervous system involvement
Möbius syndrome	Sporadic, AD	Cranial nerve VI, VII palsy; micrognathia, clubfoot

AD, Autosomal dominant; *AR*, autosomal recessive.
From Bernstein RM: Arthrogryposis and amyoplasia, *J Am Acad Orthop Surg* 10:417, 2002.

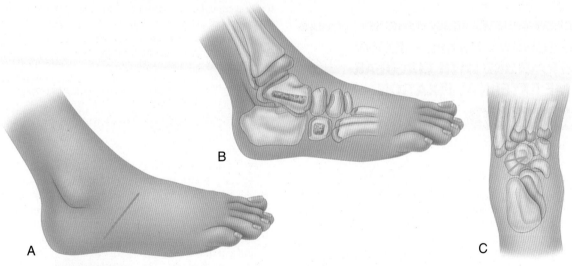

FIGURE 6.49 Cancellectomy of talus and cuboid. **A,** Incision. **B,** Windows in talus and cuboid to expose cancellous bone. **C,** Closing wedge osteotomy in cuboid.

is recommended. If the deformity recurs in a young child or is so severe that it cannot be corrected by posteromedial soft-tissue release, talectomy is indicated. Fusion of the calcaneocuboid joint at the time of talectomy may decrease the risk of progressive midfoot adduction. Gross described a technique, similar to that described by Ogston and Kopits for use in myelomeningocele, of decancellation of the talus and cuboid in which a window is created in the dorsal cortex of the cuboid and lateral cortex of the neck and body of the talus (Fig. 6.49). All cancellous bone is carefully curetted,

and the deformity is corrected by manual manipulation (see Technique 6.30). Triple arthrodesis may be performed for rigid deformity in adolescents. Gradual correction of the deformity with circular-frame external fixators is an alternative method for obtaining a plantigrade foot but is technically demanding. If the deformity recurs and is so severe that it cannot be corrected by posteromedial soft-tissue release or other methods, talectomy can be considered. Fusion of the calcaneocuboid joint at the time of talectomy may decrease the risk of progressive midfoot adduction. The long-term satisfaction rate of talectomy has been reported to be between 45% and 50%.

The two most common deformities around the knee are a flexion contracture and an extension contracture. Initial treatment of flexion contractures is by serial splinting or casting in progressive degrees of extension. Ambulation is possible with a residual knee flexion contracture of 15 to 20 degrees. If complete correction has not been obtained by 6 to 12 months of age, posterior medial and lateral hamstring lengthening and knee capsulotomies are indicated. This should be approached through vertical medial and lateral posterior incisions or an extensile posterolateral Henry incision. S-shaped incisions should be avoided because they place excessive tension on the skin after correction, causing subsequent wound breakdown. After a posterior release has been performed, an anterior release of scar tissue may need to be done to obtain correction. Supracondylar extension osteotomy of the distal femur may be required to correct a contracture and allow use of orthoses. Extension osteotomies should be done when the patient is near skeletal maturity if possible to decrease the risk of recurrent deformity with remodeling. If osteotomies are done before skeletal maturity, about 50% of correction is maintained even if the deformity recurs. Often a femoral shortening may need to be combined with an extension osteotomy to protect neurovascular structures. Gradual correction of a knee flexion contracture can be achieved with a circular-frame external fixator, with or without an associated posterior release. This technique is used most often when soft-tissue webbing is associated with a knee flexion contracture.

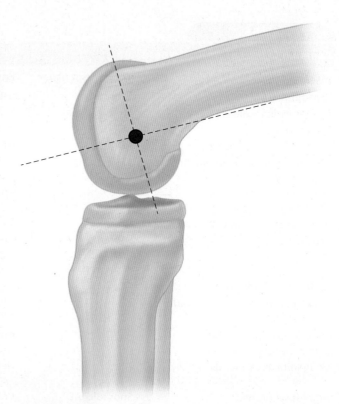

FIGURE 6.50 Estimation of the knee axis of rotation. On a true lateral projection of the knee, with the distal and posterior femoral condyles superimposed, the intersection of the posterior femoral cortex and the widest anteroposterior dimension of the femoral condyles gives the best estimate of knee axis of rotation. (Redrawn from van Bosse HJP, Feldman DS, Anavian J, Sala DA: Treatment of knee flexion contractures in patients with arthrogryposis, *J Pediatr Orthop* 27:930, 2007.) **SEE TECHNIQUE 6.42.**

CORRECTION OF KNEE FLEXION CONTRACTURE WITH CIRCULAR-FRAME EXTERNAL FIXATION

TECHNIQUE 6.42

(VAN BOSSE ET AL.)

APPROXIMATION OF KNEE CENTER OF ROTATION
- On a true lateral projection of the knee, with the distal and posterior femoral condyles superimposed, the intersection of the posterior femoral cortex and the widest anterior-posterior dimension of the femoral condyles gives the best estimate of the knee axis of motion (Fig. 6.50).

POSTERIOR KNEE RELEASE
- Approach the knee through medial and lateral incisions, 5 to 8 cm long, centered over the palpable posterior femoral condyle and parallel to the ground when both the hip and knee are on the operating table (Fig. 6.51A).
- Laterally, incise the iliotibial band in line with the incision, and release its posterior half.
- After verifying the safety of the common peroneal nerve, isolate the biceps femoris tendon and transect it proximally.
- With blunt dissection, elevate soft tissues off the knee joint capsule posteriorly until a finger can be run along

the posterior aspect of the joint capsule to at least the midpoint.
- Identify the lateral head of the gastrocnemius, running as a tight band just proximal and posterior to the joint capsule; isolate and transect its tendon.
- Make a small capsulotomy posterolaterally, and continue it anteriorly to incise the posterior half of the lateral collateral ligament (Fig. 6.51B).
- Use a Freer elevator to retract the posterior soft tissues, and cut the posterior capsule along the joint line with Mayo scissors. If the geniculate artery is cut or avulsed, obtain hemostasis by packing the wound for approximately 5 minutes.
- Medially, retract the vastus medialis obliquus anteriorly, and transect the semitendinosus and gracilis tendons.
- Deep to the tendons, transect the fascia of the semimembranosus, leaving the muscle belly intact.
- Bluntly elevate the soft tissues off the medial aspect of the posterior capsule, and transect the medial head of the gastrocnemius.
- At this point, it should be possible to pass a finger across the entire posterior joint line of the knee, even in small patients.

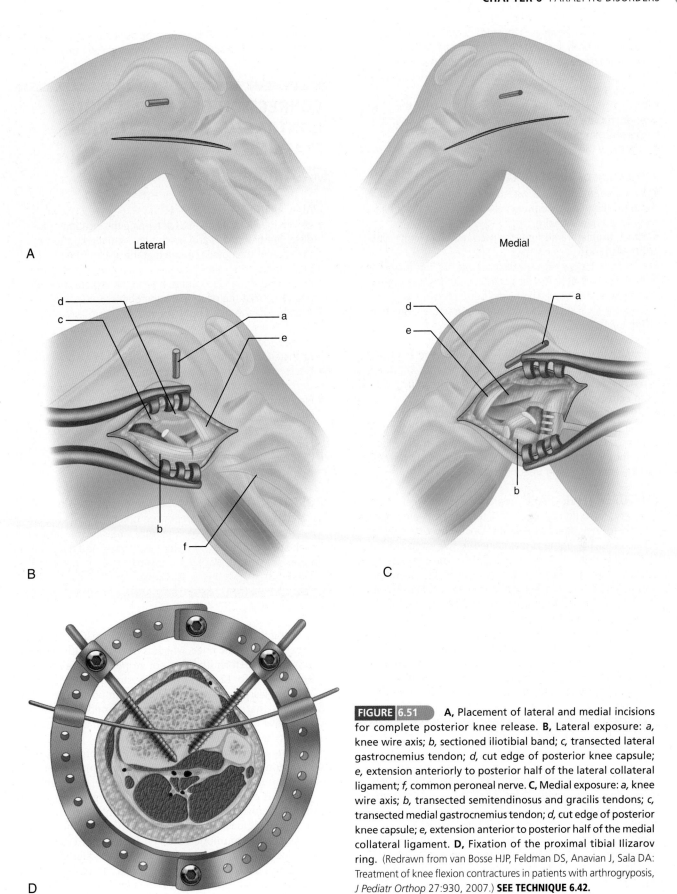

FIGURE 6.51 **A,** Placement of lateral and medial incisions for complete posterior knee release. **B,** Lateral exposure: *a,* knee wire axis; *b,* sectioned iliotibial band; *c,* transected lateral gastrocnemius tendon; *d,* cut edge of posterior knee capsule; *e,* extension anteriorly to posterior half of the lateral collateral ligament; *f,* common peroneal nerve. **C,** Medial exposure: *a,* knee wire axis; *b,* transected semitendinosus and gracilis tendons; *c,* transected medial gastrocnemius tendon; *d,* cut edge of posterior knee capsule; *e,* extension anterior to posterior half of the medial collateral ligament. **D,** Fixation of the proximal tibial Ilizarov ring. (Redrawn from van Bosse HJP, Feldman DS, Anavian J, Sala DA: Treatment of knee flexion contractures in patients with arthrogryposis, *J Pediatr Orthop* 27:930, 2007.) **SEE TECHNIQUE 6.42.**

■ Use scissors to advance a posteromedial corner capsulotomy anteriorly, incising the posterior half of the medial collateral ligament, staying cephalad to its attachments to the medial meniscus. Complete the capsulotomy with the scissors (Fig. 6.51C).

■ Verify complete release by direct palpation. If the posterior cruciate ligament can be felt as a taut band in the intercondylar notch, release it.

■ Close only the skin with absorbable sutures.

APPLICATION OF ILIZAROV FIXATOR

■ Attach a femoral frame with two full rings to the femur and position Ilizarov universal joints on either side in line with the knee axis wire.

■ Attach a tibial frame from the two universal joints with threaded rods.

■ Position a transverse transfixation wire in the proximal tibial ring so that as it is tensioned it pulls the tibia slightly anterior on the femur. This helps counter forces that cause posterior tibial subluxation during contracture correction (Fig. 6.51D).

■ Secure the tibial frame to the tibia.

■ Distract the joint 5 to 10 mm by lengthening between the universal joints and the tibial frame; this will avoid impingement and crushing of the articular cartilage during correction.

■ A telescopic rod for correction can be placed posteriorly or anteriorly; the latter is more convenient for seating purposes. Occasionally, the frame is extended to include the foot to simultaneously correct a deformity or prevent ankle equinus during treatment.

POSTOPERATIVE CARE Approximately 1 week after surgery, correction is begun at 1 to 2 degrees a day, adjusted to the patient's tolerance. Once fully corrected to 0 degrees, the frame is maintained in full extension for an additional 2 to 4 weeks, depending on the ease of initial correction. The frame is removed in the operating room, and a cast is applied with the knee in full extension; the cast is molded to prevent posterior tibial subluxation. The cast is worn for 2 weeks and then replaced with a KAFO with locking knee hinges. Physical therapy is begun for gait training and knee range of motion. The KAFO is worn in full extension for 3 months and is removed only for bathing and physical therapy. After 3 months, it is worn routinely at night and during the day as needed for ambulation.

Anterior distal femoral guided growth with staples or 8-plates has been reported by Palocaren et al. to improve flexion deformity and ambulatory capacity in arthrogrypotic patients with knee flexion contractures. This technique is less invasive than soft-tissue releases, distal femoral osteotomies, or frame distraction and is most beneficial in children with flexion contractures of less than 45 degrees. The guided growth can be done as an outpatient procedure, depending on the patient's general health, anesthetic tolerance, and need for concomitant procedures. The timing of stapling is determined by the size of the femoral condyle rather than the chronologic

age of the child: the condyle must be large enough to accommodate the smallest screw in the 8-plate set (16 mm).

CORRECTION OF KNEE FLEXION CONTRACTURE WITH ANTERIOR STAPLING

TECHNIQUE 6.43

(PALOCAREN ET AL.)

■ Use image intensification to determine the location of the distal femoral physis and make two 3-cm incisions on either side of the patella centered at the level of the physis.

■ With image intensifier guidance, place a needle into the physis and thread the central hole in the 8-plate over the needle so that the plate spans the physis.

■ Ensure that the plate rests about 2 to 3 mm away from the lateral and medial edges of the patella. If the plate is fixed too close to the patella, knee movement will be restricted and painful.

■ Insert two 1.6-mm guidewires through the screw holes in the plate, and verify their position with fluoroscopy.

■ Place two self-tapping cannulated screws over the guidewires. The screws should be sufficiently long to meet, but not penetrate, the opposite cortex. Take care not to violate the physis or the joint.

■ Close the wound in layers and apply a soft dressing. A knee immobilizer can be used for comfort.

POSTOPERATIVE CARE Ambulation is allowed as tolerated. Follow-up radiographs are obtained at 4 weeks. Patients are followed at 6-month intervals for clinical evaluation of the flexion deformity, stance, and gait. The plates are left in place until the deformity is corrected (Fig. 6.52).

Contracture of the quadriceps mechanism can cause hyperextension of the knee, which is treated initially by serial casting. If the deformity does not respond to conservative treatment by 6 to 12 months of age, surgical correction by quadricepsplasty is recommended. It is important to counsel families that although knee range of motion and function improve in the short term, both function and outcomes decline as the deformities recur with time.

The hip is involved in approximately 80% of patients with multiple congenital contractures. In general, hip deformities should be treated by passive stretching exercises, beginning in infancy. If conservative measures fail, surgical correction of the hip deformity should be delayed until deformities of the knees have been corrected. Mild hip flexion contractures may be accommodated by an increase in lumbar lordosis. Flexion contractures of more than 45 degrees should have surgical release. Van Bosse described a proximal femoral reorientational osteotomy to treat the typical hip contractures of abduction, flexion, and external rotation. This osteotomy corrects all the deformities at a single level with a posterior, medially based, wedge-shaped intertrochanteric osteotomy.

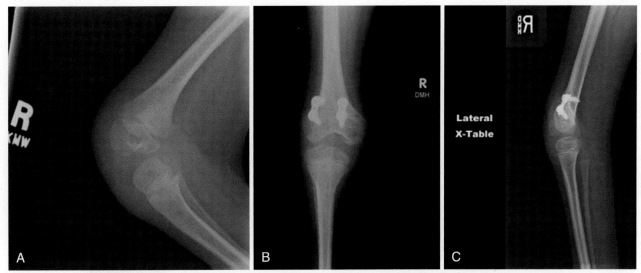

FIGURE 6.52 **A,** Preoperative lateral knee radiograph of a 4-year-old boy with arthrogryposis. **B** and **C,** Two years after anterior stapling of the distal femur with 8-plates. Lateral view shows correction of the flexion deformity and divergence of the screws with growth. (From Palocaren T, Thabet AM, Rogers K, et al: Anterior distal femoral stapling for correcting knee flexion contracture in children with arthrogryposis—preliminary results, *J Pediatr Orthop* 30:169, 2010.) **SEE TECHNIQUE 6.43.**

In a review of 65 patients with reorientational osteotomies (only six of whom were ambulatory), van Bosse and Saldana reported that, at a mean follow-up of 40 months, 36 (55%) patients were independently ambulatory and 20 (31%) were walker dependent. Nine patients were nonambulatory, of whom two had the procedure specifically to improve seating. There were 10 complications, including four fractures and three surgical site infections.

REORIENTATIONAL PROXIMAL FEMORAL OSTEOTOMY FOR HIP CONTRACTURES IN ARTHROGRYPOSIS

TECHNIQUE 6.44

(VAN BOSSE)
- Determine hip range of motion clinically, and obtain radiographs to confirm that the hips are located and there are no unusual structural abnormalities.
- Position the patient supine, with a bump at the sacrum, and drape to allow access to both hips simultaneously.
- For patients with a palpable soft-tissue flexion contracture, perform an initial anterior hip release (see Technique 6.36).
- Make a standard approach to the lateral aspect of the proximal femur.
- Make two intertrochanteric osteotomy cuts to provide cut surfaces that, when joined together, will optimally position the lower extremity (Fig. 6.53A-C).
- Impact the blade plate into the proximal fragment, and secure it to the distal fragment. (Fig. 6.53D)
- Close in routine fashion, and apply a Petrie cast.

POSTOPERATIVE MANAGEMENT. The patient is mobilized in a reclining wheelchair with elevated leg rests to gradually increase hip flexion. The family is instructed on prone positioning of the patient to maintain or increase extension. At 3 weeks, an anteroposterior radiograph is obtained and, if there is sufficient healing of the osteotomy sites, the patient is allowed to begin standing in the cast. At 6 weeks, the cast is replaced by a custom KAFO and, if radiographs show full healing, weight-bearing physical therapy is begun.

At 12 to 18 months after surgery, the blade plate is removed as an outpatient procedure through the smallest incision possible.

Developmental hip dysplasia and hip dislocation occur in about two thirds of patients with arthrogryposis. Traditional recommendations are that bilateral teratologic hip dislocations should not be reduced because reduction may not improve function. Good results have been reported, however, with early (3 to 6 months of age) open reduction through a medial approach. If surgical intervention is done between 12 and 36 months of age, a one-stage open reduction, primary femoral shortening, and possible pelvic osteotomy are recommended. Unilateral dislocation of the hip, whether flexible or rigid, should be reduced surgically and placed in a functional position to avoid potential pelvic obliquity and scoliosis. The treatment of bilateral dislocations should be individualized. Good results have been reported in bilateral hip dislocations treated with a medial or anterior approach. If the dislocated hips are treated surgically, postoperative immobilization should be limited to 6 to 8 weeks.

Traditional recommendations for treatment of the upper extremities in children with arthrogryposis have been to leave

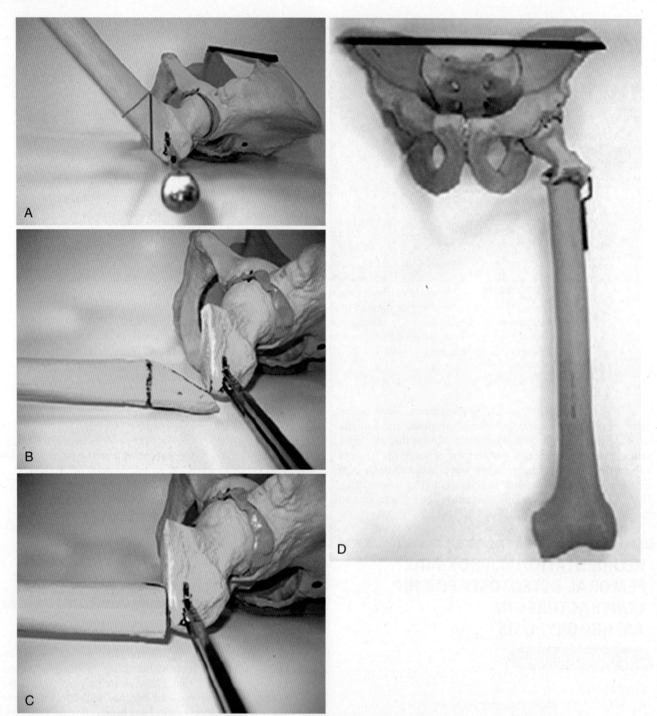

FIGURE 6.53 Creation of the proximal and distal bone cuts in the van Bosse reorientational proximal femoral osteotomies for correction of hip contractures. **A** and **B,** Proximal osteotomy is parallel and 5 to 8 mm distal to the seating chisel blade. Distal osteotomy is perpendicular to the shaft of the distal fragment so that the two cuts meet medially as the apex of the wedge. **C,** Second osteotomy cut is perpendicular to the shaft of the distal fragment. **D,** Blade plate fixation. (A and B from van Bosse HJ, Saldana RE: Reorientational proximal femoral osteotomies for arthrogrypotic hip contractures, *J Bone Joint Surg Am* 99:55, 2017. C and D from van Bosse HJP: Reorientational proximal femoral osteotomies for correction of hip contractures in children with arthrogryposis, *JBJS Essent Surg Tech* 7:e11, 2017.) **SEE TECHNIQUE 6.44.**

the shoulders internally rotated and adducted, the elbows extended, and the wrist flexed. Most of these children adapt to their disabilities and develop some form of bimanual function. Correction of upper extremity deformities should be delayed until ambulation has been achieved, usually by 3 to 4 years of age. If surgery is delayed until age 8 years, the use patterns are so well established that the child would not adapt as well to surgical correction. The goal of treatment of upper extremity deformities is to provide optimal function of the hand in activities of daily living. In most instances, this

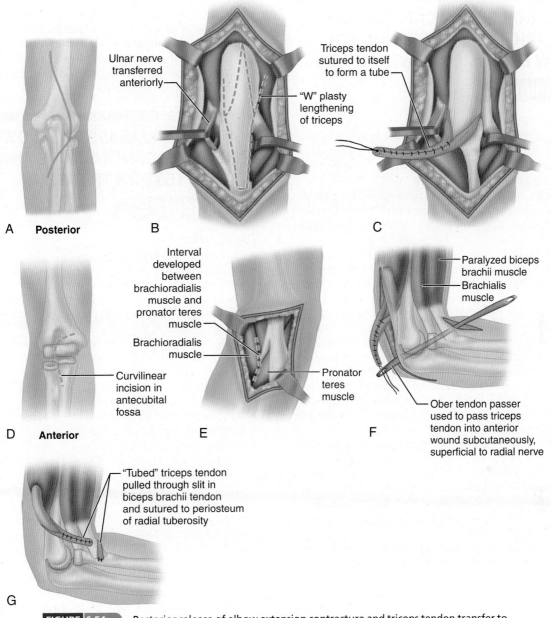

A   **Posterior**

Ulnar nerve transferred anteriorly

"W" plasty lengthening of triceps

Triceps tendon sutured to itself to form a tube

B

C

D   **Anterior**

Curvilinear incision in antecubital fossa

Interval developed between brachioradialis muscle and pronator teres muscle

Brachioradialis muscle

Pronator teres muscle

E

Paralyzed biceps brachii muscle

Brachialis muscle

Ober tendon passer used to pass triceps tendon into anterior wound subcutaneously, superficial to radial nerve

F

"Tubed" triceps tendon pulled through slit in biceps brachii tendon and sutured to periosteum of radial tuberosity

G

FIGURE 6.54 Posterior release of elbow extension contracture and triceps tendon transfer to restore flexion. (Redrawn from Herring JA, editor: *Tachdjian's pediatric orthopaedics*, ed 3, Philadelphia, 2002, Saunders.) **SEE TECHNIQUES 6.45 AND 6.46.**

involves procedures to obtain at least 90 degrees of passive elbow function, neutral wrist position, and thumb release. Function may be adequate despite severe deformity in children with arthrogryposis; the benefits of surgical intervention must be carefully weighed against the risk of surgery.

The shoulder usually is adducted and internally rotated. Weakness and stiffness around the shoulder do not significantly impair function and usually require no treatment, but the fixed internal rotation of the shoulder becomes a major obstacle for normal elbow and hand function. Proximal humeral rotation osteotomy (see Technique 6.49) may be indicated to correct this internal rotation deformity.

Deformity of the elbow usually means severe limitation of either flexion or extension. The stiff flexed elbow is not a severe impairment, and surgery is not indicated. Fixed extension elbow deformity, especially if bilateral, is a severe functional impairment. The goals for surgery for a fixed extension elbow deformity are to gain functional range of motion and achieve active elbow flexion. Surgical options available for the fixed extended elbow are release of extension contractures, tricepsplasty, triceps transfer (Fig. 6.54), flexorplasty, and pectoralis major transfer. Lengthening of the triceps mechanism and posterior capsulotomy are the most reliable and durable of available surgical procedures. This procedure is indicated when elbow flexion is limited to 45 degrees or less, with a goal to gain functional range of motion around the elbow. Zlotolow and Kozin combined posterior elbow capsular release with external rotation osteotomy of the humerus to place the forearm and hand in a better position for function and optimize hand-to-mouth activities.

POSTERIOR ELBOW CAPSULOTOMY WITH TRICEPS LENGTHENING FOR ELBOW EXTENSION CONTRACTURE

TECHNIQUE 6.45

(VAN HEEST ET AL.)

- For unilateral release, place the patient in a lateral decubitus position; for bilateral release, position the patient supine.
- Apply a tourniquet, and approach the elbow through a curvilinear posterior incision (Fig. 6.54A).
- In patients with minimal elbow movement, take care to correctly identify the posterior aspect of the olecranon; severe internal rotation of the limb may cause the medial epicondyle to be mistaken for the olecranon.
- Identify the ulnar nerve in the medial intermuscular septum. Release the cubital tunnel, trace the ulnar nerve to the flexor carpi ulnaris innervation, and place a vessel loop around it for protection during subsequent dissection.
- Once the ulnar nerve has been identified, released, and protected, remove the tourniquet.
- Isolate, mobilize medially and laterally, and lengthen the triceps with either a Z-lengthening or V-Y advancement. Most commonly, the triceps is incised in a "V" fashion so that the central tongue is based on the olecranon and the two lateral limbs include tendon over as great a length as possible, from the proximal muscular portion distally to the olecranon insertion.
- Incise the posterior aspect of the capsule at the tip of the olecranon to allow identification of the joint surface.
- Extend the arthrotomy medially and laterally to allow maximal elbow flexion with a gentle passive stretch. If necessary, extend the capsular release around the medial and lateral sides to include the posterior edges of the medial and lateral collateral ligament.
- Flex the elbow as much as possible (more than 90 degrees) while allowing contact between the distal ends of the lateral triceps limbs and the proximal end of the central tongue of triceps.
- Repair the triceps in an elongated position with nonresorbable or reinforced suture.
- Close the skin, apply a light dressing, and place the arm in a long arm cast or a prefabricated custom-hinged elbow brace.

POSTOPERATIVE CARE The elbow is immobilized in 90 degrees of flexion, with passive range of motion allowed as soon as tolerated. During the first month after surgery, physical therapy is advanced to include hand-to-mouth activities; passive flexion is limited to 90 degrees to protect the triceps lengthening during this time but is then advanced to full passive flexion. The splint or cast is worn for 4 to 6 weeks.

make the use of crutches, rising from a sitting position, and wheelchair transfers difficult. Procedures to achieve active elbow flexion in an arthrogrypotic patient are triceps transfer, flexorplasty, pectoralis major transfer, latissimus transfer, and free gracilis transfer. These procedures all have been relatively ineffective in maintaining long-term elbow flexion and have significant donor site morbidity.

POSTERIOR RELEASE OF ELBOW EXTENSION CONTRACTURE AND TRICEPS TENDON TRANSFER

TECHNIQUE 6.46

(TACHDJIAN)

- Place the patient laterally.
- Make a midline incision on the posterior aspect of the arm, beginning in its middle half and extending distally to a point lateral to the olecranon process; carry the incision over the subcutaneous surface of the shaft of the ulna for a distance of 5 cm.
- Divide the subcutaneous tissue and mobilize the wound flaps (Fig. 6.54A).
- Identify the ulnar nerve and mobilize it medially to protect it from injury.
- Expose the intermuscular septum laterally.
- Mobilize the ulnar nerve and transfer it anteriorly.
- Lengthen the triceps muscle in a W fashion, leaving a long proximal tongue (Fig. 6.54B).
- Free the triceps muscle and mobilize it proximally as far as its nerve supply permits. The motor branches of the radial nerve to the triceps enter the muscle in the interval between the lateral and medial heads as the radial nerve enters the musculospiral groove.
- Suture the distal portion of the detached triceps to itself to form a tube (Fig. 6.54C).
- Make a curvilinear incision in the antecubital fossa, and develop the interval between the brachioradialis and the pronator teres (Fig. 6.54D and E).
- With a tendon passer, pass the triceps tendon into the anterior wound subcutaneously, superficial to the radial nerve (Fig. 6.54F).
- With the elbow in 90 degrees of flexion and the forearm in full supination, either suture the triceps tendon to the biceps tendon or anchor it to the radial tuberosity by a suture passed through a drill hole (Fig. 6.54G).
- Close the wound in the routine fashion.
- Apply an above-elbow cast with the elbow in 90 degrees of flexion and full supination.

POSTOPERATIVE CARE Four weeks after surgery the cast is removed and active exercises are begun to develop elbow flexion. Gravity provides extension to the elbow.

Passive elbow flexion to a right angle is a prerequisite for considering a tendon transfer for active elbow flexion. Triceps transfer can be done to regain elbow flexion, but over time a flexion contracture often occurs. Elbow stability in extension should not be sacrificed with this procedure because it can

Steindler flexorplasty produces elbow flexion by transferring the flexor pronator origin from the medial epicondyle to the anterior humerus (Fig. 6.23). For this procedure to be beneficial, both active wrist flexors and extensors need to be present. This procedure rarely is indicated in children with

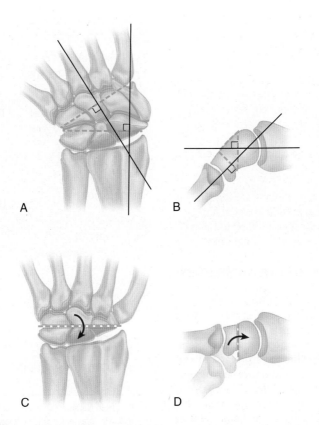

FIGURE 6.55 Carpal wedge osteotomy. Anteroposterior (**A**) and lateral (**B**) views of the location of the osteotomy, and anteroposterior (**C**) and lateral (**D**) views after wedge osteotomy. (Redrawn from Foy CA, Mills J, Wheeler L, et al: Long-term outcome following carpal wedge osteotomy in the arthrogrypotic patient, *J Bone Joint Surg Am* 95:e105[1], 2013.) **SEE TECHNIQUE 6.47.**

multiple congenital contractures because the wrist flexors usually are inactive and contracted. An active radial wrist extensor also needs to be present to prevent unacceptable wrist flexion after a flexorplasty. Triceps transfer would allow for early improvement in elbow flexion, but over time flexion contractures may occur and function deteriorates, so one must be cautious in the use of this transfer. Transfer of the long head of the triceps can be used as an alternative (Fig. 6.24). The long head of the triceps has a separate neurovascular pedicle that can be separated from the rest of the triceps. A fascia lata graft often is needed to allow for transfer into the proximal ulna. This transfer often allows for adequate elbow flexion without loss of active elbow extension. Microsurgical transfer of the gracilis muscle to the arm has been reported.

The wrist is usually flexed and in an ulnar-deviated position. Wrist stabilization in the optimal functional position probably is the most beneficial procedure in patients with multiple congenital contractures, but determination of the best position for function must be made carefully. Neutral or mild ulnar deviation and dorsiflexion between 5 and 20 degrees proves to be the most satisfactory position. Procedures described for the arthrogrypotic wrist are tendon transfers, proximal row carpectomy, dorsal radial closing wedge osteotomy of the midcarpus, and wrist fusion. Wrist palmar flexion contracture can be corrected with flexor carpi ulnaris lengthening or transfer to the wrist extensors. This transfer acts more like a tenodesis procedure than a dynamic transfer. Proximal row carpectomy is not often recommended because of the loss of correction and stiffness that occurs with

this procedure. In younger patients, a closing wedge osteotomy through the midcarpus can correct the wrist deformity. Foy et al. reported their results with carpal wedge osteotomy in 46 patients (75 wrists) (Fig. 6.55). At an average 6-year follow-up, correction of the flexion wrist posture was maintained; the arc of motion was shifted to a more useful position and range of motion was not reduced. When the patient is near skeletal maturity, a wrist fusion can be performed by traditional methods.

DORSAL CLOSING WEDGE OSTEOTOMY OF THE WRIST

TECHNIQUE 6.47

(VAN HEEST AND RODRIGUEZ, EZAKI, AND CARTER)

- Through a dorsal approach to the wrist, isolate and protect the digital and wrist extensor tendons, then make a dorsal capsulotomy.
- At the level of the midcarpus, make a dorsal wedge osteotomy sufficient to correct the wrist flexion deformity to at least a neutral position, taking care not to violate the radiocarpal joint and ensuring that finger flexor tightness is not produced by tenodesis.

- Make the proximal cut distal to the radiocarpal joint at the level of the capsular attachment of the proximal carpal row, perpendicular in two planes to the long axis of the forearm.
- Make the distal cut through the distal carpal row, perpendicular in both planes to the long axis of the metacarpus.
- If ulnar deviation correction also is required, resect more bone on the radial side of the dorsal carpal wedge to provide biplanar correction.
- Insert two crossed Kirschner wires to hold the osteotomy closed.

POSTOPERATIVE CARE The wrist is kept elevated for the first several days after surgery. The cast or splint is changed at 2 to 3 weeks. The wrist is immobilized in a cast or splint for an additional 6 weeks or until union is apparent on radiographs.

Flexion contractures of the fingers are best treated with passive stretching and splinting. Surgical procedures have not had any functional benefit over nonoperative treatment. Thumb-in-palm deformity may be difficult to treat and can involve a skin deficit, muscle/fascia contracture, flexor pollicis longus contracture, and extensor weakness. The goal is to allow the thumb to at least clear the second metacarpal. This usually is accomplished with a comprehensive thenar release.

SCOLIOSIS

Scoliosis has been reported to occur in 10% to 30% of patients with multiple congenital contractures, generally associated with neuromuscular weakness or pelvic obliquity. If the deformity is severe and progressive, early surgical intervention is warranted. The indications and techniques for treatment of scoliosis in patients with multiple congenital contractures are the same as those for patients with other neuromuscular disorders.

BRACHIAL PLEXUS PALSY

Brachial plexus palsy may be seen after injury to the brachial plexus during birth. Reported incidences range from 0.1% to 0.4% of live births. Despite advances in obstetric care, the incidence of brachial plexus palsy was believed to be increasing because of the increase in high birth weight infants, but DeFrancesco et al. found a drop in the incidence of brachial plexus palsy over a 16-year period, from 1.7 to 0.9 cases per 1000 live births. Numerous risk factors have been identified, including large birth weight, prolonged labor, difficult delivery, forceps delivery, maternal age, maternal obesity, maternal diabetes, and previous births with brachial plexopathy, but over half of patients with brachial plexus birth palsy have no identifiable risk factors. Brachial plexus palsy is thought to be caused by a mechanical traction injury during the birth process. Delivery by cesarean section does not exclude the possibility of brachial plexus birth palsy but does decrease the likelihood from 0.2% to 0.02%. Shoulder dystocia is the mechanical factor that results in an upper trunk lesion. A breech delivery often results in a stretch of the lower plexus from traction applied to the trunk with the arm abducted.

	TABLE 6.3	
Classification and Prognosis in Obstetric Palsy		
TYPE	**CLINICAL PICTURE**	**RECOVERY**
I	C5-6	Complete or almost in 1-8 wk
II	C5-6	Elbow flexion: 1-4 wk
	C7	Elbow extension: 1-8 wk
		Limited shoulder: 6-30 wk
III	C5-6	Poor shoulder: 10-40 wk
	C7	Elbow flexion: 16-40 wk
	C8-T1 (no Horner sign)	Elbow extension: 16-20 wk
		Wrist: 40-60 wk
		Hand complete: 1-3 wk
IV	C5-7	Poor shoulder: 10-40 wk
	C8	Elbow flexion: 16-40 wk
	T1 (temporary Horner sign)	Elbow extension incomplete, poor: 20-60 wk or nil
		Wrist: 40-60 wk
		Hand complete: 20-60 wk
V	C5-7	Shoulder and elbow
	C7	Wrist poor or only extension;
	C8	poor flexion or none
	T1	Very poor hand with no or
	C8-T1 (Horner sign usually present)	weak flexors and extensors; no intrinsic as above

Modified from Narakas AO: Injuries to the brachial plexus. In Bora FW Jr, editor: *The pediatric upper extremity: diagnosis and management*, Philadelphia, 1986, Saunders.

Brachial plexus birth palsy was classified by Narakas according to the location of the injury of the brachial plexus (Table 6.3). Group I includes upper plexus lesions involving C5 and C6, the classic Erb palsy. This is the most common type (46% of cases) and has the most favorable prognosis. Group II consists of lesions of C5, C6, and C7. This group is the second most common (30% of cases) but has a worse prognosis than type I. Group III is a total plexus lesion with a flail extremity. This occurs in 20% of patients. Group IV is the most severe form, characterized by global plexopathy with flail extremity and Horner syndrome, which indicates involvement of the sympathetic chain and a probable avulsion injury. Injuries isolated to the C8 and T1 nerve roots (Klumpke palsy) are rare and account for less than 1% of cases of brachial plexus birth palsy.

The likelihood of recovery also is affected by whether the level of nerve injury is preganglionic or postganglionic. The degree and type of postganglionic neural injury were defined by Sunderland as neurapraxia, axonotmesis, and neurotmesis. Neurapraxia is paralysis in the absence of peripheral degeneration. Recovery usually is complete in this type. Axonotmesis is damage to the nerve fiber with complete peripheral degeneration but intact external tissues to provide support for regeneration. Recovery depends on the degree of nerve injury and is more prolonged. Neurotmesis is disruption of the neural and supporting tissues, which carries a poor prognosis. This includes neuroma in continuity, division of the nerve, and anatomic disruption. Preganglionic avulsion injuries cannot spontaneously recover motor function because the nerve roots are avulsed from the spinal cord. These injuries also are associated with loss of motor function of other nerves that arise close to the spinal cord, which can aid in early diagnosis of these injuries. Loss of the phrenic (elevated hemidiaphragm), long thoracic, dorsal scapular, suprascapular, and thoracodorsal nerves (scapular stabilization) and the sympathetic chain with resultant Horner syndrome are suggestive of a preganglionic avulsion injury.

CLINICAL FEATURES

The diagnosis usually is evident at birth. The newborn has decreased spontaneous movement and asymmetry of infantile reflexes such as Moro reflex or asymmetric tonic neck reflex. In upper root involvement, the arm is held in internal rotation and active abduction is limited. The elbow may be slightly flexed or in complete extension. The thumb may be flexed, and occasionally the fingers do not extend. In complete paralysis, the entire arm and hand is flail. Pinching produces no reaction. Vasomotor impairment may be indicated by the relative paleness of the involved extremity. An ipsilateral Horner syndrome consisting of ptosis and a small pupil indicates injury to the T1 cervical sympathetic nerves. This is a major indication for a poor outcome. Radiographs of the shoulder may reveal fracture of the proximal humeral epiphysis or fracture of the clavicle. A clavicular fracture occurs in association with plexus palsy in 10% to 15% of patients. Pseudoparalysis from a clavicular or proximal humeral fracture should resolve within 10 to 21 days. If limited motion persists after 1 month of age, most likely a concomitant brachial plexus palsy is present. A septic shoulder in an infant also can cause a pseudoparalysis, which can be differentiated from a brachial plexus palsy by evidence of systemic illness and resolution of the pseudoparalysis after the infection is treated.

Serial physical examinations of children with brachial plexus birth palsy are needed to assess motor function and the development of joint contractures. Treatment will be determined by the return or absence of return of motor function and the development of joint contractures. Passive internal and external rotation of the shoulder should be measured with the arm adducted and also abducted to 90 degrees while stabilizing the scapula against the thorax. Assessing motor function in infants often is an approximation of function by observing spontaneous activity.

Three assessment tools have been described to aid in the clinical evaluation of patients with brachial plexus birth palsy: the Toronto Test Score, the Hospital for Sick Children Active Movement Scale, and the Mallet score (Table 6.4). All have been shown to have positive intraobserver and interobserver reliability with aggregate scores. The Toronto Test Score was designed to determine surgical indications and provide an assessment tool after nerve reconstruction procedures. The Hospital for Sick Children Active Movement Scale is a more comprehensive score that evaluates the entire brachial plexus using 15 different upper extremity movements. This scale relies on observation of the degree of movement against gravity and with gravity eliminated. The Modified Mallet Classification of Shoulder Function is the most commonly used outcome measure in patients with neonatal brachial plexus palsy (Fig. 6.56). Because this scale is heavily weighted toward external rotation of the shoulder, Abzug et al. added a sixth category—hand to belly button or navel—that adds another assessment of internal rotation. Assessing a child's ability to touch his or her belly button is important to understanding whether a child can perform activities of daily living, such as perineal care and using zippers and buttons.

Characteristic deformities usually develop promptly. The shoulder becomes flexed, internally rotated, and slightly abducted; active abduction of the joint decreases; and external rotation disappears (abduction contracture and scapular winging). Abnormal muscle forces across the shoulder lead to early changes in the glenoid. These changes include flattening of the posterior glenoid creating a pseudoglenoid (Fig. 6.57). As the deformity progresses, the glenohumeral joint center becomes more posterior and the glenoid becomes more retroverted and flattened or even convex. This leads to progressive posterior glenohumeral subluxation and eventual dislocation with the humeral head becoming flattened against the glenoid. These advanced glenohumeral changes can occur early and have been described by the age of 2 years.

Evaluation of the brachial plexus neurologic injury may include electrical diagnostic studies, ultrasound, myelography, and MRI. Combined use of MRI and electromyography is helpful because MRI may correlate better than electromyography with physical examination findings. In addition, MRI can help with anatomic localization of the nerve injury and help with surgical planning. Large diverticula and meningoceles indicate root avulsions. Plain radiography, ultrasound, arthrography, CT, and MRI, as well as diagnostic arthroscopy, have been used to determine the nature and severity of glenohumeral deformity. Often plain radiographs show delayed ossification of the proximal humerus. Bauer et al. recommended shoulder screening with ultrasound in infants who have passive external rotation in adduction of less than 60 degrees. With ultrasound they found that 29% of the infants had a dislocation during their first year of life. The clinical role of ultrasonography is more of a screening tool, and MRI remains the gold standard for fully evaluating the glenohumeral joint in patients with brachial plexus birth palsy. MRI is more commonly used than CT for evaluation of the glenohumeral joint because of its ability to demonstrate the cartilaginous anatomy, as well as the bony anatomy and lack of exposure of the patient to ionizing radiation. Waters et al. measured the glenoscapular angle (the degree of version of the glenoid) and the percentage of the humeral head anterior to it on CT and MR images (Fig. 6.58) and classified the degree of glenohumeral deformity. The degree of deformity noted on the imaging studies can help guide the surgical management of a child with brachial plexus birth palsy. Diagnostic arthrography, although invasive, is the only modality in which dynamic assessment of the joint can be obtained. Often it is performed as part of the surgical reconstruction.

TREATMENT

Varying degrees of clinical presentation and recovery correlate with the extent of injury to the brachial plexus. Most brachial plexus birth palsies are mild injuries with a good prognosis. Spontaneous neurologic recovery occurs in 66% to 92% of patients. Most authors report significant recovery within the first 3 months, with slower recovery occurring within the next 6 to 12 months. If no evidence of deltoid or biceps recovery is seen by age 3 to 6 months, surgical exploration should be considered.

The aim of treatment in the initial stages is prevention of contractures of muscles and joints. Gentle passive exercises are begun to maintain full range of passive motion of

TABLE 6.4

Clinical Evaluation of Patients with Brachial Plexus Birth Palsy

TORONTO TEST SCORE

Elbow flexion	0-2
Elbow extension	0-2
Wrist extension	0-2
Digital extension	0-2
Thumb extension	0-2
Total score	0-10

Each motor function is tested and allocated a numeric value. A score of 0 indicates no function, and a score of 2 indicates normal function. A total score of 3.5 or lower at the age of 3 months or more is considered an indication for microsurgical repair.

Adapted from Michelow BJ, Clarke HM, Curtis CG, et al: The natural history of obstetrical brachial plexus palsy, *Plast Reconstr Surg* 93:675, 1994.

HOSPITAL FOR SICK CHILDREN ACTIVE MOVEMENT SCALE

Gravity Eliminated	
No contraction	0
Contraction, no motion	1
Motion, <50% range	2
Motion, >50% range	3
Full motion	4

Against Gravity	
Motion, <50% range	5
Motion, >50% range	6
Full motion	7

Motor function tested: shoulder flexion, shoulder abduction and adduction, shoulder internal and external rotation, elbow flexion and extension, forearm pronation and supination, wrist flexion and extension, finger flexion and extension, thumb flexion and extension.

Adapted from Clarke HM, Curtis CG: An approach to obstetrical brachial plexus injuries, *Hand Clin* 11:563, 1995.

MODIFIED MALLET CLASSIFICATION OF SHOULDER FUNCTION

	Grade I	Grade II	Grade III	Grade IV	Grade V
Global abduction	None	<30°	30°-90°	>90°	Normal
Global external rotation	None	<0°	0°-20°	>20°	Normal
Hand to neck	None	Not possible	Difficult	Easy	Normal
Hand on spine	None	Not possible	S1	T12	Normal
Hand to mouth	None	Marked trumpet sign	Partial trumpet sign	<40° of abduction	Normal

Patients are asked to actively perform five different shoulder movements, and each movement is graded on a scale of 1 (no movement) to 5 (normal motion symmetric to the contralateral unaffected side.)

Adapted from Mallet J: Primaute du traitement de l'épaule—méthod d'expression des résultats, *Rev Chir Ortho* 58S:166, 1972.

all joints of the upper extremity. Scapular stabilization and passive glenohumeral mobilization in all planes are needed to prevent contractures about the shoulder. Range of motion of the elbow, wrist, and fingers also should be included. Cortical recognition and integration of the affected limb are promoted. Several authors have described the injection of botulinum toxin-A into the internal rotator muscles as an adjunct to surgery to prevent internal rotation contractures and early posterior subluxation or dislocation of the shoulder in infants with neonatal brachial plexus palsy. Even with the use of these injections, there is a high rate of relapse that requires surgery. The use of physical therapy with casting and botulism toxin injections have been shown to be effective in the treatment of elbow flexion contractures; however, recurrence is common. Functional bracing may help encourage early hand use.

The role and timing of microsurgical intervention in the treatment of brachial plexus birth palsy remain controversial. Microsurgical intervention at approximately 3 months of age is recommended in infants with global plexus palsies and Horner syndrome. These avulsion injuries have a poor prognosis of recovery. Reconstruction is limited to nerve transfers because grafting is not a viable option when the nerve root is avulsed from the spinal cord.

More controversy exists over the management of intraplexus ruptures in which there are varying degrees of injury severity and recovery. Return of antigravity elbow flexion

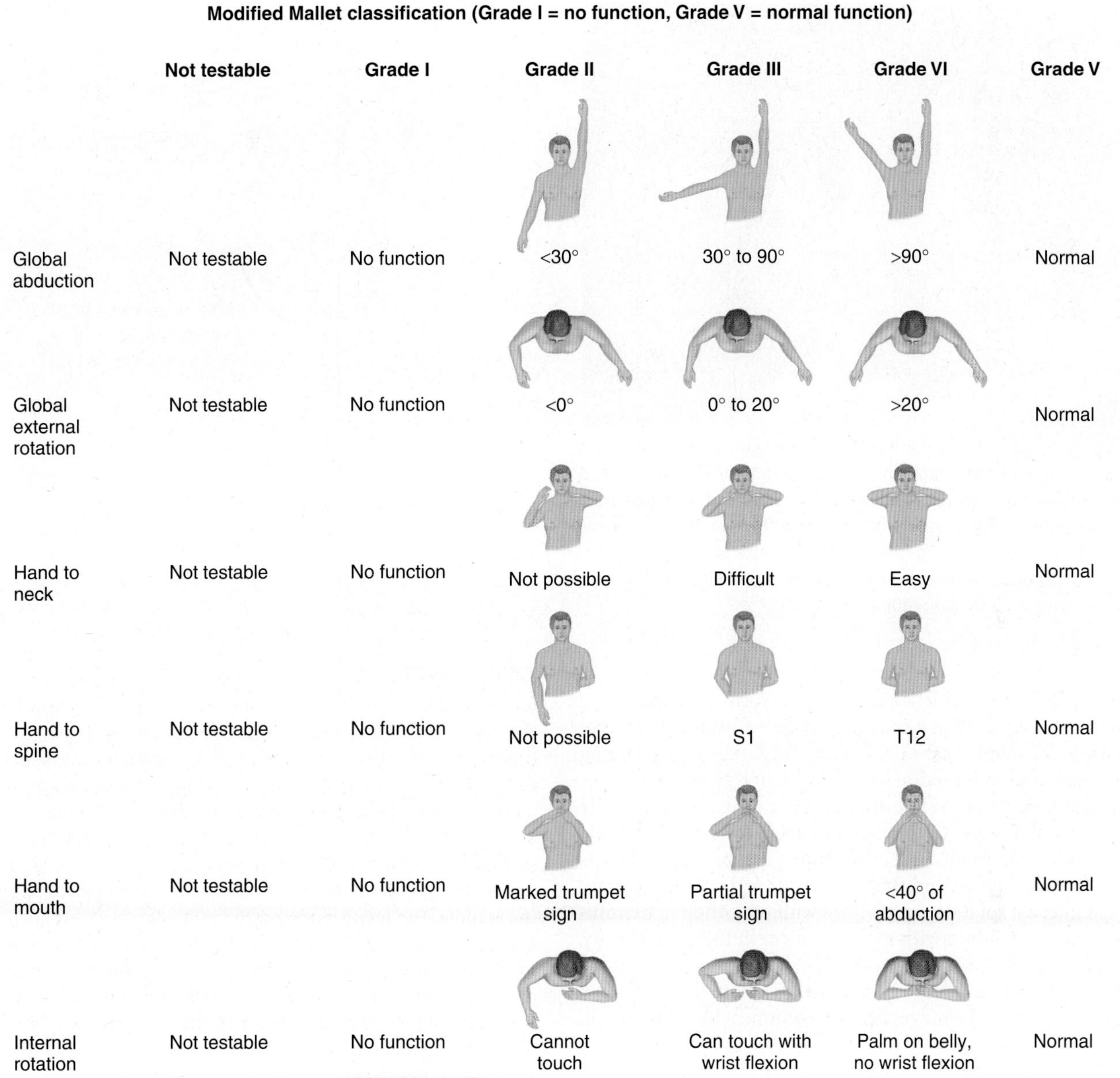

Modified Mallet classification (Grade I = no function, Grade V = normal function)

	Not testable	Grade I	Grade II	Grade III	Grade VI	Grade V
Global abduction	Not testable	No function	<30°	30° to 90°	>90°	Normal
Global external rotation	Not testable	No function	<0°	0° to 20°	>20°	Normal
Hand to neck	Not testable	No function	Not possible	Difficult	Easy	Normal
Hand to spine	Not testable	No function	Not possible	S1	T12	Normal
Hand to mouth	Not testable	No function	Marked trumpet sign	Partial trumpet sign	<40° of abduction	Normal
Internal rotation	Not testable	No function	Cannot touch	Can touch with wrist flexion	Palm on belly, no wrist flexion	Normal

FIGURE 6.56 Modified Mallet classification.

strength is the key factor in determining the need for brachial plexus exploration and nerve reconstruction. Most authors recommend microsurgical intervention if antigravity flexion has not returned by 3 to 9 months of age. Neuroma resection and nerve grafting is the most widely used technique for restoring function; however, nerve transfers are gaining popularity as an addition to or in lieu of nerve grafting. After treatment of a group of 34 infants for restoration of both elbow flexion and shoulder function, Malessy and Pondaag concluded that in neonatal patients with brachial plexus palsy lesions with neurotmesis of C5 and avulsion of C6, elbow flexion can be restored with supraclavicular intraplexal transfer of C6 to C5; however, recovery of shoulder function following suprascapular nerve reinnervation and additional grafting from C5 to the posterior division of the superior is less successful. A "triple" nerve transfer—long or lateral head of triceps branch of the radial nerve to the axillary nerve,

ulnar nerve fascicle of the flexor carpi ulnaris to the biceps motor nerve, and spinal accessory nerve to the suprascapular nerve—has been described for treatment of C5 and C6 root injuries (Erb palsy). Improvement in elbow flexion and forearm supination also has been reported with transfer of the ulnar or median nerve to the biceps motor branch.

Tendon transfers are most commonly performed about the shoulder to improve external rotation and abduction and prevent glenohumeral dysplasia and posterior humeral head subluxation or dislocation. Indications for surgical intervention involving the shoulder are infantile dislocation, persistent internal rotation contracture refractory to physiotherapy, limitation of active abduction and external rotation function with plateauing of neural recovery, and progressive glenohumeral deformity. The general problems that must be corrected are muscle imbalance, soft-tissue contractures, and joint deformity. Surgery generally involves one of four soft-tissue

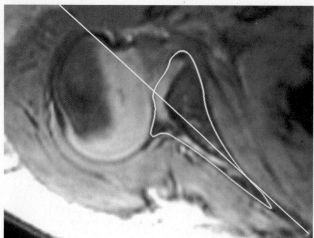

FIGURE 6.57 T2-weighted three-dimensional gradient-echo magnetic resonance image shows a pseudoglenoid. The glenoid contour and the scapular center line are enhanced with line tracings. (From Pearl ML, Edgerton BW, Kazimiroff PA, et al: Arthroscopic release and latissimus dorsi transfer for shoulder internal rotation contractures and glenohumeral deformity secondary to brachial plexus birth palsy, *J Bone Joint Surg* 88A:564, 2006.)

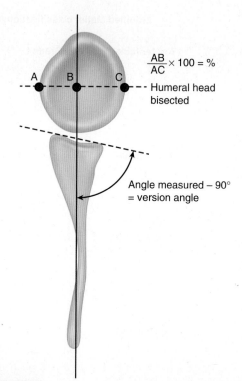

$$\frac{AB}{AC} \times 100 = \%$$

Humeral head bisected

Angle measured − 90° = version angle

FIGURE 6.58 Measurement of the glenoscapular angle (glenoid version) and the percentage of posterior subluxation of the humeral head. To measure the glenoscapular angle, a line is drawn parallel to the scapula and a second line is drawn tangential to the joint. The second line connects the anterior and posterior margins of the glenoid. On MR images, the cartilaginous margins are used. On CT scans, the osseous margins are used. The intersecting line connects the center point of the first line (approximately the middle of the glenoid fossa) and the medial aspect of the scapula. The angle in the posterior medial quadrant *(arrow)* is measured with a goniometer; 90 degrees is subtracted from this measurement to determine glenoid version. The percentage of posterior subluxation is measured by defining the percentage of the humeral head that is anterior to the same scapular line. The greatest circumference of the head is measured as the distance from the scapular line to the anterior portion of the head. This ratio (the distance to the anterior aspect of the humeral head *[AB]* divided by the circumference of the humeral had *[AC]*, multiplied by 100) is the percentage of subluxation. (Redrawn from Waters PM, Smith GR, Jaramillo D: Glenohumeral deformity secondary to brachial plexus birth palsy, *J Bone Joint Surg* 80A:668, 1998.)

procedures, all of which include some form of contracture release with or without a muscle transfer to augment external rotation: (1) anterior capsular release and Z-plasty lengthening of the subscapularis tendon with or without transfer of muscles for external rotation, (2) pectoralis major release with transfer of the latissimus and teres major as advocated by Hoffer et al., (3) subscapularis slide with or without a latissimus transfer, as described by Carlioz and Brahimi, or (4) arthroscopic release of the internal rotation contracture with or without latissimus transfer. For children with extensive glenohumeral deformity, external rotation osteotomy of the humerus is recommended to place the arm in a more functional position. Dodwell et al. described glenoid anteversion osteotomies in conjunction with tendon transfers for the treatment of established severe glenohumeral dysplasia (see Technique 6.50). They cited the procedure as being straightforward, with a low rate of complications and an infrequent need for revision.

Waters recommended that patients with grade I (normal), grade II (mild increase in glenoid retroversion), or mild grade III (slight posterior subluxation) glenohumeral deformities have an anterior musculotendinous lengthening of the pectoralis major and posterior latissimus dorsi and teres major transfer to the rotator cuff. Patients with grade V glenohumeral deformities (severe flattening of the humeral head with complete posterior dislocation) should have a humeral derotation osteotomy. Follow-up studies have shown that both tendon transfers alone and open reduction most commonly with tendon transfers improve shoulder range of motion; however, patients who have open reduction demonstrate remodeling of the glenoid retroversion and improvement of glenohumeral joint, which is not seen in patients who have tendon transfer alone.

Elbow flexion and forearm supination deformities can occur with a Klumpke palsy (C8-T1) or a mixed brachial plexus lesion. Progressive deformities occur because of weak or absent triceps, pronator teres, and pronator quadratus muscles with an intact biceps muscle. This creates progressive elbow flexion

and supination deformity from the unopposed biceps muscle. Radial head dislocation may occur with associated deformity of radius and ulna (Fig. 6.59). The wrist and hand usually are held in extreme dorsiflexion because of the unopposed wrist dorsiflexors. The biceps tendon can be Z-lengthened and rerouted around the radius to convert it from a supinator to a pronator (see Technique 6.29); this improves elbow extension and forearm pronation. In the presence of a supination contracture, a simultaneous interosseous membrane release may be effective. Bony correction of the forearm deformity can be performed more predictably. This can be achieved by forearm osteoclasis or osteotomy and internal fixation. The forearm should be positioned in 20 to 30 degrees of pronation.

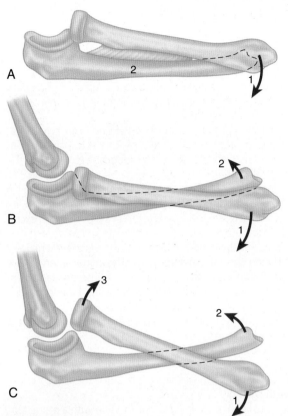

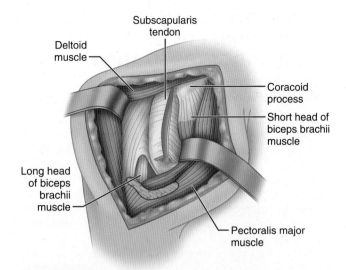

FIGURE 6.60 Anterior shoulder release for internal rotation contracture in brachial plexus palsy. **SEE TECHNIQUE 6.48.**

FIGURE 6.59 Physiopathology of supination deformity and progressive deformity with growth. **A,** Simple contracture with supination of the radius (1) and contracture of the interosseous membrane (2). **B,** Volar dislocation of the distal epiphysis of the ulna. **C,** Volar dislocation of the distal ulnar epiphysis and head of the radius.

elevate it with an elevator (Fig. 6.60), and divide it completely without incising the capsule. External rotation and abduction of the shoulder then should be almost normal.

■ A curved elongation of the acromion may interfere with abduction and with reduction of any mild posterior subluxation of the joint; in this event, either resect this obstructing part or divide the acromion and elevate this part.

POSTOPERATIVE CARE An abduction splint that holds the shoulder in abduction and mild external rotation is applied and is worn constantly for 2 weeks and intermittently for another 4 weeks. Active exercises are started early and are continued until maximal improvement has occurred.

ANTERIOR SHOULDER RELEASE

TECHNIQUE 6.48

(FAIRBANK, SEVER)

■ Make an incision on the anterior aspect of the shoulder in the deltopectoral groove distally from the tip of the coracoid process to a point distal to the tendinous insertion of the pectoralis major muscle; divide this tendon parallel to the humerus.

■ Retract the anterior margin of the deltoid laterally and the pectoralis major medially, and expose the coracobrachialis muscle.

■ With the shoulder externally rotated and abducted, trace the coracobrachialis superiorly to the coracoid process.

■ If the coracoid is elongated, resect 0.5 to 1.0 cm of its tip together with the insertions of the coracobrachialis, the short head of the biceps, and the pectoralis minor muscles; this resection increases the range of motion of the shoulder in external rotation and abduction.

■ Now locate the inferior edge of the subscapularis tendon at its insertion on the lesser tuberosity of the humerus,

ROTATIONAL OSTEOTOMY OF THE HUMERUS

TECHNIQUE 6.49

(ROGERS)

■ Approach the humerus anteriorly between the deltoid and pectoralis major muscles.

■ With the arm abducted, perform an osteotomy 5 cm distal to the joint.

■ Under direct vision, externally rotate the distal fragment of the humerus the desired amount to correct the internal rotation deformity and ensure that the fragments are then apposed.

■ Fix the osteotomy with a compression plate and screws.

■ Close the wound.

POSTOPERATIVE CARE A shoulder immobilizer or a sling is used for approximately 6 weeks with restriction of activities until radiographic healing.

DEROTATIONAL OSTEOTOMY WITH PLATE AND SCREW FIXATION

TECHNIQUE 6.50

(ABZUG ET AL.)

As an alternative, Abzug et al. described performing the derotational osteotomy and plate and screw fixation through a medial approach, which has the advantage of a more cosmetic scar.

- Make a medial incision overlying the intermuscular septum and midshaft of the humerus.
- Protect the superficial nerves, identify the intermuscular septum, and excise it.
- Retract the ulnar posteriorly and the median nerve and brachial artery anteriorly. Do not use loops around the nerves or reverse retractors than can place undue pressure on the nerve.
- Expose the humeral diaphysis.
- Choose a 6- to 8-hole plate, depending on the girth of the humerus, usually 2.7 mm or 3.5 mm. Place the plate over the humerus and insert the proximal three to four bicortical screws through the plate and humerus.
- Incise the periosteum only over the osteotomy site and place a Kirschner wire in the distal humerus below the intended osteotomy site to mark the amount of desired correction. Verify the position of the wire with a goniometer and visual assessment.
- With the wire placed in line with a hole in the plate, remove the plate and make the humeral osteotomy with an oscillating saw.
- Rotate the humerus so that the screw holes and Kirschner wire are aligned and the wire passes through a hole in the plate.
- Using the predrilled screw holes, fix the plate to the proximal fragment, close the osteotomy, and secure the distal fragment with screws using standard compression technique.
- Close the wound in standard fashion and apply a large bulky dressing from the hand to the axilla.

POSTOPERATIVE CARE No splint is used postoperatively; however, a sling must be worn to prevent stress across the osteotomy site. The dressings are removed and a humeral brace is fabricated 2 to 3 weeks after surgery. The brace is worn for about 1 month until union is confirmed radiographically and clinically.

GLENOID ANTEVERSION OSTEOTOMY AND TENDON TRANSFER

Dodwell et al. described glenoid anteversion osteotomy as an alternative to external rotation humeral osteotomy to stabilize the shoulder and improve function in older children (>4 years of age) with severe glenohumeral dysplasia (Waters type IV or V). All 32 patients in their series had improvement in active external rotation.

TECHNIQUE 6.51

(DODWELL ET AL.)

- Through an L-shaped posterior incision (Fig. 6.61A), elevate the deltoid muscle origin laterally.
- Perform a subscapularis slide by elevating the muscle belly from the anterior aspect of the scapula in an inferior-to-superolateral direction.
- Translate the humeral head anteriorly in external rotation and progressively externally rotate the shoulder to between 70 and 90 degrees in adduction to complete the muscular slide.
- Release the teres major and latissimus dorsi tendons from their insertions on the proximal part of the humerus (Fig. 6.61B). Release any adhesions to ensure adequate excursion of these muscles.
- Approach the posterior aspect of the glenohumeral joint through the infraspinatus and teres minor interval. Detach the infraspinatus tendon from its insertion, and clear the scapular neck subperiosteally, taking care to protect the suprascapular neurovascular bundle.
- Make a vertical posterior capsulotomy to visually inspect the joint.
- If the scapulohumeral angle was diminished on preoperative evaluation, indicating insufficient shoulder elevation, recess the tendon of the long head of the triceps origin at the glenoid.
- If a marked Putti sign (scapular rotation with a prominent superomedial corner at the base of the neck) is present, indicating a substantial abduction contracture, perform a lateral slide of the supraspinatus.
- Harvest a tricortical autograft from the medial aspect of the scapular spine or from the posterior aspect of the acromion. Based on preoperative templating from MR or CT images, determine the length of posterior cortical opening required to correct the glenoid retroversion to neutral, with the hinge point being the anterior cortex, and size the bone graft appropriately.
- Use an osteotome to make a scapular neck osteotomy extending from the lateral aspect of the spinoglenoid notch to the inferior aspect of the scapular neck, staying at least 5 mm medial to the glenoid rim to ensure protection of the glenoid blood supply and avoid osteonecrosis. Deepen the osteotomy to just short of the anterior cortex to retain an intact anterior hinge. Align the osteotomy parallel to the retroverted glenoid surface under direct observation.
- Use a narrow osteotome to lever open the osteotomy site and insert the bone graft (Fig. 6.61C). Gently tamp the graft into place so that it acts as a wedge, opening the cortex of the posterior aspect of the neck, and is stable.
- With the joint in the reduced position, close the capsule without capsulorrhaphy to minimize stiffness in internal rotation. Repair the infraspinatus anatomically. Suture the latissimus dorsi and teres major tendons into a longitudinal bone trough in the region of the greater humeral tuberosity, with the teres major in the inferior aspect of the trough and the latissimus, given its greater excursion, superior. Repair the deltoid to the scapular spine with sutures through bone.

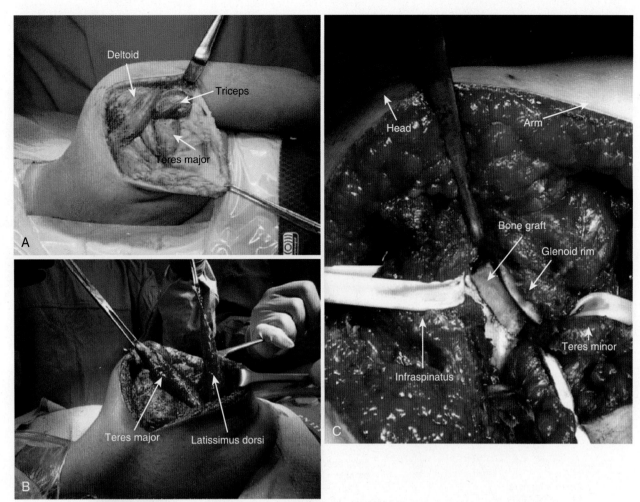

FIGURE 6.61 **A,** L-shaped posterior incision. **B,** Release of the teres major and latissimus dorsi tendons lateral to the long head of the triceps. **C,** Cortical wedge inserted in the osteotomy site. (From Dodwell E, Calaghan J, Anthony A, et al: Combined glenoid anteversion osteotomy and tendon transfers for brachial plexus birth palsy, *J Bone Joint Surg* 94A:2145, 2012.) **SEE TECHNIQUE 6.51.**

- Apply a shoulder spica cast with the shoulder in maximal external rotation (70 to 90 degrees) and limited (20 to 30 degrees) abduction.

POSTOPERATIVE CARE The cast is worn for 5 or 6 weeks, at which time a supervised physical therapy program is begun.

RELEASE OF THE INTERNAL ROTATION CONTRACTURE AND TRANSFER OF THE LATISSIMUS DORSI AND TERES MAJOR

When performed before age 6 years, the Sever-L'Episcopo procedure, as modified by Hoffer, improves external rotation of the shoulder by releasing the internal rotation contracture and transferring the latissimus dorsi and teres major posteriorly to provide active external rotation.

TECHNIQUE 6.52

(SEVER-L'EPISCOPO, GREEN)

- Place a sandbag under the upper part of the chest for proper exposure. Prepare and drape in the usual manner. An adequate amount of whole blood should be available for transfusion.
- Make an anterior incision beginning over the coracoid process and extending distally along the deltopectoral groove for 12 cm (Fig. 6.62A).
- Identify the cephalic vein and ligate or retract it with a few fibers of the deltoid muscle.
- With blunt dissection, develop the interval between the pectoral and deltoid muscles. Expose the coracobrachialis, the short head of the biceps, the coracoid process, the insertion of the tendinous portion of the subscapularis, and the insertion of the pectoralis major.
- Detach the short head of the biceps and coracobrachialis from their origin on the coracoid process and reflect downward.
- In the distal part of the wound, expose the insertion of the pectoralis major at its humeral attachment (Fig. 6.62B).

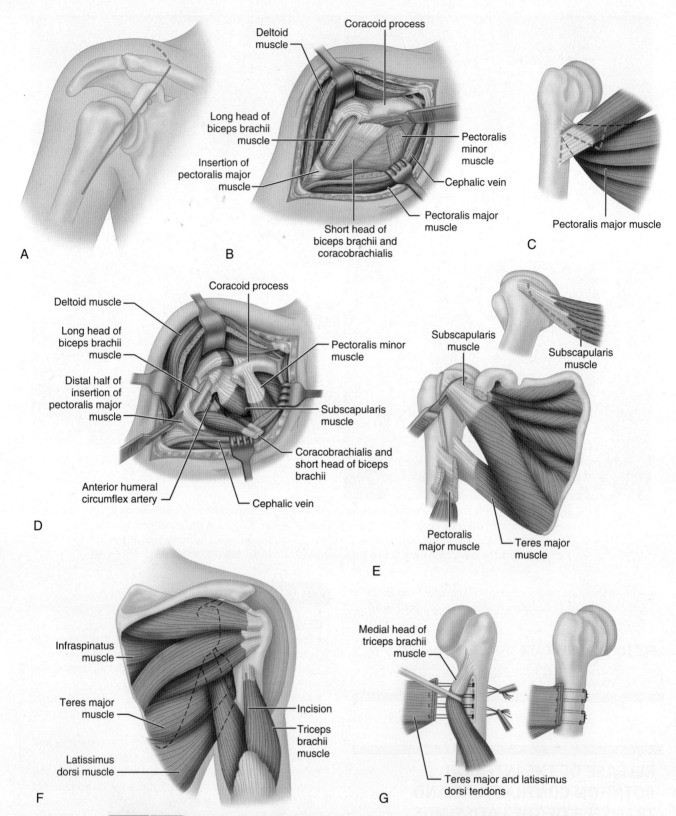

FIGURE 6.62 Sever-L'Episcopo and Green procedure. **A,** Anterior incision. **B,** Exposure of insertion of pectoralis major at humeral attachment. **C,** Incisions of tendinous insertion of pectoralis major for Z-lengthening. **D,** Distal half of tendinous insertion of pectoralis major on shaft of humerus is divided. **E,** Subscapularis is divided by oblique cut. **F,** Incision over deltoid-triceps interval *(back view)*. **G,** Teres major and latissimus dorsi tendons are attached to cleft in lateral humerus.

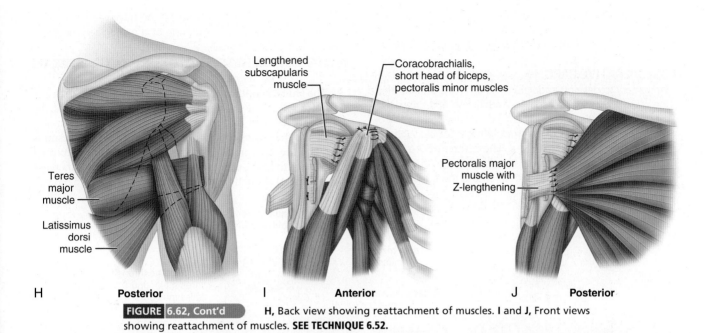

H   **Posterior**   I   **Anterior**   J   **Posterior**

FIGURE 6.62, Cont'd   **H,** Back view showing reattachment of muscles. **I** and **J,** Front views showing reattachment of muscles. **SEE TECHNIQUE 6.52.**

- With a periosteal elevator, reflect the muscle fibers of the pectoralis major medially to expose the tendinous portion of its insertion.
- To perform Z-lengthening, divide the distal half of the tendinous insertion of the pectoralis major immediately on the humeral shaft (Fig. 6.62C).
- Divide the upper half of the tendinous portion of the pectoralis major as far medially as good aponeurotic tendinous material exists, usually 4 to 5 cm from its insertion (Fig. 6.62D). Later, the distal tendon stump will be attached to the proximal tendon left inserted on the humerus, thereby providing further length to the pectoralis major. The reattachment of the tendon more proximally permits a greater degree of shoulder abduction but still allows rotary function.
- Apply whip sutures to the tendon still attached to the shaft and to the portion of the tendon attached to the muscle.
- Expose the subscapularis muscle over the head of the humerus. Starting medially with a blunt instrument, separate the subscapularis and elevate it from the capsule. Do not open the shoulder capsule. With a knife, lengthen the subscapularis tendon by an oblique cut (Fig. 6.62E).
- Starting medially, split the tendon into anterior and posterior halves, becoming more superficial laterally and completing the division at the insertion of the subscapularis into the humerus. Again, take care not to open the capsule.
- Once the subscapularis has been divided, the shoulder joint will abduct and externally rotate freely.
- If the coracoid process is elongated, hooked downward and laterally, and limits external rotation, it should be resected to its base. Likewise, if the acromion process is beaked downward and obstructs shoulder abduction, partially resect it.
- Next, identify the insertions of the latissimus dorsi and teres major and expose by separating them from adjacent tissues both anteriorly and posteriorly.

- The attachment of the latissimus dorsi is superior and anterior to that of the teres major. Divide both tendons immediately on bone and suture each tendon with a whip stitch.
- With the patient turned over on the side and with the patient's arm adducted across the chest, make a 7- to 8-cm incision over the deltoid-triceps interval (Fig. 6.62F).
- Retract the deltoid muscle anteriorly and the long head of the triceps posteriorly. Be careful not to damage the radial and axillary nerves.
- Subperiosteally expose the lateral surface of the proximal diaphysis of the humerus.
- Make a 5-cm longitudinal cleft using drills, an osteotome, and a curet.
- Drill four holes from the depth of the cleft coming out on the medial surface of the humeral shaft at the site of the former insertion of the teres major and latissimus dorsi muscles.
- Identify the tendons of the latissimus dorsi and teres major in the anterior wound, and deliver them into the posterior incision so that their line of pull is straight from their origins to the proposed site of attachment on the lateral humerus.
- Draw the latissimus dorsi and teres major tendons into the slot in the humerus, and tie securely into position with 1-0 silk sutures in the front (Fig. 6.62G and H).
- Suture the subscapularis tendon, which is lengthened "on the flat," at its divided ends to provide maximal lengthening. Suture the pectoralis major in a similar way.
- Reattach the coracobrachialis and short head of the biceps to the base of the coracoid process. If the coracobrachialis and short head of the biceps are short, lengthen them at their musculotendinous junction (Fig. 6.62I and J).
- The lengthened muscles should be of sufficient length to permit complete external rotation in abduction without undue tension.
- Close the wound in the usual manner and immobilize the upper limb in a previously prepared, bivalved shoulder spica cast that holds the shoulder in 90 degrees of abduction,

90 degrees of external rotation, and 20 degrees of forward flexion. Position the elbow in 80 to 90 degrees of flexion.
- Place the forearm and hand in a functional neutral position.

POSTOPERATIVE CARE Exercises are begun 3 weeks after surgery to develop abduction and external rotation of the shoulder, as well as shoulder adduction and internal rotation. Particular emphasis is given to developing the function and strength of the transferred muscles. When the arm adducts satisfactorily, a sling is used during the day and the bivalved shoulder spica cast is worn at night. The night support is continued for 3 to 6 more months.

Exercises are performed for many months or years to preserve functional range of motion of the shoulder and to maintain muscle control.

The Hoffer modification of the L'Episcopo procedure consists of a release of the pectoralis major and transfer of the combined tendons of the latissimus dorsi and teres major muscles to the posterior rotator cuff. Transfer of the latissimus dorsi and the teres major to the rotator cuff has been reported to have a stabilizing effect on the rotator cuff and to increase glenohumeral abduction and external rotation (Fig. 6.63).

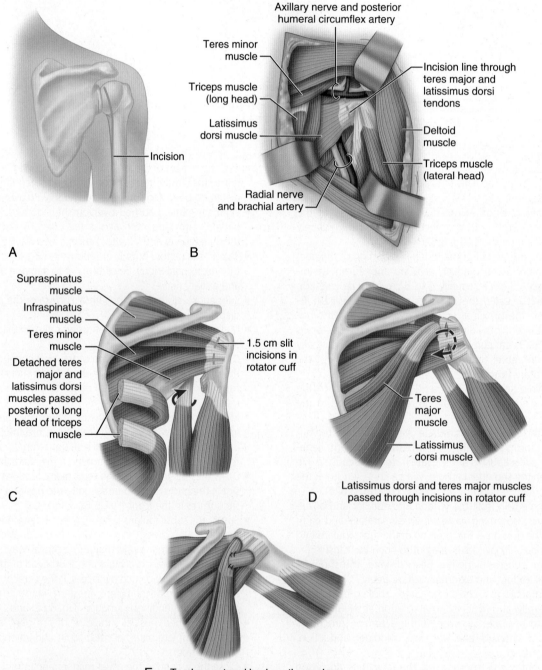

FIGURE 6.63 **Latissimus dorsi and teres major transfer to the rotator cuff.** (Redrawn from Herring JA, editor: *Tachdjian's pediatric orthopaedics*, ed 3, Philadelphia, 2002, Saunders.)

Arthroscopic techniques have been developed for release and for release combined with latissimus dorsi transfer (recommended for older children). These procedures have been reported to restore nearly normal passive external rotation and a centered glenohumeral joint at the time of surgery; however, gains in active elevation are minimal and loss of internal rotation, from moderate to severe, occurs in all children after this surgery. Pearl et al. listed the following guidelines for arthroscopic treatment of contractures and deformity secondary to brachial plexus birth palsy:

Arthroscopic release: Children younger than 3 years of age with passive external rotation of less than neutral (0 degrees) with the arm at the side

Arthroscopic release plus latissimus dorsi transfer: Children older than 3 years of age with a similar degree of contracture

Arthroscopic latissimus dorsi transfer without release: Children older than 3 years of age who have no substantial internal rotation contracture but have weakness of external rotation.

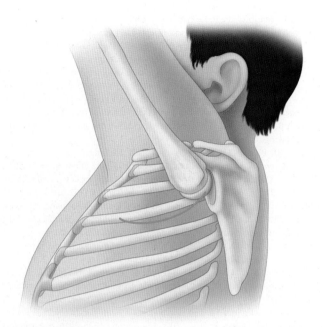

FIGURE 6.64   Curved incision in the skin lines, just medial to the posterior axillary crease toward the midline of the axilla, for latissimus dorsi transfer in conjunction with arthroscopic contracture release. (From Pearl ML, Edgerton BW, Kazimiroff PA, et al: Arthroscopic release and latissimus dorsi transfer for shoulder internal rotation contractures and glenohumeral deformity secondary to brachial plexus birth palsy, *J Bone Joint Surg* 88A:564, 2006.) **SEE TECHNIQUE 6.53.**

ARTHROSCOPIC RELEASE AND TRANSFER OF THE LATISSIMUS DORSI

TECHNIQUE 6.53

(PEARL ET AL.)

- With the patient in a lateral decubitus position, establish a posterior portal. Because of contracture and advanced deformity, it may be necessary to abduct the arm to approximately 90 degrees to allow passage of the scope across the glenohumeral joint. A surgical assistant maintains arm position while applying longitudinal traction. Make the posterior portal at the posterior glenohumeral joint line about 1 cm below the level of the posterior part of the acromion. Take care to avoid making the portal too low. A superior position makes it easier to insert the arthroscope over the top of the humeral head to avoid damage to the articular surface.
- Make an anterior portal from outside in, under direct observation through the posterior portal.
- Use an electrocautery device to release the anterior capsular ligaments, including the middle glenohumeral ligament and the anterior portion of the inferior glenohumeral ligament, at their attachment to the glenoid labrum. Basket forceps also are helpful.
- After release of the anterior soft tissues, identify the axillary nerve. Do not release the muscular portion of the subscapularis.
- Release the contracture by tenotomy of the subscapular tendon at its insertion and the overlying joint capsule. In younger children, this should allow full external rotation (70 to 90 degrees) with the arm at the side. If necessary in older children and those with more severe contractures, release the rotator interval tissue, exposing the base of the coracoid process. Release is not considered complete unless external rotation of 45 degrees or more is obtained.
- If latissimus dorsi transfer is to be done, make a 6- to 8-cm curved incision in the skin lines, just medial to the

posterior axillary crease toward the midline of the axilla (Fig. 6.64). In larger children, extend the incision to include the posterior arthroscopic portal.
- Carefully isolate the latissimus dorsi tendon from the teres major (which is left in situ), release it directly from the humerus, and transfer it under the posterior aspect of the deltoid to the greater tuberosity just adjacent to the infraspinatus tendon insertion. Secure the tendon with four No. 2 Ethibond sutures.
- Apply a shoulder spica cast to hold the arm in adduction and full external rotation.

POSTOPERATIVE CARE The shoulder spica cast is worn for 6 weeks and then modified to be used as a night splint for an additional 6 weeks.

REFERENCES

POLIOMYELITIS

Anderson GA, Thomas BP, Pallapati SC: Flexor carpi ulnaris tendon transfer to the split brachioradialis tendon to restore supination in paralytic forearms, *J Bone Joint Surg* 92B:230, 2010.

Chen D, Chen J, Liu F, Jiang Y: Tibial lengthening using a humeral intramedullary nail combined with a single-plane external fixator for leg discrepancy in sequelae of poliomyelitis, *J Pediatr Orthop B* 20:84, 2011.

Cichos KH, Lehtonen EJ, McGwin Jr G, et al.: Inhospital complications of patients with neuromuscular disorders undergoing total joint arthroplasty, *J Am Acad Orthop Surg*, 2018, https://doi.org/10.5435/JAAOS-D-18-00312, [Epub ahead of print].

Genet F, Denormandie P, Keenan MA: Orthopaedic surgery for patients with central nervous system lesions: concepts and techniques, *Ann Phys Rehabil Med*(18)31450–31457, 2018, pii: S1877-0657. [Epub ahead of print].

Godzik J, Lenke LG, Holekamp T, et al.: Complications and outcomes of complex spine reconstructions in poliomyelitis-associated spinal deformities: a single-institution experience, *Spine (Phila Pa 1976)* 39:1211, 2014.

Hopkins SE: Acute flaccid myelitis: etiologic challenges, diagnostic and management considerations, *Curr Treat Options Neurol* 19(48), 2017.

Joseph B, Watts H: Polio revisited: reviving knowledge and skills to meet the challenge of resurgence, *J Child Orthop* 9:325, 2015.

Kraay MJ, Bigach SD: The neuromuscularly challenged patient. Total hip replacement is now an option, *Bone Joint J* 96-B(11 Suppl A):27, 2014.

Lee WC, Ahn JY, Cho JH, Park CH: Realignment surgery for severe talar tilt secondary to paralytic cavovarus, *Foot Ankle Int* 34:1552, 2013.

Mach O, Tangermann RH, Wassilak SG, et al.: Outbreaks of paralytic poliomyelitis during 1996-2012: the changing epidemiology of a disease in the final stages of eradication, *J Infect Dis* 210(Suppl 1):S275, 2014.

McKay SL, Lee AD, Lopez AS, et al.: Increase in acute flaccid myelitis—United States, 2018, *MMWR Morb Mortal Wkly Rep* 67:1273, 2018.

Mehndiratta MM, Mehndiratta P, Pande R: Poliomyelitis: historical facts, epidemiology, and current challenges in eradication, *Neurohospitalist* 4:223, 2014.

Messacar K, Schreiner TL, Van Haren K, et al.: Acute flaccid myelitis: a clinical review of US cases 2012-2015, *Ann Neurol* 80:326, 2016.

Miller JD, Pinero JR, Goldstein R, et al.: Shoulder arthrodesis for treatment of flail shoulder in children with polio, *J Pediatr Orthop* 31:679, 2011.

Nathanson N, Kew OM: From emergence to eradication: the epidemiology of poliomyelitis deconstructed, *Am J Epidemiol* 172:1213, 2010.

Platt LR, Estívariz CF, Sutter RW: Vaccine-associated paralytic poliomyelitis: a review of the epidemiology and estimation of the global burden, *J Infect Dis* 210(Suppl 1):S380, 2014.

Provelengios S, Papavasiliou KA, Krykos MJ, et al.: The role of pantalar arthrodesis in the treatment of paralytic foot deformities. Surgical technique, *J Bone Joint Surg* 92A(Suppl 1):44, 2010.

Rahman J, Hanna SA, Kayani B, et al.: Custom rotating hinge total knee arthroplasty in patients with poliomyelitis affected limbs, *Int Orthop* 39:833, 2015.

Savolainen-Kopra C, Blomqvist S: Mechanisms of genetic variation in polioviruses, *Rev Med Virol* 20:358, 2010.

Shaghaghi M, Soleyman-Jahi S, Abolhassani H, et al.: New insights into physiopathology of immunodeficience-associated vaccine-derived poliovirus infection; systematic review of over 5 decades of data, *Vaccine* 36:1711, 2018.

Sierra RJ, Schoeniger SR, Millis M, Ganz R: Periacetabular osteotomy for containment of the nonarthritis dysplastic hip secondary to poliomyelitis, *J Bone Joint Surg* 92A:2917, 2010.

Tosun HB, Serbest S, Uludag A, et al.: Fixator-assisted tibial lengthening over a plate in a patient with sequelae of poliomyelitis, *Medicine (Baltimore)* 95:e5252, 2016.

Yoon BH, Lee YK, Yoo JJ, et al.: Total hip arthroplasty performed in patients with residual poliomyelitis: does in work? *Clin Orthop Relat Res* 472:933, 2014.

MYELOMENINGOCELE

Abo El-Fadl S, Sallam A, Abdelbadie A: Early management of neurologic clubfoot using Ponseti casting with minor posterior release in myelomeningocele: a preliminary report, *J Pediatr Orthop B* 25:104, 2016.

Baghdadi T, Abdi R, Bashi RZ, et al.: Surgical management of hip problems in myelomeningocele: a review article, *Arch Bone Joint Surg* 4:197, 2016.

Canaz H, Canaz G, Dogan I, et al.: Health-related quality of life in non-paraplegic (ambulatory) children with myelomeningocele, *Childs Nerv Syst* 33:1997, 2017.

Cavalheiro S, da Costa MDS, Moron AF, et al.: Comparison of prenatal and postnatal management of patients with myelomeningocele, *Neurosurg Clin N Am* 28:439, 2017.

Chambers HG: Update on neuromuscular disorders in pediatric orthopaedics: Duchenne muscular dystrophy, myelomeningocele, and cerebral palsy, *J Pediatr Orthop* 34(Suppl 1):S44, 2014.

Flanagan A, Gorzkowski M, Altiok H, et al.: Activity level, functional health, and quality of life in children with myelomeningocele as perceived by parents, *Clin Orthop Relat Res* 469:1230, 2011.

Garg S, Oetgen M, Rathjen K, Richards BS: Kyphectomy improves sitting and skin problems in patients with myelomeningocele, *Clin Orthop Relat Res* 469:1279, 2011.

Hunt KJ, Ryu JH: Neuromuscular problems in foot and ankle: evaluation and workup, *Foot Ankle Clin* 19:1, 2014.

Januschek E, Rohrig A, Kunze S, et al.: Myelomeningocele—a single institute analysis of the years 2007 to 2015, *Childs Nerv Syst* 32:1281, 2016.

Kellogg R, Lee P, Deibert CP, et al.: Twenty years' experience with myelomeningocele management at a single institution: lessons learned, *J Neurosurg Pediatr* 22:439, 2018.

Kelly SP, Bache CE, Graham HK, Donnan LT: Limb reconstruction using circular frames in children and adolescents with spina bifida, *J Bone Joint Surg* 92B:1017, 2010.

Khoshbin A, Vivas L, Law PW, et al.: The long-term outcome of patients treated operatively and non-operatively for scoliosis deformity secondary to spina bifida, *Bone Joint J* 96:1244, 2014.

Kshettry VR, Kelly ML, Rosenbaum BP, et al.: Myelomeningocele: surgical trends and predictors of outcome in the United States, 1988-2010, *J Neurosurg Pediatr* 13:666, 2014.

McDowell MM, Blatt JE, Deibert CP, et al.: Predictors of mortality in children with myelomeningocele and symptomatic Chiari type II malformation, *J Neurosurg Pediatr* 21:587, 2018.

Mednick RE, Eller EB, Swaroop VT, et al.: Outcomes of tibial derotational osteotomies performed in patients with myelodysplasia, *J Pediatr Orthop* 35:721, 2015.

Moeini Naghani I, Hashemi Zonouz T, Shahjouei S, et al.: Congenital cardiac anomalies in myelomeningocele patients, *Acta Med Acad* 43:160, 2014.

Moen TC, Dias L, Swaroop VT, et al.: Radical posterior capsulectomy improves sagittal knee motion in crouch gait, *Clin Orthop Relat Res* 469:1286, 2011.

Mundy A, Kushare I, Jayanthi VR, et al.: Incidence of hip dysplasia associated with bladder exstrophy, *J Pediatr Orthop* 36:860, 2016.

North T, Cheong A, Steinbok P, et al.: Trends in incidence and long-term outcomes of myelomeningocele in British Columbia, *Childs Nerv Syst* 34:717, 2018.

Patel J, Walker JL, Talwalkar VR, et al.: Correlation of spine deformity, lung function, and seat pressure in spina bifida, *Clin Orthop Relat Res* 469:1302, 2011.

Rowe DE, Jadhav AL: Care of the adolescent with spina bifida, *Pediatr Clin North Am* 55:1359, 2008.

Segal LS, Czoch W, Hennrikus WL, et al.: The spectrum of musculoskeletal problems in lipomyelomeningocele, *J Child Orthop* 7:513, 2013.

Shimoji K, Kimura T, Kondo A, et al.: Genetic studies of myelomeningocele, *Childs Nerv Syst* 29:1417, 2013.

Sibinski M, Synder M, Higgs ZC, et al.: Quality of life and functional disability in skeletally mature patients with myelomeningocele-related spinal deformity, *J Pediatr Orthop B* 22:106, 2013.

Spiro AS, Babin K, Lipovas S, et al.: Anterior femoral epiphysiodesis for the treatment of fixed knee flexion deformity in spina bifida patients, *J Pediatr Orthop* 30:858, 2010.

Stief F, Bohm H, Ebert C, et al.: Effect of compensatory trunk movements on knee and hip loading during gait in children with different orthopedic pathologies, *Gait Posture* 39:859, 2014.

Swaroop VT, Dias LS: Myelomeningocele. In Weinstein SL, Flynn JM, editors: *Lovell and Winter's pediatric orthopaedics*, ed 7, Philadelphia, 2014, Wolters Kluwer.

Thompson JD, Segal LS: Orthopaedic management of spina bifida, *Dev Disabil Res Rev* 16:96, 2010.

Thompson RM, Ohnow S, Dias L, et al.: Tibial derotational osteotomies in two neuromuscular populations: comparing cerebral palsy with myelomeningocele, *J Child Orthop* 11:243, 2017.

Toll BJ, Samdani AF, Janjua MB, et al.: Perioperative complications and risk factors in neuromuscular scoliosis surgery, *J Neurosrug Pediatr* 22:207, 2018.

van Bosse HJ: Syndromic feet: arthrogryposis and myelomeningocele, *Foot Ankle Clin* 20:619, 2015.

Wright JG: Hip and spine surgery is of questionable value in spina bifida: an evidence-based review, *Clin Orthop Relat Res* 469:1258, 2011.

Yamada HH, Fucs P: Long-term results of fibular-Achilles tenodesis (Westin's tenodesis) for paralytic pes calcaneus: is hypercorrection avoidable? A longitudinal retrospective study, *Int Orthop* 41:1641, 2017.

Yildirim T, Gursu S, Bayhan IA, et al.: Surgical treatment of hip instability in patients with lower lumbar level myelomeningocele: is muscle transfer required? *Clin Orthop Relat Res* 473:3254, 2015.

ARTHROGRYPOSIS MULTIPLEX CONGENITA

Astur N, Flynn JM, Flynn JM, et al.: The efficacy of rib-based distraction with VEPTR in the treatment of early-onset scoliosis in patients with arthrogryposis, *J Pediatr Orthop* 34(8), 2014.

Eldelman M, Katzman A: Treatment of arthrogrypotic foot deformities with the Taylor Spatial Frame, *J Pediatr Orthop* 31:429, 2011.

Eriksson M, Gutierrez-Farewik EM, Broström E, Bartonek A: Gait in children with arthrogryposis multiplex congenital, *J Child Orthop* 4:21, 2010.

Foy CA, Mills J, Wheeler L, et al.: Long-term outcome following carpal wedge osteotomy in the arthrogrypotic patient, *J Bone Joint Surg Am* 95:e10, 2017.

Greggi T, Martikos K, Pipitone E, et al.: Surgical treatment of scoliosis in a rare disease: arthrogryposis, *Scoliosis* 5:24, 2010.

Hall JG, Kimber E, van Bosse HJP: Genetics and classifications, *J Pediatr Orthop* 37(Suppl 1):S4, 2017.

Komolkin I, Ulrich EV, Agranovich OE, et al.: Treatment of scoliosis associated with arthrogryposis multiplex congenital, *J Pedaitr Orthop* 37(Suppl 1):S24, 2017.

Matar HE, Beirne P, Garg N: The effectiveness of the Ponseti method for treating clubfoot associated with arthrogryposis: up to 8 years follow-up, *J Child Orthop* 10:15, 2016.

Mubarak SJ, Dimeglio A: Navicular excision and cuboid closing wedge for severe cavovarus foot deformities: a salvage procedure, *J Pediatr Orthop* 31:551, 2011.

Oishi SN, Agranovich O, Pajardi GE, et al.: Treatment of the upper extremity contracture/deformities, *J Pediatr Orthop* 37(Suppl 1):S9, 2017.

Palocaren T, Thabet AM, Rogers K, et al.: Anterior distal femoral stapling for correction knee flexion contracture in children with arthrogryposis-preliminary results, *J Pediatr Orthop* 30:169, 2010.

Song K: Lower extremity deformity management in amyoplasia: when and how, *J Pediatr Orthop* 37(Suppl 2):S42, 2017.

van Bosse JHP: Reorientational proximal femoral osteotomies for correction of hip contractures in children with arthrogryposis, *JBJS Essential Surgical Techniques* 7:e11, 2017.

van Bosse HP, Ponten E, Wada A, et al.: Treatment of the lower extremity contracture/deformities, *J Pediatr Orthop* 37(Suppl 1):S16, 2017.

van Bosse HJ, Saldana RE: Reorientational proximal femoral osteotomies for arthrogrypotic hip contractures, *J Bone Joint Surg Am* 99:55, 2017.

Van Heest A, Rodriguez R: Dorsal carpal wedge osteotomy in the arthrogrypotic wrist, *J Hand Surg Am* 38:265, 2013.

Wada A, Yamaguchi T, Nakamura T, et al.: Surgical treatment of hip dislocation in amyoplasia-type arthrogryposis, *J Pediatr Orthop B* 21:381, 2012.

Yang SS, Dahan-Oliel N, Montpetit K, Hamdy RC: Ambulation gains after knee surgery in children with arthrogryposis, *J Pediatr Orthop* 30:863, 2010.

Zlotolow DA, Kozin SH: Posterior elbow release and humeral osteotomy for patients with arthrogryposis, *J Hand Surg Am* 37:1078, 2012.

BRACHIAL PLEXUS

Abid A, Accadbled F, Louis D, et al.: Arthroscopic release for shoulder internal rotation contracture secondary to brachial plexus birth palsy: clinical and magnetic resonance imaging results on glenohumeral dysplasia, *J Pediatr Orthop B* 21:305–309, 2012.

Abzug JM, Kozin SH: Evaluation and management of brachial plexus birth palsy, *Orthop Clin North Am* 45:225, 2014.

Abzug JM, Chafetz RS, Gaughan JP, et al.: Shoulder function after medial approach and derotational humeral osteotomy in patients with brachial plexus birth palsy, *J Pediatr Orthop* 30:469, 2010.

Azbug JM, Kozin SH, Waters PM: Open glenohumeral joint reduction and latissimus dorsi and teres major tendon transfers for infants and children following brachial plexus birth palsy, *Tech Hand Up Extrem Surg* 21:30, 2017.

Abzug JM, Mehlman CT, Ying J: Assessment of current epidemiology and risk factors surrounding brachial plexus birth palsy, *J Hand Surg Am*, 2018 Sep 25, https://doi.org/10.1016/j.jhsa.2018.07.020, pii: S0363-5023(17)31908-1. [Epub ahead of print].

Bauer AS, Lucas JF, Heyrani N, et al.: Ultrasound screening for posterior shoulder dislocation in infants with persistent brachial plexus birth palsy, *J Bone Joint Surg Am* 99:778, 2017.

Breton A, Mainard L, De Gaspéri M, et al.: Arthroscopic release of shoulder contracture secondary to obstetric brachial palsy: retrospective study of 18 children with an average follow-up of 4.5 years, *Orthop Traumatol Surg Res* 98:638, 2012.

Buchanan PJ, Grossman JAI, Price AE, et al.: The use of botulinum toxin infection for brachial plexus birth injuries: a systematic review of the literature, *Hand (N Y)*, 2018:1558944718760038, https://doi.org/10.1177/1558944718760038, [Epub ahead of print].

Buterbaugh KL, Shah AS: The natural history and management of brachial plexus birth palsy, *Curr Rev Musculoskelet Med* 9:418, 2016.

Chang KWC, Wilson TJ, Popadich M, et al.: Oberlin transfer compared with nerve grafting for improving early supination in neonatal brachial plexus palsy, *J Neurosurg Pediatr* 21:178, 2018.

Crouch DL, Hutchinson ID, Plate JF, et al.: Biomechanical basis of shoulder osseous deformity and contracture in a rat model of brachial plexus birth palsy, *J Bone Joint Surg Am* 97:1264, 2015.

DeFrancesco CJ, Shah DK, Rogers BH, et al.: The epidemiology of brachial plexus birth palsy in the United States: declining incidence and evolving risk factors, *J Pediatr Orthop*, 2017 Oct 9, https://doi.org/10.1097/BPO.0000000000001089, [Epub ahead of print].

Di Mascio L, Chin KF, Fox M, Sinisi M: Glenoplasty for complex shoulder subluxation and dislocation in children with obstetric brachial plexus palsy, *J Bone Joint Surg* 93B:102, 2011.

Dodwell E, O'Callaghan J, Anthony A, et al.: Combined glenoid anteversion osteotomy and tendon transfers for brachial plexus birth palsy: early outcomes, *J Bone Joint Surg* 94A:2145, 2012.

Donohue KW, Little KJ, Gaughan JP, et al.: Comparison of ultrasound and MRI for the diagnosis of glenohumeral dysplasia in brachial plexus birth palsy, *J Bone Joint Surg AM* 99:123, 2017.

Duijnisveld BJ, van Wijlen-Hempel MS, Hogendoorn S, et al.: Botulinum toxin injection for internal rotation contractures in brachial plexus birth palsy. A minimum 5-year prospective observation study, *J Pediatr Orthop* 37:e209, 2017.

Gladstein AZ, Sachleben B, Ho ES, et al.: Forearm pronation osteotomy for supination contracture secondary to obstetrical brachial plexus palsy: a retrospective cohort study, *J Pediatr Orthop* 37:e357, 2017.

Hale HB, Bae DS, Waters PM: Current concepts in the management of brachial plexus birth palsy, *J Hand Surg A* 35:322, 2010.

Ho ES, Roy T, Stephens D, Clarke HM: Serial casting and splinting of elbow contractures in children with obstetric brachial plexus palsy, *J Hand Surg* 35A:84, 2010.

Hogendoorn S, van Overvest KL, Watt I, et al.: Structural changes in muscle and glenohumeral joint deformity in neonatal brachial plexus palsy, *J Bone Joint Surg* 92A:935, 2010.

Immerman I, Valencia H, DiTaranto P, et al.: Subscapularis slide correction of the shoulder internal rotation contracture after brachial plexus birth injury:technique and outcomes, *Tech Hand Surg* 17:52, 2013.

Kozin SH: The evaluation and treatment of children with brachial plexus birth palsy, *J Hand Surg Am* 36:1360, 2011.

Kozin SH, Boardman MJ, Chafetz RS, et al.: Arthroscopic treatment of internal rotation contracture and glenohumeral dysplasia in children with brachial plexus birth palsy, *J Shoulder Elbow Surg* 19:102, 2010.

Kozin SH, Chafetz RS, Shaffer A, et al.: Magnetic resonance imaging and clinical findings before and after tendon transfers about the shoulder in children with residual brachial plexus birth palsy: a 3-year follow-up study, *J Pediatr Orthop* 30:154, 2010.

Lippert WC, Mehlman CT, Cornwall R, et al.: The intrarater and interrater reliability of glenoid version and glenohumeral subluxation measurements in neonatal brachial plexus palsy, *J Pediatr Orthop* 32:378–384, 2012.

Little KJ, Zlotolow DA, Soldado F, et al.: Early functional recovery of elbow flexion and supination following median and/or ulnar nerve fascicle transfer in upper neonatal brachial plexus palsy, *J Bone Joint Surg* 96A:215, 2014.

Louden RJ, Broering CA, Mehlman CT, et al.: Meta-analysis of function after secondary shoulder surgery in neonatal brachial plexus palsy, *J Pediatr Orthop* 33:656, 2013.

Luo PB, Chen L, Zhou CH, et al.: Results of intercostal nerve transfer to the musculocutaneous nerve in brachial plexus birth palsy, *J Pediatr Orthop* 31:884, 2011.

Malessy MJ, Pondaag W: Neonatal brachial plexus palsy with neurotmesis of C5 and avulsion of C6: supraclavicular reconstruction strategies and outcome, *J Bone Joint Surg Am* 96:e174, 2014.

Mehlman CT, DeVoe WB, Lippert WC, et al.: Arthroscopically assisted Sever-L'Episcopo procedure improves clinical and radiographic outcomes in neonatal brachial plexus palsy patients, *J Pediatr Orthop* 31:341–351, 2011.

Murison J, Jehanno P, Fitoussi F: Nerve transfer to biceps to restore elbow flexion and supination in children with obstetrical brachial plexus palsy, *J Child Orthop* 11:455, 2017.

Reading BD, Laor T, Salisbury SR, et al.: Quantification of humeral head deformity following neonatal brachial plexus palsy, *J Bone Joint Surg* 94A:131, 2012.

Sheffler LC, Lattanza L, Hagar Y, et al.: The prevalence, rate of progression, and treatment of elbow flexion contracture in children with brachial plexus birth palsy, *J Bone Joint Surg* 94A:403, 2012.

Sibbel SE, Bauer AS, James MA: Late reconstruction of brachial plexus birth palsy, *J Pediatr Orthop* 34(Suppl 1):S57, 2014.

Smith BW, Daunter AK, Yang LI, et al.: An update on the management of neonatal brachial plexus palsy—replacing old paradigms: a review, *JAMA Pediatr* 172:585, 2018.

Terzis JK, Kokkalis ZT: Restoration of elbow extension after primary reconstruction in obstetric brachial plexus palsy, *J Pediatr Orthop* 30:161, 2010.

van Alphen NA, van Doorn-Loogman MH, Maas H, et al.: Restoring wrist extension in obstetric palsy of the brachial plexus by transferring wrist flexors to wrist extensors, *J Pediatr Rehabil Med* 6:53, 2013.

The complete list of references is available online at Expert Consult. com.

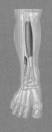

CHAPTER 7

NEUROMUSCULAR DISORDERS

William C. Warner Jr., Jeffrey R. Sawyer

Neuromuscular disease in children includes conditions that affect the spinal cord, peripheral nerves, neuromuscular junctions, and muscles. Accurate diagnosis is essential because the procedures commonly used to treat deformities in patients with neuromuscular disease such as poliomyelitis or cerebral palsy may not be appropriate for hereditary neuromuscular conditions. The diagnosis is made on the basis of clinical history, detailed family history, physical examination, laboratory testing (including serum enzyme studies, especially serum levels of creatine kinase and aldolase), genetic testing, electromyography, nerve conduction velocity studies, and nerve and muscle biopsies. Serum enzyme levels of creatine kinase are generally elevated, but the increase varies dramatically from levels of 50 to 100 times normal in patients with some dystrophic muscle conditions (e.g., Duchenne muscular dystrophy) to only slight increases (one to two times normal) in some patients with congenital myopathy or spinal muscular atrophy (SMA).

A number of advances have been made in the understanding of the genetic basis of neuromuscular disorders. Through advances in molecular biology, chromosome locations for various abnormal genes have been identified, characterized, and sequenced. In certain diseases, such as Duchenne and Becker muscular dystrophy, not only have the genes been localized, cloned, and sequenced, but the biochemical basis for these diseases is also now understood. The gene responsible for Duchenne and Becker muscular dystrophy is located in the Xp21 region of the X chromosome. This region is responsible for the coding of the dystrophin protein. Dystrophin testing (dystrophin immunoblotting) can be used as a biochemical test for muscular dystrophy; it is also useful for the differentiation of Duchenne muscular dystrophy from Becker muscular dystrophy. In addition, different types of mutations or variations can be used to predict clinical outcome. For example, Friedrich ataxia is caused by expansion of GAA nucleotide repeats in the frataxin gene intron. The amount of expansion of the GAA repeats correlates with disease severity and progression.

Due to DNA testing, nerve or muscle biopsy may not be necessary for a diagnosis, but it is often still useful for precise diagnosis. The biopsy specimen must be obtained from a muscle that is involved but still functioning—usually the deltoid, vastus lateralis, or gastrocnemius. The biopsy specimen should not be taken from the region of musculotendinous junctions because the normal fibrous tissue septa can be confused with the pathologic fibrosis. Specimens should be approximately 10 mm long and 3 mm deep and should be fixed in glutaraldehyde in preparation for electron microscopy. The muscle specimen that is to be processed for light microscopy should be frozen in liquid nitrogen within a few minutes after removal. The specimen should not be placed into saline solution or formalin. For nerve biopsy, the sural nerve is usually chosen. This nerve can be accessed laterally between the Achilles tendon and the lateral malleolus just proximal to the level of the tibiotalar joint. The entire width of the nerve should be taken for a length of 3 to 4 cm. Atraumatic technique is essential in either type of biopsy for meaningful results.

Orthopaedic treatment has been aimed at preventing the worsening of deformities and providing stability to the skeletal system to improve the quality of life for these children. Although a gene therapy cure may be possible in the future, orthopaedic treatment is still necessary to improve the quality of life for most children, no matter how severely impaired. Louis et al. reported 34 surgical procedures performed in individuals with severe multiple impairments to improve sitting posture, care, and comfort. Significant improvement was found in most patients, and no patient was made worse. The priorities of patients with severe neuromuscular diseases are the ability to communicate with other people, the ability to perform many activities of daily living, mobility, and ambulation. The role of the orthopaedic surgeon in achieving these goals includes prescribing orthoses for lower extremity control to facilitate transfer to and from wheelchairs, preventing or correcting joint contractures, and maintaining appropriate standing and sitting postures. Treatment must be individualized for each patient. The choice and timing of the procedures depend on the particular disorder, the severity of involvement, the ambulatory status of the patient, and the experience of the physician. This chapter discusses the common neuromuscular disorders in children that frequently require surgical intervention.

TREATMENT CONSIDERATIONS

BONE HEALTH—OSTEOPOROSIS AND FRACTURE MANAGEMENT

Fractures are common in children with neuromuscular disease because of disuse osteoporosis and frequent falls. Duchene muscular dystrophy patients who are on glucocorticoid therapy often develop osteoporosis. Larson and Henderson found a significant decrease in bone mineral density on dual-energy x-ray absorptiometry scans in boys with Duchenne muscular dystrophy, with 44% sustaining fractures. James et al. found that 33% of patients with Duchenne or Becker muscular dystrophy had sustained at least one fracture; full-time wheelchair use was a significant risk factor for fracture. Up to 30% of Duchenne muscular dystrophy patients develop symptomatic vertebral fractures. Most fractures are nondisplaced metaphyseal fractures that heal rapidly. Minimally displaced metaphyseal fractures of the lower limbs should be splinted so that walking can be resumed quickly. If braces are being used, they can be enlarged to accommodate the fractured limb and allow progressive weight bearing. Displaced diaphyseal fractures often require surgical stabilization to allow walking and mobilization during fracture

healing. McAdam et al. reported fat embolism syndrome following minor trauma in five patients with Duchenne muscular dystrophy, four of whom died within 36 hours of injury. The treating physician should be aware of and look for this complication. Medical treatment of disuse and steroid-induced osteopenia is beneficial in decreasing the frequency of fractures in this patient population. An algorithm for osteoporosis monitoring, diagnosis, and treatment for patients with Duchenne muscular dystrophy has been developed (Fig. 7.1).

ORTHOSES

Spinal bracing can occasionally be used to assist with sitting balance. Bracing may slow, but does not prevent, the progression of spinal deformity. Bracing is usually not well tolerated in patients with neuromuscular scoliosis. Knee-ankle-foot orthoses provide stability for patients with proximal muscle weakness. A pelvic band with hip and knee locks can be added if necessary. Ankle-foot orthoses help position the ankle and foot in a plantigrade position in an effort to prevent progressive equinus and equinovarus deformities.

SEATING SYSTEMS

For most children with severe neuromuscular disease, walking is difficult and frustrating, and a wheelchair may eventually be required. The chair—whether manual or electric—must be carefully contoured. A narrow chair with a firm seat increases pelvic support, and a firm back in slight extension supports the spine. Lateral spine supports built into the chair may help sitting balance

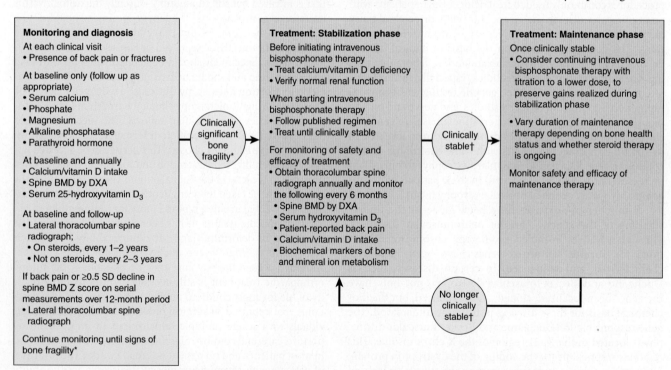

FIGURE 7.1 Osteoporosis monitoring, diagnosis, and treatment algorithm for patients with Duchenne muscular dystrophy. *BMD,* Bone mineral density; *DMD,* Duchenne muscular dystrophy; *DXA,* dual-energy x-ray absorptiometry. *Signs of clinically significant bone fragility are low-trauma fractures of long bones or vertebrae. †Clinical stability refers to absence of nonvertebral fractures, stable healed vertebra fractures, absence of new vertebral fractures in previously normal vertebral bodies, absence of bone and back pain, and BMD Z score appropriate for height Z score or higher than 2 standard deviations. (Modified from Birnkrant DJ, Bushby K, Bann CM, et al: Diagnosis and management of Duchenne muscular dystrophy, part 2: respiratory, cardiac, bone health, and orthopaedic management, *Lancet Neurol* 17:347, 2018.)

but do not usually alter the progression of scoliosis. Specialized seating clinics can provide custom-fitted chairs with numerous options for daily use. These custom-fitted chairs can accommodate most spinal deformities and pelvic obliquity that are present.

DIFFERENTIATION OF MUSCLE DISEASE FROM NERVE DISEASE

In addition to the history, physical examination, and routine laboratory studies, special tests such as electromyography, muscle tissue biopsy, serum enzyme, and molecular and genetic studies help differentiate the two diseases.

HEMATOLOGIC STUDIES

Serum enzyme assays are extremely helpful, especially the level of serum creatine kinase in the blood. Serum creatine kinase is a sensitive test for showing abnormalities of striated muscle function. Elevation of this enzyme is extremely important in the early stages of diagnosing Duchenne muscular dystrophy. Elevation of the creatine kinase parallels the amount of muscle necrosis. There is a significant elevation early in the disease process, but the elevation decreases with time as the muscle is replaced by fat and fibrous tissue. The creatine kinase levels can be elevated 20 to 200 times above normal limits. The level may decline in the later stages of the disease, when the greater muscle mass has already deteriorated and there is less breakdown of muscle mass than in the earlier stages. The levels are higher in Duchenne than in Becker muscular dystrophy; however, there is some overlap between the two diseases. This test is beneficial in detecting the carrier state of Duchenne and Becker muscular dystrophies because creatine kinase is usually elevated in the female carrier. A muscle provocation test is also beneficial in detecting the female carrier state because elevation of creatine kinase levels is greater after strenuous exercise in female carriers than in noncarrier females. Urine creatine is excessive in dystrophic patients in the active stage of muscle breakdown. Any process that causes muscle breakdown, such as excessive exercise, diabetes mellitus, and starvation in which carbohydrate intake is reduced and in the neuropathies, however, can cause an excess of creatine in the urine. In myotonic dystrophy, the level of creatine in the blood is decreased because of the reduced ability of the liver to produce creatine phosphate.

Aldolase is another enzyme that is elevated in patients with muscular dystrophy. Its course is similar to that of creatine kinase enzyme. Aspartate aminotransferase and lactate dehydrogenase values may also be elevated, but these enzymes are nonspecific for muscle disease. The diagnosis of Duchenne muscular dystrophy should be considered before liver biopsy in any male child with increased transaminases.

DNA mutation analysis (polymerase chain reaction or DNA blot analysis) can provide a definitive diagnosis of Duchenne or Becker muscular dystrophy. These tests can also help identify the carrier and may allow prenatal diagnosis in some cases. These DNA tests can be done from a small sample of blood or amniotic fluid.

ELECTROMYOGRAPHIC STUDIES

In an electromyogram of normal muscle, resting muscles are usually relatively electrosilent; on voluntary contraction of a normal muscle, the electromyogram shows a characteristic frequency, duration, and amplitude action potential (Fig. 7.2). In

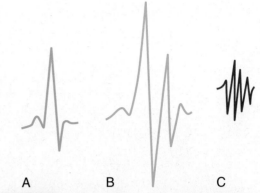

FIGURE 7.2 Motor units seen in electromyography. **A,** Normal triphasic motor unit potential. **B,** Large polyphasic motor units as seen in neurogenic disorders, such as spinal muscular atrophy, in which they also are reduced in number. **C,** Small polyphasic motor units as seen in muscular dystrophy. These are usually of normal number. (Courtesy Tulio E. Bertorini, MD.)

a myopathy, the electromyogram shows increased frequency, decreased amplitude, and decreased duration of the motor action potentials. In a neuropathy, it shows decreased frequency and increased amplitude and duration of the action potentials. In a neuropathy, nerve conduction velocities are usually slowed; in a myopathy, the nerve conduction velocities are usually normal. Myotonic dystrophy is characterized by an increase in frequency, duration, and amplitude of the action potentials on needle electrode insertion, which gradually decreases over time. When amplified, these action potentials create the "dive bomber" sound that is almost universal in this disease.

MUSCLE TISSUE BIOPSY

Interpretation of the muscle tissue biopsy differentiates not only myopathy from neuropathy but also the various types of congenital dystrophy from one another. In addition to the usual hematoxylin and eosin stain, special stains and techniques, such as the Gomori-modified trichrome stain, nicotinamide adenine dinucleotide-tetrazolium reductase (NADH-TR) stain, and the alizarin red S stain, are helpful. Electron microscopy is also beneficial.

Histopathologic study of muscle affected by myopathy shows an increased fibrosis in and between muscle spindles, with necrosis of the fibers (Fig. 7.3B). Later, deposition of fat within the fibers occurs, accompanied by hyaline and granular degeneration of the fibers. The number of nuclei is increased with migration of some nuclei to the center of the fibers. Some small groups of inflammatory cells may also be seen, and inflammatory cells are markedly increased in polymyositis. Special histochemical stains that can show muscle fiber type show a preponderance of type I fibers. In normal skeletal muscle, the ratio of type I to type II fibers is 1:2 (Fig. 7.3A). In some dystrophies other than the Duchenne type, fiber splitting is apparent. Calcium accumulation in muscle fibers has also been shown.

The microscopic picture in neuropathy is quite different (Fig. 7.3C). There is little or no increase in fibrous tissue, and small, angular, atrophic fibers are present between groups of normal-sized muscle fibers. Special stains that highlight fiber type show that 80% of the fibers are type II.

An adequate biopsy specimen must be obtained to make a correct diagnosis. An open muscle biopsy is usually

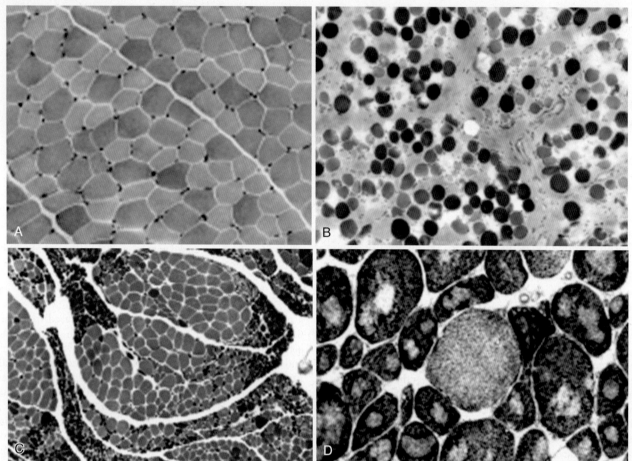

FIGURE 7.3 **A,** Normal muscle biopsy specimen (except for one small angular fiber). Note polygonal shape of myofibrils, normal distribution of type I and type II fibers, and normal connective tissue of endomysium (nicotinamide adenine dinucleotide-tetrazolium reductase [NADH-TR] stain, ×125). **B,** Muscular dystrophy. Fibers are more rounded, some fibers have internalized nuclei, and others are atrophic. One muscle fiber is necrotic and is undergoing phagocytosis. Connective tissue between fibers is increased (hematoxylin & eosin, ×295). **C,** Chronic neurogenic atrophy (juvenile spinal muscular atrophy). Notice grouping of fibers of same type and some atrophic angular fibers. Fat is increased between muscle fascicles (NADH-TR stain, ×125). **D,** Central core disease. Note pale areas of central cores in muscle fibers characteristic of this disease (NADH-TR stain ×200). (Courtesy Tulio E. Bertorini, MD.)

performed but, in some cases, a needle biopsy in small children has proved satisfactory. Muscles that are totally involved should not be used; biopsy specimens of muscles suspected of early involvement are indicated. The muscle bellies of the gastrocnemius in a patient with Duchenne muscular dystrophy are usually involved early and are a poor site to obtain material for a biopsy, whereas the quadriceps (especially the vastus lateralis at midthigh) and rectus abdominis usually show early involvement without total replacement of the muscle spindles by fibrous tissue or fat. Biopsy specimens of these muscles are usually the most reliable.

One must be careful when securing a biopsy specimen that the muscle is maintained at its normal length between clamps (Fig. 7.4) or sutures (Fig. 7.5) and that the biopsy specimen has not been violated by a needle electrode during an electromyogram or infiltrated with a local anesthetic before the biopsy. Biopsy needles should have a minimal core diameter of 3 mm.

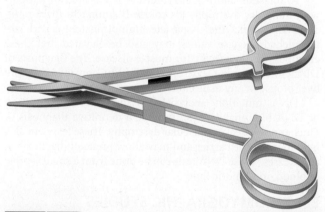

FIGURE 7.4 Two hemostats bound together to preserve length when securing muscle biopsy. (From Cruess RL, Rennie WRJ: *Adult orthopaedics*, New York, 1984, Churchill Livingstone.) **SEE TECHNIQUE 7.1.**

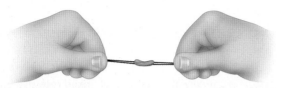

FIGURE 7.5 Muscle length maintained by muscle biopsy done on outer side of previously placed sutures. **SEE TECHNIQUE 7.1.**

A second sample of muscle tissue should be taken at the time of biopsy and sent for dystrophin analysis (dystrophin immunoblotting). Dystrophin is a muscle protein that has been found to be absent, decreased, or modified in certain types of dystrophy. The measurement and quantification of this protein combined with the clinical picture of certain types of muscular dystrophy have added significantly to the ability to diagnose various dystrophies.

Regional block anesthesia can be used for the biopsy, but a general anesthetic may be necessary. General anesthesia carries the known risk of anesthetic complications, such as acute rhabdomyolysis that can resemble malignant hyperthermia.

OPEN MUSCLE BIOPSY

TECHNIQUE 7.1

- Block the area regionally with 1% lidocaine and make a 1.5 cm incision through the skin and subcutaneous tissues.
- Carefully split the enveloping fascia to clearly expose the muscle bundles from which the biopsy specimen is to be taken.
- Using a special double clamp (Fig. 7.4) or silk sutures approximately 2 cm apart (Fig. 7.5), grasp the muscle and section around the outside of the arms of the clamp or sutures.
- Prevent bleeding within the muscle and take only small biopsy specimens.

Take more than one specimen because different stains need different preservative techniques; for example, some histochemical changes are best shown on fresh frozen sections that have had special staining. The pathologist should know in advance that a muscle biopsy is to be done so that special fixative techniques, such as freezing with liquid nitrogen, are readily available when the specimen is received.

PERCUTANEOUS MUSCLE BIOPSY

Mubarak, Chambers, and Wenger described percutaneous muscle biopsy in 379 patients. This procedure can be performed in an outpatient clinic with only local anesthesia.

TECHNIQUE 7.2

(MUBARAK, CHAMBERS, AND WENGER)
- Prepare the biopsy site with iodophor paint. Place a fenestrated adhesive drape over the site. Infiltrate the skin

and subcutaneous tissue with 5 to 8 mL of 1% lidocaine without epinephrine. When a biopsy specimen of the quadriceps is being obtained, also anesthetize the fascia.
- Check the Bergström biopsy needle to ensure a smooth sliding of the cutter within the trocar. Cut the K-50 tube at an angle and place it into the end of the cutting needle, with the other end attached to a 10 mL syringe.
- Use a No. 11 scalpel blade to make a small stab wound in the skin and fascia lata at approximately mid-thigh level.
- Insert the Bergström needle into the muscle, preferably the rectus femoris, at an oblique angle.
- Pull the needle back approximately one half of its length, and have an assistant apply suction with the 10 mL syringe. This allows muscle to be pulled into the cutting chamber.
- Cut by compressing the cutter into the trocar.
- Remove the Bergström apparatus from the thigh. Remove the muscle sample from the chamber with a fine needle and place it on saline-soaked gauze in a Petri dish.
- Through the same incision and track, reinsert the Bergström needle and repeat the procedure until five or six samples have been obtained.
- Close the small wound with ¼ inch adhesive strips.

POSTOPERATIVE CARE Dressing sponges are applied and held in place with foam tape to serve as a compressive, but not constricting, bandage for 2 days. The adhesive strips are left in place for 10 days; no perioperative antibiotics or narcotic analgesics are necessary.

MUSCULAR DYSTROPHY

The muscular dystrophies are a group of hereditary disorders of skeletal muscle that produce progressive degeneration of skeletal muscle and associated weakness (Table 7.1). The X-linked dystrophies are more common and include Duchenne muscular dystrophy, Becker muscular dystrophy, and Emery-Dreifuss muscular dystrophy. Limb-girdle muscular dystrophy and congenital muscular dystrophy are the two most common autosomal recessive muscular dystrophies. Facioscapulohumeral muscular dystrophy is inherited as an autosomal-dominant trait.

DUCHENNE MUSCULAR DYSTROPHY

Duchenne muscular dystrophy, a sex-linked recessive inherited trait, occurs in males and in females with Turner syndrome; carriers are female. It is reported to occur in one in 3500 live births. There is a family history in 70% of patients, and the condition occurs as a spontaneous mutation in approximately 30% of patients.

Duchenne muscular dystrophy is the result of a mutation in the Xp21 region of the X chromosome, which encodes the 400-kd protein dystrophin. Dystrophin is important to the stability of the cell membrane cytoskeleton. In patients with Duchenne muscular dystrophy, the total absence of this transcellular protein results in progressive muscle degeneration and loss of function.

Children with Duchenne muscular dystrophy usually reach early motor milestones at appropriate times, but independent ambulation may be delayed, and many are initially toewalkers. The disease usually becomes evident between 3 and 6 years of age. Clinical features include large, firm calf muscles;

TABLE 7.1

Characteristics of the Muscular Dystrophies

TYPE	ONSET	SYMPTOMS	PROGRESSION	INHERITANCE
Duchenne	Early childhood (2–6 years)	Generalized weakness and muscle wasting first affecting muscles of hips, pelvic area, thighs, and shoulders. Calves often enlarged.	Eventually affects all voluntary muscles, as well as heart and breathing. Survival uncommon beyond early 30s.	X-linked recessive
Becker	Adolescence or early adulthood	Similar to Duchenne, but less severe.	Progression is slow and variable but can affect all voluntary muscles. Survival usually well into mid-to-late adulthood.	X-linked recessive
Emery-Dreifuss	Childhood, usually by 10 years	Weakness and wasting of shoulder, upper arm, and calf muscles; joint stiffening; fainting caused by cardiac abnormalities.	Progression is slow; cardiac complications common and may require a pacemaker.	X-linked recessive Autosomal dominant Autosomal recessive
Limb-girdle	Childhood to adulthood	Weakness and wasting first affecting muscles around shoulders and hips	Progression is slow; cardiac complications common in later stages of disease.	Autosomal dominant Autosomal recessive
Facioscapulohumeral (Landouzy-Dejerine)	Adolescence or early adulthood, usually by age 20 years	Weakness and wasting of muscles around eyes and mouth, as well as shoulders, upper arms, and lower legs initially; later affects abdominal muscles and hip muscles	Progression is slow, with periods of rapid deterioration; may span many decades.	Autosomal dominant
Myotonic (Steinert disease)	Congenital form at birth; more common, less severe form in adolescence or adulthood	Weakness and wasting of muscles of face, lower legs, forearms, hands, and neck with delayed relaxation of muscles after contraction. Can affect gastrointestinal system, vision, heart, or respiration. Learning disabilities in some.	Progression is slow, sometimes spanning 50–60 years.	Autosomal dominant
Oculopharyngeal	Adulthood, usually 40s or 50s	Weakness of muscles of eyelids and throat, later facial and limb muscles. Swallowing problems and difficulty keeping eyes open are common.	Progression is slow.	Autosomal dominant Autosomal recessive
Distal	Childhood to adulthood	Weakness and wasting of muscles of hands, forearm, lower limbs	Progression is slow, not life-threatening.	Autosomal dominant Autosomal recessive
Congenital	At or near birth	Generalized muscle weakness, possible joint stiffness or laxity; may involve scoliosis, respiratory insufficiency, mental retardation	Progression is variable; some forms are slowly progressive, some shorten life span.	Autosomal recessive Autosomal dominant Spontaneous

Data from www.mda.org. Accessed December 30, 2008.

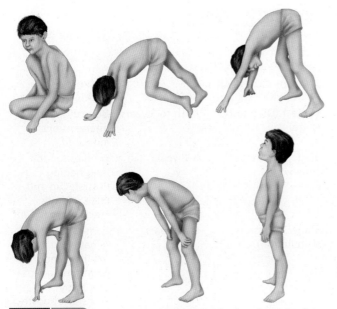

FIGURE 7.6 Gower sign. Child must use hands to rise from sitting position. (Redrawn from Siegel IM: *Clinical management of muscle disease*, London, 1977, William Heinemann.)

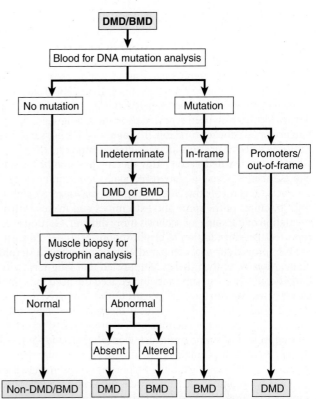

FIGURE 7.7 Flow chart of process for molecular diagnostic evaluation of patients in whom diagnosis of Duchenne muscular dystrophy *(DMD)* or Becker muscular dystrophy *(BMD)* is suspected. (From Shapiro F, Specht L: Current concepts review: the diagnosis and orthopaedic treatment of inherited muscular diseases of childhood, *J Bone Joint Surg* 75A:439, 1993.)

the tendency to toe-walk; a widely based, lordotic stance; a waddling Trendelenburg gait; and a positive Gower test indicative of proximal muscle weakness (Fig. 7.6). The diagnosis is usually obvious by the time the child is 5 or 6 years old (Fig. 7.7). A dramatically elevated level of creatine kinase (50 to 100 times normal) and DNA analysis of blood samples confirm the diagnosis. Muscle biopsy shows variations in fiber size, internal nuclei, split fibers, degenerating or regenerating fibers, and fibrofatty tissue deposition. Dystrophin testing of the muscle biopsy specimen will help confirm the type of muscular dystrophy but is not 100% confirmatory.

◼ PHYSICAL EXAMINATION

The degree of muscular weakness depends on the age of the patient. Because the proximal musculature weakens before the distal muscles, examination of the lower extremities shows an early weakness of gluteal muscle strength. The weakness in the proximal muscles of the lower extremity can be shown by a decrease in the ability to rise from the floor without assistance of the upper extremities (Gower sign). The calf pseudohypertrophy is caused by infiltration of the muscle by fat and fibrosis, giving the calves the feel of hard rubber (Fig. 7.8). The extrinsic muscles of the foot and ankle retain their strength longer than the proximal muscles of the hip and knee. The posterior tibial muscle retains its strength for the longest time. This pattern of weakness causes an equinovarus deformity of the foot. Weakness of the shoulder girdle musculature can be shown by the Meryon sign, which is elicited by lifting the child with one arm encircling the child's chest. Most children contract the muscles around the shoulder to increase shoulder stability and facilitate lifting. In children with muscular dystrophy, however, the arms abduct because of the lack of adductor muscle tone and severe shoulder girdle muscle weakness until the children eventually slide through the examiner's arms unless the chest is tightly encircled. Later in the disease process, the Thomas test shows hip flexion contracture and the Ober test shows an abduction contracture of the hip.

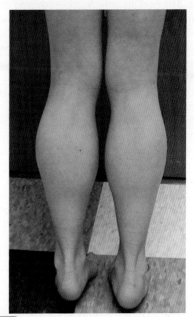

FIGURE 7.8 Calf pseudohypertrophy in muscular dystrophy.

◼ MEDICAL TREATMENT

The use of prednisone and deflazacort has been shown to preserve or improve strength, prolong ambulation, and slow the progression of scoliosis. Steroids help stabilize cell membranes and decrease inflammation and, therefore, have the potential to inhibit myocyte cell death and decrease the secondary effects associated with cell death. A group of boys treated with daily high-dose deflazacort had a substantially reduced rate of scoliosis compared with boys who elected not to take this medication. Eighty percent of untreated boys developed scoliosis of at least 20 degrees by age 18, whereas fewer than 25% of the boys in the treatment group developed scoliosis. Daily high-dose deflazacort has also been reported to result in long-term maintenance of pulmonary function. The age at which boys became full-time wheelchair users increased by several years over boys who did not use deflazacort. This therapy has significant side effects including weight gain, osteopenia, behavioral changes, cataracts, and myopathy. The osteopenia may lead to pathologic fractures of the spine and extremities and makes instrumentation of the spine for scoliosis more difficult. Gordon et al. reported that the addition of bisphosphonates to steroid treatment improved survival compared with treatment with steroid alone. More recently, Lebel et al. reported that long-term glucocorticoid treatment substantially reduced the need for spinal surgery in boys who took deflazacort (20%) compared to those who did not (92%). Other medical therapies that have been used but have not shown definite benefit are myoblast transfers, azathioprine, and aminoglycosides. Gene therapy and stem cell therapy may show promise as a treatment for muscular dystrophy but are still investigational. Eteplirsen has been shown to increase dystrophin in skeletal muscle and is under accelerated approval by the US Food and Drug Administration (FDA). This drug is indicated for patients who have a confirmed mutation of the DMD gene that is appropriate for exon 51 skipping.

ORTHOPAEDIC TREATMENT

The goals of orthopaedic treatment are to maintain functional ambulation as long as possible and enhance sitting balance in a wheelchair. The specific procedures required differ according to the age of the child and the stage of disease severity (Table 7.2). Between ages 8 and 14 years (median 10 years), children with Duchenne muscular dystrophy typically have a sensation of locking of the joints. Contractures of the lower extremity may require early treatment to prolong the child's ability to ambulate, if even for 1 to 2 years. This requires prevention or retardation of the development of contractures of the lower extremity, which would eventually prohibit ambulation. It is easier to keep patients walking than to induce them to resume walking after they have stopped. When children with Duchenne muscular dystrophy stop walking, they also become more susceptible to the development of scoliosis and severe contractures of the lower extremities. Scoliosis develops in nearly all children with Duchenne muscular dystrophy, usually when they require aided mobility or shortly after becoming wheelchair bound. The use of steroids has decreased the occurrence of scoliosis in these patients.

For surgical correction of lower extremity contractures, three approaches have been used, as follows:
1. *Ambulatory approach.* The goal of surgery during the late ambulatory phase is to correct any contractures in the lower extremity while the patient is still ambulatory. Rideau recommended early aggressive surgery. His indications for surgery were first appearance of contractures in lower extremities; a plateau in muscle strength, usually around 5 to 6 years of age; and difficulty maintaining upright posture with the feet together. Rideau recommended that surgery be performed before deterioration

TABLE 7.2

Orthopaedic Treatment of Duchenne Muscular Dystrophy

STAGE OF MUSCULAR DYSTROPHY	AGES	ORTHOPAEDIC TREATMENT
Stage 1 (Diagnostic stage)	Birth to 5 years	No orthopaedic interventions indicated
Stage 2 (Quiescent stage)	5–8 years	Achilles tendon lengthening Possible hip and knee releases Fracture treatment
Stage 3 (Loss of ambulation)	9–12 years	Contracture releases Achilles tendon lengthening or tenotomy Transfer of posterior tibial muscle to dorsum of foot
Stage 4 (Full-time sitting/development of spinal deformity)	12–16 years	Spinal fusion
Stage 5 (Complete dependence and development of respiratory insufficiency)	≥15 years	Fracture treatment

of the Gower maneuver time or time to rise from the floor. Other surgeons have recommended surgery later in the ambulatory phase, just before the cessation of ambulation.
2. *Rehabilitative approach.* Surgery is performed after the patient has lost the ability to walk but with the intention that walking will resume. Surgery during this stage usually allows for only minimal ambulation with braces.
3. *Palliative approach.* The palliative approach treats only contractures that interfere with foot wear and comfortable positioning in a wheelchair.

A comparison of ambulation and foot position in three groups of patients with Duchenne muscular dystrophy (those who had surgery to maintain ambulation, those who had surgery to correct and maintain foot position, and those who had no surgery) found that the mean age at cessation of ambulation for those who had surgery was 11.2 years, compared with 10.3 years in those who did not have surgery. Foot position was neutral in 94% of those who had surgery, and none had toe flexion deformities; 96% of those who had surgery reported being able to wear any type of shoes, compared with only 60% of those who had no surgery. In contrast, another study of full-time wheelchair users with Duchenne muscular dystrophy found no significant differences between patients who did and did not have foot surgery with respect to foot wear, hypersensitivity, or cosmesis. Hindfoot motion was significantly better, but equinus contracture was significantly worse in those who had not had surgery.

Currently, the most common approach is to correct contractures just before the patient has a significant decline in

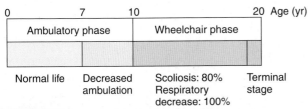

FIGURE 7.9 Graph of natural course of Duchenne muscular dystrophy: age-related stages. (From Rideau Y, Duport G, Delaubier A, et al: Early treatment to preserve quality of locomotion for children with Duchenne muscular dystrophy, *Semin Neurol* 15:9, 1995.)

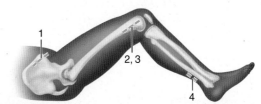

FIGURE 7.10 Tenotomy sites for release of hip flexors *(1)*, tensor fasciae latae and fascia lata *(2, 3)*, and Achilles tendon *(4)*. **SEE TECHNIQUE 7.3.**

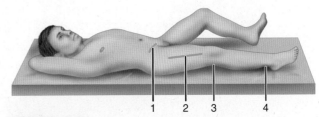

FIGURE 7.11 Surgical sites for musculotendinous releases to reduce bilaterally contractures of the hip *(1)*, thigh *(2)*, knee *(3)*, and ankle *(4)*.

ambulation and before the patient has to use a wheelchair (ambulatory approach) (Fig. 7.9).

Mild equinus contractures of the feet can help force the knee into extension, which helps prevent the knee buckling caused by severe weakness of the quadriceps. Stretching exercises and nightly bracing can be used to prevent the contractures from becoming severe. Flexion and abduction contractures of the hip impede ambulation, however, and should be minimized. Exercises to stretch the hip muscles and lower extremity braces worn at night to prevent the child from sleeping in a frog-leg position are helpful initially.

If surgery is indicated, the foot and hip contractures should be released simultaneously, usually through percutaneous incisions. Ambulation should be resumed immediately after surgery, if possible. Polypropylene braces are preferred to long-term casting. Prolonged immobilization must be avoided to prevent or limit the progressive muscle weakness caused by disuse.

PERCUTANEOUS RELEASE OF HIP FLEXION AND ABDUCTION CONTRACTURES AND ACHILLES TENDON CONTRACTURE

TECHNIQUE 7.3

(GREEN)
- With the child supine on the operating table, prepare and drape both lower extremities from the iliac crests to the toes.
- First flex and then extend the hip to be released, holding the hip in adduction to place tension on the muscles to be released; keep the opposite hip in maximal flexion to flatten the lumbar spine.
- Insert a No. 15 knife blade percutaneously just medial and just distal to the anterior superior iliac spine (Fig. 7.10).
- Release the sartorius muscle first, and then the tensor fasciae femoris muscle. Push the knife laterally and subcutaneously—without cutting the skin—to release the tensor fasciae latae completely. Bring the knife to the original insertion point and push it deeper to release the rectus femoris completely. Avoid the neurovascular structures of the anterior thigh.
- At 3 to 4 cm proximal to the upper pole of the patella, percutaneously release the fascia lata laterally through a

stab wound in its midportion. Push the knife almost to the femur to release the lateral intermuscular septum completely.
- Perform a percutaneous release of the Achilles tendon.
- Apply long-leg casts with the feet in neutral position and with the heels well padded to prevent pressure ulcers.

POSTOPERATIVE CARE The patient is mobilized immediately after surgery. If tolerated, a few steps are allowed. Walker-assisted ambulation commences as soon as possible and when transfer is achieved, the patient is placed in a regular bed and physical therapy is continued. The casts are bivalved, and bilateral polypropylene long-leg orthoses are fitted as soon as possible. Patients are discharged from the hospital as soon as they can ambulate independently with a walker.

❚ RIDEAU TECHNIQUE
Rideau et al. described a similar technique, but with an open procedure to release the hip flexor contractures and lateral thigh contractures. They also excised the iliotibial band and the lateral intermuscular septum (Fig. 7.11).

TRANSFER OF THE POSTERIOR TIBIAL TENDON TO THE DORSUM OF THE FOOT

In patients with marked overpull of the posterior tibial muscle, Greene found that transfer of the posterior tibial tendon to the dorsum of the foot combined with other tenotomies or tendon lengthening gave better results than posterior tibial tendon lengthening alone. Although transfer of the posterior tibial tendon is technically more demanding and has a higher perioperative complication rate, Greene noted that the patients retained the plantigrade posture of their

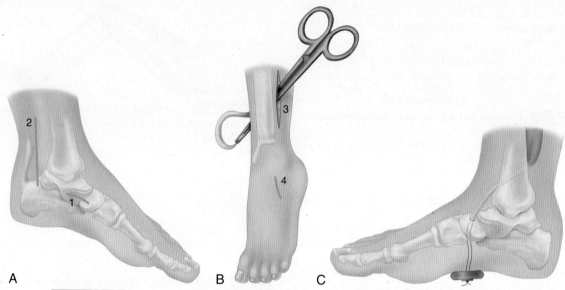

FIGURE 7.12 Posterior tibial tendon transfer to foot. **A,** First and second incisions. **B,** Third and fourth incisions and clamp placement for pulling posterior tibial tendon from posterior to anterior compartment of leg. **C,** Position of transplanted tendon and suture tied over felt pad and button on plantar aspect of foot. **SEE TECHNIQUE 7.4.**

feet, even after walking ceased. Despite the more extensive surgical procedure, early ambulation of the patients was not impeded.

TECHNIQUE 7.4

(GREENE)
- Place the patient supine; after placing a tourniquet, make a 3 cm incision starting medially at the neck of the talus and extending to the navicular (Fig. 7.12A).
- Open the sheath of the posterior tibial tendon from the distal extent of the flexor retinaculum to the navicular.
- Release the tendon from its bony insertions, preserving as much length as possible.
- Make a second incision 6 to 8 cm long vertically between the Achilles tendon and the medial distal tibia (Fig. 7.12B). The Achilles tendon can be lengthened through the same incision if necessary.
- Incise the posterior tibial tendon sheath and pull the distal portion of the tendon through the second operative wound.
- Make a third incision 6 cm long lateral to the anterior crest of the tibia and extend it to the superior extensor retinaculum (Fig. 7.12B).
- Incise the anterior compartment fascia and retract the anterior tibial tendon laterally.
- Carefully incise the interosseous membrane on the lateral aspect of the tibia adjacent to its tibial insertion for a distance of 3 cm. Enlarge the opening by proximal and distal horizontal cuts, extending halfway across the interosseous membrane.
- Pass a curved clamp close to the tibia from the anterior compartment proximally into the second incision. Keep

the curved clamp on the tibia to prevent injury to the peroneal vessels.
- After grasping the posterior tibial tendon and pulling it into the third incision, inspect the tendon through the second incision to ensure that it has neither twisted on itself nor ensnared the flexor digitorum longus tendon.
- Make a fourth incision 3 cm long on the dorsum of the foot in the region of the middle cuneiform.
- Incise the periosteum of the middle cuneiform and expose the central portion of the bone.
- Drill a hole 5 to 8 mm to insert the tendon through the middle of the cuneiform.
- Pass a Kelly clamp subcutaneously from the third incision to the fourth incision distally to create a subcutaneous track for the posterior tibial tendon. Pull the tendon through the subcutaneous track with a tendon passer.
- Holding on to the sutures tied to the end of the posterior tibial tendon, pass the tendon into the hole in the middle cuneiform, and pass the sutures through the dorsum of the foot with the aid of straight needles or it can be secured into the middle cuneiform with a suture anchor.
- Release the tourniquet, and inspect, irrigate, and close the wounds.
- After the wounds have been closed, tie the suture over a felt pad and button on the plantar aspect on the foot, with the foot in a neutral position (Fig. 7.12C).
- Apply a long-leg cast with the knee extended and the ankle in neutral position.

POSTOPERATIVE CARE Standing and walking are allowed 24 to 48 hours after surgery. A long leg cast is worn for 4 to 6 weeks, and a knee-ankle-foot orthosis is worn permanently.

TRANSFER OF THE POSTERIOR TIBIAL TENDON TO THE DORSUM OF THE BASE OF THE SECOND METATARSAL

Mubarak described transfer of the posterior tibial tendon to the dorsum of the base of the second metatarsal. Compared to the Greene technique, the more distal placement of the posterior tibial tendon increases the lever arm in dorsiflexion of the ankle and the technique allows easier plantar flexion and dorsiflexion balancing of the ankle at the time of surgery.

TECHNIQUE 7.5

(MUBARAK)

- With the patient supine and a tourniquet in place, make a 3 cm incision over the insertion of the posterior tibial tendon on the navicular.
- Open the sheath of the posterior tibial tendon from the anterior aspect of the medial malleolus to the navicular.
- Release the tendon from the bony insertions, preserving as much length as possible.
- Make a second incision in the posteromedial calf in the region of the myotendinous junction of the posterior tibial tendon. A gastrocnemius recession can be done through this incision if necessary, but excessive lengthening of the triceps surae complex should be avoided to prevent the development of a crouched gait postoperatively.
- Open the posterior tibial tendon sheath and pull the tendon through the sheath into the calf wound.
- At the myotendinous junction of the posterior tibial tendon, incise the tendon transversely halfway through its width. Extend this incision distally to within 0.5 cm of the cut insertion of the tibial tendon.
- Secure the distal aspect of the tendon with a single suture to prevent the longitudinal cut from extending out to the end of the tendon. This procedure effectively doubles the length of the posterior tibial tendon (Fig. 7.13A).
- Make a third incision 6 cm long lateral to the anterior crest of the tibia, extending it to the superior extensor retinaculum.
- Perform an anterior compartment fasciotomy and retract the anterior tibial tendon laterally.
- Incise the interosseous membrane of the lateral aspect of the tibia for a distance of 3 cm.
- Place a Kelly clamp through the anterior compartment wound across the interosseous membrane and into the deep posterior compartment. Grasp the end of the lengthened posterior tibial tendon and bring it through the interosseous membrane into the anterior compartment of the calf (Fig. 7.13B).
- Make another incision, 2 to 3 cm long, over the base of the second metatarsal. Dissect down to the base of the second metatarsal, and subperiosteally dissect around the base of the second metatarsal circumferentially.
- Take the elongated posterior tibial tendon and tunnel it subcutaneously into the incision over the dorsum of the second metatarsal. Loop the tendon around the base of the second metatarsal as a sling and suture it to itself, with the appropriate tension on the ankle to hold it in neutral plantar flexion and dorsiflexion (Fig. 7.13C).
- Release the tourniquet and inspect the tibial vessels to ensure that they are not being kinked by the transferred tendon. Irrigate the wounds and close them in a standard fashion.

POSTOPERATIVE CARE Postoperative care is the same as for transfer of the posterior tibial tendon to the dorsum of the foot (see Technique 7.4).

Equinus contractures can be corrected by a percutaneous Achilles tendon lengthening or an open Achilles tendon lengthening. If an open procedure is required because of severe contractures, lengthening or release of the posterior

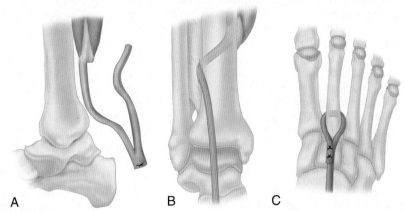

FIGURE 7.13 Posterior tibial tendon transfer to dorsum of second metatarsal base. **A,** Posterior tibial tendon removed from insertion. Length can be effectively doubled by splitting at myotendinous junction to cut end. Secure midpoint at lengthened tendon with suture. **B,** Lengthened tendon is passed through hole in interosseous membrane (posterior to anterior) and subcutaneously across anterior aspect of ankle. **C,** Lengthened tendon is pulled subcutaneously across dorsum of midfoot, looped around base of second metatarsal, and sutured to itself with enough tension to hold ankle in neutral. **SEE TECHNIQUE 7.5.**

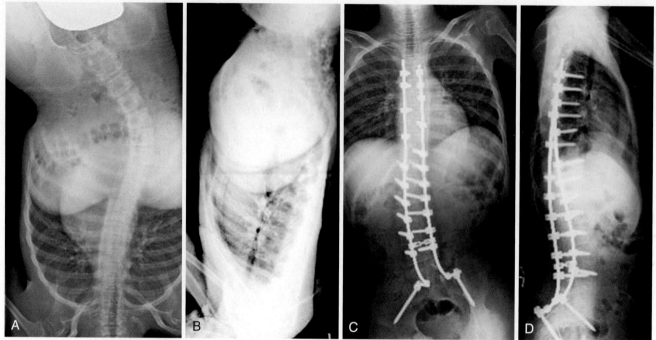

FIGURE 7.14 **A** and **B,** Radiographs of patient with Duchenne muscular dystrophy and scoliosis. **C** and **D,** Postoperative radiographs after posterior fusion and instrumentation to the pelvis.

tibial, flexor digitorum, and flexor hallucis longus tendons may also be required. When these lengthening procedures or releases are done, the child will need an ankle-foot orthosis to continue to stand or ambulate.

Although release of contractures usually allows another 2 to 3 years of ambulation, by age 12 to 13 years most children with Duchenne muscular dystrophy can no longer walk, and spinal deformity becomes the primary problem. Scoliosis affects almost all children with Duchenne muscular dystrophy, and the curve is usually progressive (Fig. 7.14); however, with the use of steroids in the medical treatment of Duchenne muscular dystrophy the frequency of scoliosis has decreased. Scoliosis produces pelvic obliquity, which makes sitting increasingly difficult. Bracing and wheelchair spinal-support systems may slow progression of the curve, but spinal fusion is ultimately required for most patients.

When a patient becomes nonambulatory, the scoliosis almost invariably worsens and significant kyphosis develops. Many authors recommend spinal arthrodesis at the onset of scoliosis when the curve is only 20 degrees. Given the natural history of the condition, delaying surgery until the curve reaches 40 or 50 degrees has no advantage and can make surgery more complicated because of the worsening of cardiac and pulmonary function during the delay. Most authors recommend that the forced vital capacity of the lungs be 50% or more of normal to reduce pulmonary complications to an acceptable level, and a forced vital capacity of less than 35% has been cited as a relative contraindication to surgery and as evidence of significant cardiomyopathy. Surgery can still be done when vital capacity is less than 50%, but the risk of pulmonary and cardiac complications increases.

Posterior spinal fusion (PSF) with segmental instrumentation is the operation of choice. The fusion and instrumentation should extend to the proximal thoracic spine to prevent postoperative kyphosis above the fusion. Facet joint

arthrodesis should be performed at every level, using autogenous or allograft bone graft as required. Most authors have recommended that fusion extend to the pelvis. Fusion to L5 can be considered if the Cobb angle is less than 40 degrees and there is less than 10 degrees of pelvic obliquity. Alman and Kim found that if the apex of the curve was at L1 or below, pelvic obliquity increased after fusion to L5.

OTHER VARIANTS OF MUSCULAR DYSTROPHY
▆ BECKER MUSCULAR DYSTROPHY

Becker muscular dystrophy is a sex-linked recessive disorder that has a later onset and a slower rate of muscle deterioration than Duchenne muscular dystrophy. The prevalence of Becker muscular dystrophy based on dystrophin analysis is 2.3 per 100,000. The affected gene in Becker muscular dystrophy is identical to that in Duchenne muscular dystrophy (located at the Xp21 locus on the X chromosome), but patients with Becker muscular dystrophy show some evidence of a functional intracellular dystrophin. The dystrophin in Becker muscular dystrophy, although present, is altered in size or decreased in amount or both. The severity of the disease depends on the amount of functional dystrophin in the muscles. Genetic studies and dystrophin testing now allow the clinician to better define severe forms of Becker muscular dystrophy. Serum creatine kinase levels are highest before muscle weakness is clinically apparent and can be 10 to 20 times normal levels. Onset of symptoms usually occurs after age 7 years, and patients may live to their mid-40s or later. Cardiac involvement is frequent in patients with Becker muscular dystrophy; a high percentage of patients with Becker muscular dystrophy have electrocardiographic abnormalities and cardiomyopathy.

The orthopaedic treatment of Becker muscular dystrophy depends on the severity of the disease. In patients with large amounts of functional dystrophin, orthopaedic procedures are frequently not required until after childhood, and in patients with more severe forms of the disease, treatment consideration is the same as for Duchenne muscular dystrophy. Contractures of the foot and overpull of the posterior tibial muscle can be treated effectively with Achilles tendon lengthening and posterior tibial tendon transfers, with good long-term results. Patients rarely need soft-tissue releases around the hip. Scoliosis is not as common in patients with Becker muscular dystrophy, and no definitive recommendations exist in the literature, so treatment must be individualized.

■ EMERY-DREIFUSS MUSCULAR DYSTROPHY

Emery-Dreifuss muscular dystrophy is an X-linked recessive disorder, with the fully developed disease seen only in boys, although milder disease has been reported in girls. The gene locus for the most common form of Emery-Dreifuss muscular dystrophy is in the Xq28 region of the X chromosome. This region encodes for a nuclear membrane protein named emerin. Muscle biopsy of patients with Emery-Dreifuss muscular dystrophy shows normal levels of dystrophin but an absence of emerin.

During the first few years of life, patients have muscle weakness, an awkward gait, and a tendency for toe-walking. The full syndrome, usually occurring in the teens, is characterized by fixed equinus deformities of the ankles, flexion contractures of the elbows, extension contracture of the neck, and tightness of the lumbar paravertebral muscles. A significant factor in the diagnosis and treatment of Emery-Dreifuss muscular dystrophy is the presence of cardiac abnormalities consisting of bradycardia and atrial ventricular conduction defects that can lead to complete heart block. It is important to recognize Emery-Dreifuss muscular dystrophy because of the cardiac abnormalities, which, initially, are almost always asymptomatic but lead to a high incidence of sudden cardiac death, which may be averted by a cardiac pacemaker. Most patients are able to ambulate until the fifth or sixth decade of life.

Orthopaedic treatment of Emery-Dreifuss muscular dystrophy involves release of the heel cord contractures and other muscles around the foot. This usually requires an Achilles tendon lengthening and a posterior ankle capsulotomy. Anterior transfer of the posterior tibial tendon may also be required. Elbow flexion contractures do not usually exceed 35 degrees, but contractures of 90 degrees have been reported. Full flexion and normal pronation and supination are maintained. Successful results of release of elbow contractures have not been reported. Contractures around the neck and back should be treated conservatively with range of motion, although full range of motion should not be expected. Scoliosis can occur with this form of muscular dystrophy but has a lower incidence of progression.

■ LIMB-GIRDLE DYSTROPHY

Limb-girdle dystrophy has been classified based on inheritance patterns into autosomal dominant, autosomal recessive, and X-linked forms. Now, with an expanding list of identified genes, there are eight dominant forms and 14 recessive forms. The clinical characteristics are sometimes indistinguishable from those of Becker muscular dystrophy, but normal dystrophin is noted on laboratory examination. The disease usually occurs in the first to fourth decades of life. The initial muscle weakness involves the pelvic or shoulder girdle (Fig.

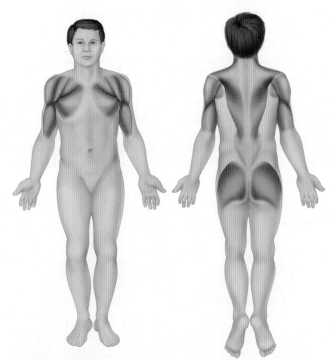

FIGURE 7.15 Pattern of weakness in limb-girdle dystrophy. (Redrawn from Siegel IM: *Clinical management of muscle disease*, London, 1977, William Heinemann.)

7.15). Lower extremity weakness usually involves the gluteus maximus, the iliopsoas, and the quadriceps. Upper extremity weakness may involve the trapezius, the serratus anterior, the rhomboids, the latissimus dorsi, and the pectoralis major. Some weakness may also develop in the prime movers of the fingers and wrists. There are two major forms of limb-girdle dystrophy: the more common pelvic girdle type and a scapulohumeral type. Surgery is seldom required in patients with limb-girdle dystrophy. Stabilization of the scapula to the ribs may be required for winging of the scapula, and in rare cases muscle transfers around the wrist may be required.

■ FACIOSCAPULOHUMERAL MUSCULAR DYSTROPHY

Facioscapulohumeral muscular dystrophy is an autosomal-dominant condition with characteristic weakness of the facial and shoulder girdle muscles (Fig. 7.16). The affected gene is located on chromosome 4q35. Onset of the disease may be in early childhood, in which case the disease runs a rapid, progressive course, confining most children to a wheelchair by age 8 to 9 years; alternatively, onset may occur in patients 15 to 35 years old, in which case the disease progresses more slowly. The most striking clinical manifestation is facial weakness with an inability to whistle, purse the lips, wrinkle the brow, or blow out the cheeks. The greatest functional impairments are the inability to abduct and flex the arms at the glenohumeral joints and winging of the scapula, both caused by progressive weakness of the muscles that fix the scapula to the thoracic wall, whereas the muscles that abduct the glenohumeral joint remain strong. As the disease progresses, weakness of the lower extremities, especially in the peroneal and the anterior tibial muscles, results in a footdrop that requires the use of an ankle-foot orthosis. Sometimes the quadriceps muscle is involved, requiring expansion of the orthosis to a knee-ankle-foot orthosis. Scoliosis is rare, although increased lumbar lordosis is common.

The inability to flex and abduct the shoulder functionally can be treated by stabilization of the scapula, with scapulothoracic arthrodesis. Scapulothoracic fusion with strut grafts or with plates and screws provides a satisfactory fusion of the medial border of the scapula to the posterior thoracic ribs (Fig. 7.17); however, it is associated with significant complications, including pneumothorax, pleural effusion, atelectasis, and pseudarthrosis. Techniques using wires for fixation have been described by Jakab and Gledhill, Twyman et al., and Diab et al. Copeland et al. described a similar fusion technique, but instead of wires they used screws to stabilize the scapula to the fourth, fifth, and sixth ribs (Fig. 7.18).

Cited indications for scapulothoracic fusion include limited shoulder abduction and flexion of more than 90 degrees, scapular winging, and shoulder discomfort; deltoid strength should be at least grade 4 of 5 at the time of surgery. In their 11 procedures in eight patients, the only complication reported by Diab et al. was prominent subcutaneous wires that required trimming in two patients. They noted that scapulothoracic fusion can relieve shoulder fatigue and pain, allow smooth abduction and flexion of the upper extremity, and improve the appearance of the neck and shoulder. Although disease progression affecting the deltoid muscle can cause a loss of abduction, other benefits of the procedure are maintained long term.

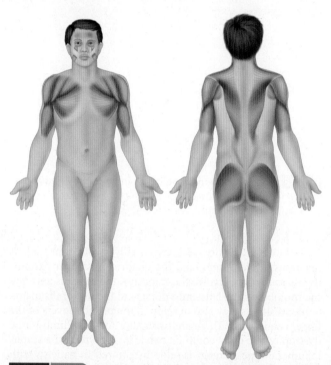

FIGURE 7.16 Pattern of weakness in facioscapulohumeral dystrophy.

SCAPULOTHORACIC FUSION

TECHNIQUE 7.6

(DIAB ET AL.)

- Place the patient prone, with the forequarter draped free. Abduct the upper limb so that the scapula lies flat against the posterior part of the thorax with its vertebral border externally rotated at an angle of 25 degrees to the midline.
- Make a linear incision over the entire vertebral border of the scapula in the reduced position.
- Cut the trapezius muscle in line with the cutaneous incision.
- Release the levator scapulae and rhomboid major and minor muscles from their sites of insertion on the vertebral border of the scapula and dissect them medially. These muscles are usually atrophic and markedly fibrotic and fatty.

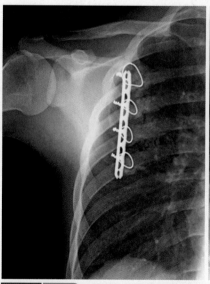
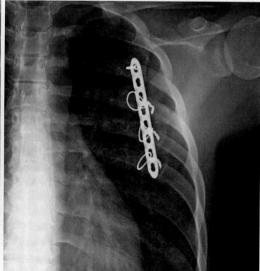

FIGURE 7.17 Bilateral scapulothoracic arthrodesis in a patient with fascioscapulohumeral dystrophy.

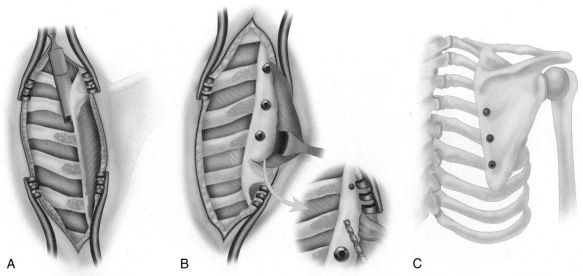

A   B   C

FIGURE **7.18**   Copeland technique of scapulothoracic fusion. **A,** Decortication of ribs. **B** and **C,** Drilling and insertion of rib screws after application of cancellous bone graft.

- Reflect the supraspinatus, infraspinatus, and teres major muscles 2 to 3 cm laterally from their sites of origin on the vertebral border of the scapula.
- Expose the posterior surface of the vertebral border of the scapula subperiosteally (Fig. 7.19A).
- Reflect a 4 to 5 cm segment of the origin of the subscapularis laterally from the anteromedial part of the scapula, also in the subperiosteal plane. Excise part of the subscapularis if necessary to expose the deep surface of the vertebral border of the scapula and to permit its apposition against the adjacent ribs.
- In the process of clearing the vertebral border of the scapula subperiosteally, free the insertion of the serratus anterior anteriorly from the whole length of the medial border of the scapula. This should allow the scapula to be placed without tension in a more medial and inferior position against the posterior part of the chest wall. It is important not to attempt to gain even further medial-inferior correction by forceful efforts because doing so might stretch adjacent neurovascular structures and cause a brachial plexus palsy.
- Expose subperiosteally, from the neck to the posterior angle, five ribs at the fusion site, typically the second to the sixth or the third to seventh ribs, taking care to protect the parietal pleura and subcostal neurovascular bundles.
- Harvest an autogenous cancellous bone graft from the posterior iliac crest.
- Use a motorized burr to partially decorticate to bleeding bone the anterior surface of the scapula and the posterior surface of the ribs.
- Place the scapula against the posterior part of the chest wall and mark the points of wire passage from the vertebral border of the scapula to the immediately adjacent ribs. Position the wires with one above the scapular spine, one at the level of the spine, and one below it, with the lowest at the most distal part of the vertebral border (Fig. 7.19B).
- Bend a doubled 16-gauge wire into a C shape and pass it under the rib subperiosteally from superior to inferior;

twist the two ends once against the posterior surface of the rib to prevent impingement against the pleura.
- Drill holes along the vertebral border of the scapula, 1.5 to 2.0 cm from its margin, opposite the selected ribs in the supraspinatus and infraspinatus fossae, and through the base of the scapular spine (Fig. 7.19B).
- Apply screws with washers or preferably a dynamic compression plate or a flattened semitubular plate to the posteromedial surface of the scapula to reinforce the thin scapular bone (Fig. 7.19C). Occasionally, if a single contoured plate is too bulky, two plates can be used, with one above and one below the scapular spine.
- Pass one end of each wire from anterior to posterior through the adjacent hole in the vertebral border of the scapula and through the hole in the overlying plate or washers.
- Sandwich the cancellous bone graft between the scapular and costal surfaces, with adjacent ribs bridged by cancellous strips (Fig. 7.19C).
- With the scapula held in its final position, pull the other end of each wire over the posterior part of the plate and tighten the wires sequentially by twisting in a clockwise direction.
- Place any remaining bone graft between the posterior surfaces of the ribs medially and the vertebral border of the scapula (Fig. 7.19D).
- Fill the operative field with crystalloid solution and perform a Valsalva maneuver to detect any relatively large pleural tears.
- Cut and twist the wires to lie flat.
- Close the posterior muscles over the posterior surface of the scapula to provide a tenodesis effect and to cover the implants. Close the thoracic and posterior iliac wounds in a routine fashion.
- In the recovery room, obtain a chest radiograph to check for a developing pneumothorax; clinical symptoms may be masked by postoperative drowsiness or pain medications.

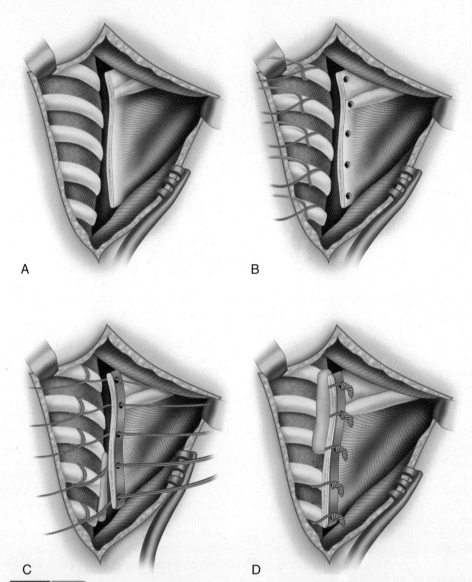

A

B

C

D

FIGURE **7.19** Technique of Diab et al. for scapulothoracic fusion (see text). **A,** Vertebral border of scapula and ribs are seen after surrounding muscles, fat, fibrous tissues, and periosteum have been cleared. **B,** Five doubled, 16-gauge wires are passed subperiosteally under the ribs and twisted on themselves to prevent impingement on the pleura. Five holes are drilled in medial aspect of scapula, adjacent to planned point of attachment to ribs. **C,** Single plate is bent to conform to shape of scapula, and one end of each wire is passed through drill hole and corresponding plate hole. Bone graft is placed between anterior border of scapula and posterior surface of ribs. **D,** Other end of each wire is pulled to posterior side of scapula and plate and tightened to firmly press scapula against ribs. (Redrawn from Diab M, Darras BT, Shapiro F: Scapulothoracic fusion for facioscapulohumeral muscular dystrophy, *J Bone Joint Surg* 87A:2267, 2005.) **SEE TECHNIQUE 7.6.**

POSTOPERATIVE CARE The shoulder and upper limb are immobilized in a sling and swathe for 4 weeks. Following this, the sling alone is used, with daily active range-of-motion exercises of the elbow, forearm, wrist, and hand, but no humeral abduction or flexion is allowed for 4 weeks. Shoulder abduction and flexion are progressed to full active range of motion with weaning from the sling over the next 4 to 8 weeks. At 3 to 4 months after surgery, when the rehabilitation program has led to pain-free clinical abduction and flexion, unrestricted activity is allowed.

■ INFANTILE FACIOSCAPULOHUMERAL MUSCULAR DYSTROPHY

An early-onset form of facioscapulohumeral muscular dystrophy has been described in which weakness is rapidly progressive and the lower extremities are also are affected. Patients become wheelchair bound by the second decade of life. Facial weakness is seen in infancy, and this is followed by sensorineural hearing loss at an average of 5 years of age. A progressive lumbar hyperlordosis develops and is almost pathognomonic for infantile facioscapulohumeral muscular dystrophy. The hyperlordosis leads to fixed hip flexion contractures. Treatment consists of accommodation of the lordosis in the wheelchair. Spinal bracing has been unsuccessful. Spinal fusion may be indicated to assist with sitting balance. Scapulothoracic fusion is usually not indicated in these patients because of the advanced weakness associated with this form of facioscapulohumeral muscular dystrophy.

CONGENITAL DYSTROPHIES

Congenital dystrophies include relatively rare conditions, such as nemaline dystrophy, central core myopathy, myotubular myopathy, congenital fiber disproportion, and multicore and minicore disease. Congenital myopathies and congenital muscular dystrophies are usually defined by the histological appearance of the muscle biopsy specimen, rather than by specific clinical or molecular criteria. Electron microscopy may be required to differentiate some of the types. Weakness and contractures at birth can cause hip dislocation, clubfeet, or other deformities. Respiratory weakness and difficulty with feeding and swallowing are common. The clinical appearance is one of dysmorphism, with kyphoscoliosis, chest deformities, a long face, and a high palate. Muscle tissue is gradually replaced with fibrous tissue, and contractures can become severe. Treatment is aimed at keeping the patient ambulatory and preventing contractures by exercises and orthotic splinting. Equinus and varus deformities of the feet may require releases if they interfere with ambulation. Congenital dislocation of the hip and clubfoot deformity are treated conventionally, but recurrence is frequent. Early rigid scoliosis may occur and need treatment.

MYOTONIC DYSTROPHY

Myotonic dystrophy is characterized by an inability of the muscles to relax after contraction. It is progressive and is usually present at birth, although it may develop in childhood. Myotonic dystrophy type I is an autosomal-dominant disorder. The genetic defect is located on chromosome 19. Myotonic dystrophy type 2 shows the typical clinic features but does not have a genetic defect on chromosome 19. In addition to the inability of the muscles to relax, muscle weakness causes the most functional impairment. Other defects include hyperostosis of the skull, frontal and temporal baldness, gonadal atrophy, dysphasia, dysarthria, electrocardiographic abnormalities, and mental retardation. The characteristic clinical appearance is a tent-shaped mouth, facial diplegia, and dull expression. Approximately half of children with myotonic dystrophy have clubfoot deformities, and hip dysplasia and scoliosis may exist. Hip dysplasia is treated conventionally, but because of capsular laxity it may not respond as readily as in other children. Serial casting can correct equinovarus deformity early on, but recurrence is likely, and extensile release is usually required; triple arthrodesis may be required at skeletal maturity because of recurrence despite extensile releases. In patients with marked clubfoot deformity, extensive posteromedial release may be insufficient to correct the deformity and a talectomy may be required. An ankle-foot orthosis, which is frequently required for weakness in dorsiflexion, can usually maintain postoperative correction. In some adolescent patients, scoliosis develops and should be treated with the same principles as the treatment of idiopathic scoliosis. The high incidence of cardiac abnormalities and decreased pulmonary function increases the risk of surgery and may prohibit surgery in these patients.

HEREDITARY MOTOR AND SENSORY NEUROPATHIES

Hereditary motor and sensory neuropathies are a large group of inherited neuropathic disorders. The most common disorder among these neuropathies is Charcot-Marie-Tooth (CMT) disease. The hereditary motor and sensory neuropathies have been classified into seven types; types I, II, and III occur most often in children, and types IV, V, VI, and VII occur in adults (Table 7.3).

CHARCOT-MARIE-TOOTH DISEASE (PERONEAL MUSCULAR ATROPHY)

Charcot-Marie-Tooth (CMT) disease is a genetically and phenotypically heterogenous group of degenerative disorders of the central and peripheral nervous systems that causes abnormal nerve conduction, muscle atrophy and loss of proprioception due to disruption of peripheral nerve myelin sheath and/or axonal structure. It is usually an autosomal-dominant trait in type I disease but can be X-linked recessive or autosomal recessive. Approximately 10% of cases are believed to be caused by spontaneous mutations. The incidence of the various forms of CMT disease ranges from 20 per 100,000 to one per 2500. Clinically, there is tremendous variability, with some patients having severe symptoms and deformity at a young age and others with only mild symptoms late in life.

Muscle atrophy is slowly and steadily progressive in most patients with the autosomal dominant form; less often, the disease arrests completely or manifests intermittently. The recessive forms have an early onset (first or second decade) and are more rapidly progressive. Initial complaints are usually general weakness of the foot and an unsteady gait. Foot problems include pain under the metatarsal heads, claw toes, foot fatigue, and difficulty in wearing regular shoes. Distal loss of proprioception and spinal ataxia are common. CMT disease should be suspected in patients with claw toes, high arches, thin legs, poor balance, and an unsteady gait. Patients may also have hand dysfunction manifested by difficulties with handwriting because of weakness, pain, and altered sensation, all of which may make the use of assistive ambulatory devices more difficult. In addition to physical examination and family history, electromyograms,

---

TABLE 7.3

Classification of Hereditary Motor Sensory Neuropathies

TYPE	NAME(S)	INHERITANCE
I	Peroneal atrophy, Charcot-Marie-Tooth disease (hypertrophic form), Roussy-Lévy syndrome (areflexic dystasia)	Autosomal dominant
II	Charcot-Marie-Tooth disease (neuronal form)	Variable
III	Dejerine-Sottas disease	Autosomal recessive
IV	Refsum disease	
V	Neuropathy with spastic paraplegia	
VI	Optic atrophy with peroneal muscle atrophy	
VII	Retinitis pigmentosa with distal muscle weakness and atrophy	

which show an increased amplitude in duration of response and slow nerve conduction velocity, typically confirm the diagnosis. Karakis et al. cited several clinical features that are helpful in differentiating CMT disease from idiopathic pes cavus deformities: weakness, unsteady gait, positive family history, sensory deficits, distal atrophy and weakness, absent ankle jerks, and gait abnormalities. In a study of 148 children with bilateral cavus feet, 78% had CMT disease; the frequency increased to 91% if there was a positive family history.

Advances in molecular biology have improved the ability to confirm the diagnosis of CMT disease and to differentiate between variants of the condition. The use of molecular biology may allow orthopaedic surgeons to make more specific treatment recommendations for patients with the variants of CMT disease. For example, patients with the most common form, CMT1A, which is caused by a duplication of the PMP22 gene, rarely require the use of a wheelchair, whereas patients with the CMT2A type caused by abnormalities in the MFN2 gene usually become nonambulatory in their 20s.

◼ CAVOVARUS FOOT DEFORMITY

Cavovarus foot deformities are the most common orthopaedic deformities in all types of CMT disease except type II, in which planovalgus foot deformities are most common. CMT disease is the most common neuromuscular cause of cavovarus foot deformity in children, but other causes should be considered when evaluating a child with a cavovarus foot deformity. This is a complex deformity of the forefoot and hindfoot. Surgery is often required to stabilize the foot. Although there is little question that the cavovarus deformity is caused by muscle imbalance, theories explaining which muscles are involved and how the imbalances produce the rigid cavovarus deformity do not completely account for the clinical deformity. It has been suggested that the neuropathic cavovarus deformity of CMT disease has been caused by a combination of intrinsic and extrinsic weakness, beginning with weakness of the intrinsic foot muscles and the anterior tibial muscle, with normal strength of the posterior tibial and peroneus longus muscles. The triceps surae is also weak and may be contracted. The forefoot is pulled into equinus relative to the hindfoot, and the first ray becomes plantarflexed (Fig. 7.20). The long toe extensors attempt to assist the weak

anterior tibial tendon in dorsiflexion but contribute to metatarsal plantarflexion, and the forefoot is pronated into a valgus position with mild adduction of the metatarsals. Initially, the foot is supple and plantigrade with weightbearing, but as the forefoot becomes more rigidly pronated, the hindfoot assumes a varus position. Weightbearing becomes a "tripod" mechanism, with weight borne on the heel and the first and fifth metatarsal heads.

◼ CLINICAL AND RADIOGRAPHIC EVALUATION

Clinical evaluation of the cavovarus deformity includes determination of the rigidity of the hindfoot varus, usually with the Coleman block test (Fig. 7.21), and assessment of individual muscle strength and overall balance. Careful examination of the peripheral and central nervous systems is required, including electromyography and nerve conduction velocity studies.

Standard anteroposterior, lateral, and oblique radiographs are the most useful methods for evaluating the child's foot; however, to determine any significant relationships between the bones, it is essential that the anteroposterior and lateral views be made with the foot in a weightbearing or simulated weightbearing position. Anteroposterior views document the degree of forefoot adduction. The degree of cavus can be estimated on the lateral view by determining the Meary angle, the angle between the long axis of the first metatarsal and long axis of the talus; the normal angle is 0 degrees. Radiographs using the Coleman block test show the correction of the varus deformity if the hindfoot is flexible.

◼ ORTHOPAEDIC TREATMENT

The management of foot deformities is important in patients with CMT. A study of more than 2700 patients with CMT found that 71% of patients had foot deformities, with pes cavus and hammer toes being the most common. Thirty percent of patients had some form of operative treatment to their feet at a median age of 15 years, and 33% had surgery more than once, highlighting the need for long-term postoperative follow-up.

Treatment is determined by the age of the patient and the cause and severity of the deformity. Medical treatment with high-dose ascorbic acid has been found to be ineffective in

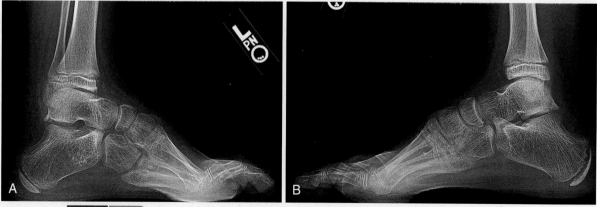

FIGURE 7.20 **A and B,** Left and right weightbearing lateral radiographs of child with Charcot-Marie-Tooth disease demonstrating high arches, clawing of toes, and plantarflexed first metatarsal. Note asymmetry in the two sides. (From Beals TC, Nickish F: Charcot-Marie-Tooth disease and the cavovarus foot, *Foot Ankle Clin North Am* 13:259, 2008.)

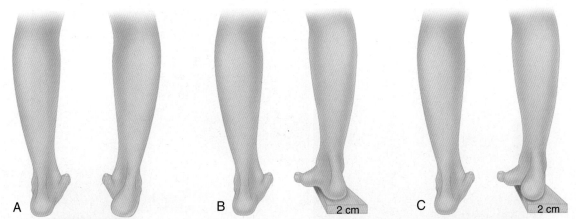

FIGURE 7.21 Coleman block test. **A,** Heel of foot and lateral border are placed on wooden block, allowing head of first metatarsal to drop into plantarflexion. **B,** If hindfoot varus is second to tripod effect of plantarflexed first ray, hindfoot will correct to neutral or valgus alignment. **C,** If hindfoot varus is rigid, it will not correct.

TABLE 7.4

Types of Foot Deformities in Charcot-Marie-Tooth Disease and Recommended Treatment

TYPE	FEATURES	PROCEDURES
A.	Normal foot	Observation
B.	Plantarflexed 1st metatarsal Mild cavovarus Fully flexible hindfoot	Soft-tissue procedures Possible 1st metatarsal osteotomy
C.	Increased plantarflexion 1st metatarsal Increased supination Stiffer hindfoot	1st metatarsal osteotomy Midfoot/hindfoot osteotomies Possible triple arthrodesis
D.	Rigid cavovarus	Triple arthrodesis

From: Louwerens JWK: Operative treatment algorithm for foot deformities in Charcot-Marie-Tooth disease, *Oper Orthop Traumatol* 30(2):130–146, 2018.

altering the natural history of this condition. Nonoperative treatment of the cavovarus foot, including the use of serial casting and botulinum toxin, has generally been unsuccessful. A randomized trial of 4 weeks of night casting found increased ankle dorsiflexion compared with no intervention, but at 8 weeks there was no significant difference. In a randomized trial of botulinum toxin to prevent pes cavus progression, although safe and well tolerated, the injections did not affect the progression of the deformity.

A multicenter task force from the Netherlands developed an expert-based consensus classification of the foot deformities in CMT to help guide treatment (Table 7.4). Surgical procedures are of three types: soft tissue for flexible deformities (plantar fascia release, tendon release or transfer), osteotomy for stiffer flexible or rigid deformities (metatarsal, midfoot, calcaneal), and joint stabilizing for completely rigid deformities (triple arthrodesis).

Experience in the treatment of foot deformities in CMT disease has shown that early, aggressive treatment when the hindfoot is flexible and early soft-tissue releases can delay the need for more extensive reconstructive procedures. Even in young patients with a fixed hindfoot deformity, limited soft-tissue release, combined with a first metatarsal, midfoot osteotomy or calcaneal osteotomy, or both, can provide a satisfactory functional outcome without sacrificing the hindfoot and midfoot joint motion that is lost after triple arthrodesis. Because of early degenerative changes in the ankle, forefoot, and midfoot, triple arthrodesis should serve as a salvage procedure for patients in whom other procedures were unsuccessful or in patients with untreated fixed deformities (Fig. 7.22).

Younger patients and patients with flexible hindfeet usually respond to plantar releases and appropriate tendon transfers. Faldini et al. reported treatment of 24 flexible cavus feet in 12 patients (age 14 to 28 years) with CMT, with a combination of plantar fascia release (Steindler stripping), closed superolateral wedge osteotomy of the cuboid and naviculocuneiform arthrodesis with closed superolateral wedge resection of articular surfaces (midtarsal osteotomy), dorsiflexion osteotomy of the first metatarsal (Fig. 7.23), and extensor hallucis transfer (Jones procedure). Results were graded as excellent in 12 feet, good in 10, and fair in two. These authors cited advantages of midtarsal osteotomy correction of the main component of the deformity (excess elevation of the plantar arch) and preservation of the overall range of motion of the foot, which results in a more normal range of motion during walking.

PLANTAR FASCIOTOMY, OSTEOTOMIES, AND ARTHRODESIS FOR CHARCOT-MARIE-TOOTH DISEASE

TECHNIQUE 7.7

(FALDINI ET AL.)

PLANTAR FASCIOTOMY

- Make a 2 cm skin incision on the medial aspect of the heel and identify the plantar fascia.

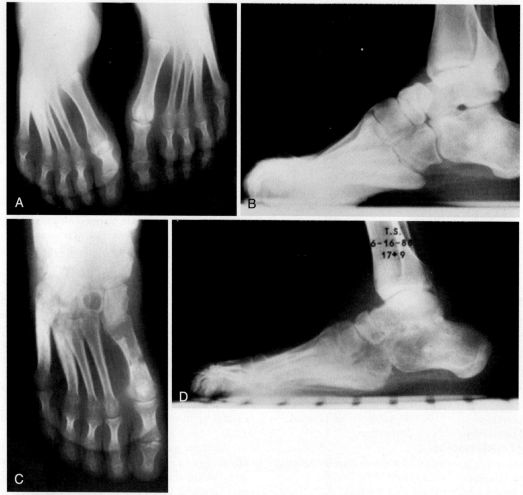

FIGURE 7.22 Cavovarus deformity in Charcot-Marie-Tooth disease. **A** and **B,** Preoperative radiographs. **C** and **D,** After triple arthrodesis, Achilles tendon lengthening, and posterior tibial tendon transfer. (Courtesy Jay Cummings, MD.)

- Apply tension by dorsiflexing the metatarsophalangeal joint and use a scalpel to completely strip the fascia from its origin. Take care to avoid damage to the lateral plantar artery and nerve and the inferior calcaneal nerve (Fig. 7.24A).

HINDFOOT CORRECTION AND STABILIZATION

- Before correction of the cavus deformity, manually reduce heel varus and stabilize the hindfoot with a 2.5 mm Kirschner wire inserted from the plantar aspect of the calcaneus into the tibia to maintain approximately 5 degrees of heel valgus and 20 degrees of ankle plantarflexion. This allows planning of the midtarsal osteotomy using the stabilized hindfoot as a fixed reference.
- Confirm the correct position of the ankle and correct insertion of the wire with fluoroscopy.

MIDTARSAL OSTEOTOMY

- Make a medial approach, approximately 3.5 cm long and centered slightly distal to the navicular prominence.
- Identify and expose the naviculocuneiform joint, with retraction of the marginal medial vein and the anterior tibial tendon.

- Use an oscillating saw to make a superolateral wedge resection of the articular surfaces.
- Through a lateral approach, also approximately 3.5 cm long, identify the cuboid and retract the extensor digitorum brevis dorsally.
- Expose the cuboid, sparing the calcaneocuboid and cuboid-metatarsal joints.
- Make a superolateral wedge resection of the cuboid to complete the midtarsal osteotomy (Fig. 7.24B).
- Close the naviculocuneiform arthrodesis and the cuboid osteotomy and fix them with a 2.5 mm Kirschner wire (Fig. 7.24C).

DORSIFLEXION OSTEOTOMY OF THE FIRST METATARSAL

- Through the medial approach, identify the base of the first metatarsal and use an oscillating saw to make a complete osteotomy of the meta-diaphysis (Fig. 7.24D).
- Displace the distal stump of the osteotomy in a plantar direction, approximating the dorsal corner of the diaphysis into the base of the metatarsal to obtain dorsiflexion of the ray.
- Fix the osteotomy with a 2-mm Kirschner wire (Fig. 7.24E).

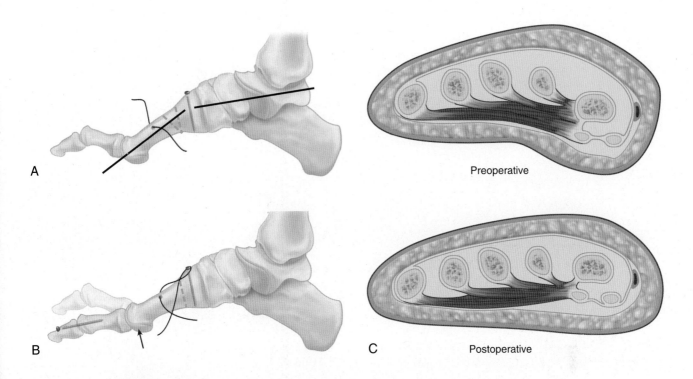

FIGURE 7.23 First metatarsal dorsiflexion osteotomy (**A** and **B**) combined with extensor hallucis longus transfer (**C**) to help correct the plantar flexion deformity of the first ray. (Modified from Louwerens JWK: Operative treatment algorithm for foot deformities in Charcot-Marie-Tooth disease. *Oper Orthop Traumatol* 30:130, 2018.)

EXTENSOR HALLUCIS TRANSFER
- Through the medial approach, expose the hallux up to the interphalangeal joint and identify the extensor hallucis longus tendon.
- Free the tendon from its retinacular attachment and detach it at the level of the first metatarsophalangeal joint.
- Drill a 3.2-mm hole at the metaphysis of the first metatarsal and pass the tendon through the hole and suture it to itself to form a loop, dorsiflexing the forefoot and applying moderate tension on the tendon transfer (Fig. 7.25A–C).
- Finally, tenodese the distal stump of the extensor longus to the extensor brevis and arthrodese the interphalangeal joint of the hallux, fixing it with a percutaneous Kirschner wire (Fig. 7.25D and E).

POSTOPERATIVE CARE A non–weight-bearing boot cast is worn for 1 month, then the cast and percutaneous Kirschner wires are removed. An ambulatory boot cast is worn for another month. After its removal, active and passive mobilization of the foot and ankle, proprioceptive exercises, and muscle strengthening commence.

In older children with rigid hindfoot deformities, radical plantar-medial release, first metatarsal osteotomy or midfoot osteotomy, and a calcaneal osteotomy usually correct the deformity. In a fixed hindfoot with a prominent calcaneus, a Dwyer lateral closing wedge osteotomy may be preferred to shorten the heel (Chapter 33). If the heel is not prominent, a sliding calcaneal osteotomy (Chapter 33) gives satisfactory results. Mubarak recommended a stepwise approach using joint-sparing osteotomies for rigid feet. These include (1) dorsal closing wedge osteotomy of the first metatarsal, (2) opening plantar wedge osteotomy of the medial cuneiform, (3) cuboid closing wedge osteotomy, and (4) accessory procedures as required, including second/third metatarsal osteotomy, calcaneal sliding osteotomy, and peroneus longus to brevis transfer. The Ilizarov method has also been used in small series to correct rigid deformities. Although patient satisfaction is improved, there was no significant improvement in pain, function, or range of motion after surgery. Further study is necessary on the use of external fixation in the correction of these deformities. Complete navicular excision and cuboid closing wedge osteotomy can also be used as a salvage procedure in severe rigid deformities where fusion is not appropriate.

Approximately 15% of patients with CMT disease require triple arthrodesis (Chapter 34). The Hoke arthrodesis or a modification of it is most often recommended. Appropriate wedge resections correct the hindfoot varus and midfoot component of the cavus deformity; soft-tissue release and muscle balancing are required for the forefoot deformity. In the most severe deformities, a Lambrinudi triple arthrodesis can produce a painless plantigrade foot. Restoration of hindfoot stability with triple arthrodesis and transfer of the posterior tibial tendon anteriorly have been recommended to eliminate the need for a postoperative footdrop brace, with a reported 88%

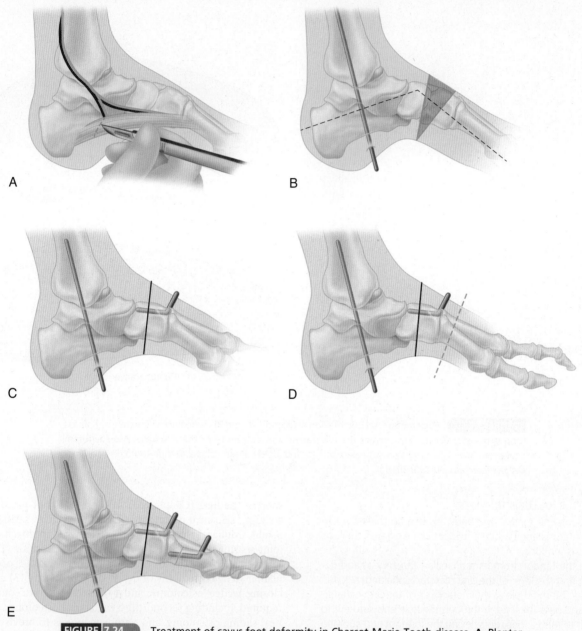

FIGURE 7.24 Treatment of cavus foot deformity in Charcot-Marie-Tooth disease. **A,** Plantar fasciotomy. **B,** Naviculocuneiform wedge resection. **C,** Fixation of arthrodesis with Kirschner wire. **D,** First metatarsal dorsiflexion osteotomy. **E,** Fixation with Kirschner wire. (Redrawn from Faldini C, Traina F, Nanni M, et al: Surgical treatment of cavus foot in Charcot-Marie-Tooth disease: a review of twenty-four cases, *J Bone Joint Surg* 97A:e30[1-10], 2015.) **SEE TECHNIQUE 7.7.**

good or excellent result. Achilles tendon lengthening with triple arthrodesis is recommended after correction of the forefoot (see Fig. 7.22). Even with surgical correction and improvement in radiographic parameters, careful examination of the feet postoperatively is essential because pedobarometric pressures can remain abnormal in feet that appear corrected radiographically.

Flexible claw toe deformity is usually corrected without additional surgery when the midfoot deformity is corrected. For clawing in a young child without severe weakness of the anterior tibial muscle, the toe extensors can be transferred to the metatarsal necks with tenodesis of the interphalangeal joint of the great toe (Jones procedure; Technique 7.9). For adolescents or children with severe weakness of the anterior tibial muscle, all the long toe extensors can

be transferred to the middle cuneiform with fusion of the interphalangeal joint (Hibbs procedure; Technique 7.10). For severe deformity, the posterior tibial tendon can be transferred anteriorly to the middle cuneiform instead of the long toe extensors.

Surgical procedures are usually staged. The initial procedure is a radical plantar or plantar-medial release, with a dorsal closing wedge osteotomy of the first metatarsal base if necessary. Achilles tendon lengthening should not be performed as part of the initial procedure because the force used to dorsiflex the forefoot would dorsiflex the calcaneus into an unacceptable position. If the hindfoot is flexible and a posterior release is unnecessary, posterior tibial tendon transfer can be done as part of the initial procedure for severe anterior tibial weakness.

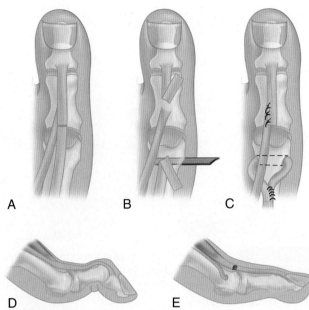

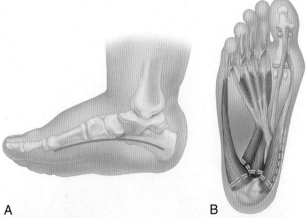

FIGURE 7.26 Radical plantar-medial release and dorsal closing wedge osteotomy for cavovarus deformity. **A,** Incision. **B,** Release of musculotendinous mass. **SEE TECHNIQUE 7.8.**

FIGURE 7.25 Treatment of cavus foot deformity in Charcot-Marie-Tooth disease. Extensor hallucis longus transfer (Jones procedure). **A** and **B,** Tendon detached at level of first metatarsophalangeal joint, passed through hole (**C**) and sutured to itself. **D** and **E,** Distal stump of extensor hallucis longus is tenodesed to extensor hallucis brevis. (Redrawn from Faldini C, Traina F, Nanni M, et al: Surgical treatment of cavus foot in Charcot-Marie-Tooth disease: a review of twenty-four cases, *J Bone Joint Surg* 97A:e30[1-10], 2015.) **SEE TECHNIQUE 7.7.**

musculotendinous mass distally and extraperiosteally as far as the calcaneocuboid joint.
- If the first metatarsal remains in plantarflexion after this release, make a dorsally based closing wedge osteotomy immediately distal to the physis, removing enough bone to correct the lateral talo-first metatarsal angle to 0 degrees.
- Fix the osteotomy with a smooth Steinmann pin or Kirschner wire.
- Close the wound in routine fashion and apply a short leg cast with the foot in the corrected position.

POSTOPERATIVE CARE If there is excessive tension on the wound, the foot can be placed in a cast in slight plantar flexion. A new cast should be applied at 2 weeks with the foot in a fully corrected position. The pins and cast are removed at 6 to 8 weeks.

RADICAL PLANTAR-MEDIAL RELEASE AND DORSAL CLOSING WEDGE OSTEOTOMY

TECHNIQUE 7.8

(COLEMAN)
- Make a curved incision over the medial aspect of the foot, extending anteriorly from the calcaneus to the base of the first metatarsal (Fig. 7.26A).
- Identify the origin of the abductor hallucis and separate it from its bony and soft-tissue attachments proximally and distally, but leave it attached at its origin and insertion.
- Identify the posterior neurovascular bundle as it divides into medial and lateral branches and enters the intrinsic musculature of the foot.
- Identify the tendinous origin of the abductor at its attachment on the calcaneus between the medial and lateral plantar branches of the nerve and artery and sever it to free the origin of the abductor hallucis.
- Identify the long toe flexors as they course along the plantar aspect of the foot and section the retinaculum of the tendons.
- Sever the origins of the plantar aponeurosis, the abductor hallucis, and the short flexors from their attachments to the calcaneus (Fig. 7.26B), and gently dissect this entire

TRANSFER OF THE EXTENSOR HALLUCIS LONGUS TENDON FOR CLAW TOE DEFORMITY

TECHNIQUE 7.9

(JONES)
- Expose the interphalangeal joint of the great toe through an L-shaped incision (Fig. 7.27).
- Retract the flap of skin and subcutaneous tissue medially and proximally and expose the tendon of the extensor hallucis longus.
- Cut the tendon transversely, 1 cm proximal to the joint and expose the joint.
- Excise the cartilage, approximate the joint surfaces, and insert a 5/64-inch intramedullary Kirschner wire or screw for fixation. Clip the wire off just outside the skin.
- Expose the neck of the first metatarsal through a 2.5 cm dorsomedial incision extending distally to the proximal extensor skin crease.

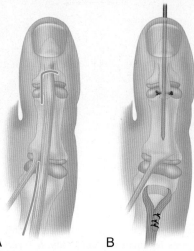

A   B

FIGURE 7.27 Transfer of extensor hallucis longus tendon for claw toe deformity (Jones procedure). **A,** Incisions. **B,** Completed procedure. **SEE TECHNIQUE 7.9.**

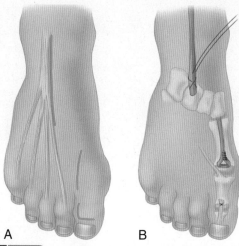

A   B

FIGURE 7.28 Transfer of extensor tendons to middle cuneiform for claw toe deformity (Hibbs procedure). **A,** Incisions. **B,** Completed procedure combined with Jones procedure. **SEE TECHNIQUE 7.10.**

- Dissect free the extensor hallucis longus tendon but protect the short extensor tendon. Cleanly and carefully excise the sheath of the long extensor tendon throughout the length of the proximal incision.
- Beginning on the inferomedial aspect of the first metatarsal neck, drill a hole transverse to the long axis of the bone to emerge on the dorsolateral aspect of the neck.
- Pass the tendon through the hole and suture it to itself with interrupted sutures.
- The same procedure can be performed on adjacent toes with clawing.
- Close the wounds and apply a short-leg walking cast with the ankle in neutral position.

POSTOPERATIVE CARE Walking with crutches is allowed in 2 to 3 days. At 3 weeks, the cast and skin sutures are removed and a short-leg walking cast is applied. At 6 weeks, the walking cast and Kirschner wire are removed and active exercises are begun.

TRANSFER OF THE EXTENSOR TENDONS TO THE MIDDLE CUNEIFORM

TECHNIQUE 7.10

(HIBBS)
- Make a curved incision 7.5 to 10 cm long on the dorsum of the foot lateral to the midline and expose the common extensor tendons (Fig. 7.28).
- Divide the tendons distally as far as feasible, draw their proximal ends through a tunnel in the third cuneiform, and fix them with a nonabsorbable suture.
- As an alternative, use a plantar button and felt with a Bunnell pull-out stitch.

- Close the wounds and apply a plaster boot cast with the foot in the corrected position.

POSTOPERATIVE CARE The cast and plantar button are removed at 6 weeks.

STEPWISE JOINT-SPARING FOOT OSTEOTOMIES

TECHNIQUE 7.11

(MUBARAK AND VAN VALIN)

FIRST RAY OSTEOTOMIES (OPENING-WEDGE OSTEOTOMY OF THE MEDIAL CUNEIFORM, DORSAL CLOSING-WEDGE OSTEOTOMY OF THE FIRST METATARSAL)
- Initial attention is focused on the first ray. Place a medial incision over the foot at the level of the first metatarsal and first cuneiform.
- Partially release the anterior tibial tendon insertion on the cuneiform.
- Place two needles to identify the midportion of the cuneiform and a position at least 1 cm distal to the first metatarsal physis. Take care not to disrupt the first metatarsal physis, which is proximal.
- Remove a 20 to 30 degree dorsal wedge from the first metatarsal and save it (Fig. 7.29A).
- Perform an opening-wedge osteotomy of the medial cuneiform (if necessary) (Fig. 7.29B) and place the bone wedge from the first metatarsal osteotomy into it and secure it with one or two Kirschner wires.

CUBOID CLOSING-WEDGE OSTEOTOMY
- Make a lateral incision over the cuboid and identify the calcaneocuboid and cuboid–fifth metatarsal joints

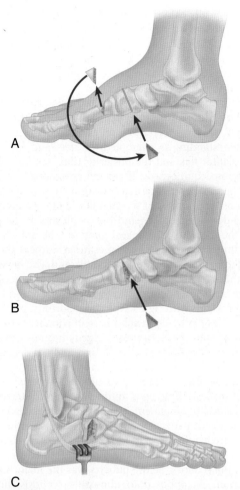

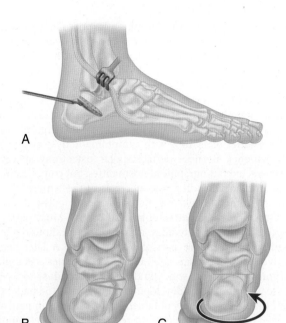

FIGURE 7.30 Stepwise joint-sparing osteotomies for cavus foot deformities (see text). **A,** Calcaneal osteotomy through lateral approach. **B,** Closing and lateral sliding wedge osteotomy. **C,** Closing and sliding wedge osteotomy. (Redrawn from Mubarak SJ, Van Valin SE: Osteotomies of the foot for cavus deformities in children, *J Pediatr Orthop* 29:294, 2009.) **SEE TECHNIQUE 7.11.**

FIGURE 7.29 Stepwise joint-sparing osteotomies for cavus foot deformities (see text). **A,** First metatarsal closing-wedge osteotomy; removed piece will be used in cuneiform. **B,** Medial cuneiform opening-wedge osteotomy. **C,** Cuboid closing-wedge osteotomy, with or without second and third metatarsal osteotomies. (Redrawn from Mubarak SJ, Van Valin SE: Osteotomies of the foot for cavus deformities in children, *J Pediatr Orthop* 29:294, 2009.) **SEE TECHNIQUE 7.11.**

■ Plantar fasciotomies are usually done through a small incision if the plantar fascia is tight after osteotomies are complete.

■ Peroneus longus-to-brevis transfer can be done after the cuboid closing–wedge osteotomy. Identify the peroneus longus on the plantar surface of the cuboid and release it. Attach the proximal end to the peroneis brevis using nonabsorbable suture.

POSTOPERATIVE CARE The patient is kept non–weight bearing in a short leg cast that is bivalved to allow for swelling. The pins are removed at approximately 4 weeks after surgery under light sedation, and a walking cast is applied. Patients can fully bear weight 8 weeks after surgery.

fluoroscopically. Remove a 5 to 10 mm dorsal wedge of the cuboid and save the wedge (Fig. 7.29C). Secure the osteotomy with a single Kirschner wire.

METATARSAL OSTEOTOMIES

■ If the second and third metatarsal heads are now prominent, dorsal closing-wedge osteotomies can be done. Place a single incision between the second and third metatarsals and remove and save dorsal wedges. These osteotomies can each be secured with a single intramedullary Kirschner wire.

ACCESSORY PROCEDURES

■ Calcaneal osteotomy, usually a lateral displacement and closing wedge, is done if there is a fixed hindfoot deformity (Fig. 7.30).

In patients with advanced CMT disease, a triple arthrodesis may be necessary to establish a plantigrade foot; however, triple arthrodesis should not be routinely done in younger patients with less severe disease because degenerative changes of the ankle may result. In patients who have not had limited procedures during early adolescence but have major hindfoot, midfoot, and forefoot deformities, a triple arthrodesis may be the only treatment option. In severe deformity, a more extensive procedure, such as a Lambrinudi or Hoke triple arthrodesis, can be performed. Techniques for triple arthrodesis are outlined in other chapter.

■ HIP DYSPLASIA

Hip dysplasia, which usually becomes apparent in the second and third decades of life, has been reported in 6% to 8% of patients with CMT disease. Dysplasia is more likely to occur in hereditary motor and sensory neuropathy type I than in type II. If hip dysplasia is present, it should be corrected. Novais et al. found that acetabular dysplasia, hip subluxation, acetabular anteversion, coxa valga, and hip osteoarthritis were more severe in patients with CMT than in those with developmental dysplasia and suggested that this should be considered in determining the appropriate surgical strategy. In a series of 19 hips with symptomatic dysplasia in 14 CMT patients, Bernese periacetabular osteotomy successfully corrected radiographic abnormalities, but complications were common, including osteonecrosis of the femoral head, transient complete bilateral peroneal nerve palsy, inferior rami fractures, and heterotopic ossification. Most patients reported improved outcomes, although seven showed signs of radiographic progression of osteoarthritis. A later comparative study by Novais et al. of the Bernese periacetabular osteotomy in patients with hip dysplasia secondary to CMT disease (27 patients) or developmental dysplasia (54 patients) found that the osteotomy obtained improvements in patient-reported outcomes scores and in redirecting the acetabulum in symptomatic CMT dysplasia; complications were much more frequent in patients with CMT (33%) than in those with developmental dysplasia of the hip (DDH; 13%).

■ SPINAL DEFORMITIES

Spinal deformities are present in approximately 25% of all patients with CMT disease. Approximately 75% of these patients have hereditary motor and sensory neuropathy type I with duplication of *PMP22* (peripheral myelin protein gene on chromosome 17). Scoliosis is uncommon in association with CMT disease, occurring in 10% to 30% of young patients, and the curve is usually mild to moderate and often does not require any treatment. In patients with CMT disease, nonoperative treatment with a brace is usually well tolerated and successfully controls the curve in many patients. Generally, spinal deformities in children with CMT disease can be managed by the same techniques used for idiopathic scoliosis. Because of the demyelination of the peripheral nerves and degeneration of the dorsal root ganglion and dorsal column of the spinal cord, somatosensory-evoked potentials may be absent.

FRIEDREICH ATAXIA

Friedreich ataxia is an autosomal-recessive condition characterized by spinocerebellar degeneration. The prevalence of Friedreich ataxia is approximately one in 50,000. The abnormal gene is located on chromosome 9, but the definitive form of Friedreich ataxia is caused by a trinucleotide repeat of GAA, which causes loss of expression of the frataxin protein. This leads to a neuronopathy of the dorsal root ganglion, leading to degeneration of peripheral nerve fibers and the dorsal spinal columns. An ataxic gait is usually the presenting symptom, with onset routinely between 7 and 15 years old. The clinical triad of ataxia, areflexia, and positive Babinski reflex suggests the diagnosis. A definitive diagnosis can be made with genetic testing. Other clinical features besides ataxia include abnormal eye movements (90%), scoliosis (74%), deformities of the feet (59%), urinary dysfunction (43%), cardiomyopathy and cardiac hypertrophy (40%), decreased visual acuity (37%), depression (14%), and diabetes (7%).

The disease is progressive, and almost all patients are wheelchair bound by the first or second decade of life.

Patients typically exhibit progressive dysarthria or weakness, decreased vibratory sense in the lower extremities, cardiomyopathy, pes cavus, and scoliosis. Knee jerk and ankle jerk reflexes are lost quite early. Patients usually die in the fourth or fifth decades of life as a result of progressive cardiomyopathy, pneumonia, and aspiration.

The primary concern of the orthopaedist is the correction of foot and spinal deformities. In patients with Friedreich ataxia, the plantar reflex is sometimes so great that when standing is attempted, the feet and toes immediately plantar flex and the posterior tibial tendon pulls the forefoot into equinovarus. If general anesthesia is contraindicated because of myocardial involvement or other medical conditions, tenotomies of the Achilles tendon, the posterior tibial tendon at the ankle, and the toe flexors at the plantar side of the metatarsophalangeal joints can be done with the patient under regional or local anesthesia. Surgery should be delayed in patients who are able to walk and who have deformities that are supple or can be controlled in braces; however, the cavovarus deformities tend to worsen and become rigid. In patients with rigid cavovarus deformity, primary triple arthrodesis provides a solid base of support with a fixed plantigrade foot. Because most patients become wheelchair bound, later development of ankle and midfoot degenerative changes is seldom clinically significant. Posterior tibial tenotomy, lengthening, or transfer should be combined with the triple arthrodesis. Bracing is routinely required after surgery.

In a study of 56 patients with Friedreich ataxia and scoliosis, the curve patterns were similar to those of idiopathic scoliosis, many curves were not progressive, no relationship existed between muscle weakness and the curvature, and the onset of the scoliosis before puberty was the major factor in progression. As opposed to idiopathic scoliosis, however, kyphosis was frequently noted in patients with Friedreich ataxia. The authors recommended that curves of less than 40 degrees should be observed, curves between 40 and 60 degrees should be treated based on the patient's age and rate of progression, and curves of more than 60 degrees should be treated surgically; a single-stage posterior arthrodesis with segmental instrumentation is the treatment of choice (Chapter 44). Intraoperatively, cardiac arrhythmias are common and somatosensory-evoked potentials are unreliable, and a wake-up test should be considered. The fusion should extend from the upper thoracic spine to the lower region of the lumbar spine.

SPINAL MUSCULAR ATROPHY

Spinal muscular atrophy (SMA) is an inherited degenerative disease of the anterior horn cells of the spinal cord that occurs in one in 20,000 births. It is generally transmitted by an autosomal-recessive gene encoding for the Survival Motor Neuron 1 (*SMN-1*) gene, but other hereditary patterns have been described. SMA has been classified into five types (Table 7.5).

Although awareness of SMA has increased, diagnostic delay is common because symptoms can vary widely in onset and severity and can resemble other diseases. Early diagnosis of SMA is important because it allows early supportive care, reduction in patient and caregiver stress, and allows for medical management before joint contractures, scoliosis and pulmonary decline occur. A systematic literature review determined that diagnostic delay averaged 6 months for

TABLE 7.5

Classification and Subtypes of Spinal Muscular Atrophy

TYPE	AGE OF ONSET	MAXIMAL MOTOR MILE-STONE	MOTOR ABILITY AND ADDITIONAL FEATURES	PROGNOSIS[a]
SMA 0	Before birth	None	Severe hypotonia; unable to sit or roll[b]	Respiratory insufficiency at birth; death within weeks
SMA I	2 weeks (1a) 3 months (1b) 6 months (1c)	None	Severe hypotonia; unable to sit or roll[c]	Death/ventilation by 2 years
SMA II	6–18 months	Sitting	Proximal weakness; unable to walk independently	Survival into adulthood
SMA III	<3 years (IIIa) >3 years (IIIb) >12 years (IIIc)	Walking	May lose ability to walk	Normal life span
SMA IV	>30 years or 10–30 years	Normal	Mild motor impairment	Normal life span

[a]Prognosis varies with phenotype and supportive care interventions.
[b]Need for respiratory support at birth; contractures and birth; reduced fetal movements.
[c]Ia joint contractures present at birth; Ic may achieve head control.
From Farrar MA, Park SB, Vucic S, et al: Emerging therapies and challenges in spinal muscular atrophy, *Ann Neurol* 81:335, 2017.

type I, 21 months for type II, and 50 months for type III. SMA should be considered in the differential diagnosis in children with any of the clinical characteristics associated with the disease (see Table 7.1), and these signs should prompt referral to a pediatric neurologist as well as for a *SMN1* gene deletion test.

In patients with SMA, the blood creatine kinase or aldolase value is normal or mildly elevated. Electromyography reveals muscle denervation. Nerve conduction velocities are normal. Genetic studies have shown the defective gene to be located on chromosome 5. In 98% of patients with SMA, deletions of either exon 7 or exon 8 have been identified in the *SMN-1* gene. A second disease-modifying gene, *SMN2*, also plays a role in the severity of the disease. Advances in molecular biology have now made a test for these genes and their potential deletions commercially available. The five types of SMA seem to result from different mutations of the same gene.

Clinical characteristics of SMA include severe weakness and hypotonia, areflexia, fine tremor of the fingers, fasciculation of the tongue, and normal sensation. Proximal muscles are affected more than distal ones, and the lower extremities are usually weaker than the upper extremities. In nonambulatory patients, variable improvement in motor function occurs up to 4 to 5 years of age, before functional ability (e.g., in upper limbs) declines between 5 and 15 years. After age 15, a relative stability in function develops with subsequent gradual decline over time. Evans, Drennan, and Russman proposed a functional classification to aid in planning long-term orthopaedic care: group I patients never develop the strength to sit independently and have poor head control; group II patients develop head control and can sit but are unable to walk; group III patients can pull themselves up and walk in a limited fashion, frequently with the use of orthoses; and group IV patients develop the ability to walk and run normally and to climb stairs before onset of the weakness.

Recent advances in the medical management of SMA include the use of a compound known as nusinersen, which was released in 2016 by the FDA. It is an antisense oligonucleotide administered intrathecally that modifies the splicing of *SMN2* and increases the number of full-length protein molecules. It has been shown to improve motor function and motor milestone development in all types of SMA, with younger and asymptomatic patients, those who have not yet developed joint contractures or scoliosis, having better outcomes. Efforts are ongoing to improve drug delivery either by implantable pumps or by orally administered medications.

Orthopaedic treatment is generally required for hip and spine problems. Fractures are frequent in these patients as well, especially nonambulators, with the femur, ankle, and humerus the most common sites. Joint contractures can also occur, especially in the upper extremities, and tend to worsen with age. Children with type I SMA are markedly hypotonic and generally die as a result of the disease early in life. In these patients, orthopaedic reconstruction is not warranted; however, patients with type I SMA may develop fractures that heal quickly with appropriate splinting. Many children with infantile SMA are never able to walk even with braces, but most patients with the juvenile form are able to walk for many years. Gentle passive range-of-motion exercises and positioning instructions can be beneficial initially. Surgical release of contractures is rarely required. Because of the absence of movement and weightbearing, coxa valga deformity of the hip is frequent and unilateral or bilateral hip subluxation may occur (Fig. 7.31). Because many of these children are sitters, a stable and comfortable sitting position is essential. Traditionally in nonambulatory patients, proximal femoral varus derotational osteotomy (Chapter 33) has been used to produce a more stable sitting base. Efforts to maintain the reduction of the hips for good sitting balance may prevent pain and pelvic obliquity. Observation instead of surgical intervention is generally recommended because of the small number of patients having symptoms or seating problems.

Among children with SMA who survive childhood, scoliosis becomes the greatest threat during adolescence. The prevalence of scoliosis is nearly 100% in children with type II SMA and in children with type III muscular atrophy who become nonambulatory. Curves typically are long and

C-shaped and are most common in the thoracolumbar spine, occurring in up to 80% of patients. Scoliosis is usually progressive and severe and can limit daily function and cause cardiopulmonary problems. Bracing may be indicated during the growing years to slow curve progression, but spinal stabilization is ultimately required in almost all adolescent patients. Several authors have emphasized the importance of early surgery before the curve becomes severe and rigid. An inverse relationship between pulmonary function and scoliosis severity has been identified: for every 10 degree increase in Cobb angle, there is a 5% decrease in predicted vital capacity and a 3% decrease in peak flow. This limits the timeframe during which patients with SMA have sufficient lung capacity to successfully undergo spinal surgery without tracheostomy and mechanical ventilation.

Growing rod constructs have been shown to improve spine height, space available for the lungs, and control of

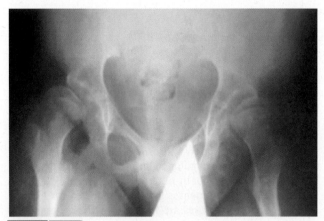

FIGURE 7.31 Coxa valga deformity and subluxation in 12-year-old child with spinal muscular atrophy.

pelvic obliquity in young patients with progressive scoliosis who are too young for definitive spinal fusion. Chandran et al. and McElroy et al. reported improvement in Cobb angles, as well as in quality of life for patients and caregivers, with few complications with the use of growing rods in patients with SMA. Use of a vertical expandable prosthetic titanium rib (VEPTR; Synthes, Westchester, PA) has been reported in children with neuromuscular scoliosis, with varying results (Fig. 7.32). Livingstone et al. compared the use of growing rods (9 children) with VEPTR (11 children) in SMA and found that neither improved "parasol rib" deformity (collapse of the rib cage), although spinal deformity was better corrected with growing rods. At least one complication occurred in 83% of those with VEPTR, compared with 41% of those with growing rods.

For most older patients, long posterior spinal fusion (PSF) to the pelvis is the treatment of choice. A 10-year follow-up of 11 patients with SMA who had PSF showed that PSF resulted in significant curve correction and an improvement in the rate of decline of forced vital capacity from 5.3%/year preoperatively to 1.3%/year postoperatively. During PSF, it is important to leave a midline "window" centrally in the fusion mass, typically at L3-L4, to allow access for intrathecal injection or port placement for the administration of nusinersen (Fig. 7.33).

Intraoperative and postoperative complications are frequent in these patients, and thorough preoperative evaluation is mandatory. Numerous studies have found the frequency of respiratory tract infections before surgery and the vital capacity of the lungs to be good indicators of the patient's ability to tolerate surgery. Tracheostomy should be considered for any patient with frequent preoperative respiratory tract infections and a vital capacity of less than 35% of normal. Techniques of surgery for the treatment of neuromuscular scoliosis are described in other chapter.

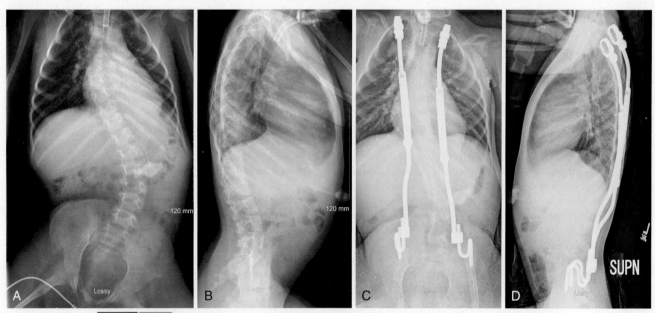

FIGURE 7.32 **A** and **B,** Spinal deformity in a young child with spinal muscular atrophy. **C** and **D,** At the age of 5 years, 2.5 years after implantation of vertical expandable prosthetic titanium rib.

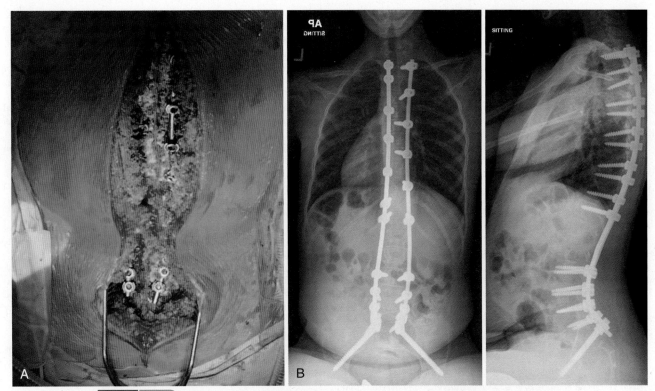

FIGURE 7.33 "Skip construct" for posterior spinal fusion in a patients with SMA-2. Operative photograph **(A)** and radiographs **(B)** show rod passage under muscle flap with uninstrumented, unfused lumbar segments to allow intrathecal nusinersen injection. (Courtesy Michael G. Vitale MD.)

REFERENCES

GENERAL

Bengtsson NE, Seto JT, Hall JK, et al.: Progress and prospects of gene therapy clinical trials for the muscular dystrophies, *Hum Mol Genet* 15:R9, 2016.

Brooks JT, Sponseller PD: What's new in the management of neuromuscular scoliosis, *J Pediatr Orthop* 36:627, 2016.

Cichos KH, Lehtonen EJ, McGwin Jr G, et al.: Inhospital complications of patients with neuromuscular disorders undergoing total joint arthroplasty, *J Am Acad Orthop Surg* 27:e535, 2019.

Conklin MJ, Pearson JM: The musculoskeletal aspects of obesity in neuromuscular conditions, *Orthop Clin North Am* 49:325, 2018.

Jirka S, Aartsma-Rus A: An update on RNA-targeting therapies for neuromuscular disorders, *Curr Opin Neurol* 28:515, 2015.

Lassche S, Janssen BH, IJzermans T, et al.: MRI-guided biopsy as a tool for diagnosis and research of muscle disorders, *J Neuromuscul Dis* 5:315, 2018.

Mary P, Servais L, Vialle R: Neuromuscular diseases: diagnosis and management, *Orthop Traumatol Surg Res* 104(1S):S89, 2018.

Mastrangelo M: Clinical approach to neurodegenerative disorders in childhood: an updated overview, *Acta Neurol Belg*, 2019 Jun 3, [Epub ahead of print].

Scoto M, Finkel R, Mercuri E, et al.: Genetic therapies for inherited neuromuscular disorders, *Lancet Child Aoles Health* 2:600, 2018.

Smitaman E, Flores DV, Mejia Gómez C, et al.: MR imaging of atraumatic muscle disorders, *Radiographics* 38:500, 2018.

Wagner S, Poirot I, Vuillerot C, Berard C: Tolerance and effectiveness on pain control of Pamidronate(r) intravenous infusions in children with neuromuscular disorders, *Ann Phys Rehabil Med* 54:348, 2011.

MUSCULAR DYSTROPHY—GENERAL

Fishman FG, Goldstein EM, Peljovich AE: Surgical treatment of upper extremity contractures in Emery-Dreifuss muscular dystrophy, *J Pediatr Orthop B* 26:32, 2017.

Griffet J, Decrocq L, Rauscent H, et al.: Lower extremity surgery in muscular dystrophy, *Orthop Traumatol Surg Res* 97:634, 2011.

Rahimov F, Kunkel LM: The cell biology of disease: cellular and molecular mechanisms underlying muscular dystrophy, *J Cell Biol* 201:499, 2013.

Whitehead NP, Kim MJ, Bible KL, et al.: A new therapeutic effect of simvastatin revealed by functional improvement in muscular dystrophy, *Proc Natl Acad Sci U S A* 112:12864, 2015.

DUCHENNE MUSCULAR DYSTROPHY

Abbs S, Tuffery-Giraud S, Bakker E, et al.: Best Practice Guidelines on molecular diagnosis in Duchenne/Becker muscular dystrophies, *Neuromuscul Disord* 20:422, 2010.

Apkon SD, Alman B, Birnkrant DJ, et al.: Orthopedic and surgical management of the patient with Duchenne muscular dystrophy, *Pediatrics* 142(Suppl 2):S82, 2018.

Birnkrant DJ, Bushby K, Bann CM, et al.: Diagnosis and management of Duchenne muscular dystrophy, part 2: respiratory, cardiac, bone health, and orthopaedic management, *Lancet Neurol* 17:347, 2018.

Bos W, Westra AE, Pinxten W, et al.: Risks in a trial of an innovative treatment of Duchenne muscular dystrophy, *Pediatrics* 136:1173, 2015.

Buckner JL, Bowden SA, Mahan JD: Optimizing bone health in Duchenne muscular dystrophy, *Int J Endocrinol*2015, 2015, 928385.

Bushby K, Finkel R, Birnkrant DJ, et al.: Diagnosis and management of Duchenne muscular dystrophy, part 1: diagnosis and pharmacologic and psychosocial management, *Lancet Neurology* 9:77, 2010.

Cheuk DK, Wong V, Wraige E, et al.: Surgery for scoliosis in Duchenne muscular dystrophy, *Cochrane Database Syst Rev* 10:CD005375, 2015.

Choi YA, Chun SM, Kim Y, et al.: Lower extremity joint contracture according to ambulatory status in children with Duchenne muscular dystrophy, *BMC Musculoskelet Disord* 19:287, 2018.

Crone M, Mah JK: Current and emerging therapies for Duchenne muscular dystrophy, *Curr Treat Options Neurol* 20:31, 2018.

Di Marco M, Joseph S, Horrocks I, et al.: Fractures and bone health in Duchenne muscular dystrophy in Scotland, *Neuromuscul Disord* 29:342, 2019.

Gordon KE, Dooley JM, Sheppard KM, et al.: Impact of bisphosphonates on survival for patients with Duchenne muscular dystrophy, *Pediatrics* 127:e353, 2011.

James KA, Cunniff C, Apkon SD, et al.: Risk factors for first fractures among males with Duchenne or Becker muscular dystrophy, *J Pediatr Orthop* 35:640, 2015.

Kim S, Campbell KA, Fox DJ, et al.: Corticosteroid treatment in males with Duchenne muscular dystrophy: treatment duration and time to loss of ambulation, *J Child Neurol* 30:1275, 2015.

Lebel DE, Corston JA, McAdam LC, et al.: Glucocorticoid treatment for the prevention of scoliosis in children with Duchenne muscular dystrophy: long-term follow-up, *J Bone Joint Surg Am* 95:1057, 2013.

McAdam LC, Rastogi A, Macleod K, et al.: Fat embolism syndrome following minor trauma in Duchenne muscular dystrophy, *Neuromuscul Disord* 22:1035, 2012.

McDonald CM, Mercuri E: Evidence-based care in Duchenne muscular dystrophy, *Lancet Neurol* 17:389, 2018.

McMillan HJ: Intermittent glucocorticoid regimes for younger boys with Duchenne muscular dystrophy: balancing efficacy with side effects, *Muscle Nerve* 59:638, 2019.

McMillan HJ, Gregas M, Darras BT, Kang PB: Serum transaminase levels in boys with Duchenne and Becker muscular dystrophy, *Pediatrics* 127:e132, 2011.

Partridge TA: Impending therapies for Duchenne muscular dystrophy, *Curr Opin Neurol* 24:415, 2011.

Sawnani H, Horn PS, Wong B, et al.: Comparison of pulmomary function decline in steroid-treated and steroid-naïve patients with Duchenne muscular dystrophy, *J Pediatr*, 2019 Apr 4, [Epub ahead of print].

Shieh PB: Duchenne muscular dystrophy: clinical trials and emerging tribulations, *Curr Opin Neurol* 28:542, 2015.

Shieh PB: Emerging strategies in the treatment of Duchenne muscular dystrophy, *Neurotherapeutics* 15:840, 2018.

Sienkiewicz D, Kulak W, Okurowska-Zawada B, et al.: Duchenne muscular dystrophy: current cell therapies, *Ther Adv Neurol Disord* 8:166, 2015.

Suk KS, Lee BH, Lee HM, et al.: Functional outcomes in Duchenne muscular dystrophy scoliosis: comparison of the differences between surgical and nonsurgical treatment, *J Bone Joint Surg Am* 96:409, 2014.

Takaso M, Nakazawa T, Imura T, et al.: Two-year results for scoliosis secondary to Duchenne muscular dystrophy fused to lumbar 5 with segmental pedicle screw instrumentation, *J Orthop Sci* 15:171, 2010.

Verhaart IEC, Aartsma-Rus A: Therapeutic developments for Duchenne muscular dystrophy, *Nat Rev Neurol*, 2019 May 30, [Epub ahead of print].

Ward LM, Hadjiyannakis S, McMillan HJ, et al.: Bone health and osteoporosis management of the patient with Duchenne muscular dystrophy, *Pediatrics* 142(Suppl 2):S34, 2018.

Wein N, Alfano L, Flanigan KM: Genetics and emerging treatments for Duchenne and Becker muscular dystrophy, *Pediatr Clin North Am* 62:723, 2015.

LIMB-GIRDLE DYSTROPHY

Angelini C, Giaretta L, Marozzo R: An update on diagnostic options and considerations in limb-girdle dystrophies, *Expert Rev Neurother* 18:693, 2018.

Chu ML, Moran E: The limb-girdle muscular dystrophies: is treatment on the horizon? *Neurotherapeutics* 15:849, 2018.

Liewluck T, Milone M: Untangling the complexity of limb-girdle muscular dystrophies, *Muscle Nerve* 58:167, 2018.

Taghizadeh E, Rezaee M, Barreto GE, et al.: Prevalence, pathological mechanisms, and genetic basis of limb-girdle muscular dystrophies: a review, *J Cell Physiol*, 2018 Dec 7, [Epub ahead of print].

Vissing J: Limb girdle muscular dystrophies: classification, clinical spectrum and emerging therapies, *Curr Opin Neurol* 29:635, 2016.

FACIOSCAPULOHUMERAL DYSTROPHY

de Greef JC, Lemmers RJ, Camano P, et al.: Clinical features of facioscapulohumeral muscular dystrophy 2, *Neurology* 75:1548, 2010.

DeSimone AM, Pakula A, Lek A, et al.: Facioscapulohumeral muscular dystrophy, *Compr Physiol* 7:1229, 2017.

DGerevini S, Scarlato M, Maggi L, et al.: Muscle MRI findings in facioscapulohumeral muscular dystrophy, *Eur Radiol* 26:693, 2016.

Goselink RJM, Mul K, van Kernebeek CR, et al.: Early onset as a marker for disease severity on facioscapulohumeral muscular dystrophy, *Neurology* 92:e378, 2019.

Goselink RJM, Schreuder THA, van Alfen N, et al.: Facioscapulohumeral dystrophy in childhood: a nationwide natural history study, *Ann Neurol* 84:627, 2018.

Hamel J, Tawil R: Facioscapulohumeral muscular dystrophy: update on pathogenesis and future treatments, *Neurotherapeutics* 15:863, 2018.

Karceski S: Diagnosis and treatment of facioscapulohumeral muscular dystrophy: 2015 guidelines, *Neurology* 85:e41, 2015.

Mah JK, Chen YW: A pediatric review of facioscapulohumeral muscular dystrophy, *J Pediatr Neurol* 16:222, 2018.

Steel D, Main M, Manzur A, et al.: Clinical features of facioscapulohumeral muscular dystrophy 1 in childhood, *Dev Med Child Neurol*, 2019 Jan 20, [Epub ahead of print].

Tawil R, Kissel JT, Heatwole C, et al.: Evidence-based guideline summary: evaluation, diagnosis, and management of facioscapulohumeral muscular dystrophy: report of the Guideline Development, Dissemination, and Implementation Subcommittee of the American Academy of Neurology and the Practice Issues Review Panel of the American Association of Neuromuscular & Electrodiagnostic Medicine, *Neurology* 85:357, 2015.

Van Tongel A, Atoun E, Narvani A, et al.: Medium to long-term outcome of thoracoscapular arthrodesis with screw fixation for facioscapulohumeral muscular dystrophy, *J Bone Joint Surg Am* 95:1404, 2013.

CONGENITAL DYSTROPHY

Chakrabarty B, Sharma MC, Gulati S, et al.: Skin biopsy for diagnosis of Ullrich congenital muscular dystrophy: an observational study, *Child Neurol* 32:1099, 2017.

Ho G, Cardamone M, Farrar M: Congenital and childhood myotonic dystrophy: current aspect of disease and future directions, *World J Clin Pediatr* 4:66, 2015.

Saade DN, Neuhaus SB, Foley AR, et al.: The use of muscle ultrasound in the diagnosis and differential diagnosis of congenital disorders of muscle in the age of next generation genetics, *Semin Pediatr Neurol* 29:44, 2019.

Takaso M, Nakazawa T, Imura T, et al.: Surgical correction of spinal deformity in patients with congenital muscular dystrophy, *J Orthop Sci* 15:493, 2010.

Theadom A, Rodrigues M, Poke G, et al.: A nationwide, population-based prevalence study of genetic muscle disorders, *Neuroepidemiology* 52:128, 2019.

MYOTONIC DYSTROPHY

Gadalla SM, Pfeiffer RM, Kristinsson SY, et al.: Brain tumors in patients with myotonic dystrophy: a population-based study, *Eur J Neurol* 23:542, 2016.

Johnson NE, Abbott D, Cannon-Albright LA: Relative risks for comorbidities associated with myotonic dystrophy: a population-based analysis, *Muscle Nerve* 52:659, 2015.

Johnston NE, Ekstrom AB, Campbell C, et al.: Parent-reported multinational study of the impact of congenital and childhood onset myotonic dystrophy, *Dev Med Child Neurol* 58:698, 2016.

Schilling L, Forst R, Forst J, Fujak A: Orthopaedic disorders in myotonic dystrophy type 1: descriptive clinical study of 21 patients, *BMC Musculoskelet Disord* 14:338, 2013.

Zapata-Aldana E, Ceballos-Sáenz D, Hicks R, et al.: Prenatal, neonatal, and early childhood features in congenital mytonic dystrophy, *J Neuromuscul Dis* 5:331, 2018.

CHARCOT-MARIE-TOOTH DISEASE

Burns J, Ryan MM, Ouvrier RA: Quality of life in children with Charcot-Marie-Tooth disease, *J Child Neurol* 25:343, 2010.

Burns J, Scheinberg A, Ryan MM, et al.: Randomized trial of botulinum toxin to prevent pes cavus progression in pediatric Charcot-Marie-Tooth disease type 1A, *Muscle Nerve* 42:262, 2010.

Cornett KMG, Menezes MP, Shy RR, et al.: Natural history of Charcot-Marie-Tooth disease during childhood, *Ann Neurol* 82:353, 2017.

Cornett KMD, Wojciechowski E, Sman AD, et al.: Magnetic resonance imaging of the anterior compartment of the lower leg is a biomarker for weakness, disability, and impaired gait in childhood Charcot-Marie-Tooth disease, *Muscle Nerve* 59:213, 2019.

Dreher T, Wolf SI, Heitzmann D, et al.: Tibialis posterior tendon transfer corrects the foot drop component of cavovarus foot deformity in Charcot-Marie-Tooth disease, *J Bone Joint Surg* 96:456, 2014.

Faldini C, Traina F, Nanni M, et al.: Surgical treatment of cavus foot in Charcot-Marie-Tooth disease: a review of twenty-four cases: AAOS exhibit selection, *J Bone Joint Surg* 97:e30, 2015.

Hoellwarth IS, Mahan ST, Spencer SA: Painful pes planovalgus: an uncommon pediatric orthopedic presentation of Charcot-Marie-Tooth disease, *J Pediatr Orthop B* 21:428, 2012.

Karakis I, Greags M, Darras BT, et al.: Clinical correlates of Charcot-Marie-Tooth disease in patients with pes cavus deformities, *Muscle Nerve* 47:488, 2013.

Kennedy RA, McGinley JL, Paterson KL, et al.: Gait and footwear in children and adolescents with Charcot-Marie-Tooth disease: a cross-sectional, case-controlled study, *Gait Posture* 62:262, 2018.

Laurá M, Singh D, Ramdharry G, et al.: Prevalence and orthopedic management of foot and ankle deformities in Charcot-Marie-Tooth disease, *Muscle Nerve* 57:255, 2018.

Lin T, Gibbons P, Mudge AJ, et al.: Surgical outcomes of cavovarus foot deformity in children with Charcot-Marie-Tooth disease, *Neuromuscul Disord*, 2019 Apr 29, [Epub ahead of print].

Louwerens JWK: Operative treatment algorithm for foot deformities in Charcot-Marie-Tooth disease, *Oper Orthop Traumatol* 30:130, 2018.

Napiontek M, Pietrzak K: Joint preserving surgery versus arthrodesis in operative treatment of patients with neuromuscular polyneuropathy: questionnaire assessment, *Eur J Orthop Surg Traumatol* 25:391, 2015.

Novais EN, Bixby SD, Rennick J, et al.: Hip dysplasia is more severe in Charcot-Marie-Tooth disease than in developmental dysplasia of the hip, *Clin Orthop Relat Res* 472:665, 2014.

Novais EN, Kim YJ, Carry PM, Millis MB: Periacetabular osteotomy redirects the acetabulum and improves pain in Charcot-Marie-Tooth hip dysplasia with higher complications compared with developmental dysplasia of the hip, *J Pediatr Orthop* 36:853, 2016.

Pouwels S, de Boer A, Leufkens HG, et al.: Risk of fracture in patients with Charcot-Marie-Tooth disease, *Muscle Nerve* 50:919, 2014.

Rose KJ, Raymond J, Regshauge K, et al.: Serial night casting increases ankle dorsiflexion range in children and young adults with Charcot-Marie-Tooth disease: a randomised trial, *J Physiother* 56:113, 2010.

Saporta AS, Sottile SL, Miller LJ, et al.: Charcot-Marie-Tooth disease subtypes and genetic testing strategies, *Ann Neurol* 69:22, 2011.

Stover MD, Podeszwa DA, De La Rocha A, Sucato DJ: Early results of the Bernese periacetabular osteotomy for symptomatic dysplasia in Charcot-Marie-Tooth disease, *Hip Int* 23(Suppl 9):S2, 2013.

VanderHave KL, Hensinger RN, King BW: Flexible cavovarus foot in children and adolescents, *Foot Ankle Clin* 18:715, 2013.

Yagerman SE, Cross MB, Green DW, Scher DM: Pediatric orthopedic conditions in Charcot-Marie-Tooth disease: a literature review, *Curr Opin Pediatr* 24:50, 2012.

FRIEDREICH ATAXIA

Ashley CN, Hoang KD, Lynch DR, et al.: Childhood ataxia: clinical features, pathogenesis, key unanswered questions, and future directions, *J Child Neurol* 27:1095, 2012.

Bodensteiner JB: Friedreich ataxia, *Semin Pediatr Neurol* 21:72, 2014.

Cook A, Giunti P: Friedreich's ataxia: clinical features, pathogenesis and management, *Br Med Bull* 124:19, 2017.

Lynch DR, Seyer L: Friedreich ataxia: new findings, new challenges, *Ann Neurol* 76:487, 2014.

Paulsen EK, Friedman LS, Myers LM, Lynch DR: Health-related quality of life in children with Friedreich ataxia, *Pediatr Neurol* 42:335, 2010.

Sival DA, Pouwels ME, Van Brederode A, et al.: In children with Friedreich ataxia, muscle and ataxis parameters are associated, *Dev Med Child Neurol* 53:529, 2011.

Tsirikos AI, Smith G: Scoliosis in patients with Friedreich's ataxia, *J Bone Joint Surg* 94:684, 2012.

Tsou AY, Paulsen EK, Lagedrost SJ, et al.: Mortality in Friedreich ataxia, *J Neurol Sci* 307:46, 2011.

Zhang S, Napierala M, Napierala JS: Therapeutic prospects for Friedreich's ataxia, *Trends Pharmacol Sci* 40:229, 2019.

SPINAL MUSCULAR ATROPHY

Cardenas J, Menier M, Heitzer MD, et al.: High healthcare resource use in hospitalized patients with a diagnosis of spinal muscular atrophy type 1 (SMA1): retrospective analysis of the Kids' Inpatient Database (KID), *Pharmaoecon Open* 3:205, 2019.

Chandran S, McCarthy J, Noonan K, et al.: Early treatment of scoliosis with growing rods in children with severe spinal muscular atrophy: a preliminary report, *J Pediatr Orthop* 31:450, 2011.

Eckart M, Guenther UP, Idkowiak J, et al.: The natural course of infantile spinal muscular atrophy with respiratory distress type I (SMRD1), *Pediatrics* 129:e148, 2012.

Fujak A, Kopschina C, Forst R, et al.: Fractures in proximal spinal muscular atrophy, *Arch Orthop Trauma Surg* 130:775, 2010.

Fujak A, Raab W, Schuh A, et al.: Natural course of scoliosis in proximal spinal muscular atrophy type II and IIIa: descriptive clinical study with retrospective data collection of 126 patients, *BMC Musculoskelet Disord* 14:283, 2013.

Funk S, Lovejoy S, Mencio G, Martus J: Rigid instrumentation for neuromuscular scoliosis improves deformity correction without increasing complications, *Spine* 41:46, 2016.

Glascock J, Sampson J, Haidet-Phillips A, et al.: Treatment algorithm for infants diagnosed with spinal muscular atrophy through newborn screening, *J Neuromuscul Dis* 5:145, 2018.

Goodkey K, Aslesh T, Maruyama Rm, et al.: Nusinersen in the treatment of spinal muscular atrophy, *Methods Mol Biol* 69:1828, 2018.

Haaker G, Fujak A: Proximal spinal muscular atrophy: current orthopedic perspective, *Appl Clin Genet* 6:113, 2013.

Halawi MJ, Lark RK, Fitch RD: Neuromuscular scoliosis: current concepts, *Orthopedics* 38:e452, 2015.

Humphrey E, Fuller HR, Morris GE: Current research on SMN protein and treatment strategies for spinal muscular atrophy, *Neuromuscul Disord* 22:193, 2012.

Humphrey E, Fuller HR, Morris GE: Current research on SMN protein and treatment strategies for spinal muscular atrophy, *Neuromuscul Disord* 22:193, 2012.

Kolb SJ, Coffey CS, Yankey JW, et al.: Natural history of infantile-onset spinal muscular atrophy, *Ann Neurol* 82:883, 2017.

Kolb SJ, Kissel JT: Spinal muscular atrophy, *Neurol Clin* 33:831, 2015.

Lawton S, Hickerton C, Archibald AD, et al.: A mixed methods exploration of families' experiences of the diagnosis of childhood spinal muscular atrophy, *Eur J Hum Genet* 23:575, 2015.

Lin CW, Kalb SJ, Yeh WS: Delay in diagnosis of spinal muscular atrophy: a systematic literature review, *Pediatr Neurol* 53:293, 2015.

Livingstone K, Zurakowski D, Snyder B: Growing Spine Study Group; Children's Spine Study Group: Parasol rib deformity in hypotonic neuromuscular scoliosis: a new radiographical definition and a comparison of short-term treatment outcomes with VEPTR and growing rods, *Spine* 40:E780, 2015.

McElroy MJ, Shaner AC, Crawford TO, et al.: Growing rods for scoliosis in spinal muscular atrophy: structural effects, complications, and hospital stays, *Spine* 36:1305, 2011.

Mercuri E, Darras BT, Chiriboga CA, et al.: Nusinersen versus sham control in later-onset spinal muscular atrophy, *N Engl J Med* 378:625, 2018.

Mesfin A, Sponseller PD, Leet AI: Spinal muscular atrophy: manifestations and management, *J Am Acad Orthop Surg* 20:393, 2012.

Modi HN, Suh SW, Jong JY, et al.: Treatment and complications in flaccid neuromuscular scoliosis (Duchenne muscular dystrophy and spinal muscular atrophy) with posterior-only pedicle screw instrumentation, *Eur J Spine* 19:384, 2010.

Strauss KA, Carson VJ, Brigatti KW, et al.: Preliminary safety and tolerability of a novel subcutaneous intrathecal catheter system for repeated outpatient dosing of nusinersen to children and adults with spinal muscular dystrophy, *J Pediatr Orthop* 38:e610, 2018.

Tisdale S, Pellizzoni L: Disease mechanisms and therapeutic approaches in spinal muscular atrophy, *J Neurosci* 35:8691, 2015.

Tobert DG, Vitale MG: Strategies for treating scoliosis in children with spinal muscular atrophy, *Am J Orthop* 42:E99, 2013.

Vai S, Bianchi ML, Moroni I, et al.: Bone and spinal muscular atrophy, *Bone* 79:116, 2015.

Wadman RI, Bosboom WM, van den Berg LH, et al.: Drug treatment for spinal muscular atrophy type I, *Cochrane Database Syst Rev* (1)CD006281, 2011.

Wadman RI, Bosboom WM, vanden Berg LH, et al.: Drug treatment for spinal muscular atrophy types II and III, *Cochrane Database Syst Rev* (1)CD006282, 2011.

White KK, Song KM, Frost N, et al.: VEPTR growing rods for early-onset neuromuscular scoliosis: feasible and effective, *Clin Orthop Relat Res* 469:1335, 2011.

Winjngaarde CA, Brink RC, de Kort FAS, et al.: Natural course of scoliosis and lifetime risk of scoliosis surgery in spinal muscular atrophy, *Neurology*, 2019 Jun 4, [Epub ahead of print].

Yuan P, Jiang L: Clinical characteristics of three subtypes of spinal muscular atrophy in children, *Brain Dev* 37:537, 2015.

Wertz MH, Sahin M: Developing therapies for spinal muscular atrophy, *Ann N Y Acad Sci* 1366:5, 2016.

Zebala LP, Bridwell KH, Baldus C, et al.: Minimum 5-year radiographic results of long scoliosis fusion in juvenile spinal muscular atrophy patients: major curve progression after instrumented fusion, *J Pediatr Orthop* 31:480, 2011.

The complete list of references is available online at Expert Consult. com.

PART III

FRACTURES AND DISLOCATIONS IN CHILDREN

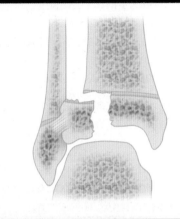

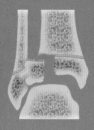

GENERAL PRINCIPLES

Fractures are common in children, occurring at a rate of 12 to 30 per 1000 children every year. The risk of sustaining a fracture between birth and 16 years of age has been reported to be 42% to 64% for boys and 27% to 40% for girls. Children and adolescents, because of their unique physiologic features, such as the presence of physes, increased elasticity of bone and other connective tissue structures, as well as decreased motor control and greater head-to-body weight ratio in younger children, have different patterns of fractures than adults. Although most fractures in children heal well without long-term complications, certain fractures, especially those involving the physis and articular surface, have the potential to cause significant morbidity.

Children, unlike adults, can remodel fractures as they grow, especially those in the plane of motion of the adjacent joint. Fractures that are angulated in the coronal plane have some remodeling potential, and those that are rotationally displaced have little to none. In the upper extremity, growth is more rapid at the proximal humerus and distal radius, whereas in the lower extremity it is primarily about the knee, at the distal femur and proximal tibia. Fractures that are closer to active physes, such as proximal humeral fractures, due to rapid growth have tremendous remodeling potential compared with fractures that occur in less active physes, such as radial neck fractures where less remodeling occurs. Understanding remodeling is essential in optimizing treatment for each patient. Because of these differences, a basic understanding of skeletal growth potential and maturation is essential in caring for children with fractures.

This chapter mainly discusses fractures that require operative management. Lateral condyle and femoral neck fractures have been called "fractures of necessity" because poor outcomes are certain without operative treatment. Some fractures, such as those of the proximal humerus, rarely require surgery. Nonunion in children is rare and if present is usually caused by factors such as open fracture, soft-tissue interposition at the fracture site, pathologic lesion, or vitamin D deficiency.

GROWTH PLATE INJURIES

It has been estimated that 30% of fractures in children involve a physis and most heal without any long-term complications. It is important to have knowledge of which fractures have a low potential for causing growth disturbance, such as those in the proximal humerus, and those that have greater potential, such as those in the distal femur and tibia. Histologically, most physeal fractures occur through the proliferative zone, which is the weakest region of the physis (Fig. 8.1); however, they can occur through any zone. Some physeal fractures may be related to endocrinologic changes that occur around the time of puberty.

The most widely used scheme to classify these injuries is that of Salter and Harris, which is based on the radiographic appearance of the fracture as it relates to the physis as described below (Fig. 8.2).

- Type I fractures occur through the physis only, with or without displacement.
- Type II fractures have a metaphyseal spike attached to the separated epiphysis (Thurston-Holland sign) with or without displacement.

- Type III fractures occur through the physis and epiphysis into the joint with joint incongruity when the fracture is displaced.
- Type IV fractures occur in the metaphysis and pass through the physis and epiphysis into the joint. Joint incongruity occurs with displaced fractures.
- Type V fractures, which are usually diagnosed only in retrospect, are compression or crush fractures of the physis, producing permanent damage and growth arrest.
- Type VI fractures are caused by a shearing injury to the peripheral aspect of the physis (perichondral ring). These fractures have been classically described in lawn mower accidents when the peripheral aspect of the physis is sheared off and have a high rate of angular deformity and growth arrest.

Although not completely prognostic, in general, Salter-Harris types III–VI fractures have a greater risk of complications than Salter-Harris types I and II injuries. An exception might be a completely displaced Salter-Harris type I fracture that has a greater potential for growth arrest than a nondisplaced Salter-Harris type IV fracture of the distal femur.

Although many Salter-Harris types I and II fractures can be treated nonoperatively, Salter-Harris types III and IV fractures usually require operative intervention, most commonly open reduction and internal fixation because of the intraarticular nature of the fracture and the potential for posttraumatic arthritis with nonanatomic reduction. Implants crossing the physis should be avoided when possible and when used should be smooth and the smallest diameter possible, and should be removed as soon as the fracture is stable (Fig. 8.3). The treatment of specific fractures and the potential for growth arrest are discussed for each specific injury. Regardless of the injury type, parents need to be educated as to the possibility of growth disturbance and the need for long-term follow-up for any physeal fracture.

When growth arrest occurs, it can result in a shortening or angular deformity or both of the limb, depending on the size and the location of the growth arrest. Growth arrest most commonly results from a bony bar that crosses the physis. Although spontaneous correction of the bar with growth resumption has been reported, it is very rare. Central bars tend to lead to shortening, and peripheral bars tend to lead to angular deformity, but in most cases there are components of each. Certain fractures, such as distal femoral and distal tibial physeal fractures, have a higher rate of growth arrest and deformity than others. Once a bony bar occurs, the size and location of the bar can be determined using three-dimensional imaging such as computed tomography (CT) or volumetric magnetic resonance imaging (MRI). Physeal bar resection has been tried using a variety of direct and indirect methods, and the results have been unpredictable with unsuccessful outcomes occurring in 10% to 40% of patients. In general, younger patients with smaller (<30% of the physis) peripheral bars have a higher rate of success with bar resection than older patients with larger central bars. Bar resection is often combined with osteotomy to correct the resultant angular deformity as well. For large bars or those that are difficult to resect, epiphysiodesis of the remaining physis with staged angular correction and/or lengthening may be the best option.

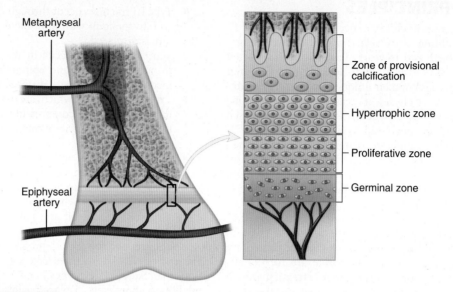

FIGURE 8.1 Physeal anatomy. Most fractures occur through the proliferative zone, which is the weakest region of the physis.

When growth across the physis ceases symmetrically, such as with large central bars or with type V fractures, the primary problem is limb shortening. In the upper extremity, the major growth centers are the proximal humerus (arm) and distal radius and ulna (forearm). In contrast, the major growth centers in the lower extremity are the distal femur (thigh) and proximal tibia and fibula (leg) (Fig. 8.4). Using either the Mosley straight-line graph or the Paley modifiers, the amount of deformity present at skeletal maturity can be predicted. The ultimate shortening that occurs is a result of the physis involved and amount of growth remaining. The relative contribution of each physis to overall limb segment growth is shown in Fig. 8.4. Shortening is much better tolerated in the upper extremity than the lower extremity, and length equalization procedures are rarely used in the upper extremity. In general, patients with a lower extremity leg-length discrepancy at maturity of up to 2 cm can be treated with a shoe lift, those 2 to 5 cm with contralateral epiphysiodesis, and those greater than 5 cm with limb lengthening. With their improvements and increased use, intramedullary lengthening nails, which are extremely accurate, have a lower complication rate and better cosmetic result than traditional external fixation-based lengthening techniques, and these guidelines, especially those for epiphysiodesis, are being questioned.

OPEN FRACTURES

The general classification and principles associated with the treatment of open fractures apply to children as well. The most common open fractures in children are in the forearm and tibia followed by the hand, femur, and humerus. It is important to remember that factors such as thick active periosteum, greater periosteal bone formation potential, and lack of comorbidities lead to faster and more reliable bone healing in children than in adults. The initial management should consist of wound irrigation and debridement, antibiotics, and stabilization of the fracture. Treatment should be individualized for each patient. Timely administration of antibiotics has been shown to decrease infection rates in patients with open fractures. A multicenter study comparing irrigation and debridement of type I open forearm fractures in the emergency room compared to the operating room demonstrated no significant difference in overall infection rates, but length of stay and costs were decreased in the emergency room group. Larger studies are necessary, however, to determine if and which grade I open fractures can be treated in the emergency room because of the considerable variability in treatment methods among surgeons and the lack of quality evidence to guide treatment.

A large multicenter review of 536 children with 554 open fractures showed an overall infection rate of 3% with no difference in infection for all Gustilo and Anderson types comparing emergent (<6 hours) with delayed (>6 hours) surgical treatment. Grade III fractures in older children and adolescents have complication rates similar to those in adults. A recent meta-analysis showed no relationship between late debridement and increased infection rates in children with open fractures as well. The treatment of specific open fractures is discussed in this chapter.

BIRTH FRACTURES

Neonates who are diagnosed with a fracture in the first week of life without any evidence of trauma are considered to have a birth fracture. The incidence is approximately 0.1/1000 live births and may be related to forced obstetric maneuvers. The most commonly fractured bones include the humerus, clavicle, and femoral shaft. Risk factors include very large or very small fetuses, breech presentation, instrumented delivery, small uterine incision (cesarean section), twin pregnancy, prematurity and prematurity-related osteopenia, and osteogenesis imperfecta. Between 60% and 80% of patients do not have positive findings on the initial newborn examination. Prenatal ultrasound may help to identify high-risk patients, such as those with osteogenesis imperfecta before delivery.

Type	Salter-Harris

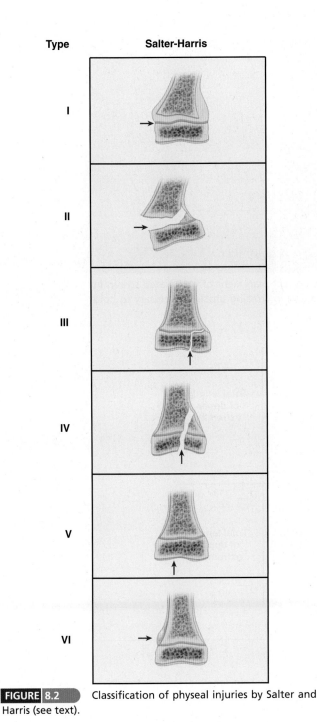

FIGURE 8.2 Classification of physeal injuries by Salter and Harris (see text).

such as arthrography or ultrasound can be used to make the diagnosis. (These specific injuries are discussed later in the chapter.)

NONACCIDENTAL TRAUMA

Musculoskeletal injuries are the second most common type of injury after soft-tissue injury, occurring 10% to 70% of the time in children with nonaccidental trauma (NAT). Because of this, 30% to 50% of these children are seen by an orthopaedic surgeon. Because there is no specific test to make the diagnosis of NAT, a careful history and physical examination must be performed and appropriate use of imaging is necessary. This usually is done using a multidisciplinary team approach. Having a high index of suspicion of NAT is essential because in up to 20% of children with NAT the diagnosis is missed on their initial medical visit. Making the diagnosis is essential because there is a high rate of reabuse and even death in children when the diagnosis is missed. It is important to be aware of risk factors for NAT and of certain injuries that are highly suggestive of this mechanism of injury. Risk factors for NAT include age younger than 2 years, children with multiple medical problems, fractures or injuries in different stages of healing, posterior rib fractures, and long bone fractures in young patients (Fig. 8.5). Other social factors, such as parental unemployment or drug abuse, lower socioeconomic status, and single parent households, have been shown to correlate with a higher risk of NAT as well. Common fractures in abused children are in the humerus, tibia, and femur. Radiographic features such as soft-tissue swelling (1 to 2 days), periosteal reaction (15 to 35 days), soft or hard callus (36 days), and bridging and remodeling (after 45 days) can be used to determine the age of the fracture. Other conditions in the differential diagnosis of NAT include metabolic bone disease and genetic conditions that can lead to bone fragility, such as osteogenesis imperfecta, rickets, renal disease, disuse osteopenia, and the use of certain medications such as corticosteroids.

Humeral shaft fractures in children younger than 3 years were at one time thought to be associated with NAT, but most are not. However, a high index of suspicion must remain for NAT in any child younger than 1 year of age with a long bone fracture. Humeral shaft fractures, although less often than clavicular fractures, can occur at birth. Risk factors include large babies, shoulder dystocia, and the use of assistive devices. These children often present with pseudoparalysis that can be confused with a brachial plexus palsy and septic arthritis.

When NAT is suspected, a skeletal survey (Box 8.1) should be ordered in children up to the age of 3 years according to the American Academy of Orthopaedic Surgery 2009 Clinical Practice Guidelines, especially when the child is younger than 1 year of age, when there is no history or an inconsistent history of injury, or in those in whom the fracture is attributed to NAT or domestic violence to look for secondary injuries. Patients with buckle fractures of the distal radius and toddlers with a fracture of the tibia do not need routine skeletal survey. It should be noted that lower extremity long bone fractures in ambulatory children rarely are caused by NAT. On skeletal survey, 50% of children have one fracture, 21% have two, 12% have three, and 17% have more than three. Controversy exists as to which studies are

Clinically, patients present with warmth, swelling, pain, and irritability with motion. Some children present with pseudoparalysis or failure to move a limb, which can be confused with differential diagnoses of osteomyelitis, septic arthritis, or brachial plexus palsy. Because it may take several days for some of these signs to develop, delayed diagnosis of 1 to 2 days is common. Most birth fractures do not require operative treatment, heal quickly, and remodel fully. Clavicular or humeral shaft fractures can be treated by pinning the baby's sleeve to the front of the shirt for 1 to 2 weeks until healed. Femoral shaft fractures can be treated with splinting or a Pavlik harness. Spica casting rarely is necessary. Physeal separations, especially at the distal femur and distal humerus, are rare but can occur with difficult delivery. Advanced imaging

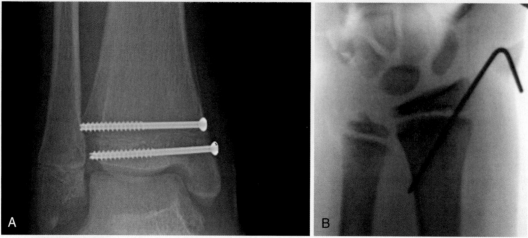

FIGURE 8.3 Fixation of physeal fracture. **A,** Correct placement of cannulated screws in metaphysis and epiphysis avoiding physis. **B,** Smooth pin crossing physis if necessary to hold reduction.

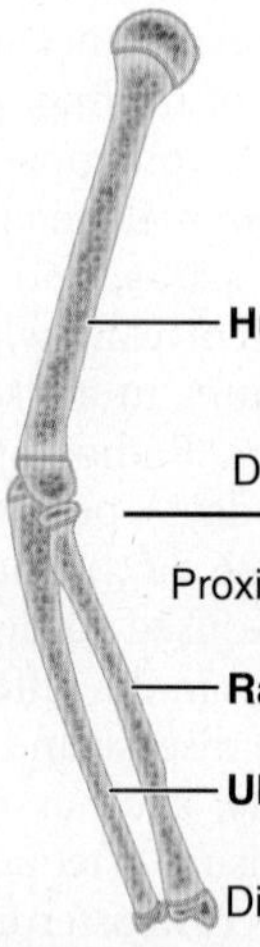

		Total length of humerus	Total length of upper extremity
Humerus	Proximal	80%	40%
	Distal physis	20%	10%
		Total length of radius and ulna	Total length of upper extremity
Radius / **Ulna**	Proximal ⌈Radius ⌊Ulna	25% 15%	11% 10%
	Distal ⌈Radius ⌊Ulna	75% 85%	39% 40%

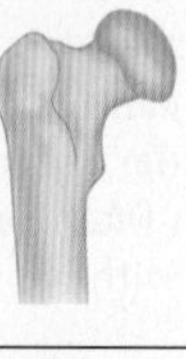

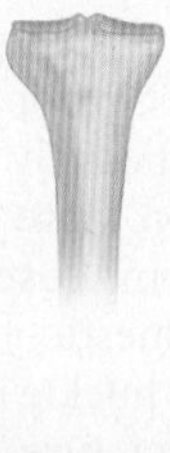

A

		Total length of the femur	Total length of lower extremity
	Proximal femur	30%	15%
	Distal femur	70%	37%
		Tibia or fibula	Total length of lower extremity
	Proximal tibia	55%	28%
	Proximal fibula	60%	
	Distal tibia	45%	20%
	Distal fibula	40%	

B

FIGURE 8.4 **A,** Approximately 80% of the growth of humerus occurs at proximal physis. **B,** Approximately 70% of growth of femur occurs at distal physis; in tibia, approximately 55% occurs in proximal physis.

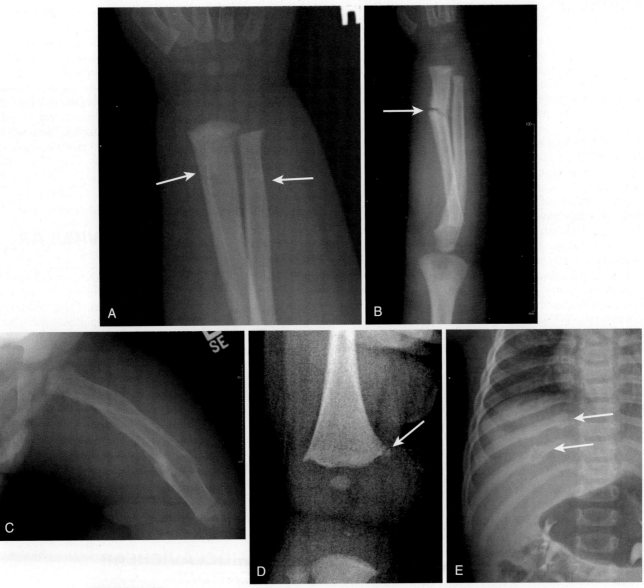

FIGURE 8.5 Child abuse. **A–C**, Six-month old child with multiple fractures at different stages of healing. **D**, Metaphyseal corner fracture. **E**, Rib fractures.

optimal to include in a skeletal survey; however, rib films are essential because of the high sensitivity and specificity for NAT. Because imaging around active physes is difficult, and with improvements in plain radiographic techniques, bone scan rarely is used in the evaluation of NAT.

Certain fracture types such as spiral femoral fractures and metaphyseal corner fractures were thought to be pathognomonic for NAT. Recent studies have shown that spiral femoral fractures actually are rare in abused children and that transverse fractures are more predictive of NAT. A recent review has shown that the metaphyseal corner fracture, once thought to be pathognomonic for NAT, is very similar to fractures seen with rickets. It is important to remember that fracture morphology gives information about the direction but not the etiology of the force applied and that the presence or absence of a fracture is probably more important than its morphology.

CLAVICLE

Fractures of the clavicle are common in children and adolescents, with a peak age for clavicular fractures being 10 to 19 years of age. Most fractures heal well with nonoperative treatment, especially in young children. Although there has been a dramatic increase in the operative treatment of clavicular fractures in all age groups, the role of operative treatment of clavicular shaft fractures in children and adolescents remains controversial. A review of members of the Pediatric Orthopaedic Society of North America showed that the majority preferred nonoperative treatment for all fracture patterns; however, older age (16 to 19 years), evidence in the adult literature, and physician years of experience (<5 years) predicted operative treatment preference. Excellent clinical and radiographic outcomes have been reported for both nonoperative and operative management of these injuries. Operatively treated patients typically have a faster return to activities but also have a higher complication rate in terms of symptomatic implants and nonunion. A recent study showed the overall complication rate following surgical treatment of 37 fractures in 36 pediatric patients to be 86%, with painful implants being the most common complication (59%), and a major complication rate of 43%, including nonunion and refracture around the plate and/or screw holes following plate removal. The rate of malunion is higher and almost exclusively associated with nonoperative treatment; however, patients with established malunions have excellent functional outcome scores. Although studies have shown good outcomes with both methods of treatment, stronger evidence is needed to determine if one method is superior to the other. The indications for operative treatment are open fracture, polytrauma, floating shoulder, fractures with skin compromise or neurovascular injury, and widely displaced or shortened fractures in older adolescents. Operative treatment of these injuries is described in other chapter.

STERNOCLAVICULAR FRACTURES AND DISLOCATIONS

The medial clavicle is one of the last growth centers to ossify, typically around 25 years of age. Fractures of the medial clavicle are usually Salter-Harris type I or II fractures, which in most cases heal with closed management and without complications (Fig. 8.6). It can be difficult to differentiate these injuries from true sternoclavicular joint dislocations because clinically they appear similar. The use of CT scan is helpful in these situations not only to determine the fracture pattern but also to evaluate the relationship between the fracture fragments and the mediastinal structures such as the brachiocephalic vein, which is the most commonly compressed structure, and innominate artery with posteriorly displaced fracture dislocation. Although injuries to the great vessels or mediastinal structures are often cited as complications of posterior sternoclavicular dislocations, a recent multicenter study of 125 such dislocations found no vascular or mediastinal injuries during reduction or fixation that required intervention. Anteriorly displaced fractures usually heal with a "bump" over the proximal clavicle but rarely are symptomatic. Up to 50% of patients with posteriorly displaced fractures may remain symptomatic. This, along with the higher complication rate in repair of longstanding sternoclavicular dislocation, leads most authors to recommend operative treatment of these acute injuries. Closed reduction under anesthesia can be attempted, but there is a high redislocation rate. Because

the epiphyseal (proximal) fragment is small, fixation is usually achieved with FiberWire (Arthrex Inc., Naples, FL) or suture repair. Care must be taken to protect the adjacent neurovascular structures and pleura. A recent meta-analysis showed that although considerable variability in the literature exists, good results can be obtained with both open and closed treatment as long as a stable reduction is achieved. It also showed that early treatment is better because patients treated less than 48 hours after injury had better results than those treated later. Patients who undergo late operative treatment for chronic posterior fracture-dislocation have been shown to do well with activities of daily living but have pain when returning to the same level of athletic participation.

LATERAL (DISTAL) CLAVICULAR FRACTURES

Injuries to the distal clavicle in young children are rare. In older children and adolescents these injuries appear very similar to acromioclavicular joint injuries. These injuries are really physeal fractures in which the epiphysis and physis maintain their normal anatomic relation to the shoulder joint, whereas the distal metaphysis is displaced superiorly, away from the underlying structures. The periosteal sleeve generally is intact inferiorly, and the ligamentous structures connecting the clavicle to the coracoid usually remain attached to the periosteal sleeve (Fig. 8.7). Because the periosteal sleeve is highly osteogenic, these fractures have a tremendous potential to remodel, and most patients do well with nonoperative treatment. Operative treatment, consisting of open reduction and internal fixation, usually is reserved for adolescent patients with significant displacement and limited remodeling potential. The operative treatment of lateral clavicular injuries is discussed in other chapter.

ACROMIOCLAVICULAR DISLOCATIONS

There are five types of acromioclavicular injuries described in children (Fig. 8.8). Type I injury is not sufficient to completely rupture the acromioclavicular or the coracoclavicular ligaments. Type II injury damages the acromioclavicular ligaments but not the coracoclavicular ligaments; a partial periosteal sleeve (tube) tear also occurs. In type III injury the acromioclavicular ligament is completely ruptured, but the coracoclavicular ligaments are intact because they are still attached to the periosteum. The clavicle is unstable and is displaced superiorly through a rent in the periosteal sleeve (pseudodislocation). Type IV injury is identical to type III except that, in addition to being displaced superiorly, the clavicle is displaced posteriorly. Type V injury is severe; the acromioclavicular ligaments are disrupted, and, although the coracoclavicular ligaments are still attached to the periosteal sleeve, the clavicle is now unstable and its lateral end is buried in the trapezius and deltoid muscles or has pierced them and is located under the skin in the posterior aspect of the shoulder.

In many type III, IV, and V dislocations, an unrecognized fracture of the distal end of the clavicle occurs, with the acromioclavicular and coracoclavicular ligaments remaining intact and attached to the empty periosteal tube

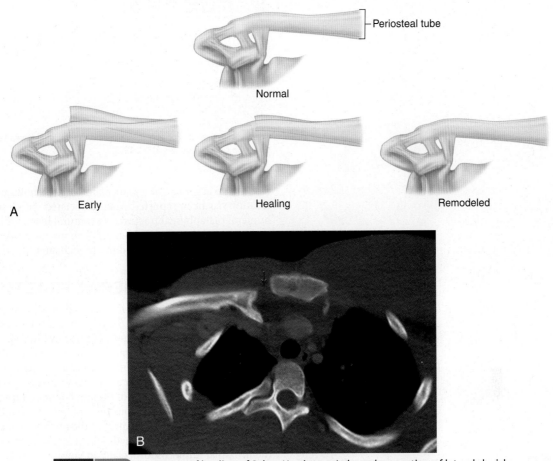

FIGURE 8.6 **A,** Stages of healing of Salter-Harris type I physeal separation of lateral clavicle. **B,** Chronic posterior displaced fracture of sternoclavicular joint (medial).

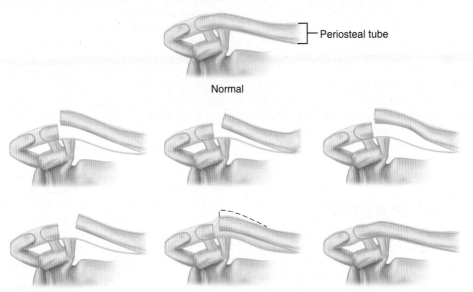

FIGURE 8.7 Distal clavicular fracture with coracoclavicular and coracoacromial ligaments still intact or at least attached to periosteal tube. Fracture in child remodels satisfactorily without surgery.

or to the most distal fragment. In children and adolescents up to age 15 years, types I, II, and III acromioclavicular separations, even with fracture of the distal third of the clavicle, can be treated by nonoperative means. In patients older than age 15 years, type III injuries may require surgery. Open reduction and internal fixation should be considered for markedly displaced types IV and V fractures.

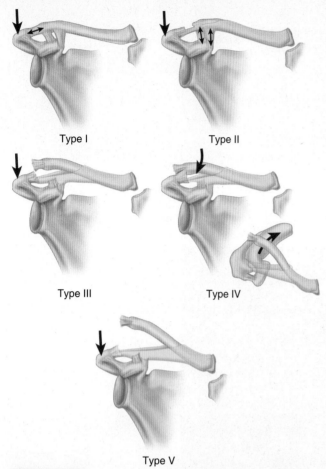

Type I

Type II

Type III

Type IV

Type V

FIGURE 8.8 Five types of acromioclavicular separation occurring in children (see text). Acromioclavicular and coracoclavicular ligaments are attached to periosteal tube, although distal end of clavicle is significantly displaced in types III, IV, and V.

In types IV and V acromioclavicular dislocations, it is important to disengage the distal clavicle from the trapezius and deltoid muscles. If this is unsuccessful by closed means, surgery is indicated to remove the clavicle from the muscles and replace it in the periosteal tube. The periosteal tube should be repaired, and the deltoid-trapezius muscle fascia should be imbricated superiorly over the clavicle. If the repair is unstable, internal fixation is required, as in adults, by acromioclavicular or coracoclavicular fixation, as described in other chapter.

SHOULDER DISLOCATIONS

Shoulder dislocations in children are rare, and proximal humeral physeal fractures are much more common. In a review of 500 glenohumeral dislocations, only eight patients were younger than 10 years of age (1.6%). Another study of 1937 patients aged 10 to 16 years who had closed reduction of a glenohumeral dislocation found that children ages 10 to 12 years composed only 6% of the cohort and had a significantly lower rate of redislocation than older children. It is thought that glenohumeral dislocations in skeletally immature patients may become more common as the level of sports participation increases. A series of 14 skeletally immature patients treated with closed reduction found a redislocation

rate of 21% at a mean of 5 years' follow-up. Glenohumeral dislocation has been reported when associated with a proximal humeral metaphyseal fracture. The natural history, diagnosis, and management of shoulder dislocations for adolescents is similar to adults, as described in other chapter.

PROXIMAL HUMERAL FRACTURES

Proximal humeral fractures are relatively rare in the pediatric population, accounting for 0.5% of pediatric fractures and 4% to 7% of all epiphyseal fractures. Of the physeal fractures, the majority are Salter-Harris type II fractures and Salter-Harris types III and IV are rare. They are most often classified by the Neer-Horowitz classification as shown in Box 8.2. A systematic review of the treatment of proximal humeral fractures in children found that nonunions did not occur and malunions were exceedingly rare, regardless of the method of treatment. This is due to the rapid growth and remodeling potential of the proximal humerus, especially in young children. In children younger than 10 years, it has been shown that angulation of up to 60 degrees can remodel completely, whereas in older children and adolescents it is closer to 20 to 30 degrees. A recent cohort-matched comparison of operative and nonoperative treatment of 32 proximal humeral fractures showed no difference in complications, functional outcome, or patient satisfaction. Within the nonoperatively treated group, there was a higher rate of dissatisfaction in patients older than 12 years treated nonoperatively. They found the odds ratio of an undesirable outcome increased 3.81 for each year of age with nonoperative treatment.

CLOSED TREATMENT

Closed treatment consisting of a sling or hanging arm cast remains the primary method of treatment for these injuries given the tremendous healing and remodeling potential of the proximal humerus. Closed reduction, when necessary, can be performed with sedation and by abducting (90 degrees) and externally rotating (90 degrees) the arm relative to the shoulder. Patients can gradually increase shoulder motion as their symptoms allow. Physical therapy rarely is needed in this population.

OPERATIVE TREATMENT

Operative treatment usually is reserved for older children and adolescents because of the excellent outcomes with nonoperative treatment seen in children younger than 10 years of age. If attempted closed reduction fails, open reduction is indicated. Other indications for open reduction using the deltopectoral approach include open fracture and skeletal maturity (or close to skeletal maturity) (Fig. 8.9A,B). The most common impediments to obtaining a successful closed reduction include the periosteum, biceps tendon, deltoid muscle, and comminuted bone fragments. Once a satisfactory reduction has been achieved, the fracture can be stabilized with Kirschner wires, cannulated screw(s), or flexible titanium elastic intramedullary nails (TEIN), all of which have been shown to have good outcomes. The use of a cannulated screw or screws, which has been shown to be biomechanically stronger than multiple Kirschner wire fixation, has increased because of the soft-tissue irritation and need for a return to the operating room for Kirschner wire removal. The use of TEIN has been shown to produce good radiographic and functional results in several studies; however, implant removal is occasionally necessary because of prominence. A comparison of percutaneous pinning and TEIN found that both techniques are effective in fracture stabilization in older children. The use of TEIN was shown to have a lower complication rate than percutaneous pinning; however, TEIN use was associated with increased blood loss, operative time, rate of reoperation for hardware removal, and cost.

tion using image intensification. This brings the fragments together satisfactorily. This maneuver should push the upper part of the shaft back through the rent in the deltoid muscle and anterior periosteum and correct the anterior angulation. Have an assistant support the proximal fragment to help achieve and maintain the reduction.
- Drill two terminally threaded Steinmann pins through the lateral shaft in a proximal direction into the humeral head to maintain the reduction. In older patients with large metaphyseal fragments, a cannulated screw can be used. The skin incision should be made fairly distal to accommodate the pin trajectory.
- In younger patients, smooth Kirschner wires can be used (Fig. 8.9C).

POSTOPERATIVE CARE Patients are placed in a sling, and gentle range-of-motion exercises are started. Pins can be irritating to the patient and are removed in 3 to 4 weeks.

CLOSED REDUCTION AND PERCUTANEOUS PINNING (OR SCREW FIXATION) OF PROXIMAL HUMERUS

TECHNIQUE 8.1

- Position the patient to allow anteroposterior and axillary lateral images of the injured shoulder. Prepare and drape the patient in a sterile manner.
- Manipulate the distal fragment into slight external rotation, 90 degrees of flexion, and 70 degrees of abduc-

CLOSED REDUCTION AND INTRAMEDULLARY NAILING OF PROXIMAL HUMERUS

TECHNIQUE 8.2

- Position the patient to allow anteroposterior and axillary lateral images of the injured shoulder. Prepare and drape the patient in a sterile manner.
- Make a lateral incision over the supracondylar ridge. Drill two holes in the lateral cortex using a drill slightly larger

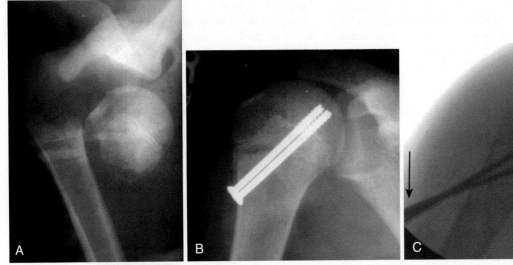

A   B   C

FIGURE 8.9   **A,** Irreducible dislocation-Salter-Harris type II fracture of proximal humerus in 15-year-old boy. **B,** After open reduction and screw fixation. **C,** Smooth Kirschner wires can also be used in younger patients. **SEE TECHNIQUE 8.1.**

than the diameter nail selected. Alternatively, one medial and one lateral hole can be drilled. If a medial nail is used, care must be taken to protect the ulnar nerve.

■ Prebend the nail and pass it retrograde to the fracture site. Gently reduce the fracture using fluoroscopic guidance and pass the first nail. Repeat for the second nail either through the lateral or second medial incision.

■ When the fracture reduction is adequate, cut the nails beneath the skin for later removal. If acceptable reduction after two attempts cannot be obtained, proceed with open reduction using the deltopectoral interval.

POSTOPERATIVE CARE Place the arm in a soft dressing with sling and begin motion. Nails are typically removed in 3 to 6 months or sooner if the implant is causing symptoms and the fracture is healed.

HUMERAL SHAFT FRACTURES

Humeral shaft fractures in children are uncommon, accounting for less than 10% of all humeral fractures in children. Most occur either in children younger than 3 years or older than 12 years, and almost all of these injuries can be treated nonoperatively because of the remodeling potential of the humerus and the ability of the glenohumeral joint to accommodate for any residual malalignment. Up to 70 degrees of angulation in children younger than 5 years and 30 degrees of angulation in children ages 12 to 13 can be accepted. Less angulation in distal fractures, especially those in varus, is acceptable because of the undesirable cosmetic appearance of the arm. Closed treatment usually consists of coaptation splinting, fracture bracing, or the use of a hanging arm cast. Operative treatment, consisting of plating or the use of TEIN, has been shown to provide good results. External fixation can be used in rare conditions in which severe soft-tissue injuries are present. Indications for operative treatment include patients with polytrauma to speed mobilization and upper extremity weight bearing, a floating elbow, a pathologic lesion, and adolescents close to skeletal maturity. Radial nerve entrapment can occur, especially with distal fractures after closed reduction maneuvers. A loss of radial nerve function after closed reduction indicates potential entrapment of the nerve between the fracture fragments, and urgent nerve exploration and internal fixation are necessary. Plating techniques for children are similar to adults as discussed in other chapter.

CLOSED/OPEN REDUCTION AND INTRAMEDULLARY NAILING OF HUMERAL SHAFT

TECHNIQUE 8.3

■ Position the patient to allow anteroposterior and axillary lateral images of the injured humerus. This can be done

on a radiolucent table or hand table. Prepare and drape the patient in a sterile manner.

■ Make a lateral incision over the supracondylar ridge. Drill two holes in the lateral cortex using a drill slightly larger than the diameter nail selected. Alternatively, one medial and one lateral hole can be drilled. If a medial nail is used, care must be taken to protect the ulnar nerve.

■ Place the nail over the skin to radiographically determine where the fracture site will be on the nail. Gently bend the nail with the apex of the bow at the fracture site. Pass both nails retrograde to the fracture site. Gently reduce the fracture using fluoroscopic guidance and pass the first nail 1 to 2 cm across the fracture site. Repeat for the second nail either through the lateral or a second medial incision. Once both nails have crossed the fracture site, advance them to their final positions.

■ When the fracture reduction is adequate, cut the nails beneath the skin for later removal. If acceptable reduction cannot be obtained after two attempts, proceed with open reduction.

POSTOPERATIVE CARE Place the arm in a soft dressing with sling and begin motion. Nails typically are removed in 4 to 6 months or sooner if the implant is causing symptoms.

SUPRACONDYLAR HUMERAL FRACTURES

A review of over 63,000 supracondylar humeral fractures in the United States over a 5-year period showed the rate of injury to be 60 to 70 per 100,000 children. The mean age of patients with closed fractures was 5.5 years (52% male), with 54% of them occurring in children 4 to 6 years of age. Older patients (mean age, 9.1 years) were more likely to sustain open fractures and neurologic injuries. Almost all (98%) are extension-type injuries, which usually are caused by a fall onto an outstretched hand. Flexion-type fractures, although rarer, are more difficult to reduce, have worse outcomes, and are associated with ulnar nerve injury (Fig. 8.10). Approximately 5% to 10% of children have an associated ipsilateral distal radial fracture. The most commonly used classification is that by Gartland in which type I fractures are nondisplaced, type II fractures have an intact posterior hinge, and type III fractures have complete displacement. A type IV injury has been described in which there is complete loss of the anterior and posterior periosteal hinge, making it unstable in both flexion and extension. Type IV fractures usually are the result of high-energy injury. Care must be taken when reducing a type III fracture to avoid tearing the periosteal hinge, making it a type IV injury. The diagnosis can be made in most cases using plain radiographs. Advanced imaging, such as CT, occasionally is used in an adolescent when there are concerns about a coronal split in the distal fragment or T-condylar fracture.

A careful neurologic examination is essential because 10% to 15% of patients have a nerve injury, with the anterior interosseous nerve being the most frequently injured in extension-type fractures. The ulnar nerve is most frequently injured in flexion-type injuries in 10% of patients. Obese children have been shown to have a higher rate of both pre-operative and postoperative nerve palsy and higher rate of open reduction. A loss of neurologic function after reduction is concerning for nerve entrapment at the time of reduction, and urgent open exploration of the nerve is necessary. Most nerve injuries are a result of neurapraxia and resolve within 6 to 12 weeks; electromyography is indicated if there is no return of nerve function within 3 months. A recent long-term follow-up study of patients with neurologic injuries showed that at an average follow-up of 8 years most patients had excellent function; 100% of patients with radial nerve, 88% of patients with median nerve, and only 25% of patients with ulnar nerve injuries fully recovered.

Urgent assessment of the vascular status of the limb also is essential to minimize complications. A vascular injury,

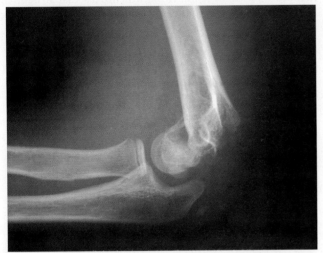

FIGURE 8.10 Flexion type supracondylar humeral fracture.

typically to the brachial artery, can occur in up to 10% to 20% of patients with a type III fracture (Fig. 8.11). Because of the rich collateral blood supply about the elbow, the hand may be well perfused even with complete disruption of the brachial artery. The vascular status of the limb can be classified as normal—pulseless but with a warm pink (perfused) hand—or pulseless, pale (nonperfused) hand. Treatment of patients with a pulseless warm hand remains controversial in terms of the need for brachial artery exploration (Fig. 8.12). A supracondylar fracture with a nonperfused hand is a surgical emergency to prevent reperfusion injury and compartment syndrome leading to Volkmann ischemic contracture. Compartment syndrome occurs in approximately 0.1% to 0.3% of patients with supracondylar humeral fractures and is more common with concurrent fracture of the forearm or wrist. In pediatric patients, the 3 A's—*a*gitation, *a*nxiety, and increasing *a*nalgesia requirements—are sensitive and reliable indicators of impending compartment syndrome.

In patients with vascular compromise, urgent reduction in the operating room should be performed and the vascular status of the hand assessed. Arteriography should not be used unless the level of vascular injury is unclear in patients with polytrauma and should never delay closed reduction of a supracondylar humeral fracture. If perfusion is not restored, urgent exploration of the brachial artery with release of entrapping structures and direct repair with vein grafting if necessary should be performed by a surgeon with experience in the repair of small vessels. Prophylactic forearm and hand fasciotomies are necessary in patients with prolonged ischemia time. This is especially important in patients with concomitant nerve injuries in which the ability to detect a compartment syndrome clinically is impaired. Most patients in whom perfusion is restored (pink hand) even in the absence of a radial pulse have good long-term outcomes with observation.

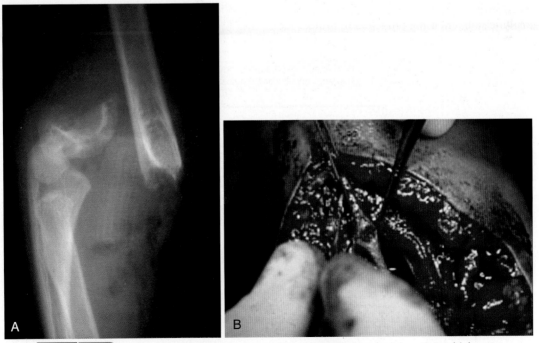

FIGURE 8.11 **A,** Type III supracondylar humeral fracture with vascular injury. **B,** Brachial artery occlusion with supracondylar humeral fracture.

Treatment of supracondylar humeral fractures is based on the Gartland type. Type I fractures are treated with long arm cast immobilization for 3 weeks followed by a brief period of protected activity. Patients with the presence of a posterior fat pad on radiographs should be presumed to have a type I fracture and treated in this fashion.

Treatment of type II injuries is somewhat controversial. Wilkins subdivided type II injuries into A and B with type IIA fractures being stable and type IIB fractures having some degree of rotation or translation making them unstable. Closed reduction and casting can be used in patients with type IIA injuries. Closed reduction and percutaneous pinning typically with two or three lateral pins has become the main form of treatment for type IIB injuries and for those in which the stability is in question. Pinning is preferred for most type II fractures because of concerns about the ability to maintain reduction in a splint or cast, poor patient compliance with barriers to timely follow-up, and difficulty in differentiating between type IIA and B fractures. Type III and IV fractures are treated with closed reduction and pinning (Fig. 8.13).

Complications of percutaneous pinning occur in approximately 5% of patients, with pin migration or irritation being the most common followed by infection (1%) and elbow stiffness. The ideal pin configuration remains controversial; however, although crossed medial and lateral pins are more stable than two lateral pins in vitro, use of two or three lateral pins appears to be equal to crossed pins in vivo. A comparison study of medial crossed pins and lateral entry pins showed equal maintenance of reduction in both groups, but the crossed pin group had a 7.7% rate of iatrogenic nerve injury. This rate of iatrogenic nerve injury with crossed pins has been shown in other studies as well. If lateral pinning is used, it is important to engage both fragments and have bicortical fixation with at least two pins and at least 2 mm of pin separation at the fracture site. Most centers use two or three lateral pins for most type III fractures and use a medial pin for fractures that are very unstable (Figs. 8.14 and 8.15). If a medial pin is used, making a small incision and using retractors to protect the

ulnar nerve, as well as avoiding pinning these fractures in maximal elbow flexion, can reduce the rate of ulnar nerve injury. It is difficult to maintain reduction of type IV fractures because of the loss of the periosteal hinges. For this reason, it may be necessary to hold the arm stable and rotate the C-arm for imaging rather than rotating the arm. A transolecranon pin placed retrograde from the proximal ulna into the humeral shaft can be used to provisionally control these highly unstable fractures during pinning (Fig. 8.16A,B). The indications for open reduction, which occurs approximately 10% of the time, include irreducible fractures, open fractures, and those with suspected or confirmed neurovascular injuries. A direct anterior approach can be used in most patients with posterior displaced fracture because it provides the best access to the neurovascular structures and fracture site. Because of the muscle stripping that occurs with these injuries, the neurovascular structures are typically in a subcutaneous position (Fig. 8.17).

CLOSED REDUCTION AND PERCUTANEOUS PINNING OF SUPRACONDYLAR FRACTURES (TWO LATERAL PINS)

TECHNIQUE 8.4

- Position the patient supine and position the elbow on an inverted image intensifier (see Fig. 8.15A).
- For the more common extension type of supracondylar fracture, with countertraction on the humerus, apply traction to the forearm and examine the fracture with image intensification. With the elbow in extension, correct rotational malalignment and medial and lateral translation. Once this is corrected, maintain traction on the elbow

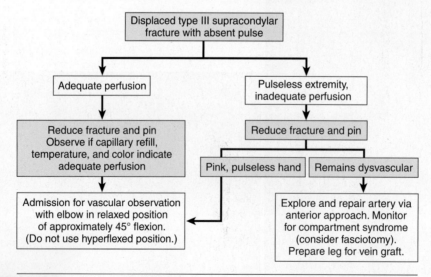

FIGURE 8.12 Management of pulseless supracondylar humeral fracture. (From Abzug JM, Herman MJ: Management of supracondylar humerus fractures in children: current concepts, *J Am Acad Orthop Surg* 20:69, 2012.)

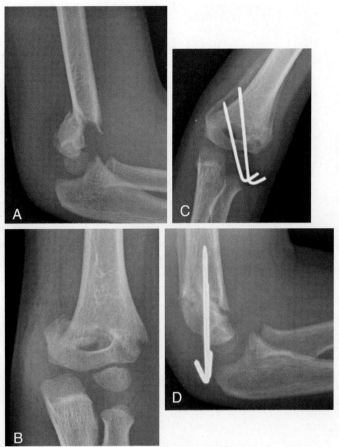

FIGURE 8.13 Fixation of supracondylar fracture. **A** and **B,** Severely displaced type III supracondylar fracture. **C** and **D,** Closed reduction and percutaneous pinning were performed.

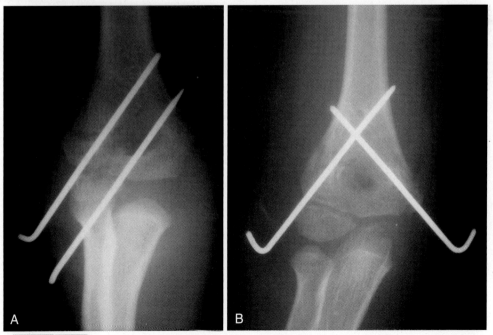

FIGURE 8.14 Fixation of supracondylar humeral fractures is most commonly done with **(A)** two lateral pins or **(B)** two crossed pins.

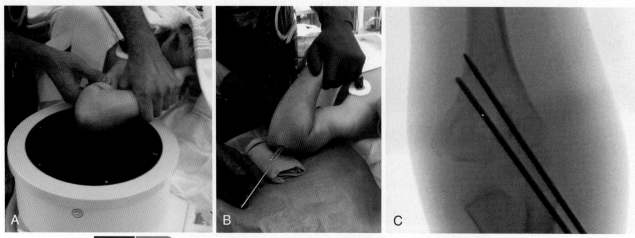

FIGURE 8.15 Pinning of supracondylar humeral fracture. **A,** Positioning of arm on image intensifier. **B,** Confirm that lateral pins engage fracture fragments. **C,** Final fluoroscopic imaging. **SEE TECHNIQUE 8.4.**

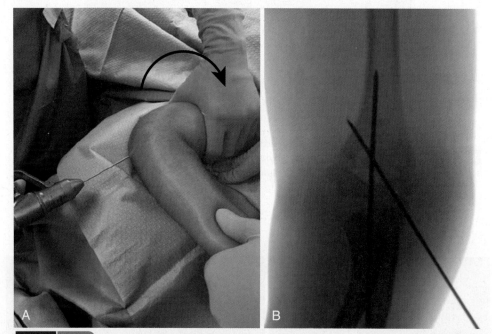

FIGURE 8.16 Transolecranon pin placed retrograde from proximal ulna to humeral shaft can be used to provisionally control unstable flexion-type supracondylar fractures during pinning. **A,** Proximal humerus must be manually externally rotated (*arrow*) to avoid rotational malalignment. **B,** Fluoroscopic image shows transolecranon and laterally based Steinmann pin. (From Green BM, Stone JD, Bruce RW Jr, et al: The use of a transolecranon pin in the treatment of pediatric flexion type supracondylar humerus fractures, *J Pediatr Orthop* 37:e347, 2017.)

and gently flex the elbow to 120 degrees. Use anteriorly directed pressure on the olecranon as the elbow is flexed to correct extension of the distal fragment. Maximally flex the elbow and pronate the forearm to lock the posterior and medial soft-tissue hinges. It is important to correct rotation and translation before flexing the elbow.
- For the rarer flexion-type injury, flexing the elbow will further displace the fragment because of the disruption of the posterior periosteal hinge. In this case the elbow will need to be pinned in extension. This can be difficult, and posterior open reduction often is needed. Alternatively,

a "push-pull" technique (Fig. 8.18) can be used to help achieve reduction.
- Confirm the anteroposterior reduction with image intensification, aiming the beam through the forearm and rotating the humerus from medial to lateral to assess the medial and lateral column reduction. Confirm lateral reduction by externally rotating the shoulder to obtain a lateral view of the elbow.
- Maintain reduction while performing closed percutaneous pinning with image intensification to verify that the two lateral pins engage both fracture fragments (see

Fig. 8.15B). The pins should be divergent and not cross at the fracture site.

- If a medial pin is used, make a 1 cm incision over the medial epicondyle. Spread the soft tissues so that the epicondyle can be seen and ensure that the ulnar nerve is protected. Alternatively, a small soft-tissue drill sleeve can be used. It is not necessary to expose or explore the ulnar nerve in patients without ulnar nerve symptoms. Once the pin is placed, it can be cut outside the skin and the incision closed with absorbable suture.
- After the pins are inserted, extend the elbow as far as possible without bending the pins. With the aid of im-

age intensification, check the stability of the reduction by rotating and stressing the elbow to determine if a third (medial or lateral) pin is necessary. Compare the carrying angle with that of the normal extremity. Cut and bend the pins outside of the skin and check final fluoroscopic images to ensure no displacement occurred during bending (Fig. 8.15C).

POSTOPERATIVE CARE Place the patient in a well-padded posterior splint or bivalved cast with the elbow flexed at 75 degrees to allow for swelling and convert to a long arm cast with the elbow flexed 90 degrees at 1 week. Patients are treated in a cast for 3 to 4 weeks. The pins are then removed, and gentle range of motion is started.

See also Video 8.1.

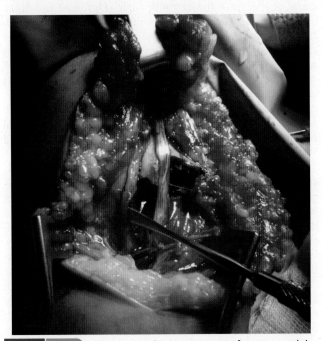

FIGURE 8.17 Neurovascular structures of supracondylar humerus. Medial nerve and brachial artery under Freer elevator. **SEE TECHNIQUE 8.5.**

ANTERIOR APPROACH

See Figure 8.17

TECHNIQUE 8.5

- If an anterior approach is to be used, make a transverse incision over the antecubital space. This can be extended proximally and distally if necessary. The proximal extension should be performed (medial or lateral) over the proximal fragment because this is usually the site of neurovascular injury. Note that in high-energy injuries the anterior soft tissues may be stripped and the neurovascular bundle may be subcutaneous.

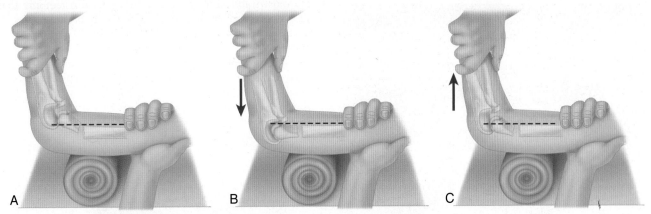

FIGURE 8.18 "Push-pull" reduction method. **A,** Before attempted reduction rolled towel is placed to be used as fulcrum. **B,** The "push" maneuver is used to over-reduce fracture into extension. **C,** Then fracture is "pulled" back to align anterior humeral line with middle of capitellum. (Redrawn from Chukwunyerenwa C, Orlik B, El-Hawary R, et al: Treatment of flexion-type supracondylar fractures in children: the "push-pull" method for closed reduction and percutaneous K-wire fixation, *J Pediatr Orthop B* 25:412, 2016.) **SEE TECHNIQUE 8.4.**

- Develop a plane between the biceps and brachialis tendons. Release the biceps aponeurosis while protecting the brachial artery. Retract the biceps and brachialis muscle medially and the brachioradialis laterally. Protect the radial nerve and posterior interosseous artery.
- Observe the supracondylar fragment and note its alignment with the proximal fragment. Use a small curet to remove any hematoma at the fracture site. Note any interdigitations on the ends of the bone, and by matching them reduce the fracture.
- Use two or three Steinmann pins in a manner similar to that described for percutaneous pinning. Image intensification simplifies pin placement. Cut the pins off outside the skin for removal later.

POSTOPERATIVE CARE Close the incision and place the patient in a well-padded posterior splint with the elbow in 60 degrees of flexion to allow for swelling and convert to a long arm cast to 90 degrees of flexion in 5 to 7 days. The pins are removed in 3 to 4 weeks, and gentle range-of-motion exercises are begun.

The timing of reduction for type III fractures remains controversial; however, recent studies have shown no difference in complication rates between patients treated in an urgent (<12 hours) or delayed (later than 12 hours) fashion. Delayed treatment requires a conscious, cooperative patient without neurovascular compromise and the ability to proceed with surgery in a timely fashion if their neurovascular examination changes with monitoring. Type II fractures can be treated safely in a delayed fashion.

Postoperatively, patients are placed either in a long arm posterior splint or a bivalved cast with the elbow in 60 degrees of flexion to allow for swelling. Follow-up radiographs are obtained at 1 week, and the cast or splint is removed and changed to a long arm cast with the elbow in 90 degrees for an additional 2 to 3 weeks. The pins are removed in the office, and most patients regain motion without the need for physical therapy. Most children, unlike adults, have good mid-term

and long-term functional outcomes after supracondylar humeral fracture.

Cubitus varus is the most common angular deformity that results from supracondylar fractures in children (Fig. 8.19). Cubitus valgus, although mentioned in the literature as causing tardy ulnar nerve palsy, rarely occurs and is more often caused by nonunion of lateral condylar fractures. Because the normal carrying angle increases from childhood to adulthood, an increase in valgus is not as cosmetically noticeable as a complete reversal to a varus position.

Several causes for cubitus varus have been suggested. Medial displacement and rotation of the distal fragment have been cited most often, but experimental studies showed that varus tilting of the distal fragment was the most important cause of change in the carrying angle (Figs. 8.20 and 8.21). This can occur with relatively benign-appearing type II fractures, with medial column instability leading to collapse when the fracture is treated with cast immobilization. Osteonecrosis and delayed growth of the trochlea, with relative overgrowth of the normal lateral side of the distal humeral epiphysis, is an extremely rare cause of progressive cubitus varus deformity after supracondylar fracture. This progressive growth abnormality cannot be prevented by stabilization of the distal fragment because it probably is related to injury to the blood supply of the trochlea at the time of fracture.

Rotational malalignment may occur but is not a significant deformity as malrotation of the distal humerus is compensated for to a large degree by motion of the shoulder joint. As a result, the rotational component in cubitus varus deformities is of little consequence and all that is usually necessary for correction is a lateral closing wedge osteotomy. Occasionally, a hyperextension deformity requires the addition of a flexion component.

Three basic types of osteotomies have been described: a lateral closing wedge osteotomy, a medial opening wedge osteotomy with a bone graft, and an oblique osteotomy with derotation. Uchida et al. described a three-dimensional osteotomy for correction of cubitus varus deformity in which medial and posterior tilt and rotation of the distal fragment can be corrected if necessary.

A lateral closing wedge osteotomy is the easiest, safest, most stable, and most commonly used osteotomy that allows correction in both the sagittal and coronal planes. A review of 18 patients who had lateral humeral closing wedge osteotomy and ulnar nerve release at a mean age of 8 years found improvement in mean elbow flexion from 101 to 126 degrees. Supracondylar osteotomy for cubitus varus should

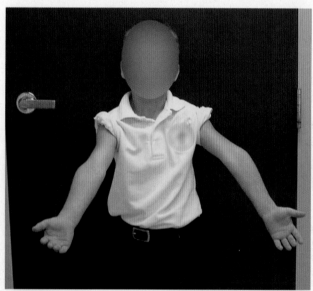

FIGURE 8.19 Cubitus varus deformity of left elbow.

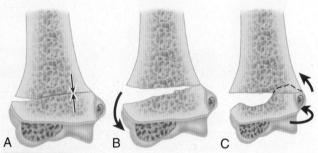

FIGURE 8.20 Mechanism of coronal tilting. **A,** Impaction of fracture medially. **B,** Tilting of fragment medially. **C,** Horizontal rotation.

be viewed as a reconstructive procedure and not as fracture management. The fixation used can be tailored to the age of the child and degree of deformity (Fig. 8.22). A combination of screws and Kirschner wires may be needed for younger patients, whereas plate-and-screw fixation is more appropriate for adolescents.

DeRosa and Graziano reported good results with a step-cut osteotomy technique fixed with a single cortical screw (Fig. 8.23). While this technique is technically more challenging, they reported no ulnar or radial nerve injuries, infections, nonunions, or hypertrophic scars, and all patients retained preoperative ranges of motion. They concluded that this osteotomy with single-screw fixation is a safe procedure that can correct multiple planes of deformity, but they emphasized the importance of careful preoperative planning and special attention to surgical detail. If a more extensive osteotomy is needed,

a step-cut translation osteotomy and fixation with a Y-shaped humeral plate that allows early movement of the joint may be used.

LATERAL CLOSING WEDGE OSTEOTOMY FOR CUBITUS VARUS

TECHNIQUE 8.6

- After standard preparation and draping and inflation of the tourniquet, approach the elbow through a lateral incision.

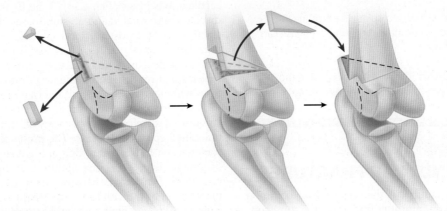

FIGURE 8.21 Three-dimensional osteotomy for correction of cubitus varus deformity. Medial and posterior tilt is corrected. After osteotomy, distal fragment is compacted with proximal fragment by adding external rotation using wedge of humeral cortex. Bone graft is added if necessary. (From Uchida Y, Ogata K, Sugioka Y: A new three-dimensional osteotomy for cubitus varus deformity after supracondylar fracture of the humerus in children, *J Pediatr Orthop* 11:327, 1991.)

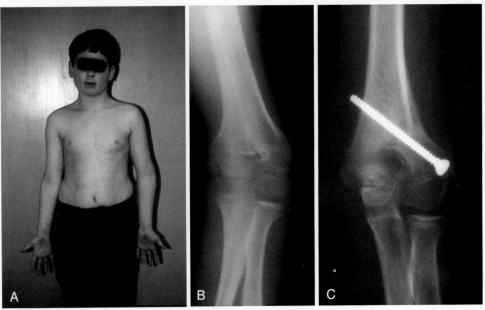

FIGURE 8.22 **A** and **B,** Cubitus varus deformity of left elbow after cast treatment of supracondylar humeral fracture. **C,** After osteotomy and screw fixation.

- With fluoroscopic guidance, insert two Kirschner wires into the lateral condyle before osteotomy and advance them just distal to the planned distal cut. Alternatively, guide pins in preparation for cannulated screw placement can be used. Be prepared to advance these proximally after the closing wedge osteotomy has been made.
- Make a closing wedge osteotomy laterally, leaving the medial cortex intact. The saw or osteotome cuts can be angled in the sagittal plane to correct any flexion deformity as well.
- Weaken the medial cortex using drill holes. Apply a valgus stress to complete the osteotomy with the forearm in pronation and the elbow flexed.
- Close the osteotomy and advance the Kirschner wires or guidewires from the lateral condyle into the medial cortex of the proximal fragment.
- Stabilize the osteotomy with either Kirschner wires or cannulated screws.
- Close the wound in layers and splint the arm in 90 degrees of flexion and full pronation. A long arm cast can be applied in 5 to 7 days.

POSTOPERATIVE CARE The wires, if used, are removed at approximately 6 weeks after surgery, and a range-of-motion exercise program is started.

LATERAL CONDYLAR FRACTURES

Fracture of the lateral condyle is the second most common (17%) pediatric elbow fracture after fracture of the supracondylar humerus, usually occurring between the ages of 4 and 6 years. The most common mechanism of injury is a fall onto an outstretched arm with the elbow in varus, which causes avulsion of the lateral humeral condyle. Alternatively, these injuries can occur, although less commonly, during a fall onto a flexed elbow. Unlike supracondylar humeral fractures, lateral condylar fractures are rarely associated with neurovascular injuries.

These injuries can be classified either anatomically or by displacement. Historically, the Milch classification was used to determine whether the fracture passed through (type I) or around (type II) the capitellum. The Milch type II fracture, which is really a Salter-Harris type II fracture, is the most common type (95%) (Fig. 8.24). More often the fractures are classified by displacement because the amount of displacement determines the method of treatment. A recent displacement-based classification system by Weiss et al. has been shown to be prognostic for complications. Type I fractures are displaced less than 2 mm, type II fractures are displaced more than 2 mm with an intact cartilaginous hinge, and type III fractures are displaced more than 2 mm without an intact cartilaginous hinge (Fig. 8.25). Type III fractures tend to be displaced and rotated and, in some cases, if enough trochlear stability is lost, a posterolateral subluxation of the radius and ulna can occur (Fig. 8.26). This classification also helps guide treatment, because type I fractures can be treated with a cast, type II fractures with percutaneous pinning, and type III fractures with open reduction and internal fixation.

Radiographically, it can be difficult to determine the amount of displacement because of the large amount of unossified epiphysis present. The presence of a metaphyseal fragment on the lateral radiograph is helpful in making the diagnosis (Fig. 8.27). The addition of an internal oblique radiograph is necessary to assess the true amount of displacement. It can be difficult to determine the stability of the cartilaginous hinge on plain radiographs, and it may be necessary to perform stress radiographs or arthrography under anesthesia for full assessment. Advanced imaging such as MRI can be used when the diagnosis is in question or to evaluate the stability of the cartilaginous hinge; however, this may require sedation to obtain satisfactory high-resolution images in this age group.

Nondisplaced or minimally displaced fractures can be treated in a long arm cast for 4 to 6 weeks depending on the age of the patient. These fractures need to be watched closely because late displacement can occur in 5% to 10% of fractures. For type II fractures or fractures in which there is concern about the integrity of the cartilaginous hinge, a stress examination under anesthesia with or without arthrography may be performed. In patients with a large metaphyseal fragment, percutaneous pinning using smooth Kirschner wires or a cannulated screw is performed. Displaced fractures or those with unclear reduction require open reduction and internal

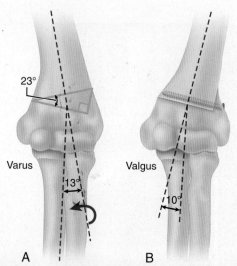

FIGURE 8.23 **A,** Osteotomy designed to correct cubitus varus deformity of 13 degrees. Distal fragment can be rotated to correct additional deformity. **B,** After wedge removal and closure, screw is used for fixation. **SEE TECHNIQUE 8.6.** (Redrawn from DeRosa GP, Graziano GP: A new osteotomy for cubitus varus, *Clin Orthop Relat Res* 236:160, 1988.)

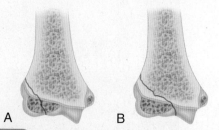

FIGURE 8.24 Lateral humeral condylar fractures. **A,** Milch type I fracture, which is Salter-Harris type IV epiphyseal fracture. **B,** Milch type II fracture, which is Salter-Harris type II epiphyseal fracture.

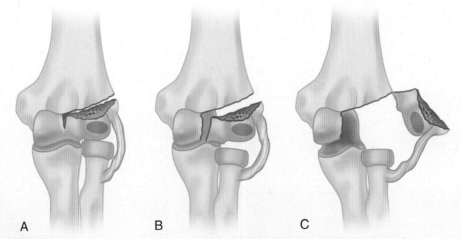

FIGURE 8.25   Weiss classification of lateral condylar fractures. **A**, Type 1 fracture, less than 2 mm displacement. **B**, Type 2 fracture, 2 mm or more displacement and congruity of articular surface. **C**, Type 3 fracture, 2 mm or more displacement and lack of articular congruity.

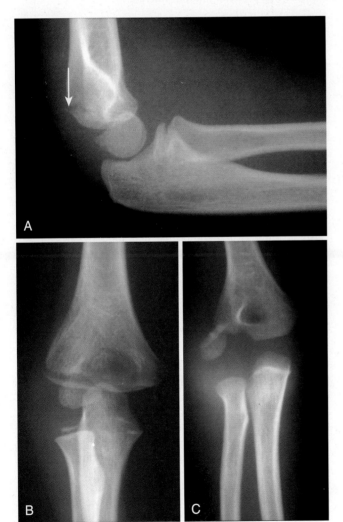

FIGURE 8.26   Fractures of lateral humeral condyle. **A**, Type I, stable fracture with minimal lateral gap *(arrow)*. **B**, Type II, fracture to epiphyseal cartilage with a lateral gap; displacement risk undefined. **C**, Type III, fracture gap as wide laterally as medially; high risk of later displacement.

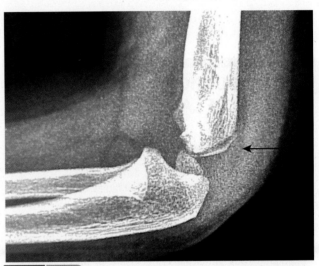

FIGURE 8.27   Metaphyseal fragment on lateral radiograph.

fixation (Fig. 8.28). This is done most commonly through a lateral approach, taking care to avoid dissection posteriorly that may injure the blood supply to the trochlea, which enters posteriorly, and cause osteonecrosis. Alternatively, in rare cases when a lateral approach is not possible, a posterior approach protecting the posterior blood supply has been described. Fixation using smooth Kirschner wires and cannulated screws has been described with good results. The use of cannulated screws is becoming more common as they allow for fracture-site compression, leading to faster time to union and earlier mobilization and avoiding the risk of pin site infections with Kirschner wires. If Kirschner wires are used, typically in younger patients, they can safely be left outside the skin for 3 to 4 weeks to avoid a second surgical procedure to remove buried wires.

The most common complication after fracture of the lateral condyle is loss of reduction. Therefore close follow-up is necessary for these patients. Even fractures with less than 2 mm of initial displacement can displace late.

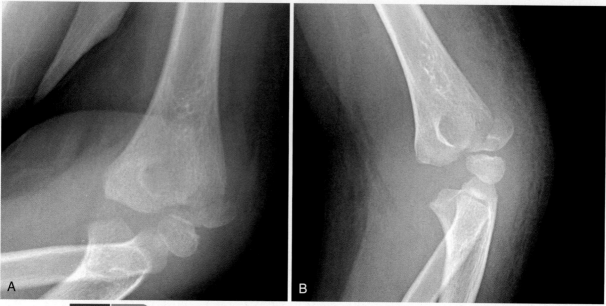

FIGURE 8.28   **A** and **B,** Radiographs showing displaced type III lateral condylar fracture.

OPEN REDUCTION AND INTERNAL FIXATION OF LATERAL CONDYLAR FRACTURE

TECHNIQUE 8.7

- Expose the elbow through a Kocher lateral approach and carry the dissection down to the lateral humeral condyle. A headlamp often is helpful to improve visualization. In some patients, especially with type III fractures, the distal fragment is rotated and the articular cartilage is subcutaneous, and care is necessary to prevent iatrogenic articular cartilage injury. The soft-tissue dissection is between the brachioradialis and the triceps, although often the capsule is already torn. Expose the anterior surface of the joint. It is important that no dissection be performed posteriorly to prevent injury to the trochlear blood supply.
- The displacement and the size of the fragment are always greater than is apparent on radiographs because much of the fragment is cartilaginous. The fragment usually is rotated and displaced. Irrigate the joint to remove blood clots and debris, reduce the articular surface accurately, and confirm the reduction by observing the articular surface, particularly at the trochlear ridge. Because of the plastic deformation that often occurs, there may be some metaphyseal displacement, even with anatomic articular surface reduction. The fracture should be stabilized in the position of anatomic joint reduction regardless of the metaphyseal deformity.
- Insert two smooth Kirschner wires across it into the medial cortex of the distal humerus in a divergent fashion.

Alternatively, a cannulated screw, typically 4.5 mm, can be used if the metaphyseal fragment is large enough.
- Check the reduction and the position of the internal fixation by stress fluoroscopy before closing the wound. Cut off the ends of the wires outside the skin for removal in the clinic (Fig. 8.29).
- Place the arm in a bivalved long arm cast or splint with the elbow flexed 90 degrees.

POSTOPERATIVE CARE   Immobilization should continue 4 weeks with the arm in a cast followed in some cases by splinting. At the end of that time the pins can be removed if union is progressing. Gentle active motion of the elbow usually is resumed intermittently out of the splint. These fractures need to be monitored for late and delayed union, and some require immobilization with intermittent range-of-motion exercises for more than 6 weeks.

COMPLICATIONS AFTER LATERAL CONDYLAR FRACTURE

Complications from lateral condylar fractures include physeal arrest, physeal stimulation, osteonecrosis, and nonunion with resultant cubitus valgus (Fig. 8.30). Lateral condylar overgrowth, radial prominence, and variation in the carrying angle of the elbow have been attributed to transient stimulation of the lateral column of the elbow. Osteonecrosis of the capitellum (Fig. 8.31) or a small growth arrest in the central physis occurs with "fishtail" deformity (deepening of the trochlear groove) and rare varus deformity (see Fig. 8.30). Because of the lack of cases, data concerning prevention, treatment, and long-term follow-up are limited.

Nonunion with resultant cubitus varus probably is the most significant complication (Fig. 8.32). The most common

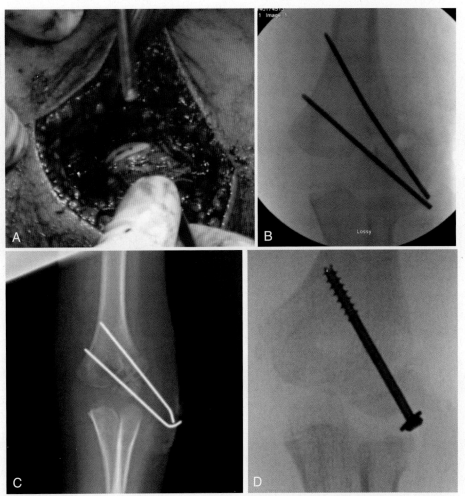

FIGURE 8.29 **A,** Open reduction and internal fixation of lateral condylar fracture shown in Fig. 8.28. **B,** After open reduction and fixation with smooth wires. **C,** After open reduction with Kirschner wires. **D,** After screw fixation. **SEE TECHNIQUE 8.7.**

risk factors for nonunion include type III fractures and fractures that are more difficult to reduce. Nonunion must be differentiated from delayed union. A delay in union may result from inadequate external immobilization or internal fixation. If union is not achieved at 12 weeks, a small wedge-shaped bone graft can be placed across the metaphyseal fragment with supplemental smooth pin or screw fixation (Fig. 8.33). If the elbow is stable and is not painful and all that is present is a lucent line with no motion of the fracture fragment on stress views, observation and prolonged immobilization may be all that are necessary. If motion is present or a nonunion seems to be developing, however, early surgery is indicated. Surgery for well-established nonunions is difficult, and the goals should be to restore a more anatomic alignment of the elbow. Arthrotomy and realignment of the articular surface should be avoided because of the high risk of further elbow stiffness and osteonecrosis; osteotomy generally is a better option (Figs. 8.34 and 8.35). Rigid internal fixation should be used to promote early motion. Tardy ulnar nerve palsy can accompany lateral condyle nonunions and can be treated with ulnar nerve transposition and correction of the cubitus valgus.

OSTEOTOMY FOR ESTABLISHED CUBITUS VALGUS SECONDARY TO NONUNION OR GROWTH ARREST

TECHNIQUE 8.8

- Place the patient prone with the forearm supported on an arm board.
- Use a posterior muscle-splitting incision, exposing the distal humerus, but do not open the elbow joint. Take care to protect the radial nerve proximally.
- Split the fibers of the triceps muscle, retract them, and identify the ulnar nerve. When indicated for treatment of tardy ulnar nerve palsy, transpose the nerve anteriorly.
- As a landmark, note the upper limit of the condylar fragment. Perform a transverse osteotomy at the level of the intersection of the forearm axis with the lateral cortex of the humerus (Fig. 8.35A,B).

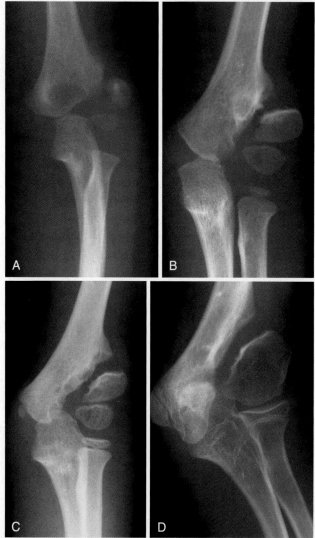

FIGURE **8.30** **A,** Fracture of lateral humeral condyle in 5-year-old boy. **B,** Established valgus nonunion 1 year after nonoperative treatment (observation only). **C,** Apparent proximal migration of capitellum and condyle at 3 years. **D,** Severe cubitus valgus 9 years after fracture.

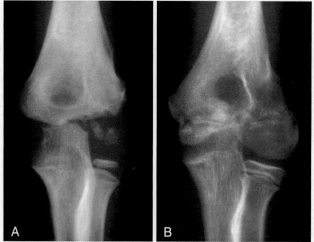

FIGURE **8.31** **A,** Fracture of lateral humeral condyle through ossific nucleus. **B,** Development of osteonecrosis of capitellum with subsequent overgrowth.

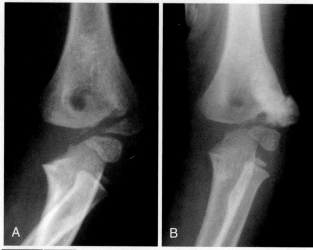

FIGURE **8.32** **A** and **B,** Varus nonunion of lateral condylar fracture after closed treatment.

■ Notch the inferior surface of the proximal fragment to receive the apex of the superior surface of the distal fragment, which is moved laterally (Fig. 8.35C,D). Adduct the distal fragment until the excessive angle of abduction (valgus) has been reduced to the normal carrying angle, controlling the amount of correction by radiographs made with the extremity and the fragments in extension.

■ When correction is satisfactory, stabilize the fragments by inserting two smooth crossed Kirschner wires or cannulated screw(s), carefully flex the elbow to 90 degrees, and immobilize it in a long arm cast.

POSTOPERATIVE CARE The cast is left on for 4 to 6 weeks, depending on the age of the child and evidence of bony union. The wires are removed, and motion is encouraged at that time.

MEDIAL CONDYLAR FRACTURES

Fractures of the medial humeral condyle in children are rare, accounting for 1% of pediatric elbow fractures. They usually occur in slightly older children than fractures of the lateral condyle, around the ages of 3 to 8 years. They are caused by a direct fall onto the elbow or a fall onto an outstretched hand with the elbow in a varus position. Medial condylar fractures in younger children can be associated with nonaccidental trauma. Kilfoyle described three types based on displacement: type I, a greenstick or impacted fracture; type II, a fracture through the humeral condyle into the joint with little or no displacement (Fig. 8.36); and type III, an epiphyseal fracture that is intraarticular and involves the medial condyle with the fragment displaced and rotated (Fig. 8.37). Type III fractures, which occur in older children, account for 25% of all medial condylar fractures. In type III fractures the flexor pronator mass, which is attached to the distal fragment, causes the distal fragment to rotate anteriorly and medially, causing the articular surface to face posteriorly and laterally (Fig. 8.38). This injury often is confused

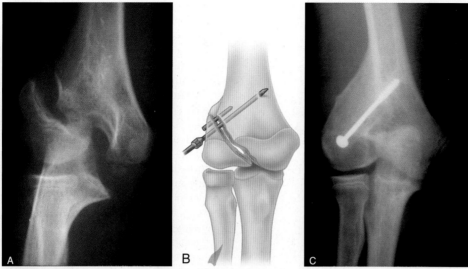

FIGURE 8.33 **A,** Nonunion of lateral condyle with distal fragment in acceptable position for bone grafting and internal fixation. **B** and **C,** Transfixed, freshened, bone-grafted nonunion; physis of condylar fragment is not violated by pin or graft.

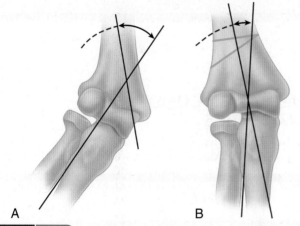

FIGURE 8.34 Correction of cubitus valgus by osteotomy. **A,** Cubitus valgus secondary to nonunion of lateral humeral condyle. **B,** Opening wedge osteotomy laterally to restore alignment.

with medial epicondylar fracture, which is more common but occurs in older children. Making a radiographic diagnosis can be difficult, especially in younger patients in whom the trochlea has not yet ossified, which occurs around the age of 8 years. MRI and elbow arthrography can be used to make the diagnosis in unclear cases. Medial epicondylar fractures often occur with elbow dislocations and, because of the intraarticular nature of the medial condyle, patients with medial condylar fractures, unlike those with medial epicondylar fractures, have fat pad changes evident on radiographs.

For nondisplaced fractures treatment consists of 4 to 6 weeks of cast immobilization. These fractures heal more slowly than supracondylar fractures and are more like lateral condylar fractures because of the intraarticular nature of the fracture site. The treatment for displaced fractures is open reduction and internal fixation to ensure joint congruity. This

is best done through a posteromedial incision, which provides excellent exposure of the fracture site and allows for protection of the ulnar nerve. Care must be taken not to extend the dissection posteriorly to avoid injury to the trochlear blood supply. Fixation consists typically of two smooth Kirschner wires in younger children and screw fixation in older children to control rotation and prevent nonunion that can occur with inadequate fracture fixation (see Fig. 8.38).

COMPLICATIONS AFTER MEDIAL CONDYLAR FRACTURE

The most common complication with this fracture is failing to make the correct diagnosis (see Fig. 8.38). Once the correct diagnosis is made, nonunion is rare and usually results from inadequately stabilized fractures. Complications usually consist of nonunion with resultant cubitus varus, trochlear osteonecrosis, and loss of reduction, and the complication rate can be as high as 33%. Nonunion can be treated with revision open reduction and internal fixation and bone grafting. Many patients with osteonecrosis of the trochlea are asymptomatic and require only observation. Cubitus varus caused by growth delay or arrest of the trochlea and cubitus valgus caused by fracture-simulated overgrowth can occur with these injuries. Corrective osteotomy can be used to treat these deformities if they become painful or interfere with function.

OPEN REDUCTION AND INTERNAL FIXATION OF MEDIAL CONDYLAR FRACTURE

TECHNIQUE 8.9

- Begin a medial incision just distal to the medial condyle and extend it proximally parallel to the long axis of the

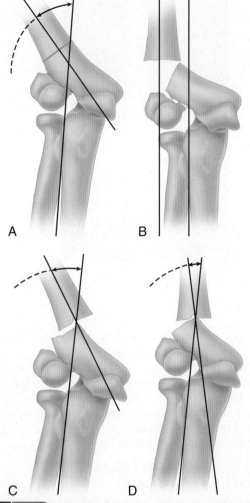

A

B

C

D

FIGURE 8.35 **A,** Malunion of Milch II fracture. **B,** Simple osteotomy results in unaccetable alignment. **C,** Osteotomy with lateral translation of distal fragment in addition to angulation. **D,** Final acceptable result. **SEE TECHNIQUE 8.8.**

humerus. Carry the dissection down to bone, isolating the ulnar nerve, and retract it posteriorly. The capsule usually is ruptured and need not be incised for exposure of the fracture. The capsule can be released anteriorly if more exposure is desired.

■ Carefully examine the detached condyle and remove all hematoma. The fragment is surprisingly large, and often a part of the capitellum is included.

■ Gently reduce the fracture and hold it with a bone tenaculum without disturbing the soft-tissue attachments of the fragment. Some metaphyseal plastic deformation may occur, so it is essential to restore the normal contour of the articular surface rather than the medial column.

■ Insert two smooth Kirschner wires through the condylar fragment and into the humerus in a proximal and lateral direction. Two wires are necessary to prevent rotation of the fragment. Use smooth Kirschner wires rather than screws if the child is young and cannulated screw fixation in older children. Before closing the incision, verify the position of the fragment by stress fluoroscopy. Cut off the wires outside the skin, leaving them long enough to allow easy removal.

■ Close the wound and apply a splint or bivalve cast with the elbow flexed 90 degrees.

MEDIAL EPICONDYLAR FRACTURES

Medial epicondylar fractures account for approximately 10% of pediatric elbow fractures, with a peak age at occurrence of 11 to 12 years. Between 30% and 50% occur with elbow dislocations, and it is important to ensure that the

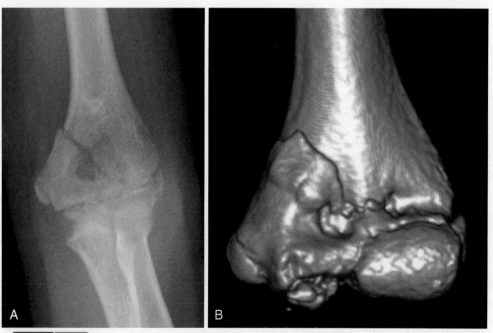

A

B

FIGURE 8.36 Anteroposterior radiograph **(A)** and CT scan **(B)** of type II medial condylar fracture.

medial epicondyle is not entrapped after reduction of the dislocation.

The most common mechanism of injury is an avulsion that can occur as a result of a valgus stress being placed on the extended elbow, usually after a fall. The medial epicondylar apophysis is the origin of the ulnar collateral ligament, which, if under valgus stress, avulses it. It can also occur as a result of a pure avulsion by the forearm flexors and rarely with a direct blow to the elbow. In complete fractures, the avulsed apophysis displaces distally from pull of the forearm flexor mass originating on it. Standard radiographic studies have shown that accurately measuring the true amount of displacement in all planes is difficult compared to CT scanning. A newer radiographic view, the distal humerus axis (axial) view, has been shown to be more accurate and reliable while reducing the need for advanced imaging (Fig. 8.39).

Nondisplaced fractures can be treated with 2 to 3 weeks of immobilization in a long arm cast or brace followed by gradual resumption of activity. The absolute indication for operative treatment is an entrapped intraarticular apophyseal fragment in an elbow dislocation, which can be performed urgently and not emergently unless ulnar nerve injury is present. Other indications include fractures associated with elbow dislocations to allow early range of motion and fractures displaced more than 1 cm. A relative indication is a minimally displaced fracture in a high-demand throwing athlete. Treatment of mildly displaced fractures, less than 1 cm, remains controversial because of the difficulty in measuring true displacement, the good results being reported in small series of patients treated both operatively and nonoperatively, and the lack of comparison studies.

Surgery can be performed with the patient supine or prone in the "hammerlock position," which provides relaxation to the forearm flexor musculature, making reduction easier (Fig. 8.40). Careful dissection is necessary if the epicondyle is entrapped to prevent injury to the ulnar nerve (Fig. 8.41). Typically a single 4.0- or 4.5-mm cannulated screw is used for fixation, and a long arm cast is worn for 2 to 3 weeks before beginning physical therapy. In comminuted fractures, which are rare, smooth Kirschner wires, suture anchors, or both can be used to stabilize the fragments. Patients are treated with a long arm cast or brace for 2 to 3 weeks followed by physical therapy.

COMPLICATIONS AFTER MEDIAL EPICONDYLAR FRACTURE

Complications associated with medial epicondylar fractures are rare and most often associated either with missed incarcerated intraarticular fragments or elbow stiffness related to an elbow dislocation and ulnar nerve palsy. Nonunion of these fractures is rare and can be associated with long-term elbow instability leading to a tardy ulnar nerve palsy. Ulnar nerve dysesthesia is common after operative treatment especially with removal of incarcerated intraarticular fragments, which usually resolves. Ulnar nerve transposition is reserved for late palsies and not for acute ulnar nerve symptoms. Because of the subcutaneous location of the medial epicondyle, screw prominence and pain can occur and can be treated with hardware removal once satisfactory healing has occurred.

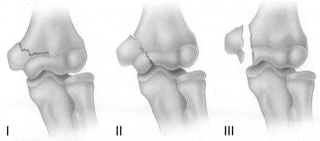

I	II	III

FIGURE 8.37 Three types of medial condylar fractures described by Kilfoyle: type I, impacted; type II, epiphyseal and intraarticular; and type III, displacement of entire medial condyle.

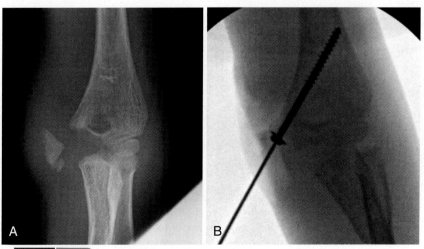

FIGURE 8.38 **A** and **B,** Screw fixation of displaced medial condylar fracture.

OPEN REDUCTION AND INTERNAL FIXATION FOR DISPLACED OR ENTRAPPED MEDIAL EPICONDYLE

TECHNIQUE 8.10

- Position the patient prone with a nonsterile tourniquet and place the elbow on a sterile-draped image intensifier. Mark the course of the ulnar nerve on the skin.
- Make a medial incision centered on the medial epicondyle approximately 5 cm in length.
- The ulnar nerve is posterior and should be protected for the entire procedure. For displaced fractures without entrapment, the fracture site can be viewed directly. Irrigate the fracture site thoroughly. Use a small curet to remove any remaining apophyseal cartilage on the displaced fragment to promote bony healing.
- If the fragment is entrapped within the elbow joint when the fracture site is exposed, only the bony surface of the condyle is seen; no loose fragment is visible. The medial capsule, musculotendinous origin of the long flexor muscles, and epicondyle are folded within the joint, covering the lower part of the coronoid fossa and process. With a small tenaculum, remove the epicondyle with its soft-tissue attachments from within the joint.

- Reduce the epicondyle and secure it with a screw and washer if possible, which allows for early motion. If the fracture is comminuted or the patient is very young, smooth Kirschner wires and/or a suture anchor(s) can be used.
- Suture the tear in the capsule and forearm muscles, close the wound, and apply a posterior splint or a bivalved cast.

POSTOPERATIVE CARE A splint or cast is worn for 2 to 3 weeks. Alternatively, if good stability is obtained, a hinged elbow brace can be used in compliant patients to begin gentle immediate early range-of-motion exercises. Early motion is especially important when the fracture is associated with an elbow dislocation.

CHRONIC MEDIAL EPICONDYLE APOPHYSITIS (LITTLE LEAGUE ELBOW)

This chronic injury is related to overuse in young athletes, primarily baseball players. Excessive throwing places repetitive tension on the medial epicondylar apophysis. Overuse is a major contributor to this as the incidence is relatively low when established age-related pitch counts are followed. Patients have pain directly over the medial epicondyle, which is increased with valgus stress. Some patients have a loss of elbow extension as well. Radiographically, the apophysis is widened compared with the opposite side, and comparison views can be helpful but are not necessary to make the diagnosis.

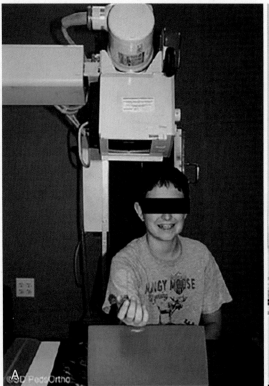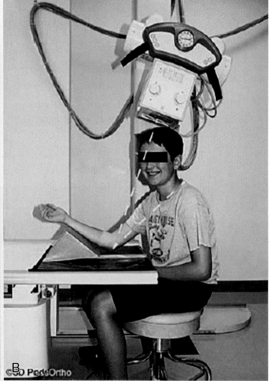

FIGURE 8.39 Distal humeral axial view. **A,** Position of patient and x-ray beam. **B,** X-ray beam is projected 25 degrees anterior to long axis of humerus (*dashed lines*). (From Sounder CD, Farnsworth CL, McNeil NR, et al: The distal humerus axial view: assessment of displacement in medial epicondyle fractures. *J Pediatr Orthop* 35:449, 2015.)

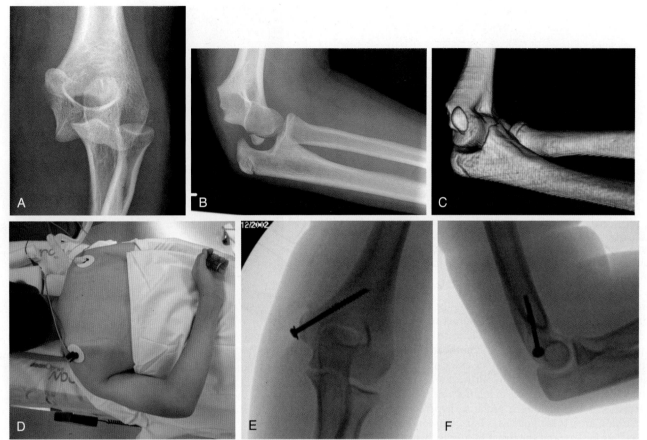

FIGURE 8.40 Anteroposterior (**A**) and lateral (**B**) radiographs of patient with elbow dislocation and associated fracture of medial epicondyle. **C,** Postreduction CT showing true displacement of epicondyle. **D,** Hammerlock position allows for relaxation of forearm flexors attached to displaced fragment. Anteroposterior (**E**) and lateral (**F**) radiographs after fixation with cannulated screw and washer.

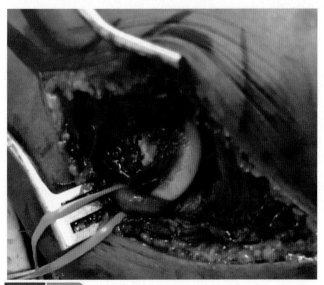

FIGURE 8.41 Fracture of the medial epicondyle with entrapped ulnar nerve. Note the close proximity of the ulnar nerve *(vessel loop)* to the entrapped fragment *(arrow).*

The most important treatment is rest followed by a gradual resumption of activity. Antiinflammatory medications, splinting, and ice may be helpful for symptomatic relief. Patients, families, and coaches need to be educated about the overuse nature of this injury. Once the patient is pain free, activity can be gradually progressed, ensuring proper throwing mechanics are followed. Although this can be very debilitating in terms of sports participation, no long-term complications from this have been reported.

DISTAL HUMERAL FRACTURES

Fracture of the entire distal humeral physis, which occurs more distally than a supracondylar fracture (Fig. 8.42), most commonly occurs during a fall and most frequently in young children (mean age, 5 years). This injury has historically been underreported because making the diagnosis was difficult. With increased awareness and advanced imaging techniques such as MRI, ultrasound, and arthrography, this injury is being diagnosed with greater frequency.

The distal humeral epiphysis extends across to include the secondary ossification of the medial epicondyle until about 6 to 7 years of age in girls and 8 to 9 years in boys. Most fractures involving the entire distal humeral physis occur before

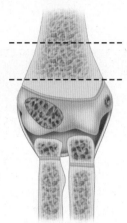

FIGURE 8.42 *Dashed horizontal lines* indicate proximal area, where supracondylar fracture occurs, and distal area, where physeal fracture-separation occurs in wider part of distal humerus in younger age group.

the age of 6 or 7 and usually younger. The younger the child, the greater the volume of distal humerus occupied by cartilaginous epiphysis. As children mature, the volume of the epiphysis decreases, which some authors believe is protective of injury. This may explain the association between distal humeral physeal fractures and birth trauma, as well as NAT. In addition, the physeal line in infants is near the center of the olecranon fossa, making it prone to hyperextension injury. Malunion after these injuries is less common because of the broad surface area of the distal humerus. Because the blood supply to the medial trochlea courses through the physis, osteonecrosis of the trochlea can occur.

These fractures are classified into three groups based on the degree of ossification of the lateral condylar epiphysis. Group A fractures occur in infants up to 12 months of age, before the secondary ossification center of the lateral condylar epiphysis appears (and are usually Salter-Harris type I physeal injuries) (Fig. 8.43). These often are missed because the lateral condylar epiphysis lacks an ossification center. Group B fractures occur most often in children 12 months to 3 years of age in whom there is definite ossification of the lateral condyle. Group C fractures occur in older children, from 3 to 7 years of age, and result in a large metaphyseal fragment.

In an infant younger than 18 months of age whose elbow is swollen secondary to trauma or suspected trauma, a fracture involving the entire distal humeral physis should be considered. In a young infant or newborn, swelling may be minimal with little crepitus because the fracture fragments are covered in cartilage (physis) rather than bone.

Radiographic diagnosis can be difficult, especially if the ossification center of the lateral condyle is not visible. The only relationship that can be determined is that of the primary ossification centers of the distal humerus to the proximal radius and ulna (Fig. 8.44). The proximal radius and ulna maintain an anatomic relationship to each other but are displaced posteriorly and medially in relation to the distal humerus. Comparison views of the opposite uninjured elbow may be helpful to determine the presence of displacement.

Once the lateral condylar epiphysis becomes ossified, displacement of the entire distal epiphysis is much more obvious. The anatomic relationship of the lateral condylar epiphysis with the radial head is maintained, even though the

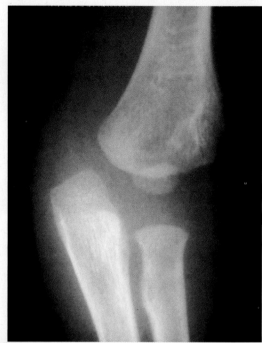

FIGURE 8.43 Transphyseal dislocation in neonate. Note loss of normal relationship between ulna and distal humerus.

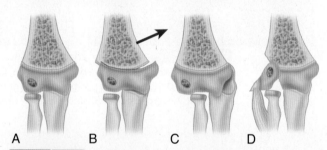

FIGURE 8.44 Elbow injuries that may be confused clinically. **A,** Normal elbow before three centers of ossification appear. **B,** Separation of entire distal humeral epiphysis. **C,** Dislocation of elbow. **D,** Lateral condylar fracture.

distal humeral epiphysis is displaced posterior and medial in relation to the metaphysis of the humerus.

Because they have a large metaphyseal fragment, type C fractures may be confused with either a low supracondylar fracture or a fracture of the lateral condylar physis. The key diagnostic point is the smooth outline of the distal metaphysis in fractures involving the total distal physis. With supracondylar fractures, the distal portion of the distal fragment has a more irregular border.

A lateral condylar physeal fracture in an infant can be differentiated from the rare elbow dislocation by radiograph. With a displaced fracture of the lateral condylar physis, the relationship between the lateral condylar epiphysis and the proximal radius usually is disrupted. If the lateral crista of the trochlea is involved, the proximal radius and ulna may be displaced posterolaterally. Elbow dislocations are rare in the peak age group for fractures of the entire distal humeral physis. With elbow dislocations, the displacement of the proximal radius and ulna is almost always posterolateral, and the relationship between the proximal radius and lateral condylar

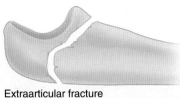

Extraarticular fracture

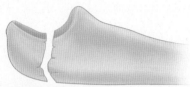

Intraarticular fracture

FIGURE 8.45 Two types of olecranon fractures. Regardless of type, if displacement is significant, open reduction and internal fixation probably are indicated.

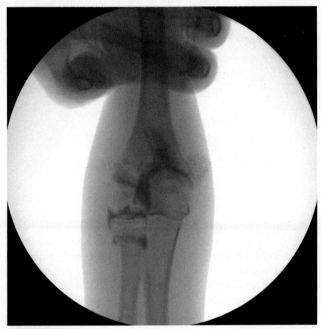

FIGURE 8.46 Arthrogram helps to define cartilaginous distal fragment.

epiphysis is disrupted. Comparison views are helpful in making this diagnosis. Ultrasound can also be used to make the diagnosis and avoid the use of general anesthesia in infants.

TREATMENT

Treatment is first directed toward prompt recognition. Because this injury may be associated with child abuse, the parents may delay seeking treatment and ossification may already be present on the initial radiographs. These injuries, when recognized in a timely fashion, can be treated with closed reduction and percutaneous pinning (Fig. 8.45). Arthrography can be helpful to define the cartilaginous distal fragment (Fig. 8.46). Missed untreated fractures may remodel completely without any residual deformity if the distal fragment

is only medially translocated and not tilted. In older children, these injuries can be stabilized with either percutaneous pinning or TEIN. The more proximal the fracture and the closer to the metaphyseal-diaphyseal junction, the more difficult and less biomechanically stable percutaneous pinning becomes, making TEIN the better option.

CAPITELLAR FRACTURES

Fractures of the capitellum, which make up less than 1% of pediatric elbow fractures, involve only the true articular surface of the lateral condyle, including in some instances the articular surface of the lateral crista of the trochlea. Unlike in adults, these fractures are rare in children and usually occur in adolescents. Murthy et al. classified capitellar fractures into three types: type I are anterior shear fractures and are the most common, type II are posterior shear fractures, and type III are chondral shear fractures (Fig. 8.47). The diagnosis can often be made using plain radiographs; MRI can be helpful, especially when the fragment is primarily cartilaginous, and in types II and III injuries, which often are missed on plain radiographs (Fig. 8.48).

Excision of the fragment, if small, and open reduction and reattachment are the two most common forms of treatment. However, because of the intraarticular nature of the injury, closed reduction is not likely to be successful. Many small fragments can be excised through either a lateral open or arthroscopic approach. This eliminates the need for postoperative immobilization and accompanying elbow stiffness. Open reduction and internal fixation can be performed if the fragments are large enough; however, osteonecrosis of the attached fragment can occur. Compression screws have been shown to provide stable fixation (Fig. 8.49). Alternatively, a suture repair can be performed if the fragment is primarily cartilaginous, which allows for follow-up MRI examination and eliminates the need for implant removal (Fig. 8.50). Regardless of the treatment method used, patients and parents should be counseled that elbow motion will be lost after this injury, especially in patients with large osteochondral fragments that involve the trochlea, and that up to 40% of patients require a secondary procedure because of stiffness, painful or prominent implants, and osteonecrosis.

OLECRANON FRACTURES

Isolated physeal fracture of the olecranon in children is uncommon due in part to the broad-based insertion of the triceps. When it does occur, it typically is the result of an avulsion force being applied to the olecranon with the elbow flexed. Although rare in the general population, these fractures, especially bilateral ones, are well described in children with osteogenesis imperfecta in whom refracture also is common. Apophyseal stress injuries can occur in high-level athletes, especially gymnasts and throwing athletes, and if left untreated can result in a painful nonunion. The most common fractures of the olecranon are metaphyseal, either isolated or associated with other elbow injuries. The peak age is 5 to 10 years, and olecranon fractures account for approximately 5% of pediatric elbow fractures. Isolated olecranon fractures are classified by the mechanism of injury: flexion, extension, or shear. Isolated flexion fractures most commonly occur in a fall directly onto a flexed elbow. A fall onto a hyperextended elbow is the usual mechanism of injury in supracondylar

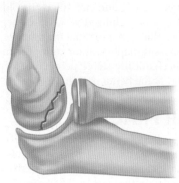 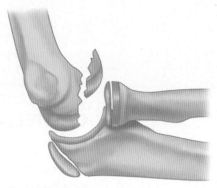

Type Ia: Nondisplaced anterior shear   Type Ib: Displaced anterior shear

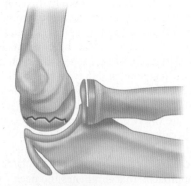 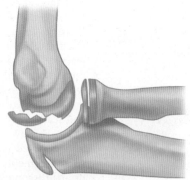 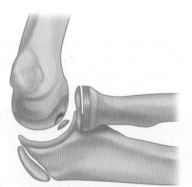

Type IIa: Nondisplaced
posterolateral shear

Type IIa: Displaced
posterolateral shear

Type III: Acute chondral shear fracture

FIGURE 8.47 **Classification of capitellar fractures.** (From Murthy PG, Vuillerman C, Naqvi MN, et al: Capitellar fractures in children and adolescents: classification and early results of treatment. *J Bone Joint Surg Am* 99:1282, 2017.)

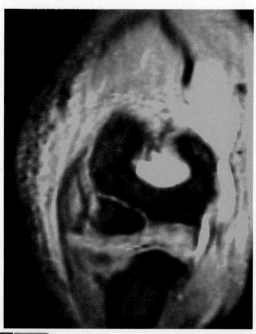

FIGURE 8.48 T2-weighted MRI shows large cartilaginous shear fracture.

humeral fractures; however, if there is a significant varus or valgus stress applied simultaneously, a metaphyseal olecranon fracture can occur. Shear injuries, which typically produce an oblique fracture line, are rare and can occur either in flexion

or extension. Associated fractures occur in 50% to 75% of children with an olecranon fracture, the most common being a proximal radial fracture and type I Monteggia injury.

Treatment for stress fractures includes time away from the causative activity followed by gradual resumption of activity. Cannulated screw fixation is used for rare patients with symptomatic delayed unions or nonunions. Most olecranon fractures are nondisplaced and can be treated for 3 to 4 weeks in a long arm cast with the elbow in 70 to 80 degrees of flexion. Late displacement can occur, so these fractures need to be monitored carefully. For fractures that are displaced or that had an unsatisfactory closed reduction, open reduction and internal fixation is indicated. A variety of fixation techniques, such as percutaneous pinning, tension banding, and screw and plate fixation, have been described with good outcomes (Fig. 8.51). Tension banding using bioabsorbable suture can be used in younger, smaller children to eliminate the need for implant removal. These techniques are discussed in other chapter. Elbow stiffness is a common complication after olecranon fracture in children, and stable fixation is essential to start early range of motion to prevent this.

RADIAL HEAD AND NECK FRACTURES

Isolated radial head fractures in children are rare because the immature radial head is cartilaginous. When they do occur, they usually are Salter-Harris type IV injuries in

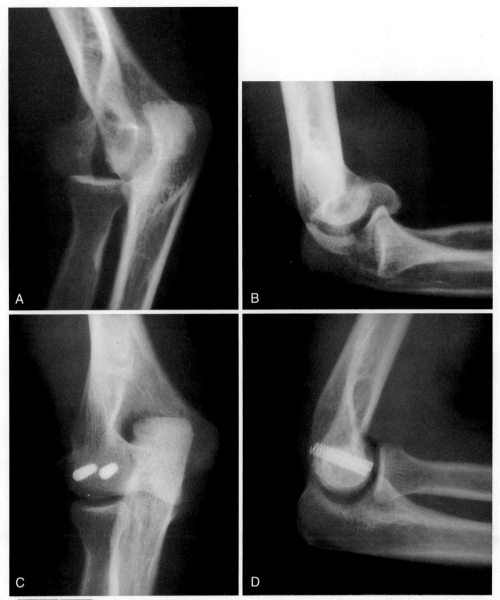

FIGURE 8.49   **A** and **B,** Capitellar fracture in adolescent. **C** and **D,** After reduction and fixation with cannulated screws.

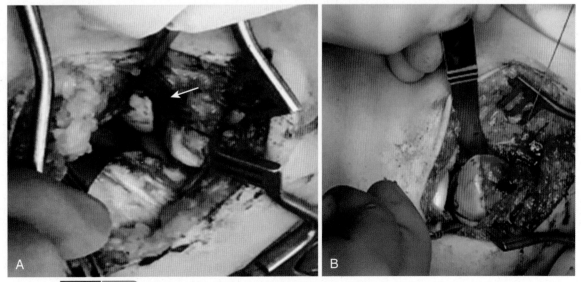

FIGURE 8.50   **A,** Anterior capitellar shear fracture (type 1B) with displaced fragment *(arrow).* **B,** After reduction and suture repair.

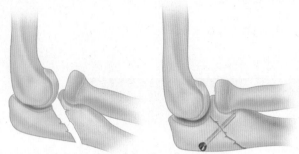

FIGURE 8.51 Metaphyseal intraarticular olecranon fracture that is unstable and requires open reduction and internal fixation, here with oblique screw.

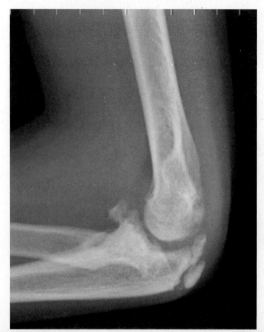

FIGURE 8.52 Posttraumatic radiocapitellar arthritis in 10-year-old girl after missed Salter-Harris type II fracture of radial head.

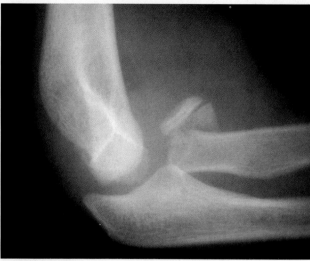

FIGURE 8.53 Displaced Salter-Harris type II fracture of the radial head and neck.

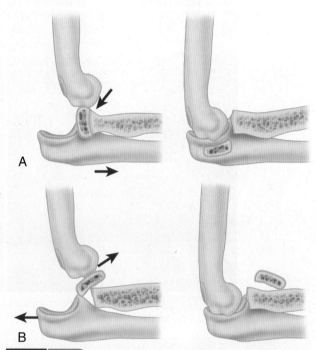

FIGURE 8.54 **A,** Fractures occurring at time of elbow dislocation. **B,** Fracture occurring when elbow dislocation is reduced.

children 10 to 12 years of age. Patients with true radial head fractures are at increased risk of progressive radial head subluxation, osteonecrosis, and radiocapitellar arthrosis and need to be followed long term (Fig. 8.52). Most children sustain fractures of the radial neck, which account for approximately 1% of all children's fractures and 5% of pediatric elbow fractures.

The majority of radial neck injuries occur during a fall onto an outstretched upper extremity with the elbow in a valgus position. They typically occur in the metaphysis but can extend into the proximal radial physis producing a Salter-Harris type II pattern (Fig. 8.53). Many of these fractures are angulated, with the most common direction being lateral, followed by anterior, then posterior. Radial neck fractures also can occur in conjunction with an elbow dislocation, either at the time of dislocation or during reduction (Fig. 8.54). The fracture may be completely displaced or intraarticular and may block reduction. For this reason the radial neck must be thoroughly evaluated before and after reduction of a pediatric elbow dislocation.

Making the diagnosis, especially in young children, can be difficult because of the unossified radial head. In these patients the only sign of a fracture may be a small metaphyseal fragment. A radiocapitellar view can be helpful in making the diagnosis.

Due to the remodeling potential of the proximal radius, fractures with less than 30 degrees of angulation can be treated nonoperatively as long as there is no loss of forearm rotation. Patients are placed in a long arm cast for 3 weeks and then allowed to resume range-of-motion exercises. Patients with displaced, significantly angulated or displaced fractures require reduction. This consists of a stepwise approach starting with closed reduction, progressing to percutaneous-assisted reduction, and finally open reduction and internal fixation if satisfactory reduction cannot be obtained. Because there is great potential for elbow stiffness after open reduction and internal fixation, a closed reduction with slight malalignment is preferable to an open reduction and internal fixation with anatomic alignment. The loss of motion in patients with open treatment may reflect selection of most displaced fractures for open reduction and internal fixation.

Closed reduction can be performed using a variety of techniques based on the direction of displacement of the radial neck with the help of image intensification (Fig. 8.55). One very useful technique is that described by Patterson. With the use of general anesthesia if needed and fluoroscopy (image intensification), an assistant stabilizes the radius distal to the fractured radial neck. With the elbow in extension and forearm rotated in the position of maximal tilt, the surgeon applies a varus stress with one hand on the elbow and lateral pressure directly over the radial head with the thumb of the other hand (see Fig. 8.60). Other reduction techniques have been described with the elbow in flexion. In addition, the wrapping of the arm with an Esmarch bandage has been shown to occasionally improve fracture reduction, and this maneuver should be attempted with all radial neck reduction techniques.

A percutaneous-assisted technique is used when closed techniques have failed. The most commonly used technique involves the percutaneous manipulation of the fracture with a Kirschner wire. The wire is cut, and the blunt end is used to reduce the radial neck and head to the shaft (Fig. 8.56). The reduced radial neck can be stabilized by percutaneous pinning (Fig. 8.57). Alternatively, a flexible intramedullary nail can be introduced retrograde from the distal radius using the technique described

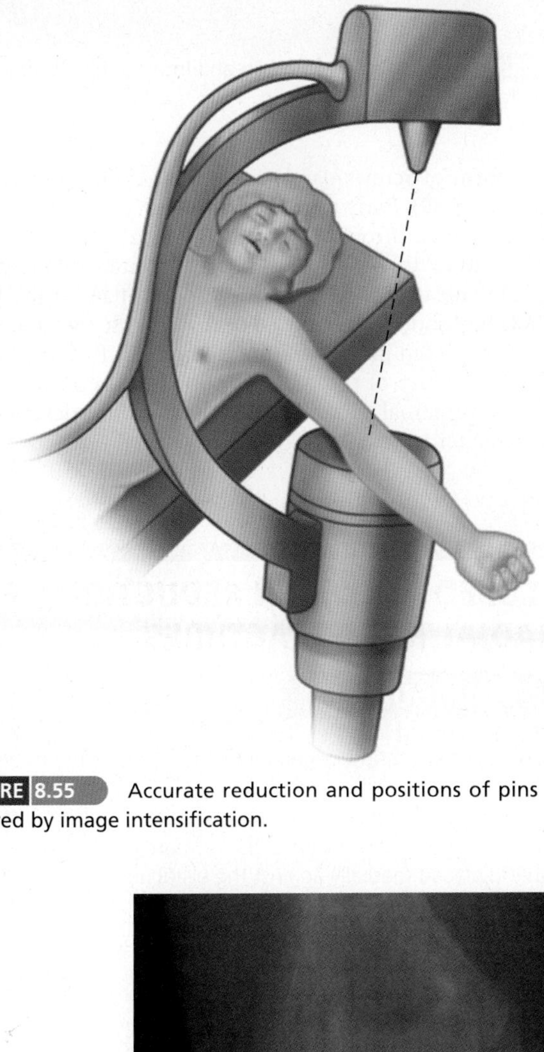

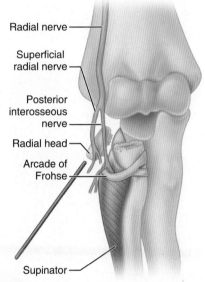

FIGURE 8.56   Radial neck fracture in relation to radial nerve and its branches. During percutaneous reduction, wire should be introduced on ulnar side of radius to avoid deep branch of radial nerve.

FIGURE 8.55   Accurate reduction and positions of pins are ensured by image intensification.

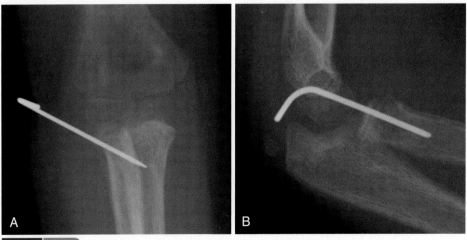

FIGURE 8.57   **A** and **B**, Anteroposterior and lateral views of radial neck pin.

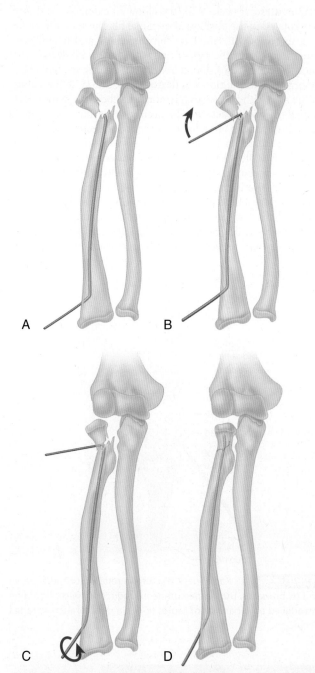

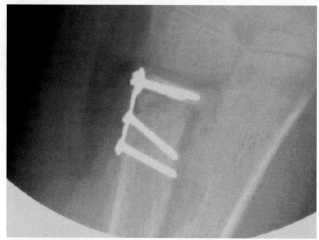

FIGURE 8.59   Open reduction and internal fixation of radial neck fracture.

in the form of screws or plates in older children or adolescents (Fig. 8.59). Early rigid fixation allows early motion. This should be done through a lateral approach with the forearm in supination to protect the posterior interosseous nerve. Impediments to reduction such as capsular flaps or the annular ligament should be removed or repaired. Screws and plates should be placed in the "safe zone," which is the 100 degrees of circumference of the radial head that does not articulate with the proximal ulna. These techniques are described in other chapter.

FIGURE 8.58   A–D, Reduction of radial head by leverage method and retrograde intramedullary pinning with Kirschner wire. Note slightly bent tip first pointing laterally. After it is placed in radial head, it is rotated 180 degrees along its axis.   (Redrawn from Stiefel D, Meuli M, Altermatt S: Fractures of the neck of the radius in children: early experience with intramedullary pinning. *J Bone Joint Surg* 83B:536, 2001. Copyright British Editorial Society of Bone and Joint Surgery.) **SEE TECHNIQUE 8.11.**

by Metaizeau. Using this technique, a flexible intramedullary nail is passed retrograde from the radial metaphysis proximally to the fracture site. Once engaged in the proximal fragment, the nail is rotated until the optimal reduction is obtained (Fig. 8.58). The fracture is then stabilized with the nail until healing has occurred.

In open reduction and internal fixation, most surgeons use smooth pin fixation in younger children and rigid fixation

CLOSED AND OPEN REDUCTION OF RADIAL NECK FRACTURES

TECHNIQUE 8.11

- After administering general anesthesia, place the patient supine.
- Use the manipulative technique as described by Patterson. Have an assistant hold the arm proximally, with one hand placed medially against the distal humerus, and apply straight longitudinal distal traction. Apply a varus force to the forearm and digital pressure directly over the tilted radial head to complete the reduction (Fig. 8.60). Hold the forearm in 90 degrees of flexion and in pronation. If this manipulation reduction is unsuccessful, have the assistant hold the arm with the shoulder abducted to 90 degrees and the forearm held in supination. With the use of an image intensifier and in a sterile operating field, introduce a Kirschner wire through the skin on the radial side of the elbow down to the angulated and displaced radial head and neck. Disimpact and push the radial head into anatomic position with the Kirschner wire. Remove the wire and flex the elbow to 90 degrees. The fracture can be pinned percutaneously from lateral to medial, taking care to protect the posterior interosseous nerve (see Fig. 8.58).

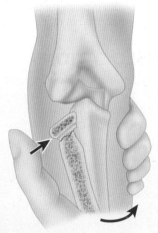

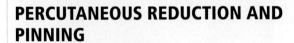

FIGURE 8.60 Mechanism of reduction of radial neck fracture. **SEE TECHNIQUE 8.11.**

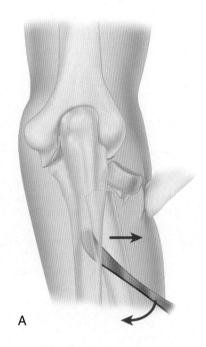

A

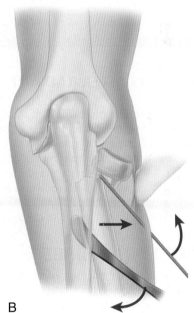

B

FIGURE 8.61 Radial head reduction technique. **A,** Periosteal elevator is used to lever distal fragment laterally while thumb pushes proximal fragment medially. **B,** Kirschner wires are used to assist reduction if necessary. (Redrawn from Erickson M, Frick S: Fractures of the proximal radius and ulna. In Beaty JH, Kasser JR, editors: *Rockwood and Wilkins' fractures in children,* ed 7, Philadelphia, 2010, Wolters Kluwer.) **SEE TECHNIQUE 8.12.**

PERCUTANEOUS REDUCTION AND PINNING

TECHNIQUE 8.12

- With the patient under general anesthesia, prepare and drape the upper limb.
- With fluoroscopy in the anteroposterior projection, determine the forearm rotation that exposes the maximal amount of deformity of the fracture and mark the level of the bicipital tuberosity of the proximal radius.
- Make a 1-cm dorsal skin incision at the marked level just lateral to the subcutaneous border of the ulna.
- Gently insert a periosteal elevator between the ulna and the radius, taking care not to disrupt the periosteum of the radius or ulna (Fig. 8.61A). The radial shaft usually is much more ulnarly displaced than expected, and the radial nerve is lateral to the radius at this level.
- While counter-pressure is applied against the radial head, lever the distal fragment away from the ulna (Fig. 8.61C). An assistant can aid in this maneuver by gently applying traction and rotating the forearm back and forth to disimpact the fracture fragments.
- If necessary to correct angulation, insert a percutaneous Kirschner wire into the fracture site, parallel to the radial head, and use it to lever the epiphysis perpendicular to the radial axis (Fig. 8.61B).
- Once adequate reduction has been obtained, insert an oblique Kirschner wire to provide fracture fixation.

POSTOPERATIVE CARE A posterior splint or bivalved cast is applied and worn for 3 to 4 weeks, and the Kirschner wire is removed once fracture callus is present.

If these maneuvers are unsuccessful, reduction can be attempted using a retrograde flexible intramedullary nail.

CLOSED INTRAMEDULLARY NAILING

TECHNIQUE 8.13

- With the patient under general anesthesia, prepare and drape the upper limb.

- Expose the radial aspect of the distal radial metaphysis through a short radial incision 1 cm proximal to the radial physis, avoiding injury to the cutaneous branch of the radial nerve.
- Drill the cortex, starting perpendicular to the radius and then in a more proximal direction.
- Introduce the nail into the medullary canal. Advance the wire using gentle taps of the mallet to avoid perforation of the ulnar cortex of the distal radius.
- If a lateral displacement of the distal fragment remains, rotate the nail 180 degrees around its long axis so that its point faces inward. This produces a medial shift of the radial head and reduces it. The tension produced in the lateral intact periosteum prevents overcorrection medially.
- Cut the lower metaphyseal end of the pin and close the skin.
- When the epiphysis is impossible to reach, tilting of more than 80 degrees by external manipulation or by percutaneous pinning makes it possible to obtain at least a partial reduction, which is maintained with an intramedullary nail.

POSTOPERATIVE CARE The arm is immobilized in a long arm cast for 2 to 3 weeks. The Kirschner wire is removed in 3 to 4 weeks once callus is present on radiographs.

COMPLICATIONS AFTER RADIAL NECK FRACTURE

Complications of treatment include loss of motion, which is most common in pronation and supination rather than flexion and extension. Malunion and nonunion can occur; however, this is rare. Patients with asymptomatic nonunions can be observed (Fig. 8.62). Radial neck three-dimensional computer-assisted osteotomies have been used on a small number of patients with moderate success, and radial head excision is reserved for a very select, small group of salvage cases.

CORONOID FRACTURES

Regan and Morrey classified fractures of the coronoid process as type I, a small chip fracture; type II, a fracture involving less than 50% of the process; and type III, a fracture involving more than 50% of the process (Fig. 8.63). They recommended closed treatment for types I and II fractures and open reduction and internal fixation for type III fractures if possible. Operative

treatment of these injuries is more common in adolescent and adult patients. This is described in other chapter.

ELBOW DISLOCATIONS

Acute elbow dislocation in children is rare, accounting for approximately 5% of all children's elbow injuries. The most common type is posterior but, as in adults, dislocations can be anterior, medial, or lateral. In rare cases a proximal radioulnar

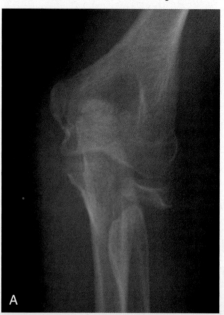

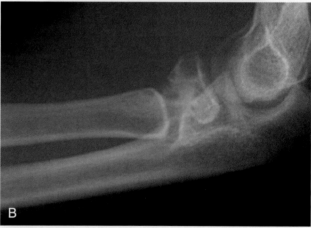

FIGURE 8.62 Radial neck nonunion.

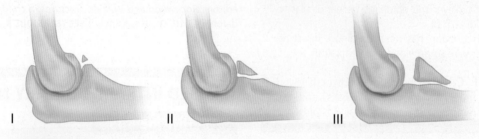

FIGURE 8.63 Classification of coronoid fractures. *Type I*, small fragment avulsion. *Type II*, involvement of less than 50% of coronoid process. *Type III*, involvement of more than 50% of coronoid process.

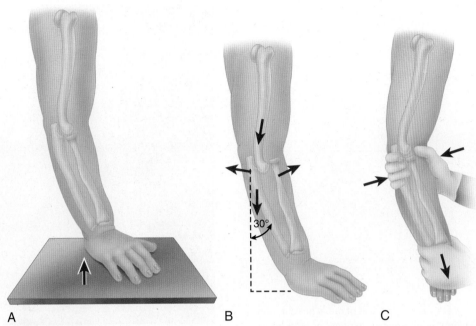

FIGURE 8.64 **A** and **B,** Mechanism of injury in a fall on outstretched hand with elbow in approximately 30 degrees of flexion. There is separation of all three articulations, with humerus acting as wedge between proximal radius and ulna **(B)**. **C,** Mechanism of reduction aims to reverse deforming forces with longitudinal traction and compression of radius and ulna together. (Redrawn from Altuntas AO, Balakumar J, Howells RJ, et al: Posterior divergent dislocation of the elbow in children and adolescents: a report of three cases and review of the literature, *J Pediatr Orthop* 25:317, 2005.)

joint disruption can occur (Fig. 8.64). Elbow dislocations often occur in conjunction with fractures of the medial epicondyle and radial neck.

Most patients can be treated with closed reduction, a brief period of immobilization, followed by progressive protected range of motion in a splint or brace to prevent redislocation. Indications for operative treatment include entrapped intraarticular fragments (medial epicondyle, radial neck), open fracture, or associated elbow injury that will require open reduction and internal fixation.

COMPLICATIONS AFTER ELBOW DISLOCATION

The most common complications are elbow stiffness and loss of motion, especially extension. Other rare complications include redislocation, myositis ossificans after open fractures, and neurovascular injuries. It is essential to perform a thorough neurovascular examination before and after closed or open reduction to ensure that nerve or vessel entrapment did not occur at the time of reduction.

RADIAL HEAD DISLOCATIONS (MONTEGGIA FRACTURE-DISLOCATIONS)

Monteggia fractures are relatively rare, accounting for less than 1% of all pediatric elbow dislocations, with a peak age of 4 to 10 years. Although rare, they receive considerable interest because they are often missed, resulting in poor outcomes. Radial nerve injury has been reported to occur in 10% to 20% of patients, especially those with anterior and lateral

dislocations because of the proximity of the radial head to the posterior interosseous nerve.

The diagnosis of Monteggia fracture can be made with standard anteroposterior and lateral radiographs of the elbow, and it is essential that the elbow be viewed in both planes for all patients with forearm fractures. A line drawn through the center of the radial neck should extend through the central portion of the capitellum regardless of elbow position (Fig. 8.65). In rare instances when radiographs are equivocal, advanced imaging, such as CT, MRI, or ultrasound, should be used. The absence of trauma and changes such as a hypoplastic capitellum and a flattened convex radial head (Fig. 8.66) should raise suspicion for a congenital radial head dislocation, which often is bilateral.

The most commonly used classification system is that of Bado, which is based on the direction of radial head dislocation (Fig. 8.67). The most common is a fracture of the proximal third of the ulna, anterior angulation of the fracture, and anterior dislocation of the radial head (type I). The second most common is a fracture of the proximal ulna, posterior angulation of the fracture, and posterior dislocation of the radial head (type II). Lateral angulation of a proximal ulnar fracture may result in a third type with lateral dislocation of the radial head (type III), and a rare fourth type may occur with a proximal both-bone fracture and anterior dislocation of the radial head (type IV) (Fig. 8.68). Although it is descriptive and straightforward, the Bado classification is not prognostic. Classification systems by Letts and Ring, based on the pattern of ulnar injury, may be more prognostic in terms of outcome given the fact that successful reduction of the ulna typically provides stability to the radiocapitellar joint (Box 8.3). A study of 112 Monteggia fractures at two

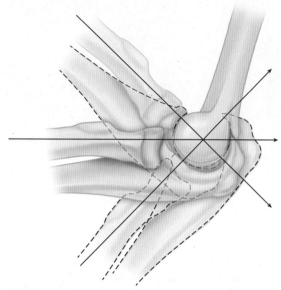

FIGURE 8.65 On lateral radiograph, axis of radial head should bisect center of capitellum on all views, regardless of amount of elbow flexion.

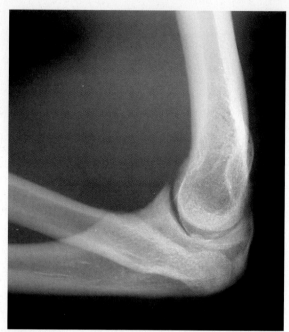

FIGURE 8.66 Congenital radial head dislocation. Note convexity of radial head indicative of congenital rather than traumatic radial head dislocation.

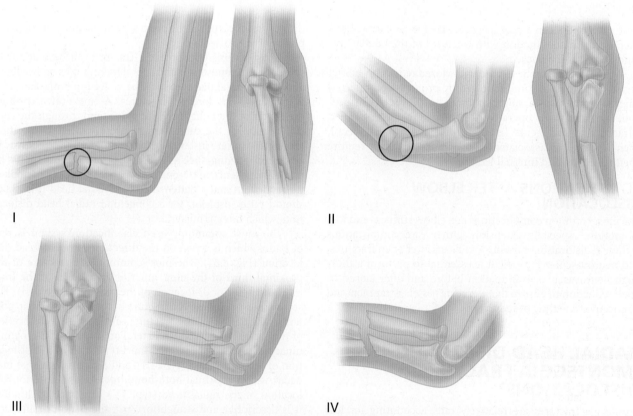

I

II

III

IV

FIGURE 8.67 Types of Monteggia fractures. *Type I* with anterior dislocation of radial head and anterior angulation of ulnar fracture. *Type II* with posterior dislocation of radial head and posterior angulation of ulnar fracture. *Type III* with lateral dislocation of radial head and lateral angulation of ulnar fracture. Rare *Type IV* with fractures of radial and ulnar shafts and dislocation of radial head.

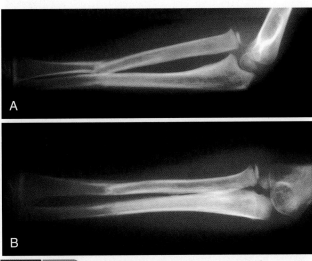

FIGURE 8.68 Type IV Monteggia fracture with fractures of radial and ulnar shafts and dislocation of radial head.

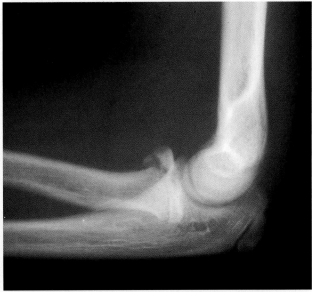

FIGURE 8.69 Monteggia equivalent fracture of anterior third of radial head with subsequent dislocation.

BOX 8.3

Classification of Monteggia Fracture-Dislocations in Children According to Ulnar Injury

Type of Ulnar Injury	Treatment
Plastic deformation	Closed reduction of the ulnar bow and cast immobilization
Incomplete (greenstick or buckle) fracture	Closed reduction and cast immobilization
Complete transverse or short oblique fracture	Closed reduction and intramedullary Kirschner wire fixation
Long oblique or comminuted fracture	Open reduction and internal fixation with plate and screws

Modified from Ring D, Jupiter JB, Waters PM: Monteggia fractures in children, *J Am Acad Orthop Surg* 6:215, 1998.

---

high-volume trauma centers found that all treatment failures, which affected 19% of patients, occurred when a less rigorous strategy than that proposed by Ring was used. In addition, there have been numerous reports of "Monteggia equivalents," including the three most common: (1) isolated radial head dislocation (see "Isolated Dislocations of Radial Head") (Fig. 8.69), (2) fracture of the proximal ulna with fracture of the radial neck, and (3) both-bone proximal third fractures with the radial fracture more proximal than the ulnar fracture (Fig. 8.70).

An isolated radial head dislocation is very rare (see Fig. 8.69). This is because many children thought to have an isolated radial head fracture have subtle plastic deformation of the ulna, which when corrected leads to stable radial head reduction (Fig. 8.71). This must be differentiated from nursemaid's elbow in which the radiographs are completely normal.

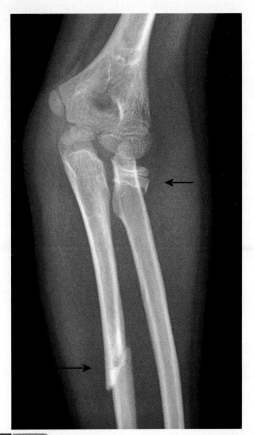

FIGURE 8.70 Monteggia variant: both-bone proximal-third fractures with radial fracture more proximal than ulnar fracture.

Successful treatment of a Monteggia fracture is dependent on correcting and stabilizing the ulnar deformity, which in turn provides stability for the radiocapitellar joint. Closed reduction and cast treatment is indicated for patients with either stable or greenstick fractures of the ulna, as well as those with plastic deformation of the ulna and satisfactory reduction of the radial head.

Patients should be immobilized in a long arm cast in 90 to 100 degrees of flexion and supination and followed closely radiographically for 2 to 3 weeks to ensure maintenance of radial head reduction. Operative stabilization of the ulna is necessary with either an intramedullary nail for transverse or short oblique fractures or a plate for long oblique or comminuted fracture to provide ulnar length stability (Fig. 8.72). Open reduction of the radial head combined with annular ligament reconstruction is indicated for patients with irreducible radial head dislocations caused by interposition of the annular ligament. Patients need to be followed closely postoperatively for redislocation of the radial head (Fig. 8.73). Pinning of the radiocapitellar joint should be avoided when possible to prevent intraarticular pin breakage. A radiocapitellar joint unstable enough to require pinning should raise the suspicion of inadequate ulnar reduction or entrapped soft tissue.

Controversy exists as to when an acute Monteggia fracture becomes chronic. Some patients are asymptomatic while others complain of pain, decreased range of motion, or deformity. Many authors believe that, although treatment of chronic Monteggia fractures is difficult and the results unpredictable, it is better than the natural history of untreated fractures (Fig. 8.74). Generally, operative treatment is more successful in symptomatic younger patients without radial head deformity. Principles of surgical reconstruction include correction of the ulnar deformity with an ulnar osteotomy and annular ligament reconstruction. The ulnar osteotomy should be stabilized in the position of maximal stability of the radiocapitellar joint, which often creates a secondary ulnar deformity that is clinically insignificant (Fig. 8.75, Technique 8.14). Most authors recommend reconstruction of the annular ligament, either with the native ligament itself or a strip of triceps tendon or fascia as advocated by Boyd, Lloyd-Roberts, and Bell-Tawse (Fig. 8.76). Radial head resection should be avoided in younger patients because of the risk of late deformity and should only be used as a salvage procedure.

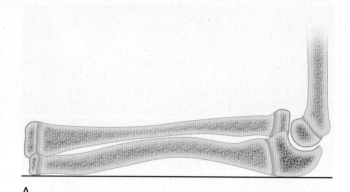

A

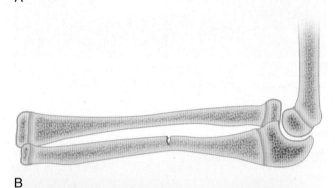

B

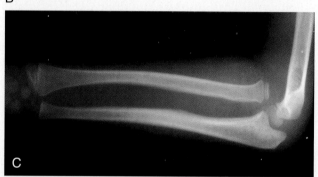

C

FIGURE 8.71 Plastic deformation of ulna. **A,** Anterior bend. **B,** Anterior greenstick. **C,** Radiographic appearance.

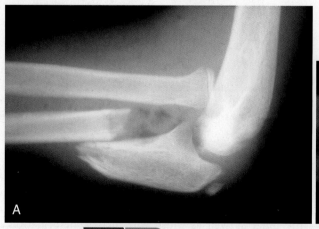

A

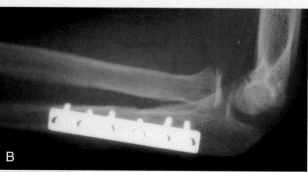

B

FIGURE 8.72 **A,** Monteggia fracture. **B,** After open reduction and plate fixation.

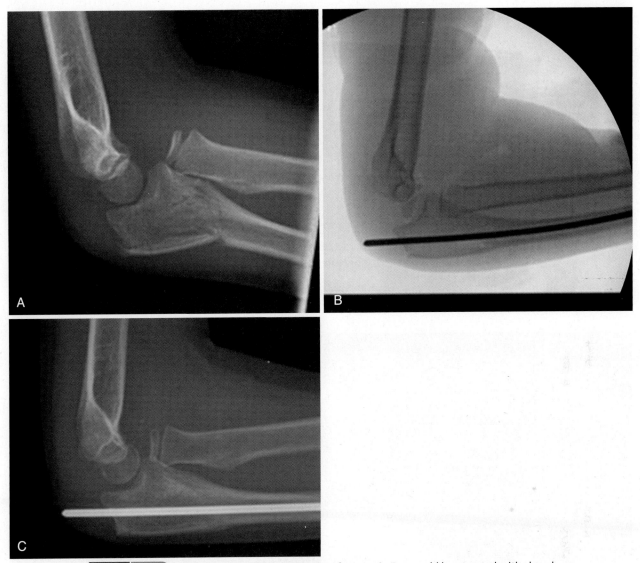

FIGURE 8.73 **A** and **B,** Bado type I Monteggia fracture in 7-year-old boy treated with closed reduction and intramedullary nail fixation of ulna. **C,** At 2-week follow-up, radiograph shows redislocation.

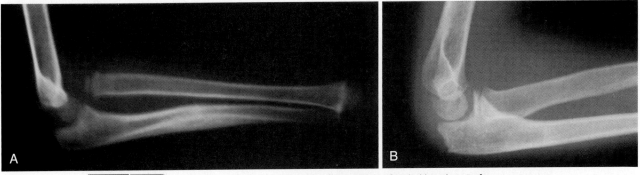

FIGURE 8.74 Malunion of ulna and anterior dislocation of radial head. **A,** Before treatment. **B,** At 3 years after surgery, showing maintenance of radial head reduction.

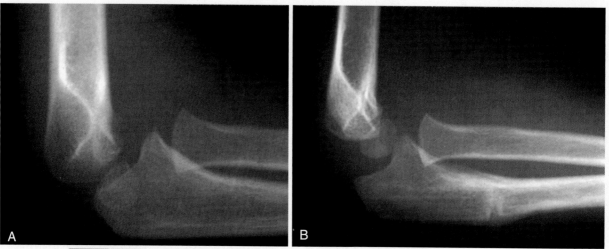

FIGURE 8.75 **A,** Deformity after Monteggia fracture. **B,** After overcorrection osteotomy (see text).

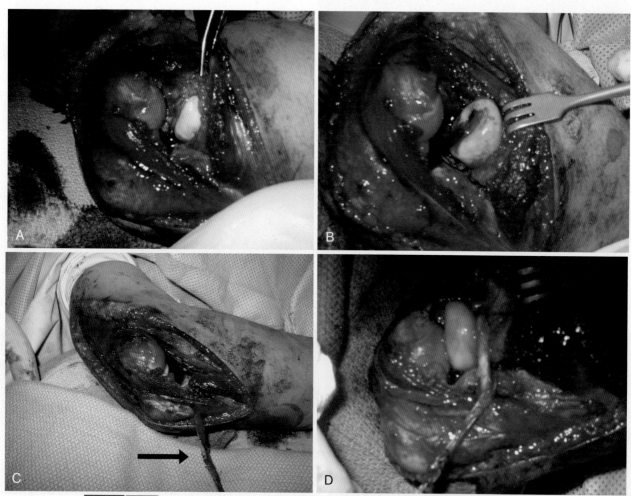

FIGURE 8.76 Lateral approach to the elbow shows incongruent radiocapitellar joint (**A**) and changes in radial head morphology (**B**). The triceps fascia has been harvested (**C,** *arrow*) and is used to reconstruct the annular ligament (**D**).

OVERCORRECTION OSTEOTOMY AND LIGAMENTOUS REPAIR OR RECONSTRUCTION

TECHNIQUE 8.14   *Figure 8.77*

(SHAH AND WATERS)

- Make a curvilinear incision to allow for possible triceps tendon harvesting and to perform an ulnar opening wedge osteotomy (Fig. 8.77B). Initially, open only the proximal portion.
- Identify the radial nerve between the brachialis and brachioradialis in the distal humerus. Dissect the nerve distal to its motor (posterior interosseous nerve) and sensory branches.
- Mobilize and protect the nerves throughout the remainder of the procedure.
- Expose the joint through the anconeus–extensor carpi ulnaris interval. Carry the dissection proximal and elevate the extensor-supinator mass and capsule as a single tissue plane off the distal humerus (Fig. 8.77C).
- Debride the elbow joint of synovitis and pulvinar. Pay particular attention to the proximal radioulnar joint so that it will fit anatomically into place.
- At this point, it must be determined if the native annular ligament can be used for reconstruction. Identify the central perforation in the capsular wall that separates the dislocated radial head from the joint. This is the site of opening of the original ligament. Extend the incision from the center outward to enlarge this opening. This will allow the native annular ligament to be reduced over the radial neck (Fig. 8.77D).
- Remove capsular adhesions from the radial head for reduction back into the joint. Reattach the native ligament to the ulna using the large periosteal sleeve.
- If the native ligament cannot be used, prepare to harvest the triceps fascia for ligament reconstruction.
- Attempt radial head reduction, carefully scrutinizing congruity between the radial head and capitellum. If satisfactory, proceed with ligamentous repair or reconstruction. If the radius cannot be reduced, perform an ulnar osteotomy at the site of maximal deformity, which will involve a more distal ulnar exposure (Fig. 8.77E).
- Perform periosteal dissection under fluoroscopic guidance.
- Make an opening wedge osteotomy using a laminar spreader to allow the radial head to align with the capitellum without pressure. The goal is partial overcorrection of the ulnar alignment. Alternatively, temporary anatomic pinning of the radiocapitellar joint can be done to allow opening of the ulnar osteotomy.
- Once reduced, partially fix the ulnar osteotomy proximally and distally using a plate and screws. No bone graft is necessary.
- Remove the temporary pin from the radiocapitellar joint. To ascertain radiocapitellar and radioulnar alignment, rotate the radial head, testing for a complete stable arc.
- Repair the periosteum and return attention to the ligamentous repair or reconstruction.
- If the native annular ligament can be used, repair this with mattress sutures through the ulnar periosteal tunnels. Do not tighten these sutures until all have been placed.
- If the annular ligament cannot be used, develop a 6- to 8-cm strip of triceps fascia from proximal to distal, elevating the periosteum from the proximal ulna to the level of the radial neck. Take care not to amputate the fascia.
- Pass the strip of tendon through the periosteum, around the radial neck, bringing it back and suturing it to itself and the ulnar periosteum. Passing and securing the tendon through the periosteum is similar to the drill holes described by Seel and Peterson.
- Repair the capsule and extensor supinator origin back to the lateral epicondylar area of the humerus.
- Before complete closure, obtain final radiographs and fluoroscopy to make sure there is a stable arc of motion in flexion and extension and pronation and supination.
- Prophylactically perform forearm fasciotomies and inspect the radial nerve before subcutaneous and skin closure.
- Apply a long arm, bivalved cast with the forearm in 60 to 90 degrees of supination and the elbow flexed 80 to 90 degrees.

POSTOPERATIVE CARE The cast is worn for 4 to 6 weeks and then changed to a removable bivalved cast to allow active pronation and supination. Flexion and extension of the elbow are usually the first to return, with full rotary motion returning over 6 months.

GALEAZZI FRACTURES

Galeazzi fractures, or fractures of the radius with dislocation of the distal radioulnar joint (DRUJ), are rare in children. Most fractures of the distal forearm are associated with anterior displacement of the distal ulna unlike proximal forearm fractures, which are associated with posterior dislocations. True lateral radiographs are essential in making the diagnosis. Reduction of the radial fracture will reduce the DRUJ in most patients. In patients with irreducible fractures, open reduction and internal fixation of the distal radius should be performed and the DRUJ reassessed. If the DRUJ remains dislocated, then open reduction and internal fixation of the DRUJ should be performed to remove interposed structures, most commonly periosteum, extensor carpi ulnaris, or extensor digiti quinti tendon, and the triangular fibrocartilage complex (TFCC). The DRUJ may be pinned with the forearm supinated to provide additional stability.

Although this injury usually occurs in adolescents, a pediatric variant consisting of a Salter-Harris type II fracture of the distal ulna occurs before rupture of the TFCC can occur in a younger child. The treatment principles are the same as for adolescents; however, periosteal entrapment may block reduction rather than the TFCC.

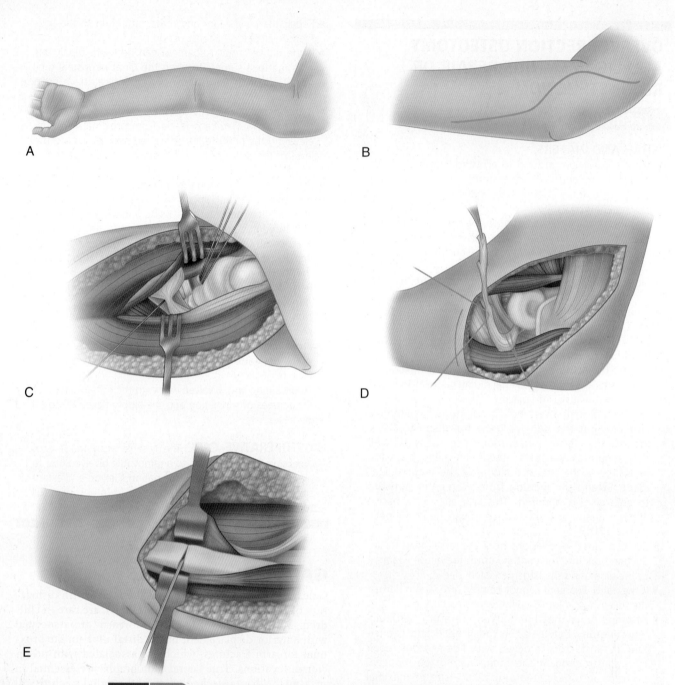

FIGURE **8.77** Reconstruction of late or chronic Monteggia fracture-dislocation. **A,** Clinical deformity of chronic Monteggia lesion with increased cubitus valgus. **B,** Extensile incision for annular ligament reconstruction and ulnar osteotomy. **C,** Exposure of radiocapitellar and radioulnar joint with elevation of extensor-supinator origin from lateral epicondyle, protection of radial nerve, and thorough joint debridement. **D,** Radial head with osteochondral change from chronic dislocation. Annular ligament has been reduced around radial neck, and sutures are in place for reconstruction to annular ligament. **E,** Ulnar opening wedge osteotomy at site of maximal deformity. (Redrawn from Shah AS, Waters PM: Monteggia fracture-dislocations in children. In Flynn JM, Skaggs DL, Waters PM, editors: *Rockwood and Wilkins' fractures in children*, ed 8, Philadelphia, 2015, Wolters Kluwer.) **SEE TECHNIQUE 8.14.**

NURSEMAID'S ELBOW

Nursemaid's elbow is a subluxation of the annular ligament over the radial head, most commonly occurring in children 2 to 3 years of age when longitudinal traction is placed on the upper extremity with the elbow extended and forearm supinated. Despite the well-known mechanism of injury, 30% to 40% of patients with nursemaid's elbow present without any history of a traction injury. Radiographs are normal in this condition, unlike Monteggia variants in which there is plastic deformation of the ulna. A variety of closed reduction techniques have been reported to be successful. A combination of forearm flexion and supination or forced hyperpronation will reduce most nursemaid's elbows. Immobilization with a sling has been used for several days for symptomatic relief. Recurrence is high, and parents need to be counseled to avoid traction on the child's upper limbs. Patients in which the diagnosis is unclear should be reexamined in 7 to 10 days to ensure the correct diagnosis. This usually resolves around the age of 5 years when the ligamentous structures about the elbow mature and give it more stability.

FOREARM FRACTURES

Forearm fractures are the most common fractures in children and account for up to 40% of all pediatric fractures and, unlike in adult patients, the rate of segmental fracture is around 1%. The forearm can be divided into three regions: proximal, middle, and distal based on unique physiologic differences such as muscle forces and growth potential. Ninety percent of the growth of the forearm occurs at the distal third, giving it tremendous remodeling capacity, unlike the proximal third where very little growth and remodeling capacity exists.

PROXIMAL THIRD FOREARM FRACTURES

Fractures of the proximal third of the forearm without radial head subluxation or dislocation are uncommon. Because of the possibility of an associated radial head dislocation, radiographs of the elbow should be obtained in any proximal forearm fracture. Many proximal fractures are unstable in flexion, making operative treatment often necessary, especially in older children and adolescents. When surgical fixation is necessary, good results can be obtained with intramedullary nailing or plate fixation. Radioulnar synostosis is rare and can occur during forearm fracture at any level but is most common in proximal third fractures. Risk factors for radioulnar synostosis include severe initial injury, displaced fractures at the same level, operative treatment, and radial head excision.

MIDDLE THIRD FOREARM FRACTURES

Diaphyseal fractures of the forearm are the third most common pediatric fracture, behind the distal radius and supracondylar humerus. The most common mechanism of injury is a fall onto an outstretched hand. Many of the fractures of the midforearm in children can be treated nonoperatively, especially in young children because of the remodeling potential. The unique physiologic characteristics of pediatric bone, including its increased elasticity, increases the potential for incomplete or greenstick fractures and plastic deformation. These fractures have no remodeling potential and reduction is necessary.

Despite increased interest in operative treatment of these injuries, closed reduction with cast application remains an essential method of treatment, especially for minimally displaced fractures in younger children. Meticulous casting technique, including an intraosseous mold, straight ulnar border, three-point molding, and close follow-up to watch for late displacement or angulation, is essential for a good outcome. The cast index, defined as the sagittal cast width divided by the coronal cast width, of less than 0.7 is predictive of successful outcome (Fig. 8.78). Although this was initially described

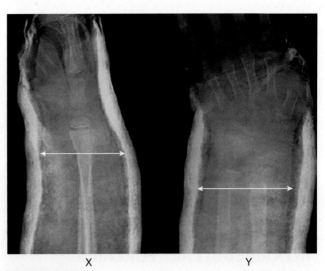

FIGURE 8.78 Cast index is X/Y (sagittal width divided by coronal width). Arrows demonstrate that cast index is calculated from inner surface of plaster cast on both coronal and sagittal views of plain film. (From Kamat AS, Pierse N, Devane P, et al: Redefining the cast index: the optimum technique to reduce redisplacement in pediatric distal forearm fractures. *J Pediatr Orthop* 32:787, 2012.)

for distal radial fractures, it is a good guideline for diaphyseal fractures as well.

Indications for operative treatment include open fracture, fracture in older children, loss of reduction in a cast, malunion, irreducible fracture caused by soft-tissue interposition, unstable fracture pattern, shortening more than 1 cm, and refracture after cast treatment. The need for operative stabilization of the forearm with an ipsilateral supracondylar humeral fracture has been called into question by a recent report of 17 patients treated with closed reduction and casting of their forearm fractures and had no loss of reduction. A dramatic increase in operative treatment of diaphyseal fractures in children between the ages of 5 and 12 years has been the result of the use of intramedullary nailing. The most common procedures use stable elastic intramedullary nailing of the radius and ulna, as described by Metaizeau, or plating. Studies, including a Cochrane review and meta-analysis comparing nailing with plating, showed that there was no significant difference in outcomes between the two techniques and outcomes were good in 90% of patients. Patients with intramedullary nailing had better cosmetic results but did require a second procedure to remove the implant. The Metaizeau nailing technique involves prebending of the nails to allow for restoration of the radial bow and to facilitate optimal reduction. It is important to avoid the distal radial physis and insert the nail in the radial side of the distal radius proximal to the physis. This approach avoids nail placement in Lister's tubercle, which has been shown to have a high rate of extensor pollicis brevis tendon injury. The ulna usually is nailed antegrade either through or proximal to the proximal ulnar physis. Transphyseal nail placement is technically easier and has not been shown to cause growth arrest but is associated with a higher rate of minor implant irritation. The pins are buried below the skin, and most authors recommend a brief period of immobilization, with nail removal between 4 and 12 months after fracture when the bone is healed radiographically. Other authors have shown good results with single-bone fixation of the ulna. The advantages of this technique include decreased operative time and ease of implant removal. It is not recommended for open fractures because of the higher rate of radial malunion. Repeated attempts at closed reduction and nailing increase the risk of compartment syndrome; therefore, an open reduction should be performed after two or three unsuccessful closed attempts. The rate of delayed union primarily in the ulna using this technique is 8% to 15% and higher in boys, adolescents, those with increased fracture displacement, and those who had open reduction of the ulna.

INTRAMEDULLARY FOREARM NAILING

TECHNIQUE 8.15

- Place the child supine with the affected arm on a radiolucent table and apply, but do not inflate, a pneumatic tourniquet if open reduction is required.
- Identify the distal radial physis and fracture site with fluoroscopy and mark these on the skin.
- Make a 5-mm longitudinal incision on the lateral (radial) side of the distal metaphysis proximal to the distal radial physis, taking care to protect the radial sensory nerve.
- Drill a hole in the bone 5 to 10 mm proximal to the physis, first perpendicularly and then obliquely toward the elbow.
- Depending on the diameter of the bone, choose a titanium or stainless steel nail of the appropriate size, which is typically 2.0 to 3.0 mm. Introduce the nail into the radius proximally, taking care not to pass it out the medial (ulnar) cortex of the radius (Fig. 8.79).
- Reduce the fracture and pass the nail into the proximal diaphysis.
- The ulna can be nailed antegrade or retrograde, although antegrade nailing is technically straightforward. To do this, mark the course of the ulnar nerve as it crosses the elbow on the skin for reference. Make a 5-mm longitudinal incision over the posterior olecranon and drill a small entry hole, taking care to protect the ulnar nerve. Pass the nail across the fracture site in an antegrade fashion. An alternative proximal lateral entry portal can be created on the lateral side of the olecranon just distal to the olecranon apophysis.
- Alternatively, retrograde nailing can be done in a fashion to that used for the radial nail. To do this, place a small drill hole just proximal to the distal ulnar physis. Pass the nail retrograde, taking care to prevent cutout of the lateral (radial) cortex. Once the fracture is reduced and the nail is in good position, cut the nail approximately 5 mm from the entry point, irrigate, and close the soft tissues. Avoid multiple passes with the nail because this increases the risk of compartment syndrome. Open reduction should be performed if it is difficult or impossible to pass the nail in a closed fashion.
- Close all wounds. Apply a long arm, bivalved cast or splint.

POSTOPERATIVE CARE After intramedullary nail fixation, the cast is removed after 4 to 6 weeks. The nails are removed at 6 months after fracture. Participation in sports is avoided for 2 months.

Patients treated with intramedullary nailing for open or closed forearm fractures have been reported to have an increased incidence of compartment syndrome compared with patients treated with closed reduction and casting. Also, patients with longer operative times, increased use of intraoperative fluoroscopy, and multiple attempts at closed percutaneous nailing are at higher risk of developing compartment syndrome. Close observation and monitoring of all patients with both-bone forearm fractures is recommended, but especially of those at risk.

Plate fixation is indicated for patients with length unstable or comminuted fractures and fractures with delayed or nonunion in which the medullary canal may be inaccessible to an intramedullary nail. Although plates provide better length and rotational stability, as well as restoration of the radial bow, they require longer operative time and larger incisions. Single bone plating of the radius or ulna has been reported as well, but there is a risk of malunion of the unplated bone. Refracture after plate removal is well documented in adults, but no clear data exist in children. Adolescents at or near skeletal maturity need to be counseled as to the risk of refracture after implant removal.

PLASTIC DEFORMATION AND GREENSTICK FRACTURES

Plastic deformation occurs due to the increased porosity and elasticity of a child's bone. Plastic deformation occurs as a result of microfracture along the bow. These fractures have little to no remodeling potential, especially in older children, and should be reduced to prevent cosmetic and functional complications. These can be reduced gradually under sedation either with direct manipulation or over a fulcrum. Outcomes are good as long as the injury is recognized.

Greenstick fractures are unique to children and most commonly occur in the mid-diaphysis of the radius and ulna. Fractures at the same level can be treated with closed reduction and cast application. Fractures at different levels indicate a rotational component that needs to be corrected at the time of reduction. Important features of greenstick fractures are that they have little remodeling potential and a high rate of refracture. For this reason, most authors recommend completing the greenstick fracture before casting, which allows for more abundant callus formation.

DISTAL THIRD FOREARM FRACTURES

The distal radius is the most commonly fractured bone in childhood, with a peak age of 10 years. This is typically caused by a fall onto an outstretched upper extremity. Approximately half of children with a distal radial fracture have an associated ulnar fracture. Other associated injuries, although rare, can occur and include ipsilateral scaphoid and supracondylar humeral fracture. Isolated ulnar fractures are very rare in children. The diagnosis of these injuries usually can be

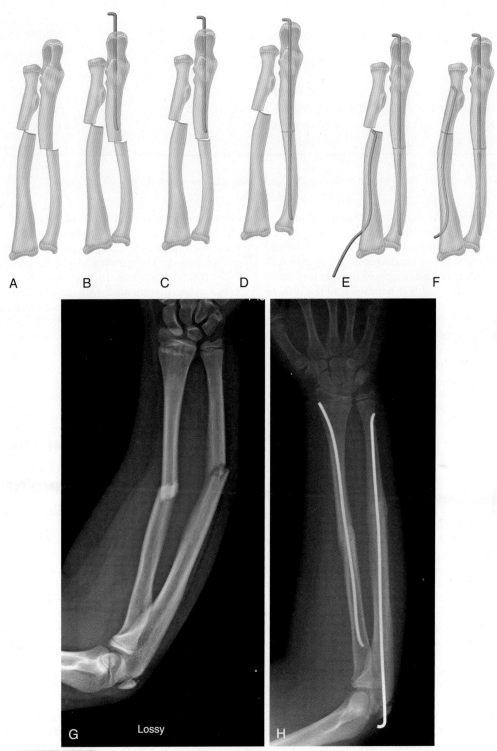

A   B   C   D   E   F

G   Lossy   H

FIGURE 8.79   Intramedullary nailing of both-bone fractures of forearm. **A** and **G,** Displaced both-bone fractures. **B,** Pin is introduced into least displaced bone. **C,** Pin is advanced to fracture site. **D,** Fracture is reduced by external manipulation, and pin is advanced into proximal metaphysis. **E,** Fracture of other bone is reduced and fixed in same manner. **F** and **H,** Both pins in place. **SEE TECHNIQUE 8.15.**

TABLE 8.1				
Recommended Acceptable Alignment Parameters for Pediatric Forearm Fracture by Age				
SOURCE	**AGE**	**ANGULATION**	**MALROTATION**	**BAYONETTE APPOSITION/ DISPLACEMENT**
Price (2010)	<8 yr	<15 degrees (MS) <15 degrees (DS) <10 degrees (PS)	<30 degrees	100% displacement
Noonan, Price (1998)	<9 yr	<15 degrees	<45 degrees	<1 cm short
Tarmuzi et al. (2009)	<10 yr	<20 degrees		No limits
Qairul et al. (2001)	<12 yr	<20 degrees		

DS, Distal shaft; *MS*, mid-shaft; *PS*, proximal shaft.
From Vopat ML, Kane PM, Christino MA, et al: Treatment of diaphyseal forearm fractures in children, *Orthop Rev (Pavia)* 6:5325, 2014.

made with plain radiographs alone, and the elbow should be included in all imaging of distal third fractures to rule out an associated elbow injury. Advanced imaging, such as MRI and CT, is not routinely used unless the diagnosis is in question or an associated wrist injury such as scaphoid fracture is present. Ultrasound can be used to diagnose nondisplaced fractures in young children; however, it is user dependent and not readily available in all centers.

Because of its frequency, the management of distal radial fractures is one of the cornerstones of pediatric orthopaedic care. Although there has been an increase in operative treatment of these injuries, especially in older children, closed treatment is still the most common method of treatment. Because 90% of the growth of the forearm occurs distally, there is tremendous remodeling potential for these fractures, especially in young children. An age-based approach in determining acceptable alignment and need for operative treatment can be used (Table 8.1). Fundamentals of closed treatment include reduction using the periosteal hinge, well-molded cast, and close early follow-up. It has been shown that the cast index, as described by Chess, of less than 0.7 is predictive of successful cast treatment. A recent study showed that 80% of fractures that lost reduction did so in the first 2 weeks, emphasizing the need for close, early follow-up. The optimal time of cast immobilization remains controversial but ranges from 3 to 4 weeks for children 5 years of age or younger and from 4 to 6 weeks for older children. Buckle (torus) fractures are common, and well-designed randomized studies show that removable splint treatment without further radiographic follow-up is well tolerated, safe, and cost-effective for these injuries. Considerable interest exists in minimizing radiation exposure in children in general and specifically in those with distal radial fractures. The use of routine radiographs for evaluation of buckle and other stable fractures is becoming less common; however, radiographs are warranted if there is any concern about loss of reduction. Risk factors for loss of reduction include open fractures, obese patients, residual translation of more than 50% in any plane, age greater than 9 years, and angulation of the radius of more than 15 degrees on the lateral view and of the ulna more than 10 degrees on the anteroposterior view.

Physeal fractures are common, accounting for a third of all distal radial fractures. Most are Salter-Harris types I and II injuries; Salter types III to VI injuries are very rare. The risk of growth arrest is 1% to 7%. This can be treated by epiphysiodesis of the remaining physis and ulnar shortening osteotomy. Distal

ulnar growth arrest is rare and can be treated with radial epiphysiodesis and ulnar lengthening osteotomy.

Closed reduction with percutaneous pinning with single or dual pins has been shown to provide good outcomes with a low complication rate. In a randomized study of percutaneous pinning compared with cast treatment, the authors found a higher rate of loss of reduction in the cast group than the pinning group. However, 38% of patients in the pinning group had mild complications related to the pin, which resolved with removal. The pins can be left outside the skin, and pin removal can be performed in the outpatient setting. The use of open reduction and internal fixation is reserved for older children who are near or at skeletal maturity.

CLOSED REDUCTION AND PERCUTANEOUS PINNING OF FRACTURES OF THE DISTAL RADIUS

TECHNIQUE 8.16

- Position the patient on the operating table with the wrist over a sterilely draped inverted image intensifier.
- Reduce the fracture using traction and gentle manipulation, especially for a physeal fracture.
- While holding the wrist in a flexed position to stabilize the fracture, use a Kirschner wire and the image intensifier to mark the trajectory of the pin on the skin.
- Start the pin at the tip of the radial styloid and pass it proximally and ulnarly across the fracture site.
- Once the fracture is pinned, cut and bend the pin and obtain final images. It is important to leave the pin long so that it does not become buried under the skin during cast treatment.
- Place the arm in a well-padded short arm splint or bivalved cast.

POSTOPERATIVE CARE The short arm cast is worn for 3 to 4 weeks, and the pin is then removed. Range-of-motion exercises are started, and the patient is placed in a removable splint for an additional 4 weeks.

WRIST DISLOCATIONS

Because of the proximity of the distal radial and ulnar physes to the wrist joint, wrist dislocations are extremely rare in children. When they do occur, it is usually in a skeletally mature adolescent. Treatment is similar to that in adults.

SCAPHOID AND CARPAL FRACTURES

The carpal bones ossify relatively late in childhood; therefore fractures of the carpal bones are rare and when present can be overlooked. A recent study of MRI examination of 90 consecutive wrist injuries in patients younger than 18 years found that of the carpal fractures the most common were scaphoid fractures (83%), followed by fractures of the capitate (12%) and triquetrum (5%). Scaphoid fractures are the most common carpal injuries in children and adolescents, with peak age of 15 to 19 years. They have become more common as more children participate in competitive sports.

The scaphoid is the largest bone in the proximal row of the carpus, and ossification begins between age 5 and 6 years and is completed between the ages of 13 and 15 years corresponding with the peak incidence of fracture. Fractures of other carpal bones generally follow their times of ossification: triquetrum, 12 to 13 years; trapezium, 13 to 14 years; trapezoid, 13 to 14 years; and hamate, 15 years. The most common mechanism of injury is a fall onto the outstretched hand with the forearm pronated. This usually produces a middle third fracture. Distal third fractures usually are caused by direct trauma or avulsion and are the most common. Proximal pole fractures are the least common.

An age-based classification that is predictive of the type of injury has been developed. Type I injuries occur in children younger than 8 years and usually are chondral. Type II injuries that occur between 8 and 11 years usually are osteochondral, and type III injuries that occur in children older than 12 years are more "adult-like" because the scaphoid is ossified. Pediatric scaphoid fractures also can be classified by location: tuberosity, transverse distal pole, avulsion of the distal pole, waist, or proximal pole. In children, fractures of the distal third of the scaphoid (transverse distal pole and tuberosity) are the most common.

The most common clinical signs of scaphoid fracture are dorsal swelling of the wrist, tenderness in the anatomic snuffbox and over the distal part of the radius, and painful dorsiflexion of the wrist or extension of the thumb. Radiographs should include anteroposterior, lateral, and scaphoid views with the wrist in ulnar deviation; however, normal radiographs do not preclude the presence of a scaphoid fracture. Plain radiography is approximately 50% sensitive for the detection of a scaphoid fracture and less than 50% for the other carpal bones. If a scaphoid fracture is suggested but radiographs are negative, the wrist should be immobilized and reevaluated in 2 weeks because up to 30% of patients may have positive follow-up radiographs. MRI, which is more sensitive than CT, is useful in making the diagnosis, and a normal study as early as 2 days after injury has a negative predictive value of 100%.

Fractures of the proximal pole, although rare, seem to heal uneventfully when treated by prolonged immobilization.

Avulsion fractures in the distal third of the scaphoid are common in children and usually require only cast immobilization, with healing rates approaching 95% for nondisplaced fractures. Healing times of scaphoid fractures have been described as 3 to 4 weeks for tuberosity fractures, 4 to 16 weeks for waist fractures, 4 to 8 weeks for distal scaphoid fractures, and 3 to 6 weeks for distal avulsions. Indications for operative treatment of scaphoid fractures in pediatric patients at or near skeletal maturity are similar to those for scaphoid fractures in adults. Smooth wires rather than compression screws have been used in young children to prevent growth arrest.

A painful nonunion of the proximal scaphoid, which in children is extremely rare, may occur after a delay in treatment generally because of an incorrect diagnosis or lack of immobilization. An established nonunion in a child may be treated operatively as in an adult. A meta-analysis of 176 surgically treated scaphoid nonunions found the healing rate to be 95%, with improvement in functional outcomes including range of motion and grip strength. A dorsal or volar approach can be used. Some authors have speculated that bipartite scaphoid may be an ununited waist fracture that has taken on the characteristics of a bipartite bone. Bipartite scaphoid usually is bilateral, asymptomatic, and not related to trauma.

Fractures of the triquetrum in children often are subtle flake avulsion or impingement fractures that require good oblique radiographs for recognition. The incidence of these fractures probably is much higher than currently known because many are misdiagnosed as wrist sprains or type I physeal injuries of the distal radius and ulna. Three weeks of cast immobilization usually is sufficient treatment.

METACARPAL FRACTURES

Fractures of the metacarpals can occur at any location; however, the most common site of metacarpal fractures in children is the metacarpal neck (75%), usually in the small and ring fingers. The peak incidence is 13 to 16 years of age. The most common mechanisms of injury are contact sports and striking an object (e.g., boxer's fracture). Metacarpal shaft fractures usually are the result of trauma such as a direct blow.

Most fractures of the metacarpals in children can be treated closed with cast immobilization. Metacarpal shaft fractures are usually stable because of the presence of intermetacarpal ligaments and can be treated with cast immobilization. Percutaneous pinning either intramedullary or to adjacent stable metacarpals can be performed for displaced or unstable fractures. Occasionally, open reduction and internal fixation is necessary for long oblique length unstable fractures as in adults. Metacarpal neck fractures usually can be treated with closed reduction and cast immobilization. Because of the mobility of the fourth and fifth metacarpals and the excellent remodeling capacity, up to 30 to 40 degrees of residual angulation can be accepted with closed treatment. Between 10 and 20 degrees of angulation generally is thought to be acceptable in the second and third metacarpal necks. Reduction can be done using the Jones technique of flexing the metacarpophalangeal joint 90 degrees and placing a dorsally directed force on the proximal phalanx with counter pressure on the metacarpal shaft. Occasionally, a metacarpal neck fracture in a noncompliant patient or an unstable fracture requires treatment with closed reduction and percutaneous pinning.

TABLE 8.2

Fractures of the Thumb Metacarpal Base in Children

TYPE	DESCRIPTION	TREATMENT
A	Between physis and junction of proximal and middle thirds of bone Often transverse or slightly oblique Often some medial impaction Angulated in apex lateral direction	Closed reduction + cast Residual angulation of 20-30 degrees is acceptable depending on age of child and clinical appearance of thumb If unstable after reduction, percutaneous pinning required
B	Salter-Harris type II physeal fracture with metaphyseal fragment on medial side More common than type C	Mild angulation—no reduction, cast Moderate angulation—closed reduction + cast Severe angulation—closed reduction + percutaneous pinning; open reduction and fixation if closed reduction unsuccessful
C	Salter-Harris type II physeal fracture with metaphyseal fragment on lateral side	
D	Salter-Harris type III or IV fracture Resembles Bennett fracture in adults	Closed or open reduction and internal fixation

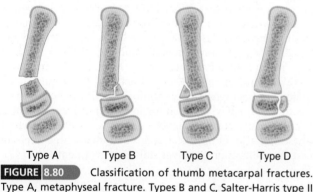

Type A   Type B   Type C   Type D

FIGURE 8.80 Classification of thumb metacarpal fractures. Type A, metaphyseal fracture. Types B and C, Salter-Harris type II physeal fractures with lateral or medial angulation. Type D, Salter-Harris type III fracture.

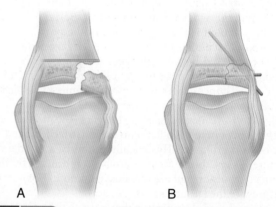

A   B

FIGURE 8.81 **A,** Type III physeal fracture. **B,** After open reduction and internal fixation with pins.

The most important goal in treatment of these injuries is restoration of normal rotation. Normal rotation should be confirmed by the ability to flex the fingers into the palm. Even a small amount (<10 degrees) of rotational malalignment can create overlap of the digits during flexion and cause functional limitations; corrective osteotomy to align the digit often is necessary. If troublesome malrotation persists, the fracture will not remodel and either percutaneous pinning or open reduction and internal fixation is indicated. A displaced intraarticular metacarpal head fracture, which usually is seen in older children or adolescents, may also require open reduction and internal fixation.

THUMB METACARPAL FRACTURES

Most thumb metacarpal fractures in children occur proximally near the physis rather than the distal metacarpal as in the other metacarpals (Table 8.2). As a rare variant, the thumb metacarpal may have a physis at the proximal and distal ends, and comparison views are helpful in making this diagnosis. A fracture of the thumb metacarpal base usually can be treated for 3 to 4 weeks in an abduction thumb spica cast (Fig. 8.80A). The physeal fracture that occurs most often in this area is a Salter-Harris type II injury, and it can be treated by closed reduction (Fig. 8.80B, C). Pediatric Bennett fractures can occur, however, and are Salter-Harris type III fractures (Fig. 8.80D). This fracture is intraarticular, and in a

child it can result in a physeal disturbance if not treated properly. Closed reduction and percutaneous pin fixation or open reduction and internal fixation with smooth pins, as in an adult Bennett fracture, is indicated. Occasionally, in an older adolescent, a fracture of the base of the first metacarpal that does not involve the physis (Rolando fracture) can be satisfactorily reduced and pinned percutaneously with the aid of image intensification.

PHALANGEAL FRACTURES

Phalangeal fractures are common in children, with the most common mechanism being sports activity. Up to two thirds occur in the proximal phalanx at a peak age of 12 years. They can involve the shaft, physis, neck, and condyles. The majority of proximal and middle phalangeal shaft fractures can be treated with cast immobilization for 3 to 4 weeks with closed reduction being performed for displaced fractures. Ensuring proper rotation as described previously for metacarpal fractures is essential to ensure a good outcome. Many of these fractures are physeal, and Salter-Harris type II fractures of the proximal phalanx are the most common. Growth arrest, however, is uncommon. Salter-Harris type III fractures of the base of the proximal

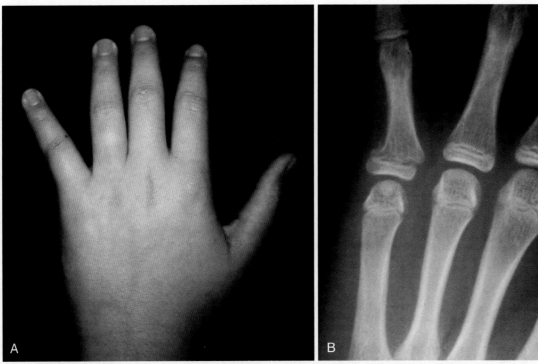

FIGURE 8.82   Extra-octave phalangeal fracture. **A,** Clinical appearance. **B,** Radiographic appearance.

or middle phalanx do occur and because of their intraarticular nature often require open reduction and internal fixation Fig. 8.81. The "extra-octave fracture," or an angulated apex radial base of the fifth proximal phalanx fracture (Fig. 8.82), can occur and is treated by placing a bolster in the fourth web space to act as a fulcrum for reduction followed by casting. Irreducible fractures require open reduction and internal fixation. Fractures of the phalangeal neck and condyles usually are unstable and often require operative treatment. Nondisplaced intraarticular fractures can be treated closed with close follow-up. Open reduction and internal fixation with small diameter wires is indicated for displaced intraarticular fractures (Fig. 8.83).

OPEN REDUCTION AND INTERNAL FIXATION OF PHYSEAL FRACTURES OF PHALANGES AND METACARPALS

TECHNIQUE 8.17

- Make a straight midlateral incision over the involved physis. After soft-tissue dissection and retraction, mobilize the neurovascular structures and lateral bands. Expose the physis, but take care not to damage it or the perichondral ring or periosteum overlying it.
- Carefully mobilize the fragments; clean out any small fragments or hematoma and reduce the fracture anatomically. Ensure that the reduction is satisfactory at the physis and joint surface.

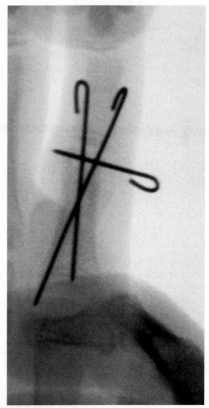

FIGURE 8.83   Pinning for phalangeal neck fracture.

- With a power drill (low torque, high speed), transfix the fracture with two smooth parallel pins, preferably in the metaphysis or epiphysis. Crossed pins and pins that cross the physis generally should be avoided, but sometimes small fracture fragments cannot be adequately transfixed and held otherwise. Cut off the pins beneath the skin but leave them long enough to be removed easily as an outpatient procedure.

- Close the soft tissues appropriately and apply a splint or cast.

POSTOPERATIVE CARE The pins are removed at 3 to 4 weeks, and a range-of-motion exercise program is started at that time or shortly thereafter. This program should be taught to the parents and the patient and should concentrate on active range of motion only. (Passive range-of-motion exercises in a child will cause the child to withdraw or guard against any motion at all.) The parents should be warned of the possibility of growth arrest with subsequent angular deformity.

DISTAL PHALANGEAL FRACTURE

Distal phalangeal fractures, unlike other fractures of the hand, occur most commonly in younger children, at a mean age of 7.5 years. They can be classified as physeal or extraphyseal. Extraphyseal fractures usually are the result of crush injuries and heal uneventfully. Meticulous nailbed exploration and repair are necessary for severe injuries to prevent late nail deformity. Displaced physeal fractures are mallet finger equivalents in children because of the attachment of the flexor digitorum profundus (FDP) tendon on the distal fragment. The Seymour fracture is a Salter-Harris type I or II fracture of the distal phalanx that is associated with a nailbed injury. These injuries often are overlooked and have a high rate of infection when treatment consisting of irrigation and debridement is initiated more than 24 hours after injury. They usually are irreducible because of the interposed sterile matrix in the physis. Operative stabilization occasionally is necessary and can be done with a small smooth Kirschner wire.

COMPLICATIONS OF PHALANGEAL FRACTURES

Complications of pediatric phalangeal fractures are uncommon, but stiffness, nonunion, malunion, infection, osteonecrosis, and growth disturbance may occur. Fractures at high risk for complications include Salter-Harris type IV (100%), Seymour (62%), and mallet fractures (52%). Nonunion is rare except in severe injuries in which the fracture fragments are devascularized. Malunion is more common and can result in angulation or rotational deformities and limited motion (Fig. 8.84). Although most malunions remodel satisfactorily, especially in young children, considerable deformity may require osteotomy for realignment. Waters et al. described a percutaneous technique for reduction of malunion of phalangeal neck fractures with partial bony healing (Fig. 8.85). An obliquely inserted Kirschner wire (0.9 to 1.6 mm, depending on the size of the child) is used to break down the callus and partially healing bone and lever the dorsally displaced and rotated condylar fragment back into the correct anatomic position. One or two percutaneous wires (0.7 to 1.1 mm) are used to hold the reduction. Growth disturbance can result from any injury that involves the physes but is uncommon after phalangeal fracture.

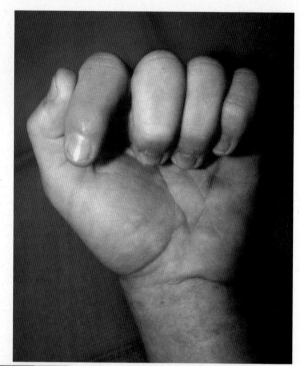

FIGURE 8.84 Malunion of phalangeal neck fracture producing malalignment of fingers.

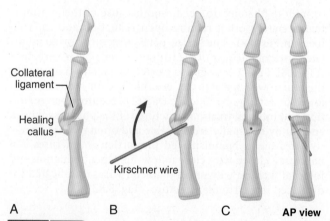

FIGURE 8.85 **A,** Percutaneous reduction of malunion of phalangeal neck fracture with partial bony healing. **B,** Kirschner wire is used to break down the callus and partial bony healing and lever the fragment into anatomic position. **C,** One or two percutaneous wires are used to hold the reduction.

PEDIATRIC SPINE FRACTURES AND DISLOCATIONS

Spine fractures and dislocations are relatively uncommon in children, accounting for 1% to 3% of pediatric fractures; however, they are associated with a high rate of other injuries and morbidity and mortality. In older children, they are most commonly caused by motor vehicle accidents and sports. A recent review of pediatric spine fractures from a high-volume center showed that 80% of injuries occurred in older children (ages 13 to 19 years) and 60% of all patients had an associated injury, most often intrathoracic. Multiple spinal-level injuries were seen in 45% of patients, of which a third were in a different region of the spine. Therefore examination of the entire spine is essential in a child with a spine injury. NAT should always be considered in young children with a cervical spine injury, especially in patients with multiple associated injuries, including retinal hemorrhages and subdural hematomas and those requiring cardiopulmonary resuscitation (CPR). Children younger than 3 years have a higher rate of spinal cord injury and mortality than older children and adolescents.

CERVICAL SPINE

Cervical spine fractures are less common in children than in adolescents or adults. They may occur at any age as a result of trauma, with motor vehicle accident being the most common mechanism in a recent large series. Because of the large head-to-body weight ratio and increased ligamentous laxity in young children, upper cervical spine injuries are more common, and lower cervical spine injuries are most often seen in adolescents. The initial radiographic examination of a child with a suspected cervical spine injury consists of anteroposterior, lateral, and odontoid radiographs, which have been shown to be more sensitive than a cross-table lateral image alone. The use of CT is becoming more prevalent, especially in the adult population, but does have an increased radiation exposure. It is important to note that small children, because of their greater relative head size, need to be positioned by elevating the torso to avoid inadvertent flexion of the cervical spine. Supervised flexion-extension radiographs can be used in an awake, cooperative patient to assess cervical spine stability. The role of MRI continues to evolve; however, it is useful in detecting ligamentous injury in patients who cannot perform flexion or extension radiographs. It also is useful in detecting disc herniation and the status of the spinal cord in patients with neurologic deficits.

■ ATLANTOOCCIPITAL FRACTURES AND INSTABILITY

Occipital condyle fractures in children are extremely rare. The majority are stable and can be treated with a cervical orthosis. Atlantooccipital dislocation (AOD) was once thought to be uniformly fatal; however, with advanced trauma care more children are surviving. A recent report of 14 patients found that most were injured in automobile accidents, and complications including spinal cord and brain injury were common (Fig. 8.86). Cranial nerve injuries also can be present. At our institution over a 20-year period, we had 14 AODs that were treated with posterior occipitocervical fusion with internal fixation. All fusions united, but at the time of the most recent follow-up, half of the patients had residual neurologic impairment. The most common postoperative complication was hydrocephalus, which should be suspected with postoperative neurologic decline.

A variety of imaging radiographic measurements has been described to aid in making the diagnosis. One helpful reproducible measurement is the Wackenheim line. The Wackenheim line drawn along the clivus should intersect tangentially the tip of the odontoid. A shift in this line either anteriorly or posteriorly from the odontoid tip is indicative of AOD (Fig. 8.87). MRI, which shows disruption of the tectorial membrane, is helpful in making this diagnosis. It is also helpful in assessing the degree of soft-tissue disruption at adjacent caudal levels. Operative stabilization, in most instances, is an

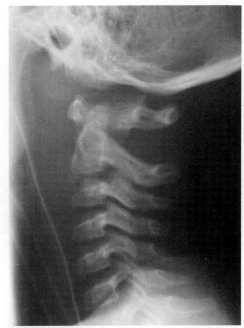

FIGURE 8.86 Atlantooccipital dislocation.

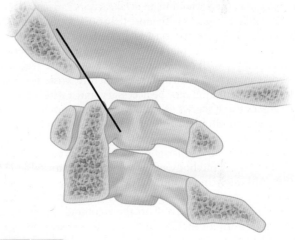

FIGURE 8.87 Wackenheim line. (Redrawn from Astur N, Sawyer JR, Klimo P Jr, et al: Traumatic atlantooccipital dislocation in children. *J Am Acad Orthop Surg* 22:274, 2014.)

occiput-to-C2 fusion using wires or screws depending on the size and anatomy of the patient. Acute hydrocephalus related to changes in cerebrospinal fluid flow is common in the early postoperative period.

■ UPPER CERVICAL SPINE (C1–C2) INJURIES

C1 fractures are extremely uncommon in children. Often the normal synchondrosis is mistakenly identified as a fracture (Fig. 8.88)—fractures are relatively common cervical spine fractures in children, with a peak incidence at 4 years. These fractures usually result from high-energy trauma such as a motor vehicle accident or fall. They typically occur through the odontoid synchondrosis at the base of the odontoid and displace anteriorly. Because of this, the diagnosis usually can be made on plain radiographs, especially the lateral view. CT with sagittal reconstruction also is helpful in confirming

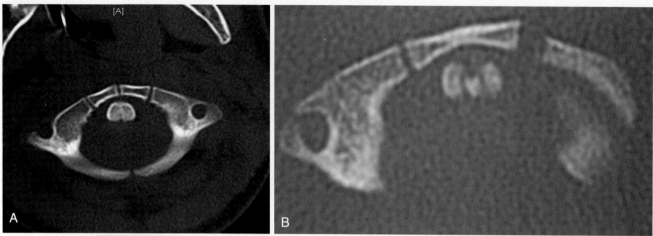

FIGURE 8.88 **A,** Normal C1 synchondrosis. **B,** Left C1 fracture. Note widening of normal synchondrosis on right compared to left and normal individual in **A**.

the diagnosis and evaluating for other associated injuries (Fig. 8.89). Physician-supervised flexion-extension radiographs can be performed in an awake, cooperative patient to assess stability. Patients with more than 50% opposition of the odontoid can be treated with an extension Minerva cast or halo for 6 to 8 weeks followed by an orthosis. Many patients cannot comply with or tolerate this, and operative treatment is necessary. In patients with C1–C2 fracture, posterior fusion with instrumentation may be necessary, and a wide variety of techniques using screws or wires has been reported.

An os odontoideum describes a range of deficiencies of the odontoid from complete absence to mild hypoplasia. It most commonly consists of an accessory ossicle that is separated from the body of C2, rendering it unstable (Fig. 8.90). Although most authors believe this is a congenital deformity, some have suggested this may occur as a result of a minor traumatic event to the odontoid. Presentation can range from an incidental finding to a displaced injury after a traumatic event. The diagnosis usually can be made on a lateral radiograph because the ossicle usually is smaller and more sclerotic than the normal odontoid. Supervised flexion-extension radiographs can be performed to assess the stability of the os, which correlates to the likelihood of developing neurologic symptoms from spinal cord compression. CT with sagittal reconstruction can aid in confirming the diagnosis and in operative planning. It can detect the presence of other associated cervical spine abnormalities such as a hypoplastic ring of C1. Indications for surgery include progressive or significant instability, pain, or neurologic compromise, and there is no role for nonoperative treatment in these patients. C1–C2 fusion can be performed using a variety of techniques including wiring or transarticular screw fixation depending on the surgeon's ability and patient's anatomy.

■ ROTATORY SUBLUXATION

Rotatory subluxation between C1 and C2 occurs most frequently after an acute upper respiratory tract infection

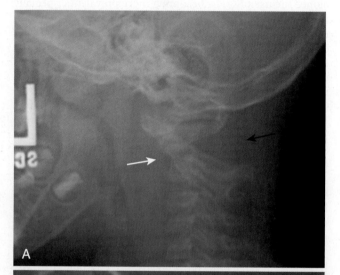

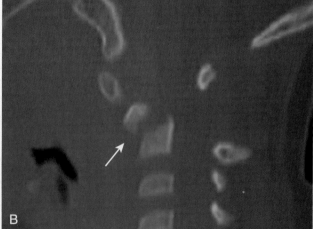

FIGURE 8.89 Lateral radiograph (**A**) and sagittal CT scan (**B**) of displaced odontoid fracture (white arrows). Note widening of the posterior elements consistent with significant injury and widening of the posterior ligamentous structures (black arrow).

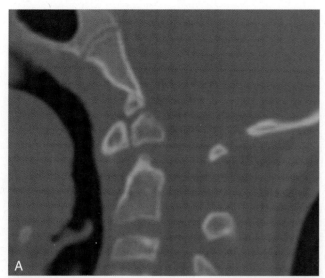

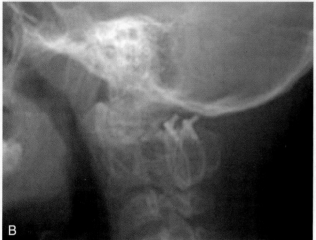

FIGURE 8.90 A, Os odontoideum, preoperative sagittal CT reconstruction. B, After C1-C2 wiring and arthrodesis.

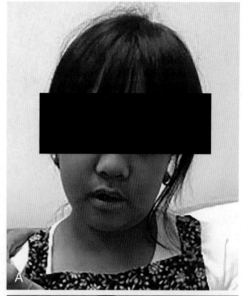

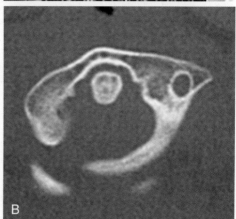

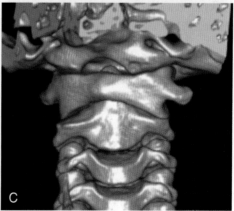

FIGURE 8.91 Torticollis. **A,** Typical "cock-robin" clinical appearance. **B,** Axial CT shows asymmetry of C1-C2 facets. **C,** 3-D reconstruction shows subluxed C1-C2 facet.

or after low-grade trauma. It is thought that the inflammation associated with an upper respiratory tract infection increases the blood supply to the region, inducing laxity of the capsular and ligamentous structures. Patients typically present with a torticollis or "cock robin" position to their neck (Fig. 8.91A). Pain is common in the acute stage and is usually associated with sternocleidomastoid spasm as the child attempts to stabilize the head. In late cases the pain subsides and fixed deformity persists. Diagnosis can be made on plain films, especially the odontoid view, which shows asymmetry of the distance between the odontoid and lateral masses. CT, either dynamic or with three-dimensional reconstruction, can be used to confirm the diagnosis (Fig. 8.91B,C). Rotatory subluxation has been classified by Fielding and Hawkins: type I is a unilateral facet subluxation and an intact transverse ligament, type II is a unilateral facet subluxation with transverse ligament involvement resulting in 3 to 5 mm of anterior displacement, type III is a bilateral facet subluxation with greater than 5 mm anterior displacement, and type IV is displacement of the atlas posteriorly rather than anteriorly. Types III and IV injuries are

exceedingly rare but are associated with a high rate of neurologic injury.

Most acute subluxations can be treated nonoperatively. Patients can be placed in a soft collar and given antiinflammatory medication and diazepam for muscle spasm. If it does not resolve within a week, hospitalization and halter traction are indicated. Halo traction also can be used in severe cases. Operative treatment consisting of reduction and C1–C2

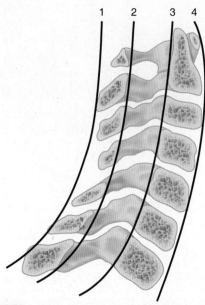

FIGURE 8.92 Spinal lines. Normal relationships in the lateral cervical spine: 1, spinous processes; 2, spinolaminar line; 3, posterior vertebral body line; 4, anterior vertebral body line. (Redrawn from Copley LA and Dormans JP: Cervical spine disorders in infants and children. *J Am Acad Orthop Surg* 6:204, 1998.)

fusion is reserved for the rare acute cases that do not resolve with nonoperative treatment or those with neurologic deficits. Often it is necessary in patients with chronic subluxations to correct the head and neck deformity operatively with posterior spinal fusion and instrumentation.

■ LOWER CERVICAL SPINE (C3–C7) INJURIES

Subaxial cervical spine injuries occur more commonly in older children and adolescents and are usually the result of high-energy injuries and sporting accidents. Both clinical and radiographic evaluation of the entire spine is necessary in these patients because of the high rate of secondary spine injuries that frequently occur at noncontiguous levels. Subaxial cervical spine injury can be a pure ligamentous disruption, facet dislocation(s), or fracture; it is similar to an adult injury. An understanding of normal developmental anatomy is helpful, as pseudosubluxation or apparent anterior translation, most commonly of C2 on C3, is a normal finding in children and adolescents. In addition, anterior wedging of the vertebral bodies is also a normal finding related to the ossification pattern of the vertebral body.

Plain radiographs are the standard initial step in the radiographic evaluation of the pediatric cervical spine. The anterior and posterior vertebral and spinolaminar lines (Fig. 8.92) are helpful in assessing the normal and pathologic anatomic relationships. CT has been shown to have improved sensitivity in making the diagnosis of cervical spine fracture but does have a higher radiation exposure. MRI is helpful in assessing the amount of ligamentous and soft-tissue disruption and detecting subtle compression fractures that may be missed on plain radiographs or CT.

One unique injury in pediatric patients is spinal cord injury without radiographic abnormality (SCIWORA), first described by Pang and Wilberger. This condition is characterized by a spinal cord injury, either complete or incomplete, in the absence of any radiographic abnormalities. A meta-analysis found that in half the patients, MRI was normal, which carries a better long-term prognosis as well. It is hypothesized to be related to a severe flexion distraction injury of the cervical spine. Cadaver studies have shown that, due to ligamentous laxity, the spinal column in children can undergo 4 to 5 cm of distraction before disruption compared with 4 mm to 5 mm for the spinal cord. A stretch-related vascular mechanism has also been proposed. Delayed neurologic compromise can occur in 50% of patients, and some demonstrate transient warning signs. Recovery is unpredictable, and there is no treatment available when this occurs.

The operative techniques for treatment of these specific injuries are similar to adults and are discussed in other chapter. It should be noted that the use of intraoperative neuromonitoring including transcranial motor-evoked potentials (tcMEP), when possible, is essential. In a series of 77 pediatric patients undergoing surgical treatment of spine injuries, 10% had significant loss of tcMEP during the procedures, despite somatosensory-evoked potentials (SSEP) remaining normal.

THORACOLUMBAR SPINE

Thoracolumbar fractures are rare in young children and can be the result of NAT in neonates. They are more common in older children and adolescents and are usually the result of motor vehicle accidents, sports injuries, and falls. Thoracolumbar spine fractures in the absence of trauma can be associated with infection and osteopenia in conditions such as juvenile osteoporosis, corticosteroid use, and certain genetic syndromes. Associated injuries, both spine and non-spine, are common and a thorough examination of the entire patient is necessary to evaluate and treat these appropriately. One such injury is the lap belt injury, in which a child receives a hyperflexion injury from the lap belt causing anterior spinal compression, posterior spinal distraction, and compression of the intraabdominal structures between the lap belt and the spine. This often is diagnosed by the presence of seat belt abrasions on the patient's skin. The risk of intraabdominal injury is 42% with this injury. The role of corticosteroids in children with thoracolumbar fractures and spinal cord injuries remains controversial.

Initial radiographic evaluation should consist of anteroposterior and lateral radiographs of the entire spine and odontoid views. CT with sagittal and coronal reconstructions is helpful in making the diagnosis and evaluating spinal canal compromise (axial view) and posterior element injuries. MRI has been shown to be beneficial in assessing soft-tissue structures including the disc, spinal cord, and posterior ligamentous structures. The assessment of the posterior ligamentous structures is essential in assessing spinal stability and guiding treatment. These fractures are typically classified similarly to adult fractures based on mechanism: compression, burst, flexion distraction, and ligamentous disruption (Fig. 8.93). The Thoracolumbar Injury Classification and Severity Score (TLICS), which has been used in adults, has been shown to have good intra- and inter-observer reliability and may help guide treatment in pediatric patients. Using this scoring system, a score of 1 to 3 suggests nonoperative treatment is best, a score of 4 indicates either operative or nonoperative treatment, and a score of more than 5 indicates that operative treatment is best. It should be noted that this system is based on CT scan findings and that the use of MRI, which is more

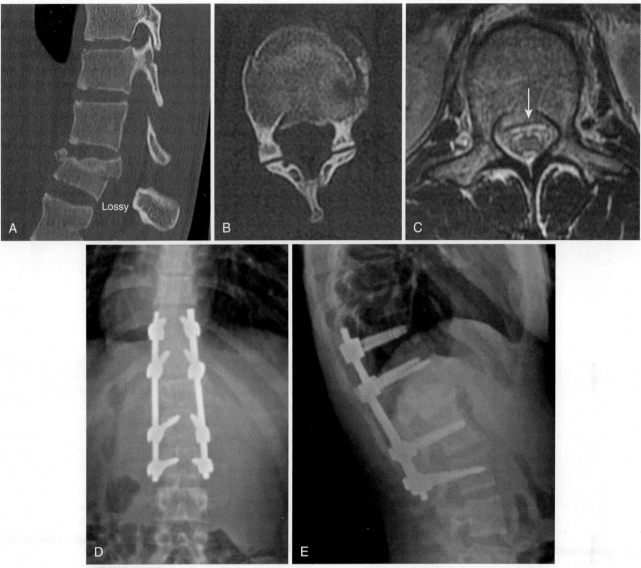

FIGURE 8.93 Burst fracture. **A**, Coronal CT. **B**, Sagittal CT. **C**, Axial MRI. **D** and **E**, Postoperative anteroposterior and lateral radiographs.

prone to false-positive diagnosis of PCL injuries, may produce falsely elevated TLICS scores, leading to a greater rate of operative treatment. Treatment usually is similar to adults, which is described in other chapter.

The Chance, or flexion distraction, fracture commonly is seen in children and is a result of a flexion distraction force usually applied by a lap belt (Fig. 8.94). In children these can be bony, usually through the endplate, ligamentous, or both. Historically, some of these fractures, especially the isolated bony injury, were treated in braces. Several outcome studies have shown that operative treatment is superior in terms of return to function and better long-term sagittal alignment than nonoperative treatment, especially in those with abdominal injuries or significant posterior ligamentous disruption as seen on MRI (Fig. 8.95). In a multicenter study, Arkader et al. reported better clinical outcomes in patients treated operatively for Chance fractures.

Another fracture unique to pediatric patients is the endplate fracture, which is a flexion-type injury that usually occurs in an older child. A displaced fragment of a lumbar vertebral ring epiphysis in adolescents may simulate disc rupture (Fig. 8.96). The finding at surgery usually is a displaced bony fragment from the apophyseal ring, which is deficient posteriorly. This fragment can occasionally be seen on plain radiographs and can readily be seen on CT. MRI is the diagnostic imaging procedure of choice and has been reported to be able to differentiate endplate physeal fractures from herniated discs in children. In symptomatic patients, treatment consists of removal of the avulsed bony fragment.

PELVIC FRACTURES

Fractures of the pelvis in children are uncommon. Surgical fixation rarely is necessary for these fractures. Generally, the long-term results of conservative treatment are satisfactory because of the remodeling potential of the pelvis in children. However, recent literature has questioned the true remodeling potential of the immature pelvis, leading to an increase in surgical stabilization of pelvic fractures in this age group. Pelvic fractures may be associated with high-energy mechanisms, and soft-tissue

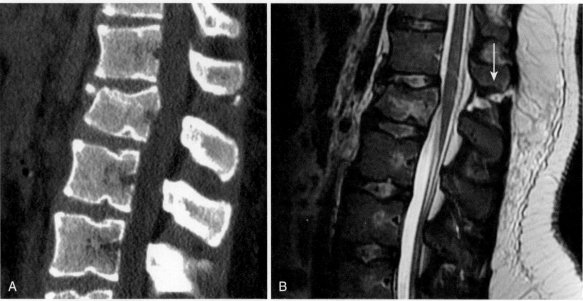

FIGURE 8.94 Chance fracture. **A,** Preoperative sagittal CT. **B,** MRI. Note significant intraspinous ligament edema and disruption *(arrow)*.

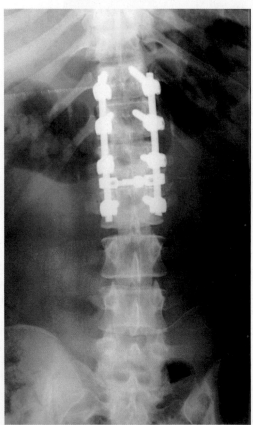

FIGURE 8.95 Chance fracture after spinal fixation.

injuries occurring in conjunction with pelvic fractures may be severe and require emergency treatment. Associated injuries include skull, cervical, facial, and long bone fractures; subdural hematomas, cerebral contusions, and concussions; lung contusions; hemothorax; hemopneumothorax; ruptured diaphragm;

and lacerations of the spleen, liver, and kidney. Injuries that may be associated with and adjacent to pelvic fractures include damage to major blood vessels, retroperitoneal bleeding, rectal tears, and rupture or laceration of the urethra or bladder. The location and number of pelvic fractures are strongly associated with the probability of abdominal injury: 1% for isolated pubic fractures, 15% for iliac or sacral fractures, and 60% for multiple fractures of the pelvic ring. Because of these other injuries, mortality in children is high (9% to 18%). In a study of 54 patients with major pelvic fractures, 87% had associated pelvic or extrapelvic (soft-tissue) injuries; 14.8% died. Most patients (70.4%) were treated conservatively. This suggests that the principles of management in children should not differ greatly from those in adults. Serious associated pelvic or extrapelvic injuries may pose more treatment problems than the actual pelvic fractures. The death rate from pelvic fractures alone is quite low (0% to 2.3%). Torode and Zieg reported 11 deaths in 141 patients with pelvic fractures, and 40% of patients with type IV injuries required laparotomy because of other injuries. Frequently, a child who has what radiographically appears to be a minor pelvic fracture also has had significant and possibly life-threatening soft-tissue injuries around the pelvis.

The initial evaluation of pelvic fractures usually is dictated by the mechanism of injury and associated injuries, and if a high-energy mechanism was the cause, the pediatric advanced life support protocol should be followed. This should include a thorough history, careful physical examination, laboratory tests when indicated, and appropriate imaging. If there is a high suspicion of pelvic trauma, an anteroposterior radiograph of the pelvis should be obtained. Additional radiographs, such as inlet and outlet views and Judet views of the pelvis, also may be of benefit. CT should be obtained in any patient suspected of having pelvic instability, anterior disruption, or posterior ring involvement. If a patient with a pelvic fracture becomes hemodynamically unstable, a pelvic binder should be placed. If the patient remains unstable, angiography or surgical packing should be considered based on institutional guidelines. For patients

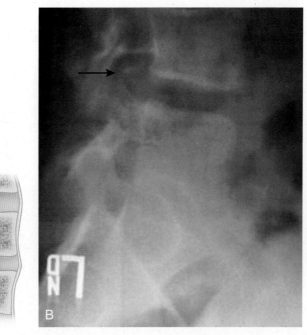

FIGURE 8.96   A, Posterior physeal injury that can mimic ruptured disc. B, Avulsion of ring apophysis has produced displaced fracture *(arrow)* that has pressed on nerve root.

with a vertically unstable pelvis or hip joint instability, skeletal traction should be placed.

The pelvis in children differs from that in adults in that (1) more malleability is present because of the nature of the bone itself, the increased elasticity of joints, and the ability of the cartilaginous structures to absorb energy; (2) the elasticity of the joints around the pelvis is greater, which may allow for significant displacement and result in fracture of only one area rather than the traditional double break in the pelvic ring seen in adults; (3) the cartilage at the apophyses is inherently weak compared with bone, so avulsion fractures occur more frequently in children and adolescents than in adults; and (4) fractures into the triradiate cartilage can occur, causing growth arrest, which results in leg-length inequality and faulty development of the acetabulum.

In children and adolescents with pelvic fractures, isolated pubic rami and iliac wing fractures occur more often in an immature pelvis (open triradiate cartilage), whereas acetabular fractures and pubic or sacroiliac diastasis occur more often in a mature pelvis (closed triradiate cartilage). In patients with an immature pelvis, treatment of pelvic fractures should focus on associated injuries (e.g., head, abdominal) that often are the cause of mortality.

Numerous classification systems have been devised for pelvic fractures in children. The most widely used classification was proposed by Torode and Zieg and describes a four-part classification of pelvic fractures: type I, avulsion of the bony elements of the pelvis; type II, iliac wing fractures; type III, simple ring fractures, including fractures involving the pubic rami or disruptions of the pubic symphysis; and type IV, including unstable injuries such as ring disruption fractures, hip dislocations, disruption of the sacroiliac joint, and fractures involving the acetabular portion of the pelvic ring. More recently, Shore et al. proposed a modification of the Torode and Zieg classification that subdivided type III injuries into

type III-A (simple, stable anterior ring fractures) and type III-B (stable pelvic fractures involving the anterior and posterior ring). Shore et al. demonstrated that type III-B injuries were associated with increased blood product use, intensive care requirement, and length of hospital stay (Fig. 8.97).

This classification does not subdivide acetabular fractures. Quinby and Rang classified pelvic fractures into three categories: uncomplicated fractures, fractures with visceral injuries requiring surgical exploration, and fractures associated with immediate massive hemorrhage. Although this classification is useful concerning the patient's ultimate outcome, its emphasis is on associated soft-tissue injuries, rather than on the pelvic fracture itself. Moreno et al. described four types of "fracture geometry" based on radiographic appearance and used to identify patients at risk for severe hemorrhage. Adult classifications such as the AO/ASIF group and the Young and Burgess should be applied to a pelvis with a closed triradiate cartilage and emphasize fracture stability and direction of force: lateral compression, anteroposterior compression, vertical shear, and combined mechanisms (Fig. 8.98). Key and Conwell's classification of pelvic fractures in adults is based on the number of breaks in the pelvic ring. Their system, which includes acetabular fractures, also is applicable in children. We have evaluated 134 pelvic fractures in children; the percentages of the individual bones and types of fractures are given in Table 8.3. The Orthopaedic Trauma Association devised a classification scheme that consists of three main types and numerous subtypes: A, lesion sparing (or with no displacement of) posterior arch; B, incomplete disruption of posterior arch, partially stable; and C, complete disruption of posterior arch, unstable.

Comparison among studies using different systems is difficult. The most useful information is whether a fracture is stable or unstable. Most pelvic fractures in children are stable.

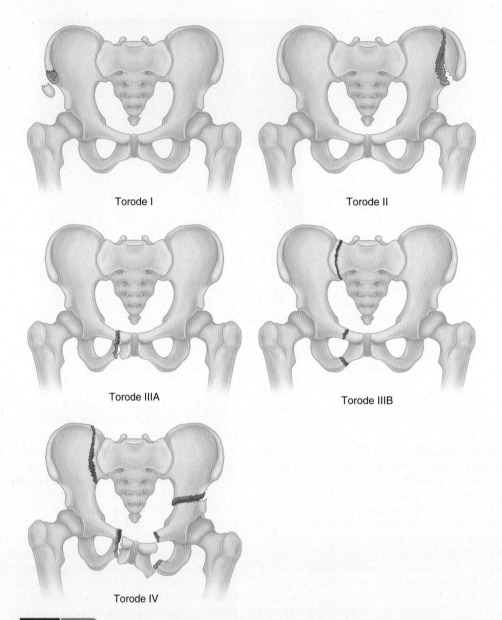

Torode I

Torode II

Torode IIIA

Torode IIIB

Torode IV

FIGURE 8.97 Shore et al. modification of Torode classification. *Torode I,* avulsion of bony elements of pelvis and separation through or adjacent to cartilaginous physis. *Torode II,* iliac wing fracture resulting from direct lateral force against pelvis causing disruption of iliac apophysis or infolding fracture of wing of ilium. *Torode IIIA,* simple stable anterior ring fracture involving pubic rami or pubic symphysis. *Torode IIIB,* stable anterior and posterior ring fracture. *Torode IV,* unstable ring disruption fracture, including ring disruptions, hip dislocations, and combined pelvic and acetabular fractures. (Redrawn from Shore BJ, Palmer CS, Bevin C, et al: Pediatric pelvic fracture: a modification of a preexisting classification. *J Pediatr Orthop* 32:162, 2012.)

Three physical signs are commonly associated with pelvic fractures: (1) Destot sign, a large superficial hematoma formation beneath the inguinal ligament or in the scrotum; (2) Roux sign, a decrease in the distance of the greater trochanter to the pubic spine on the affected side in lateral compression fractures; and (3) Earle sign, a bony prominence or large hematoma and tenderness on rectal examination, indicating a significant pelvic fracture. Posterior pressure on the iliac crest causes pain at the fracture site as the pelvic ring is opened, and compression of the pelvic ring at the iliac crest from lateral to medial causes pain and possibly crepitation. Downward pressure on the symphysis pubis and posteriorly

on the sacroiliac joints causes pain and motion if a break in the pelvic ring is present. Pain in the inguinal area can be elicited by flexion and extension of the hips.

As already noted, most pelvic fractures in children can be treated closed, usually with protected weight bearing and activity restriction. Minor residual deformity usually is inconsequential and may remodel with growth. However, significant displacement or an unstable fracture pattern should be treated operatively. Occasionally, if the child is young and has significant diastasis of the symphysis, a spica cast alone may be used to maintain a reduced position during healing. In older children or those with unstable fracture patterns, the management of pelvic fractures should closely follow adult principles with surgical fixation that does not disrupt or alter the growth of the triradiate cartilage. If the triradiate cartilage is closed, operative techniques are the same as in adults.

AVULSION FRACTURES

Avulsion fractures occur most commonly in adolescent athletes. These fractures occur due to rapid and forceful contraction of muscles that attach to apophyses of a developing pelvis. The force required to disrupt the cartilaginous apophysis is typically less than that required for musculotendinous disruption; therefore apophyseal fractures occur more often than musculotendinous injury in the adolescent population. The most common injuries as reported in a recent meta-analysis are the anterior inferior iliac spine (AIIS) from the pull of the rectus femoris, the ischial tuberosity (IT) from the pull of the hamstrings, the anterior superior iliac spine (ASIS) from the pull of the sartorius, the iliac crest from the pull of the tensor fasciae latae, the lesser trochanter from the pull of the iliopsoas, and the superior corner of the pubic symphysis from the pull of the rectus abdominis (Fig. 8.99). CT scans are rarely required in this subset of pelvic injuries. Operative treatment of these injuries is rarely indicated, regardless of the amount of displacement; however, recent studies have suggested that operative results may lead to slightly improved results particularly with displacement of 2 cm or more. Sundar and Carty described 32 avulsion fractures of the pelvis in adolescents (average age 13.8 years) seen at an average 44-month follow-up; 10 patients had disability persisting into adulthood and limitation of sports activity, and six patients continued to have persistent symptoms. Although they advocated surgical exploration and removal of ununited fragments, Sundar and Carty cautioned that operative treatment does not guarantee

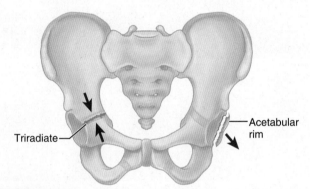

FIGURE 8.98 Small acetabular rim fracture and triradiate cartilage compression fracture.

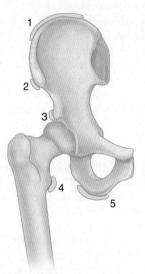

FIGURE 8.99 Iliac crest, 1; anterior superior iliac spine, 2; anterior inferior iliac spine, 3; lesser trochanter, 4; ischium or ischial apophysis, 5.

TABLE 8.3

Distribution of Pelvic Fractures in Children, Campbell Clinic Series (134 Patients)

I—INDIVIDUAL BONES 66.5%				II—SINGLE BREAK 11.9%			III—DOUBLE BREAK 11.9%			IV—ACETABULUM 9.7%			
A	B	C	D	A	B	C	A	B	C	A	B	C	D
13.4%	33.6%	18%	1.5%	8.2%	3%	0.7%	3%	8.2%	0.7%	0.7%	6%	0	3%

COMPARISON WITH OTHER SERIES

	DUNN* (115 PATIENTS)	PELTIER* (186 PATIENTS)	REED* (84 PATIENTS)	HALL, KLASSEN, ILSTRUP† (204 PATIENTS)	CAMPBELL CLINIC† (134 PATIENTS)
I—Individual bones		10%	60.5%	24.5%	66.5%
II—Single break	70%	39%	2.5%	18.6%	11.9%
III—Double break	30%	27%	32%	31.9%	11.9%
IV—Acetabulum	Not included	24%	5%	7.8% (17.2% acetabulum and pelvis)	9.7%

Classification of Key and Conwell.
*Adult series.
†Children's series.
From Rockwood CA Jr, Wilkins KD, King RE, editors: *Fractures in children,* ed 3, Philadelphia, 1991, Lippincott.

the return of the athlete to the same standard as before the injury.

Rarely, excessive callus formation or myositis ossificans occurs after a displaced IT fracture. In two of our patients it was necessary to excise the fragment and the callus, rather than reattach the fragment. Recurrence of some excessive callus or myositis ossificans occurred, but these two patients continued their athletic activity. Any of these avulsion injuries, especially in the area of the ischium, can be confused with infection, myositis ossificans, and sarcoma. If there is any question of diagnosis, appropriate imaging and laboratory workup should be performed.

ACETABULAR FRACTURES

Acetabular fracture-dislocations in children make up 4% to 20% of pelvic fractures in the pediatric population. Damage to the triradiate cartilage in a child may cause growth arrest and a shallow, dysplastic acetabulum (Fig. 8.100). CT may help determine the extent of acetabular involvement and femoral head stability. However, in an immature pelvis, radiographs and CT may underestimate the extent of the injury; therefore, MRI should be considered to evaluate the cartilaginous portion of the acetabulum, labrum, and triradiate cartilage. The Watts classification of acetabular fractures is based on the extent of acetabular involvement: (1) small fragments most often associated with dislocation of the hip (see Fig. 8.98), (2) linear fractures associated with pelvic fractures without displacement, (3) large linear fractures with hip joint instability, and (4) central fracture-dislocations.

Initial treatment should focus on a reduced hip joint. Hip reduction requires optimal sedation and muscle relaxation. Although this can be performed safely in the emergency department, many institutions prefer this maneuver to be done in the operating room to avoid femoral head displacement. It is important, however, for a dislocated hip to be reduced immediately to minimize further vascular insult to the femoral head. Hip stability should be assessed at the time of reduction, and radiographs of the contralateral hip should be obtained for comparison of joint congruency. Radiographs before reduction may reveal an occult fragment more readily than films taken after the reduction. If an incongruence is found or suspected, a CT or MRI should be obtained to evaluate the cause and for operative planning purposes.

The treatment of many pediatric acetabular fractures is nonoperative. Stable linear fractures with less than 1 mm of displacement and a negative stress test require only conservative treatment with a minimum of 6 to 8 weeks of non–weight bearing. Linear fractures producing hip joint instability often require a period of skeletal traction followed by definitive fixation to ensure an accurate reduction. This injury usually occurs in older children, and treatment should be the same as for adults. A review of 38 adolescents with acetabular fractures demonstrated open reduction and fixation to be safe and effective at obtaining bony union with low complication rates. As expected, articular involvement was predictive of higher rates of degenerative arthritis. Central fracture-dislocations in children should be reduced promptly because the triradiate cartilage may be involved. Because injury to the triradiate cartilage is easily missed on initial radiographs, all patients with pelvic trauma should be followed clinically and radiographically for at least 1 year. Two main patterns of physeal disruption have been identified in patients with triradiate cartilage

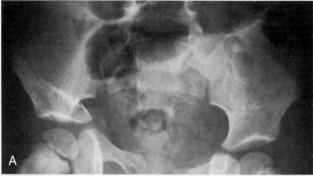
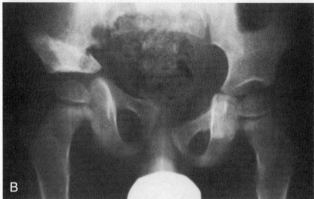
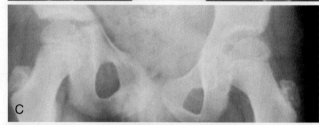
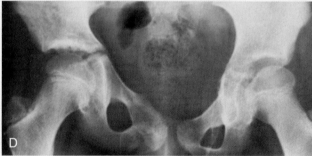

FIGURE 8.100 Premature closure of triradiate cartilage. **A,** Fracture of right ilium is visible. Fracture on left was not identified. **B,** At 4 months, fracture on right is seen again. At left, acetabulum shows increased sclerosis caused by ischial fracture into acetabulum. **C,** At 5 years, premature closure of left triradiate cartilage. **D,** At 6 years, premature closure of left triradiate cartilage and subluxation of femoral head caused by shallow acetabulum.

injuries: a Salter-Harris type I or II injury, which has a favorable prognosis for continued normal acetabular growth, and a Salter-Harris type V crushing injury, which has a poor prognosis because of premature closure of the triradiate physes secondary to formation of a medial osseous bridge (Fig. 8.101). In both patterns, the prognosis depends on the age of the patient at the time of injury. In young children, especially those younger than 10 years, abnormal acetabular growth can result in a shallow acetabulum. By skeletal maturity, disparate

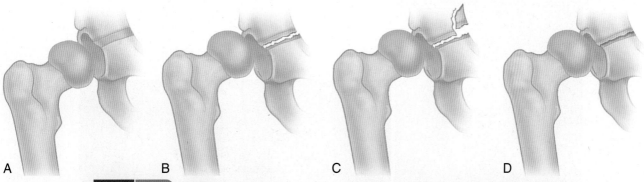

FIGURE 8.101 Types of injuries to the pelvis and triradiate cartilage. **A,** Normal hemipelvis. **B,** Salter-Harris type I fracture. **C,** Salter-Harris type II fracture. **D,** Salter-Harris type V fracture.

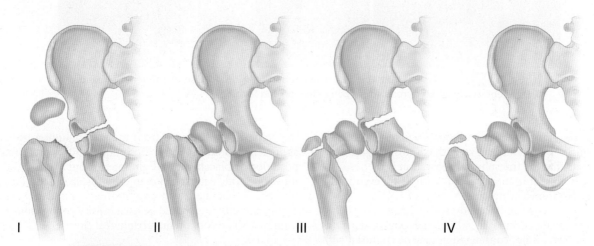

FIGURE 8.102 Delbet classification of hip fractures in children. *Type I,* transepiphyseal, with or without dislocation from acetabulum. *Type II,* transcervical. *Type III,* cervicotrochanteric (basicervical). *Type IV,* intertrochanteric.

growth may increase the incongruity of the hip joint and lead to progressive subluxation. Acetabular reconstruction may be indicated for correction of the gradual subluxation of the femoral head with associated dysplasia.

HIP FRACTURES

Hip fractures include fractures of the head, neck, and intertrochanteric region of the femur and account for less than 1% of all pediatric and adolescent fractures. Different hip morphology and the presence of a physis produce hip fracture patterns that are different in children from those in adults. Complications of both the injury and treatment are frequent and should be considered during the treatment course. Late complications include osteonecrosis, coxa vara, nonunion, and premature physeal closure. Appropriate treatment of hip fractures in children is necessary to minimize these late complications. Diagnosis of a hip fracture is based on history, physical examination, and radiographs. Hip fractures in children most commonly result from a high-energy mechanism followed by pathologic fracture. As in adults, the index of suspicion for hip fracture should be high to facilitate urgent management. A standard anteroposterior radiograph of the pelvis and lateral of the hip should be obtained, as well as imaging of the entire femur. Advanced imaging

may be helpful to rule out an occult injury or to evaluate the extent of the fracture.

The most widely used classification for hip fractures in the pediatric population was proposed by Delbet. This classification groups fractures according to their location: type I, transepiphyseal separations with or without dislocation of the femoral head from the acetabulum; type II, transcervical fractures, displaced and nondisplaced; type III, cervicotrochanteric fractures, displaced and nondisplaced; and type IV, intertrochanteric fractures (Fig. 8.102). The Delbet classification has proved to have prognostic value in regard to risk of osteonecrosis, healing rates, and malunion.

TYPE I, TRANSEPIPHYSEAL SEPARATIONS

Type I fractures occur when the epiphysis separates from the metaphysis. They are further subdivided into type IA, in which the epiphysis remains in the acetabulum, and type IB, in which the epiphysis is dislocated from the acetabulum. In our experience, the outcomes after type IB fractures have been the worst of any of the fracture types, with an incidence of osteonecrosis of 100% in some series. Type 1A fractures may be difficult to differentiate from an unstable slipped capital femoral epiphysis (SCFE). Fractures tend to occur in younger children as the result of high-energy mechanisms, whereas SCFE is mostly seen in patients between the ages of

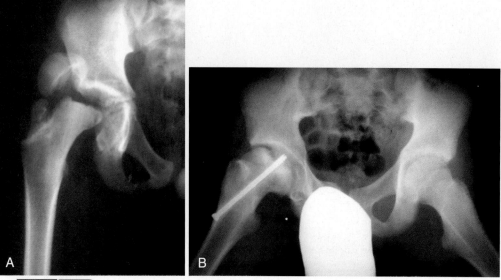

FIGURE **8.103** **A,** Type I, transepiphyseal separation with dislocation of the femoral head. **B,** Development of osteonecrosis after open reduction and fixation.

10 to 16 years after minor or no trauma. The presence of posterior medial callus on imaging or at the time of surgical fixation suggests that the transphyseal separation is the result of SCFE and is present in most patients with SCFE even in the absence of prodromal symptoms.

In newborns, an entity called *proximal femoral epiphysiolysis* occasionally occurs in which the physis separates probably at birth. If not considered, it may be confused with congenital dislocation or infection of the hip. Ultrasound, arthrography, or MRI is generally necessary to make the diagnosis early. At approximately 2 weeks after the separation, callus may be seen along the medial border of the femoral neck. Operative treatment with internal fixation is not needed for this separation. Clinical signs, such as pseudoparalysis of the lower extremity, and laboratory studies should aid in differentiating proximal femoral epiphysiolysis from infection.

The management of transepiphyseal separations depends on the age of the patient, displacement of the fracture, and presence of a dislocated epiphysis. All type I fractures should be managed urgently to minimize the vascular insult sustained by the injury (Fig. 8.103). In children younger than 2 years with a nondisplaced or minimally displaced fracture, spica cast application alone may be sufficient. If the fracture is displaced at any age and the epiphysis is located within the acetabulum, we advocate a gentle closed reduction attempt with fixation. Smooth pins are used in young patients and cannulated screws in older patients. An arthrogram may help evaluate the quality of the reduction in young patients. We routinely perform a capsulotomy to evacuate the hemarthrosis, although evidence is inconclusive that this decreases the incidence of osteonecrosis. If a gentle closed reduction does not yield a satisfactory reduction, then an open reduction should be performed through a Watson-Jones or Smith-Peterson approach (see Techniques 1.62 and 1.63), Alternatively, a surgical dislocation approach may be used; however, we have used this technique only in the setting of delayed fixation with the presence of early callus formation or in the presence of femoral head fracture (Fig. 8.104). If

the epiphysis is displaced from the acetabulum, a posterior approach (modified Gibson, Technique 1.80) is preferred for posterior displacement and an anterior approach (Watson-Jones or Smith-Peterson) for anterior displacement. Fixation typically is obtained with two or three cannulated screws. Again, smooth pins should be used in very young children to minimize the risk of premature physeal closure.

TYPE II, TRANSCERVICAL FRACTURES

Transcervical fractures are the most common hip fractures in children. Most of these are displaced, and the amount of displacement seems to be directly related to the development of osteonecrosis. We believe that displacement of the fracture is the leading variable in vascular insufficiency and that the maximal amount of displacement probably occurs at the time of injury. Capsular distention and subsequent tamponade of the vessels have been suggested to increase the incidence of osteonecrosis, and evacuation of the hematoma early by aspiration or capsular release and early internal fixation have been recommended to decrease the rate of osteonecrosis. In one report of 70 femoral neck fractures in children, however, early ORIF of type II fractures still resulted in an incidence of osteonecrosis of 35%. Type II fractures have an increased risk of varus malunion, hardware failure, and physeal arrest than more distal fractures. Internal fixation is recommended for all transcervical and basicervical fractures because of their inherent instability. A gentle closed reduction, similar to that for adult femoral neck fractures, should be done with longitudinal traction, abduction, and internal rotation, followed by fixation with pins or cannulated hip screws. Multiple closed reduction attempts should be avoided. For unsatisfactory closed reductions, open reduction through an anterior Watson-Jones approach or Smith-Peterson approach is used. Percutaneous screw placement can be done with the use of an image intensifier, and a capsulotomy should be performed. The head and neck of a child's femur are extremely hard, and the use of triflanged nails or other similar devices should be avoided for fear of distraction of the fracture and

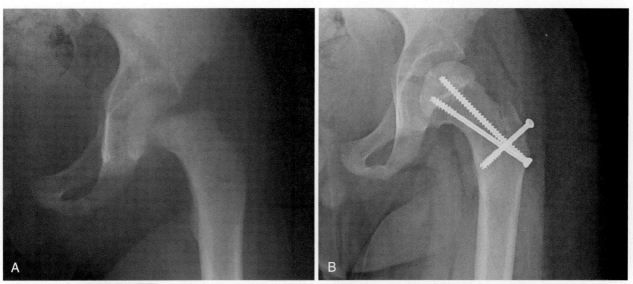

FIGURE 8.104 Surgical fixation in setting of late presenting femoral neck fracture with presence of early callus formation with modified Dunn approach.

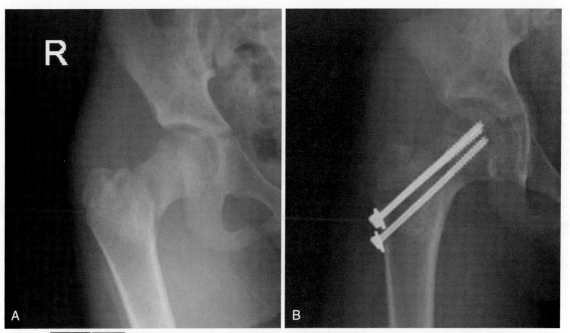

FIGURE 8.105 **A,** Displaced type III (cervicotrochanteric) fracture in 6-year-old child. **B,** After closed reduction, capsular decompression, and fixation across physis for additional stability.

possible separation of the capital femoral epiphysis. In small children, two or three pins may suffice but should be backed up with a spica cast. We routinely use two or three cannulated screws with the largest diameter that the femoral neck will accommodate. Alternatively, a pediatric or an adolescent hip screw or proximal femoral locking plate may be used for basicervical fractures. Swiontkowski and Winquist recommended 4.5-mm AO cortical screws inserted short of the physis and overdrilled in the proximal fragment for a lag effect. In young children, we try to avoid crossing the physis with fixation; however, in older children or when additional stability is required, fixation is advanced across the physis (Figs. 8.105 and 8.106). Postfixation SCFE has been reported when fixation abuts the proximal femoral physis. The priority

of treatment should be achieving stable fixation instead of preservation of growth because the sequelae of failed fixation or osteonecrosis are more challenging problems than subsequent growth arrest. A spica cast with the hip in abduction is used for 6 weeks for patients with questionable fixation, young age, or questionable compliance.

TYPE III, CERVICOTROCHANTERIC FRACTURES

Type III fractures (cervicotrochanteric) are similar to fractures occurring at the base of the femoral neck in adults, although osteonecrosis after this fracture in children is more common than in adults. A fracture in this location often allows for more stable fixation without crossing the physis;

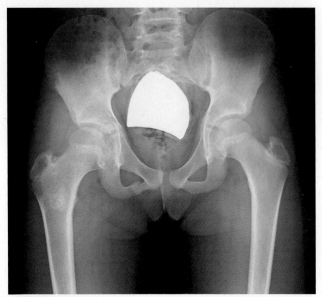

FIGURE 8.106 Displaced type III cervicotrochanteric fracture. Same pattern as in Figure 8.105 after screw removal.

however, nonunion, malunion, premature physeal closure, and hardware failure can still occur in this subset of patients. Treatment is recommended as for type II fractures with the goal of anatomic reduction and stable fixation.

TYPE IV, INTERTROCHANTERIC FRACTURES

In our experience, type IV fractures (intertrochanteric) result in fewer complications than the other types. Because of the child's osteogenic potential in the trochanteric area, rapid union almost always occurs, usually within 6 to 8 weeks (Fig. 8.107). These fractures are generally extracapsular, making osteonecrosis less common, with a reported incidence of 0% to 10%.

Because intertrochanteric fractures are extracapsular, they are not treated with the same sense of urgency. However, the quality of the fracture reduction and stability of the fixation are still important to preserve the biomechanics of the hip and optimize healing. In children 3 years of age and younger, nondisplaced fractures may be treated with spica cast application alone. In the presence of displacement or age older than 3 years, internal fixation is recommended. Reduction and fixation are achieved through a lateral approach to the hip and placement of a pediatric or adolescent compressive hip screw or proximal femoral locking plate. Fixation does not need to cross the physis, and a capsulotomy does not need to be routinely performed. Stronger implants often allow for early motion without cast immobilization; however, a spica cast is recommended if noncompliance is a concern.

COMPLICATIONS

Complications after femoral neck fractures are frequent. The most serious complication of hip fractures in children is osteonecrosis. As Trueta described, the blood supply to the femoral head transitions from metaphyseal during infancy toward the lateral epiphyseal vessels during childhood with the formation of the physis, which acts as a barrier for metaphyseal blood supply. During preadolescence the artery of the ligamentum teres anastomoses to the lateral epiphyseal vessels, and finally in late adolescence and into adulthood, the metaphyseal blood supply is restored. Osteonecrosis has been demonstrated to directly correlate with worse outcomes after femoral neck fractures. Spence et al. reviewed 70 femoral neck fractures at a single institution and found an overall incidence of osteonecrosis of 29%. The only independent predictors of osteonecrosis were displacement and fracture location. Yeranosian et al. reviewed 30 studies and found an overall incidence of 23%, with the fracture location and timing of reduction being the only predictors. Moon and Mehlman reviewed 390 patients as part of a meta-analysis

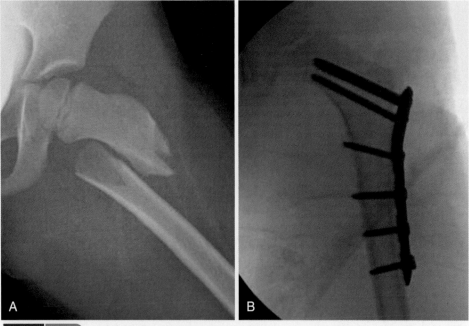

FIGURE 8.107 **A,** Type IV (intertrochanteric) fracture in 5-year-old child. **B,** After fixation with proximal femoral locking plate. **SEE TECHNIQUE 8.22.**

and found fracture type and patient age to be the strongest predictors of osteonecrosis, with rates of osteonecrosis of 38% for type I fractures, 28% for type II fractures, 18% for type III fractures, and 5% for type IV fractures.

Ratliff described three types of osteonecrosis: type I, whole head involvement; type II, partial head involvement; and type III, an area of osteonecrosis from the fracture line to the physis (Fig. 8.108). Although osteonecrosis usually is diagnosed radiographically within 12 months of injury, it may not be clinically evident for several years. The prognosis and treatment options for osteonecrosis depend on the extent of the osteonecrosis, the degree of deformity and collapse, and the age at which symptoms begin (Fig. 8.109). In general, restricted weight bearing has not produced acceptable results in the treatment of osteonecrosis; reports in the literature indicate that it is successful in fewer than 25% of patients. Operative treatment options include core decompression, with or without cancellous bone grafting; nonvascularized and vascularized bone grafting; various osteotomies to rotate the necrotic segment of the femoral head out of the weight-bearing area; and even resurfacing or total hip arthroplasty in older adolescents. Some preliminary reports indicate that the addition of osteoinductive or angiogenic factors may improve the results of core decompression.

Coxa vara occurs less often when internal fixation is used. In our experience, if the neck-shaft angle is more than 120 degrees in a young child, remodeling will occur to some degree, and even if not the deformity causes little disability. If the neck-shaft angle is between 100 and 110 degrees, however, the coxa vara deformity generally does not remodel. Significant coxa vara causes a shortened extremity and an abductor or gluteal lurch and delayed degenerative joint changes. For these reasons we have routinely used a subtrochanteric valgus osteotomy for persistent coxa vara deformity and for nonunion (Fig. 8.110). A closing wedge osteotomy just distal to the greater trochanter, using a pediatric lag screw

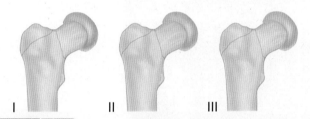

FIGURE 8.108 Three types of osteonecrosis described by Ratliff. Type I, total head involvement. Type II, segmental involvement. Type III, involvement from fracture line to physis.

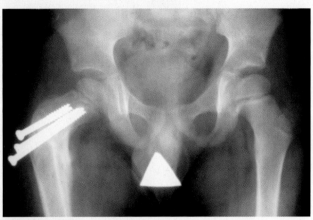

FIGURE 8.110 Coxa vara deformity after type III fracture. Fixed-angle locking plates can be used to minimize the risk of coxa vara.

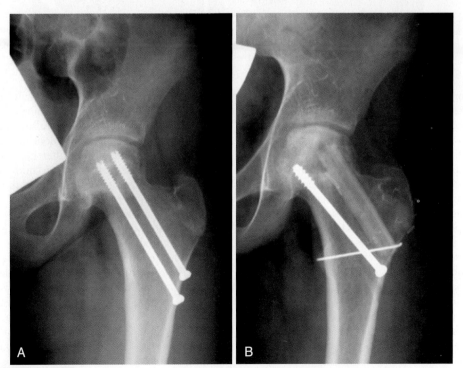

FIGURE 8.109 **A,** Osteonecrosis after type III fracture in an 11-year-old girl. The fracture was treated with urgent open reduction and internal fixation and capsular decompression. **B,** One year after vascularized fibular grafting.

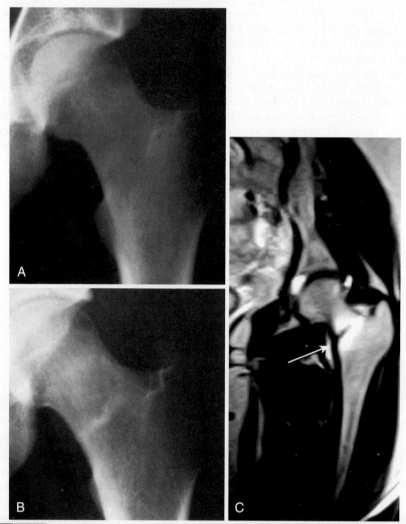

FIGURE 8.111 Stress fracture of femoral neck. **A,** Radiograph showing possible faint inferior femoral neck fracture. **B,** Radiograph made 3 weeks later revealing callus formation in inferior neck at stress fracture. **C,** MR image shows stress fracture.

with a side plate or proximal femoral locking plate for internal fixation, is preferred. Although nonunion of the osteotomy is rare, a one and one-half spica cast may be applied if there are concerns about the quality of the fixation or compliance of the patient.

Internal fixation also decreases the rate of nonunion, but when nonunion occurs, operative treatment should be undertaken as soon as possible. We have used a valgus subtrochanteric osteotomy to make the nonunion more horizontal and allow compressive vertical forces to aid in union. This osteotomy can be augmented, if necessary, with bone grafts. Internal fixation is routinely used across the nonunion site, with or without the use of a spica cast. A modification of the Pauwels intertrochanteric osteotomy using a 120-degree double-angle osteotomy plate has been described for the treatment of nonunion or coxa vara or both (see Technique 8.21).

Although premature physeal closure can occur, because the capital femoral physis contributes 15% of the growth of the entire lower extremity and normally closes earlier than most of the other lower extremity physes, shortening generally is less than 2 cm. The discrepancy usually is more than 2 cm only in children in whom osteonecrosis also develops. Nevertheless, we try

to avoid penetrating the physis, especially in a young child. Leg-length inequality should be determined with scanograms and correlated with bone age and carefully recorded. Epiphysiodesis in the opposite extremity can be done if necessary.

Infection is uncommon after hip fractures in children. Chondrolysis after hip fractures in children has been reported, but most investigators have not found this complication.

Stress fractures of the femoral neck can occur in children, especially in adolescents. Devas noted two types: (1) a transverse type in the superior portion of the femoral neck, which may become displaced and cause severe morbidity, and (2) a compression stress fracture in the inferior portion of the femoral neck, which rarely becomes displaced, although mild varus deformity has occurred in young patients (Fig. 8.111). Internal fixation with a screw or pin is recommended for the transverse type, whereas the compression type may be treated by non–weight bearing and limitation of the child's activity; however, a stress fracture can progress to a complete fracture if proper treatment is not begun and the child is allowed to continue the same activity. The technique for closed reduction and percutaneous pin or screw fixation is described in the section on SCFE (see Technique 8.23).

CLOSED REDUCTION AND INTERNAL FIXATION

TECHNIQUE 8.18

- Place the child supine on a fracture table and place the appropriately padded feet in the traction stirrups.
- Perform a gentle closed reduction by applying longitudinal traction, abduction, and internal rotation. Check the reduction with anteroposterior and lateral radiographs or with an image intensifier.
- With the use of an image intensifier, make a stab wound percutaneously or a small incision just distal to the greater trochanter and dissect through the fascia lata. Reflect the vastus lateralis anteriorly, exposing the proximal femoral shaft. Elevate the periosteum and place reverse retractors around the proximal femur to aid in exposure.
- With an image intensifier, determine the correct placement for a guide pin in the lateral shaft of the femur. Drill a guide pin across the fracture site and proximally into the femoral neck. In young children, avoid penetrating the physis, if possible. Verify the correct position of the guide pin with the image intensifier.
- Measure the exact length of the portion of the guide pin in the bone. Drill a pin or a cannulated hip screw the same length as the measured length of the guide pin parallel to or over it across the fracture site.
- Remove the guide pin and place a second pin or cannulated screw parallel to the first through the guide pin hole. Use a minimum of two pins or one 6.5-mm cannulated screw. We generally use three pins or two 6.5-mm cannulated screws, depending on the size of the child and the femoral neck. Place the pins or screws parallel and in a "cluster" or inverted triangle formation.
- Close the incision and, if there is concern about the stability of fixation or compliance with weight-bearing restrictions, apply a long leg cast with pelvic band.

POSTOPERATIVE CARE If required, the cast is worn for 6 weeks. If a cast is not required, the patient should remain touch-down weight bearing for 6 weeks. The patient progresses to weight bearing on crutches during the next 6 weeks. The pins or screws can be removed at 1 year when the fracture has united or when there is evidence of osteonecrosis. Implant removal is generally recommended in young patients with significant growth remaining or if the screws cross an open physis.

OPEN REDUCTION AND INTERNAL FIXATION

TECHNIQUE 8.19

(WEBER ET AL., BOITZY)

- Place the patient supine and drape the limb so that it can be moved freely during the operation.

- Use a Watson-Jones approach to the hip joint (see Technique 1.63).
- Incise the hip joint capsule longitudinally and evacuate and flush out the hematoma, which usually is under pressure.
- Reduce the fracture with a periosteal elevator. This can be made easier by appropriate traction and internal rotation of the extremity.
- Temporarily stabilize the fracture with Kirschner wires and check the reduction in the region of the calcar. Fix the fracture permanently with cancellous screws fitted with washers. The screw threads should be in the proximal fragment only and not across the physis of the femoral head unless needed for fixation.
- Confirm the reduction radiographically and close the hip capsule.

An anterior approach, such as the Watson-Jones, can be used for displaced types II and III fractures and for type I transepiphyseal separations when the femoral head is dislocated from the acetabulum anteriorly. If the femoral head is dislocated posteriorly, a modified Gibson approach (see Technique 1.68) is used. The femoral head may be devoid of all blood supply. It should be replaced in the acetabulum, however, ensuring there are no cartilaginous or osseous fragments in the joint, and fixed to the femoral neck with cancellous screws.

POSTOPERATIVE CARE If internal fixation is stable, touch-down weight bearing on crutches is maintained for 6 weeks. If stability is questionable, a spica cast or a long leg cast with a pelvic band should be used for 6 weeks.

VALGUS SUBTROCHANTERIC OSTEOTOMY FOR ACQUIRED COXA VARA OR NONUNION

TECHNIQUE 8.20

- Place the patient on a fracture table with an image intensifier or radiographic equipment in place to obtain anteroposterior and lateral radiographs. Prepare and drape the hip in the usual fashion. If bone grafts are to be used, prepare and drape the iliac crest also.
- Make a straight lateral longitudinal incision beginning at the greater trochanter and extending distally for 8 to 10 cm. Carry the dissection down to the lateral aspect of the femur. Elevate the periosteum and insert reverse retractors around the femur subperiosteally to expose the lateral aspect of the bone.
- Determine preoperatively the amount of valgus necessary to align the hip properly by comparing radiographs with those of the contralateral hip. We have used trigonometric functions to evaluate the effect of proximal femoral osteotomy. If a varus or a valgus osteotomy is performed in the subtrochanteric or trochanteric area, the length of the femoral head and neck fragment does not change;

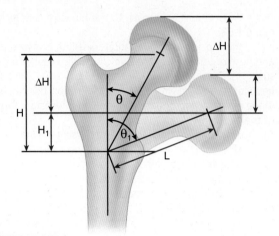

FIGURE 8.112 Illustration of constant head-neck length L, change in angles θ to θ_1, and ultimately change in height, ΔH. Formula is used to determine change in height; H = head-neck segment; $H_1 = L \cos \theta_1$; $\Delta H = L(\cos \theta_1 - \cos \theta)$. **SEE TECHNIQUE 8.20.**

only the angles and the leg length change (Fig. 8.112). The amount of change in leg length can be computed by determining the change in the two angles. The change in leg length (ΔH) is equal to the length of the point from the middle of the osteotomy site to the middle of the femoral head (L) times the cosine of one angle minus the cosine of the new angle:

$$\Delta H = L\,(\cos \theta_1 - \cos \theta)$$

Going from a varus position to a valgus position increases the leg length and, conversely, going from a valgus position to a varus position decreases the leg length, or ΔH. The original angle is given for femoral head-neck segments of 2, 3, and 4 cm. The estimated increase or decrease in leg length is given for the "desired angle" obtained by a varus or valgus osteotomy.

- When the angle of correction is determined, the appropriate laterally based closing wedge osteotomy can be determined. First determine the diameter of the bone by drilling a guide pin transversely through the femur. Determine the correct size of the wedge by using a template, tangent tables (W = tangent of the angle × the diameter), or the formula $W = 0.02 \times$ diameter × angle. Outline the appropriate closing wedge osteotomy in the subtrochanteric area.
- After preparation of the osteotomy site, attention should be turned to placement of an intermediate hip compression screw or proximal femoral locking plate. Drill a hole just distal to the greater trochanter and check its placement with the image intensifier. Place an appropriate guide pin of the proper length in the femoral neck with the aid of an adjustable angle guide (Fig. 8.113A,B). If the child is young, avoid crossing the physis if possible. If the nonunion is proximal, crossing the physis may be necessary to gain union. The proximal femoral physis contributes 30% to the growth of the femur and only 15% to the entire lower extremity. Often it is preferable to obtain union of the femoral neck and manage about minor to moderate leg-length inequality afterward. Check the placement of the guide pin with image intensification.
- After the guide pin is placed, use a percutaneous direct measuring gauge to determine the lag screw length. Set

the adjustable positive stop on the combination reamer for the lag screw length determined by a percutaneous direct measuring gauge. Place the reamer over the guide pin and ream until the positive stop reaches the lateral cortex (Fig. 8.113C). It is prudent to check the fluoroscopic image periodically during reaming to ensure that the guide pin is not inadvertently advancing proximally into the epiphysis.

- Set the adjustable positive stop on the lag screw tap to the same length that was reamed. Tap until the positive stop reaches the lateral cortex. Screw the appropriate intermediate compression screw over the guide pin (Fig. 8.113D,E).
- Take the plate chosen during preoperative planning and insert its barrel over the barrel guide and onto the back of the lag screw. The plate angle ultimately determines the final hip angle. Remove the barrel guide and insert a compression screw to prevent the plate from disengaging during the reduction maneuver. Use the slotted screwdriver for the pediatric compression screw or the hex screwdriver for the intermediate compression screw. If the plate obscures the osteotomy site, loosen the screw and rotate the side plate.
- Make the appropriate angled osteotomy using a power saw, remove the wedge, and align the two fragments.
- Reduce the osteotomy and secure the plate to the femur using the plate clamp. Check the rotational position of the lower extremity in extension.
- To achieve compression, insert a drill or tap guide into the distal portion of the most distal compression slot. Drill through the medial cortex. If less compression is required, follow the same steps detailed previously in the distal portion of the second or third distal slots for 2.5 mm of compression.
- Select the appropriate-length bone screw and insert it using the hex screwdriver. Use the self-holding sleeve to keep the screw from disengaging from the screwdriver (Fig. 8.113F). Finally, in the most proximal slot, the intermediate combination drill/tap guide can be angled proximally so that the drill and, ultimately, the bone screw cross the osteotomy line. Positioning the proximal bone screw in this way can provide additional stability at the osteotomy site. Insert screws into any remaining screw holes.
- The lag screw can be inserted farther to apply compression across the nonunion. To insert the lag screw for approximately 5 mm of compression, stop when the lateral cortex is midway between the two depth calibrations (Fig. 8.113G). To insert the lag screw for approximately 10 mm of compression, stop when the second depth calibration meets the lateral cortex (Fig. 8.113H).
- Close the wound in layers. Insert a suction drainage tube and apply a one and one-half spica cast with the hip in 30 to 40 degrees of abduction.
- For fixation of a nonunion, the intermediate compression hip screw should cross the nonunion site. The nonunion seems to heal better if it is made more horizontal by placing the hip in a valgus position at the subtrochanteric osteotomy site. The fibrous tissue need not be removed from the nonunion. A cancellous or cortical bone graft placed across the nonunion site may be helpful in

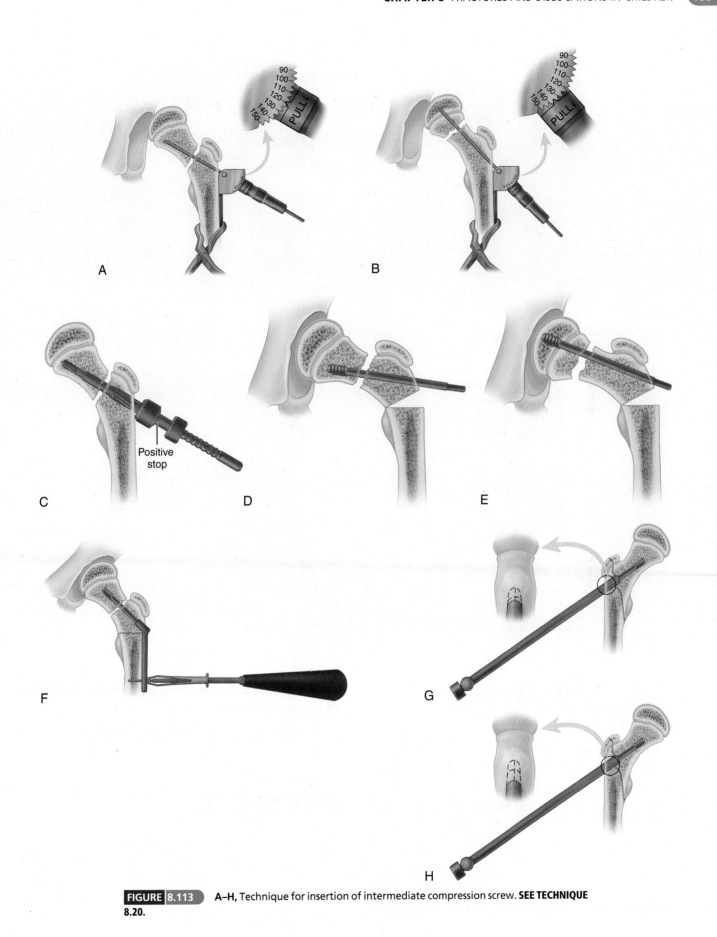

FIGURE 8.113 **A–H,** Technique for insertion of intermediate compression screw. **SEE TECHNIQUE 8.20.**

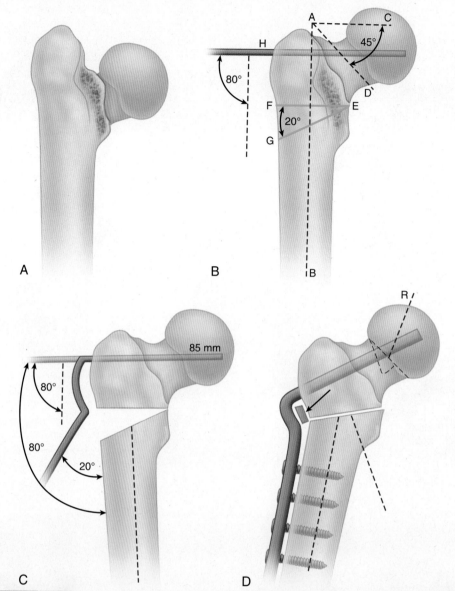

FIGURE **8.114** A–D, Modified Pauwels intertrochanteric osteotomy for acquired coxa vara or nonunion. (Redrawn from Magu NK, Rohilla R, Singh R, et al: Modified Pauwels' intertrochanteric osteotomy in neglected femoral neck fracture. *Clin Orthop Relat Res* 467:1064, 2009.) **SEE TECHNIQUE 8.21.**

older children. The graft is inserted by drilling a hole the size of the graft up through the femoral neck adjacent and parallel to the fixation device. Care should be taken not to loosen the device. A cortical graft from the tibia or fibula can be used, but we prefer cancellous bone from the iliac crest. We have not used bone graft routinely in this procedure. In younger children with good internal fixation, making the nonunion more horizontal has been all that is necessary. A smaller version of the compression hip screw is available for younger patients.

POSTOPERATIVE CARE The spica cast should be worn for approximately 12 weeks, depending on the age of the child. When the cast is removed, touch-down weight bearing on crutches is begun.

MODIFIED PAUWELS INTERTROCHANTERIC OSTEOTOMY FOR ACQUIRED COXA VARA OR NONUNION

TECHNIQUE 8.21

(MAGU ET AL.)

- On a tracing of a radiograph of the normal hip, determine the correct point of entry of the chisel for seating of the blade in the femoral neck, the appropriate blade length, the osteotomy line, and the appropriate intertrochanteric wedge (Fig. 8.114A,B). In a patient with open physes, make sure the blade length chosen avoids penetration of the proximal femoral physis.

- Contour a semi-tubular plate into a 120-degree double-angle plate (Fig. 8.114C).
- Attempt closed reduction through skeletal traction (if a proximal tibial pin is already in place) or manual traction.
- With image intensifier guidance, make a standard lateral approach to the hip joint and provisionally stabilize the hip with two 2-mm Kirschner wires to prevent rotation of the femoral head when the seating chisel is used to create a track for the implant blade.
- Make the two osteotomy cuts as determined on the normal hip radiograph to create a laterally based 15- to 30-degree intertrochanteric wedge of bone (Fig. 8.114B). Remove this wedge of bone to place the femoral head into a valgus position as defined by preoperative planning.
- Insert the seating chisel through the previously determined entry point, keeping the flap of the chisel parallel to the femoral shaft. Advance the chisel into the inferior half of the femoral neck for a length equal to that of the blade length of a 120-degree contoured osteotomy plate (usually 65 mm).
- Remove the chisel and insert the blade portion of the osteotomy plate into its track (Fig. 8.114C).
- Abduct the distal fragment to close the osteotomy and stabilize the plate to the femur with screws (Fig. 8.114D).

POSTOPERATIVE CARE A hip spica cast is worn for 6 to 10 weeks, depending on the healing of the osteotomy. The cast is removed, and touch-down weight bearing on crutches is begun, followed by graduated partial and full weight bearing between 12 and 20 weeks.

TRAUMATIC HIP DISLOCATIONS

Traumatic hip dislocations in children are more common than hip fractures, although they are also rare. Trivial injury may cause a hip dislocation in young children primarily because their immature cartilage is pliable and their ligaments are lax. The reported age distribution of traumatic hip dislocations has varied among authors, with some suggesting that over half occur between the ages of 12 and 15 years, some reporting no peak age group, and some identifying two distinct groups: children 2 to 5 years old and children 11 to 15 years old. As in adults, posterior dislocations are more common than anterior ones. Factors that influence the ultimate result after dislocations of the hip are (1) the severity of the injury, (2) the interval between injury and reduction, (3) the type of treatment, (4) the period of non–weight bearing, (5) whether recurrent dislocation develops, (6) whether osteonecrosis develops, and (7) whether reduction was incomplete because of the interposition of an object in the joint. Hip dislocation with spontaneous incomplete reduction probably occurs more often than previously thought, and the diagnosis of hip subluxation may be missed initially.

Hips left unreduced for more than 24 hours usually have poor results, and osteonecrosis of the femoral head develops more frequently than in hips reduced promptly. Closed reduction often is successful if a congruous joint is obtained. Open reduction may be necessary, however, for more severe injuries or to remove any entrapped structures. Contrary to previous reports, the period of non–weight bearing does not appear to influence the development of osteonecrosis of the femoral head.

Recurrent dislocation also is more common in children than in adults because of cartilaginous pliability and ligamentous laxity. Recurrent dislocations are more frequent in children with hyperlaxity syndromes, especially Down syndrome, and may require posterior plication of the capsule and bony intervention, such as an innominate or varus osteotomy. Recurrent dislocations may be involuntary and posttraumatic and should be differentiated from voluntary dislocations, which may be habitual or nonhabitual. Additionally, Manner et al. suggested a possible association between femoroacetabular impingement (FAI) and recurrent hip dislocation and advocated operative treatment of underlying FAI to optimize outcomes.

Osteonecrosis of the femoral head occurs after simple dislocation of the hip in an estimated 10% to 26% of adults and 8% to 10% of children (Fig. 8.115). Delays in reduction and the severity of the injury probably influence the development of osteonecrosis. Sciatic nerve palsy, heterotopic ossification, and coxa magna also have been reported as complications of hip dislocation in children.

Complete reduction may be prevented by interposition of the capsule, labrum, other soft tissue, or an osteocartilaginous fragment. An anteroposterior radiograph of the pelvis and a lateral radiograph of both hips should be made after closed reduction to compare the width of the joint spaces. If the involved joint space is wider or the Shenton line is broken, an incongruous reduction should be suspected (Fig. 8.116). If an incongruous joint is suspected, then advanced imaging with CT or MRI is obtained; however, a recent study concluded that MRI is more sensitive than CT at detecting injury, particularly posterior labral entrapment and posterior unossified acetabular fractures. If interposed structures are found, we recommend open reduction and removal of the offending material. For posterior dislocations, a posterior approach, such as a modified Gibson (see Technique 1.68) or Moore (see Technique 1.70) approach, should be used. For anterior dislocations, an anterior approach, such as the Smith-Petersen or Watson-Jones (see Techniques 1.60 and 1.63) approach, is used. If the direction of dislocation cannot be determined, MRI is helpful in localizing a soft-tissue injury. A posterior approach is frequently used because this is the more common direction of dislocation. A surgical dislocation approach may be used if more extensive work is required as in the case of a femoral head fracture. At open reduction, the hip should be distracted and the acetabulum should be checked for loose bony fragments or an inverted labrum or other soft tissue. Reduction should be confirmed under direct inspection and radiographically in the operating room, ensuring that the width of the joint space has returned to normal. The technique for open reduction of an incongruous closed reduction is the same as for irreducible hip dislocation and is described in other chapter. For late complications, such as persistent mechanical symptoms or pain, hip arthroscopy may be useful with the most common findings being loose bodies, chondral damage, labral tears, and ligamentum teres injuries. Hip arthroscopy technique and indication are discussed further in other chapter.

Rarely, a neglected traumatic dislocation may require open reduction in a child or adolescent. In a report of eight chronic dislocations, traction failed to obtain reduction in all eight and

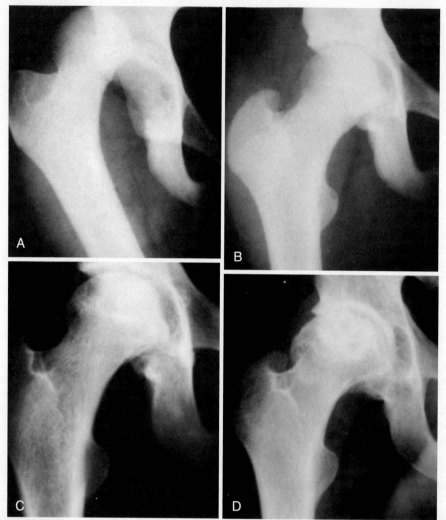

FIGURE 8.115 Osteonecrosis of femoral head after hip dislocation. **A,** Traumatic dislocation in older child. **B,** After satisfactory closed reduction. **C,** At 1 year after reduction, suggestion of early osteonecrosis. **D,** At 8 years after reduction, cystic appearance of osteonecrosis.

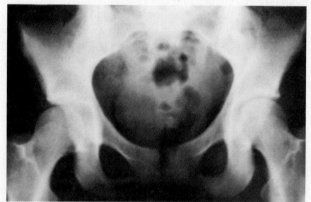

FIGURE 8.116 Incongruous reduction of hip. Radiograph of both hips after what was thought to be successful closed reduction of traumatic dislocation of the right hip in adolescent. Reduction is incongruous, however, as shown by break in Shenton line and increase in width of joint space.

open reduction was required because of pain and gait disturbances. At an average follow-up of almost 8 years, six of the hips remained reduced; all had evidence of osteonecrosis. Although these results are not particularly good, they are, according to the authors, preferable to those obtained with other treatment methods or with no treatment. Other authors have recommended open reduction of neglected dislocations, even with the likelihood of osteonecrosis, because an anatomically placed femoral head maintains the stimulus for growth of the pelvis and femur, prevents deformity, and maintains limb length.

Occasionally, an ipsilateral femoral fracture occurs at the time of hip dislocation. The treatment of this combination of injuries is described in other chapter.

SLIPPED CAPITAL FEMORAL EPIPHYSIS

A type I transepiphyseal fracture-separation and SCFE are epiphyseal separations, but controversy over their natural histories and pathogenesis separates the two disorders. Type I transepiphyseal separations generally are caused by high-energy trauma, whereas SCFE can occur insidiously and minor trauma can cause acute separation or a chronic slip. Type I transepiphyseal separations are most common in young children, whereas SCFE occurs in a distinct older age group (age 10 to 16 years); 78% of patients with SCFE are adolescents in the rapid growth phase. SCFE occurs more frequently in obese children and is almost twice as common in boys as in girls. It occurs approximately twice as often in children of African descent than in children of European descent. The left hip is affected twice as often as the right, and bilateral involvement is reported to occur in 25% to 40% of children. When bilateral slips occur, the second slip usually occurs within 12 to 18 months of the initial slip. Patients with open triradiate cartilage are at higher risk.

Several etiologic factors have been suggested for SCFE, including local trauma, mechanical factors (especially obesity, growth spurts, and puberty), inflammatory conditions, endocrine disorders (e.g., hypothyroidism, hypopituitarism, and chronic renal disease), genetic factors, Down syndrome, and seasonal variations. Although shear forces generally are cited as causative factors, torsional forces also play a role in SCFE. Sankar et al. also demonstrated increased acetabular retroversion and overcoverage in the unaffected hip with SCFE. Moreover, in the proximal femur throughout childhood and culminating in adolescence, several pathophysiologic changes occur that increase the vulnerability of the physis, including a decrease in the neck-shaft angle, increase in the obliquity of the physis, thinning of the perichondrial ring, and change in the cellular anatomy of the physis. Liu et al. also noted that the epiphyseal tubercle may be protective at an early age until it decreases in size during adolescence. Physeal widening at this age may then allow the epiphysis to internally rotate around the tubercle. The reliable orientation of the lateral epiphyseal vessels adjacent to the tubercle might explain the low rate of osteonecrosis in chronic, stable slips. The true cause of SCFE, however, is likely multifactorial: a physis that is weakened by some underlying condition fails when it is subjected to more than normal stress, resulting in slipping of the proximal femoral epiphysis.

The clinical symptoms and radiographic signs of SCFE vary according to the type of slip, but usually include pain in the groin, hip, medial thigh, or knee and limitation of hip motion, especially internal rotation. Georgiadis and Zaltz described the medial thigh pain in SCFE as being referred by a reflex arc involving somatic sensory nerves ending at the same spinal level as opposed to being caused by irritation of the obturator nerve branches. Often when the hip is flexed the leg externally rotates in a frog-leg position because of the abnormal contact between the displaced femoral neck and the acetabular rim. SCFE should be suspected in patients age 10 to 16 years who complain of vague knee pain, which may be referred pain from the hip. Patients with chronic slips may have mild or moderate shortening of the affected extremity, the leg may be in fixed external rotation leading to an outward foot progression angle compared with the uninvolved side, and a Trendelenburg gait may be present. Unfortunately, the diagnosis is frequently delayed, which may result in more severe deformity and worse long-term outcomes. Kocher reported that delays in diagnosis occur primarily in patients with knee or distal thigh pain, patients with Medicaid coverage, and patients with stable slips.

The diagnosis of SCFE usually is apparent from anteroposterior and frog-leg pelvic radiographs, but special views may be helpful. The Klein line is a line along the superior aspect of the femoral neck that normally is intersected by the

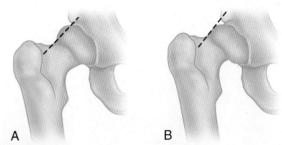

FIGURE **8.117**   The Klein line: in early slips, the epiphysis is flush with or below this line. **A,** Normal hip. **B,** Slipped capital femoral epiphysis.

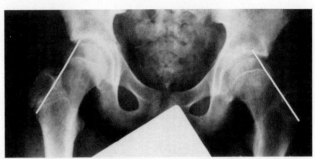

FIGURE **8.118**   "Blanch" sign in slipped capital femoral epiphysis. Double density can be seen at the metaphysis of the left hip. (From Steel HH: The metaphyseal blanch sign of slipped capital femoral epiphysis, *J Bone Joint Surg* 68A:920, 1986.)

epiphysis. In early slips, the epiphysis is flush with or below this line (Fig. 8.117). A modification of this measurement considered a slip to have occurred if the maximal width of the epiphysis lateral to the Klein line differed 2 mm or more from the contralateral hip. This modification was reported to improve sensitivity from 40% to almost 80%. Often a double density is seen at the metaphysis on the anteroposterior radiograph as compared with the contralateral hip when the metaphysis is translated anteriorly and externally rotated relative to the epiphysis; this has been called a *metaphyseal blanch sign* (Fig. 8.118). Although not routinely used in our practice, advanced imaging may add benefit in some cases. MRI can be used for diagnosis of a subtle or "preslip" condition suggested by edema around the physis on T2-weighted images, which should be a sign that a slip is present. It also is useful in ruling out additional hip pathology or assessing femoral head perfusion. CT is helpful in determining if the physis is closed or for preoperative planning before complex osteotomies.

SCFE traditionally has been classified according to the duration of symptoms and the stability of the slip. Acute SCFE presents within 3 weeks of the onset of symptoms, whereas a chronic SCFE has a more gradual onset of symptoms of more than 3 weeks' duration. A third subset of patients may be symptomatic from a longer period and then develop more acute symptoms resulting in acute-on-chronic SCFE. Radiographs of a chronic SCFE usually show the epiphyseal displacement with evidence of bone healing or remodeling with possible secondary changes to the acetabulum and femoral neck, depending on the duration of symptoms and degree of the slip. This temporal classification of SCFE is descriptive

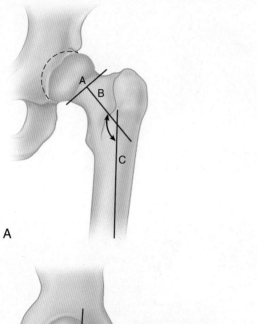

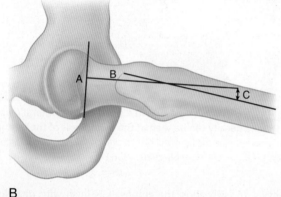

FIGURE 8.119   **A** and **B,** Measurement of head-shaft angle on anteroposterior and lateral radiographs. Line *A* connects peripheral portions of physis. Line *B* is perpendicular to line *A,* and line *C* is in long axis of femoral shaft. Intersection of lines *B* and *C* forms head-shaft angle in both views.

but has little prognostic value. The most widely accepted classification of SCFE was introduced by Loder et al. and is based on the stability of the physis. A slip is classified as unstable if severe pain prevents walking, even with crutches, regardless of the duration of symptoms. With a stable slip, walking is possible, with or without crutches. Satisfactory results were obtained in 96% of stable slips compared with 47% of unstable slips. In addition, the osteonecrosis rate for the stable slips was 0% compared with 47% in the unstable group with operative intervention.

SCFE can be graded based on the severity of the slip. A preslip condition is present if there is symptomatic weakening of the physis without loss of the normal epiphyseal-metaphyseal orientation. Radiographs may demonstrate irregularity, widening, and indistinctness of the physis, and MRI demonstrates abnormal edema surrounding the physis. Mild slipping (grade I) exists when the neck is displaced less than one third of the diameter of the femoral head or when the head-shaft angle deviates from normal by 30 degrees or less on either projection as described by Southwick (Fig. 8.119). In moderate slipping (grade II), the neck is displaced between one third and one half of the diameter of the femoral head or the head-shaft angle deviates between 30 and 60 degrees from normal on either view. Severe slipping (grade

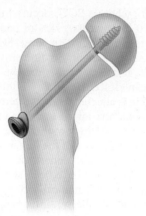

FIGURE 8.120   Principle of dynamic screw fixation. Short screw thread (10 mm) in epiphysis only, and screw and washer are left long for continued growth.

III) is characterized by neck displacement of more than half the diameter of the head or deviation of the head-shaft angle of more than 60 degrees. In most large series of SCFE, 60% to 90% of slips are classified as chronic and more than half are classified as mild slips.

SCFE also can be idiopathic or atypical (associated with renal failure, radiation therapy, hypogonadism, Down syndrome, and various endocrine disorders). Children younger than 10 years old or older than 16 have been reported to be 4.2 times more likely to have atypical SFCE and 8.4 times more likely if their weight was below the 50th percentile. Slips occurring in children with underlying endocrinopathies or other risk factors may be susceptible to failure of screw fixation, progressive slipping, or contralateral slipping. When symptoms of pain continue (average 5 months) in such patients, close follow-up with radiographs or prophylactic pinning is necessary. Some authors have advocated treatment with pins that are smooth proximally and threaded distally to engage the anterolateral femoral cortex with no threads crossing the physis to allow continued growth in younger patients with renal osteodystrophy. A single cannulated 7-mm diameter screw with 10-mm threads also can be used. The screw should be placed in the centerline of the femoral head so that all screw threads are within the femoral head and not in the joint. The screw is left protruding 15 to 20 mm to allow further physeal growth (Fig. 8.120).

TREATMENT

The ideal treatment of SCFE would restore the biomechanics of the hip, prevent additional slipping of the epiphysis, and stimulate early physeal closure while avoiding the complications of osteonecrosis, chondrolysis, and osteoarthritis. Stabilization of the slip and closure of the physis are relatively easy to obtain by a variety of methods; however, restoration of hip biomechanics and prevention of complications has proved more difficult.

Methods of operative treatment of SCFE have included percutaneous and open in situ pinning, ORIF, epiphysiodesis, osteotomy, and reconstruction by arthroplasty, arthrodesis, or cheilectomy. Each technique has its proponents and opponents, and the choice of treatment must be individualized for each child, depending on age, type of slip, and severity of displacement.

■ IN SITU PIN OR SCREW FIXATION

Percutaneous in situ screw fixation currently is the most commonly used treatment for both stable and unstable SCFE regardless of the severity of the slip. Modern cannulated screw systems allow more accurate placement of screws and have become the implant of choice for fixation. Although earlier reports indicated that two or three pins were necessary for stability, several studies have failed to demonstrate a clinical or biomechanical advantage to multiple pins and advocate the use of a single, larger-diameter screw inserted into the center-center position of the epiphysis. Occasionally, a second screw is used at our institution if a high-grade slip is present and a single screw does not achieve adequate stability in the unstable SCFE. Alternatively, an open procedure may be performed to restore the epiphyseal alignment and achieve stability. For unstable slips, a gentle or "incidental" reduction may be applied by simply positioning the patient in the appropriate position on the operative table, but forceful manipulation of the hip should be avoided because of the high association between a manipulative reduction and osteonecrosis.

Our techniques for determining the entry point for screw fixation and placement of the cannulated screw into the epiphysis are described in Techniques 8.22 and 8.23, respectively. Obtaining the appropriate starting point to allow passage of the screw perpendicular to the physis and into the center-center position is important; however, Merz et al. noted that a screw passed obliquely across the physis into the center-center position does not significantly alter the biomechanical stability of the construct. This may be helpful when trying to avoid screw placement that results in dynamic impingement of the screw head.

Persistent screw penetration has been the most serious disadvantage of in situ fixation. Adverse effects attributed to unrecognized implant penetration include joint sepsis, localized acetabular erosion, synovitis, postoperative hip pain, chondrolysis, and late degenerative osteoarthritis. As a practical clinical guide, placing the screw in the center of the femoral head no closer than 4 mm from the subchondral bone helps to decrease the prevalence of screw penetration (Fig. 8.121). Additionally, multiple radiographic views should be obtained to ensure persistent penetration has not occurred. Other methods such as the passage of the blunt end of the guidewire or injection of contrast dye through the cannulated screw have been described.

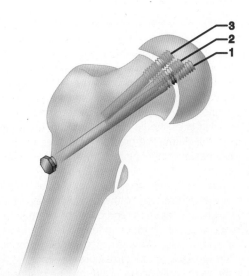

FIGURE 8.121 Screw positions in proximal femur. Position *1*, central axis of screw is located over center line of femoral head or within distance equal to one-half diameter of screw (ideal position). Position *2*, distance between axis of screw and center line of femoral head is between one half and one screw diameter. Position *3*, axis of screw is more than one screw diameter from center line. Position is given as two numbers: first for position of screw on anteroposterior radiograph and second for position as seen on lateral view. Ideal position is 1.

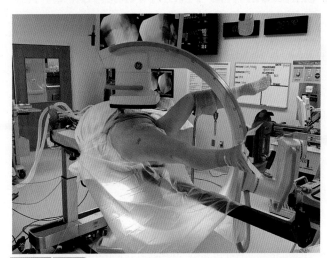

FIGURE 8.122 Patient positioning and C-arm placement for fluoroscopy. **SEE TECHNIQUE 8.22.**

DETERMINING THE ENTRY POINT FOR CANNULATED SCREW FIXATION OF A SLIPPED EPIPHYSIS

TECHNIQUE 8.22

(CANALE ET AL.)

- Place the patient supine so that anteroposterior and lateral fluoroscopic views can be obtained without repositioning the patient or the extremity; a fracture table, or alternatively a radiolucent flat top table, can be used. The entire proximal femoral epiphysis and hip joint space should be clearly visible on both views. Prepare and drape the extremity to allow free access to the entire anterior surface of the thigh and as far medially as the pubis in the inguinal area. A fluoroscopic C-arm is used for an anteroposterior and an exact lateral image (Fig. 8.122). On the lateral view, the femoral neck should be parallel to the femoral shaft.
- Place a guidewire on the anterior aspect of the thigh so that the anteroposterior image shows it in the desired varus-valgus position and mark the position of the guidewire on the anterior surface of the thigh with a marking pen.

- Place the guidewire along the lateral aspect of the thigh so that it is in the correct anteroposterior position on fluoroscopic image and mark the position of the wire on the skin. In SCFE, the epiphysis is displaced posteriorly relative to the femoral neck, and this lateral guidewire angles from anterior to posterior and appears on the fluoroscopic image to enter at the anterior femoral neck. The two skin lines should intersect on the anterolateral aspect of the thigh. The greater the degree of the slip (the more posterior the epiphysis), the more anterior the intersection.
- Place a guidewire, drill, or pin through a small lateral incision at the intersection of the two skin lines. Monitor proper alignment, position, and depth of insertion in the proximal femoral epiphysis on anteroposterior and lateral fluoroscopic images. Take care not to bend, kink, or notch the guidewire for fear of interosseous breakage.
- Insert the cannulated screw in the routine manner; the threads of the screw at the tip should traverse the physis (see Fig. 8.107F).

DETERMINING THE ENTRY POINT FOR CANNULATED SCREW FIXATION OF A SLIPPED EPIPHYSIS

TECHNIQUE 8.23

(MORRISSY)
- Place the patient on the fracture table with the affected leg abducted 10 to 15 degrees and internally rotated as far as possible without force. This brings the femoral neck as close as possible to parallel to the floor to assist in obtaining true anterior and lateral image views. Position the image intensifier between the legs so that anteroposterior and lateral views can be obtained by moving the tube around the arc of the machine (Fig. 8.123).
- After standard preparation and draping and under image control, insert a Kirschner wire percutaneously through the anterolateral area of the thigh down to the femoral neck (Fig. 8.124), adjusting the guidewire on the anteroposterior projection to determine the axis of the femoral neck. Obtain a lateral view to determine the amount of posterior inclination necessary.
- When the starting point on the femoral neck and amount of posterior inclination have been estimated, insert the guide assembly through a small puncture wound. Advance the guide assembly to the physis and confirm placement in the central axis of the femoral head by image intensification. If the position is correct, advance the guide assembly across the plate. (If positioning is incorrect, insert a second guide assembly using the first to determine what correction in the starting point or angulation is necessary.) When the proper depth is reached (at least 0.5 cm from subchondral bone), remove the cannula and leave the guidewire in the bone.

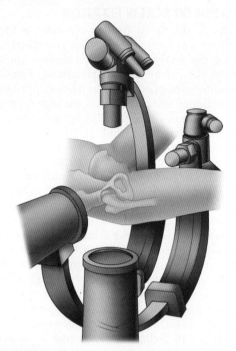

FIGURE 8.123 Percutaneous in situ fixation of slipped capital femoral epiphysis. Positioning of image intensifier to allow rotation necessary to obtain lateral and anteroposterior views. (From Morrissy RT: Slipped capital femoral epiphysis: technique of percutaneous in site fixation, *J Pediatr Orthop* 10:347, 1990.) **SEE TECHNIQUE 8.23.**

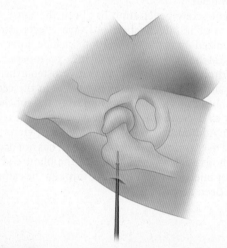

FIGURE 8.124 Kirschner wire passed percutaneously to estimated starting point on the femur. **SEE TECHNIQUE 8.23.**

- Determine the correct screw length by passing a guidewire of identical length along the one in the bone and measuring the difference. Advance the correct-length screw over the guide pin and remove the pin.
- Remove the leg from the traction device and move it in multiple directions, using anteroposterior and lateral views to confirm that the screw does not penetrate the joint. If two screws are deemed necessary for an acute, unstable slip, the first screw should lie in the central axis of the femoral head and the second below it, avoiding the

superolateral quadrant. The second screw should stop at least 5 mm from the subchondral bone.

■ Close the stab wound with a single subcuticular suture.

See also Video 8.2.

POSTOPERATIVE CARE Range-of-motion exercises are begun the day after surgery. For stable slips, patients are allowed to bear weight as tolerated with an assistive device the first day after surgery and are discharged the same day. Crutches are used until all signs of synovitis are gone and motion is free and painless (usually 2 to 3 weeks). For unstable slips, partial weight bearing is maintained with crutches for 6 to 8 weeks. All rigorous sports and other activities are limited until the physes have closed. Screw removal is not necessary, but the screws can be removed after physeal closure has been shown radiographically. The easiest method of removal is to pass a guidewire into the cannula of the screw under image control to allow the screwdriver to be guided into the head of the screw over the guidewire. However, we routinely do not remove the screws.

CONTRALATERAL SLIPS

Bilateral slips are present in 20% to 30% of patients at initial presentation; the reported frequency of a subsequent, contralateral slip during the remaining growth period has ranged from 20% to 40%. Castro et al. estimated that patients with unilateral SCFE are 2335 times more likely to develop a contralateral slip than those who have never had SCFE are to have an initial slip. Even with this very high prevalence of bilateral slips, prophylactic pinning of the contralateral hip in a patient with a unilateral slip remains controversial. Because of the risks associated with prophylactic pinning of a radiographically and clinically normal hip, emphasis has been placed on trying to predict which patients with a unilateral slip will ultimately develop a second, contralateral slip.

Age appears to be one predictive factor. Females younger than 10 years of age and males younger than 12 years of age have a substantially increased incidence of contralateral SCFE, and prophylactic in situ fixation probably is indicated for these patients to prevent problems with leg-length inequality and long-term degenerative joint disease. Prophylactic fixation also may be indicated in patients with endocrine abnormalities or other processes related to their SCFE, those for whom reliable follow-up is not feasible, and those who have high risk factors for developing osteonecrosis or chondrolysis, such as obesity in younger children. A "posterior sloping" angle of more than 12 degrees (Fig. 8.125) has been described as predictive of the development of a contralateral slip. The use of a cannulated screw with a shorter threaded length that does not engage the physis has been recommended in young children to maintain stability without causing physeal closure and extremity shortening. Kocher et al. in a decision analysis found the optimal decision to be observation but advocated for contralateral fixation in patients with added risk factors or in patients in whom reliable follow-up was not feasible. Other recent studies have advocated for more routine fixation of the contralateral hip when a unilateral slip is present, especially in younger children with an open triradiate cartilage.

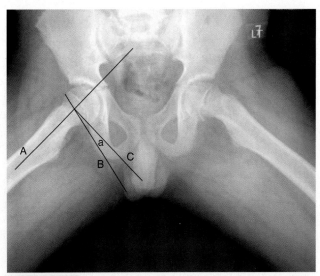

FIGURE 8.125 Posterior sloping angle of more than 12 degrees is described as predictive of development of contralateral slip. Line *A* is drawn along femoral neck (diaphyseal axis). Line *B* is drawn along plane of the physis. Line *C* is drawn perpendicular to line *A*. *a* is posterior sloping angle. (From Park S, Hsu JE, Rendon N, et al: The utility of posterior sloping angle in predicting contralateral slipped capital femoral epiphysis, *J Pediatr Orthop* 30:683, 2010.)

■ OPEN TECHNIQUES

Several modern open techniques for the treatment of SCFE have been developed in an attempt to improve on the high rates of complications seen with in situ fixation by addressing the acquired deformity of a slipped epiphysis and minimizing the vascular insult. The ideal treatment of a slip remains controversial but should take into account the degree of deformity, stability of the slip, risk of osteonecrosis, and an honest assessment of the skill set of the surgeon. For mild or stable slips that result in impingement or functional loss, limited open, surgical dislocation, and arthroscopic osteochondroplasty have been reported after in situ fixation with good results and are described in other chapter (femoroacetabular impingement). For acute, unstable slips, some advocate an open approach to the hip through a Smith-Peterson or Watson-Jones approach with wide capsulotomy, gentle "finger" reduction, and fixation with cannulated screws. Alternatively, in moderate-grade or high-grade slips, where posterior callus formation and a contracted retinaculum may result in a block to anatomic reduction or an increase in the tension on the epiphysis vessels, a subcapital wedge resection of the femoral neck with reduction of the epiphysis may be performed with the modified Dunn technique (Technique 8.25). Ziebarth et al. reported 40 patients from two centers with moderate or severe SCFE who underwent capital realignment with the modified Dunn procedure. In their series, there were no cases of osteonecrosis at short-term follow-up, and the anatomy was restored to a slip angle of 4 to 8 degrees. The average alpha angle in their series was 40.6 degrees, and the incidence of cartilage damage, especially in stable slips, was very high. Navais et al. retrospectively compared 15 patients with severe, stable SCFE treated with the modified Dunn technique to 15 patients with severe, stable SCFE treated with in situ fixation. They found that the modified Dunn procedure resulted in better morphologic features of the femur, a higher rate of good and excellent

Heyman and Herndon clinical outcome, a lower reoperation rate, and a similar occurrence of complications, which included an osteonecrosis risk of 7%. Alternatively, Sankar et al. reported 27 patients who had restoration of their capital alignment with the modified Dunn technique, but had a 15% incidence of implant failure requiring revision and 26% incidence of osteonecrosis at 22-month follow-up. Additional studies are needed to accurately assess the outcomes of this procedure for both unstable and stable slips.

Historically, several other corrective osteotomies have been described and can be divided into femoral neck and intertrochanteric osteotomies. Because moderately or severely displaced slips produce permanent irregularities in the femoral head and acetabulum, some form of realignment procedure often is indicated to restore the normal relationship of the femoral head and neck and possibly delay the onset of degenerative joint disease; however, in long-term follow-up, patients with osteotomies have been reported to have worse scores on the Iowa hip rating with each passing decade than patients without hip realignment procedures. Suggested indications for osteotomy have included problems with gait, sitting, pain, or cosmetic appearance. Often these procedures were performed more than 1 year after stabilization because of the belief that the femoral head may have the capacity to remodel. More recent data and a better understanding of SCFE-induced impingement call into question the ability of a significant deformity to remodel and raise concern that any "remodeling" may come at the cost of repetitive trauma to the labrum, chondrolabral junction, and weight-bearing acetabular cartilage. Historically, poor results with osteotomy techniques may have been partially related to a poor understanding of the blood supply to the head and intervention after irreparable damage has occurred to the articular surface.

The two basic types of corrective osteotomy are closing wedge osteotomy through the femoral neck, usually near the physis to correct the deformity, and compensatory osteotomy through the trochanteric region to produce a deformity in the opposite direction (Fig. 8.126). The advantage of osteotomy through the femoral neck is that the deformity itself is corrected, but incidences of osteonecrosis ranging from 2% to 100% and of chondrolysis from 3% to 37% have been associated with this procedure. Advocates of the modified Dunn procedure have proposed this technique as a viable option for patients with moderate or severe deformity; however, it does introduce a risk of osteonecrosis, and long-term results are needed before it should be widely adopted. With the exception of the modified Dunn technique, femoral neck osteotomies have been abandoned at our institution.

Trochanteric osteotomies can produce an opposite deformity to correct the coxa vara, hyperextension, and external rotation produced by a slipped epiphysis. Southwick described a biplanar osteotomy at the level of the lesser trochanter to correct the varus and hyperextension and dynamically correct the external rotation. Alternatively, the Imhaüser osteotomy can be used to primarily correct the hyperextension and secondarily to correct the varus and external rotation, as described in Technique 8.28. If the physis is not yet fused, then fixation of the physis should be achieved with a screw before the osteotomy. Trochanteric osteotomies have the advantage of low osteonecrosis rates but the disadvantage of incomplete correction of the deformity. Outcomes of trochanteric osteotomies are largely

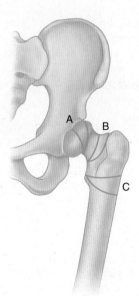

FIGURE 8.126 Osteotomies for slipped capital femoral epiphysis. *A,* Through neck near epiphysis. *B,* Through base of neck. *C,* Through trochanteric region.

dependent on the degree of correction achieved and the extent of the underlying articular damage. Trochanteric osteotomies also have been combined at our institution with femoral neck osteochondroplasty through a surgical dislocation or limited anterior approach.

POSITIONAL REDUCTION AND FIXATION FOR SCFE

TECHNIQUE 8.24

(CHEN, SCHOENECKER, DOBBS ET AL.)

- After induction of general endotracheal anesthesia, place the patient on a fracture table with the involved extremity in gentle traction and the hip in extension, neutral rotation, and neutral abduction.
- Flex the uninvolved hip into the lithotomy position to allow an image intensifier to adequately access the pelvis. Obtain anteroposterior and lateral fluoroscopic images before making the incision. Often simple positioning results in reduction and can be determined by the remodeling of the femoral neck, particularly on the lateral view.
- If reduction is not obtained by positioning, apply minimal internal rotation (generally no more than 10 degrees) with slightly more traction; make no attempt at forceful reduction past the preacute position. This reduction reestablishes the preacute length of the retinacular vessels that supply the femoral head.
- If decompression of an intraarticular hematoma is needed, perform a capsulotomy through an anterior iliofemoral approach between the tensor fascia lata and sartorius muscles, taking care not to sacrifice the ascending branch of the lateral femoral circumflex artery.

- Once the hip joint is exposed, apply gentle flexion and internal rotation to confirm reduction under direct observation.
- Use a triangulation technique with a guidewire under fluoroscopic vision to determine the skin entry point on the anterolateral aspect of the hip.
- Advance the guidewire through the anterior aspect of the femoral neck and direct it perpendicular to the physis, slightly superiorly and anteriorly to the center of the physis.
- Place a second guidewire parallel to the first and slightly inferior and posterior to the center of the physis.
- Advance a cannulated drill over each guidewire and insert two appropriate-sized cannulated screws over the guidewires. When position of the screws is confirmed, remove the guidewires.

PERCUTANEOUS CAPSULOTOMY TO DECOMPRESS THE INTRAARTICULAR HEMATOMA

- Place long Metzenbaum scissors on the anterior femoral neck just distal to the physis under fluoroscopic confirmation.
- Use tactile confirmation to locate the generally tough hip capsule overlying the anterior femoral neck and carefully advance the scissors to perforate the capsule. Confirm this with fluoroscopy.
- Alternatively, advance a drill bit through the capsule and into the epiphysis under image intensifier guidance.

POSTOPERATIVE CARE Patients are restricted to non–weight bearing on crutches or in a wheelchair for approximately 2 months.

SUBCAPITAL REALIGNMENT OF THE EPIPHYSIS (MODIFIED DUNN) FOR SCFE

Leunig, Slongo, and Ganz described a subcapital realignment procedure in which the femoral head is dislocated, an osteotomy of the greater trochanter is made, and the capital epiphysis is realigned and internally fixed. The rationale behind this technique is that the blood supply to the femoral head is preserved with the dislocation technique, thus avoiding osteonecrosis of the femoral head and avoiding FAI by aligning the physis to the femoral neck. This is a complex procedure that should be done only by experienced hip surgeons.

TECHNIQUE 8.25

(LEUNIG, SLONGO, AND GANZ)

- Place the patient in the lateral decubitus position, with the leg draped free and placed on a sterile bag fixed to the front of the operating table.
- Make a Gibson approach (see Technique 1.68), posteriorly retracting the gluteus maximus. This approach allows exposure similar to that obtained with a Kocher-Langenbeck approach but produces a more acceptable cosmetic result.
- Retract the fascial layer between the gluteus maximus and medius along with the gluteus maximus to preserve optimal innervation and blood supply to the muscle.
- Internally rotate the leg and identify the posterior border of the gluteus medius by dissecting the overlying adipose tissue.
- Mark the level and direction of the trochanteric osteotomy with a knife, creating a line from the posterosuperior edge to the posterior border of the vastus lateralis. Place this line anterior to the trochanteric crest to avoid injury to the insertion of the external rotators. After the osteotomy, the gluteus medius, the vastus lateralis, and the long tendon of the gluteus minimus will remain attached to the trochanteric fragment. The maximal thickness of the trochanteric fragment should not exceed 1.5 cm, and the osteotomy should exit proximally just anterior to the most posterior inserting fibers of the gluteus medius to keep most of the piriformis insertion on the femur and not on the fragment.
- Expose the hip joint capsule by further dissection between the piriformis tendon and gluteus minimus, an interval that offers the best protection for the blood supply to the femoral head and allows preservation of the constant anastomosis between the inferior gluteal artery and the deep branch of the medial femoral circumflex artery.
- Flip the greater trochanteric fragment anteriorly by elevating the vastus lateralis along its posterior border to the middle of the gluteus maximus tendon insertion on the femoral shaft.
- Proximally, cut the few gluteus medius fibers remaining on the stable trochanter to allow further anterior mobilization of the trochanteric fragment.
- Flex and externally rotate the leg to increase exposure of the capsule within the gap between the piriformis and the gluteus minimus.
- Release the anterosuperior capsular insertion of the gluteus minimus muscle while preserving the long tendon of the gluteus minimus that inserts anterior on the trochanteric fragment. Up to this point in the procedure, all external rotators remain attached to the stable trochanter and protect the medial femoral circumflex artery.
- Incise the capsule close to the anterosuperior edge of the stable trochanter in a direction axial to the neck. Make a perpendicular extension along the anterior neck insertion to create a flap that can be lifted to create an inside-out capsulotomy that provides protection from cutting into cartilage and labrum.
- Extend the Z-shaped capsulotomy (for the right side) along the posterior border of the acetabulum. Direct the anteroinferior extension of the capsulotomy toward the anteroinferior border of the acetabulum. This extension must remain anterior to the lesser trochanter to avoid damage to the main branch of the medial femoral circumflex artery, which is located in the vicinity of the femur just superior and posterior to the lesser trochanter.
- Retract the anteromedial capsular flap with a small, spiked Hohmann retractor that is driven into the supraacetabular bone just lateral to the anterior inferior iliac spine.

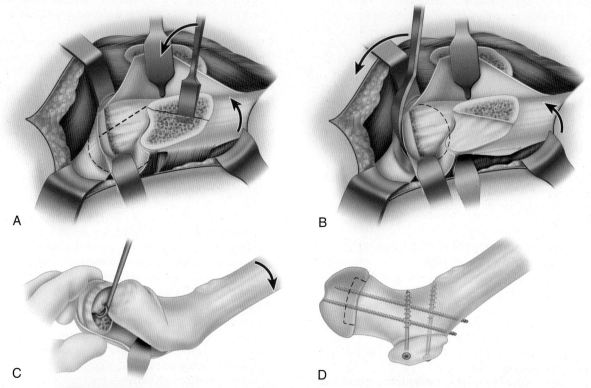

A   B

C   D

FIGURE 8.127 **A–D, Subcapital realignment of epiphysis.** Redrawn from Leunig M, Slongo T, Ganz R: Subcapital realignment in slipped capital femoral epiphysis: surgical hip dislocation and trimming of the stable trochanter to protect the perfusion of the epiphysis, *Instr Course Lect* 57:499, 2008.) **SEE TECHNIQUE 8.25.**

■ Use two additional Langenbeck retractors to provide exposure for inspection of the joint for synovitis, color and quantity of synovial fluid, degree of femoral head tilt, and stability of the epiphysis on the metaphysis. If the epiphysis is mobile or stability is questionable, prophylactic pinning is recommended; however, any attempt at reducing a mobile epiphysis anatomically should be avoided at this time because there is a high risk of pathologic stretching of the retinaculum before removal of the posterior callus.

■ Before surgical dislocation, drill a 2-mm hole in the femoral head to document blood perfusion. Laser Doppler flowmetry can provide dynamic control of the perfusion throughout the operation.

■ Flex and externally rotate the hip and place the leg into a sterile bag over the anterior side of the table to sublux the femoral head. Use a bone hook around the femoral calcar to improve exposure of the joint.

■ Document the damage pattern to the labrum and cartilage of the acetabulum and recreate the damage by the anterior metaphysis above the level of the epiphyseal contour by reducing the femoral head and moving it through flexion and internal rotation. If the epiphyseal tilt is small (<30 degrees) in a stable situation, and if trimming of the anterior metaphysis would be sufficient without creating a too thin femoral neck, full dislocation is not necessary. Create a normal offset by trimming the metaphyseal contour and pinning the epiphysis in situ.

■ If slippage is more severe, dislocate the femoral head. With the head subluxed, section the round ligament with curved scissors. With manipulation of the leg and the use of special retractors on the acetabular rim and teardrop area, inspect the entire acetabulum (360 degrees).

■ Rotate the leg to make visible the difference in surfaces of the femoral head and record the actual amount of epiphyseal slip. The retinaculum protecting the terminal branches of the medial femoral circumflex artery to the femoral epiphysis is clearly visible on the posterosuperior contour of the femoral neck as a somewhat mobile layer of connective tissue. Constantly moisten the femoral head cartilage during exposure.

■ Reduce the femoral head into the acetabulum for creation of the soft-tissue flap consisting of the retinaculum and external rotators and containing the blood supply for the epiphysis.

■ With an osteotome, carefully mobilize the area of the stable trochanter proximal to the visible physis (Fig. 8.127A) and then excise this fragment subperiosteally in an inside-out fashion.

■ Incise the periosteum of the neck anterior to the visible retinaculum from the anterosuperior edge of the trochanter physis toward the femoral head. Elevate the periosteum from the posterior neck with a knife and sharp periosteal elevators, taking care to avoid suture of the anterior insertion of the retinaculum near the femoral epiphysis.

■ Extend the periosteal release distally to the base of the lesser trochanter and level the remaining osseous ledge of the trochanteric base.

- In a similar manner, free the anteromedial periosteum (this is easier with the head dislocated), taking care to prevent disruption of the periosteal tube from the epiphysis (Fig. 8.127B).
- With the femoral head dislocated, use two blunt retractors to expose the femoral neck medially and laterally, avoiding any stretching of the retinaculum.
- Mobilize the epiphysis in a stepwise fashion with a curved 10-mm osteotome placed anteriorly into the physis.
- The physis is located proximal to the distal border of the epiphyseal joint cartilage. Normally, no wedge resection is necessary. With simultaneous levering with the osteotome and controlled external rotation of the leg, deliver the metaphyseal stump from the periosteal tube while the epiphysis remains in the posteromedial position. Removal of a posteromedial callus bridge in flexion-external rotation may facilitate this step.
- Spontaneous reduction of the isolated epiphysis into the acetabulum may occur at this time. Redislocation is difficult even with Kirschner wires inserted into the epiphysis. To help avoid this complication, place a small swab in the acetabulum.
- Remove visible or palpable callus formation on the posterior and posteromedial aspect of the neck. To provide a large contact area with the epiphysis, carefully round the front surface of the metaphyseal stump. Use controlled rotational maneuvers of the shaped femoral neck to allow manual fixation of the epiphysis while curettage of the remainder of the physis is performed (Fig. 8.127C). Normally, the exposed epiphyseal bone shows clear bleeding as a sign of intact perfusion.
- After removal of all callus particles, reduce the epiphysis onto the neck under visual control of the retinacular tension; reduction is easier with internal rotation of the leg. If any tension in the retinaculum occurs during this maneuver, immediately stop the reduction. Check to see that parts of the posterior soft-tissue flap are not inverted and need to be unfolded. The height of the metaphysis rarely requires reduction.
- Carefully determine the correct spatial orientation of the epiphysis. Use a palpating instrument or fluoroscopy to ensure that the border of the epiphysis has an equal distance to the neck in all planes. Visually check correct rotation relative to the location of the retinaculum and the fovea capitis. Use fluoroscopy to obtain the correct varus-valgus position.
- When the correct position is obtained, temporarily fix the epiphysis in place with a fully threaded Kirschner wire inserted in a retrograde direction through the fovea capitis, perforating the lateral cortex of the femur just distal to the vastus lateralis.
- Pull this wire back so far that its tip is level with the articular head cartilage and reduce the head into the acetabulum to allow final control of alignment with fluoroscopy. If perfect alignment of the epiphysis is achieved, insert one or two additional fully threaded Kirschner wires from the lateral cortex of the subtrochanteric bone. Check the correct wire length visually or with fluoroscopy. The wires should be optimally distributed within the epiphysis.
- Close the periosteal tube with a few stitches, avoiding any tension. Close the capsule, also without any tension. If the tendon of the piriformis muscle is producing tension on the capsule, release it.

- Fix the trochanteric fragment with two 3.5-mm screws (Fig. 8.127D).
- Carefully close the subcutaneous adipose tissue in several layers; suction drainage usually is not necessary.

POSTOPERATIVE CARE Continuous passive motion is used during the postoperative hospital stay. Crutches are used for toe-touch walking. Deep venous thrombosis prophylaxis with low-dose heparin is administered to obese patients only. Full weight bearing is allowed at 8 to 10 weeks if radiographs show healing of the trochanteric osteotomy. Strengthening of the gluteus medius is begun at 6 to 8 weeks, and full muscle strength should be achieved at 10 to 12 weeks. If implant removal is required, it should not be done until at least 1 year after surgery.

COMPENSATORY BASILAR OSTEOTOMY OF THE FEMORAL NECK

A compensatory osteotomy of the base of the femoral neck that corrects the varus and retroversion components of moderate or severe chronic SCFE has been suggested to be safer than an osteotomy made near or at the physis because the line of the osteotomy is distal to the major blood supply in the posterior retinaculum. Threaded pins are used for fixation of the osteotomy and the epiphysis. Not only is the anatomic relationship of the proximal femur restored, but also further slipping is prevented.

TECHNIQUE 8.26

(KRAMER ET AL.)
- Determine preoperatively the size of wedge to be removed by measuring the degree of the slip. Determine on anteroposterior radiographs the head and neck angle. Use paper tracings of the anteroposterior and lateral radiographs and cut with scissors the wedge on the tracing paper to determine the amount of bone to be removed and the results to be obtained.
- Approach the hip laterally. Begin the skin incision 2 cm distal and lateral to the ASIS and curve it distally and posteriorly over the greater trochanter and then distally along the lateral surface of the femoral shaft to a point 10 cm distal to the base of the trochanter. Incise longitudinally the fascia lata. Develop the interval between the gluteus medius and tensor fasciae latae. Carry the dissection proximally to the inferior branch of the superior gluteal nerve, which innervates the latter muscle. Incise the capsule of the hip joint longitudinally along the anterosuperior surface of the femoral neck. Release widely the capsular attachment along the anterior intertrochanteric line. Reflect distally the vastus lateralis to expose the base of the greater trochanter and the proximal part of the femoral shaft.
- With the capsule of the hip joint open, identify the junction between the articular cartilage of the femoral head and the callus and the junction of the callus with the nor-

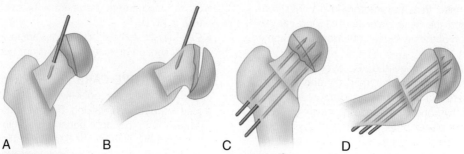

FIGURE 8.128 **A** and **B,** Widest part of wedge (at base of neck) is in line with widest part of slip, correcting varus and retroversion components, and Steinmann pin is inserted into femoral neck to control proximal fragment. If wedge is too wide anteriorly, retroversion is overly corrected. Most common mistake is to make wedge too narrow superiorly, resulting in incomplete correction of varus. **C** and **D,** Osteotomy is closed, and 5-mm threaded Steinmann pins are inserted from outer cortex of femoral shaft through femoral neck, across osteotomy site, and into femoral head. Pins fix osteotomy; because they cross the physis, they prevent any further slip. **SEE TECHNIQUE 8.26.**

mal cortex of the femoral neck. Compare the distance between these two junctions with the calculations made from the paper cutouts of the radiographs. The widest part of the wedge is in line with the widest part of the slip, in the anterior and superior aspects of the neck (Fig. 8.128A,B).

- Make the more distal osteotomy cut first, perpendicular to the femoral neck and following the anterior intertrochanteric line from proximal to distal. Extend this osteotomy cut to the posterior cortex but leave this cortex intact. Make the second osteotomy cut with the blade of the osteotome directed obliquely so that its cutting edge stays distal to the posterior retinacular blood supply. The capsule with the blood supply reaches to the intertrochanteric line anteriorly, but posteriorly the lateral third of the neck is extracapsular. According to Kramer et al., an osteotomy made through the region of the anterior intertrochanteric line lies distal to the posterior retinacular vessels.

- Drill one or two 5-mm threaded Steinmann pins into the femoral neck proximally to ensure that the proximal portion of the femur is kept under control before completing the osteotomy (Fig. 8.128A,B). During the osteotomy, ensure that the osteotome does not fully penetrate the posterior cortex. Insert several 5-mm threaded Steinmann pins from the outer cortex of the femoral shaft through the femoral neck. Complete the osteotomy by greensticking the posterior cortex and removing the wedge of bone. Advance the threaded Steinmann pins across the osteotomy site and the physis to prevent further slipping (Fig. 8.128C,D).

- Close the capsule of the hip with interrupted sutures. Clip off the pins close to the femoral shaft and close the wound in layers. If epiphysiodesis of the greater trochanter is necessary, do it at this time.

POSTOPERATIVE CARE Bed rest is prescribed for 2 to 3 weeks, followed by non–weight bearing. Partial weight bearing is allowed depending on the stability of the osteotomy and the weight of the patient. The threaded Steinmann pins should be removed only after the physis has fused.

EXTRACAPSULAR BASE-OF-NECK OSTEOTOMY

Extracapsular base-of-neck osteotomy has been recommended as safe and effective in preventing further slipping and improving hip range of motion in patients with severe chronic slips; however, it does not affect limb-length discrepancy. With severe slips the amount of correction of varus and posterior tilt of the femoral head is limited, and complete restoration of a normal head-shaft angle may not be possible or necessary. Removal of a wedge larger than 20 mm compromises femoral neck length and may increase greatly femoral anteversion. Also, pinning across the osteotomy site becomes more difficult when correction of more than 55 degrees of varus or valgus is attempted. These same restrictions also are applicable to intracapsular base-of-neck osteotomies and to the Southwick procedure (trochanteric osteotomy).

TECHNIQUE 8.27

(ABRAHAM ET AL.)

- Before surgery, the head-shaft angle is determined on lateral radiographs by measuring the angle formed by the epiphyseal line and the femoral shaft in the affected limb (Fig. 8.129) and comparing it with the contralateral side (or to 145 degrees). The head-shaft angle for posterior tilt or retroversion is determined on a frog-leg view and compared with the contralateral side (or to 10 degrees). The differences between the abnormal and normal angles are used to determine the size of the wedges removed during osteotomy.

- Secure the anesthetized patient on a fracture table and maximally internally rotate the involved limb by gently moving the footplate. Widely abduct the contralateral leg to make placement of fluoroscopic equipment easier. Obtain permanent anteroposterior and "shoot-through" lateral radiographs to confirm the chronicity of the slip and to outline the femoral head better. Prepare and drape the hip and patellar areas appropriately.

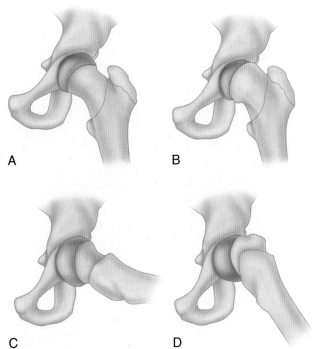

FIGURE 8.129 Extracapsular base-of-neck osteotomy: measurement of head-shaft angles on radiograph. **A,** Normal anteroposterior angle compared with slipped capital femoral epiphysis (SCFE). **B,** Moderate SCFE shows decrease in anteroposterior head-shaft angle. **C,** Normal acute angle. **D,** Severe slip shows increase in frog-leg lateral head-shaft angle. (From Abraham E, Garst J, Barmada R: Treatment of moderate to severe slipped capital femoral epiphysis with extracapsular base-of-neck osteotomy, *J Pediatr Orthop* 13:294, 1993.) **SEE TECHNIQUE 8.27.**

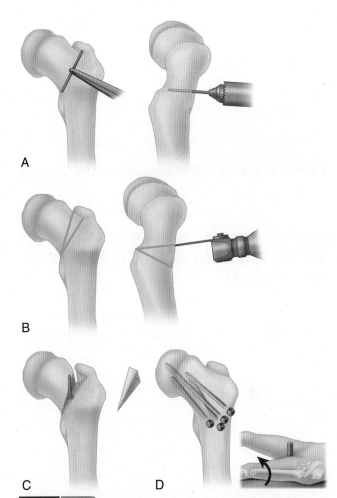

FIGURE 8.130 Extracapsular base-of-neck osteotomy (see text). **A,** Determination of proximal osteotomy cut. **B,** Osteotomy cuts. **C,** Removal of bony wedge. **D,** Fixation with cannulated screws. (From Abraham E, Garst J, Barmada R: Treatment of moderate to severe slipped capital femoral epiphysis with extracapsular base-of-neck osteotomy, *J Pediatr Orthop* 13:294, 1993.) **SEE TECHNIQUE 8.27.**

- Make a standard anterolateral approach and place a Charnley retractor deep to the iliotibial band. Locate the anterior joint tissue or intertrochanteric line between the gluteus medius and the vastus lateralis muscles. With a periosteal elevator, carefully elevate the anterior iliofemoral ligament. Place a narrow-tipped Hohmann retractor around the femoral neck superiorly and deep to the ischiofemoral ligament. Place another retractor deep to the iliofemoral ligament proximal to the lesser trochanter.
- Delineate a triangle on the anterior surface of the femoral neck to indicate the two-plane wedge osteotomy. Locate the proximal cut by placing a 3-cm long Kirschner wire on the anterior surface of the femur from the lesser to the greater trochanter at the base of the neck along the edge of the capsule (Fig. 8.130A). Confirm this position by fluoroscopy.
- Use a wide osteotome to mark the bone along the wire. Externally rotate the leg and drill a second Kirschner wire in the anteroposterior plane just distal to the guidewire (Fig. 8.130B). Place this wire vertical to the anterior surface of the femoral neck. Rotate the limb internally and obtain a lateral fluoroscopic view to confirm correct wire placement.
- Begin the second distal osteotomy line from the lesser trochanter to the growth plate of the greater trochanter. The angle at which this line is made from the first osteotomy line depends on the amount of correction needed. Usually

a 15-mm-wide wedge, measured superiorly to the baseline of the triangle, is needed. Make the osteotomy cuts with a saw, converging them posteriorly to make a single osteotomy along the posterior cortex. Completely remove the wedge of bone, especially superiorly, for maximal correction (Fig. 8.130C).
- While maintaining traction to prevent proximal migration of the femur, internally rotate the leg until the wedge closes completely. Abducting the leg also helps to close the osteotomy. When the patella can be internally rotated 15 degrees, adequate correction has been achieved. Remove additional bone from the metaphyseal side if necessary but remove a maximum of 20 mm in the bony wedge.
- Fix the osteotomy with three or four cannulated screws (Fig. 8.130D). Use the first guidewire to hold the osteotomy temporarily in the desired position. Use only one screw to span the physis of the femoral head, avoiding the superolateral quadrant.
- Check alignment and screw placement on permanent radiographs before closing the wound. Usually the iliofemoral ligament and capsule are not reattached, but if they

are excessively elevated from the bone, suture or staple them back to the anterior femur to preserve anterior joint stability.

■ Close the wound in routine fashion and apply a sterile dressing.

POSTOPERATIVE CARE Partial weight bearing with crutches is allowed for 6 to 8 weeks, and then full weight bearing is allowed. Weight bearing as tolerated is permitted after bilateral osteotomies.

INTERTROCHANTERIC OSTEOTOMY (IMHÄUSER)

The Imhäuser osteotomy is similar to the Southwick osteotomy but is technically easier. This trochanteric osteotomy primarily corrects posterior angulation with secondary correction of external rotation and varus; thus, the osteotomy wedge is simply a closing wedge anteriorly. In theory, this reduces the varus and external rotation and allows more flexion while avoiding anterior impingement with the acetabulum. The results of intertrochanteric osteotomies have been variable, but they do appear to lessen the chance of chondrolysis and osteonecrosis that occur with osteotomies at other locations, and they do correct impending FAI. A study of 47 hips in 39 patients demonstrated a cumulative 39 years' survivorship free from total hip arthroplasty of 68.5%, but the age at surgery, presence of osteonecrosis, and presence of chondrolysis negatively affected the outcome.

TECHNIQUE 8.28

■ Through a straight lateral approach to the hip, stabilize the SCFE with a 7.3-mm cannulated, terminally threaded cancellous screw placed centrally and perpendicular to the proximal femoral physis or with Kirschner wires.

■ Make the angle of insertion equal to the angle of posterior inclination of the capital epiphysis; this angle is equal to the degree of flexion of the femoral shaft that is necessary to position the epiphysis to the long axis of the femur and serves as a guide for the slotted chisel.

■ Place the slotted chisel for a 90-degree angled blade plate at the base of the greater trochanter and rotate it until the anticipated anterior inclination of the side plate matches the desired degree of flexion (Fig. 8.131A). Alternatively, a proximal femoral locking plate may be used.

■ Make a transverse osteotomy 2 cm distal to the chisel entry site and proximal to the lesser trochanter (Fig. 8.131B).

■ Flex the distal fragment and fix it to the side plate.

■ If the posterior periosteum prevents flexion of the distal fragment, release it. With increasing slip severity, increasing flexion is necessary. The flexion is accompanied by anterior translation to bring the femoral shaft in line with the proximal femoral epiphysis. This combi-

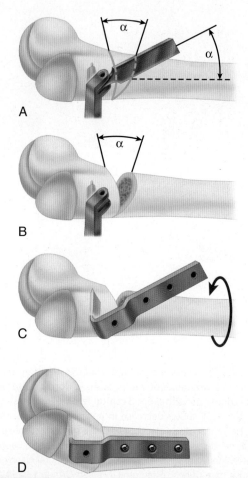

FIGURE 8.131 Intertrochanteric osteotomy (Imhäuser). **A,** Seating chisel is inserted into neck at right angles to shaft axis. **B,** Femoral osteotomy removes ventral wedge. **C,** Chisel is exchanged for blade plate, and femur is derotated. **D,** Blade plate is fixed to femur with screws. (Redrawn from Parsch K, Zehender H, Bühl T, Weller S: Intertrochanteric corrective osteotomy for moderate and severe chronic slipped capital femoral epiphysis, *J Pediatr Orthop B* 8:223, 1999.) **SEE TECHNIQUE 8.28.**

nation of movements counteracts the secondary zigzag deformity produced by a compensatory osteotomy at a site other than the primary site of deformity (the site of the slip).

■ Perform an anterior capsulotomy to allow full extension of the hip after fixation of the distal fragment.

■ Rotate the distal fragment medially to balance internal and external rotation of the hip and to match the uninvolved hip as determined by preoperative examination (Fig. 8.131C).

■ Fix the osteotomy with a 90-degree angled and 10-mm recessed blade plate (Fig. 8.131D).

POSTOPERATIVE CARE A spica cast is applied with the hip in appropriate flexion, slight abduction, and internal rotation and worn for 8 to 12 weeks. Depending on the amount of healing of the osteotomy on radiograph, weight bearing is slowly increased on the operated leg. The blade plate usually is removed approximately 1 year after surgery.

COMPLICATIONS

■ OSTEONECROSIS

Osteonecrosis has been reported to occur in 10% to 40% of patients with acute unstable SCFE, although more recent reports of in situ pinning with cannulated screws generally report lower incidences (0% to 5%). Osteonecrosis is rare in chronic, stable slips and probably results from interruption of the retrograde blood supply by the original injury and is more common in acute, unstable slips. Further insult to the blood supply may result from forceful manipulations, delay in treatment in unstable slips, tamponade of the vessels, or technical errors during open procedures.

Superolateral placement of pins also has been associated with the development of osteonecrosis or at least with exacerbation of the process.

Herman et al. and Loder et al. suggested that instability may be the best predictor of osteonecrosis after acute slips, and others have confirmed that unstable slips are more likely to result in osteonecrosis than stable slips. It has been estimated that up to 50% of patients with unstable SCFE will develop osteonecrosis.

Controversy exists in the recent literature not only about the natural history of osteonecrosis after SCFE but also about treatment to alter the natural history. Although the natural history is not known for certain, treatment plans are based on these theories of cause. Those who believe that osteonecrosis occurs at the time of maximal instability recommend urgent reduction, whereas those who believe osteonecrosis is caused by a tamponade effect advocate capsulotomy, especially if manipulation is done. Hip pressures in the affected side have been shown to be double those in the unaffected side and to be higher than those of compartment syndromes after manipulation. If a significant effusion is suspected, ultrasound can be used to determine the amount of fluid and the necessity of a capsulotomy. If immediate (within 24 hours) stabilization of an acute slip cannot be accomplished because of delayed presentation, a delay of at least 7 days has been recommended by some authors to avoid the "unsafe window" during which surgical intervention may increase the risk of osteonecrosis. At our institution, however, we advocate urgent reduction, stable fixation, and routine capsulotomy for all acute, unstable slips.

Ballard and Cosgrove coined the term *physeal separation,* which is defined as the amount of separation of the anterior lip of the epiphysis from the metaphysis on a frog-leg lateral radiograph (Fig. 8.132). Of the eight hips that developed osteonecrosis in their study of 110 hips, seven had anterior physeal separation. It was concluded that anterior physeal separation is associated with a high incidence of subsequent osteonecrosis after SCFE.

The role of early detection of osteonecrosis with advanced imaging also remains controversial. A recent study by Napora et al. suggests that early MRI detection followed by closed bone graft epiphysiodesis may improve outcomes in patients who have developed osteonecrosis following an unstable SCFE. Further research is needed in this area to determine optimal screening methods and the role of early surgical intervention.

■ CHONDROLYSIS

The diagnosis of chondrolysis requires a joint space less than 3 mm wide (normal 4 to 6 mm) and a decreased range of motion of the hip joint (Fig. 8.133). Persistent pin penetration

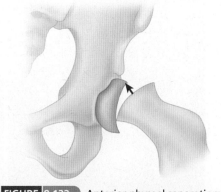

FIGURE 8.132 Anterior physeal separation.

into the joint has been the most frequently cited cause of chondrolysis, but it has been suggested that some other factor is necessary to produce chondrolysis, such as slip or an immune response.

Although fibrous ankylosis of the hip joint often occurs after chondrolysis, spontaneous partial cartilage recovery has been reported. Bed rest, traction, salicylates, nonsteroidal anti-inflammatory drugs, steroids, and physical therapy have not modified the course of chondrolysis. We have had some success with intraarticular cortisone injection and operative manipulation, followed by a vigorous physical therapy program. If severe joint space narrowing persists with limitation of joint motion, arthrodesis or arthroplasty should be considered.

■ FEMORAL NECK FRACTURE

Femoral fractures have been reported infrequently as a complication of in situ fixation of SCFE, although several authors have reported subtrochanteric fractures. We have treated a few patients with subtrochanteric fractures through unused drill holes below screw fixation (Fig. 8.134). After trying various methods of treatment for the subtrochanteric fracture, we now recommend immediate open reduction of the fracture and internal fixation with a hip screw and a long side plate while maintaining the reduction of SCFE.

Femoral neck fracture after in situ pinning of SCFE is even less common. We have treated two patients with displaced femoral neck fractures after in situ fixation of SCFE. In both patients, treatment of the femoral neck fractures was operative and difficult and the results were less than satisfactory.

As more reports are accumulated, femoral fractures after in situ fixation of SCFE may be found to be more frequent than currently appreciated. The likelihood of this complication perhaps can be decreased by avoiding drilling unnecessary holes in the bone during surgery and by avoiding overzealous reaming of the femoral neck.

The necessity of pin removal after fixation of SCFE remains an area of controversy. Pin removal is not without costs and risks, and the question of whether a pin must be removed at the end of treatment remains unanswered. We currently are leaving pins and screws in place after treatment of SCFE.

■ CONTINUED SLIPPING

Continued slipping (Fig. 8.135) has occurred in patients who refused treatment, were not compliant with postoperative restrictions, and in whom stable fixation was not

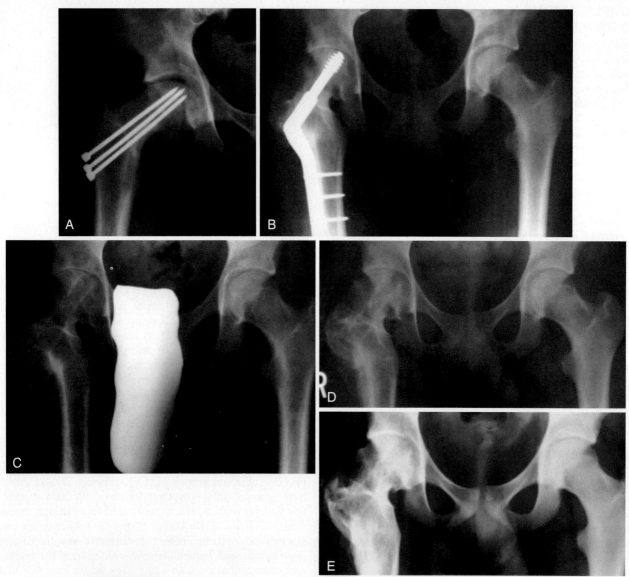

FIGURE 8.133 **A–E,** Chondrolysis 24 months after flexion internal rotation osteotomy for severe slipped capital femoral epiphysis.

achieved. Progressive slipping may also occur if osteonecrosis develops and fixation is lost before physeal closure.

■ FEMOROACETABULAR IMPINGEMENT

Recent interest in FAI, which has become a frequently reported and described entity that causes pain, decreased range of motion, and early osteoarthritis of the hip joint, has led to a better understanding of SCFE-induced impingement. Anterolateral displacement of the femoral neck in relation to the femoral epiphysis produces a reduced head-neck offset, elevated alpha angle (Fig. 8.136), and cam type lesion. One study reported a high proportion (32% to 38%) of young adults with signs of clinical impingement after SCFE. Although extreme posterior angulation (slippage) obviously may cause impingement, the real question is how little angular deformity will cause impingement. This is key to in situ pinning, after which generally good early results can be expected. The literature is unclear about how much posterior angulation can be accepted during initial treatment or even how much angulation later will cause symptomatic FAI.

According to most series, the grade of slip in adolescence cannot be used as a predictor of the development of symptomatic FAI and ultimately osteoarthritis in adulthood.

The cam effect in which the femoral head or screw head abuts the acetabular labrum (Fig. 8.137) and the pincer effect in which the acetabular rim impinges on the femoral neck (Fig. 8.138) have both been described in adults who had treatment of SCFE as adolescents. FAI can be identified by arthroscopy and MRI; plain cross-table lateral radiographs dramatically demonstrate cam and pincer impingement described by Nötzli as "jamming rim" impingement (Fig. 8.139).

Femoral osteochondroplasty, valgus osteotomy, or the Imhäuser procedure (see Technique 8.28) has been recommended after in situ pinning to avoid acetabular impingement.

FEMORAL FRACTURES

Femoral fracture is a common injury. The annual rate of femoral shaft fractures in children is 20 per 100,000. With regard to age, the distribution appears to be bimodal, with peaks at

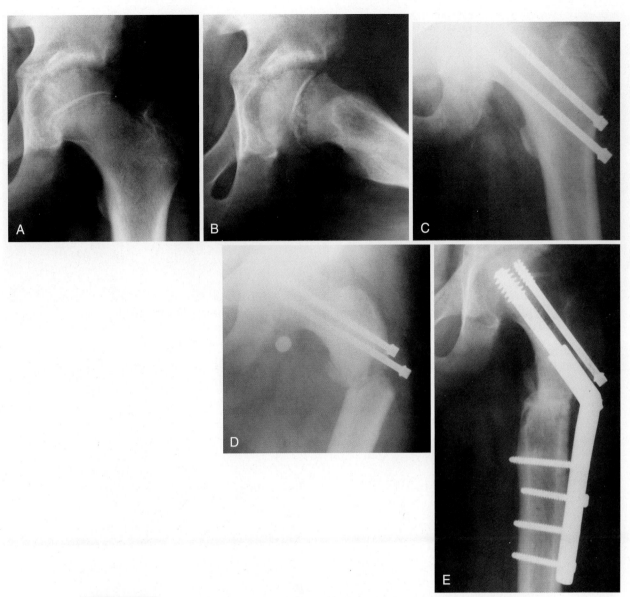

FIGURE 8.134 **A** and **B,** Slipped capital femoral epiphysis. **C,** After pin fixation, several unnecessary drill holes remain distal to last pin. **D,** After pathologic fracture through drill hole. **E,** One year after open reduction and internal fixation with compression hip screw; note evidence of union of subtrochanteric fracture. Cannulated hip screw was left in place to prevent further slipping of capital femoral epiphysis at the time of hip screw insertion.

2 and 17 years. Boys have higher rates of fracture than girls at all ages. The primary mechanisms of fracture are age dependent and include falls for children younger than 6 years old, motor vehicle–pedestrian accidents for children 6 to 9 years old, and motor vehicle accidents for teenagers.

Fractures of the femur usually are classified according to location as subtrochanteric, shaft (proximal, middle, and distal thirds), supracondylar, and distal femoral physeal. Additionally, femoral fractures are classified by being open or closed, comminuted or noncomminuted, and by fracture pattern (transverse, spiral, or oblique). Fractures occur most commonly in the middle third of the shaft as a closed, non-comminuted, transverse fracture.

Historically, most femoral fractures in children are closed injuries and traditionally have been treated by closed methods. However, management of pediatric femoral fractures has

evolved toward operative approaches because of a desire for more rapid recovery and reintegration of the patients, with the recognition that prolonged immobilization can have negative effects even in children. External fixation, submuscular plating, and intramedullary nailing all have been advocated.

Besides the usual mechanisms of injury, femoral fractures can occur at birth, can be caused by child abuse, or can be pathologic. In children younger than 1 year of age, 70% of femoral fractures are abuse related. Abuse should be suspected if any of the following are present: (1) unreasonable history; (2) inappropriate delay in coming to the hospital; (3) previous history of abuse; (4) evidence of other fractures in various stages of healing; (5) multiple acute fractures; and (6) characteristic fracture patterns. A recent study from our institution demonstrated that a transverse fracture pattern is more closely associated with abuse and should raise the index of suspicion for abuse.

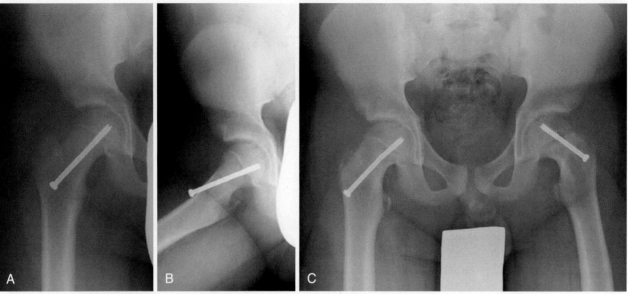

FIGURE 8.135 **A,** Slipped capital femoral epiphysis fixed with partially threaded cannulated screw. **B and C,** One month after return to sports, broken screw is seen; no lucency or "windshield wiping" visible. (From Murphy RE, Beaty JH, Kelly DM, et al: Implant failure in slipped capital femoral epiphysis: a report of two cases, *JBJS Case Connect* 3:e138, 2013.)

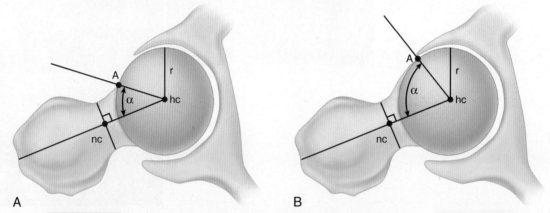

FIGURE 8.136 Anterior head-neck offset (Nötzli) angle. Point *A,* anterior point where distance from center of the head (*hc*) exceeds radius (*r*) of subchondral surface of femoral head. α is then measured as angle between *A-hc* and *hc-nc*, with *nc* being center of neck at narrowest point. **A,** Hip in normal individual. **B,** Typical deformation. The greater anterior head-neck offset angle, the smaller arc of motion required to cause cam-type impingement on acetabular rim.

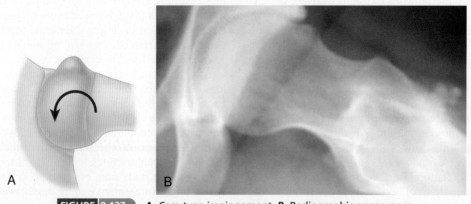

FIGURE 8.137 **A,** Cam-type impingement. **B,** Radiographic appearance.

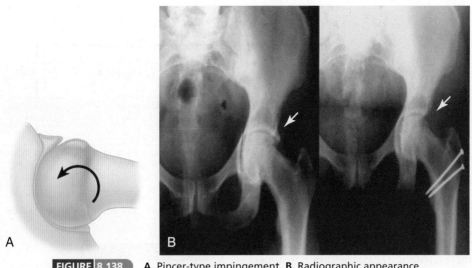

FIGURE 8.138 **A,** Pincer-type impingement. **B,** Radiographic appearance.

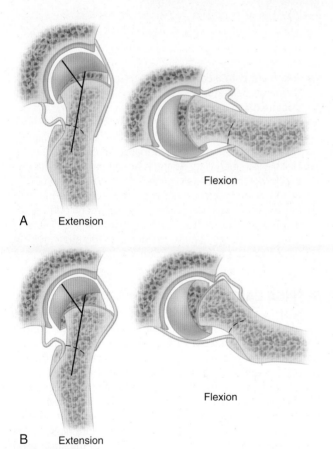

FIGURE 8.139 "Jamming rim" impingement. **A,** Mild to moderate slipped capital femoral epiphysis (SCFE) causes jamming of femoral metaphysis against acetabular cartilage in flexion. **B,** Severe SCFE causes impingement of femoral neck against acetabular rim in flexion.

In the setting of a femoral fracture, a thorough evaluation should be performed and concomitant injury ruled out. If a child sustains enough trauma to fracture the largest bone in his or her body, the child may have occult abdominal or other injuries. A careful secondary survey should be performed. Ipsilateral knee instability has been reported to occur in 4% of children with femoral fractures and may be difficult to assess at the time of injury.

FEMORAL SHAFT FRACTURES (DIAPHYSEAL FEMORAL FRACTURES)

Understanding the deforming forces applied by various structures around the femur helps in selecting the appropriate treatment of a femoral fracture. In proximal shaft and subtrochanteric fractures, the proximal fragment usually is in a position of flexion, abduction, and external rotation because of the unopposed pull of the iliopsoas, abductor, and short external rotator muscles. The adductors and extensors are intact in midshaft fractures, and the distal fragment usually is in satisfactory alignment except for some external rotation. In supracondylar fractures, the distal fragment is in a position of hyperextension because of the overpull of the gastrocnemius. The muscle imbalances are important when aligning the distal fragment to the proximal fragment whether closed or open treatment strategies are selected.

Staheli defined the ideal treatment of femoral shaft fractures in children as one that controls alignment and length, is comfortable for the child and convenient for the family, and causes the least negative psychologic impact possible. Determining the ideal treatment for each child depends on the age of the child, the location and type of fracture, the family environment, the knowledge and ability of the surgeon, and, to a lesser degree, financial considerations. Heyworth et al. reviewed femoral fractures in children 6 to 17 years old from a national database of pediatric inpatient admissions from 1997 to 2000 in about half of the United States. The frequency of operative treatment, most often consisting of internal fixation, increased significantly over this period, whereas the use of spica casting declined. This change in practice was significantly greater at pediatric hospitals than general hospitals. Sanders et al. surveyed members of the Pediatric Orthopedic Society of North America to determine their current preferences in treating femoral fractures in four age groups. For each fracture pattern, operative treatment was increasingly preferred over nonoperative treatment as patient age increased and the preferred treatments within operative and nonoperative categories changed significantly as patient age increased. There was a trend by pediatric orthopaedists to

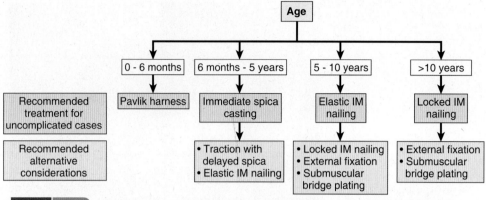

FIGURE 8.140 Algorithm for treatment of femoral fractures in children. *IM,* Intramedullary.

treat femoral fractures operatively in older children and non-operatively in younger children. The consensus on treatment was that it is age dependent (Fig. 8.140).

The AAOS, after extensive review of the literature, made 14 evidence-based recommendations concerning fracture of the femur in children. Five of the recommendations with enough evidence to support a grade of recommendation (grade A or B, supported by good evidence; grade C, supported by poor evidence) are listed in Box 8.4.

Our general treatment recommendations are listed in Table 8.4.

Several authors have evaluated the comparative economics of nonoperative and operative treatment. The charges or cost included hospital and physician charges (orthopaedists, radiologists, and anesthesiologists). Table 8.5 gives the cost or charges in different series of patients. The differences seen among series are not comparable because of many variables. On average, however, immediate or early spica casting (traction spica) cost less than prolonged traction with spica casting, intramedullary rods, or external fixation. Prolonged skeletal traction and spica casting, intramedullary rods, and external fixation frequently cost the same. The cost of reoperations for malrotation or removal of implants also was similar for the three groups.

In a very young child (birth to 6 months), a Pavlik harness can be used instead of a spica cast with cited advantages of ease of application without anesthesia; minimal hospitalization (<24 hours); easy reduction; ability to adjust the harness; minimal costs; and ease in diaper changing, nursing, and bonding. Our institution investigated the use of a Pavlik harness for femoral fractures in children under 6 months of age and found excellent clinical results with minimal complication rates. Parent reliability and compliance, however, must be carefully considered before using this method of treatment.

Immediate spica casting of femoral shaft fractures in children has been recommended by several authors; best results with this method seem to be obtained in infants and young children with low-energy, length-stable fracture. Although rare, a compartment syndrome secondary to spica casting also can occur. The primary problems with immediate spica casting are shortening and angulation of the fracture in high-energy femoral shaft fractures. In young children, a higher degree of angulation and shortening is accepted; these parameters become stricter with increasing age (Table 8.6).

BOX 8.4

Treatment Recommendations for Diaphyseal Femoral Fractures

- We recommend that children younger than 36 months with a diaphyseal femoral fracture be evaluated for child abuse (A).
- Treatment with a Pavlik harness or spica cast is an option for infants 6 months and younger with a diaphyseal femoral fracture (C).
- We suggest early spica casting or traction with delayed spica casting for children age 6 months to 5 years with a diaphyseal femoral fracture with less than 2 cm of shortening (B).
- Flexible intramedullary nailing is an option to treat diaphyseal femoral fractures in children 5-11 years of age (C).
- Rigid trochanteric entry nailing, submuscular plating, and flexible intramedullary nailing are treatment options for diaphyseal femoral fractures in children age 11 years to skeletal maturity, but piriformis or near piriformis entry rigid nailing is not a treatment option (C).

▓ SPICA CASTING

Early spica casting in the 90-90 position has been recommended to avoid shortening and angulation in children younger than 6 years old with a closed femoral shaft fracture stemming from low-energy trauma. Alternatively, for low-energy femoral fractures, a walking spica or single leg spica can be applied with the hip and knee flexed to 45 degrees and the cast ending above the ankle. Flynn et al. performed a prospective study comparing a walking spica with a traditional spica cast and found similar outcomes with significantly lower burden of care to the family. The walking spica group did, however, have a higher early loss of reduction requiring cast wedging in the outpatient setting.

Good results also have been reported with 90-90 skeletal traction and spica casting, although the current indication for this technique at our institution is for length-unstable fractures or concomitant injuries that prevent the patient from having a spica cast in place or from being safely sedated. If this treatment course is selected, pins for skeletal traction should be placed parallel to the axis of the knee joint (Fig. 8.141).

Adolescents do not tolerate prolonged immobilization as well as younger children, and knee pain, angulation at

TABLE 8.4

General Treatment Guidelines in Children With Femoral Shaft Fractures

AGE	<6 MO	6 MO TO 5 YR	5 TO 11 YR	11 YR TO ADULT
PREFERRED TREATMENT Alternate treatment because of: Head injury High velocity (comminuted) Floating knee Difficult location (proximal third and distal third) Obesity Surgical risk (multiple trauma)	Pavlik harness	Early spica casting Traction and spica casting	Elastic intramedullary nail Traction and spica casting Submuscular plating Antegrade locked intramedullary nail	Antegrade locked intramedullary nail Submuscular plating
OPEN FRACTURES		External fixation	External fixation	External fixation

TABLE 8.5

Cost of Treatment of Femoral Shaft Fractures

SERIES	IMMEDIATE (EARLY SPICA)	TRACTION SPICA	INTRAMEDULLARY ROD	EXTERNAL FIXATION
Newton and Mubarak	—	$5494	$21,093	$21,359
Clinkscales and Peterson	$5490	$16,273	$16,056	$16,394
Stans et al.	$5264	$15,980	$15,495	$14,478
Yandow et al.	$1867	$11,171	—	—
Nork and Hoffinger	$22,396	$11,520	—	—
Coyte et al.	$5970*	$7626*	—	—

*Canadian $.

TABLE 8.6

Acceptable Angulation in Femoral Shaft Fractures

AGE	VARUS/VALGUS (DEGREES)	ANTERIOR/POSTERIOR (DEGREES)	SHORTENING (MM)
Birth to 2 years	30	30	15
2-5 years	15	20	20
2-10 years	10	15	15
11 years to maturity	5	10	10

From Flynn JM, Skaggs DL: Femoral shaft fractures. In Flynn JM, Skaggs DL, Waters PM, editors: *Rockwood and Wilkins' fractures in children*, ed 8, Philadelphia, 2015, Wolters Kluwer.

the fracture, and difficulty in maintaining length have been reported when 90-90 traction was used in children older than 10 years, as well as limb shortening and leg-length discrepancy, malunion, pin track infection, loss of joint motion, and muscle atrophy. As a result, internal fixation is preferred in this age group.

At our institution, if skeletal or skin traction is applied in children younger than 6 years old, longitudinal traction or traction at a 45-degree angle with up to 5 lb of weight is recommended. Overhead skin traction should not be used for femoral fractures in this age group because of the increased risk of neurovascular compromise. Neurovascular status and

skin condition should be monitored carefully while the child is in traction. When length and alignment are achieved, the patient is medically stable; once appropriate callus formation is noted, a spica cast is applied.

In older or larger children who require traction because they are too unstable for more definitive treatment, a 5/64-inch Steinmann pin can be inserted into the distal femur or proximal tibia. If a tibial pin is used, it should be placed distal to the tibial tubercle and the proximal tibial physis to minimize the risk of growth disturbance and genu recurvatum deformity. A distal femoral traction pin may be necessary for a distal supracondylar fracture because of posterior

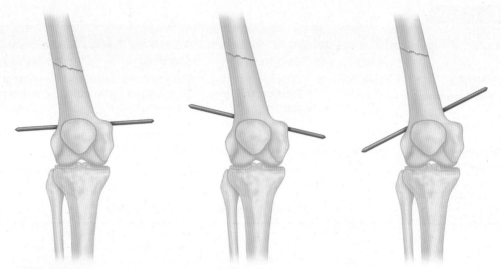

FIGURE 8.141 Position of pin in traction is either horizontal (optimal) or oblique. Oblique pins are either "to varus" or "to valgus," reflecting resultant pull of traction bow.

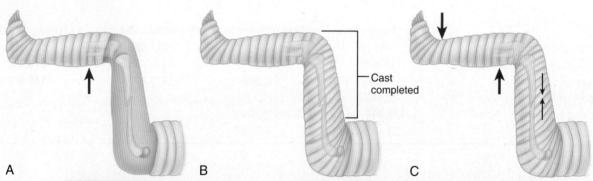

A   B   C

Cast completed

FIGURE 8.142 Pathogenic factors of traction, elevation, and pressure during application of short leg cast used for traction can cause compartment syndrome. **A,** Below-knee cast is applied while patient is on spica frame. **B,** Traction is applied to short leg cast to produce distraction at fracture site. The remainder of cast is applied, fixing relative distance between leg and torso. **C,** After child awakens from general anesthesia, there is shortening of femur from muscular contraction, which causes thigh and leg to slip somewhat back into spica. This causes pressure at corners of cast *(arrows).* (Redrawn from Mubarak SJ, Frick S, Sink E, et al: Volkmann contracture and compartment syndromes after femur fractures in children treated with 90/90 spica casts, *J Pediatr Orthop* 26:567, 2006.)

angulation or for 90-90-degree traction in a proximal femoral fracture with anterior displacement of the proximal fragment. A femoral pin generally should not be used if intramedullary nailing is being contemplated in the course of treatment.

Peroneal nerve palsy is a rare complication of skin or skeletal traction and casting. Two of our patients younger than 2 years old developed peroneal nerve palsies after skin traction and spica casting. Spontaneous recovery occurs in most patients.

Mubarak et al. described the development of a compartment syndrome in the lower leg after application of a short leg cast used for traction to reduce femoral fractures during the application of a 90-90 spica cast. They cited as pathogenic factors traction, elevation, and pressure (Fig. 8.142). Because of the possibility of this potentially devastating complication, the use of a short leg cast for applying traction should be avoided during application of a 90-90 spica cast and alternative cast application methods should be used.

SPICA CAST APPLICATION
TECHNIQUE 8.29

- After general anesthesia, remove the skeletal traction pin and sterilely clean the wound sites if traction was used.
- Apply a well-padded long leg cast with the knee flexed 45 or 90 degrees, depending on whether a traditional or walking spica is being applied. Mold the proximal part to help avoid angulation with a strong valgus mold. To avoid compartment syndrome, do not apply traction through a short leg cast to effect reduction.

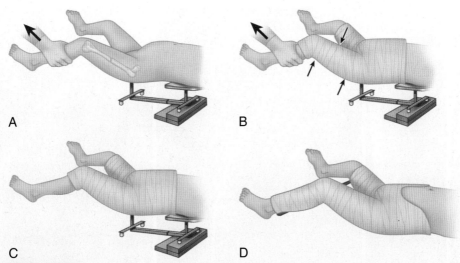

FIGURE 8.143 Technique of spica cast application. **A,** Patient is placed on child's fracture spica table. Leg is held in about 45 degrees of flexion at hip and knee, with traction applied to proximal calf. **B,** One and one-half spica cast is applied down to proximal calf. Molding of thigh is done during this phase. **C,** Radiographs of femur are obtained, and any necessary wedging of cast can be done at this time. **D,** Leg portion of cast and cross-bar are applied. Belly portion of spica cast is trimmed to umbilicus. (Redrawn from Mubarak SJ, Frick S, Sink E, et al: Volkmann contracture and compartment syndromes after femur fractures in children treated with 90/90 spica casts, *J Pediatr Orthop* 26:567, 2006.) **SEE TECHNIQUE 8.29.**

- Place the child on a "spica table" or fracture table, depending on the size of the child, and check the reduction. Apply a one and one-half spica cast or full spica cast with the hip or hips flexed at 45 or 90 degrees (Fig. 8.143), with approximately 15 degrees of external rotation and 30 degrees of hip abduction. Children younger than 3 years tolerate the 90-90-degree spica cast well. This position helps prevent shortening and aids in transporting the child. (According to Flynn, automobile restraint laws in many states make it difficult or impossible to legally transport a child casted in full extension.) Knee flexion of less than 50 degrees may result in a 20% incidence of loss of reduction.
- Apply the spica to a level between the umbilicus and nipple line with a ¼ to ½ inch thick towel over the thorax and under the Webril (Kendall Healthcare, Mansfield, MA), which is to be removed later to allow for chest and abdominal expansion.
- Reinforce the groin, inguinal, and buttocks areas with splints to avoid breakage.
- After trimming the cast and after satisfactory radiographs are obtained, apply a wooden bar spanning the extremities and incorporate it in the cast if additional cast stability is required.

EXTERNAL FIXATION

External fixation with both monolateral and circular frames has been recommended for treatment of femoral shaft fractures in children and adolescents, with good results reported by a number of authors in patients ranging in age from 3 years to skeletal maturity. Complications, however, also have been frequent with this method of fixation. Ramseier et al., in a comparison of four fixation methods (elastic stable intramedullary nail, rigid intramedullary nail, plate, and external fixator), found that external fixation was associated with the highest number of complications. Major complications associated with external fixation of femoral fractures in children and adolescents include loss of reduction, refracture, and deep infection. The most common minor complication is pin site or pin track infection. Refracture has been reported in 2% to 33% of patients treated with external fixation. Refracture has been suggested to occur because of the detrimental effect of prolonged rigidity imposed by the external fixator. An association has been noted between the number of cortices showing bridging callus (on anteroposterior and lateral views) at the time of fixator removal and the rate of refracture. Kesemenli et al. reported a refracture rate of only 1.8% in closed femoral fractures and a 20% rate of refracture in open fractures or in patients who had ORIF. They concluded that external fixation itself was not a risk factor for refracture. Other suggested risk factors include open fractures and bilateral fractures with the increase of time in the fixator. Factors that appear to have an inconclusive effect on refracture include fracture pattern, dynamization status, fixator type, pin size, and number of pins.

Open fractures of the femur have traditionally been stabilized with external fixation. A comparison of the results of external fixation and intramedullary nailing (both rigid and flexible nails) found that intramedullary nailing was associated with fewer complications, especially varus malunion and refracture. Infection rates appeared to be the same. Intramedullary fixation should be considered, especially for grade I open fractures. If external fixation is chosen as the method of treatment for pediatric femoral fractures, careful attention must be paid to operative technique and postoperative treatment to minimize complications.

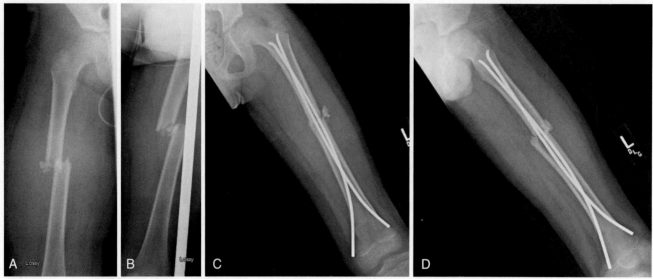

FIGURE 8.144 **A** and **B,** Femoral shaft fracture. **C** and **D,** After fixation with flexible intramedullary nails, avoiding proximal and distal physes.

At our institution, in a young child with polytrauma, open fracture with significant soft-tissue injury, pathologic fracture, metadiaphyseal fracture, or severe head injury, external fixation is considered as a fixation option. The technique of external fixation of fractures of the femur is described in other chapter.

■ INTRAMEDULLARY NAILING

Good results using flexible stainless steel or titanium intramedullary rods have been reported with suggested advantages of less disruption of family life, shorter hospitalization, earlier independent ambulation, and earlier return to school (Fig. 8.144). With the overall trend to more frequent internal fixation of femoral fractures, it is not surprising that the indications have expanded to include younger children. The lower age limit for flexible intramedullary nailing has not been definitively established (see AAOS Guidelines, Box 8.4), but certainly there is an age at which any type of immobilization (e.g., Pavlik harness, spica cast) will produce a good result without the risk of surgical complications. Several reports have documented good results with few complications in preschool (18 months to 6 years of age) children treated with flexible intramedullary nailing. Heffernan et al. reviewed 215 patients between the ages of 2 and 6 years who were treated with either elastic nails or a spica cast and found similar complication and healing rates, with an earlier return to independent ambulation and full activities in the elastic nail group. They concluded that elastic nails were a reasonable treatment option in this age group and should be considered, especially when high-energy mechanisms are present. Long-term follow-up (at least 24 months) is recommended to monitor overgrowth, and the child's activity must be closely monitored. Malalignment and leg-length discrepancy are frequently reported complications of flexible intramedullary nailing of femoral fractures in children, but these seldom cause functional problems. Increased complication rates have been reported in unstable fractures, older patients, and overweight patients treated with titanium elastic nails. One study found that the complication rate was improved from 52% to 23% when the use of titanium elastic nailing was limited to

stable fractures. Additional studies have found that the use of stainless steel nails can significantly lower the malunion rate, major complication rate, and overall cost when compared with titanium nails.

Rigid intramedullary fixation of femoral shaft fractures in adolescents has been reported to result in high rates of union with short hospital stays and brief periods of immobilization that may have psychologic, social, educational, and some economic advantages over conservative treatment. In a review of our early results of intramedullary nailing of 31 femoral fractures in 30 adolescents, ranging in age from 10 to 15 years (average 12.3 years), we found that all 31 fractures united without evidence of trochanteric overgrowth, coxa valga deformity, or narrowing of the femoral neck. Two patients had bony overgrowth of more than 2 cm (2.5 and 2.8 cm). Other complications included one superficial distal wound infection that resolved after intravenous antibiotic therapy and decreased sensation in the distribution of the deep peroneal nerve in one patient and in the distribution of the pudendal nerve in another; both neurologic problems resolved spontaneously. Mild heterotopic ossification over the nail proximally was found in three patients. Asymptomatic segmental osteonecrosis developed in one patient when a piriformis entry site was used and was not visible on radiographs until 15 months after fracture. A subsequent study of femoral shaft fractures in children 12 years and under treated with a rigid, locked, antegrade nailing inserted from a trochanteric entry point was conducted at our institution and demonstrated no malunion, leg-length difference, osteonecrosis, or hardware failure at final follow-up. A subsequent report by Crosby et al. on a 20-year experience with trochanteric rigid intramedullary nails in pediatric and adolescent femoral fractures demonstrated acceptable complication rates with no cases of osteonecrosis. Because of the few complications and high rate of union in our patients and other reports, we believe trochanteric rigid intramedullary nailing is the treatment of choice for femoral shaft fractures in older adolescents (12 to 16 years old) and is a reasonable option for children with risk factors for malunion, such as obesity or unstable fracture patterns.

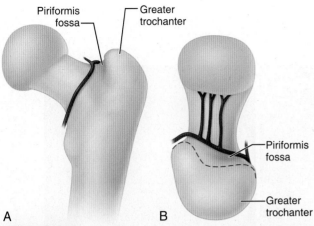

FIGURE 8.145 **A and B,** Proximal femoral anatomy. (Redrawn from Keeler KA, Dart B, Luhmann SJ, et al: Antegrade intramedullary nailing of pediatric femoral fractures using an interlocking pediatric femoral nail and a lateral trochanteric entry point, *J Pediatr Orthop* 29:345, 2009.)

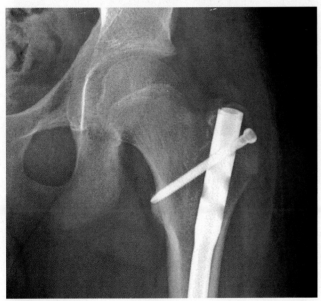

FIGURE 8.146 Proximal end of nail is left long (≤1 cm) to make later removal easier.

To minimize the risk of osteonecrosis, it is important that the dissection during placement and removal not extend medial to the greater trochanter, with care to avoid extension to the capsule or the piriformis fossa. The tip of the greater trochanter in adolescents or a more lateral starting point in younger children should be used for the entry site. Only one instance of osteonecrosis has been reported when the tip of the trochanter has been used as the entry point, and no cases of osteonecrosis have been reported to our knowledge with a lateral entry point. This prevents dissection near the piriformis fossa and the origin of the lateral ascending cervical artery, which is medial to the piriformis fossa (Fig. 8.145). The proximal end of the nail should be left long (≤1 cm) to make later removal easier (Fig. 8.146). Nails can be removed 9 to 18 months after radiographic union to prevent bony overgrowth over the proximal tip of the nail.

The length and diameter of the intramedullary nail may limit the use of this technique, but the development of a smaller (7 mm diameter) pediatric nail expands its application. We use a pediatric nail that has a transverse proximal interlocking screw that can be dynamized and avoids the greater trochanter and has more distal screw holes in the nail to avoid the physis (Fig. 8.147). Most small-diameter nails are solid, making passage through the fracture site a challenge. The technique of locked intramedullary nailing of the femur is described in other chapter.

Although mechanical studies have demonstrated equal or superior fixation with titanium nails compared with stainless steel nails, and the biomechanical properties of titanium have been suggested to be superior to those of stainless steel for intramedullary fixation, a comparison of the two devices found a malunion rate nearly four times higher with the use of titanium nails (23%) than with stainless steel nails (6%). Overall, major complications were more frequent with the titanium nails (36%) than with stainless steel nails (17%).

FLEXIBLE INTRAMEDULLARY NAIL FIXATION

Biomechanical testing of flexible intramedullary nails using synthetic bone models has shown that (1) retrograde nail fixation has significantly less axial range of motion and more torsional stiffness than antegrade fixation in comminuted and transverse fracture models; (2) there is no significant difference between the mechanical properties of three different retrograde nail constructions (two C-shaped and two S-shaped and two straight flexible nails were tested), suggesting that any of the three constructs could be used to treat femoral fractures in children; and (3) length and rotation control with two divergent flexible nails of comminuted midshaft femur fractures may be sufficient for early mobilization (Fig. 8.148). Most femoral shaft fractures in children can be stabilized using retrograde fixation. Usually, medial and lateral insertion sites are used, but a single insertion site, either medial or lateral, can be used in the distal femoral metaphysis. Two divergent C-configuration nails or one C-configuration and one S-configuration nail (bent by the surgeon at a point approximately 5 cm distal to the eyelet) are routine; additional nails can be added if necessary. Special expertise is needed to stabilize subtrochanteric fractures and fractures of the distal third of the femur; antegrade insertion commonly is used for the latter. Most agree that fixation of some proximal and distal long spiral fractures may lack stability as far as rotation and angulation, and testing for stability after nailing at surgery is indicated. If instability is present, a long leg cast with a pelvic band is used short term. A prospective comparison of titanium elastic nail fixation and spica casting for treatment of femoral shaft fractures in children found that children treated with flexible nails achieved recovery milestones significantly faster than those treated with traction and spica casting. Hospital charges for the two methods were similar, and the complication rate after flexible nailing (21%) was lower than after traction and spica casting (34%).

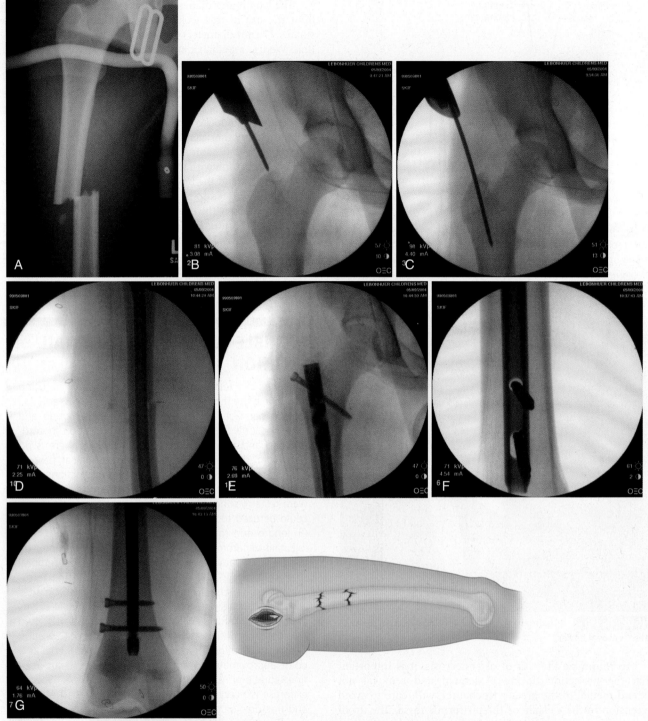

FIGURE 8.147   Pediatric TriGen intramedullary nailing. **A,** Midshaft femoral fracture in a 15-year-old. **B,** Entry at tip of greater trochanter (inset shows approach). **C,** Channel reamer and guide placement. **D,** A 9-mm nail placed across fracture site. **E,** Locking of proximal screw. **F and G,** Concentric circle technique for distal locking.

TECHNIQUE 8.30

- Place the patient on an orthopaedic table and reduce the fracture partially by traction guided by fluoroscopy (Fig. 8.149A,B).
- Use blunt-ended nails of quality steel (cold-hammered at 140 degrees) or titanium. The nails should be 45 cm long

with diameters of 2.5, 3.0, 3.5, or 4.0 mm, depending on the child's weight and age.
- Prepare the nails preoperatively by angling them at 45 degrees about 2 cm from one end to facilitate penetration of the medullary canal and bend them into an even curve over their entire length.

- With the help of a T-handle and by rotation movements of the wrist, introduce the nails through a longitudinal drill hole made in the distal femoral metaphysis just above the physis. Use two nails, one lateral and one medial, to stabilize the fracture. Carefully impact both up the medullary canal to the fracture site. After touching the opposite internal cortex, the nails bend themselves in the direction of the long bone's axis. The nails should cross distal to the fracture site (normally 4 to 6 cm distal) (Fig. 8.149C).
- With the fracture held reduced, rotate the T-handle or manipulate the limb to direct the pins into the opposite fragment. If the first is impeded, try the second with the aid of an image intensifier. Ensure both nails are in the

canal across the fracture site. When they pass the fracture level, release traction, pushing the nails farther and fixing their tips in the spongy tissue of the metaphysis, without their passing through the physis (Fig. 8.149D). Small distractions can be corrected by rotation of the pins. Avoid residual angulation by ensuring that the nails are introduced at the same level and that the tips of the nail oppose each other in both planes so that they have identical curvatures (Fig. 8.149E). Leave the distal portion of the nails slightly protruding for ease of removal (Fig. 8.149F).

- If the technique is performed correctly, the fracture is finally stabilized by two nails, each with three points of fixation. The fixation is elastic but sufficiently stable to allow automatic small position corrections by limited movements during the limb's loading.

POSTOPERATIVE CARE Postoperatively, the limb is rested on a pillow. A knee immobilizer may give more comfort. Mobilization using crutches without weight bearing is allowed as soon as the fracture causes no pain. A spica cast can be used if rotation or angulation is evident after the procedure. At the beginning of the third week, partial weight bearing is allowed. After the appearance of calcified external callus, full weight bearing is allowed. Nails are removed when the surgeon is positive that healing has occurred, usually 6 to 12 months postoperatively.

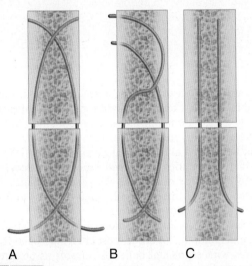

FIGURE 8.148 **A,** Midshaft diaphyseal fracture model stabilized with two C-shaped nails. **B** and **C,** Midshaft diaphyseal fracture stabilized with S-shaped and C-shaped nails **(B)** and two straight nails **(C).**

▉ PLATING

Plating of femoral fractures in children and adolescents has been reported by several authors, primarily for patients with severe head injury, multiple trauma, proximal or distal fractures, or length-unstable fractures (Fig. 8.150). Although open plating techniques have been used in the past, a less

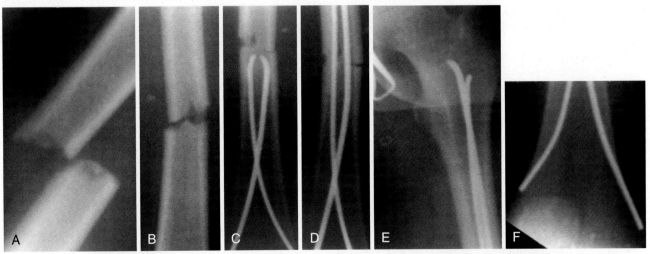

FIGURE 8.149 Flexible intramedullary nail technique. **A** and **B,** Radiographs of femoral fracture before **(A)** and after **(B)** reduction on fracture table. **C,** Both nails are placed (medial and lateral) to cross well below fracture site and stopped temporarily at fracture site for ease of passage. **D,** Both nails are driven past fracture site by manipulating distal fragment, hugging wall of intramedullary canal as necessary. **E,** Nails are driven into greater trochanteric and cervical area. **F,** Distal portions of nails are left slightly protruding for ease of removal but not too long to prevent knee motion. **SEE TECHNIQUE 8.30.**

invasive submuscular technique has been advocated by many to decrease operative time, blood loss, unsightly scars, and disruption of fracture biology. Several studies demonstrated equal or superior results of submuscular plating to elastic nails in the management of subtrochanteric, distal femoral, or length-unstable femoral fractures in regard to healing time, major or minor complication rates, and time to return to activity. Reported complications include leg-length discrepancy, refracture, hardware breakage, hypertrophic scarring, and rotational malalignment. Additionally, in a review of 85 skeletally immature diaphyseal femoral fractures treated with submuscular plate fixation, 30% of distal fractures and 12% of all fractures developed a late distal femoral valgus deformity. The authors advocated close follow-up and routine hardware removal once fracture union has occurred.

■ COMPLICATIONS

The most common complication after femoral shaft fractures in children is leg-length discrepancy, usually resulting from "overgrowth" of the injured femur. The exact cause of this overgrowth is unknown, but it has been attributed to age, gender, fracture type, fracture level, handedness, and amount of overriding of the fracture fragments. Age seems to be the most constant factor, but fractures in the proximal third of the femur and oblique comminuted fractures also have been associated with relatively greater growth acceleration. According to Staheli, shortening is more likely in patients older than 10 years of age and overgrowth is more likely in patients 2 to 10 years old, especially if traction has been used. Treatment with a spica cast with or without traction can result in significant shortening. This occurs when more than 2 cm of shortening is accepted and if "traction time" has not been long enough at the time of casting when excessive shortening is present at the time of initial presentation.

Although some angular deformity occurs after femoral shaft fractures in children, it usually remodels with growth. The acceptable amount of angular deformity is controversial; Table 8.6 presents our general guideline of acceptable angulation based on age. Genu recurvatum deformity of the proximal tibia has been reported after traction pin or wire

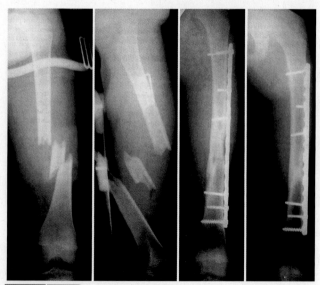

FIGURE 8.150 Submuscular bridge plating of severely comminuted segmental femoral fracture.

placement through or near the anterior aspect of the proximal tibial physis, excessive traction, pin track infection, and prolonged cast immobilization. Occasionally, a significant angular deformity requires corrective osteotomy, but this should be delayed at least a year unless function is impaired. Torsional deformities have been reported to occur in one third to two thirds of children with femoral shaft fractures; however, most of these are mild (<10 degrees) and asymptomatic, rarely requiring treatment.

Delayed union and nonunion of femoral shaft fractures are rare in children and occur most often after open fractures, fractures with segmental bone loss or soft tissue interposed between the fragments, and subtrochanteric fractures that have been poorly aligned with inadequate stabilization. Delayed union in a young child whose femoral fracture has been treated with casting probably should be treated by continuing cast immobilization until bridging callus forms. Rarely, bone grafting and internal fixation may be required for nonunion in an older child; an interlocking intramedullary nail usually is preferred for fixation in children older than 10 to 12 years of age. With the increased use of flexible intramedullary nails, we have noted, as expected, an increase in complications. Besides the usual complications of delayed or malunion and leg-length discrepancy, operative complications include implant failure with resulting varus deformity, protruding nails with and without skin erosion, knee stiffness, and septic arthritis. Narayanan et al. reported complications in 45 (58%) of 78 fractures treated with flexible intramedullary nailing (Box 8.5); most were minor and caused no serious sequelae.

Risk factors suggested to be associated with complications of flexible nailing include:

- Age older than 10 or 11 years and weight exceeding 49 kg
- Obesity, related to wound site complications or failure at the fracture site (40% complication rate in obese children)
- Titanium nails, compared with stainless steel nails; malunions are more frequent with flexible titanium nails
- Subtrochanteric fractures
- Comminution, more than 25% of shaft
- Open fracture
- Multiple injuries

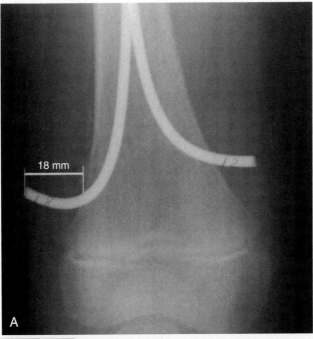

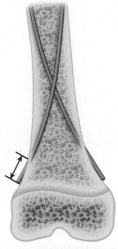

FIGURE 8.151   **A,** Bending of the nails at insertion site can lead to postoperative irritation and pain, which may require reoperation to advance, trim, or remove nails. **B,** Optimal position of distal nail ends against supracondylar flare of metaphysis leaves nails sufficiently out of cortical entry site for subsequent retrieval if necessary. (From Narayanan UG, Hyman JE, Wainwright AM, et al: Complications of elastic stable intramedullary nail fixation of pediatric femoral fractures, and how to avoid them, *J Pediatr Orthop* 24:363, 2004.)

Many of the complications associated with flexible intramedullary nailing can be prevented by careful attention to operative technique and careful follow-up.

- Pain at the insertion site can be avoided by not bending the nails at the insertion site (Fig. 8.151). Nails should be cut close to the bone, leaving less than 10 mm protruding but with enough length left to allow nail retrieval. If prominent nail migration distally occurs, it can be managed by either removing the nail at union or impacting the nail farther into the bone at reoperation.
- Malunion can be minimized by using stainless steel nails and avoiding nails that are mismatched in terms of size, determining that comminution is less than 25% of the shaft, using postoperative immobilization if necessary, and paying careful attention to the location of the fracture and final position of the nails (nails can be placed farther proximally in subtrochanteric fractures).
- Loss of reduction is a serious complication requiring reoperation and consideration of another fixation method.
- Neurologic deficits can be prevented by careful attention to traction, especially with the use of a fracture table.
- Superficial wound infections can be minimized by using perioperative antibiotics and avoiding prominent nails at the insertion site.

FRACTURES OF THE DISTAL FEMORAL PHYSIS

Fractures of the distal femoral physis are not as common as physeal injuries elsewhere, accounting for only 7% of physeal injuries of the lower extremity. At the distal femur, Salter-Harris type II physeal fractures cause more severe physeal arrests than in other parts of the skeleton. Occult

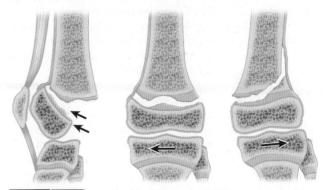

FIGURE 8.152   Various angulations of distal femoral physeal fractures, including posterior angulation, varus angulation, and valgus angulation.

Salter-Harris type V compression fractures with premature closure of the physis also occur more frequently in this location.

Salter-Harris type I fractures of the distal femoral physis rarely need operative treatment unless they are displaced. These fractures are caused more often by motor vehicle accidents or by a varus or valgus force encountered in athletic activities, and many are undisplaced (Fig. 8.152). Gentle stress radiographs may be helpful in differentiating a tear of a collateral ligament from a type I epiphyseal separation. Salter-Harris type II fractures are most common and occur in older children. Displacement usually is in the coronal plane, although it can be in the anteroposterior plane. Physeal arrest is more frequent after this fracture than after type II fractures in many other locations.

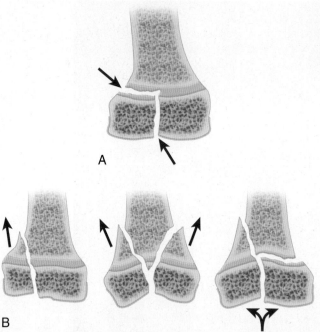

FIGURE 8.153 **A,** Salter-Harris type III distal femoral physeal fracture that requires anatomic reduction. **B,** Various types of Salter-Harris type III and IV fracture-separations, including unicondylar, bicondylar, and combination of types III and IV, which is triplane fracture.

In an experimental study in rabbits, Mäkelä et al. found that destruction of 7% of the cross-sectional area of the distal femoral physis caused permanent growth disturbance and shortening of the femur. The portion of the physis beneath the metaphyseal fracture spike (Thurston-Holland sign) usually is spared. If the metaphyseal spike is medial, valgus deformity may occur because of lateral closure of the physis. If the spike is lateral, varus angulation may follow.

Salter-Harris type III fractures rarely occur. The amount of displacement is important because joint incongruity results if anatomic alignment is not restored and a bony bridge develops if the physis is not realigned exactly (Fig. 8.153A). A Salter-Harris type IV fracture is even more uncommon. It likewise requires accurate reduction. The metaphyseal spike of bone that occurs with this type of fracture is worrisome because of the increased possibility of physeal arrest from bony bridge formation (Fig. 8.153B).

When late premature physeal closure occurs, a retrospective diagnosis of a Salter-Harris type V compression injury is made. Whether this is a true compression injury, with premature closure uniformly across the distal femoral physis, was questioned by Peterson and Burkhart, who speculated whether this uniform premature physeal closure could be caused by some other mechanism, such as prolonged immobilization or an undiscovered mechanism.

An avulsion injury can occur at the edge of the physis, especially on the medial side. A small fragment, including a portion of the perichondrium and underlying bone, may be torn off the femur when the proximal attachment of a collateral ligament is avulsed. This uncommon injury, although assumed to be benign, can lead to localized premature physeal arrest. If physeal arrest from a bony bridge is located at the most peripheral edge of a physis, severe angular deformity can occur.

The value of the Salter-Harris classification as an indicator of the mechanism of injury and the prognosis of distal femoral physeal injuries is debatable, with some authors noting that most types I and II fractures do well, whereas others have reported unsatisfactory results and frequent measurable growth disturbances in types I and II fractures. In a study of 73 patients with distal femoral physeal fractures, Arkader et al. found that both the Salter-Harris classification and displacement of the fractures were significant predictors of the final outcome.

Types I and II fractures usually are reduced with the patient under general anesthesia, and the reduction is maintained in a long leg cast with a pelvic band and pin or screw fixation in unstable fractures. These fractures are noted for redisplacement, especially if they are initially displaced anteriorly (Fig. 8.154). Closed reduction can be made easier by the use of a traction bow on a Kirschner wire in the proximal tibia. Reduction should be 90% by traction or distraction and only 10% by leverage or manipulation. Most types I and II physeal fractures do not require anatomic reduction because the fracture occurs through the zone of provisional calcification of the physis, leaving the cells responsible for growth with the ossified epiphysis, although Salter-Harris types I and II fractures in the distal femur may be an exception. If a less than anatomic reduction results, but acceptable general alignment and position are obtained, union and satisfactory growth and remodeling can be expected, especially in children younger than 10 years old in whom 20 degrees of posterior angulation would remodel. In older patients nearer skeletal maturity, only slight anteroposterior displacement and no more than 5 degrees of varus-valgus angulation are acceptable. According to Salter, it is better to accept a less than anatomic reduction with the possibility of an osteotomy later than to use forceful or repeated manipulation. In older children, a closed reduction can be done, but because of inherent instability, percutaneous cross-wire fixation with the aid of image intensification may be necessary

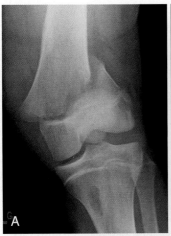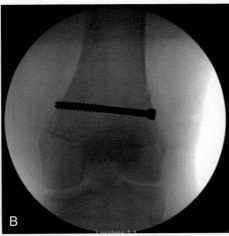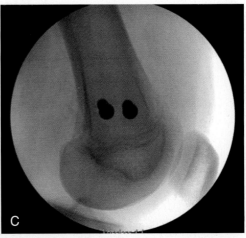

FIGURE 8.154 **A,** Displaced Salter-Harris type II fracture of distal femoral physis. **B** and **C,** Fixation with cannulated screws.

to maintain reduction (Fig. 8.155). The pins should cross the metaphysis to prevent rotation of the epiphysis. Rarely, a Salter-Harris type I or II fracture cannot be satisfactorily reduced closed because of interposition of soft tissue, and ORIF becomes necessary.

In adolescents, a large metaphyseal spike (Thurston-Holland fragment) can be stabilized with two cannulated screws. Salter-Harris types III and IV fractures require anatomic reduction. If this cannot be achieved by closed methods, ORIF is indicated. The amount of displacement that is acceptable in type III fractures has not been determined conclusively, but most authors report 2 mm or less as acceptable for closed reduction. We believe that if the surgeon thinks realistically that the amount of displacement can be decreased by performing an open reduction, this should be done. CT or MRI may be helpful when there is suspicion of injury without radiographic abnormality for evaluating articular displacement and for operative planning purposes.

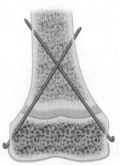

FIGURE 8.155 Cross wire fixation with aid of image intensifier. Smooth pins should be used and should penetrate opposite cortex. **SEE TECHNIQUE 8.31.**

- If the Salter-Harris type I or II fracture cannot be reduced closed, expose the epiphysis through a lateral or medial longitudinal incision, as described in other chapter for intercondylar fractures.
- Reduce the separation as gently and completely as possible by manual traction and minimal leverage. If the use of instruments is necessary, avoid injury to the physis. Remove any interposed soft tissue and gently maneuver the epiphysis into position.
- After reduction is achieved, drill 2.4-mm unthreaded pins through the medial and lateral condyles so that they cross near the center of the physis and enter the metaphysis. Cut the pins off beneath the skin.
- If the pins are inserted as described and removed at 4 to 6 weeks, they are unlikely to cause any growth disturbance. If a type II or IV fracture has a large metaphyseal spike, rather than using smooth crossed pins, drill two 2.4-mm threaded pins or a cancellous screw (Fig. 8.156) through the metaphysis of the spike into the proximal metaphyseal portion of the fracture. This should provide good stability and avoids crossing the physis. If the fragment is too small, cross the physis with smooth crossed pins.

CLOSED OR OPEN REDUCTION

TECHNIQUE 8.31

CLOSED REDUCTION OF SALTER-HARRIS TYPES I AND II FRACTURES
- Perform closed reduction for Salter-Harris types I and II fractures.
- If the reduction is satisfactory, apply a single spica or long leg cast, depending on the direction of the original displacement.

OPEN REDUCTION OF SALTER-HARRIS TYPES I AND II FRACTURES
- If reduction cannot be maintained, insert crossed, smooth 2.4-mm ({3/32}-inch) Steinmann pins through the medial and lateral condyles and into the metaphysis (see Fig. 8.155). If a large metaphyseal spike (Salter-Harris type II) is present after closed reduction, horizontal percutaneous pins or cannulated screws can be used.

OPEN REDUCTION OF SALTER-HARRIS TYPE III FRACTURES
- If the injury is a displaced Salter-Harris type III fracture, expose the displaced condyle through an anteromedial or anterolateral incision, depending on which condyle is involved.

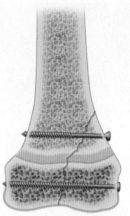

FIGURE 8.156 Salter-Harris type IV fracture. Metaphyseal spike is secured transversely with cancellous screws. **SEE TECHNIQUE 8.31.**

- An arthrotomy is necessary to ensure an anatomic reduction of the articular surface.
- Drill a large smooth pin, a cancellous screw, or a guide pin for cannulated cancellous screws into the displaced condyle to manipulate it. Gently and carefully reduce the displaced condyle into position with the pin or screw. Insert the pin or screw transversely into the intact opposite condyle without crossing the physis. Confirm the reduction by radiographs. Threaded or cancellous screws can be used across the epiphysis, as long as they do not involve, penetrate, or cross the physis.

OPEN REDUCTION OF SALTER-HARRIS TYPE IV FRACTURES

- Growth disturbance occurs frequently after type IV fractures if an anatomic reduction is not achieved and fixation is not secure. Arthrotomy usually is required to ensure anatomic reduction at the articular surface.
- Approach the fracture anteromedially or anterolaterally, depending on which condyle is involved or on which side the metaphyseal spike is present.
- Reduce the articular surface and the physis precisely with smooth pins or cancellous screws. Secure the fragment to the intact condyle with transverse fixation, without crossing the physis if possible.
- If, as in type II fractures, a large displaced metaphyseal spike is present, reduce the fracture anatomically with traction and secure the metaphyseal spike to the proximal metaphyseal fragment with threaded pins, screws, or cancellous bone screws (Fig. 8.157). If the metaphyseal spike is not large enough to ensure rigid fixation, or if transverse fixation of the epiphysis cannot be secured, smooth pins can be inserted across the physis.

POSTOPERATIVE CARE When the initial displacement is anterior, a long leg or single spica cast, depending on the stability, is applied with the knee in 45 degrees of flexion. These fractures are comparable to supracondylar fractures of the humerus in that the quadriceps and flexed knee are comparable to the triceps and flexed elbow in the maintenance of reduction. If the initial displacement is posterior, the knee should be immobilized in extension. Union usually occurs at 4 to 6 weeks. The cast and any temporary pins can be removed and an exercise program begun. Weight bearing can be permitted at 8 to 10 weeks.

■ COMPLICATIONS

The immediate complications of closed or open reduction include vascular impairment, peroneal nerve palsy, and recurrent displacement and angulation. Late complications include joint stiffness and physeal arrest. A meta-analysis that included 564 distal femoral physeal fractures found that 52% had growth disturbances, 36% in type I fractures, 58% in type II fractures, 49% in type III fractures, and 64% in type IV fractures. Leg-length discrepancies of more than 1.5 cm developed in 52%. Although growth disturbance was more frequent in those treated with fixation than those without fixation, clinically significant leg-length discrepancy was less frequent with fixation (27%) than without fixation (37%). Children with fractures of the distal femoral physis should be observed periodically until skeletal maturity. Epiphysiodesis of the contralateral extremity may be necessary because of premature physeal arrest with shortening or angulation or both. Angular deformity caused by bony bridge formation is common in distal femoral physeal fractures. Bony bridge resection and epiphysiodesis of the opposite extremity and osteotomy may be necessary to equalize leg lengths and correct angular deformity (Fig. 8.158; see other chapter).

KNEE FRACTURES AND DISLOCATIONS
PATELLAR DISLOCATIONS

Acute traumatic patellar dislocations usually occur in adolescents involved in athletic activities. Patients often report a twisting injury and seeing or feeling the patella dislocate and then spontaneously reduce with knee flexion. In younger children, patellofemoral dysplasia generally is an underlying cause. Less commonly, a direct blow to the medial aspect of the patella results in patellar dislocation. Factors associated with patellar dislocation include patella alta, trochlear dysplasia, hyperlaxity, an increased Q angle from torsional deformities of the femur or tibia, female sex, and a positive family history.

Diagnosis of patellar dislocation, even with spontaneous reduction, generally is easily made by clinical symptoms: diffuse tenderness and swelling around the patella, worse on the medial side; positive apprehension test with lateral translation of the patella; and hemarthrosis. Radiographs should be obtained to detect an osteochondral fracture; MRI or CT also may be valuable for evaluation of an osteochondral fracture. Stress radiographs may be needed if physeal fracture or ligament injury is suspected.

Treatment of first-time patellar dislocations usually is nonoperative, consisting of a short period of immobilization, followed by bracing and rehabilitation with return to sports activities at 6 to 12 weeks. Nonoperative management of patellar dislocations is further outlined in other chapter. Operative treatment is most often needed for an associated osteochondral fracture but has been recommended to reduce the risk of redislocation, which has been reported in 15% to 75% of patients. Risk factors for redislocation include young age (<15 years of age), presence of trochlear dysplasia, elevated tibial tuberosity–trochlear groove (TT-TG) distance, and patella alta.

Operative treatment is most often indicated for recurrent patellar dislocations that cause functional disability

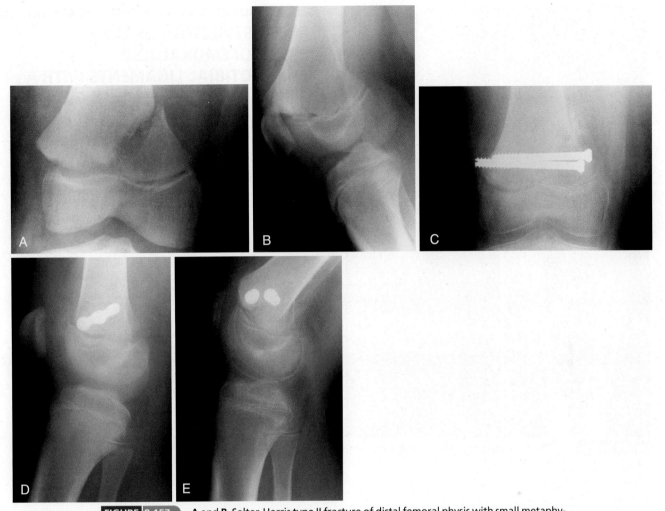

FIGURE 8.157 **A** and **B,** Salter-Harris type II fracture of distal femoral physis with small metaphyseal spike. **C** and **D,** After closed reduction and percutaneous pinning. **E,** Two weeks after surgery, loss of reduction occurred because of inadequate fixation through metaphyseal spike only. **SEE TECHNIQUE 8.31.**

and patellar dislocations with large femoral osteochondral fractures that require fixation. Operative stabilization may occasionally be considered for high-demand athletes with a primary patellar dislocation, particularly if multiple risk factors are present.

Chronic recurrent subluxation or dislocation is a difficult problem. For management in a skeletally mature patient, see other chapter. Additional challenges are encountered in children with open physes because bony procedures at the tibial tubercle and medial patellofemoral ligament reconstruction techniques that encroach on the distal femoral physis should be avoided so as not to cause growth arrest. With this in mind, procedures have been described to correct patellar instability using soft-tissue advancement (vastus medialis), lateral release, and when needed some soft-tissue restraining procedure, such as transfer of the medial or lateral third of the patellar tendon to the medial collateral ligament (Fig. 8.159), reconstruction of the medial patellofemoral ligament, and transfer of the semitendinosus tendon through a patellar tendon (Galeazzi). Nietosvaara et al. compared operative treatment (direct repair of damaged medial structures and lateral release)

to nonoperative treatment in a randomized trial involving 74 dislocations without large loose bodies in 71 patients younger than 16 years of age. Initial operative repair of the medial structures combined with lateral release did not improve the long-term outcome. Subjective results were good or excellent in 75% of those treated nonoperatively compared with 66% in those treated operatively; rates of recurrent dislocation were 71% after nonoperative treatment and 67% after operative treatment. A positive family history was identified as a risk factor for recurrence and for contralateral patellar instability.

If medial patellofemoral ligament reconstruction is selected as part of the proximal realignment, then care must be taken to avoid damage to the distal femoral physis. This can be accomplished with careful placement of the femoral tunnel distal to the physis in older adolescents or alternatively with suture or suture anchor fixation distal to the physis in younger patients. The selection of a graft is similar to that for skeletally mature patients and includes a hamstring autograft, allograft, or partial quadriceps graft. For medial patellofemoral ligament reconstruction techniques, refer to Chapter 45.

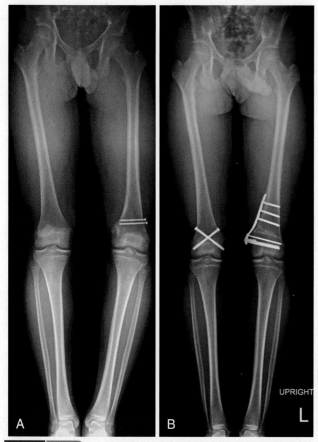

FIGURE 8.158 **A,** Distal femoral physeal fracture. **B,** After open reduction and fixation.

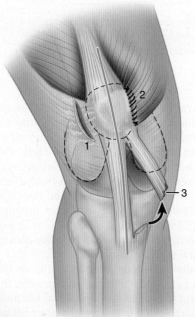

FIGURE 8.159 Schematic view of 3-in-1 procedure: *1,* lateral release; *2,* vastus medialis muscle advancement; *3,* transfer of medial third of patellar tendon to medial collateral ligament, sutured using two metal anchor sutures. (Redrawn from Oliva F, Ronga M, Longo UG, et al: The 3-in-1 procedure for recurrent dislocation of the patella in skeletally immature children and adolescents, *Am J Sports Med* 37:1814, 2009.) **SEE TECHNIQUE 8.33.**

RECONSTRUCTION OF THE PATELLOFEMORAL AND PATELLOTIBIAL LIGAMENTS WITH A SEMITENDINOSUS TENDON GRAFT

TECHNIQUE 8.32

(NIETOSVAARA ET AL.)

- Place the patient supine on a standard operating room table. After induction of general anesthesia, examine both knees, including patellofemoral tracking, before sterile preparation and draping of the limb. Apply and inflate a thigh tourniquet (pressure of 250 mm Hg).
- Through standard portals, arthroscopically examine the knee to evaluate patellar tracking, depth of the femoral trochlea, and condition of the patellofemoral joint surfaces. Remove any loose bodies.
- Make a longitudinal 4-cm skin incision medial to the tibial tubercle.
- Identify the semitendinosus and harvest its tendon with a tendon stripper, leaving the distal insertion intact.
- Place a running 2-0 Vicryl crisscross suture (Ethicon, Sommerville, NJ) in the proximal end of the tendon.
- Make two additional 2-cm incisions at the inferomedial and superomedial borders of the patella.
- With a 3.2-mm cannulated drill, create a longitudinal intraosseous tunnel in the medial quadrant of the patella; enlarge the tunnel with a 4-mm drill.
- Create a subfascial tunnel between the semitendinosus insertion and the inferomedial patellar incision.
- Pass the tendon graft through this tunnel and through the patella from distal to proximal, exiting at the superomedial pole.
- From its exit at the superior aspect of the patella, tunnel the graft in a subfascial plane to the adductor tubercle and make a 3-cm incision.
- Tension the graft with the knee in 30 to 45 degrees of flexion, making sure that the patella is well seated in the trochlea. Check the tension with the knee fully extended (the graft should allow little lateral movement of the patella, only up to one-fourth of patellar width). Proper graft tension also allows congruent smooth tracking of the patella.
- Test patellar tracking and stability throughout the range of knee motion.
- Drill a 7-mm hole at the adductor tubercle and secure the graft with an absorbable 8 × 23-mm Biotenodesis screw (Arthrex, Naples, FL).
- In skeletally immature patients, do not use a Biotenodesis screw; instead, pass the graft around the adductor magnus tendon and suture it to this tendon and to itself with 0 Vicryl.
- If tightness of the lateral retinaculum does not allow congruent patellar tracking, perform a lateral retinacular release through an extended anterolateral arthroscopic portal to allow 45 degrees of rotation of the patella above the horizontal.
- In skeletally mature patients with a Q angle of more than 20 degrees, transfer the tibial tubercle 8 to 12 mm medially and fix it with two 6.5-mm lag screws.
- Release the tourniquet and close the incisions in the standard manner.

POSTOPERATIVE CARE Weight bearing and active range-of-motion exercises are allowed immediately. Patients with tibial tubercle transfer are allowed only partial weight bearing on crutches for the first 6 weeks. Return to participation in sports is allowed after 4 to 6 months after completion of a return-to-sport program.

3-IN-1 PROCEDURE FOR RECURRENT DISLOCATION OF THE PATELLA: LATERAL RELEASE, VASTUS MEDIALIS OBLIQUUS MUSCLE ADVANCEMENT, AND TRANSFER OF THE MEDIAL THIRD OF THE PATELLAR TENDON TO THE MEDIAL COLLATERAL LIGAMENT

TECHNIQUE 8.33

(OLIVA ET AL.)

- Place the patient supine on a standard operating-room table and apply a tourniquet to the thigh.
- After induction of general anesthesia, examine the knee clinically and arthroscopically.
- Make a 10-cm incision from the midpoint of the patella inferiorly to the medial aspect of the tibial tuberosity (see Fig. 8.159) to expose the lateral and medial retinacula, the patellar tendon, and the superomedial aspect of the patella in the area of insertion of the vastus medialis obliquus (VMO) tendon.
- Section the lateral retinaculum proximal to the superior pole of the patella (lateral release), taking care not to breach the synovium.
- Expose the medial patellar tendon by division of the medial retinaculum and expose and release the vastus medialis obliquus (VMO) insertion.
- Prepare the medial third of the patellar tendon by detaching it as distally as possible from its tibial insertion; leave it attached to the patella proximally. Alternatively, detach the lateral third to half of the patella tendon and pass it underneath the intact medial portion.
- With the knee flexed 30 degrees, transfer the patellar tendon medially with an angle of 45 degrees with the main body of the patellar tendon. Incise the periosteum, insert two suture anchors, and suture the patellar tendon to the medial aspect of the proximal tibia and to the medial collateral ligament.
- Advance the VMO insertion 10 mm distally and laterally and secure it with continuous no. 1 Vicryl suture on the surface of the patella, which has been gently scarified with a burr.
- Close the wound in layers and apply routine dressings, bandages, and a straight-knee splint.

POSTOPERATIVE CARE Partial weight bearing is allowed in a controlled-motion brace, progressing to full weight bearing after 2 weeks. Range of motion is slowly increased in increments with the goal of 90 degrees of flexion at 6 weeks. Gentle concentric training and proprioception training also are begun. At 12 weeks, sport-specific rehabilitation is begun. Progressive return to daily activities is allowed over the next 3 months, with return to sports activities usually possible at 6 months.

PATELLAR FRACTURES

It is estimated that only 1% of all fractures occur in the patella and that only 1% of these occur in the immature skeleton, so fractures of the patella in children are rare. They usually occur in older children. Some fractures, especially osteochondral and small peripheral fractures and sleeve-type fractures, can be caused by acute dislocation of the patella, which is common in children. In adolescents, "jumper's knee" and Sinding-Larsen-Johansson syndrome occur frequently. These are avulsion injuries of the proximal and distal poles of the patella and should be considered chronic repetitive ligamentous injuries. Bipartite patella should not be confused with a patellar fracture, although it can be misleading because bipartite patella occasionally is painful in adolescent athletes. In bipartite patella, the edges of the defect usually are rounded, the condition is bilateral in approximately 50% of children, and it is almost always in the superolateral quadrant of the bone. Congenital absence of the patella or congenital hypoplasia may be seen in onychoosteodysplasia or nail-patella syndrome. Fractures of the distal pole of the patella and even transverse fractures of the patella occur often in children with cerebral palsy and spasticity of the quadriceps muscle.

A sleeve type of fracture of the distal pole of the patella has been described. Often only a fleck of bone is seen on the radiograph, giving a falsely benign appearance; however, a large, cartilaginous "sleeve" is often attached to the patellar tendon that, if not replaced properly, when healed and ossified becomes malaligned and produces an abnormally elongated patella and patellar mechanism (Fig. 8.160). If this fracture occurs in conjunction with dislocation or subluxation of the patella, the elongation of the patellar mechanism makes the dislocation more unstable. MRI is helpful for evaluating the extent of the sleeve fracture and ruling out concomitant injury (Fig. 8.161).

Patellar fractures should be classified according to location, type, and amount of displacement (Fig. 8.162).

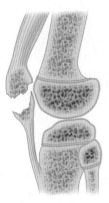

FIGURE 8.160 Substantial sleeve of avulsed cartilage when seen on radiograph appears as only "fleck" of bone and looks benign.

A review of 67 patellar fractures in 66 children (average age of 12.4 years) at our institution determined that 19 fractures were comminuted, 18 were transverse fractures, 15 were chip fractures, 6 were vertical fractures, and 2 were sleeve fractures; 7 fractures could not be classified from the available radiographs. Treatment followed guidelines generally accepted for patellar fractures in adults, but numerous ipsilateral lower extremity fractures often dictated that treatment be determined according to the associated injury. Overall results were good in only 50% of patients.

Some general trends were evident: (1) restoration of the extensor mechanism is essential, and results were less than optimal when this was not accomplished; (2) ORIF produced good results with no growth disturbance after the use of cerclage wires in patients near skeletal maturity; and (3) displaced, comminuted fractures and fractures associated with ipsilateral tibial or femoral fractures had the poorest results.

Because of the possibility of growth disturbance, and because of frequent breakage of wires in children, we routinely remove wires, pins, and screws, preferably before they break. If the fracture occurs in conjunction with an acute or recurrent dislocation of the patella, a limited lateral release and medial reefing of the retinaculum may be indicated. An osteochondral fracture of the patella or lateral femoral condyle should be suspected when acute patellar dislocation occurs.

Because in a sleeve fracture a large cartilaginous fragment usually is attached to the fleck of bone, anatomic reduction is required with displaced fractures. Malunion of the fracture may be painful and require excision of the distal fragment. If the sleeve fracture was caused by dislocation of the patella, healing in an elongated position may contribute to chronic recurrent dislocation.

The technique for ORIF of patellar fractures in children is the same as in adults. Because the sleeve fracture of the patella is unique to children, however, the technique of reduction and fixation is described here.

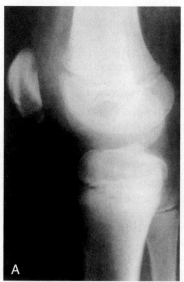
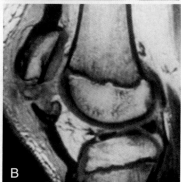

FIGURE 8.161 **A,** Apparent minor inferior pole patellar fracture. **B,** MRI reveals extent of sleeve fracture.

OPEN REDUCTION AND INTERNAL FIXATION OF SLEEVE FRACTURE

TECHNIQUE 8.34

(HOUGHTON AND ACKROYD)

- Place the patient supine on the operating table and prepare the leg in the usual fashion; use a tourniquet.
- Approach the inferior pole of the patella through a medial parapatellar or direct anterior incision. Expose the distal pole patellar fracture.

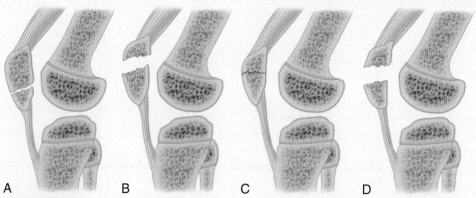

FIGURE 8.162 Types of patellar fracture. **A,** Inferior pole. **B,** Superior pole. **C,** Transverse undisplaced midsubstance. **D,** Transverse displaced midsubstance.

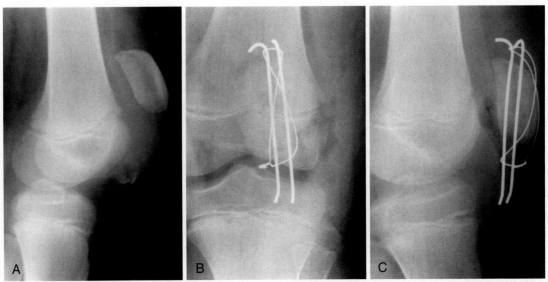

FIGURE 8.163 **A,** Patellar "sleeve" fracture. **B** and **C,** After reduction and fixation with Kirschner wires and tension band wiring. **SEE TECHNIQUE 8.34.**

- Irrigate the fracture copiously with saline and with a small curet remove any clots and loose cancellous bone. Reduce the fragment with a small bone holder. Observe the fracture fragments anteriorly and try to observe the reduction posteriorly on the articular surface. If this is impossible, use a gloved finger to feel for any angulation or offset on the articular surface. Perform a tension band wiring with two Kirschner wires or cannulated screws.
- After reduction of the fracture, place two parallel longitudinal Steinmann pins across the fracture site. Leave them protruding approximately ¼ inch (0.5 cm) distally for easy removal. Place a tension band wire from the superior to the inferior pole of the patella, crossing itself and incorporating the parallel pins (Fig. 8.163). Tighten the wire sufficiently but not enough to overly compress and angulate the fracture fragments.
- Alternatively, a suture repair can be done through vertical tunnels in the patella in a manner similar to repair of a proximal patellar tendon rupture.
- A careful retinacular closure adds additional stability to the repair and may improve patellar tracking after healing is achieved.
- Close the wound in layers and apply an appropriate cast with the knee in slight flexion. Alternatively, if a gravity stress test demonstrates sufficient stability, a controlled-motion brace can be used to allow early motion.

POSTOPERATIVE CARE At 3 to 4 weeks, the cast is removed and range-of-motion exercises are started.

FRACTURES OF THE INTERCONDYLAR EMINENCE OF THE TIBIA

Tibial intercondylar eminence fractures account for 2% to 5% of knee injuries associated with knee effusion in children and adolescents. Tibial eminence fractures are most commonly classified according to the modified Meyers and McKeever system, which describes four types: type I, little or no displacement of the fragment; type II, fragment elevated anteriorly and proximally, with some displacement but with a cartilaginous hinge posteriorly; and type III (intact fragment) and type IV (comminuted fragment), with complete displacement of the fragment (Fig. 8.164). The goal of treatment is to achieve near-anatomic reduction to restore appropriate tension of the attached anterior cruciate ligament. This has been done traditionally by closed treatment with knee extension for types I and II and by open or arthroscopic reduction and fixation for types III and IV.

The mechanism of action for tibial eminence fractures is similar to that of an anterior cruciate ligament injury, with many occurring in low-energy, noncontact activities. This injury has also been reported with higher energy mechanisms such as motor vehicle accidents, pedestrian–motor vehicle accidents, or falls from bicycles. The workup includes a careful physical examination and routine knee radiographs. Although the injury usually is detected with plain radiographs, CT and MRI may be used to better evaluate the extent of the injury, rule out associated injury, and for preoperative planning purposes. At our institution, we routinely use MRI to evaluate the degree of displacement, assess barriers to reduction, and evaluate associated injuries. Nonoperative management often is adequate for type I and many type II fractures if adequate reduction is achieved. If adequate reduction of the fracture is noted or restored with extension of the knee, then a cylinder or long leg cast should be applied with the knee in slight flexion. Some authors advocate the aspiration of the hemarthrosis before cast application. The fracture should be closely followed with serial radiographs. Typically, the cast can be removed by 6 weeks and the patient transitioned into a control-motion brace with progression of range of motion to full by 10 to 12 weeks.

Operative intervention is reserved for type II or III fractures that do not reduce with closed manipulation and for type IV fractures (Fig. 8.165). Kocher et al. demonstrated that meniscal or intermeniscal ligament entrapment with block to reduction is present in 26% of type II and 65% of type III fractures, necessitating open or arthroscopic reduction. Several open and arthroscopic techniques have

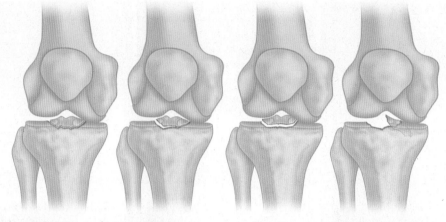

Type I   Type II   Type III   Type III with rotation

FIGURE 8.164   Meyers and McKeever classification of tibial eminence fractures.

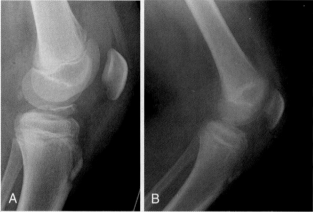

FIGURE 8.165   **A,** Type III tibial eminence fracture that could not be reduced closed. **B,** Lateral radiograph after open reduction and fixation with nonabsorbable sutures. Entrapped meniscus that prevented closed reduction was found at the time of surgery.

been described for surgical repair of a displaced tibial eminence fracture. Regardless of technique, the knee should be systematically evaluated for concomitant injury, the fracture bed debrided, the fracture reduced under direct vision, and stable fixation achieved. A systematic review failed to show which of the many described techniques is superior. Whether open or arthroscopic, fixation is commonly achieved with suture fixation or screw placement. If suture fixation is selected, the suture is passed through the distal attachment of the anterior cruciate ligament and passed through drill tunnels placed in the proximal tibia and tied over a bony bridge. For screw fixation, the fragment is held reduced and a screw or bioabsorbable screw is passed across the fracture with care not to cross the physis. If additional fixation is required, some authors advocate crossing the physis with a metallic screw and then removing the screw once union has been achieved. Potential complications include nonunion, malunion, persistent laxity of the anterior cruciate ligament, loss of motion, and arthrofibrosis. Nonunion is uncommon but may be a challenge to treat, especially in very young patients in whom further growth has occurred, preventing adequate reduction of the fragment. Nonunion is more commonly encountered with nonoperative management. Malunion is a more common

problem and is more commonly seen when there is a delay in diagnosis until healing has occurred. Malunion may result in a block to extension and can be treated with debridement of the elevated fragment or femoral notchplasty. A significant malunion also may result in ligamentous laxity and knee instability. If this occurs, then revision surgery or anterior cruciate ligament reconstruction should be considered. Laxity also may occur in spite of union in good position because of injury of the anterior cruciate ligament at the time of initial injury. This is encountered more frequently in types III and IV fractures, likely as a result of higher forces applied to the anterior cruciate ligament at the time of injury. Intraoperatively, the fracture bed may be gently recessed to increase the tension applied to the anterior cruciate ligament. In addition to malunion, loss of motion may occur as a result of postoperative muscle tightness or arthrofibrosis. Patel et al. found that early posttreatment range-of-motion rehabilitation significantly improved time of return to full activity independent of age, fracture type, and operative or nonoperative management. In operatively treated fractures, arthrofibrosis occurred in 36% of knees if range of motion was initiated after 4 weeks compared with 0% in knees when early range of motion was initiated.

OPEN REDUCTION AND INTERNAL FIXATION OF TIBIAL EMINENCE FRACTURE

TECHNIQUE 8.35

- Expose the knee through the distal portion of an anteromedial parapatellar incision (see Technique 1.38). Open the capsule medially to expose the fracture fragments and the defect in the proximal tibia.
- Examine the menisci and intermeniscal ligament to ensure that they are not impeding the reduction. Place the knee in less than 30 degrees of flexion and reduce the fragment after any clots and cancellous bone have been removed from the defect.

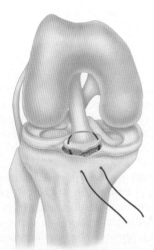

FIGURE 8.166 Repair of intercondylar eminence fracture with absorbable suture. (Redrawn from Owens BD, Crane GK, Plante T, et al: Treatment of type III tibial intercondylar eminence fractures in skeletally immature athletes, *Am J Orthop* 2:103, 2003.) **SEE TECHNIQUE 8.35.**

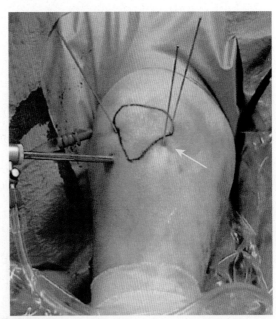

FIGURE 8.167 Arthroscopic reduction of tibial eminence fracture. (From Liljeros K, Werner S, Janarv PM: Arthroscopic fixation of anterior tibial spine fractures with bioabsorbable nails in skeletally immature patients, *Am J Sports Med* 37:923, 2009.) **SEE TECHNIQUE 8.36.**

Alternatively, the inspection and reduction can be done with arthroscopic assistance.

■ Drill two holes from distal to proximal through the tibial epiphysis. Take care to drill the holes proximal to the physis. The holes should enter the joint (1) just medial and lateral to the fracture fragments or (2) into the defect and into the fragment itself if it is large enough. Pass a 1-0 nonabsorbable suture through the most distal portion of the anterior cruciate ligament just proximal to the fracture fragment (Fig. 8.166). With suture carriers, pass the ends of the suture through the drill holes and tie them onto themselves after the reduction is satisfactory.

■ Flex and extend the knee to ensure the reduction is stable. Irrigate and close the wound.

POSTOPERATIVE CARE If stable fixation is achieved, the leg is placed in a controlled-motion brace with gradual increase in range of motion to full by 6 to 8 weeks. If a cast is used for additional stability, it should be discontinued by 4 weeks to initiate range-of-motion exercises. The patient is released to full activity only after healing has occurred and full, painless range of motion has been achieved with good strength.

ARTHROSCOPIC REDUCTION OF TIBIAL EMINENCE FRACTURE AND INTERNAL FIXATION WITH BIOABSORBABLE NAILS

TECHNIQUE 8.36

(LILJEROS ET AL.)

■ With a thigh tourniquet applied and inflated, perform standard knee arthroscopic examination through anteromedial and anterolateral portals.

■ Remove the ligamentum mucosum and part of the infrapatellar fat pad to better expose the injured area.

■ Remove fibrin clots and small fracture fragments from underneath the anterior tibial spine fragment and from the tibial crater.

■ If the intermeniscal ligament is trapped in the fracture, interfering with reduction, free it with a probe.

■ With the knee flexed to 45 degrees, reduce the fragment with a probe and temporarily fix it with a 1.6-mm AO wire introduced through a midpatellar entrance close to the medial margin of the patella (Fig. 8.167).

■ Keeping as close as possible to the patella and slightly proximal to the AO wire, insert the drill guide into the joint and secure the fragment.

■ Close the portals in standard fashion and apply a cast or brace with the knee in slight flexion.

POSTOPERATIVE CARE If stable fixation is achieved, the leg is placed in a controlled-motion brace with gradual increase in range of motion to full by 6 to 8 weeks. If a cast is used for additional stability, it should be discontinued by 4 weeks to initiate range-of-motion exercises. The patient is released to full activity only after healing has occurred and full, painless range of motion has been achieved with good strength.

TIBIAL TUBEROSITY FRACTURES

Fractures of the tibial tuberosity usually occur in older children, often during jumping sports such as basketball (Fig. 8.168). These fractures were classified by Watson-Jones as type I, a small fragment that is displaced superiorly; type II, a larger fragment involving the secondary center of ossification and the proximal tibial physis, which is hinged upward; and type III, a fracture that passes proximally and

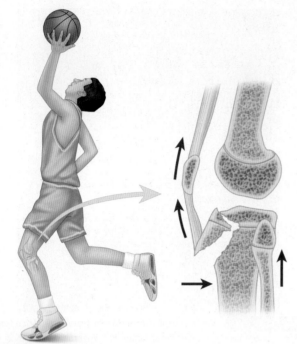

FIGURE 8.168 Mechanism of injury of flexion-avulsion injuries. These injuries are most common in adolescent boys and most often occur when attempting to push off for a jump in basketball.

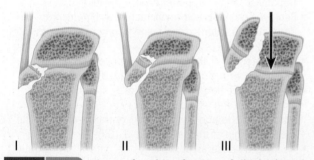

I   II   III

FIGURE 8.169 Types of avulsion fracture of tibial tuberosity. *Type I*, through secondary ossification center. *Type II*, at junction of primary and secondary ossification centers. *Type III*, across primary ossification center (Salter-Harris type III) with physis near closing posteriorly. (Redrawn from Roberts JM: Fractures and dislocations of the knee. In Rockwood CA Jr, Wilkins KE, King RE, editors: *Fractures in children*, Philadelphia, 1984, Lippincott.)

posteriorly across the physis and proximal articular surface of the tibia (Salter-Harris type III physeal fracture) (Fig. 8.169). Ogden et al. classified type III fractures further as to whether there is a rotational, comminuted, or epiphyseal component. This classification is important because type III fractures in younger children, if not anatomically reduced and held, can result in bony bridge formation, causing anterior growth arrest and hyperextension deformity; however, this complication is unlikely because these fractures usually occur in older adolescents (Fig. 8.170). Frankl described a type I-C injury as a tibial tuberosity avulsion fracture with a patellar tendon rupture from its proximal insertion. Further modifications to the classification scheme were added to include injuries to the entire proximal tibial physis. Ryu and Debenham suggested the addition of a type IV injury, in which the anterior tubercle fracture line extends completely across the tibial physis in a

Salter-Harris type I pattern. Donahue et al. subdivided type IV injuries into type IV-A injuries, a strictly physeal injury, and type IV-B injuries, those with a posterior metaphyseal fragment, consistent with a Salter-Harris type II injury. Finally, a type V injury was described by Curtis and later classified by McKoy et al. with an intraarticular Salter-Harris type III extension and an associated type IV fracture, giving the fracture a Y configuration (Fig. 8.171). We have seen a number of patients, all adolescent males, with anterior tuberosity fractures combined with a posterior metaphyseal fragment (Fig. 8.172).

Differentiating between Osgood-Schlatter disease and tibial tuberosity fractures can be difficult because they both present with pain over the tibial tuberosity in jumping athletes. Osgood-Schlatter disease is a chronic traction injury at the distal attachment of the patellar tendon that results in insidious onset of inflammation along the anterior aspect of the tuberosity. A tibial tuberosity fracture, however, is an acute failure of the underlying physis. Although Osgood-Schlatter disease has been known to precede tibial tuberosity fractures, this is likely related to the strong correlation between the age and activities that result in these injuries. With Osgood-Schlatter disease, symptomatic and supportive treatment is all that is necessary, the prognosis is good, and only occasionally are symptoms prolonged by a persistent ossicle. Conversely, tibial tuberosity fractures result in an incompetent extensor mechanism and require urgent treatment to restore function.

Imaging workup consists of standard radiographs of the knee. Historically, the incidence of concomitant knee injury or intraarticular pathology was thought to be low because of the mechanism of action; however, several more recent studies that used preoperative MRI demonstrated a higher incidence of intraarticular findings, commonly meniscal pathology and osteochondral injury, than previously reported. As a result, some authors advocate routine use of MRI as part of the preoperative workup, whereas others conclude that a careful inspection of the joint at time of surgery through an arthrotomy or arthroscopic assessment is sufficient.

The role of nonoperative management of tibial tuberosity fractures is limited to nondisplaced type I or type II fractures with little to no displacement. Closed treatment consists of cast immobilization in near full extension for 4 to 6 weeks followed by progressive range of motion and strengthening. Serial lateral radiographs are obtained to ensure that proximal displacement does not occur because of the pull of the quadriceps. For displacement of more than 3 mm, or for type III or greater fractures, surgical stabilization is recommended. If the fracture is reducible by closed manipulation, percutaneous fixation can be placed to maintain the reduction and allow early range of motion. If acceptable reduction is not obtained, then formal open reduction and fixation should be performed. Fixation typically is with cannulated screws; however, if the tuberosity fragment is comminuted or small, alternative methods of fixation may be used including suture, wires, suture anchors, or even plate fixation. Typically a large periosteal flap is present and, if repaired, provides addition stability to the fracture. It is hoped that with healing, fusion occurs across the traction apophysis only. We have found anterior tuberosity fractures combined with a posterior metaphyseal fragment to have a high risk of refracture after conservative treatment, and we treat these with ORIF that includes both anterior and posterior fragments (Fig. 8.173).

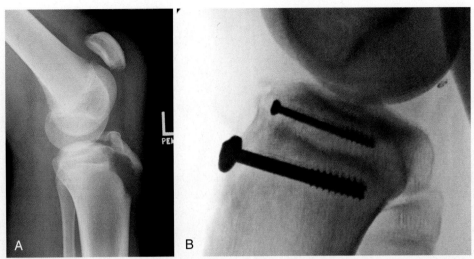

FIGURE 8.170 Tibial tuberosity fracture. **A,** Watson-Jones type III fracture (Salter-Harris type III) extending into knee joint. **B,** After open reduction and screw fixation.

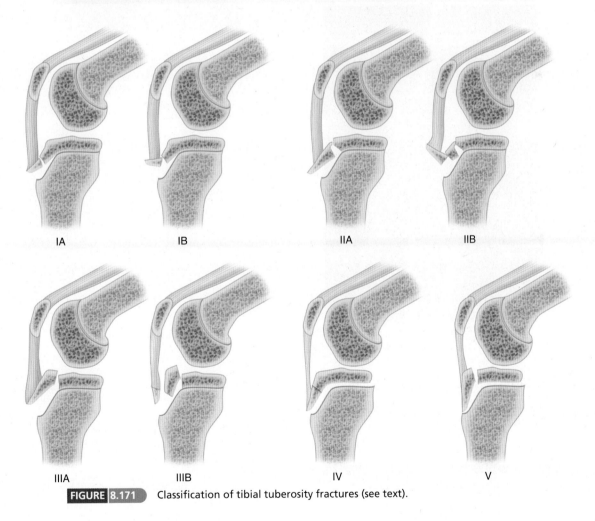

FIGURE 8.171 Classification of tibial tuberosity fractures (see text).

Complications related to tibial tuberosity fractures are uncommon. Acute compartment syndrome has been reported and often attributed to disruption of the anterior tibial recurrent vessels. We routinely admit patients with displaced tuberosity fractures overnight for observation regardless of treatment. Growth disturbance can occur but is rare because this fracture occurs most often toward the end of growth. If growth arrest does occur, then it may result in genu recurvatum and require surgical correction. Implant prominence is the most common complication and can be minimized by avoiding washers or using smaller, low profile implants. Our preference, however, is to use appropriate fixation to achieve a stable construct and to remove the implants once healing has occurred only

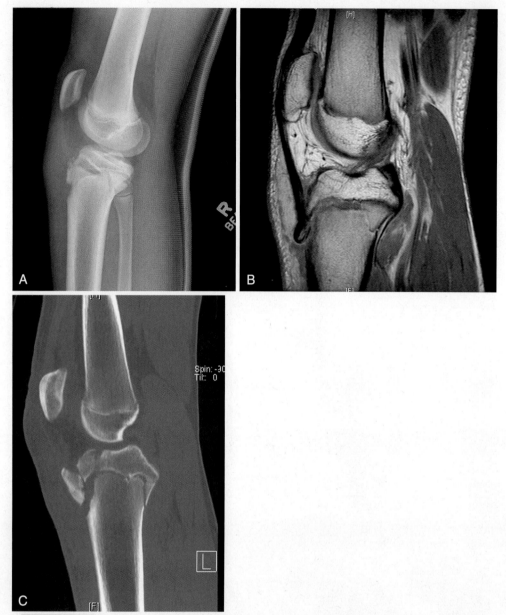

FIGURE 8.172 Anterior tibial tuberosity fracture combined with posterior metaphyseal fracture in adolescent male. **A,** Radiograph. **B,** MRI. **C,** CT scan.

if implant-related pain persists. Finally, loss of motion has been reported, but similar to tibial eminence fractures it can be minimized with stable fixation and early range of motion.

OPEN REDUCTION AND INTERNAL FIXATION

TECHNIQUE 8.37

- Make an anterior, midline incision adjacent to the tibial tuberosity and parallel to the patellar tendon. Carry the dissection laterally over the tibial tuberosity and the insertion of the patellar tendon.

- Identify any large periosteal flap, which may be avulsed medially, laterally, bilaterally, or distally. If it is frayed, resect some of it. If it is not frayed, retain it for stability.
- Expose the fracture and clean its base with a curet. Do not dissect completely free the attachments of the tibial tuberosity.
- Reduce the fracture with the knee in full extension.
- Insert guidewires for cannulated screws across the fracture. Once placed, confirm the reduction and guidewire position. If satisfactory, then place the cannulated screws in standard fashion. If the fragment is comminuted or small, tension band, suture repair, or suture anchors can be placed to achieve fixation. Confirm the final reduction with radiographs. Suture any periosteal flap and close the wound in layers.

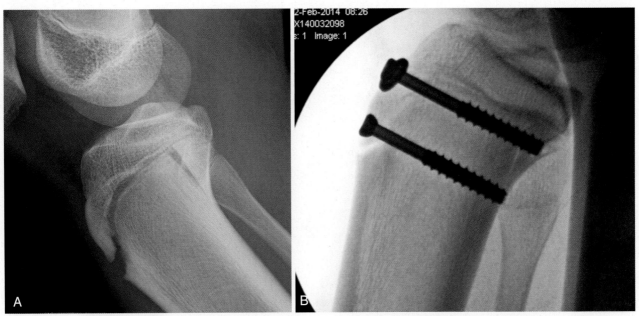

FIGURE 8.173 **A,** Anterior tibial tuberosity combined with a posterior metaphyseal fracture. **B,** Fixation with screws that includes anterior and posterior fragments.

A   B   C

FIGURE 8.174 Three locations of osteochondral fractures caused by dislocation of patella. **A,** Inferior surface of patella. **B,** Femoral condyle. **C,** Medial surface of patella.

> **POSTOPERATIVE CARE** A cylinder cast or long leg cast has historically been applied with the knee in full extension for 4 to 6 weeks. If stable fixation is achieved, however, a controlled-motion brace can be used to allow for early range of motion.

OSTEOCHONDRAL FRACTURES

Osteochondral fractures of the knee occur primarily on the cartilaginous surfaces of the medial or lateral femoral condyle or the patella (Fig. 8.174). They may be caused by direct forces applied against the femur or patella or by dislocation of the patella itself (Fig. 8.175). Osteochondral fractures have been reported in over half of acute patellar dislocations, with equal numbers of capsular avulsions of the medial patellar margin and loose intraarticular fragments detached from the patella or the lateral femoral condyles (Fig. 8.176). Intraarticular fragments may be identified only after spontaneous relocation of the patella. Femoral fractures usually involve the edge of the articular surface and the middle third of the condylar arc. Usually a significant hemarthrosis follows the traumatic episode. If ligamentous instability is not present and the aspirate of the knee is sanguineous (hemarthrosis), an osteochondral fracture should be suspected, although often the fragment is not bony and cannot be seen on standard radiographs. Occasionally, just a faint density or fleck of subchondral bone can be identified. This small osseous fragment

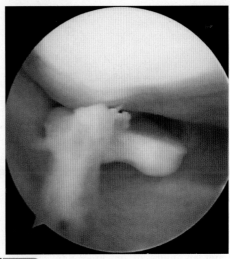

FIGURE 8.175 Osteochondral loose body from lateral femoral condyle secondary to acute patellar dislocation.

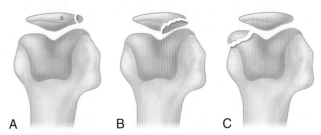

A   B   C

FIGURE 8.176 Most common types of osteochondral fractures in acute patellar dislocations. **A,** Medial marginal patellar avulsions. **B,** Inferomedial patellar facet. **C,** Lateral femoral condyle.

usually is part of an osteocartilaginous loose body that at surgery is surprisingly large. Additional views, such as the tunnel view, may improve exposure, but one study demonstrated that standard radiographs failed to identify an osteochondral fragment in 36% of children who had a loose body found at

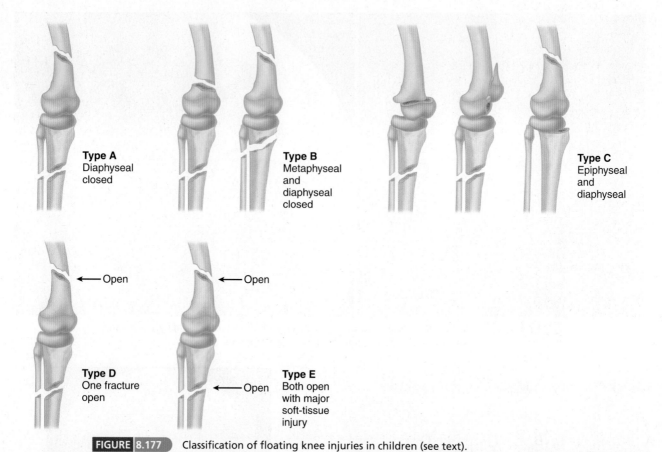

Type A
Diaphyseal
closed

Type B
Metaphyseal
and
diaphyseal
closed

Type C
Epiphyseal
and
diaphyseal

← Open

← Open

Type D
One fracture
open

← Open

Type E
Both open
with major
soft-tissue
injury

FIGURE 8.177 Classification of floating knee injuries in children (see text).

time of surgery. MRI is indicated if there is a high suspicion of osteochondral fracture. Arthroscopy is indicated to locate, identify, and remove the loose body. The defect in the patella or femur also should be identified. Small fragments or cartilaginous loose bodies can be excised, but larger fragments, particularly in weight-bearing portions of the joint, should be repaired when possible. For a more thorough discussion of osteochondral fractures, refer to Chapter 32.

FLOATING KNEE INJURIES

Although not an injury of the knee joint, "floating knee" describes the flail knee joint segment resulting from a fracture of the shafts or adjacent metaphyses of the ipsilateral femur and tibia. This is an uncommon injury in children; it most often results from motor vehicle accidents and usually is associated with major soft-tissue damage, open fractures, and head injuries. Letts et al. proposed a five-part classification of these injuries (Fig. 8.177): type A, femoral and tibial fractures are closed diaphyseal fractures; type B, one fracture is diaphyseal, one is metaphyseal, and both are closed; type C, one fracture is diaphyseal, and the other is an epiphyseal displacement; type D, one fracture is open with major soft-tissue injury; and type E, both fractures are open with major soft-tissue injury. Their basic recommendation for treatment of these injuries is that at least one fracture (usually the tibial) must be rigidly fixed by ORIF. If mobilization of the child is essential, internal fixation of both fractures is indicated in most patients. In older children, intramedullary nailing may be more appropriate than plate fixation. Open fractures with major soft-tissue injury should be left open and stabilized with external fixation (Fig. 8.178). Outcomes of these fractures appear to be age related, with successful closed

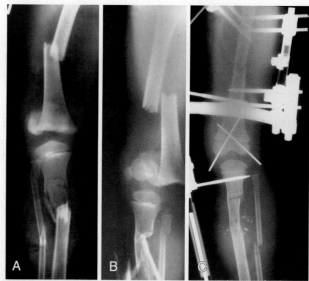

FIGURE 8.178 **A** and **B,** Severe floating knee injury with midshaft fracture of femur, Salter-Harris type I fracture of distal femoral physis, and comminuted fracture of tibial shaft. **C,** After internal fixation of distal femoral physeal fracture with crossed pins and external fixation of fractures of femoral and tibial shafts.

treatment of children younger than 10 years, but frequent complications and concomitant ligamentous injuries have been reported in children older than 10 years treated with reduction and fixation (intramedullary rods, plates, external fixator) of the femoral fracture. Poor results have been reported to be as high as 50% of older children because of limb-length discrepancy, angular deformity, or instability of the knee, particularly ligamentous instability. A multicenter study evaluated 130 patients with an average age of 10.2 years who had floating knee injuries and found that, with modern fixation techniques, 93% of patients had good to excellent results with shorter length of stays than previously reported.

TIBIAL AND FIBULAR FRACTURES

Fractures of the tibia and fibula are common across all age groups and represent the third most common long bone injury in children and adolescents. They are more common in males and occur from many different mechanisms. The most common location of fracture is in the distal third of the tibia followed by the middle and then proximal thirds. Sheffer et al. reported a 4.3% incidence of concurrent ipsilateral tibial shaft and distal tibial fractures, so care must be taken to image the entire bone appropriately when evaluating a tibial fracture. Many tibial and fibular fractures can be managed nonoperatively; however, these fractures require careful monitoring and management to avoid complications. Fracture patterns and potential complications vary according to location, so each anatomic site will be discussed separately. Otherwise, fractures of the tibia and fibula can be treated closed. A worrisome fracture is incomplete metaphyseal fracture of the proximal tibia. Fractures of the distal tibial and fibular physes also are of special concern because, if not treated properly, varus and valgus angulation may occur in older children and a bony bridge may form causing angular deformity in younger children.

PROXIMAL TIBIAL PHYSEAL FRACTURES

Fractures of the proximal tibial physis are uncommon fractures largely because of the anatomic stability at this location and the energy required to produce such an injury. The proximal tibial physis is partially protected by the ligamentous attachments around the knee, the fibula laterally, and the tibial tuberosity anteriorly. There also are fewer ligamentous attachments directly to the epiphysis when compared with the distal femoral epiphysis. Fractures of the epiphysis, however, deserve special attention because of the proximity to the popliteal artery, which is tethered to the proximal tibia and may be injured when the tibial metaphysis is posteriorly displaced (Fig. 8.179). There are few dedicated studies about injuries at this location because many authors have included tibial tuberosity fractures in their series. We believe that, although there are many correlations between these two injuries, they ought to be considered separately because of some inherent differences. For type IV tibial tuberosity fractures, the proximal tibial physis also is disrupted and should be considered a true physeal injury.

Proximal tibial physeal fractures are commonly classified by the Salter-Harris classification. They can be further classified by the amount of displacement and the direction of displacement. Mubarak et al. found that by grouping fractures of the proximal tibia, including the eminence, tuberosity, and metaphyseal fractures, by direction of force and fracture pattern, there were several age-related correlations. In early childhood (ages 3 to 6 years), metaphyseal fractures were most common. In prepubescent children (ages 4 to 9 years), varus and valgus forces were the predominate mechanisms of fracture. During preadolescence (around ages 10 to 12 years), a fracture mechanism involving extension forces predominated. During adolescence (after age 13 years), the flexion-avulsion pattern consisting primarily of tibial tuberosity fracture was most common. Furthermore, tibial spine fractures occurred at age 10 years, Salter-Harris types I and II fractures at age 12 years, and Salter-Harris types III and IV physeal injuries at around age 14 years as tibial plateau equivalents.

Management of proximal tibial physeal fractures closely follows the Salter-Harris recommendations discussed earlier. Most types I and II injuries can be managed closed with cast

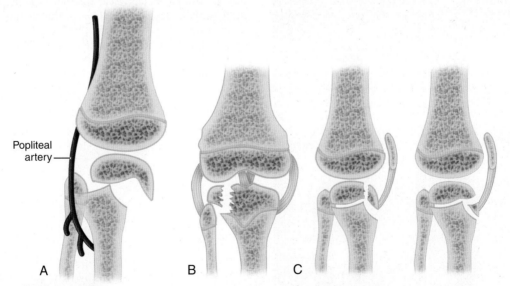

Popliteal
artery

A   B   C

FIGURE 8.179 **A**, Salter-Harris types I and II fractures with posterior displacement of tibial shaft may injure popliteal artery. **B**, Salter-Harris type III fracture of proximal tibia. Analogous to a tibial plateau fracture. **C**, Fracture through tibial tuberosity and across epiphysis into knee joint similar to avulsion of epiphysis of tibial tuberosity.

immobilization if an adequate reduction is obtained. Gentle reduction with adequate sedation should be performed to minimize additional trauma to the physis. If the reduction is unsuccessful and there is persistent instability after reduction, vascular compromise, or impending compartment syndrome, then we prefer surgical stabilization with smooth pins across the physis or cannulated screws across the metaphyseal component. For types III or IV injuries, we accept only minimal articular displacement and have a low threshold for surgical stabilization (Fig. 8.180). Many of these fractures occur near the end of skeletal maturity and can be managed with adult techniques and implants to optimize stability and facilitate early range of motion. There is a high association between types III and IV fractures and associated intraarticular pathology. Advanced imaging with CT or MRI is helpful in determining displacement, identifying intraarticular injuries, and for preoperative planning.

Variants of Salter-Harris types III and IV fractures have been described as "triplane fractures of the proximal tibial epiphysis." These are similar to fractures that occur in the ankle in adolescent patients. Generally, these are two-part fractures that are type IV fractures and three-part fractures that are type III (Tillaux component) or type II fracture combinations. If displaced, both variants require ORIF (Fig. 8.181).

In a review of 39 proximal tibial physeal injuries at our institution, several complications occurred, including anterior compartment syndrome, transient and permanent peroneal nerve palsy, arterial thrombosis, angular deformity, and leg-length inequality. Any suggestion of ischemic changes, a compartment syndrome, or peroneal nerve palsy

requires that immediate action be taken in the emergency department. Leg-length inequality of more than 1 inch (2.5 cm) occurred in 2 of the 39 children requiring additional treatment. Two children had joint incongruity and angular deformity.

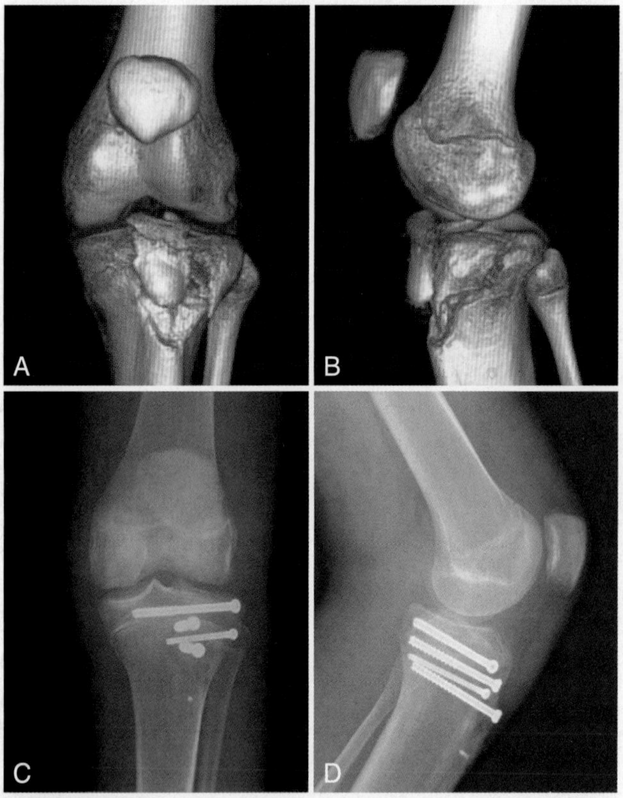

PROXIMAL TIBIAL METAPHYSEAL FRACTURES

Fractures of the proximal tibial metaphysis occur most commonly between the ages of 3 and 8 years. The most common fracture pattern is a minimally displaced fracture created by a valgus moment to the leg from a medially directed force. Another common fracture pattern is an impaction fracture of the proximal metaphysis classically created by a trampoline injury with a young child bouncing with an older child or adult. Displaced fractures of the proximal tibial metaphysis are uncommon and are usually caused by a high-energy mechanism. Displaced fractures in this location are of concern because of their proximity to the posterior tibial artery and the possibility of damaging the vasculature of the leg.

Children with minimally displaced, low-energy fractures often present with the inability to walk. Children may describe pain in their knee or leg and have tenderness and swelling along the metaphysis. With high-energy trauma, the location of the fracture is more obvious, and careful attention should be placed on the neurovascular examination and serial compartment checks. An ankle-brachial index (ABI) test should be performed and compared with the contralateral side to rule out arterial injury if significant displacement is present.

For minimally displaced fractures, a long leg cast should be applied with the knee in slight flexion and a slight varus mold applied at the level of the fracture. For significantly angulated fractures, a reduction under sedation should be performed at the time of cast application. Displaced, high-energy fractures should be urgently reduced and surgically stabilized with age-appropriate techniques.

An uncommon but well-described complication of a proximal tibial metaphyseal fracture is a late valgus deformity. Initially described by Cozen, this phenomenon occurs in fractures of the proximal tibial metaphysis, even when nondisplaced. Radiographs often reveal a benign "greenstick"

FIGURE 8.180 A and B, Salter-Harris type III fracture of proximal tibial physis. **C** and **D**, After open reduction and internal fixation.

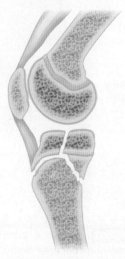

FIGURE 8.181 Sagittal view of knee depicting epiphyseal fracture pattern. Anterior and posterior fracture fragments are shown.

nondisplaced fracture pattern in a young child. Frequently, the fracture is treated in a straight or bent-knee cast and heals uneventfully with apparently satisfactory alignment. Later the tibia is noted to have a significant valgus angulation compared with the opposite tibia. This excess valgus may not have been preventable, and for this reason, parents should be told at the beginning of treatment about the possibility of this complication.

At what point the valgus angulation occurs and why it occurs are unknown. Numerous explanations have been advanced, however, including the following:

1. Asymmetric growth stimulation of the proximal tibial physis has been suggested. Houghton and Rooker surgically lacerated the proximal tibial periosteum medially in animals and noted a resultant valgus angulation.

2. Asymmetric growth stimulation of the medial proximal metaphysis from asymmetric vascular response has been suggested by several authors who postulated that an unbalanced vascular healing response occurs after injury to the metaphysis, causing the medial side of the tibia to outgrow the lateral side.

3. The tibial physis is stimulated more or for a longer period than the fibular physis, which may or may not have been fractured. This would cause a tethering effect, with the tibia overgrowing more medially than the fibula laterally, pulling the extremity into a valgus position.

4. Valgus angulation occurs at the time of fracture. Too often, radiographs of these fractures are taken in a cast with the knee flexed and the valgus angulation is not apparent. Radiographs of the contralateral extremity are not taken for comparison, and the amount of valgus is not appreciated. Weight bearing before solid union of the fracture also has been suggested to produce the valgus angulation.

5. Soft tissue, such as the pes anserinus, is interposed between the fragments, preventing an adequate reduction and complete healing of the fracture, which causes an exaggerated stimulation of the physis on the medial side of the tibia, resulting in overgrowth and valgus deformity (Fig. 8.182). Open reduction is recommended, especially when the fracture fragments are mildly to moderately separated medially, as is removal of the interposed material.

6. A physeal injury occurs, causing premature closure of the physis laterally, leaving the physis open medially with resultant valgus angulation.

Because the incidence, etiology, and prognosis of this deformity are uncertain, prevention and treatment are controversial. The fractures usually occur between age 3 and 8 years, when the normal physiologic valgus is at its maximum. In a retrospective study of 181 patients between 1 and 8 years of age with proximal tibial fractures, Yang et al. found that 14% of patients who initially had less than 4 degrees of angulation developed angulation of more than 4 degrees at some point during follow-up. Of the 120 patients who developed progressive angulation, only four had persistent valgus at final follow-up; none required surgical correction. A review of patients with this fracture at our institution revealed similar findings. Like others, we are uncertain of the exact cause of the deformity or how to prevent it. The fracture should be treated precisely, however. First, parents should be warned before treatment is begun of the possibility of valgus deformity both during treatment and after healing has occurred. Second, a long leg cast in 5 to 10 degrees of flexion should be applied and radiographs of the fractured tibia and the

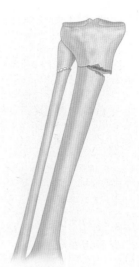

FIGURE 8.182 Opening of fracture gap medially showing that periosteum or pes anserinus could be interposed.

opposite tibia should be taken frequently and compared. If any valgus angulation does occur, the cast should be wedged into a corrected position. Reduction, with the patient under general anesthesia, is recommended of any fracture with a break in the medial cortex and even minimal valgus deformity. Third, we have tried, when appropriate, to put the fractured tibia in slightly less valgus than the opposite tibia.

Of the children we reviewed at our institution, the deformity increased in some children 12 months after treatment. In some, the deformity improved spontaneously for 3 years after injury (Fig. 8.183). This improvement may have been caused by the normal correction of physiologic valgus seen in children 2 to 9 years old. Proximal tibial osteotomy or guided growth for significant deformity should be delayed because the deformity may correct spontaneously. Osteotomy corrects the deformity, but it also can stimulate the medial side of the tibia and cause the deformity to recur later, as noted in some of our children. Guided growth with compression of the medial physis may be the best treatment option in the rare patient who does not obtain spontaneous correction with growth.

OPEN REDUCTION AND REMOVAL OF INTERPOSED TISSUE

If interposition of soft tissue is strongly suspected or is confirmed by appropriate valgus stress radiographs with gapping of the fracture, and if the fracture is not a stress fracture, operative removal of the tissues, including the periosteum and pes anserinus, from the fracture may be necessary.

TECHNIQUE 8.38

(WEBER ET AL.)

- Place the patient supine on the operating table and prepare and drape the involved area in the usual fashion. Approach the fracture site medially through a 6-cm vertical incision.

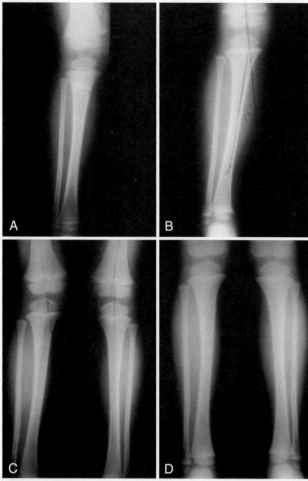

FIGURE 8.183 Spontaneous correction of valgus deformity. **A,** Proximal metaphyseal fracture at time of injury with no valgus angulation while standing. **B,** At 8 months, valgus angulation of 15 degrees is present. **C,** At 16 months, some spontaneous correction of angulation has occurred. **D,** At 2-year follow-up, valgus angulation has almost disappeared.

- Carry the soft-tissue dissection down to the medial surface of the tibia and identify the fracture. Notice if the periosteum is stripped away from the medial surface of the tibia and, together with the pes anserinus, is trapped in the transverse fracture gap (Fig. 8.184A,B). Clean all debris away from the fracture, including the hematoma.
- Slide a periosteal elevator under the interposed tissues and extract them from the fracture. Hold the periosteum back with forceps (Fig. 8.184C,D) and irrigate the fracture.
- Suture the periosteum and the pes anserinus in their original positions if possible.
- Observe the fracture before closing to ensure that the gap is closed and that no further interposition of periosteum has occurred.
- Close the wound in layers and apply a long straight-leg cast.

POSTOPERATIVE CARE Radiographs of both lower extremities in full extension should be made to ensure that no increased valgus is present in the injured tibia compared with the opposite tibia.

MIDDLE AND DISTAL TIBIAL SHAFT FRACTURES

Fractures of the shaft of the tibia, with or without associated fibular fractures, usually can be treated by closed reduction and casting. This also applies to distal tibial metaphyseal fractures. In a large series of tibial shaft fractures treated with above-knee casts, (1) initial shortening of 10 mm was compensated wholly or partially by growth acceleration; (2) mild varus deformities corrected spontaneously; (3) valgus deformity and posterior angulation persisted to some degree; and (4) rotational deformities persisted, especially internal rotation.

In general, transverse isolated fractures are less likely to displace early or late while in a cast, but spiral and oblique fractures are prone to displacement into varus or valgus for 2 to 3 weeks after injury and require careful follow-up. Fractures manipulated at 2 weeks have been found to be still mildly malleable, but fractures left for 3 weeks may not. With fractures that involve both the tibial and fibular shafts, valgus angulation is common because of the pull of the anterior and lateral compartment musculature. If the fibula is intact, the pull of the anterior compartment musculature tends to result in varus angulation as the fibula maintains the length of the lateral cortex. Posterior angulation (recurvatum) of distal tibial metaphyseal fractures can occur, especially when the ankle is held in dorsiflexion.

Spontaneous correction of angular deformity after tibial fractures has been reported to occur in boys up to age 10 years and in girls up to age 8 years; however, other reports indicate that little spontaneous correction occurs regardless of the age of the child.

Because of the possibility of compartment syndromes, long bone fractures of the lower extremity should not be treated casually. A retrospective review of 515 patients with tibial shaft fractures from our institution demonstrated a 1.7% incidence of acute compartment syndrome, with age greater than 14 years, elevated BMI, high-energy mechanisms, and associated injuries all being risk factors. A careful clinical examination should be performed and documented followed by serial examinations to monitor for signs of impending compartment syndrome. If vascular injury is suspected, an ABI or arteriogram should be obtained at the direction of a vascular surgeon. If there is high suspicion or risk of compartment syndrome based on a thorough workup, a splint with soft-tissue dressing should be applied instead of a circular cast, and the extremity should be monitored with a suitable compartment-pressure measuring device. If compartment syndrome is anticipated or developing, surgical stabilization of the fracture should be considered and a very low threshold for compartment releases should be maintained. The treatment of impending and established compartment syndromes is described elsewhere.

Although most tibial fractures can be managed with closed treatment, there has been a trend toward expanding the indications for operative intervention of tibial fractures. The indications for operative treatment of tibial and fibular fractures in a child are:

1. Unstable fractures that cannot be adequately aligned or maintained by closed methods.
2. Open tibial fractures, which should be treated as emergencies with irrigation and debridement. If

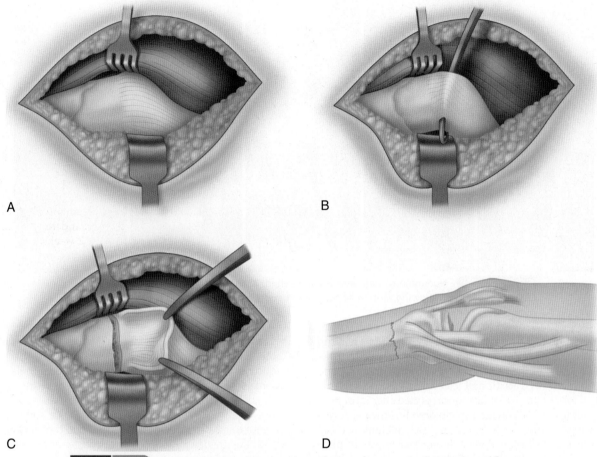

FIGURE 8.184 Weber technique for removing soft tissue from proximal metaphyseal fracture. **A,** Exposure of fracture. **B–D,** Removal of pes anserinus and periosteum from fracture with periosteal elevator and forceps. **SEE TECHNIQUE 8.38.**

soft-tissue damage is extensive, an external fixator is used as in adults. Care should be taken not to cross the physis with pins when applying the fixator.

3. Fractures in which surgical stabilization facilitates mobilization or nursing care, such as floating knees, polytrauma, or multiple long bone injuries.

4. Nonunions of tibial fractures, which are rare in children and are probably more serious and more difficult to manage than in adults. We have treated several children with obvious nonunions of the tibia with no other pathologic or congenital anomaly in whom internal fixation and bone grafting were required to achieve union (Fig. 8.185).

The general assumption that even grades II and III open diaphyseal fractures in children heal readily was refuted in a large series of these fractures: 55% healed primarily, 30% had delayed unions, 7.5% were classified as nonunions, and 7.5% (all with Gustilo grade IIIC fractures) required early amputation. The same factors that predispose to these complications in adults (degree of displacement, comminution, soft-tissue damage, and periosteal stripping) also contribute to delayed union and nonunion in children. Reported incidences of compartment syndrome, vascular injury, infection, and delayed union are similar to those in adults. Two complications are unique to children: late angular deformities and tibial overgrowth. Laine et al. reported eight patients with open (type IIIB or IIIC) tibial fractures who all required soft-tissue

flaps and had an average bone loss of 5.4 cm. They found that with the use of a circular external fixator and the application of an algorithm based on bone loss and the ability to acutely shorten the construct, seven out of eight limbs could be salvaged, and of the seven in whom the fracture healed, all were ambulatory without assistive devices at time of final follow-up in spite of a high rate of secondary procedures.

Intramedullary nailing may be indicated because of an inability to obtain or maintain reduction in an older or larger child with an unstable fracture pattern that is at high risk of displacement or for multiple pathologic fractures in a young child, such as occur in osteogenesis imperfecta or congenital pseudarthrosis of the tibia. The ever-expanding indications for femoral intramedullary nailing in children have been extrapolated to tibial nailing, and tibial fractures in children as young as 4 years of age have been treated with flexible intramedullary nailing. A retrospective review of tibial fractures in 31 patients with open physes found shorter times to union and better functional outcomes in those treated with intramedullary nailing than in those treated with external fixation.

If intramedullary nailing is done, the proximal and distal physes should be avoided. Intramedullary nailing has been reported to be successful in stabilizing severely comminuted tibial fractures so that union is obtained without angular deformity. If possible, closed techniques of nail insertion should be used, with a small incision over the fracture

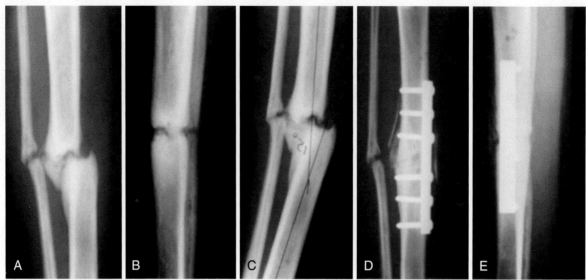

FIGURE 8.185 Nonunion of tibia and fibula in child. **A** and **B,** Nonunion before treatment. **C,** Stress radiograph showing motion at fracture. **D** and **E,** Early union after bone grafting and compression plate fixation.

if necessary for adequate reduction of the fracture. Titanium or stainless elastic intramedullary nails can be used, but the medullary canal of the tibia must be measured carefully and the appropriate-sized elastic nail selected based on the criteria described for femurs. Complications reported after intramedullary nailing of tibial fractures in children include neurovascular complications (8%), infection (8%), malunion (8%), and leg-length discrepancy (4%). In another review of tibial fractures treated with elastic intramedullary nails, delayed union occurred at a rate of 18%.

ELASTIC STABLE INTRAMEDULLARY NAILING OF TIBIAL FRACTURE

TECHNIQUE 8.39

(O'BRIEN ET AL.)

- After induction of general anesthesia and placement of a well-padded tourniquet on the proximal thigh, prepare and drape the affected leg. The tourniquet usually is not inflated.
- With the use of fluoroscopy, mark on the skin the fracture site, the proximal tibial physis, and the starting points for nail entry. The starting point for the nail entry hole is 1.5 to 2.0 cm distal to the physis.
- Make lateral longitudinal 2-cm incisions over the proximal tibial metaphysis just proximal to the starting points.
- Select two appropriately sized nails (2, 3, or 4 mm) based on the width of the medullary canal, choosing the largest possible diameter nails that will fit the medullary canal; for example, if the canal measured 6 mm, use two 3-mm nails.
- The nails come with a beveled blunt tip. Bend the very tip of the nail to 45 degrees to facilitate passage along the opposite cortex and aid in fracture reduction.

- Contour the entire length of the nail to a gentle curve such that the apex will rest at or near the fracture site after reduction. The depth of the curve should be approximately three times the diameter of the canal to achieve the optimal balance between ease of insertion and stability.
- Use a drill 0.5 cm larger than the nail in a soft-tissue sleeve to create the entry hole, confirming the entry hole with fluoroscopy in both the anteroposterior and lateral planes. Take care to avoid the tibial tubercle apophysis.
- Drill the hole in the midpoint of the anteroposterior dimension, starting perpendicular to the physis. Under fluoroscopic guidance, angle the drill caudad until it is 45 degrees from the long axis of the tibia, taking care not to drill out the far cortex or migrate toward the physis.
- Place the prebent nail on an inserter and insert it from the side opposite the distal displacement in an antegrade fashion.
- Under fluoroscopic guidance, slide the nail along the opposite cortex until the fracture is reached.
- Reduce the fracture and advance the nail across the fracture. Embed the nail in the distal tibial metaphysis without violating the cortex or the physis.
- Place the second nail from the other side in a similar fashion.
- If necessary, rotate the bent tips of the nails after passing the fracture site to effect an anatomic reduction, taking care not to distract the fracture site.
- Bend the proximal nail ends and cut them 1 cm from the cortical surface so that the nail ends will sit deep to the compartment fascia but be proud enough for easy retrieval.
- Close the wounds with an absorbable fascial and subcuticular stitch and apply a short leg cast.

POSTOPERATIVE CARE Weight bearing is begun when evidence of bridging callus is present, usually at about 5 weeks. Nails are removed at 6 to 12 months after fracture; no immobilization is required after nail removal (Fig. 8.186).

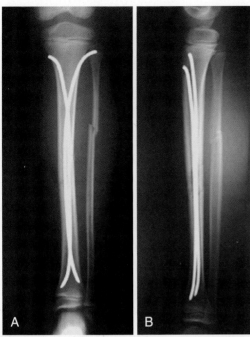

FIGURE 8.186 Grade II open fracture in 7-year-old boy. **A** and **B,** Postoperative anteroposterior and lateral radiographs of tibia and fibula. (From O'Brien T, Weisman DS, Ronchetti P, et al: Flexible titanium nailing for the treatment of the unstable pediatric tibial fracture, *J Pediatr Orthop* 24:601, 2004.) **SEE TECHNIQUE 8.39.**

DISTAL TIBIAL AND FIBULAR EPIPHYSEAL FRACTURES

Carothers and Crenshaw described the mechanism of injury of distal tibial physeal fractures using a classification of abduction, external rotation, and plantarflexion; adduction; and axial compression. Abduction, external rotation, and plantarflexion frequently produce Salter-Harris type I or II physeal fractures (Fig. 8.187); adduction produces type III or IV fractures (Fig. 8.188); and axial compression produces type V fractures. Since this original study, we have reviewed 100 ankle fractures in children. The most common were Salter-Harris type II fractures (26). Type III fractures were more common than anticipated (19), and type I fractures (9) and type IV fractures (6) were relatively rare. Also studied were six triplane and six Tillaux fractures. The remaining were distal fibular fractures, and all were Salter-Harris type I or II fractures except for one Salter-Harris type IV fracture. Most fractures of the fibular physis occur in conjunction with distal tibial fractures; Salter-Harris type III fractures usually are isolated injuries.

Fibular physeal fractures are treated for 3 to 6 weeks in a short leg cast. Salter-Harris types I and II fractures of the distal tibial physis usually are treated by closed reduction and the application of a bent-knee, long leg cast. In young children, moderate displacement after closed reduction, especially in the anteroposterior plane, can be accepted. Varus or valgus angulation in older children with type I or II fractures does not correct spontaneously, however, and excessive angulation should not be accepted (Fig. 8.189). Because the foot tolerates these positions poorly, the result is unacceptable. Two of our patients had open reduction because such a deformity could not be reduced closed. Residual gaps in the physis after closed reduction of Salter-Harris types I and II fractures may represent entrapped periosteum, which can lead to premature

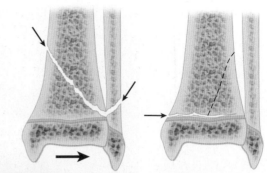

FIGURE 8.187 Salter-Harris type II physeal fractures are produced by external rotation, abduction, and plantarflexion forces.

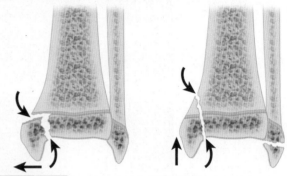

FIGURE 8.188 Salter-Harris types III and IV fractures are produced by adduction forces (supination-inversion).

physeal closure. Open reduction and removal of the entrapped periosteum may be beneficial in a younger child.

In a series of 91 types I and II distal tibial physeal fractures, Rohmiller et al. reported premature physeal closure in 40%. They found a difference in the rates of premature physeal closure between fractures caused by a supination-external rotation mechanism (35%) and those caused by a pronation-abduction mechanism (54%). The most significant predictor of premature physeal closure was not initial fracture displacement but postreduction displacement. Anatomic reduction is recommended, regardless of treatment method, to decrease the risk of premature physeal closure (Fig. 8.190). In spite of treatment methods, the rate of premature physeal closure after distal tibial physeal fractures remains quite high.

Most Salter-Harris type III and IV fractures, including triplane and Tillaux fractures, require ORIF. Internal fixation methods include smooth pins or wires if the physis must be crossed, cannulated cancellous screws, and, more recently, bioabsorbable screws. Bioabsorbable screws have the advantage of not requiring second surgery for removal, but care must be taken not to damage the physis during their insertion. The amount of displacement acceptable for closed treatment has not been defined. If after a closed reduction the surgeon believes that the amount of displacement can be reduced operatively, ORIF is justified (Fig. 8.191). Surgery traditionally has been recommended for 2 to 3 mm or more of displacement. For the most part, standards for acceptable displacement using CT techniques have not been refined or defined. The amount of displacement, the extent of comminution, and proper placement of screw fixation (at right angle to the fracture fragments) can be determined, however (Fig. 8.192).

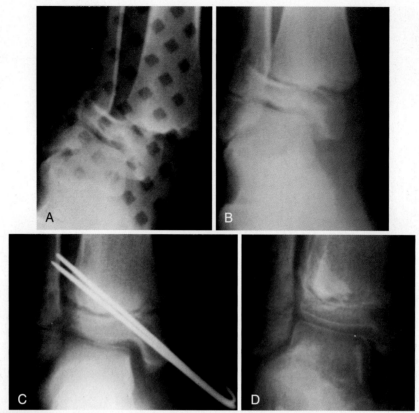

FIGURE 8.189 Open reduction of Salter-Harris type I fracture. **A,** Before treatment. **B,** After closed reduction, residual angulation is 17 degrees in this older child. **C,** After open reduction and internal fixation with smooth pins, flap of periosteum was found caught in fracture. **D,** At early follow-up, no evidence of bony bridge is seen.

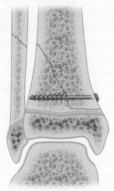

FIGURE 8.190 Cancellous screw fixing large metaphyseal spike of Salter-Harris type II fracture.

Salter-Harris types III and IV fractures are almost always medial and occur at the plafond, with the exception of Tillaux and triplane fractures. Often a tiny triangular piece of bone is present on the metaphyseal side in a type IV fracture (Fig. 8.193). At the time of open reduction, this piece of bone can be removed to better expose the physis and to try to prevent the formation of a peripheral bony bridge in this area. Symptomatic ossification centers in the medial malleolus should not be mistaken for Salter-Harris type III fractures.

It is best not to cross the physis with any kind of pin unless absolutely necessary for fixation to minimize the risk

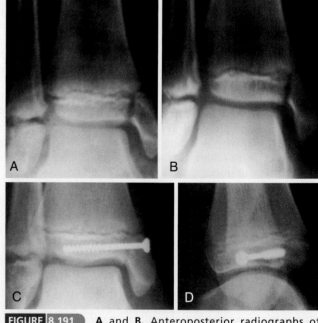

FIGURE 8.191 **A** and **B,** Anteroposterior radiographs of displaced Salter-Harris type III fracture of medial malleolus and Salter-Harris type I fracture of lateral malleolus. **C** and **D,** After open reduction and internal fixation of medial malleolar fracture with threaded screw through epiphysis.

of a bony bridge developing where the pins cross the physis. The perichondral ring can be avulsed in this area, just as from the distal femoral physis, from a minor fracture or ligamentous or other injury and may cause peripheral growth arrest with resultant angular deformity.

Of our 100 ankle fractures, the result was poor in four type III tibial injuries and one type IV tibial injury because of varus or valgus deformity secondary to growth arrest and in one type II tibial injury because of refracture. Supramalleolar osteotomy was necessary in two injuries.

The development of a sclerotic line of growth disturbance (Park or Harris line) that appears 6 to 12 weeks after fracture has been suggested to predict the likelihood of growth arrest from the presence and displacement of the line. If the line extends across the whole width of the metaphysis in both planes, and if the line continues to grow away from the physis remaining parallel to it, growth disturbance is not likely to occur. An absence of this formation and displacement of the line may indicate abnormal growth that will result in varus or valgus angulation. Letts et al. proposed a classification of

pediatric pilon fractures similar to the adult classification but amended it to include articular surface displacement of more than 5 mm and physeal displacement (Table 8.7). These types II and III fractures seem to be more severe and involve comminution of the articular surface and should be considered more complex than Salter-Harris types II, III, and IV fractures and triplane fractures.

High-velocity motor vehicle accidents or lawn mower injuries often produce severe open ankle fractures. These injuries may involve the distal tibial physis; a shearing fracture of the body of the talus also can be present. The result is physeal arrest and joint roughening. After an open fracture, infection can develop. External fixators can be used in the initial management until the wound is clean. Bony bridge resection and osteotomy for angular deformity may be necessary later. If infection develops or joint involvement is severe, ankle fusion may be necessary (Fig. 8.194). At the time of fusion, the physis should be preserved, and compression clamps should be used to hasten fusion. An interposed iliac bone graft can be used.

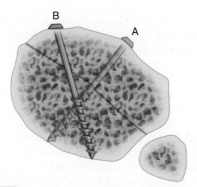

FIGURE 8.192 Distal tibial physeal fractures. Difference in entry point and direction of screw between ideal position (A) and observed position (B). (Redrawn from Cutler L, Molloy A, Dhukuram V, et al: Do CT scans aid assessment of distal tibial physeal fractures? *J Bone Joint Surg* 86B:239, 2004. Copyright British Editorial Society of Bone and Joint Surgery.)

OPEN REDUCTION AND INTERNAL FIXATION

TECHNIQUE 8.40

- Place the patient supine on the operating table; prepare and drape the involved area in the usual fashion and use a tourniquet.
- Make a straight longitudinal incision over the medial malleolus, anteriorly and slightly laterally, for approximately 4 cm. Carry the soft-tissue dissection down to the fracture. Clear all soft tissue from the area but preserve the periosteum if possible. Gently expose the fracture. Remove any interposed soft tissue from within the fracture, especially periosteum and small bony fragments.

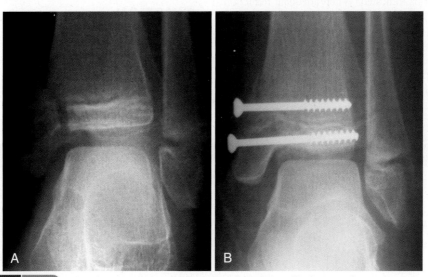

FIGURE 8.193 **A,** Salter-Harris type IV fracture of medial malleolus. **B,** After open reduction and internal fixation with threaded cancellous screws in metaphysis and epiphysis, avoiding physis.

■ Expose the ankle joint anteriorly and, with the aid of a bone holder, reduce the fracture anatomically. If the fracture is a Salter-Harris type IV with a small metaphyseal spike, remove the spike to see the reduction better and prevent a later bony bridge at the periphery.
■ Insert small, parallel, smooth Steinmann pins horizontally across the fracture. Do not cross the physis unless necessary. Use a cannulated or cancellous screw if desired, ensuring, however, that the threads do not damage the physis and the screw is horizontal across the fracture (Fig. 8.195). Check the reduction and pin or screw placement with radiographs.
■ Reduce manually any fibular fracture.
■ Close the wound and apply a long leg, bent-knee cast with the ankle in neutral position.

POSTOPERATIVE CARE Weight bearing is not permitted for 4 to 6 weeks, depending on the age of the patient. A short leg, weight-bearing cast is worn for 3 weeks.

TRIPLANE FRACTURES

Triplane fractures are caused by an external rotational force and are considered a combination of Salter-Harris types II and III fractures. Marmor first coined the term *triplane fracture of the distal part of the tibia* in 1970 in his description of lesions consisting of three fragments: (1) the anterolateral portion of the distal tibial epiphysis; (2) the remainder of the epiphysis (anteromedial and posterior portions) with an attached posterolateral spike of the distal tibial metaphysis; and (3) the remainder of the distal tibial metaphysis and tibial shaft.

The triplane fracture has been reported to be a two-part rather than a three-part fracture. This fracture is caused by an external rotational force, and if it is a three-part fracture, it is considered a combination of Salter-Harris types II and III fractures. If it is a two-part fracture, it is a Salter-Harris type IV fracture (Figs. 8.196 and 8.197). CT evaluation has been recommended as an adjunct to radiographs to better classify the fracture, assess displacement, and formulate a treatment plan. Usually, closed reduction can be achieved by internal rotation of the foot and immobilization in a long leg cast. If a closed reduction cannot be achieved, ORIF is indicated. When adequate reduction (<2 mm displacement) is not achieved, degenerative changes are likely to occur. If it is a three-part fracture, open reduction of the Salter-Harris type II and type III components may be necessary and adequate exposure is required. Triplane fractures frequently occur in older children, and although physeal arrest and angular deformity can occur, they are rare.

The operative technique for triplane fractures depends on whether it is a two-part or a three-part fracture. Most two-fragment triplane fractures can be treated by closed reduction. The closed reduction should be satisfactory because this is a Salter-Harris type IV fracture with possible joint incongruity and physeal arrest. When an open reduction of this intraarticular fracture is necessary, it usually is a three-part fracture. We approach the Salter-Harris type III component laterally first. If adequate open reduction can be achieved, the Salter-Harris type II component (medially) can be treated closed; if not, both components require open reduction. The trend has been for limited incisions and cannulated screw fixation of intraarticular fragments.

TILLAUX FRACTURES

A special fracture occurring in older adolescents originally was described by Tillaux. The mechanism of injury is an external rotational force with stress placed on the anterior tibiofibular ligament, causing avulsion of the distal tibial physis anterolaterally (Fig. 8.198). This occurs after the medial part of the physis has closed (Fig. 8.199) but before the lateral part closes. The resultant fracture through the physis runs across the epiphysis and distally into the joint, creating a Salter-Harris type III or IV fracture. If nondisplaced, these fractures can be treated conservatively with close observation to ensure a nonunion or delayed union does not occur. If there is any doubt, however, a CT is recommended to evaluate the extent of articular displacement. ORIF is indicated if the fracture is displaced (Fig. 8.200). Fracture displacement of more than 2 mm generally is considered an indication for fracture reduction and fixation.

The fracture fragment, because it is pulled off by the anterior tibiofibular ligament, is almost always anterior. Generally, Tillaux fractures occur in adolescents just before the entire physis (not just the medial part) closes, and there is little worry about using fixation across the physis as in Fig. 8.201. If the child is young or there is any doubt, either smooth pins or a transverse screw across the epiphysis should be used (see Fig. 8.195).

OPEN REDUCTION AND INTERNAL FIXATION

TECHNIQUE 8.41

■ Expose the type III or IV fracture anterolaterally through a 3-cm anterolateral incision.

TABLE 8.7

Pediatric Classification of Pilon Fracture

TYPE	ARTICULAR SURFACE DISPLACEMENT (MM)	PHYSEAL DISPLACEMENT (MM)	COMMINUTION	ADJACENT INJURIES
I	>5	None	None	None
II	>5	<5	2-3 fragments	None
III	>5	>5	Multiple fragments	Ipsilateral tibial shaft fracture and/or ankle dislocation

From Letts M, Davidson D, McCaffrey M: The adolescent pilon fracture: management and outcome, *J Pediatr Orthop* 21:20, 2001.

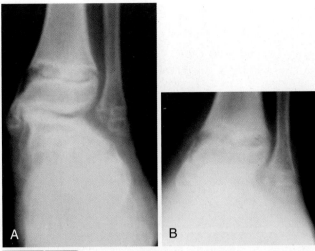

FIGURE 8.194 Severe physeal injury caused by lawn mower. **A,** Severe injury with loss of talar dome and part of distal tibia and separation of distal tibial physis. **B,** Solid fusion with physis still open.

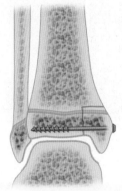

FIGURE 8.195 Salter-Harris type III or IV fracture should be fixed by horizontal pins or cancellous bone screws not involving the physis. **SEE TECHNIQUE 8.40.**

- Gently clean and observe the fracture fragments. Take care not to disrupt the periosteum but to remove it from within the fracture.
- Use a bone holder to reduce the fracture gently. Check the reduction by examining the fragment in the ankle joint.
- Insert a small cancellous screw transversely or obliquely across the fracture but not penetrating the physis in a young child.
- Check the reduction with radiographs.
- Close the wound and apply a short leg cast.

POSTOPERATIVE CARE Weight bearing is prohibited for 3 to 4 weeks.

FOOT FRACTURES
TALAR FRACTURES
■ TALAR NECK FRACTURES

Fractures of the talus have three basic types: (1) fractures of the talar neck, (2) fractures of the talar body and dome, and (3) transchondral (osteochondral) fractures.

Be aware of the retrograde blood supply, which is present in a sling fashion around the talar head and neck. This blood supply enters the bone through three primary arteries: (1) artery of the tarsal sinus, (2) artery of the tarsal canal, and (3) the deltoid artery. We use the fracture classification proposed by Hawkins, which is based on the amount of disruption of the blood supply to the talus. A type I lesion is a fracture through the neck of the talus with minimal displacement and minimal damage to the blood supply of the talus, theoretically damaging only one vessel, the one entering through the talar neck. In type II lesions, the subtalar joint is subluxated or dislocated and at least two of the three sources of blood supply may be disrupted through the talar neck and entering the tarsal canal and sinus tarsi. In type III lesions, the body of the talus is dislocated from the tibia and from the calcaneus and all three of the sources of blood supply may be disrupted. The incidence of osteonecrosis is high in type III fractures.

We have described a type IV fracture that is not related to the blood supply, in which the body of the talus is dislocated or subluxated at the subtalar joint, the body of the talus is dislocated at the ankle joint, the talar neck is fractured, and the head of the talus is dislocated at the talonavicular joint. Most of the fractures in our series were types I, II, or III.

We use the treatment recommended by Boyd and Knight. Closed reduction followed by non–weight bearing is the preferred treatment for type I mildly or nondisplaced fractures. If an adequate reduction cannot be obtained or maintained, ORIF is recommended. A reduction of less than 3 mm of displacement and less than 5 degrees of malalignment is considered adequate. Most of the closed reductions are done on type I fractures. In types II, III, and IV fractures, open reduction with or without internal fixation is used frequently because of the difficulty of maintaining an adequate reduction by closed methods in significantly displaced fractures. Open fractures require a thorough irrigation and debridement, and internal fixation is done only if required for stability of reduction. If the soft-tissue envelope is compromised, temporary stabilization may be achieved with a spanning external fixator until definitive fixation can be performed.

Varus malalignment is a frequent problem. A special radiographic technique is used to determine the amount of varus angulation in the anteroposterior plane. A cassette is placed directly under the foot, and the ankle is placed in maximal equinus position, the usual position after reduction of the fracture of the talar neck. This position can be maintained more easily by maximal flexion of the hip and knee. The foot is pronated 15 degrees, and the x-ray tube is directed cephalad at a 75-degree angle from the horizontal tabletop. This technique has enabled us to detect any offset or varus deformity of the head and neck of the talus.

For open reduction, an anteromedial approach is often used, retracting the neurovascular bundle laterally. Alternatively, a dual approach can be performed. Fixation is usually performed with cannulated screws from a medial to a lateral direction or small modular plates. As an alternative, cancellous lag screws can be inserted percutaneously from posterior to anterior. Techniques for talar fracture fixation are discussed further in other chapter.

Complications include osteonecrosis of the talar body, malunion, traumatic arthritis of the ankle and subtalar joint, and infection. Subchondral lucency present 12 weeks after injury (Hawkins line) is an indication that osteonecrosis

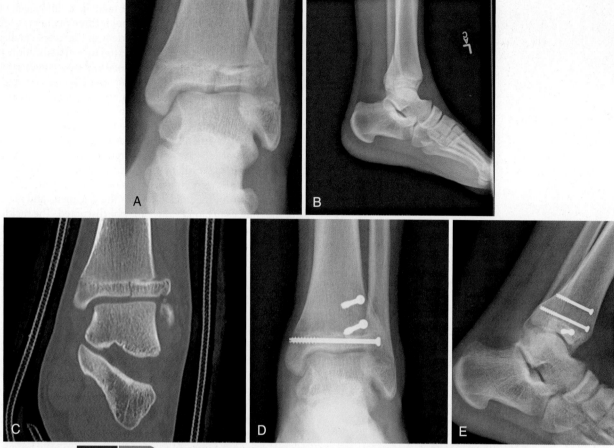

FIGURE 8.196   Distal tibial triplane fracture. **A,** Anteroposterior view showing triplane fracture. **B,** Lateral view of fracture, Salter-Harris type IV (two parts of three-part fracture, type II plus type III). **C,** Preoperative coronal CT. **D** and **E,** After open reduction and internal fixation.

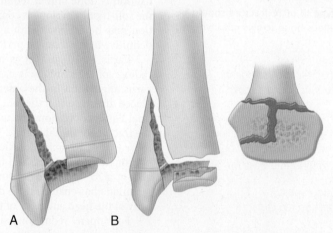

FIGURE 8.197   **A,** Example of two-fragment triplane fracture, which is Salter-Harris type IV fracture. **B,** Example of three-fragment triplane fracture, consisting of Salter-Harris types II and III fractures.

will not occur, but this is not an absolute prognosticator. Conversely, lack of a subchondral lucency at 3 months suggests that osteonecrosis has occurred (Fig. 8.202), and advanced imaging with MRI or bone scan may confirm the diagnosis (Fig. 8.203).

We evaluated a series of pediatric and adult patients for a Hawkins line to determine early if osteonecrosis was present. Osteonecrosis did not occur in any patient in whom a

Hawkins line was present. A large percentage of patients in whom a Hawkins line was absent at 12 weeks developed osteonecrosis. A few patients who were immobilized for only a short time did not have a Hawkins line, however, and did not develop osteonecrosis. Not all the patients who developed osteonecrosis required operative treatment. Some did satisfactorily with patellar tendon-bearing braces. Of the 12 children, osteonecrosis developed in five, and all five healed

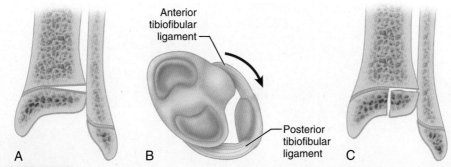

FIGURE 8.198   Mechanism of injury in Tillaux fracture. **A,** Physis in older child closing medially but still open laterally. **B,** External rotational force causes anterior tibiofibular ligament to avulse physis anterolaterally. **C,** Avulsion produces Salter-Harris type III fracture because medial part of physis is closed.

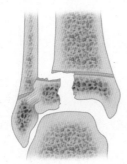

FIGURE 8.199   Tillaux fracture. See Figure 8.198 for mechanism of injury.

uneventfully. The osteonecrosis process in these children was different from that in adults. They developed a sclerotic lesion in the dome and body of the talus that became a cystic lesion on radiographs; over a 2- to 3-year period, the area resolved and all but one at long-term follow-up were asymptomatic (Fig. 8.204). Most children with osteonecrosis do not require surgery, and consequently, a prolonged period of non–weight bearing or the use of a patellar tendon-bearing, weight-relieving brace should be tried before surgery is considered. According to several reports, children younger than 12 years of age have better results and osteonecrosis has a more favorable outcome than in older children.

Malunions of talar fractures were frequent in adults; however, only 2 of the 12 children reviewed in our series had malunion. Malunion usually occurs with the distal fragment dorsiflexed or in a varus position and with the fibula rotated more anteriorly than normal. Most of our adult patients bore an excessive amount of weight on the lateral side of the foot, and many developed traumatic arthritis in the ankle and subtalar joint. The only infection in our series occurred after an open talar neck fracture. Because the talus is composed almost entirely of cancellous bone, and because fracture through the neck may seriously disrupt the blood supply, an established osteomyelitis of the talus may be resistant to treatment. Repeated sequestrectomy or attempted excision and drainage of the sinus track are not indicated in established osteomyelitis of the talus. The results of talectomy without fusion have been poor. The preferred treatment for fractures of the talus complicated by infection is excision of the affected bone followed by arthrodesis, even in children. Operations, when necessary for osteonecrosis, malunion, or infection, include triple arthrodesis, ankle fusion, and talocalcaneal fusion, all of which produce better results than talectomy alone.

■ FRACTURES OF THE DOME AND LATERAL PROCESS OF THE TALUS

Fractures of the dome and body of the talus are rare in children but do occur in shearing injuries, especially lawn mower, bicycle spoke, and "degloving" injuries. Often severe, open shearing injuries from lawn mowers and other power equipment require excision of a portion of the talus. The wound should be irrigated, debrided, and left open; delayed closure and skin grafting, if necessary, can be performed later. The primary goal of treatment is to salvage as much length and function of the foot and ankle as possible. A large, nondisplaced, closed talar dome or body fracture can be treated satisfactorily by closed methods, especially in a child, and good results can be expected. If the fracture is significantly displaced, is intraarticular, and has cancellous bone attached to the fragment, ORIF through an anterior approach (see Technique 1.19) usually is necessary. Only rarely is osteotomy of the medial malleolus necessary for exposure. Care should be taken to avoid the physis in this area. Oblique or transverse cancellous screws inserted across the body of the talus, usually without medial malleolar osteotomy, are all that is necessary. Smaller displaced fragments often can be removed and handled in much the same manner as osteochondral fragments. A CT scan may be necessary to make the diagnosis when persistent lateral subtalar pain is present. Nondisplaced fragments can be treated closed. Large displaced fragments may need ORIF, whereas small displaced fragments can be excised to prevent subtalar arthritis (Fig. 8.205).

■ OSTEOCHONDRAL FRACTURES OF THE TALUS

In our experience, symptoms of osteochondral talar fractures most often begin in the second decade of life, suggesting that this is a lesion of adolescence progressing into early adulthood. We use the classification of Berndt and Harty: stage I, a small area of subchondral compression; stage II, a partially detached fragment; stage III, a completely detached fragment remaining in the crater; and stage IV, a fragment that is detached and loose in the joint (Fig. 8.206). Medial and lateral lesions appear to occur with almost equal frequency, whereas central lesions are rare.

Most lateral lesions are caused by trauma. Morphologically, lateral lesions are thin and wafer shaped and resemble osteochondral fractures. Most medial lesions are deep and

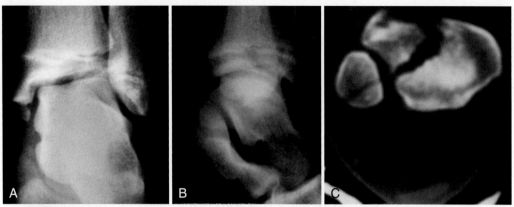

FIGURE 8.200 Tillaux fracture. **A** and **B,** Seemingly undisplaced Tillaux type of Salter-Harris type III fracture. **C,** CT scan revealing significant displacement.

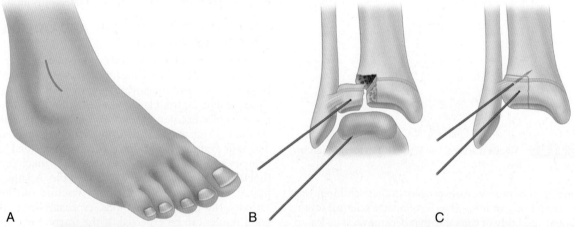

FIGURE 8.201 Percutaneous reduction and fixation of displaced Tillaux fracture. **A,** Skin incision. **B,** Steinmann pin used to reduce fracture. **C,** While fracture is held reduced with Steinmann pin, Kirschner wire is inserted in fragment and across fracture.

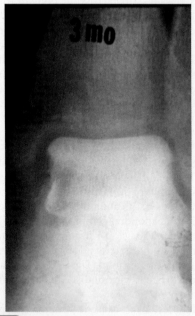

FIGURE 8.202 Hawkins line is not visible in sclerotic (latent osteonecrosis) talar dome 3 months after injury.

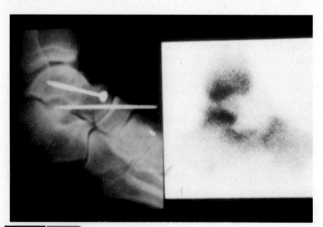

FIGURE 8.203 Bone scan 8 days after open reduction of type IV talar neck fracture with talonavicular dislocation shows decreased uptake indicating area of osteonecrosis.

morphologically cup shaped, not resembling a traumatic fracture (Fig. 8.207).

Surgery usually is required because of persistent symptoms or a loose body in the ankle joint, most often in lateral stage III or IV lesions. Stage I and II lesions generally can be

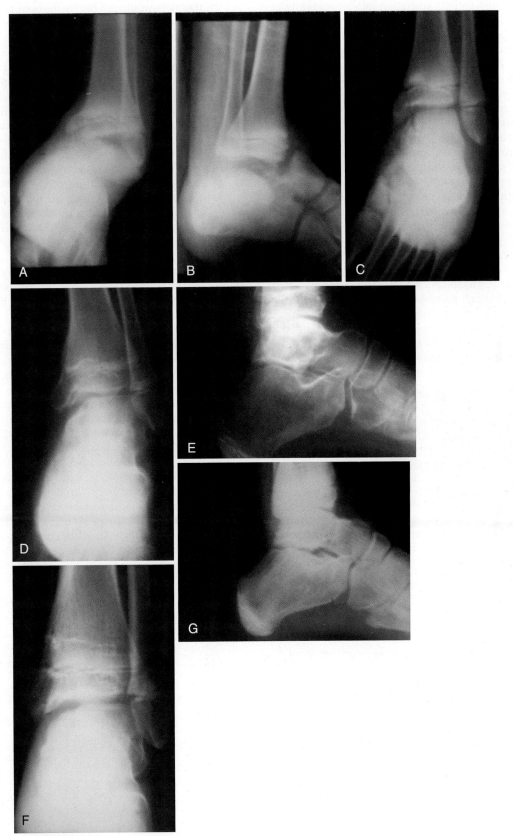

FIGURE 8.204 A and B, Type III talar neck fracture with posteromedial displacement in 9-year-old child. C, After closed reduction and cast immobilization. D and E, At 9 months after injury, there is evidence of healing but osteonecrosis of talus with sclerotic and cystic changes is evident. F and G, At 6 years after injury, physes are still open and some healing of osteonecrosis of talus has occurred; patient has no symptoms.

treated successfully without operation. Nonoperative treatment of stage III medial lesions compares favorably with the results of operative treatment; most are asymptomatic after conservative treatment. Conversely, lateral stage III lesions generally have better results after surgical excision than after conservative treatment. We recommend operative treatment of stage III lateral lesions and all stage IV lesions; all stage I and II lesions and stage III medial lesions can be observed for healing, especially in young children and adolescents.

Histologic analysis has shown that, although morphologically the lesions were wafer shaped on the lateral side and cup shaped on the medial side, histologically they were the same. We cannot say definitely that lateral lesions are osteochondral fractures and that medial lesions are true osteochondritis dissecans. In our experience, lateral lesions have more persistent symptoms and degenerative changes than the medial lesions and require surgery more often.

Three technical operative points should be made:

1. If the osteochondral fragment appears on radiographs to be floating in its crater and riding high, with a flake of bone proximally that appears to be in the joint, the fragment probably is inverted in the crater. This means that the subchondral bone is proximal in the ankle joint and the cartilaginous portion is in the crater (Fig. 8.208). In this position, the cartilaginous

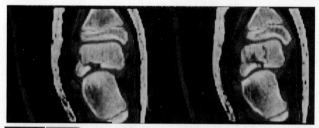

FIGURE 8.205 Coronal CT reconstruction highlighting intraarticular nature of talar lateral process fracture. (From Leibner ED, Simanovsky N, Abu-Sneinah K, et al: Fractures of the lateral process of the talus in children, *J Pediatr Orthop* 10B:68, 2001.)

fragment would not heal to the bone in the crater, and excision is indicated. This elevated, apparently "floating" fragment is pathognomonic of an inverted fragment within the crater.

2. Advanced imaging with CT is helpful in identifying the exact location and extent of the bony lesion and is important for operative planning (Fig. 8.209).

3. Because the fibula is more posterior than the medial malleolus, osteotomy rarely is needed to reach the lateral lesions. If a CT scan shows the medial lesion to be in the middle or posterior part of the talus, however, a medial malleolar osteotomy often is necessary in skeletally mature patients. We osteotomize the medial malleolus at the plafond horizontally or obliquely. The malleolus should be predrilled to accept a cancellous screw. The malleolar fragment can be displaced with a towel clip, and the lesion is seen quite readily.

We have replaced several large fragments and held them with subchondral pins (Fig. 8.210), similar to the technique described for osteochondritis dissecans of the knee. The short-term results have been variable.

The lesions in types I, II, and III are often difficult to see at surgery and can only be palpated or "ballotted" to determine their location. Using a Keith needle or a hemostat to "ballotte" helps outline the extent of the lesion. Good results have been reported with arthroscopic excision of osteochondral lesions of the talus, but it is sometimes difficult to find and define the margins of occult lesions. With newer arthroscopy techniques and equipment, posterior and especially posteromedial lesions can be seen more easily. Often, type III lesions, if not completely detached, can be drilled, especially in children. The drilling can be done arthroscopically, percutaneously, or transmalleolarly (through the malleolus). Large fragments can be reattached, and osteochondral grafts can be inserted. Concomitant use of an image intensifier, although complex, may be of benefit. Also, computer-assisted minimally invasive treatment has been described. See the discussion of arthroscopy of the ankle joint in other chapter.

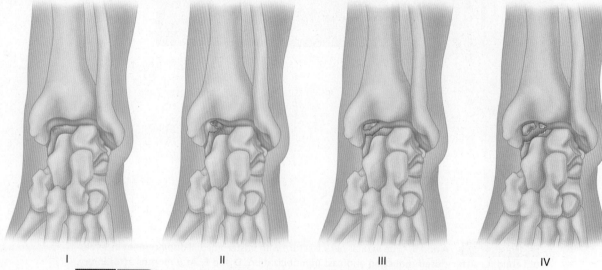

I	II	III	IV

FIGURE 8.206 Four types or stages of osteochondral fractures (osteochondritis dissecans of talus). Stage I, "blister"; stage II, elevated fragment but attached; stage III, fragment detached but still in crater; stage IV, displaced fragment.

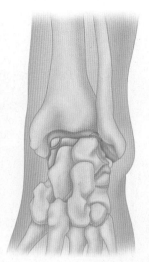

FIGURE 8.207 Morphology of medial and lateral lesions (see text).

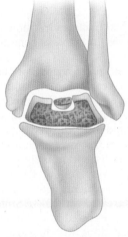

FIGURE 8.208 "Floating" fragment in reality is loose fragment turned upside down in crater.

EXCISION OF OSTEOCHONDRAL FRAGMENT OF THE TALUS

If osteotomy of the medial malleolus is necessary, surgery on the medial side should be delayed until after closure of the physis.

TECHNIQUE 8.42

- Place the patient supine.
- Make a longitudinal incision 7 cm long over the antero-medial aspect of the ankle. Place the incision far enough medially to allow an osteotomy of the medial malleolus to be made if necessary and to allow inspection of the medial aspect of the joint. Carry the soft-tissue dissection down to the ankle joint; retract the neurovascular bundle, the anterior tibial tendon, and the common extensor tendons. Incise the capsule and expose the ankle joint. Plantarflex the foot as much as possible to try to see the lesion. If the lesion is posterior, an osteotomy usually is necessary.
- Predrill for a cancellous screw from distal to proximal through the medial malleolus into the distal tibia and remove the screw.
- Make an osteotomy obliquely across the medial malleolus at the ankle joint level perpendicular to the predrilled hole for the cancellous screw.
- With a towel clip, turn the medial malleolus distally. Evert the ankle until the medial and posterior aspects of the talar dome can be seen.
- Ballotte for any occult lesion with a Keith needle; with a small curet, remove the central necrotic area and determine the margins of the lesion. The fragment often is loose, and the subchondral bone is yellowish and hard. Remove the crater and the fragment and copiously irrigate the joint.
- With a small drill, make four or five holes in the subchondral crater for vascular ingrowth.

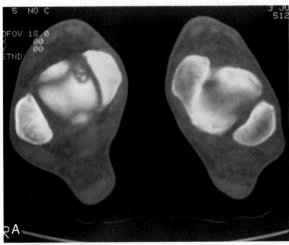
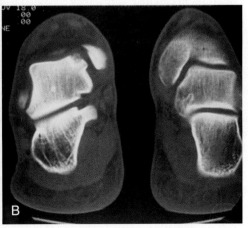

FIGURE 8.209 Osteochondral lesion in anteromedial dome of talus. **A,** CT scan in axial plane shows crater and fragments. **B,** Coronal CT scan locates lesion whether anterior, middle, or posterior, which often is difficult to determine on radiograph.

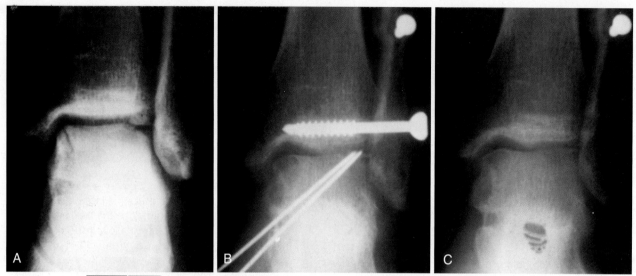

FIGURE 8.210 **A,** Large osteochondral fragment in lateral talus. **B,** After retrograde pinning of fragment; osteotomy of lateral malleolus was performed for better exposure. **C,** Healed lesion after removal of syndesmosis screw.

- Realign the medial malleolar osteotomy and insert a cancellous bone screw in the predrilled hole. Take radiographs to check for anatomic alignment of the screw and the osteotomy.
- Close the wound in layers and apply a short leg cast.

POSTOPERATIVE CARE The patient should wear a cast or patellar tendon-bearing brace for 6 to 8 weeks, preferably non–weight bearing for a total of 8 to 12 weeks, while fibrocartilaginous tissue in the crater fills in the defect.

CALCANEAL FRACTURES

Calcaneal fractures are rare in children. They differ from calcaneal fractures in adults because (1) they occur much less frequently; (2) they do not exhibit the same fracture patterns, having less intraarticular involvement; (3) they are less serious because of the elasticity of structures in children; and (4) they remodel (Fig. 8.211). Schmidt and Weiner reported 62 calcaneal fractures in children, which they classified using a system similar to that of Essex-Lopresti. They included physeal fractures at the tuberosity and a fracture almost unique to children that involves the posterior aspect of the calcaneus with significant loss of bone that occurs in lawn mower injuries. Of the fractures, 63% were extraarticular and only 37% were intraarticular, which is the reverse of the adult fracture pattern. Displacement of the intraarticular fractures was minimal compared with adult fractures, and only two required ORIF. In several older children, the subtalar joint was obviously involved and incongruous, however, similar to the Essex-Lopresti type II fracture, with a decreased "crucial" angle and the presence of a joint compression fracture. Open fractures of the calcaneus occur more often in children than in adults, probably because of the increased incidence of lawn mower injuries.

Because displacement is uncommon in extraarticular and intraarticular fractures, most calcaneal fractures in children are expected to heal without any functional loss. The prognosis of calcaneal fractures in children is good unless a lawn mower injury results in loss of bone and soft tissue from the heel.

Harris views (ski-jump views) of the heel should be obtained, and a CT scan can be helpful because the diagnosis can be obscure secondary to minimal disturbance in the bony architecture and the high percentage of cartilage in the calcaneus of children compared with adults. Operative treatment of calcaneal fractures in children is not indicated unless subtalar joint disruption is significant. A CT scan is mandatory in operative planning. Good clinical outcomes have been reported in patients with displaced intraarticular calcaneal fractures treated with ORIF. Stress fractures of the calcaneus have been reported in children, and a bone scan may be helpful in making the diagnosis. Trott noted that cysts in the triangular space of the calcaneus become large enough for ordinary activities to produce stress or pathologic fractures.

TARSAL FRACTURES

Fractures of the tarsal bones are uncommon in children because of the flexibility of the foot. Fractures, especially of the navicular, cuboid, or cuneiform bones, usually are part of a severe injury to the foot, such as a wringer, severe compression, or lawn mower injury. The second metatarsal has been described as the cornerstone of the foot, and strong ligamentous attachments are present between the metatarsals themselves and between the cuneiforms. The most relevant anatomic features are the fixed mortise position of the base of the second metatarsal and the ligamentous attachments at this base. If there is a fracture of the base of the second metatarsal, with or without a "buckle" fracture of the cuboid, significant tarsometatarsal joint injury, although occult, has occurred. Treatment recommendations include closed reduction for gross displacement or instability, with open reduction if needed to restore anatomic relationships. Because of inherent instability, however, percutaneous Kirschner wire or screw fixation can be used to maintain the reduction and the alignment after open or closed reduction. The wires

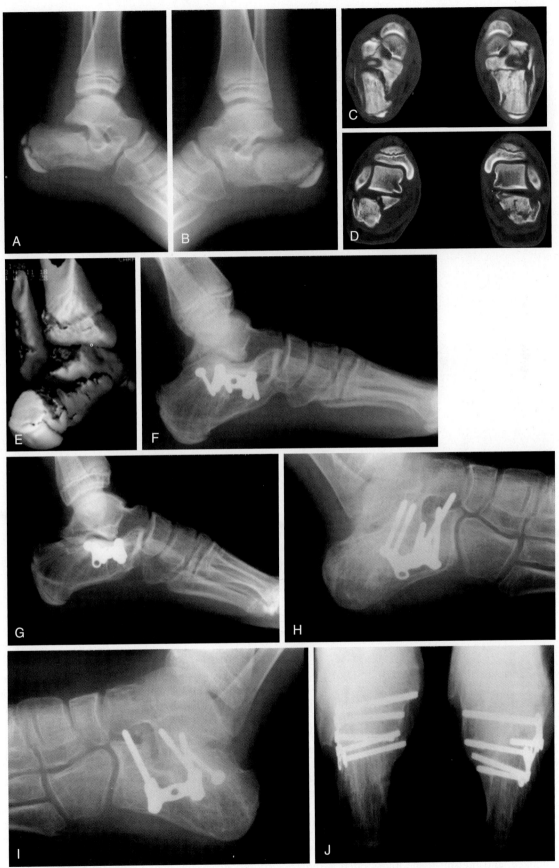

FIGURE 8.211 **A** and **B,** Lateral radiographs of bilateral severe calcaneal fractures with depression of crucial angle in child who also had T12 compression fracture resulting from a fall. **C** and **D,** CT scan at two different levels, revealing severe comminution and displacement. **E,** Three-dimensional reconstruction of lateral calcaneal fractures. **F** and **G,** Lateral radiographs after open reduction and internal fixation with contoured plates and screws. **H–J,** Bilateral oblique and anteroposterior radiographs at follow-up.

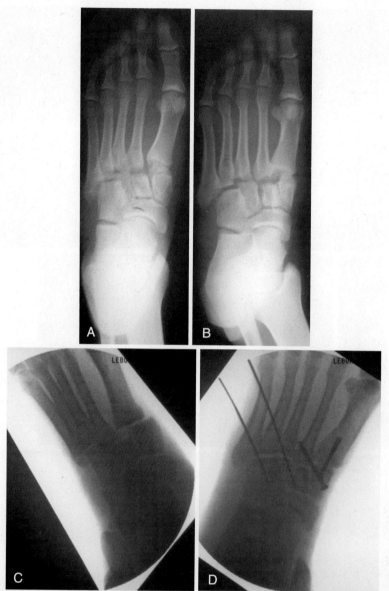

FIGURE 8.212 **A,** Anteroposterior radiograph appears normal. **B,** Oblique radiograph reveals subtle subluxation of metatarsocuneiform joint. **C,** At surgery, image intensification reveals extent of involvement. **D,** Open and percutaneous reduction and fixation of Lisfranc dislocation. Physis of first metatarsal is closed.

are removed after approximately 4 weeks and the screws at around 16 weeks.

In our experience, a persistent dorsal dislocation, even in a child, produces a painful hypertrophic osseous area on the dorsum of the foot. Also, varus angulation often is present. With the patient under general anesthesia, any dislocated tarsometatarsal joints should be reduced. If this cannot be accomplished closed, ORIF of the dislocation is indicated (Fig. 8.212). Care should be taken not to violate the proximal physis of the first metatarsal.

Pediatric Lisfranc injuries consist of a fracture or ligamentous injury involving the first and second tarsometatarsal area. This injury may produce a subtle deformity that can be overlooked, and the soft-tissue injury often is more severe than is indicated by the bony injury seen on the radiographs. Often a fracture-dislocation or a fracture-subluxation of the first tarsometatarsal joint occurs or the first and second

metatarsals may be involved (Fig. 8.213). A study of 56 children with Lisfranc injuries demonstrated that most were sports-related, and, unlike adults, only 34% required ORIF, with few (4%) complications noted.

Cuboid "nutcracker" fractures have been described in four children, all of whom were injured while horseback riding. The mechanism of injury is forced abduction of the forefoot, usually in combination with an axial force. Compression cuboid fractures rarely are isolated injuries, usually occurring with other midfoot fractures or dislocations. The identification of a cuboid nutcracker fracture on radiograph should prompt CT evaluation to rule out or identify other injuries. Minimally displaced isolated cuboid nutcracker fractures can be treated conservatively, but poor results are common after nonoperative treatment of displaced fractures, and operative treatment is recommended to avoid alterations in foot mechanics and function, leading to foot stiffness and pain.

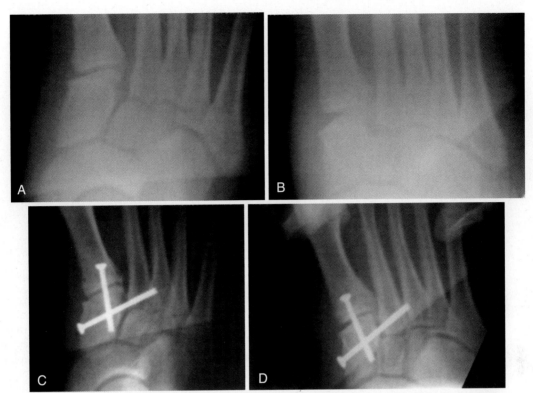

FIGURE 8.213 Anteroposterior and stress radiographs of foot with subtle Lisfranc dislocation. **A,** Radiograph appears normal. **B,** With stress into everted position, metatarsals sublux laterally. **C,** Postreduction radiograph reveals satisfactory reduction and internal fixation. **D,** Reduction maintained on eversion stress radiograph.

OPEN REDUCTION AND INTERNAL FIXATION OF CUBOID COMPRESSION (NUTCRACKER) FRACTURE

TECHNIQUE 8.43

(CERONI ET AL.)

- Make a lateral incision along the axis from the tip of the fibula to the tip of the fifth metatarsal.
- Retract the peroneus tendons plantarly and partially elevate the extensor digitorum brevis muscle.
- Elevate the extruded lateral wall of the cuboid and inspect the fracture and adjacent joint.
- Elevate depressed fragments with a laminar spreader until the adjacent joint surfaces are congruent.
- When the shape of the cuboid is restored, fill the large corticocancellous defect with a large allograft bone block to provide stable bony support. Cut the allograft bone block overly large so that it fits into the defect with some resistance.
- This construct is stable enough that no fixation is required.
- Obtain an oblique radiograph to confirm the articular reconstruction and reestablishment of lateral column length.
- Close the wound in layers and apply a short leg cast.

POSTOPERATIVE CARE The non–weight bearing cast is worn for 6 weeks, followed by a walking cast for another 6 weeks. Unprotected full weight bearing is allowed at 12 weeks after surgery.

METATARSAL AND PHALANGEAL FRACTURES

Although metatarsal and phalangeal fractures in children are common, little has been written about these fractures. Perhaps this is because they usually heal uneventfully and rarely need operative treatment. Because of their strong interosseous ligaments, fractures of the proximal metatarsals usually do not become displaced significantly. Displaced fractures usually are produced by severe trauma. In addition to the fractures, the soft tissues usually are damaged considerably and swelling may be excessive. These severe injuries should be treated by elevation and observation and not by a circumferential cast. When the swelling has resolved, a displaced fracture can be reduced closed, if necessary, by longitudinal traction. For severe trauma producing multiple fractures with significant displacement, when the swelling has subsided, open reduction and smooth pin fixation are performed if necessary. This is occasionally needed in the first metatarsal of older children, where little remodeling can be expected (Fig. 8.214). Most displaced fractures of the metatarsal neck heal and usually remodel nicely in young children; however, if displacement and deformity are significant, especially in the

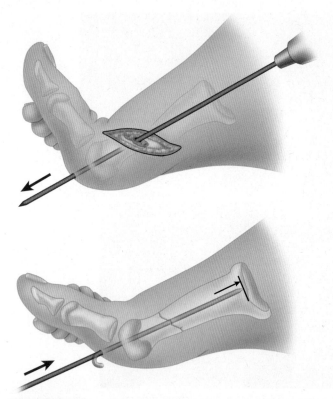

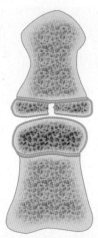

FIGURE 8.215 Fissuring (not fracture) of physis of proximal phalanx of great toe.

FIGURE 8.214 Method of open pinning of metatarsal shaft or neck fractures in retrograde fashion through first metatarsal head.

anteroposterior plane, and multiple neck fractures are present, occasionally ORIF with longitudinal wires is necessary, especially in older children.

Stress fractures of the metatarsal shaft or neck occur in children. MRI may be helpful in diagnosis, and these fractures should be treated expectantly. We have seen a 10-year-old child with a metatarsal stress fracture, and although these fractures occur less frequently in children than in adults, they can be produced by chronic repetitive, stressful activity. Nonoperative treatment is usually appropriate combined with vitamin D supplementation. Fractures of the base of the fifth metatarsal in children and adults traditionally have been called Jones fractures, although Jones' original description from 1896 appears to be that of a diaphyseal fracture rather than an avulsion fracture of the base of the fifth metatarsal caused by overpull of the peroneus brevis muscle. Several studies have noted the uncertainty of healing of this diaphyseal fracture and recommended ORIF with a medullary screw in high-performance athletes, recreational athletes, and nonathletes with delayed union. A more recent study also suggested that fixation of Jones fractures in active adolescents should be considered to allow faster return to regular activities and prevent refracture. Avulsions of the most proximal base of the fifth metatarsal also occur in children and heal uneventfully except for some bony hypertrophy at the fracture site. This injury should be differentiated from a secondary ossification center seen on oblique views in a 10- to 13-year-old child that when painful is termed *Iselin disease*.

Fractures of the phalanges are caused primarily by hitting a hard object or compressing the toe with a heavy weight.

Open fractures of the great toe distal phalanx (stubbed toe) can be worrisome. Dislocations of the phalanges usually are dorsal and can be reduced easily. Certain developmental disorders of the phalanges should not be confused with fractures. Fragmentation of the proximal epiphysis of the hallux occurs frequently (Fig. 8.215). The epiphysis may be fissured, compressed, or fragmented. Usually the physis is not fractured.

Fractures and dislocations of the phalanges should be reduced by longitudinal traction and held by "buddy" taping to the next toe. ORIF is only rarely indicated. If fracture of a phalanx is caused by a penetrating wound, as in stepping on a nail, *Pseudomonas* infection should be suspected. If the wound becomes infected, it should be irrigated and debrided and intravenous antibiotic therapy should be administered. For infected phalangeal fractures, debridement, wet dressing, intravenous administration of antibiotics, and delayed closure save some toes, especially the great toe, when impending infection or gangrene has suggested amputation. Severe open fractures occur in the forefoot and the phalanges, primarily in bicycle spoke or rotary lawn mower injuries. Treatment consists of adequate debridement of the wounds, leaving the wounds open, and delayed closure. The operative treatment of these injuries is similar to that for the digits of adults.

REFERENCES

GROWTH INJURIES, BIRTH INJURIES, AND NONACCIDENTAL TRAUMA

Anton C, Podberesky DJ: Little League shoulder: a growth plate injury, *Pediatr Radiol* 40(Suppl 1):S54, 2010.

Ariyawatkul T, Worawuthangkul K, Chotigavanichaya C, et al.: Potential risk factors for birth fractures: a case-control study, *Int Orthop* 41:2361, 2017.

Baldwin K, Pandya NK, Wolfgruber H, et al.: Femur fractures in the pediatric population: abuse or accidental trauma? *Clin Orthop Relat Res* 469:798, 2011.

Baldwin KD, Scherl SA: Orthopaedic aspects of child abuse, *Instr Course Lect* 62:399, 2013.

Banerjee J, Asamoah FK, Singhvi D, et al.: Haemoglobin level at birth is associated with short term outcomes and mortality in preterm infants, *BMC Med* 13:16, 2015.

Basha A, Amarin Z, Abu-Hassan F: Birth-associated long-bone fractures, *Int J Gynaecol Obstet* 123:127, 2013.

Blatz AM, Gillespie CW, Katcher A, et al.: Factors associated with nonaccidental trauma evaluation among patients below 36 months old presenting with femur fracture at a Level-1 pediatric trauma center, *J Pediatr Orthop* 39:175, 2019.

Clarke NM, Shelton FR, Taylor CC, et al.: The incidence of fractures in children under the age of 24 months – in relation to non-accidental injury, *Injury* 43:762, 2012.

Duffy SO, Squires J, Fromkin JB, Berger RP: Use of skeletal surveys to evaluate for physical abuse: analysis of 703 consecutive skeletal surveys, *Pediatrics* 127:347, 2011.

Garrett BR, Hoffman EB, Carrara H: The effect of percutaneous pin fixation in the treatment of distal femoral physeal fractures, *J Bone Joint Surg* 93:689, 2011.

Gkiokas A, Brilakis E: Spontaneous correction of partial physeal arrest: report of a case and review of the literature, *J Pediatr Orthop B* 21:369, 2012.

Havranek P, Pesl T: Salter (Rang) type 6 physeal injury, *Eur J Pediatr Surg* 20:174, 2010.

Ho-Fung VM, Zapala MA, Lee EY: Musculoskeletal traumatic injuries in children: characteristic imaging findings and mimickers, *Radiol Clin North Am* 55:785, 2017.

Jayakumar P, Barry M, Ramachandran M: Orthopaedic aspects of paediatric non-accidental injury, *J Bone Joint Surg* 92B:189, 2010.

Jha P, Stein-Wexler R, Coulter K, et al.: Optimizing bone surveys performed for suspected non-accidental trauma with attention to maximizing diagnostic yield while minimizing radiation exposure: utility of pelvic and lateral radiographs, *Pediatr Radiol* 43:668, 2013.

Kamaci S, Danisman M, Marangoz S: Neonatal physeal separation of distal humerus during cesarean section, *Am J Orthop* 43:E279, 2014.

Kang HG, Yoon SJ, Kim JR: Resection of a physeal bar under computer-assisted guidance, *J Bone Joint Surg* 92:1452, 2010.

Karmazyn B, Lewis ME, Jennings SG, et al.: The prevalence of uncommon fractures on skeletal surveys performed to evaluate for suspected abuse in 930 children: should practice guidelines change? *AJR Am J Roentgenol* 197:W159, 2011.

Karmazyn B, Miller EM, Lay SE, et al.: Double-read of skeletal surveys in suspected non-accidental trauma: what we learned, *Pediatr Radiol* 47:584, 2017.

Leaman L, Hennrikus W, Nasreddine AY: An evaluation of seasonal variation of nonaccidental fractures in children less than 1 year of age, *Clin Pediatr (Phila)* 56:1345, 2017.

Linder N, Linder I, Friedman E, et al.: Birth trauma—risk factors and short-term neonatal outcome, *J Matern Fetal Neonatal Med* 26:1491, 2013.

Loraas EK, Schmale GA: Endoscopically aided physeal bar takedown and guided growth for the treatment of angular limb deformity, *J Pediatr Orthop B* 21:348, 2012.

Luri B, Koff MF, Shah P, et al.: Three-dimensional magnetic resonance imaging of physeal injury: reliability and clinical utility, *J Pediatr Orthop* 34:239, 2014.

Marine MB, Corea D, Steenburg SD, et al.: Is the new ACR-SPR practice guideline for addition of oblique views of the ribs to the skeletal survey for child abuse justified? *AJR Am J Roentgenol* 202:868, 2014.

Mulpuri K, Slobogean BL, Tredwell SJ: The epidemiology of nonaccidental trauma in children, *Clin Orthop Relat Res* 469:759, 2011.

Murphy R, Kelly DM, Moisan A, Thompson NB: Transverse fractures of the femoral shaft are a better predictor of nonaccidental trauma in young children than spiral fractures are, *J Bone Joint Surg* 97A:106, 2015.

Pandya NK, Baldwin K, Kamath AF, et al.: Unexplained fractures: child abuse or bone disease? A systematic review, *Clin Orthop Relat Res* 469:805, 2011.

Pandya NK, Baldwin KD, Wolfgruber H, et al.: Humerus fractures in the pediatric population: an algorithm to identify abuse, *J Pediatr Orthop B* 19:535, 2010.

Powell-Doherty RD, Raynor NE, Goodenow DA, et al.: Examining the role of follow-up skeletal surveys in non-accidental trauma, *Am J Surg* 213:606, 2017.

Prosser I, Lawson Z, Evans A, et al.: A timetable for the radiologic features of fracture healing in young children, *AJR Am J Roentgenol* 1014:198, 2012.

Ranade SC, Allen AK, Deutsch SA: The role of the orthopaedic surgeon in the identification and management of nonaccidental trauma, *J Am Acad Orthop Surg* 28:53, 2020.

Ravichandiran N, Schuh S, Bejuk M, et al.: Delayed identification of pediatric abuse-related fractures, *Pediatrics* 125:60, 2010.

Sink EL, Hyman JE, Matheny T, et al.: Child abuse: the role of the orthopaedic surgeon in nonaccidental trauma, *Clin Orthop Relat Res* 469:790, 2011.

Sonik A, Stein-Wexler R, Rogers KK, et al.: Follow-up skeletal surveys for suspected non-accidental trauma: can a more limited survey be performed without compromising diagnostic information? *Child Abuse Negl* 34:804, 2010.

Wood JN, Fakeye O, Feudtner C, et al.: Development of guidelines for skeletal survey in young children with fractures, *Pediatrics* 134:45, 2014.

Wood JN, Fakeye O, Mondestin V, et al.: Development of hospital-based guidelines for skeletal survey in young children with bruises, *Pediatrics* 135:e312, 2015.

Zhao C, Starke M, Tompson JD, et al.: Predictors for nonaccidental trauma in a child with a fracture—a National Inpatient Database study, *J Am Acad Orthop Surg*, 2019 Jun 11, [Epub ahead of print].

OPEN AND PATHOLOGIC FRACTURES

Bazzi AA, Brooks JT, Jain A, et al.: Is nonoperative treatment of pediatric type I open fractures safe and effective? *J Child Orthop* 8:467, 2014.

Godfrey J, Choi PD, Shabtai L, et al.: Management of pediataric type I open fractures in the emergency department or operating room: a multicenter persective, *J Pediatr Orthop* 39:372, 2019.

Ibrahim T, Riaz M, Hegazy A, et al.: Delayed surgical debridement in pediatric open fractures: a systematic review and meta-analysis, *J Child Orthop* 8:135, 2014.

Iobst CA, Spurdle C, Baitner AC, et al.: A protocol for the management of pediatric type I open fractures, *J Child Orthop* 8:71, 2014.

Rapp M, Svoboda D, Wessel LM, Kaiser MM: Elastic stable intramedullary nailing (ESIN), Orthoss® and Gravitational Platelet Separation—system (GPS®): an effective method of treatment for pathologic fractures of bone cysts in children, *BMC Musculoskelet Disord* 12:45, 2011.

Trionfo A, Cavanaugh PK, Herman MJ: Pediatric open fractures, *Orthop Clin North Am* 47:565, 2016.

Wang KK, Rademacher ES, Miller PE, et al.: Management of Gustilo-Anderson type II and IIIA open long bone fractures in children: which wounds require a second washout?, *J Pediatr Orthop*, 2019 Sep 4, [Epub ahead of print].

Wetzel RJ, Minhas SV, Patrick BC, et al.: Current practice in the management of type I open fractures in children: a survey of POSNA membership, *J Pediatr Orthop* 35:762, 2015.

FRACTURES AND DISLOCATIONS INVOLVING THE CLAVICLE, HUMERAL SHAFT, PROXIMAL END OF THE HUMERUS, AND SHOULDER

Bae DS, Shah AS, Kalish LA, et al.: Shoulder motion, strength, and functional outcomes in children with established malunion of the clavicle, *J Pediatr Orthop* 33:544, 2013.

Canavese F, Athlani L, Marengo L, et al.: Evaluation of upper-extremity function following surgical treatment of displaced proximal humerus fractures in children, *J Pediatr Orthop B* 23:144, 2014.

Canavese F, Margeno L, Cravino M, et al.: Outome of conservative versus surgical treatment of humeral shaft fracture in children and adolescents: comparison between nonoperative treatment (Desault's banage), external fixation, and elastic stable intramedullary nailing, *J Pediatr Orthop* 37:e156, 2017.

Carry PM, Koonce R, Pan Z, Polousky JD: A survey of physician opinion: adolescent midshaft clavicle fracture treatment preferences among POSNA members, *J Pediatr Orthop* 31:44, 2011.

Chaus GW, Carry PM, Pishkenari AK, Hadley-Miller N: Operative versus nonoperative treatment of displaced proximal humeral physeal fractures: a matched cohort, *J Pediatr Orthop* 35:234, 2015.

Eisenstein ED, Misenhimmer JJ, Kotb A, et al.: Management of displaced midshaft clavicle fractures in adolescents patients using intramedullary flexible nails: a case series, *J Clin Orthop Trauma* 9(Suppl 1):S97, 2018.

Franklin CC, Weiss JM: The natural history of pediatric and adolescent shoulder dislocation, *J Pediatr Orthop* 39(Issue 6, (Suppl 1):S50, 2019.

Gladstein AZ, Schade AT, Howard AW, et al.: Reducing resource utilization during non-operative treatment of pediatric proximal humeral fractures, *Orthop Traumatol Surg Res* 103:115, 2017.

Hannonen J, Hyvönen H, Korhonen L, et al.: The incidence and treatment trends of pediatric proximal humerus fractures, *BMC Musculoskelet Disord* 20:571, 2019.

Hariharan AR, Ho C, Bauer A, et al.: Transphyseal humeral separations: what can we learn? A retrospective multicenter review of surgically treated patients over a 25-year period, *J Pediatric Orthop*, 2019 Sep 12, [Epub ahead of print].

Hohloch L, Eberbach H, Wagner FC, et al.: Age- and severity-adjusted treatment of proximal humerus fractures in children and adolescents: a systematical review and meta-analysis, *PloS One* 12:e0183157, 2017.

Hong S, Nho JH, Lee CJ, et al.: Posterior shoulder dislocation with ipsilateral proximal humerus type 2 physeal fracture: case report, *J Pediatr Orthop B* 24:215, 2015.

Hutchinson PH, Bae DS, Waters PM: Intramedullary nailing versus percutaneous pin fixation of pediatric proximal humerus fractures: a comparison of complications and early radiographic results, *J Pediatr Orthop* 31:617, 2011.

Khan A, Athlani L, Rousset M, et al.: Functional results of displaced proximal humerus fractures in children treated by elastic stable intramedullary nail, *Eur J Orthop Surg Traumatol* 24:164, 2014.

King EC, Ihnow SB: Which proximal humerus fractures should be pinnedd? Treatment in skeletally immature patients, *J Pediatr Orthop* 36(Suppl 1):S44, 2016.

Li Y, Helvie P, Farley FA, et al.: Complictions after plate fixation of displaced pediatric midshaft clavicle fractures, *J Pediatr Orthop* 38:350, 2018.

Lin KM, James EW, Spitzer E, et al.: Pediatric and adolescent anterior shoulder instability: clinical management of first-time dislocators, *Curr Opin Pediaatr* 30:49, 2018.

Luo TD, Ashraf A, Larson AN, et al.: Complications in the treatment of adolescent clavicle fractures, *Orthopedics* 38:e287, 2015.

McIntosh AL: Surgical treatment of adolescent clavicle fractures: results and complications, *J Pediatr Orthop* 36(Suppl 1):S41, 2016.

Miller MC, Redman CN, Mistovich RJ, et al.: Single-screw fixation of adolescent Salter-II proximal humeral fractures: biomechanical analysis of the "one pass door lock" technique, *J Pediatr Orthop* 37:e342, 2017.

Namdari S, Ganley TJ, Baldwin K, et al.: Fixation of displaced midshaft clavicle fractures in skeletally immature patients, *J Pediatr Orthop* 31:507, 2011.

Nenopoulous SP, Gigis IP, Chytas AA, et al.: Outcome of distal clavicular fracture separations and dislocations in immature skeleton, *Injury* 42:376, 2011.

O'Shaughnessy MA, Parry JA, Liu H, et al.: Management of paediatric humeral shaft fractures and associated nerve palsy, *J Child Orthop* 13:508, 2019.

Pahlavan S, Bladwin KD, Pandya NK, et al.: Proximal humerus fractures in the pediatric population: a systematic review, *J Child Orthop* 5:187, 2011.

Pandya NK, Behrends D, Hosalkar HS: Open reduction of proximal humerus fractures in the adolescent population, *J Child Orthop* 6:111, 2012.

Parry JA, Van Straaten M, Luo TD, et al.: Is there a deficit after nonoperative versus operative treatment of shortened midshaft clavicular fractures in adolescents? *J Pediatr Orthop* 37:227, 2017.

Pavone V, de Cristo C, Cannavo L, et al.: Midterm results of surgical treatment of displaced proximal humeral fractures in children, *Eur J Orthop Surg Traumatol* 26:461, 2016.

Pavone V, de Cristo C, Testa G, et al.: Does age affect outcome in children with clavicle fracture treated conservatively? QuickDash and MRC evaluation of 131 consecutive cases, *Minerva Pediatr*, 2018 Apr 12, [Epub ahead of print].

Pennock AT, Edmonds EW, Bae DS, et al.: Adolescent clavicle nonunions: potential risk factors and surgical management, *J Shoulder Elbow Surg* 27:29, 2018.

Pogorelic Z, Kadic S, Milunovic KP, et al.: Flexible intramedullary nailing for treatment of proximal humeral and humeral shaft in children: a retrospective series of 118 cases, *Orthop Traumatol Surg Res* 103:765, 2017.

Popkin CA, Levine WN, Ahmad CS: Evaluation and management of pediatric proximal humerus fractures, *J Am Acad Orthop Surg* 23:77, 2015.

Randsborg PH, Fuglesang HF, Røtterfud JH, et al.: Long-term patient-reported outcome after fractures of the clavicle in patients aged 10 to 18 years, *J Pediatr Orthop* 34:393, 2014.

Schulz J, Moor M, Roocroft J, et al.: Functional and radiographic outcomes of nonoperative treatment of displaced adolescent clavicle fractures, *J Bone Joint Surg* 95A:1159, 2013.

Shannon SF, Hernandez NM, Sems SA, et al.: High-energy pediatric scapula fractures and their associated injuries, *J Pediatr Orthop* 39:377, 2019.

Song MH, Yun YH, Kang K, et al.: Nonoperative versus operative treatment for displaced midshaft clavicle fractures in adolescents: a comparative study, *J Pediatr Orthop B* 28:45, 2019.

Suppan CA, Bae DS, Donohue KS, et al.: Trends in the volume of operative treatment of midshaft clavicle fractures in children and adolescents: a retrospective, 12-year, single-institution analysis, *J Pediatr Orthop B* 25:305, 2016.

Sykes JA, Ezetendu C, Sivitz A, et al.: Posterior dislocation of sternoclavicular joint encroaching on ipsilateral vessels in 2 pediatric patients, *Pediatr Emerg Care* 27:327, 2011.

Tennent TD, Pearse EO, Eastwood DM: A new technique for stabilizing adolescent posteriorly displaced physeal medial clavicular fractures, *J Shoulder Elbow Surg* 21:1734, 2012.

Tepolt F, Carry PM, Taylor M, Hadley-Miller N: Posterior sternoclavicular joint injuries in skeletally immature patients, *Orthopedics* 37:e174, 2014.

Tepolt F, Carry PM, Heyn PC, Miller NH: Posterior sternoclavicular joint injuries in the adolescent population: a meta-analysis, *Am J Sports Med* 42:2517, 2014.

Ting BL, Bae DS, Waters PM: Chronic posterior sternoclavicular joint fracture dislocations in children and young adults: results of surgical management, *J Pediatr Orthop* 34:542, 2014.

Van Tassel D, Owens BD, Pointer L, Moriatis Wolf J: Incidence of clavicle fractures in sports: analysis of the NEISS Database, *Int J Sports Med* 35:83, 2014.

Vander Have KL, Perdue AM, Caird MS, Farley FA: Operative versus nonoperative treatment of midshaft clavicle fractures in adolescents, *J Pediatr Orthop* 30:307, 2010.

Xie F, Wang S, Jiao Q, et al.: Minimally invasive treatment for severely displaced proximal humeral fractures in children using titanium elastic nails, *J Pediatr Orthop* 31:839, 2011.

Yang S, Werner BC, Gwathmey Jr FW: Treatment trends in adolescent clavicle fractures, *J Pediatr Orthop* 35:229, 2015.

SUPRACONDYLAR FRACTURES

Abbott MD, Buchler L, Loder RT, Caltoum CB: Gartland type III supracondylar humerus fractures: outcome and complications as related to operative timing and pin configuration, *J Child Orthop* 8:473, 2014.

Abzug JM, Herman MJ: Management of supracondylar humerus fractures in children: current concepts, *J Am Acad Orthop Surg* 20:69, 2012.

Acosta AM, Li YJ, Bompadre V, et al.: The utility of the early postoperative follow-up and radiographs after operative treatment of supracondylar humerus fractures in children, 2018 Jul 29, [Epub ahead of print].

Altay MA, Erturk C, Altay M, et al.: Ultrasonographic examination of the radial and ulnar nerves after percutaneous cross-wiring of supracondylar humerus fractures in children: a prospective, randomized controlled study, *J Pediatr Orthop B* 20:334, 2011.

Babal JC, Mehlman CT, Klein G: Nerve injuries associated with pediatric supracondylar humeral fractures: a meta-analysis, *J Pediatr Orthop* 30:253, 2010.

Bales JG, Spencer HT, Wong MA, et al.: The effects of surgical delay on the outcome of pediatric supracondylar humeral fractures, *J Pediatr Orthop* 30:786, 2010.

Bauer JM, Stutz CM, Schoenecker JG, et al.: Internal rotation stress testing improves radiographic outcomes of type 3 supracondylar humerus fractures, *J Peditr Orthop* 39:8, 2019.

Belthur MV, Iobst CA, Bor N, et al.: Correction of cubitus varus after pediatric supracondylar elbow fracture: alternative method using the Taylor Spatial Frame, *J Pediatr Orthop* 36:608, 2016.

Choi PD, Melikian R, Skaggs DL: Risk factors for vascular repair and compartment syndrome in the pulseless supracondylar humerus fracture in children, *J Pediatr Orthop* 30:50, 2010.

Chukwunyerenwa C, Orlik B, El-Hawary R, et al.: Treatment of flexion-type supracondylar fractures in children: the "push-pull" method for closed reduction and percutaneous K-wire fixation, *J Pediatr Orthop B* 25:412, 2016.

Eberl R, Eder C, Smolle E, et al.: Iatrogenic ulnar nerve injury after pin fixation and after antegrade nailing of supracondylar humeral fractures in children, *Acta Orthop* 82:606, 2011.

Ernat J, Ho C, Wimberly RL, et al.: Fracture classification does not predict functional outcomes in supracondylar humerus fractures: a prospective study, *J Pediatr Orthop* 37:e233, 2017.

Farr S, Ganger R, Girsch W: Distal humeral flexion osteotomy for the treatment of supracondylar extension-type malunions in children, *J Pediatr Orthop B* 27:115, 2018.

Flynn K, Shah AS, Brusalis CM, et al.: Flexion-type supracondylar humeral fractures: ulnar nerve injury increases risk of open reduction, *J Bone Joint Surg* 99:1485, 2017.

Frick SL: Should you explore the brachial artery in children who have a perfused hand but no palpable radial pulse after sustaining a supracondylar humeral fracture? Commentary on articles by Amanda Weller, MD, et al: "Management of the pediatric pulseless supracondylar humeral fracture: is vascular exploration necessary?" and Brian P. Scannell, MD, et al.: "The perfused, pulseless supracondylar humeral fracture: intermediate-term follow-up of vascular status and function, *J Bone Joint Surg* 95A:e168, 2013.

Gaston RG, Cates TB, Devito D, et al.: Medial and lateral pin versus lateral-entry pin fixation for type 3 supracondylar fractures in children: a prospective, surgeon-randomized study, *J Pediatr Orthop* 30:799, 2010.

Green BM, Stone JD, Bruce Jr RW, et al.: The use of a transolecranon pin the treatment of pediatric flexion-type supracondylar humerus fracutres, *J Pediatr Orthop* 37:e347, 2017.

Hamdi A, Poitras P, Louati H, et al.: Biomechanical analysis of lateral pin placements for pediatric supracondylar humerus fractures, *J Pediatr Orthop* 30:135, 2010.

Ho CA, Podeszwa DA, Riccio AI, et al.: Soft tissue injury severity is associated with neurovascular injury in pediatric supracondylar humerus fractures, *J Pediatr Orthop* 38:443, 2018.

Holt JB, Glass NA, Bedard NA, et al.: Emerging U.S. national trends in the treatment of pediatric supracondylar humeral fractures, *J Bone Joint Surg Am* 99:681, 2017.

Holt JB, Glass NA, Shah AS: Understanding the epidemiology of pediatric supracondylar humeral fractures in the United States: identifying opportunities for intervention, *J Pediatr Orthop* 38:e245, 2018.

Howard A, Mulpuri K, Abel MF, et al.: The treatment of pediatric supracondylar humerus fracture, *J Am Acad Orthop Surg* 20:320, 2012.

Isa AD, Furey A, Stone C: Functional outcome of supracondylar elbow fractures in children: a 3- to 5-year follow-up, *Can J Surg* 57:241, 2014.

Joiner ER, Skaggs DL, Arkader A, et al.: Iatrogenic nerve injuries in the treatment of supracondylar humerus fractures: are we really just missing nerve injuries on preoperative examination? *J Pediatr Orthop* 34:388, 2014.

Karalius VP, Stanfield J, Ashley P, et al.: The utility of routine postoperative radiographs after pinning of pediatric supracondylar humeral fractures, *J Pediatr Orthop* 37:e309, 2017.

Kronner JMJR, Legakis JE, Kovacevic N, et al.: An evaluation of supracondylar humerus fractures: is there a correlation between postponing treatment and the need for open surgical intervention, *J Child Orthop* 7:131, 2013.

Lacher M, Schaeffer K, Boehm R, Dietz HG: The treatment of supracondylar humeral fractures with elastic stable intramedullary nailing (ESIN) in children, *J Pediatr Orthop* 31:33, 2011.

Larson AN, Garg S, Weller A, et al.: Operative treatment of type II supracondylar humerus fractures: does time to surgery affect complications, *J Pediatr Orthop* 34:382, 2014.

Lee BJ, Lee SR, Kim ST, et al.: Radiographic outcomes after treatment of pediatric supracondylar humerus fractures using a treatment-based classification system, *J Orthop Trauma* 25:18, 2011.

Lewine E, Kim JM, Miller PE, et al.: Closed versus open supracondylar fractures of the humerus in children: a comparison of clinical and radiographic presentation and results, *J Pediatr Ortojp* 38:77, 2018.

Li NY, Bruce WJ, Joyce C, et al.: Obesity's influence on operative management of supracondylar humerus fractures, *J Pediatr Orthop* 38:e118, 2018.

Martus JE, Hilmes MA, Grice JV, et al.: Radiation exposure during operative fixation of pediatric supracondylar humerus fractures: is lead shielding necessary, *J Pediatr Orthop* 38:249, 2018.

Meyer CL, Kozin SH, Herman MJ, et al.: Complications of pediatric supracondylar humeral fractures, *Instr Course Lect* 64:483, 2015.

North D, Held M, Dix-Peek S, et al.: French osteotomy for cubitus varus in children: a long-term study over 27 years, *J Pediatr Orthop* 36:19, 2016.

Novais EN, Carry PM, Mark BJ, et al.: Posterolaterally displaced and flexion-type supracondylar fractures are associated with a higher risk of open reduction, *J Pediatr Orthop B* 25:406, 2016.

Or O, Weil Y, Simanovsky N, et al.: The outcome of early revision of malaligned pediatric supracondylar humerus fractures, *Injury* 46:1585, 2015.

Pesenti S, Ecalle A, Gaubert L, et al.: Operative management of supracondylar humeral fractures in children: comparison of five fixation methods, *Orthop Traumatol Surg Res* 103:771, 2017.

Ramesh P, Avadhani A, Shetty AP, et al.: Management of acute "'pink pulseless'" hand in pediatric supracondylar fractures of the humerus, *J Pediatr Orthop B* 20:124, 2011.

Roberts L, Strelzow J, Schaeffer EK, et al.: Nonperative treatment of type IIA supracondylar humerus fractures: comparing 2 modalities, *J Pediatr Orthop* 38:521, 2018.

Robertson AK, Snow E, Browne TS, et al.: Who gets compartment syndrome?:a retrospective analysis of the national and local incidence of compartment syndrome in patients with supracondylar humerus fractures, *J Pediatr Orthop* 38:e252, 2018.

Schlechter JA, Dempewolf M: The utility of radiographs prior to pin removal after operative treatment of supracondylar humerus fractures in children, *J Child Orthop* 9:303, 2015.

Schroeder NO, Seeley MA, Hariharan A, et al.: Utility of posterative antibiotics after percutaneous pinning of pediatric supracondylar humerus fractures, *J Pediatr Orthop* 37:363, 2017.

Seeley MA, Gagnier JJ, Srinivasan RC, et al.: Obesity and its effects on pediatric supracondylar humeral fractures, *J Bone Joint Surg* 96A:e18, 2014.

Sharma A, Sethi A: Multidirectionally unstable supracondylar humeral fractures in children, *JBJS Rev* 7:e3, 2019.

Shore BJ, Gillespie BT, Miller PE, et al.: Recovery of motor nerve injuries associated with displaced, extension-type pediatric supracondylar humerus fractures, 39:e652, 2019.

Silva M, Cooper SD, Cha A: The outcome of surgical treatment of multidirectionally unstable (type IV) pediatric supracondylar humerus fractures, *J Pediatr Orthop* 35:600, 2015.

Silva M, Delfosse EM, Park H, et al.: Is the "Appropriate Use Criteria" for type II supracondylar humerus fractures really appropriate? *J Pediatr Orthop* 39:1, 2019.

Silva M, Pandarinath R, Garng E, et al.: Inter- and intra-observer reliability of the Baumann angle of the humerus in children with supracondylar humeral fractures, *Int Orthop* 34:553, 2010.

Sinikumpu JJ, Victorzon S, Pokka T, et al.: The long-term outcome of childhood supracondylar humeral fractures: a population-based follow up study with a minimum follow up of ten years and normal matched comparisons, *Bone Joint Lett J* 98-B:1410, 2016.

Slobogean BL, Jackman H, Tennant S, et al.: Iatrogenic ulnar nerve injury after the surgical treatment of displaced supracondylar fractures of the humerus: number needed to harm, a systematic review, *J Pediatr Orthop* 30:430, 2010.

Smuin DM, Hennrikus WL: The effect of the pucker sign on outcomes of type III extension supracondylar fractures in children, *J Pediatr Orfthop* 37:e229, 2017.

Spencer HT, Wong M, Fong YJ, et al.: Prospective longitudinal evaluation of elbow motion following pediatric supracondylar humeral fractures, *J Bone Joint Surg* 92A:904, 2010.

Srikumaran U, Tan EW, Erkula G, et al.: Pin size influences sagittal alignment in percutaneously pinned pediatric supracondylar humerus fractures, *J Pediatr Orthop* 30:792, 2010.

Teo TL, Schaeffer EK, Habib E, et al.: Assessing the reliability of the modified Gartland classification system for extension-type supracondylar humerus fractures, *J Child Orthop* 13:569, 2019.

Valencia M, Moraleda L, Diez-Sebastian J: Long-term functional results of neurological complications of pediatric humeral supracondylar fractures, *J Pediatr Orthop* 35:606, 2015.

Wang JH, Morris WZ, Bafus BT, et al.: Pediatric supracondylar humerus fractures: AAOS Appropriate Use Criteria versus actual management at a pediatric Level 1 trauma center, *J Pediatr Orthop* 39:e578, 2019.

Wegmann H, Eberl R, Kraus T, et al.: The impact of arterial vessel injuries associated with pediatric supracondylar humeral fractures, *J Trauma Acute Care Surg* 77:381, 2014.

Weiss JM, Kay RM, Waters P, et al.: Distal humerus osteotomy for supracondylar fracture malunion in children: a study of perioperative complications, *Am J Orthop (Belle Mead NJ)* 39:22, 2010.

Weller A, Garg S, Larson AN, et al.: Management of the pediatric pulseless supracondylar humeral fracture: is vascular exploration necessary? *J Bone Joint Surg* 95A:2013, 1906.

White L, Mehlman CT, Crawford AH: Perfused, pulseless, and puzzling: a systematic review of vascular injuries in pediatric supracondylar humerus fractures and results of a POSNA questionnaire, *J Pediatr Orthop* 30:328, 2010.

Woratanarat P, Angsanuntsukh C, Rattanasiri S, et al.: Meta-analysis of pinning in supracondylar fracture of the humerus in children, *J Orthop Trauma* 26:48, 2011.

Zusman NL, Barney NA, Halsey MF, et al.: Utility of follow-up radiographs after pin removal in supracondylar humerus fractures: a retrospective cohort study, *J Am Acad Orthop Surg*, 2019 May 29, [Epub ahead of print].

LATERAL CONDYLAR FRACTURES

Beaty JH: Fractures of the lateral humeral condyle are the second most frequent elbow fracture in children, *J Orthop Trauma* 24:438, 2010.

Bernthal NM, Hoshino CM, Dichter D, et al.: Recovery of elbow motion following pediatric lateral condylar fractures of the humerus, *J Bone Joint Surg* 93A:871, 2011.

Bland DC, Pennock AT, Upasani VV, et al.: Measurement reliability in pediatric lateral condyle fractures of the humerus, *J Pediatr Orthop* 38:e439, 2018.

Conaway WK, Hennrikus WL, Ravanbakhsh S, et al.: Surgical treatemt of displaced pediatric lateral condyle fractures of the humerus by the posterior approach, *J Pediatr Orthop B* 27:128, 2018.

Franks D, Shatrov J, Symes M, et al.: Cannulated screw versus Kirschner-wire fixation for Milch II lateral condyle fractures in a paediatric sawbone model: a biomechanical comparison, *J Child Orthop* 12:29, 2018.

Greenhill DA, Funk S, Elliott M, et al.: Minimally displaced humeral lateral condyle fractures: immobilize or operate when stability is unclear? *J Pediatr Orthop* 39:e349, 2019.

Knapik DM, Gilmore A, Liu RW: Conservative management of minimally displaced (≤2 mm) fractures of the lateral humeral condyle in pediatric patients: a systematic review, *J Pediatric Orthop* 37:e83, 2017.

Koh KH, Seo SW, Kim KM, Shim JS: Clinical and radiographic results of lateral condylar fracture of distal humerus in children, *J Pediatr Orthop* 30:425, 2010.

Pace JL, Arkader A, Sousa T, et al.: Incidence, risk factors, and definition for nonunion in pediatric lateral condyle fractures, *J Pediatr Orthop* 38:e257, 2018.

Shabtai L, Lightdale-Miric N, Rounds A, et al.: Incidence, risk factors and outcomes of avascular necrosis occurring after humeral lateral condyle fractures, *J Pediatr Orthop B*, 2019 Dec 9, [Epub ahead of print].

Silva M, Paredes A, Sadlik G: Outcomes of ORIF >7 days after injury in displaced pediatric lateral condyle fractures, *J Pediatr Orthop* 37:234, 2017.

Sinikumpu JJ, Pokka T, Victorzon S, et al.: Paediatric lateral humeral condylar fracture outcomes at twelve years follow-up as compared with age and sex matched paired controls, *Int Orthop* 41:1453, 2017.

Song KS, Shin YW, Oh CW, et al.: Closed reduction and internal fixation of completely displaced and rotated lateral condyle fractures of the humerus in children, *J Orthop Trauma* 24:434, 2010.

Stein BE, Ramji AF, Hassanzadeh H, et al.: Cannulated lag screw fixation of displaced lateral humeral condyle fractures is associated with lower rates of open reduction and infection than pin fixation, *J Pediatric Orthop* 37:7, 2017.

Tan SHS, Dartnell J, Lim AKS, et al.: Paediatric lateral condyle fractures: a systematic review, *Arch Orthop Trauma Surg* 138:809, 2019.

Thévenin-Lemoine C, Salanne S, Pham T, et al.: Relevance of MRI for management of non-displaced lateral humeral condyle fractures in children, *Orthop Traumatol Surg Res* 103:777, 2017.

Wormald JCR, Park CY, Eastwood DM: A systematic review and meta-analysis of adverse outcomes following non-buried versus buried Kirschner wires for paediatric lateral condyle elbow fractures, *J Child Ortho* 11:465, 2017.

Zale C, Winthrop ZA, Hennrikus W: Rate of displacement for Jakob type 1 lateral condyle fractures treated with a cast, *J Child Orthop* 12:117, 2018.

MEDIAL EPICONDYLAR AND MEDIAL HUMERAL CONDYLAR FRACTURES

Biggers MD, Bert TM, Moisan A, et al.: Fracture of the medial humeral epicondyle in children: a comparison of operative and nonoperative management, *J Surg Orthop Adv* 24:188, 2015.

Cao J, Smetana BS, Carry P, et al.: A pediatric medial epicondyle fracture cadaveric study comparing standard AP radiographic view with the distal humerus axial view, *J Pediatr Orthop* 39:e205, 2019.

Dodds SD, Flanagin BA, Bohl DD, et al.: Incarcerated medial epicondyle fracture following pediatric elbow dislocation: 11 cases, *J Hand Surg Am* 39:1739, 2014.

Edmonds EW: How displaced are "nondisplaced" fractures of the medial humeral epicondyle in children? Results of a three-dimensional computed tomography analysis, *J Bone Joint Surg* 92A:2785, 2010.

Fernandez FF, Vatlach S, Wirth T, et al.: Medial humeral condye fracture in childhood: a rare but often overlooked injury, *Eur J Trauma Emerg Surg* 45:757, 2019.

Gottschalk HP, Bastrom TP, Edmonds EW: Reliability of internal oblique elbow radiographs for measuring displacement of medial epicondyle humerus fractures: a cadaveric study, *J Pediatr Orthop* 33:26, 2013.

Haflah NH, Ibrahim S, Sapuan J, Abdullah S: An elbow dislocation in a child with missed medial epicondyle fracture and late ulnar nerve palsy, *J Pediatr Orthop B* 19:459, 2010.

Hughes M, Dua K, O'Hara NN, et al.: Variation among pediatric orthopaedic surgeons when treating medial epicondyle fractures, *J Pediatr Orthop* 39:e592, 2019.

Knapik DM, Fausett CL, Gilmore A, et al.: Outcomes of nonoperative pediatric medial humeral epicondyle fractures with and without associated elbow dislocation, *J Pediatr Orthop* 37:e224, 2017.

Osbahr DC, Chalmers PN, Frank JS, et al.: Acute avulsion fractures of the medial epicondyle while throwing in youth baseball players: a variant of Little League elbow, *J Shoulder Elbow Surg* 19:951, 2010.

Pace GI, Hennrikus WL: Fixation of displaced medial epicondyle fractures in adolescent, *J Pediatr Orthop* 37:e80, 2017.

Pappas N, Lawrence JT, Donegan D, et al.: Intraobserver and interobserver agreement in the measurement of displaced humeral medial epicondyle fractures in children, *J Bone Joint Surg* 92A:322, 2010.

Park KB, Kwak YH: Treatment of medial epicondyle fracture without associated elbow dislocation in older children and adolescents, *Yonsei Med J* 53:1190, 2012.

Rigal J, Thelen T, Angelliaume A, et al.: A new procedure for fractures of the medial epicondyle in children: Mitek* bone suture anchor, *Orthop Traumatol Surg Res* 102:117, 2016.

Souder CD, Faarnsworth CL, McNeil NP, et al.: The distal humerus axial view: assessment of displacement in medial epicondyle fractures, *J Pediatr Orthop* 35:449, 2015.

Stepanovich M, Bastrom TP, Munch 3rd J, et al.: Does operative fixation affect outcomes of displaced medial epicondyle fractures? *J Child Orthop* 10:413, 2016.

Vuillermin C, Donohue KS, Miller P, et al.: Incarcerated medial epicondyle fractures with elbow dislocation: risk factors associated with morbidity, *J Pediatr Orthop* 39:e647, 2019.

ELBOW JOINT FRACTURES AND DISLOCATIONS

Ackerson R, Nguyen A, Carry PM, et al.: Intra-articular radial head fractures in the skeletally immature patient: complications and management, *J Pediatr Orthop* 35:443, 2015.

Badoi A, Frech-Dörfler M, et al.: Influence of immobilization time of functional outcome in radial neck fractures in children, *Eur J Pediatr Surg* 26:514, 2016.

Bexkens R, Washburn FJ, Eygendaal D, et al.: Effectiveness of reduction maneuvers in the treatment of nursemaid's elbow: a systematic review and meta-analysis, *Am J Emerg Med* 35:159, 2017.

Choi WS, Han KJ, Lee DH, et al.: Stepwise percutaneous leverage technique to avoid posterior interosseous nerve injury in pediatric radial neck fracture, *J Orthop Trauma* 31:e151, 2017.

Dizdarevic I, Low S, Currie DW, et al.: Epidemiology of elbow dislocations in high school athletes, *Am J Sports Med* 44:202, 106.

Eberl R, Singer G, Fruhmann J, et al.: Intramedullary nailing for the treatment of dislocated pediatric radial neck fractures, *Eur J Pediatr Surg* 20:250, 2010.

Ek ET, Paul SK, Hotchkiss RN: Outcomes after operative treatment of elbow contractures in the pediatric and adolescent population, *J Shoulder Elbow Surg* 25:2066, 2016.

Elanti P, O'Farrell D: Iatrogenic radial neck fracture on closed reduction of elbow dislocation, *CJEM* 15:389, 2013.

Falciglia F, Giordano M, Aulisa AG, et al.: Radial neck fractures in children: results when open reduction is indicated, *J Pediatr Orthop* 34:756, 2014.

Furushima K, Itoh Y, Iwabu S, et al.: Classification of olecranon stress fractures in baseball players, *Am J Sports Med* 42:NP44, 2014.

Fuller CB, Guillen PT, Wongworawat MD, et al.: Bioabsorbable pin fixation in late presenting pediatric radial neck fractures, *J Pediatr Orthop* 36:793, 2016.

Gutiérrez-de la Iglesia D, Pérez-López LM, Cabrera-González M, Knörr-Giménez J: Surgical techniques for displaced radial neck fractures: predictive factors of functional results, *J Pediatr Orthop* 37:159, 2017.

Guyonnet C, Martins A, Marengo L, et al.: Functional outcome of displaced radial head fractures in children treated by elastic stable intramedullary nailing, *J Pediatr Orthop B* 27:296, 2018.

Jo AR, Jung ST, Kim MS, et al.: An evaluation of forearm deformities in hereditary multiple exostoses: factors associated with radial head dislocation and comprehensive classification, *J Hand Surg Am* 42:292, 2017.

Kalem M, Sahin E, Kocaoglu H, et al.: Comparison of two closed surgical techniques at isolated pediatric radial neck fractures, *Injury* 49:618, 2018.

Modi P, Dhammi IK, Rustagi A, Jain AK: Elbow dislocation with ipsilateral diaphyseal fractures of radius and ulna in an adult-is it type 1 or type 2 Monteggia equivalent lesion? *Chin J Traumatol* 15:303, 2012.

Murphy RF, Vuillermin C, Naqvi M, et al.: Early outcomes of pediatric elbow dislocation—risk factors associated with morbidity, *J Pediatr Orthop* 37:440, 2017.

Nussberger G, Schädelin S, Mayr J, et al.: Treatment strategy and long-term functional outcome of traumatic elbow dislocation in childhood: a single centre study, *J Child Orthop* 12:129, 2018.

Paci JM, Dugas JR, Guy JA, et al.: Cannulated screw fixation of refractory olecranon stress fractures with and without associated injuries allows a return to baseball, *Am J Sports Med* 41:306, 2013.

Rosenbaum AJ, Leonard GR, Uhl RL, et al.: Radiologic case study. Diagnosis: congenital posterior dislocation of the radial head, *Orthopedics* 37:62, 2014.

Shabtai L, Arkader A: Percutaneous reduction of displaced radial neck fractures achieves better results compared with fractures treated by open reduction, *J Pediatr Orthop* 36:S63, 2016.

Silva M, Cooper SD, Cha A: Elbow dislocation with an associated lateral condyle fracture of the humerus: a rare occurrence in the pediatric population, *J Pediatr Orthop* 35:329, 2015.

Singh V, Dey S, Parikh SN: Missed diagnosis and acute management of radial head dislocation with plastic deformation of ulna in children, *J Pediatr Orthop*, 2020 Jan 7, [Epub ahead of print].

Su Y, Xie Y, Qin J, et al.: Internal fixation with absorbable rods for the treatment of displaced radial neck fractures in children, *J Pediatr Orthop* 36:797, 2016.

Van Zeeland NL, Bae DS, Goldfarb CA: Intra-articular radial head fracture in the skeletally immature patient: progressive radial head subluxation and rapid radiocapitellar degeneration, *J Pediatr Orthop* 31:124, 2011.

Weigelt L, Fürnstahl P, Schweizer A: Computer-assisted corrective osteotomy of malunited pediatric radial neck fractures—three-dimensional postoperative accuracy and clinical outcome, *J Orthop Trauma* 31:e436, 2017.

Wong K, Troncoso AB, Calello DP, et al.: Radial head subluxation: factors associated with its recurrence and radiographic evaluation in a tertiary pediatric emergency department, *J Emerg Med* 51:621, 2016.

Yoon HK, Seo GW: Proximal radioulnar translocation associated with elbow dislocation and radial neck fracture in child: a case report and review of the literature, *Arch Orthop Trauma Surg* 133:1425, 2013.

FOREARM FRACTURES/MONTEGGIA FRACTURES

Abraham A, Kumar S, Chaudhry S, Ibrahim T: Surgical interventions for diaphyseal fractures of the radius and ulna in children, *Cochrane Database Syst Rev* 11:CD007907, 2011.

Acree JS, Schlechter J, Buzin S: Cost analysis and performance in distal pediatric forearm fractures: is a short-arm cast superior to a sugar-tong splint? *J Pediatr Orthop B* 26:424, 2017.

Asadollahi S, Pourale M, Heidari K: Predictive factors for re-displacement in diaphyseal forearm fractures in children—role of radiographic indices, *Acta Ortho* 88:101, 2017.

Auer RT, Mazzone P, Robinson L, et al.: Childhood obesity increases the risk of failure in the treatment of distal forearm fractures, *J Pediatr Orthop* 36:e86, 2016.

Bae DS, Valim C, Connell P, et al.: Bivalved versus circumferential cast immobilization for displaced forearm fractures: a randomized clinical trial to assess efficacy and safety, *J Pediatr Orthop* 37:239, 2017.

Baldwin K, Morrison 3rd MJ, Tomlinson LA, et al.: Both bone forearm fractures in children and adolescents, which fixation strategy is superior – plates or nails? A systematic review and meta-analysis of observational studies, *J Orthop Trauma* 28:38, 2014.

Baldwin 3rd PC, Han E, Parrino A, et al.: Valve or no valve: a prospective randomized controlled trial of casting options for pediatric forearm fractures, *Orthopedics* 40:e849, 2017.

Blumberg TJ, Bremjit P, Bompadre V, et al.: Forearm fixation is not necessary in the treatment of pediatric floating elbow, *J Pediatr Orthop* 38:82, 2018.

Bowman EN, Mehlman CT, Lindsell CJ, Tamai J: Nonoperative treatment of both-bone forearm shaft fractures in children: predictors of early radiographic failure, *J Pediatr Orthop* 31:23, 2011.

Chen HY, Wu KW, Dong ZR, et al.: The treatment of chronic radial head dislocation in Monteggia fracture without annular ligament reconstruction, *Int Orthop* 42:2165, 2018.

Devendra A, Velmurugesan PS, Dheenadhayalan J, et al.: One-bone forearm reconstruction: a salvage solution for the forearm with massive bone loss, *J Bone Joint Surg Am* 101:e74, 2019.

Dietz JF, Bae DS, Reigg E, et al.: Single bone intramedullary fixation of the ulna in pediatric both bone forearm fractures: analysis of short-term clinical and radiographic results, *J Pediatr Orthop* 30:420, 2010.

Douma-den Hamer D, Blanker MH, Edens MA, et al.: Ultrasound for distal forearm fracture: a systematic review and diagnostic meta-analysis, *PLoS Oe* 11:e0155659, 2016.

Dua K, Stein MK, O'Hara NN, et al.: Variation among pediatric orthopaedic surgeons when diagnosing and treating pediatric and adolescent distal radius fractures, *J Pediatr Orthop* 39:306, 2019.

Eismann EA, Parikh SN, Jain VV: Rereduction for redisplacement of both-bone forearm shaft fractures in children, *J Pediatr Orthop* 36:405, 2016.

Fernandez FF, Langendörfer M, Wirth T, Eberhardt O: Failures and complications in intramedullary nailing of children's forearm fractures, *J Child Orthop* 4:159, 2010.

Flynn JM, Jones KJ, Garner MR, Goebel J: Eleven years experience in the operative management of pediatric forearm fractures, *J Pediatr Orthop* 30:313, 2010.

Foran I, Upasani VV, Wallace CD, et al.: Acute pediatric Monteggia fractures: a conservative approach to stabilization, *J Pediatr Orthop* 37:e335, 2017.

Goodman AD, Zonfrillo M, Chiou D, et al.: The cost and utility of postreduction radiographs after closed reduction of pediatric wrist and forearm fractures, *J Pediatr Orthop* 39:e8, 2019.

Goyal T, Arora SS, Banerjee S, Kandwal P: Neglected Monteggia fracture dislocations in children: a systematic review, *J Pediatr Orthop B* 24:191, 2015.

Heare A, Goral D, Belton M, et al.: Intramedullary implant choice and cost in the treatment of pediataric diaphyseal forearm fractures, *J Orthop Trauma* 31:e334, 2017.

Ho CA, Jarcis DL, Phelps JR, Wilson PL: Delayed union in internal fixation of pediatric both-bone forearm fractures, *J Pediatr Orthop B* 22:383, 2013.

Kang SB, Mangwani J, Ramachandran M, et al.: Elastic intramedullary nailing of paediatric fractures of the forearm: a decade of experience in a teaching hospital in the United Kingdom, *J Bone Joint Surg* 93B:262, 2011.

Katzer C, Wasem J, Eckert K, et al.: Ultrasound in the diagnostics of metaphyseal forearm fractures in children: a systematic review and cost calculation, *Pediatr Emerg Care* 32:401, 2016.

Kim CY, Gentry M, Sala D, et al.: Single-bone intramedullary nailing of pediatric both-bone forearm fractures: a systematic review, *Bull Hosp Jt Dis* 75:227, 2017.

Ko C, Baird M, Close M, et al.: The diagnostic accuracy of ultrasound in detecting distal radius fractures in a pediatric population, *Clin J Sport Med* 29:426, 2019.

Kruppa C, Bunge P, Schildhauer TA, et al.: Low complication rate of elastic stable intramedullary nailing (ESIN) of pediatric forearm fractures: a retrospective study of 202 cases, *Medicine (Baltimore)* 96:e6669, 2017.

Kuba MHM, Izuyka BH: One brace: one visit: treatment of pediatric distal radius buckle fractures with a removable wrist brace and no follow-up visit, *J Pediatr Orthop* 38:e338, 2018.

Kutsikovich JI, Hopkins CM, Gannon 3ed EW, et al.: Factors that predict instability in pediatric diaphyseal both-bone forearm fractures, *J Pediatr Orthop B* 27:304, 2018.

Luther G, Miller P, Waters PM, et al.: Radiographic evaluation during treatment of pediatric forearm fractures: implications on clinical care and cost, *J Pediatr Orthop* 36:465, 2016.

Nørgaard SL, Riber SS, Danielsson FB, et al.: Surgical approach for elastic stable intramedullary nail in pediatric radius shaft fracture: a systematic review, *J Pediatr Orthop B* 27:309, 2018.

Okoroafor UC, Cannada LK, McGinty JL: Obesity and failure of nonsurgical manaqgement of pediatric both-bone forearm fractures, *J Hand Surg Am* 42:711, 2017.

Paneru SR, Rijal R, Shrestha BP, et al.: Randomized controlled trial comparing above- and below-elbow plaster casts for distal forearm fractures in children, *J Child Orthop* 4:233, 2010.

Park H, Park KW, Park KB, et al.: Impact of open reduction on surgical strategies for missed Monteggia fracture in children, *Yonsei Med J* 58:829, 2017.

Price CT: Acceptable alignment of forearm fractures in children: open reduction indications, *J Pediatr Orthop* 30:S82, 2010.

Ramski DE, Hennrikus WP, Bae DS, et al.: Pediatric Monteggia fractures: a multicenter examination of treatment strategy and early clinical and radiographic results, *J Pediatr Orthop* 35:115, 2015.

Runyon RS, Doyle SM: When is it ok to use a splint versus case and what remodeling can one expect for common pediatric forearm fractures, *Curr Opin Pediatr* 29:46, 2017.

Saglam Y, Kizildag H, Toprak G, et al.: Prevalence of vitamin D insufficiency in children with forearm fractures, *J Child Orthop* 11:180, 2017.

Saul T, Ng L, Lewis RE: Point-of-care ultrasound in the diagnosis of upper extremity fracture-dislocation. A pictorial essay, *Med Ultrason* 15:230, 2013.

Sferopoulos NK: Monteggia type IV equivalent injury, *Open Orthop J* 5:198, 2011.

Sferopoulos NK: Segmental forearm bone injuries in children: classification and treatment, *J Orthop Traumatol* 17:215, 2016.

Shah AS, Lesniak BP, Wolter TD, et al.: Stabilization of adolescent both-bone forearm fractures: a comparison of intramedullary nailing versus open reduction and internal fixation, *J Orthop Trauma* 24:440, 2010.

Sinikumpu JJ, Pokka T, Serlo W: The changing pattern of pediatric both bone forearm shaft fractures among 86,000 children from 1997 to 2009, *Eur J Pediatr Surg* 23:289, 2013.

Ting ML, Kalish LA, Waters PM, et al.: Reducing cost and radiation exposure during the treatment of pediatric greenstick fractures of the forearm, *J Pediatr Orthop* 36:816, 2016.

Tisosky AJ, Werger MM, McPartland TG, et al.: The factors influencing the refracture of pediatric fractures, *J Pediatr Orthop* 35:677, 2015.

Van Tongel A, Ackerman P, Liekens K, Berghs B: Angulated greenstick fractures of the distal forearm in children: closed reduction by pronation or supination, *Acta Orthop Belg* 77:21, 2011.

Varga M, Józsa G, Fadgyas B, et al.: Short, double elastic nailing of severely displaced distal pediatric radial fractures: a new mthod for stable fixation, *Medicine (Baltimore)* 96:e6532, 2017.

Zhao L, Wang B, Bai X, et al.: Plate fixation versus intramedullary nailing for both-bone forearm fractures: a meta-analysis of randomized controlled trials and cohort studies, *World J Surg* 41:722, 2017.

Zheng W, Tao Z, Chen C, et al.: Comparison of three surgical fixation methods for dual-bone forearm fractures in older children: a retrospective cohort study, *Int J Surg* 51:10, 2018.

HAND AND WRIST FRACTURES, DISLOCATIONS, AND FRACTURE-DISLOCATIONS

Abzug JM, Kozin SH: Seymour fractures, *J Hand Surg Am* 38:2267, 2013.

Abzug JM, Little K, Kozin SH: Physeal arrest of the distal radius, *J Am Acad Orthop Surg* 22:381, 2014.

Al-Qattan MM, Al-Qattan AM: A review of phalangeal neck fractures in children, *Injury* 46:935, 2015.

Bae DS, Gholson JJ, Zurakowski D, et al.: Functional outcomes after treatment of scaphoid fractures in children and adolescents, *J Pediatr Orthop* 36:13, 2016.

Chew EM, Chong AK: Hand fractures in children: epidemiology and misdiagnosis in a tertiary referral hospital, *J Hand Surg Am* 37:1684, 2012.

Davison PG, Boudreau N, Burrows R, et al.: Forearm-based ulnar gutter versus hand-based thermoplastic splint for pediatric metacarpal neck fractures: a blinded, randomized trial, *Plast Reconstr Surg* 137:908, 2016.

Dua K, Stein MK, O'Hara NN, et al.: Variation among pediatric orthopaedic surgeons when diagnosing and treating pediatric and adolescent distal radius fractures, *J Pediatr Orthop* 39:306, 2019.

Gholson JJ, Bae DS, Zurakowski D, Waters PM: Scaphoid fractures in children and adolescents: contemporary injury patterns and factors influencing time to union, *J Bone Joint Surg* 93A:1210, 2011.

Johnson BK, Brou L, Fields SK, et al.: *Hand and wrist injuries among US high school athletes: 2005/06-2015/16, Pediatrics* 140: pii:e20171255, 2017.

Jørgsholm P, Thomsen N, Besjakov J, et al.: MRI shows a high incidence of carpal fractures in children with posttraumatic radial-sided wrist tenderness, *Acta Orthop* 87:533, 2016.

Kadar A, Morsy M, Sur YJ, et al.: Capitate fractures: a review of 53 patients, *J Hand Surg Am* 10:e359, 2016.

Korhonen L, Victorzon S, Serlo W, et al.: Non-union of the ulnar styloid process in children is common but long-term morbidity is rare: a population-based study with mean 11 years (9-15) follow-up, *Acta Orthop* 90:383, 2019.

Krusche-Mandl I, Köttstorfer J, Thalhammer G, et al.: Seymour fractures: retrospective analysis and therapeutic considerations, *J Hand Surg Am* 38:258, 2013.

Offiah AC, Burke D: The diagnostic accuracy of cross-sectional imaging for detecting acute scaphoid fractures in children: a systematic review, *Br J Radiol* 91:20170883, 2018.

Park KB, Lee KJ, Kwak YH: Comparison between buddy taping with a short-arm splint and operative treatment for phalangeal neck fractures in children, *J Pediatr Orthop* 36:736, 2016.

Porter J, Porter R, Chan KJ: Scaphoid fractures in children: do we need to x-ray? A retrospective chart review of 144 wrists, *Pediaatr Emerg Care*, 2018 Mar 12, [Epub ahead of print].

Reyes BA, Ho CA: The high risk of infection with delayed treatment of open Seymour fractures: Salter-Harris I/II or juxta-epiphyseal fractures of the distal phalanx with associated nailbed laceration, *J Pediatr Orthop* 37:247, 2017.

Shah NS, Buzas D, Zinberg EM: Epidemiologic dynamics contributing to pediatric wrist fractures in the United States, *Hand (N Y)* 10:266, 2015.

Shaterian A, Santos PJF, Lee CJ, et al.: Management modalities and outcomes following acute scaphoid fractures in children: a quantitative review and meta-analysis, *Hand (N Y)* 14:305, 2019.

SPINE FRACTURES AND DISLOCATIONS

Andras LM, Skaggs KF, Badkoobehi H, et al.: Chance fractures in the pediatric population are often misdiagnosed, *J Pediatr Orthop* 39:222, 2019.

Arkader A, Warner Jr WC, Tolo VT, et al.: Pediatric Chance fractures: a multicenter perspective, *J Pediatr Orthop* 31:741, 2011.

Astur N, Sawyer JR, Klimo Jr P, et al.: Traumatic atlanto-occipital dislocation in children, *J Am Acad Orthop Surg* 22:274, 2014.

Astur N, Klimo Jr P, Sawyer JR, et al.: Traumatic atlanto-occipital dislocation in children: evaluation, treatment, and outcomes, *J Bone Joint Surg* 95A:e194, 2013.

Boese CK, Oppermann J, Siewe J, et al.: Spinal cord injury without radiologic abnormality in children: a systematic review and meta-analysis, *J Trauma Acute Care Surg* 78:874, 2015.

Copley PC, Tilliridou V, Kirby A, et al.: Management of cervical spine trauma in children, *Eur J Trauma Emerg Surg* 45:777, 2019.

Dauleac C, Beuriat PA, Di Rocco F, et al.: Surgical management of pediatric spine trauma: 12 years of experience, *World Neurosurg* 126:e1494, 2019.

Falavigna A, Righesso O, Gaurise da Silva P, et al.: Epidemiology and management of spinal trauma in children and adolescents <18 years old, *World Neurosurg* 110:e479, 2018.

Franklin 3rd DB, Hardaway AT, Sheffer BW, et al.: The role of computed tomography and magnetic resonance imaging in the diagnosis of pediatric thoracolumbar compression fractures, *J Pediatr Orthop* 39:e520, 2019.

Jeszensky D, Fekete TF, Lattig F, Bognár L: Intraarticular atlantooccipital fusion for the treatment of traumatic occipitocervical dislocation in a child: a new technique for selective stabilization with nine years follow-up, *Spine* 35:E421, 2010.

Kempen DHR, Delawi D, Altena MC, et al.: Neurological outcome after traumatic transverse sacral fractures: a systematic review of 521 patients reported in the literature, *Spine* 44:17, 2019.

Knox JB, Schneider JE, Cage JM, et al.: Spine trauma in a very young children: a retrospective study of 206 patients presenting to a level 1 pediatric trauma center, *J Pediatr Orthop* 34:698, 2014.

Leonard JC, Browne LR, Ahmad FA, et al.: Cervical spine injury risk factors in children with blunt trauma, *Pediatrics* 144. Pii:3e201183221, 2019.

Murphy RF, Davidson AR, Kelly DM, et al.: Subaxial cervical spine injuries in children and adolescents, *J Pediatr Orthop* 35:136, 2015.

Rush JK, Kelly DM, Astur N, et al.: Associated injuries in children and adolescents with spinal trauma, *J Pediatr Orthop* 33:393, 2013.

PELVIC AND HIP FRACTURES AND DISORDERS

Amorosa LF, Kloen P, Helfet DL: High-energy pediatric pelvic and acetabular fractures, *Orthop Clin North Am* 45:483, 2014.

Clohisy JC, Oryhon JM, Seyler TM, et al.: Function and fixation of total hip arthroplasty in patients 25 years of age or young, *Clin Orthop Relat Res* 468:3207, 2010.

de ridder VA, Olson SA: Operative treatment of pediatric pelvic and acetabulum fractures, *J Orthop Trauma* 33(Suppl 8):S33, 2019.

Eberbach H, Hohloch L, Feucht MJ, et al.: Operative versus conservative treatment of apophyseal avulsion fractures of the pelvis in the adolescents: a systematical review with meta-analysis of clinical outcome and return to sports, *BMC Musculoskelet Disord* 18:162, 2017.

Finnegan MA, Insights® CORR: Delayed slipped capital femoral epiphysis after treatment of femoral neck fracture in children, *Clin Orthop Relat Res* 473:2718, 2015.

Ganz R, Horowitz K, Leunig M: Algorithm for femoral and periacetabular osteotomies in complex hip deformities, *Clin Orthop Relat Res* 468:3168, 2010.

Guillaume JM, Pesenti S, Jouve JL, et al.: Pelvic fractures in children (pelvic ring and acetabulum), *Orthop Traumatol Surg Res* 106:S125, 2020.

Guimaraes JA, Mendes PH, Vallim FC, et al.: Surgical treatment for unstable pelvic fractures in skeletally immature patients, *Injury* 45(Suppl 5):S40, 2014.

Harding RJ, Moideen AN, Carpenter EC, et al.: Trochanteric fractures in young children, *Pediatr Emerg Care* 35:e84, 2019.

Herrera-Soto JA, Price CT: Core decompression and labral support for the treatment of juvenile osteonecrosis, *J Pediatr Orthop* 31(Suppl 2):S212, 2011.

Ilizaliturri Jr VM, Gonzalez-Gutierrez B, Gonazalez-Ugalde H, Camacho-Galindo J: Hip arthroscopy after traumatic hip dislocation, *Am J Sports Med* 39(Suppl):50S, 2011.

Kruppa CG, Khoriaty JD, Sietsema DL, et al.: Does skeletal maturity affect pediatric pelvic injury patterns, associated injuries, and treatment intervention? *Injury* 49:1562, 2018.

Manner HM, Mast NH, Ganz R, Leunig M: Potential contribution of femoroacetabular impingement to recurrent traumatic hip dislocation, *J Pediatr Orthop B* 21:574, 2012.

Papalia R, Torre G, Maffulli N, et al.: Hip fractures in children and adolescents, *Br Med Bull* 129:117, 2019.

Rao RD, Berry C, Yoganandan N, et al.: Occupant and crash characteristics in thoracic and lumbar spine injuires resulting from motor vehicle collisions, *Spine J* 14:2355, 2014.

Sen MK, Warner SJ, Sama N, et al.: Treatment of acetabular fractures in adodlescents, *Am J Orthop (Belle Mead MJ)* 44:465, 2015.

Shore BJ, Palmer CS, Bevin C, et al.: Pediatric pelvic fracture: a modification of a preexisting classification, *J Pediatr Orthop* 32:162, 2012.

Spence D, DiMauro JP, Miller PE, et al.: Osteonecrosis after femoral neck fractures in children and adolescents: analysis of risk factors, *J Pediatr Orthop* 36:111, 2015.

Tanaka R, Yasunaga Y, Fujii J, et al.: Transtrochanteric rotational osteotomy for various hip disorders, *J Orthop Sci* 24:463, 2019.

Thanacharoenpanich S, Bixby S, Breen MA, et al.: MRI is better than CT scan for detection of structural pathologies after traumatic posterior hip dislocation in children and adolescents, *J Pediatr Orthop* 40:86, 2020.

Yeranosian M, Horneff JG, Baldwin K, Hosalkar HS: Factors affecting the outcome of fractures of the femoral neck in children and adolescents: a systematic review, *Bone Joint Lett J* 95B:135, 2013.

SLIPPED CAPITAL FEMORAL EPIPHYSIS

Allen MM, Rosenfeld SB: Treatment for post-slipped capital femoral epiphysis deformity, *Orthop Clin North Am* 51:37, 2020.

Azzopardi T, Sharma S, Bennet GC: Slipped capital femoral epiphysis in children aged less than 10 years, *J Pediatr Orthop B* 19:13, 2010.

Daley E, Zaltz I: Strategies to avoid osteonecrosis in unstable slipped capital femoral epiphysis: a critical analysis review, *JBJS Rev* 7:e7, 2019.

Davis 2nd RL, Samora 3rd WP, Persinger F, et al.: Treatment of unstable versus stable slipped capital femoral epiphysis using the modified Dunn procedure, *J Pediatr Orthop* 39:411, 2019.

Georgiadis AG, Zaltz I: Slipped capital femoral epiphysis: how to evaluate with a review and update of treatment, *Pediatr Clin North Am* 61:1119, 2014.

Ghijselings S, Touquet J, Himpe N, et al.: Degenerative changes of the hip following *in situ* fixation for slipped capital femoral epiphysis: a minimum 18-year follow-up study, *Hip Int* Aug 4, 2019, [Epub ahead of print].

Herngren B, Stenmarker M, Enskär K, et al.: Outcomes after slipped capital femoral epiphysis: a population-based study with three-year follow-up, *J Child Orthop* 12:434, 2018.

Lang P, Panchal H, Delfosse EM, et al.: The outcome of in-situ fixation of unstable slipped capital femoral epiphysis, *J Pediatr Orthop B* 28:452q, 2019.

Liu RW, Armstrong DG, Levine AD, et al.: An anatomic study of the epiphyseal tubercle and its importance in the pathogenesis of slipped capital femoral epiphysis, *J Bone Joint Surg* 95A:e341, 2013.

Matthew SE, Larson AN: Natural history of slipped capital femoral epiphysis, *J Pediatr Orthop* 39(6 (Suppl 1):S23, 2019.

Merz MK, Amirouche F, Solitro GF, et al.: Biomechanical comparison of perpendicular versus oblique in situ screw fixation of slipped capital femoral epiphysis, *J Pediatr Orthop* 35:816, 2014.

Napora JK, Gilmore A, Son-Hing JP, et al.: Early MRI detection and closed bone graft epiphysiodesis may alter the course of avascular necrosis following unstable slipped capital femoral epiphysis, *J Pediatr Orthop* 38:202, 2018.

Novais EN, Hill MK, Carry PM, Heare TC, Sink EL: Modified Dunn procedure is superior to in situ pinning for short-term clinical and radiographic improvement in severe stable SCFE, *Clin Orthop Relat Res* 473:2108, 2015.

Obana KK, Siddiqui AA, Broom AM, et al.: Slipped capital femoral epiphysis in children without obesity, *J Pediatr*, 2020 Jan 16, [Epub ahead of print].

Palocaren T, Holmes L, Rogers K, Kumar SJ: Outcome of in situ pinning in patients with unstable slipped capital femoral epiphysis: assessment of risk factors associated with avascular necrosis, *J Pediatr Orthop* 30:31, 2010.

Perry DC, Metcalfe D, Lane S, et al.: Childhood obesity and slipped capital femoral epiphysis, *Pediatrics* 142:e20181067, 2018.

Sankar WN, Brighton BK, Kim YJ, et al.: Acetabular morphology in slipped capital femoral epiphysis, *J Pediatr Orthop* 31:254, 2011.

Sankar WN, Novais EN, Lee C, et al.: What are the risks of prophylactic pinning to prevent contralateral slipped capital femoral epiphysis? *Clin Orthop Relat Res* 471:2118, 2013.

Sankar WN, Vanderhave KL, Matheney T, et al.: The modified Dunn procedure for unstable slipped capital femoral epiphysis: a multicenter perspective, *J Bone Joint Surg* 95A:585, 2013.

Shank CF, Thiel EF, Klingele KE: Valgus slipped capital femoral epiphysis: prevalence, presentation, and treatment options, *J Pediatr Orthop* 30:140, 2010.

Swarup I, Goodbody C, Goto R, et al.: Risk factors for contralateral slipped capital femoral epiphysis: a meta-analysis of cohort and case-control studies, *J Pediatr Orthop*, 2019 Dec 10, [Epub ahead of print].

Trisolino G, Pagliazzi G, De Gennaro GL, et al.: Long-term results of combined epiphysiodesis and Imhauser intertrochanteric osteotomy in SCFE: a retrospective study on 53 hips, *J Pediatr Orthop* 37:409, 2017.

Woelfle JV, Fraitzl CR, Reichel H, et al.: The asymptomatic contralateral hip in unilateral slipped capital femoral epiphysis: morbidity of prophylactic fixation, *J Pediatr Orthop B* 21:226, 2012.

Ziebarth K, Leunig M, Slongo T, et al.: Slipped capital femoral epiphysis: relevant pathophysiological findings with open surgery, *Clin Orthop Relat Res* 471:2156, 2013.

FEMORAL FRACTURES

American Academy of Orthopaedic Surgeons: Guideline on the treatment of pediatric diaphyseal femur fractures. www.aaos.org/research/guidelines/PDFFguideline.asp.

Anastasopoulos J, Petratos D, Konstantoulakis C, et al.: Flexible intramedullary nailing in paediatric femoral shaft fractures, *Injury* 41:578, 2010.

Baldwin K, Hsu JE, Wenger DR, Hosalkar HS: Treatment of femur fractures in school-aged children using elastic stable intramedullary nailing: a systematic review, *J Pediatr Orthop B* 20:303, 2011.

Barreto Rocha DF, Horwitz DS, Sintenie JB: Femoral neck fractures in children: issues, challenges, and solutions, *J Orthop Trauma* 33(Suppl 8):S27, 2019.

Crosby SN, Kim EJ, Koehler DM, et al.: Twenty-year experience with rigid intramedullary nailing of femoral shaft, *J Bone Joint Surg* 96A:1080, 2014.

Flynn JM, Garner MR, Jones KJ, et al.: The treatment of low-energy femoral shaft fractures: a prospective study comparing the "walking spica" with the traditional spica, *J Bone Joint Surg* 93A:2196, 2011.

Garner MR, Bhat SB, Khujanazarov I, et al.: Fixation of length-stable femoral shaft fractures in heavier children: flexible nails vs rigid locked nails, *J Pediatr Orthop* 31:11, 2011.

Garrett BR, Hoffman EB, Carrara H: The effect of percutaneous pin fixation in the treatment of distal femoral physeal fractures, *J Bone Joint Surg* 93B:689, 2011.

Heffernan MJ, Gordon JE, Sabatini CS, et al.: Treatment of femur fractures in young children: a multicenter comparison of flexible intramedullary nails to spica casting in young children aged 2 to 6 years, *J Pediatr Orthop* 35:126, 2015.

Heyworth BE, Hedequist DJ, Nasreddine AY, et al.: Distal femoral valgus deformity following plate fixation of pediatric femoral shaft fractures, *J Bone Joint Surg* 95A:526, 2013.

Hosalkar HS, Pandya NK, Cho RH, et al.: Intramedullary nailing of pediatric femoral shaft fracture, *J Am Acad Orthop Surg* 19:472, 2011.

Hubbard EW, Thompson RM, Jo CH, et al.: Retrograde stainless steel flexible nails have superior resistance to bending in distal third femoral shaft fractures, *J Pediatr Orthop* 39:e258, 2019.

MacNeil JA, Francis A, El-Hawary R: A systematic review of rigid, locked intramedullary nail insertion sites and avascular necrosis of the femoral head in the skeletally immature, *J Pediatr Orthop* 31:377, 2011.

Memeo A, Panuccio E, D'Amato RD, et al.: Retrospective, multicenter evaluation of complications in the treatment of diaphyseal femur fractures in pediatric patients, *Injury* 50(Suppl 4):S60, 2019.

Murphy R, Kelly DM, Moisan A, et al.: Transverse fractures of the femoral shaft are a better predictor of nonaccidental trauma in young children than spiral fractures are, *J Bone Joint Surg* 97A:106, 2015.

Patterson JT, Tangtiphaboontana J, Pandya NK: Management of pediatric femoral neck fracture, *J Am Acad Orthop Surg* 26:411, 2018.

Ramseier LE, Janicki JA, Weir S, Narayanan UG: Femoral fractures in adolescents: a comparison of four methods of fixation, *J Bone Joint Surg* 92A:1122, 2010.

Roaten JD, Kelly DM, Yellin JL, et al.: Pediatric femoral shaft fractures: a multicenter review of the AAOS Clinical Practice Guidelines before and after 2009, *J Pediatr Orthop* 39:394, 2019.

Rush JK, Kelly DM, Sawyer JR, et al.: Treatment of pediatric femur fractures with the Pavlik harness: multiyear clinical and radiographic outcomes, *J Pediatr Orthop* 33:614, 2013.

Sagan ML, Datta JC, Olney BW, et al.: Residual deformity after treatment of pediatric femur fractures with flexible titanium nails, *J Pediatr Orthop* 30:638, 2010.

Sargent MC: Single-leg spica cast application for treatment of pediatric femoral fracture, *JBJS Essent Surg Tech* 7:e26, 2017.

Siddiqui AA, Abousamra O, Compton E, et al.: Titanium elastic nails are a safe and effective treatment for length unstable pediatric femur fractures, *J Pediatr Orthop* Nov 22, 2019, [Epub ahead of print].

Sink EL, Faro F, Polousky J, et al.: Decreased complications of pediatric femur fractures with a change in management, *J Pediatr Orthop* 30:633, 2010.

Wang WT, Li YQ, Guo YM, et al.: Risk factors for the development of avascular necrosis after femoral neck fractures in children: a review of 239 cases, *Bone Joint Lett J* 101-B:1160, 2019.

KNEE FRACTURES AND DISLOCATIONS

Adams AJ, Talathi NS, Gandhi JS, et al.: Tibial spine fractures in children: evaluation, management, and future directions, *J Knee Surg* 31:374, 2018.

Ares O, Seijas R, Cugat R, et al.: Treatment of fractures of the tibial tuberosity in adolescent soccer players, *Acta Orthop Belg* 77:78, 2011.

Baldwin K, Anari J, Shore B, et al.: The pediatric "floating knee" injury: a state-of-the-art multicenter study, *J Bone Joint Surg Am* 101:1761, 2019.

Davis JT, Rudloff MI: Posttraumatic arthritis after intra-articular distal femur and proximal tibia fractures, *Orthop Clin North Am* 50:445, 2019.

Mayo MH, Mitchell JJ, Axibal DP, et al.: Anterior cruciate ligament injury at the time of anterior tibial spine fracture in young patients: an observational cohort study, *J Pediatr Orthop* 39:e668, 2019.

Patel NM, Park MJ, Sampson NR, Ganley TJ: Tibial eminence fractures in children: earlier posttreatment mobilization results in improved outcomes, *J Pediatr Orthop* 32:139, 2012.

Riccio AI, Tulchin-Francis K, Hogue GD, et al.: Functional outcomes following operative treatment of tibial tubercle fractures, *J Pediatr Orthop* 39:e108, 2019.

Schmal H, Strohm PC, Niemeyer P, et al.: Fractures of the patella in children and adolescents, *Acta Orthop Belg* 76:644, 2010.

Scrimshire AB, Gawad M, Davies R, et al.: Management and outcomes of isolated paediatric tibial spine fractures, *Injury* 49:437, 2018.

Vander Have KL, Ganley TJ, Kocher MS, et al.: Arthrofibrosis after surgical fixation of tibial eminence fractures in children and adolescents, *Am J Sports Med* 38:298, 2010.

TIBIAL AND FIBULAR FRACTURES

Bauer JM, Lovejoy SA: Toddler's fractures: time to weight-bear with regard to immobilization type and radiographic monitoring, *J Pediatr Orthop* 39:314, 2019.

Connors JC, Hardy MA, Ehredt Jr DJ, et al.: The use of pediatric flexible intramedullary nails for minimally invasive fibular fracture fixation, *J Foot Ankle Surg* 57:844, 2018.

Kinney MC, Nagle D, Bastrom T, et al.: Operative versus conservative management of displaced tibial shaft fracture in adolescents, *J Pediatr Orthop* 36:661, 2016.

Kozaci N, Ay MO, Avci M, et al.: The comparison of point-of-care ultrasonography and radiography in the diagnosis of tibia and fibula fractures, *Injury* 48:1628, 2017.

Laine JC, Cherkashin A, Samchukov M, et al.: The management of soft tissue and bone loss in type IIIB and IIIC pediatric open tibia fractures, *J Pediatr Orthop* 36:453, 2015.

Sheffer BW, Villarreal ED, Ochsner 3rd MG, et al.: Concurrent ipsilateral tibial shaft and distal tibial fractures in pediatric patients: risk factors, frequency, and risk of missed diagnosis, *J Pediatr Orthop* Apr 8, 2019, [Epub ahead of print].

Villarreal ED, Wrenn JO, Sheffer BW, et al.: Do patient-specific or fracture-specific factors predict the development of acute compartment syndrome after pediatric tibial shaft fractures?, *J Pediatr Orthop* May 29, 2019, [Epub ahead of print].

FOOT AND ANKLE FRACTURES

Beck JJ, VandenBerg C, Cruz AI, et al.: Low energy, lateral ankle injuries in pediatric and adolescent patients: a systematic review of ankle sprains and nondisplaced distal fibula fractures, *J Pediatr Orthop* Aug 12, 2019, [Epub ahead of print].

Binkley A, Mehlman CT, Freeh E: Salter-Harris II ankle fractures in children: does fracture pattern matter? *J Orthop Trauma* 33:e190, 2019.

Chauvin NA, Jaimes C, Khwaja A: Ankle and foot injuries in the young athlete, *Semin Musculoskelet Radiol* 22:104, 2018.

Eismann EA, Stephan ZA, Mehlman CT, et al.: Pediatric triplane ankle fractures: impact of radiographs and computed tomography on fracture classification and treatment planning, *J Bone Joint Surg Am* 97:995, 2015.

Oestreich AE, Bhojwani N: Stress fractures of ankle and wrist in childhood: nature and frequency, *Pediatr Radiol* 40:1387, 2010.

Ruffing T, Rückauer T, Bludau F, et al.: Cuboid nutcracker fracture in children: management and results, *Injury* 50:607, 2019.

Shirley ED, Maguire KJ, Mantica AL, et al.: Alternatives to traditional cast immobilization in pediatric patients, *J Am Acad Orthop Surg* 28:e20, 2020.